Dewhurst's Textbook of Obstetrics & Gynaecology

EDITED BY

D. KEITH EDMONDS

FRCOG, FRACOG
Consultant Obstetrician and Gynaecologist
Queen Charlotte's and Chelsea Hospital
Goldhawk Road
London, UK

SEVENTH EDITION

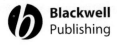

Blackwell
Publishing

© 2007 by Blackwell Publishing
© 1972, 1976, 1981, 1986, 1995, 1999 Blackwell Science
Blackwell Publishing, Inc., 350 Main Street, Malden, Massachusetts 02148-5020, USA
Blackwell Publishing Ltd, 9600 Garsington Road, Oxford OX4 2DQ, UK
Blackwell Publishing Asia Pty Ltd, 550 Swanston Street, Carlton, Victoria 3053, Australia

First published 1972
Second edition 1976
Third edition 1981
Fourth edition 1986
Fifth edition 1995
Sixth edition 1999
Seventh edition 2007

1 2007

Library of Congress Cataloging-in-Publication Data

Dewhurst's textbook of obstetrics and gynaecology. – 7th ed. / edited by D. Keith Edmonds. – 7th ed.
    p. ; cm.
  Rev. ed. of: Dewhurst's textbook of obstetrics and gynaecology for postgraduates. 6th ed. 1999.
  Includes bibliographical references and index.
  ISBN-13: 978-1-4051-3355-5 (hardback: alk. paper)
  ISBN-10: 1-4051-3355-4 (hardback: alk. paper)
  ISBN-13: 978-1-4051-3355-5 (pbk.: alk. paper)
  ISBN-10: 1-4051-3355-4 (pbk.: alk. paper)
  1. Gynecology. 2. Obstetrics. I. Edmonds, D. Keith. II. Dewhurst, John, Sir, 1920- . III. Dewhurst's textbook of obstetrics and gynaecology for postgraduates. IV. Title: Textbook of obstetrics and gynaecology.
  [DNLM: 1. Genital Diseases, Female. 2. Obstetrics. WP 100 D5193 2006]
RG101.D5573 2006
618–dc22

                                                        2005032517
ISBN: 978-1-4051-3355-5 (hardback)
ISBN: 978-1-4051-5667-7 (paperback)

A catalogue record for this title is available from the British Library

Set in 9.5/12.5pt Palatino by
Newgen Imaging Systems Pvt Ltd
Printed and bound in India by Replika Press Pvt Ltd, Haryana, India

Commissioning Editor: Stuart Taylor
Editorial Assistant: Jennifer Seward
Development Editor: Fiona Pattison
Production Controller: Debbie Wyer

For further information on Blackwell Publishing, visit our website: http://www.blackwellpublishing.com

The publisher's policy is to use permanent paper from mills that operate a sustainable forestry policy, and which has been manufactured from pulp processed using acid-free and elementary chlorine-free practices. Furthermore, the publisher ensures that the text paper and cover board used have met acceptable environmental accreditation standards.

Contents

Plate section can be found facing p. 562

Contributors

S. Arulkumaran
Professor and Head, St George's Hospital Medical School, Cranmer Terrace, London, SW17 0RE, UK

Adam H. Balen
Professor of Reproductive Medicine and Surgery, Department of Obstetrics and Gynaecology, Clarendon Wing, Leeds General Infirmary, United Leeds Teaching Hospitals, Leeds, LS2 9NS, UK

Phillip Bennett
Professor of Obstetrics and Gynaecology, Parturition Research Group, Faculty of Medicine, Imperial College London; and Institute of Reproductive and Developmental Biology, Hammersmith Hospital Campus, Du Cane Road, London, W12 0NN, UK

Siladitya Bhattacharya
Senior Lecturer, Department of Obstetrics and Gynaecology, University of Aberdeen, Aberdeen Maternity Hospital, Foresterhill, Aberdeen, AB25 2ZL, UK

Fiona Broughton-Pipkin
Professor of Perinatal Physiology, School of Human Development, Nottingham University Hospital, Queen's Medical Centre, Derby Road, Nottingham, NG7 2UH, UK

A.A. Calder
Professor of Obstetrics and Gynaecology, University of Edinburgh, Reproductive and Developmental Sciences, Simpson Centre for Reproductive Health, 51 Little France Crescent, Edinburgh, EH16 4SA, UK

L. Cardozo
Department of Urogynaecology, Kings College Hospital, London, UK

P. Clark
Consultant Haematologist, Ninewells Hospital Dundee; and Honorary Senior Lecturer, University of Dundee, UK

John A. Crowhurst
Consultant Anaesthetist, Mercy Hospital for Women, Melbourne, Australia; and Formerly Reader in Obstetric Anaesthesia, Imperial College; and Director of Obstetric Anaesthesia, Queen Charlotte's and Chelsea Hospital, London, UK

Patricia Crowley
Department of Obstetrics and Gynaecology, Trinity College Dublin, Coombe Women's Hospital, Dublin 8, Ireland

Maureen Dalton
Consultant Obstetrician and Gynaecologist, Royal Devon and Exeter Hospital, Barrack Road, Exeter, EX2 5DW, UK

John Davison
Consultant Obstetrician, Department of Obstetrics and Gynaecology, Directorate of Women's Services, Royal Victoria Infirmary, Queen Victoria Road, Newcastle upon Tyne, NE1 4LP, UK

Anne Dornhorst
Consultant Physician and Honorary Senior Lecturer, Metabolic Medicine, Imperial College London, Du Cane Road, London, W12 0NN, UK

D. Keith Edmonds
Consultant Obstetrician and Gynaecologist, Queen Charlotte's and Chelsea Hospital, Goldhawk Road, London, W6 0XG, UK

A.D. Edwards
Consultant Paediatrician, Department of Paediatrics, Hammersmith Hospital, Du Cane Road, London, W12 0HS, UK

Roy G. Farquarson
Clinical Director, Liverpool Women's Hospital, Crown Street, Liverpool, L8 7SS, UK

Alan Farthing
Consultant Gynaecological Surgeon, West London Gynaecological Cancer Centre, Queen Charlotte's and Chelsea Hospital, Du Cane Road, London, W12 0HS, UK

Nicholas M. Fisk
Professor of Obstetrics and Gynaecology, Institute of Reproductive and Developmental Biology, Imperial College, London; and Centre for Fetal Care, Queen Charlotte's and Chelsea Hospital, London, UK

Gillian Flett
Consultant, Sexual and Reproductive Health, 13 Golden Square, Aberdeen, AB10 1RH, UK; and Gynaecology Department, Aberdeen Royal Infirmary, Foresterhill, Aberdeen, UK

Hani Gabra
Professor of Medical Oncology and Head of Section of Molecular Therapeutics, Imperial College London; and Director of the Helene Harris Memorial Trust Ovarian Cancer Action Research Unit; and Chief of Service, West London Gynaecological Cancer Centre, Hammersmith Hospitals NHS Trust, London, UK

Jason Gardosi
West Midlands Perinatal Institute, Crystal Court, Aston Cross, Birmingham, B6 5RQ, UK

Anna Glasier
Director of NHS Lothian Family Planning and Well Women Service; and Honorary Professor University of Edinburgh Clinical Sciences and Community Health; and University of London, School of Hygiene and Tropical Medicine Department of Public Health Policy, UK

I.A. Greer
Regius Professor of Obstetrics and Gynaecology, University of Glasgow, Reproductive and Maternal Medicine, Glasgow Royal Infirmary, 10 Alexandra Parade, Glasgow, G31 2ER, UK

G. Justus Hofmeyr
Consultant, East London Hospital Complex; and Director, Effective Case Research Unit, Eastern Cape Department of Health; and University of the Witwatersrand/University of Fort Hare, South Africa

Berthold Huppertz
University Professor of Cell Biology, Department of Cell Biology, Histology and Embryology, Center of Molecular Medicine, Harrachgasse 21/7, Medical University of Graz, 8010 Graz, Austria

Davor Jurkovic
Consultant Obstetrician and Gynaecologist, Head Early Pregnancy and Gynaecology Assessment Unit, King's College Hospital, Denmark Hill, London, SE5 9RS, UK

Stephen Kennedy
Clinical Reader, Nuffield Department of Obstetrics and Gynaecology, University of Oxford, UK

John C.P. Kingdom
Department of Obstetrics and Gynecology, Samuel Lunenfeld Research Institute, Mount Sinai Hospital, University of Toronto, Canada

Henry C. Kitchener
Professor of Gynaecological Oncology, University of Manchester, Academic Unit of Obstetrics/Gynaecology, St Mary's Hospital, Whitworth Park, Manchester, M13 0JH, UK

Philippe Koninckx
Nuffield Department of Obstetrics and Gynaecology, University of Oxford; and Department of Obstetrics and Gynecology, University of Leuven, Belgium

Sailesh Kumar
Consultant in Fetal Medicine, Obstetrics and Gynaecology, Centre for Fetal Care, Queen Charlotte's and Chelsea Hospital, Du Cane Road, London, W12 0HS, UK

William L. Ledger
Professor of Obstetrics and Gynaecology, Academic Unit of Reproductive and Developmental Medicine, The Jessop Wing, Tree Root Walk, Sheffield, S10 2SF, UK

C. C. Lees
Consultant in Obstetrics and Maternal and Fetal Medicine, The Rosie Hospital, Addenbrookes NHS Trust, Cambridge, CB2 2QQ, UK

Bertie Leigh
Solicitor, Senior Partner at Hempsons, Hempsons House, 40 Villiers Street, London, WC2N 6NJ, UK

James A. Low
Department of Obstetrics and Gynaecology, Queen's University, Kingston, Ontario, K7L 3N6, Canada

David M. Luesley
Lawson-Tait Professor of Gynaecological Oncology, City Hospital, Dudley Road, Birmingham, B18 7QH, UK

Mary Ann Lumsden
Professor of Gynaecology and Medical Education, Division of Developmental Medicine, University of Glasgow, Queen Elizabeth Building, 10 Alexandra Parade, Glasgow, G31 2ER, UK

Adam Magos
Minimally Invasive Therapy Unit and Endoscopy Training Centre, University Department of Obstetrics and Gynaecology, The Royal Free Hospital, Pond Street, Hampstead, London, NW3 2QG, UK

Andrew McCarthy
Consultant Obstetrician, Hammersmith and Queen Charlotte's and Chelsea Hospital, Du Cane Road, London, W12 0HS, UK

Catherine Nelson-Piercy
Consultant Obstetric Physician, Guy's and St Thomas' Hospitals Foundation Trust, and Queen Charlotte's Hospital, London, UK

P.M.S. O'Brien
Consultant Obstetrician and Gynaecologist, Academic Unit of Obstetrics and Gynaecology, Keele University Medical School, University Hospital of North Staffordshire NHS Trust, Stoke on Trent, ST4 6QG, UK

Timothy G. Overton
Consultant in Obstetrics and Fetal Medicine, Honorary Senior Clinical Lecturer, University of Bristol, St Michael's Hospital, Southwell Street, Bristol, BS2 8EG, UK

Nick Panay
Consultant Obstetrician and Gynaecologist, Queen Charlotte's and Chelsea Hospital, Hammersmith Hospitals NHS Trust; and Honorary Senior Lecturer, Imperial College, London, UK

Sara Paterson-Brown
Consultant Obstetrician and Gynaecologist, Queen Charlotte's and Chelsea Hospital, Du Cane Road, London, W12 0HS, UK

Raj Rai
Senior Lecturer/Consultant Gynaecologist, Sub-specialist in Reproductive Medicine, Imperial College London, Mint Wing, St Mary's Hospital, London, W2 1PG, UK

Fran Reader
Consultant in Reproductive Health, Ipswich Hospital, Heath Road, Ipswich, Suffolk, IP4 5PD, UK

Margaret C.P. Rees
Reader in Reproductive Medicine, Nuffield Department of Obstetrics and Gynaecology, John Radcliffe Hospital, Oxford, OX3 9DU, UK

D. Robinson
Department of Urogynaecology, Kings College Hospital, London, UK

Jonathan D.C. Ross
Professor of Sexual Health and HIV, Whittall Street Clinic, Birmingham, UK

Philip Savage
Department of Medical Oncology, Charing Cross Hospital, Fulham Palace Road, London, W6 8RF, UK

Michael Seckl
Director, Charing Cross Hospital Trophoblastic Disease Centre, Fulham Palace Road, London, W6 8RF, UK

Mahmood I. Shafi
Consultant Gynaecological Surgeon and Oncologist, Addenbrooke's Hospital, Hills Road, Cambridge, CB2 2QQ, UK

Andrew Shennan
Professor of Obstetrics, King's College London, Guy's, King's and St. Thomas' School of Medicine, Lambeth Palace Road, London, SE1 7EH, UK

Anthony R.B. Smith
Consultant Urogynaecologist, The Warrell Unit, St Mary's Hospital, Hathersage Road, Manchester, M13 0JH, UK

G.C.S. Smith
Head of Department and Consultant in Maternal–Fetal Medicine, Department of Obstetrics and Gynaecology, The Rosie Hospital, Robinson Way, Cambridge, CB2 2QQ, UK

Richard Staughton
Consultant Dermatologist, Chelsea and Westminster Hospital, 369 Fulham Road, London, SW10 9NH, UK

Peter Stewart
Consultant Obstetrician and Gynaecologist, Royal Hallamshire Hospital, Sheffield, UK

Gordon M. Stirrat
Emeritus Professor of Obstetrics and Gynaecology, and Senior Research Fellow in Ethics in Medicine, Centre for Ethics in Medicine, University of Bristol, 73 St Michael's Hill, Bristol, BS2 8BH, UK

R. William Stones
Senior Lecturer in Obstetrics and Gynaecology, University of Southampton, Southampton, SO16 5YA, UK

Allan Templeton
Gynaecology Department, Aberdeen Royal Infirmary, Forresterhill, Aberdeen, UK

A.J. Thomson
Consultant Obstetrician and Gynaecologist/Honorary Senior Lecturer, University of Glasgow, UK

M.A. Thomson
University of Glasgow, Reproductive and Maternal Medicine, Glasgow Royal Infirmary, 10 Alexandra Parade, Glasgow, G312ER, UK

Jim G. Thornton
Professor of Obstetrics and Gynaecology, Division of Obstetrics and Gynaecology, City Hospital, Hucknall Road, Nottingham, NG5 1PB, UK

Joanne Topping
Consultant in Obstetrics and Early Pregnancy Care, Liverpool Women's Hospital, Crown Street, Liverpool, L8 7SS, UK

Geoffrey Trew
The Hammersmith Hospital, Du Cane Road, W12 0HS, UK

Catherine Williamson
Senior Lecturer in Obstetric Medicine, Institute of Reproductive and Developmental Biology, Imperial College, Hammersmith Hospital, Du Cane Road, London, W12 0NN, UK

R.C. Wimalasundera
Consultant Obstetrician and Fetal Medicine Specialist, Centre for Fetal Care, Queen Charlotte's and Chelsea Hospital, Du Cane Road, London W12 0HS, UK

Professor Sir John Dewhurst

Professor Sir John Dewhurst died on the 1st December 2006. Jack, as he was known to all his colleagues, was a doyen amongst obstetricians and gynaecologists of the twentieth century. His reputation was internationally renowned and he became a worldwide expert in paediatric and adolescent gynaecology for which he received due accolade. He was also an outstanding teacher of obstetrics and gynaecology and as such this textbook that he began in the 1970s is testament to his dedication to the passing on of knowledge to others. In 1976 he became President of the Royal College of Obstetricians and Gynaecologists, a post he held for three years, for which he was subsequently knighted. He retired in 1986 after a long and distinguished career but his legacy lives on and he will be remembered by all who knew him with great affection and professional respect.

D. KEITH EDMONDS

Preface to the Seventh Edition

As I write this Preface in 2006, the specialty of obstetrics and gynaecology worldwide is going through a crisis of recruitment. It seems to all the contributors to this book a strange and sad time as the fascination of obstetrics and gynaecology remains unchallenged. Since the 6th edition, many advances have occurred and these have led to improvements in healthcare throughout the world. The efforts with regard to maternal and fetal health and to the gynaecological care of women remains a triumph of modern medicine. We hope that the reader will enjoy being stimulated by the fascination and intellectual stimulation that comes from the study of obstetrics and gynaecology.

I wish to thank all the contributors who have submitted chapters for the readers' pleasure, to impart their knowledge and to hopefully see this translated into high quality clinical practice.

I would like to thank all of the contributors whose contributions span the breadth of obstetrics and gynaecology and we hope that these individual chapters will stimulate the reader to a greater understanding and thereafter a healthy appetite for more knowledge.

The obstetrics and gynaecology of the future will almost certainly be different from the practice that has occurred over the last 150 years and as the future beckons more specialized individuals, a basic knowledge of obstetrics and gynaecology will still underpin the training of young doctors for the future. I hope this book will continue to provide that wealth of knowledge and stimulate young doctors to join the specialty and become contributors in the future.

I would like to thank my secretary, Liz Manson, without whom many of the contributors in this book would have slept very soundly. Her incessant efforts to obtain the chapters have been remarkable and I am indebted to her. I would also like to thank Fiona Pattison at Blackwell Publishing and the editorial team for their support in the publication of this volume.

D. KEITH EDMONDS
2006

Preface to the First Edition

Our purpose in writing this book has been to produce a comprehensive account of what the specialist in training in obstetrics and gynaecology must know. Unfortunately for him, he must now know a great deal, not only about his own subject, but about certain aspects of closely allied specialties such as endocrinology, biochemistry, cytogenetics, psychiatry, etc. Accordingly we have tried to offer the postgraduate student not only an advanced textbook in obstetrics and gynaecology but one which integrates the relevant aspects of other subjects which nowadays impinge more and more on the clinical field.

To achieve this aim within, we hope, a reasonable compass we have assumed some basic knowledge which the reader will have assimilated throughout his medical training, and we have taken matters on from there. Fundamental facts not in question are stated as briefly as is compatible with accuracy and clarity, and discussion is then devoted to more advanced aspects. We acknowledge that it is not possible even in this way to provide all the detail some readers may wish, so an appropriate bibliography is provided with each chapter. Wherever possible we have tried to give a positive opinion and our reasons for holding it, but to discuss nonetheless other important views; this we believe to be more helpful than a complete account of all possible opinions which may be held. We have chosen moreover to lay emphasis on fundamental aspects of the natural and the disease processes which are discussed; we believe concentration on these basic physiological and pathological features to be important to the proper training of a specialist. Clinical matters are, of course, dealt with in detail too, whenever theoretical discussion of them is rewarding. There are, however, some clinical aspects which cannot, at specialist level, be considered in theory with real benefit; examples of these are how to palpate a pregnant woman's abdomen and how to apply obstetric forceps. In general these matters are considered very briefly or perhaps not at all; this is not a book on *how*

things are done, but on how correct treatment is chosen, what advantages one choice has over another, what complications are to be expected, etc. Practical matters, we believe, are better learnt in practice and with occasional reference to specialized textbooks devoted solely to them.

A word may be helpful about the manner in which the book is set out. We would willingly have followed the advice given to Alice when about to testify at the trial of the Knave of Hearts in Wonderland, 'Begin at the beginning, keep on until you come to the end and then stop'. But this advice is difficult to follow when attempting to find the beginning of complex subjects such as those to which this book is devoted. Does the beginning lie with fertilization; or with the events which lead up to it; or with the genital organs upon the correct function of which any pregnancy must depend; or does it lie somewhere else? And which direction must we follow then? The disorders of reproduction do not lie in a separate compartment from genital tract disease, but each is clearly associated with the other for at least part of a woman's life. Although we have attempted to integrate obstetrics with gynaecology and with their associated specialties, some separation is essential in writing about them, and the plan we have followed is broadly this—we begin with the female child *in utero*, follow her through childhood to puberty, through adolescence to maturity, through pregnancy to motherhood, through her reproductive years to the climacteric and into old age. Some events have had to be taken out of order, however, although reiteration has been avoided by indicating to the reader where in the book are to be found other sections dealing with different aspects of any subject under consideration. We hope that our efforts will provide a coherent, integrated account of the field we have attempted to cover which will be to the satisfaction of our readers.

SIR JOHN DEWHURST
1972

Chapter 1: Clinical anatomy of the pelvis and reproductive tract

Alan Farthing

Introduction

This chapter aims to summarize the important aspects of the anatomy of the abdomen and the pelvis, which should be known to the Obstetric or Gynaecological specialist. Many of the investigations and treatments we order on a daily basis require good anatomical knowledge in order to be properly understood.

Surface anatomy

The anterior abdominal wall can be divided into four quadrants by lines passing horizontally and vertically through the umbilicus (Fig. 1.1). In the upper abdomen is the epigastrium, which is the area just inferior to the xiphisternum, and in the lower abdomen lie the right and left iliac fossae and the hypogastrium.

The cutaneous nerve supply of the anterior abdominal wall arises from the anterior rami of the lower thoracic and lumbar vertebrae. The dermatomes of significant structures on the anterior abdominal wall are:

T7 xiphisternum
T10 umbilicus
L1 symphysis pubis

The blood supply is via the superior epigastric (branch of the internal thoracic artery) and the inferior epigastric (branch of the external iliac artery) vessels. During laparoscopy, the inferior epigastric vessels can be seen between the peritoneum and rectus muscle on the anterior abdominal wall and commence their journey superiorly from approximately two thirds of the way along the inguinal ligament closer to the symphysis pubis. Care needs to be taken to avoid them while using accessory trochars during laparoscopy and to ensure that they are identified when making a Maylard incision of the abdominal wall.

The anterior abdominal wall

Beneath the skin and the fat of the superficial anterior abdominal wall lies a sheath and combination of muscles including the rectus abdominus, external and internal oblique and tranversalis muscles (Fig. 1.2). Where these muscles coalesce in the midline, the linea alba is formed. Pyramidalis muscle is present in almost all women originating on the anterior surface of the pubis and inserting into the linea alba. The exact configuration of the muscles encountered by the surgeon depends on exactly where any incision is made.

The umbilicus

The umbilicus is essentially a scar made from the remnants of the umbilical cord. It is situated in the linea alba and in a variable position depending on the obesity of the patient. However the base of the umbilicus is always the thinnest part of the anterior abdominal wall and is the commonest site of insertion of the primary port in laparoscopy. The urachus is the remains of the allantois from the fetus and runs from the apex of the bladder to the umbilicus.

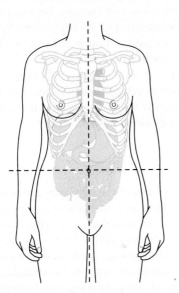

Fig. 1.1 The abdomen can be divided into quadrants.

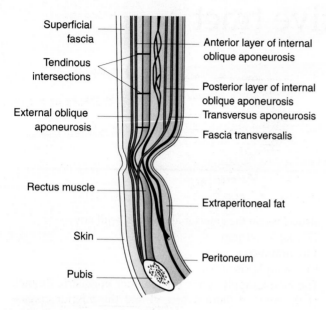

Fig. 1.2 The layers of the anterior abdominal wall in tranverse section.

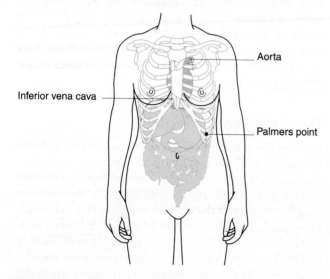

Fig. 1.3 The umbilicus in relation to the underlying vasculature in a thin patient.

Occasionally this can remain patent in newborns. In early embryological life, the vitelline duct also runs through the umbilicus from the developing midgut. Although the duct is severed long before delivery, a remnant of this structure is found in 2% of the population as a Meckels diverticulum.

The aorta divides into the common iliac arteries approximately 1–2 cm below the umbilicus in most slim women (Fig. 1.3). The common iliac veins combine to form the inferior vena cava just below this and all these structures

are a potential hazard for the laparoscopist inserting ports at the umbilicus.

Epithelium of the genital tract

The anterior abdominal wall including the vulva, vagina and perineal areas are lined with squamous epithelium. The epithelium lining the endocervix and uterine cavity is columnar and the squamocolumnar junction usually arises at the ectocervix in women of reproductive age. This is an important site as it is the area from which cervical intraepithelial neoplasia (CIN) and eventually cervical malignancy arises. The bladder is lined by transitional epithelium which becomes columnar. The anal verge is still squamous epithelium but this changes to columnar immediately inside the anus and into the rectum.

The genital tract, from the vagina, through the uterus and out through the fallopian tubes into the peritoneal cavity, is an open passage. This is an essential route for the traversing of sperm in the process of fertilization but unfortunately it also allows the transport of pathologic organisms which may result in ascending infection.

The peritoneum

The peritoneum is a thin serous membrane which lines the inside of the pelvic and abdominal cavities. In simplistic terms it is probably best to imagine a pelvis containing the bladder, uterus and rectum (Fig. 1.4) and note that the peritoneum is a layer placed over these organs in a single sheet. This complete layer is then pierced by both the fallopian tubes and the ovaries on each side. Posteriorly the rectum also pierces the peritoneum connecting to the sigmoid colon and the area between the posterior surface of the uterus and its supporting ligaments and the rectum is called the Pouch of Douglas. This particular area is important in gynaecology as the place where gravity dependent fluid collects. As a result this is where blood is found in ectopic pregnancies, pus in infections and endometriosis which has been caused by retrograde menstruation (Sampsons theory).

Vulva

The vulva is the area of the perineum including the Mons pubis, labia majora and minora and the opening into both the vagina and urethra (Fig. 1.5). The labia majora are areas of skin with underlying fat pads which bound the vagina. Medial to these are the labia minora which consist of vascular tissue which reacts to the stimulation of sexual arousal. Anteriorly they come together to form the prepuce of the clitoris and posteriorly they form the forchette.

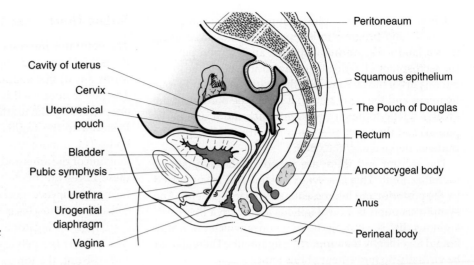

Fig. 1.4 Transverse view of the pelvic organs.

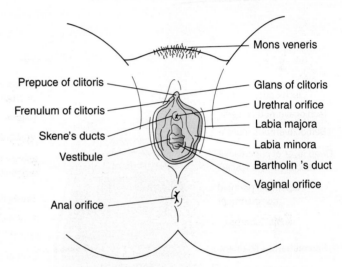

Fig. 1.5 Surface anatomy of the vulva.

The hymen is a fold of vaginal mucosa at the entrance to this organ. It usually has a small opening in virgins and is only seen as an irregular remnant in sexually active women.

To each side of the introitus are the ducts of the vestibular glands commonly known as Bartholin's glands which produce much of the lubrication at sexual intercourse.

The vulval blood supply comes from the pudendal artery and lymphatic drainage is through the inguinal lymph nodes. The nerve supply comes mostly from the pudendal nerve and pelvic plexus with branches of the perineal nerves and posterior cutaneous nerve of the thigh important in the posterior region.

The clitoris

The clitoris corresponds to the male penis consisting of the same three masses of erectile tissue (Fig. 1.6). The bulb

of the vestibule is attached to the underlying urogenital diaphragm and split into two because of the presence of the vagina. The right and left crura become the corpora cavernosa and are covered by the ischiocavernosus muscles.

Bony pelvis

The bony pelvis consists of two hip bones (consisting of the ileum and ischium) which are joined together by the sacrum posteriorly and the symphysis pubis anteriorly (Figs. 1.7 and 1.8). In addition, the coccyx lies on the inferior aspect of the sacrum. A plane drawn between the sacral promontory and the superior aspect of the symphysis pubis marks the pelvic inlet and a similar plane drawn from the tip of S5 to the inferior aspect of the symphysis pubis marks the pelvic outlet.

Clinically the ischial spine is important as it can be felt vaginally and progress in labour can be measured using it as a landmark. Additionally it is an insertion point of the sacrospinous ligament which also attaches to the lower lateral part of the sacrum. Together with the sacrotuberous ligament and the bony pelvis, it forms the borders of the greater sciatic foramen (through which the sciatic nerve passes) and the lesser sciatic foramen (through which the pudendal nerve enters the pelvis).

The sacrum and ilium are joined by the very strong sacroiliac joint. This is a synovial joint and is supported by the posterior and interosseous sacroiliac ligaments. The symphysis pubis is a cartilaginous joint with a fibrocartilaginous disc separating the two bones which are firmly bound together by the supporting ligaments. There should be virtually no movement of this joint.

Pelvic floor (Figs. 1.9 and 1.10)

The obturator internus muscle sits on the medial side of the ischial bone and, together with the body of the pubis, forms a wall that supports the origins of the pelvic floor. The pelvic floor itself is a sling of various muscles which are pierced by the urethra, the vagina and the anal canal. Posterior to the vagina these muscles form the perineal body. The puborectalis muscle forms a sling around the junction of the anus and rectum and posterior to the anus, these fibres are made up by the pubococcygeus which forms the anococcygeal body in the midline (Fig. 1.9). The collection of muscles is variously referred to as the pelvic diaphragm or levator ani muscles (Fig. 1.10). These muscles support the pelvic organs, holding them in position and resisting the forces created when the intraperitoneal

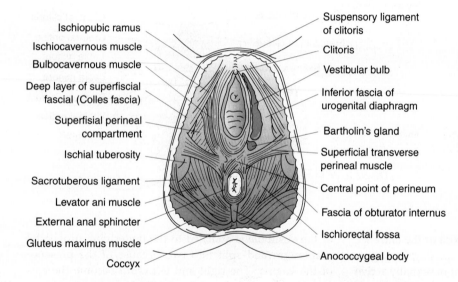

Ischiopubic ramus
Ischiocavernous muscle
Bulbocavernous muscle
Deep layer of superfiscial fascial (Colles fascia)
Superfisial perineal compartment
Ischial tuberosity
Sacrotuberous ligament
Levator ani muscle
External anal sphincter
Gluteus maximus muscle
Coccyx

Suspensory ligament of clitoris
Clitoris
Vestibular bulb
Inferior fascia of urogenital diaphragm
Bartholin's gland
Superficial transverse perineal muscle
Central point of perineum
Fascia of obturator internus
Ischiorectal fossa
Anococcygeal body

Fig. 1.6 The deeper vulval tissues.

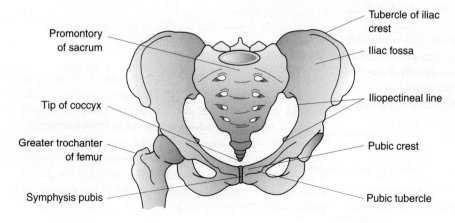

Promontory of sacrum
Tip of coccyx
Greater trochanter of femur
Symphysis pubis

Tubercle of iliac crest
Iliac fossa
Iliopectineal line
Pubic crest
Pubic tubercle

Fig. 1.7 Bony pelvis.

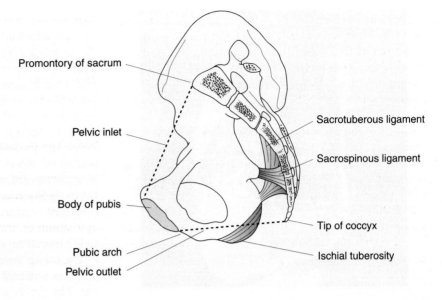

Promontory of sacrum

Pelvic inlet

Body of pubis

Pubic arch

Pelvic outlet

Sacrotuberous ligament

Sacrospinous ligament

Tip of coccyx

Ischial tuberosity

Fig. 1.8 Bony pelvis.

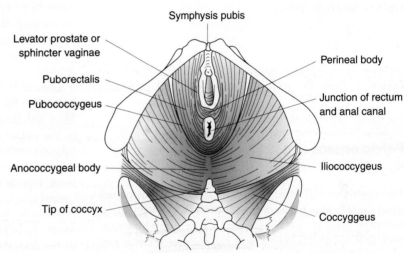

Symphysis pubis

Levator prostate or sphincter vaginae

Puborectalis

Pubococcygeus

Anococcygeal body

Tip of coccyx

Perineal body

Junction of rectum and anal canal

Iliococcygeus

Coccyggeus

Fig. 1.9 Pelvic floor muscles.

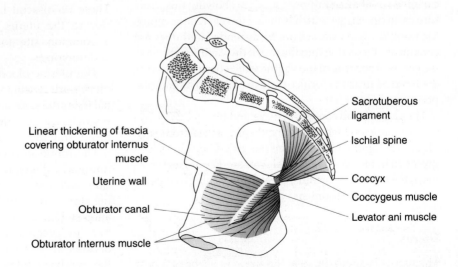

Linear thickening of fascia covering obturator internus muscle

Uterine wall

Obturator canal

Obturator internus muscle

Sacrotuberous ligament

Ischial spine

Coccyx

Coccygeus muscle

Levator ani muscle

Fig. 1.10 Transverse view of the pelvic floor muscles.

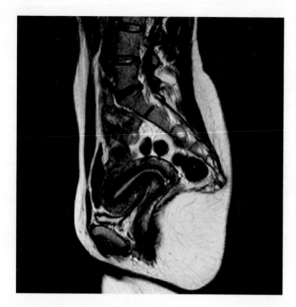

Fig. 1.11 MRI of the pelvis.

pressure is raised as in coughing or straining. The nerve supply is from the fourth sacral nerve and pudendal nerve.

Pelvic organs (Fig. 1.11)

Vagina

The vagina is a distensible muscular tube which passes from the introitus to the cervix. It pierces the pelvic floor and then lies flat on its posterior surface using it as support. It is approximately 8 cm long and the anterior and posterior walls oppose each other. Anatomical text books can give a confusing impression when showing this structure as an open tube with a lumen. However, on imaging, the normal vagina should not be distended and does not contain air. Projecting into the top of the vagina is the uterine cervix. The areas of the vagina which border the cervix are referred to as the fornices and are labelled as anterior, posterior, right or left.

The vaginal wall consists of outer and inner circular layers of muscles which cannot be distinguished from each other. The epithelium contains no glands but is rich in glycogen in the premenopausal woman. The normal commensal, Doderleins bacillus, breaks down this glycogen to create an acid environment.

Uterus

The uterus is approximately the size and shape of a pear with a central cavity and thick muscular walls (Fig. 1.12).

The serosal surface is the closely applied peritoneum beneath which is the myometrium which is a smooth muscle supported by connective tissue. The myometrium is made up of three layers of muscle, external, intermediate and internal layers. Clinically this is important as fibroids leave the layers intact and removal through a superficial incision leaves the three layers intact. The three layers run in complimentary directions which encourage vascular occlusion during contraction, an important aspect of menstrual blood loss and postpartum haemostasis. The mucous membrane overlying the myometrium to line the cavity is the endometrium. Glands of the endometrium pierce the myometrium and a single layer of columnar epithelium on the surface changes cyclically in response to the menstrual cycle.

The uterus consists of a fundus superiorly, a body, an isthmus (internal os) and inferiorly the cervix (external os). The cervix is a cylindrical structure which is muscular in its upper portions but this gives way to fibrous connective tissue as the cervix sits at the top of the vagina. The cervix is lined by columnar epithelium, which secretes alkaline mucus neutralizing the effects of vaginal acidity.

The cervix and uterus do not always sit in the same plane and when the uterine body rotates anteriorly it is referred to as anteflexed and posteriorly as retroflexed. The axis of the entire uterus can be anteverted or retroverted in relation to the axis of the vagina (Fig. 1.13).

The uterus is supported by the muscles of the pelvic floor together with three supporting condensations of connective tissue. The pubocervical ligaments run from the cervix anteriorly to the pubis, the cardinal ligaments pass laterally from the cervix and upper vagina to the lateral pelvic side walls and the uterosacral ligaments from the cervix and upper vagina to the sacrum. These uterosacral ligaments can be clearly seen posterior to the uterus in the Pouch of Douglas and are a common site for superficial and deep infiltrating endometriosis.

The uterine blood supply is derived mainly from the uterine artery, a branch of the anterior division of the internal iliac artery. An anastamosis occurs with the blood supply delivered through the ovarian ligament and derived direct from the ovarian artery.

The round ligament is the remains of the gubernaculum and extends from the uterus laterally to the pelvic side wall and then into the inguinal canal before passing down into the labia majora. It holds the uterus in anteversion, although it is a highly distensible structure in pregnancy. It is usually the first structure divided at hysterectomy allowing the surgeon to open the overlying folds of peritoneum known as the broad ligament.

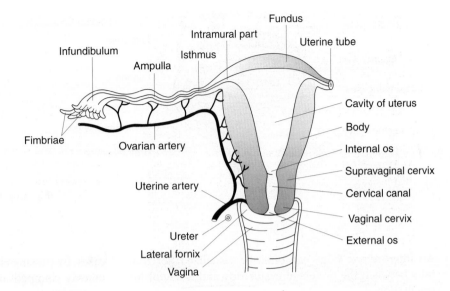

Fig. 1.12 Uterus and fallopian tubes.

Fallopian tubes

The fallopian tubes are delicate tubular structures which carry the ovum or sperm between the ovary and uterine cavity. The tubes are divided into named regions, most medially the cornu and interstial portion within the uterine wall, then the isthmus followed by the infundibulum, ampulla and finally fimbrial ends. They are lined by columnar epithelium and cilia which together with the peristaltic action of the surrounding smooth muscle propel the fertilized ovum towards the uterine cavity. The blood supply of the fallopian tubes arises from both the uterine and ovarian arteries through the mesosalpinx which is covered by peritoneum.

Ovaries

The ovaries vary in size depending on age and their function. They are approximately $2 \times 4\,\text{cm}^2$ with the long axis running vertically and are attached to the posterior leaf of the broad ligament by the mesovarium. In addition they are fixed in position by the ovarian ligament (to the uterus medially) and the infundibulopelvic ligament which contains the ovarian blood supply direct from the aorta. Venous drainage is to the ovarian veins which drain direct into the inferior vena cava on the right and into the renal vein on the left. The aortic nerve plexus also accompanies the ovary in its descent from around the level of the first lumbar vertebra.

The lateral pelvic side wall is covered by peritoneum which is folded to form the ovarian fossa. Pathological adhesions around the ovary will often cause it to be

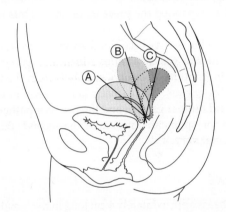

Fig. 1.13 The axis of the uterus in relation to the vagina.

fixed into the ovarian fossa causing cyclical pain or dyspareunia.

The ovary is not covered by peritoneum but is surrounded by a thin membranous capsule, the tunica albuginea, which in turn is covered by the germinal epithelium.

Bladder

The urinary bladder is situated immediately behind the pubic bone and anterior to the uterine cervix and upper vagina. It has a strong muscular wall consisting of three layers of interlacing fibres which are known together as the detrusor muscles (Fig. 1.14). The trigone is the only smooth part of the bladder as it is fixed to the underlying muscle. At the superior margins of the trigone lie the ureteric openings and at the inferior aspect the urethra.

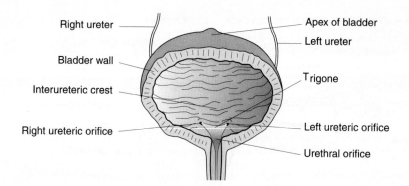

Right ureter

Bladder wall

Interureteric crest

Right ureteric orifice

Apex of bladder

Left ureter

Trigone

Left ureteric orifice

Urethral orifice

Fig. 1.14 The bladder.

An interureteric ridge can often be visualized horizontally between the ureters at cystoscopy and is useful for orientation.

The rest of the bladder is highly distensible ensuring that as it is expanded the pressure of its contents remains the same.

The bladder receives its blood supply from the superior and inferior vesical arteries which originate from the internal iliac artery. The nerve supply is from the inferior hypogastric plexus. Sympathetic nerves arise in the first and second lumbar ganglia and the parasympathetic supply from the splanchnic nerves of the second, third and fourth sacral nerves.

URETHRA

The urethra is approximately 4 cm long in the female adult starting at the internal meatus of the bladder and passing through the pelvic floor to the vestibule. The epithelium is squamous near the external meatus and changes to transitional epithelium about two thirds of the way to the bladder. The deeper tissue is muscular and this maintains the urethral tone. There are no anatomical sphincters but the muscle fibres of the bladder at the internal meatus act as an 'internal sphincter' and the pelvic floor as a voluntary external sphincter.

URETERS

The ureters run from the renal hilum to the trigone of the bladder and are approximately 30 cm in length. They enter the pelvis by passing over the common iliac bifurcation at the pelvic brim. They then pass along the lateral pelvic side wall before passing anteriorly and medially under the uterine artery as it originates from the internal iliac artery and into the base of the bladder. The ureter comes close to the ovarian artery and vein and can be adherent to these vessels or the overlying ovary in pathological

cases. By passing close to the uterine artery it can be mistakenly clamped and divided as a rare complication of hysterectomy.

The ureters are muscular tubes lined by transitional epithelium. The blood supply varies during its course but small vessels along the surface of the ureter require careful preservation when dissecting it free from other structures.

Rectum

The rectum is approximately 12 cm in length and starts at the level of S3 as a continuation of the sigmoid colon. The puborectalis part of the pelvic floor forms a sling around the lower end at the junction with the anal canal. The rectum is commonly depicted in anatomic drawing as being dilated, causing the other pelvic organs to be pushed forward. This is because the original drawings were taken from cadavers but in the live patient the rectum is often empty allowing the other structures to lie supported on the pelvic floor.

The mucosa of the rectum is columnar and this is surrounded by inner circular and outer longitudinal fibres of smooth muscle. The serosal surface is covered by peritoneum.

The blood supply is from the superior rectal artery from the inferior mesenteric artery, and the middle and inferior rectal arteries arise from the posterior division of the internal iliac artery. The nerve supply is from the inferior hypogastric plexus and ensures the rectum is sensitive to stretch only.

Conclusion

A clear knowledge of anatomy is required for many gynaecological diagnoses and certainly for surgery. Many clinicians do not gain a full understanding of pelvic anatomy until they start operating and then rarely refer back to anatomical textbooks. The advent of more sophisticated pelvic floor surgery and especially minimal access surgery has modified the skills required of a gynaecological surgeon which necessitates the need for greater practical anatomical knowledge.

Further reading

Shah Farthing & Richardson Lennard (2003) *The Interactive Pelvis & Perineum: Female.* Primal Pitures Ltd, www.primalpictures.com

Snell R. *Clinical Anatomy for Medical Students.* London: Little Brown & Co.

Chapter 2: Maternal physiology

Fiona Broughton-Pipkin

The physiological changes of pregnancy are strongly proactive, not reactive, with the luteal phase of every ovulatory menstrual cycle 'rehearsing' for pregnancy [1]. Most pregnancy-driven changes are qualitatively in place by the end of the first trimester, only maturing in magnitude thereafter. This chapter gives a brief overview of the major changes.

The cardiovascular system

There is a significant fall in total peripheral resistance by 6 weeks gestation to a nadir of ~40% by mid-gestation, resulting in a fall in afterload. This is 'perceived' as circulatory underfilling, which activates the renin-angiotensin-aldosterone system and allows the necessary expansion of the plasma volume (PV; Fig. 2.1) [2,3]. By the late third trimester, the PV has increased from its baseline by about 50% in a first pregnancy and 60% in a second or subsequent pregnancy. The bigger the expansion is, the bigger, on average, the birthweight of the baby. The total extracellular fluid volume rises by about 16% by term, so the percentage rise in PV is disproportionate to the whole. The plasma osmolality falls by ~10 mOsm/kg as water is retained.

The heart rate rises synchronously, by 10–15 b.p.m., so the cardiac output begins to rise [4]. There is probably a fall in baroreflex sensitivity as pregnancy progresses and heart rate variability falls. Stroke volume rises a little later in the first trimester. These two factors push the cardiac output up by 35–40% in a first pregnancy, and ~50% in later pregnancies; it can rise by a further third in labour (Fig. 2.2). Table 2.1 summarizes the percentage changes in some cardiovascular variables during pregnancy.

Measuring systemic arterial blood pressure in pregnancy is notoriously difficult, but there is now broad consensus that Korotkoff 5 should be used with auscultatory techniques [5]. However measured, there is a small fall in systolic and a greater fall in diastolic blood pressure during the first half of pregnancy resulting in an increased pulse pressure. The blood pressure then rises steadily and, even in normotensive women, there is some late overshoot of non-pregnant values. Supine hypotension occurs in ~8% of women in late gestation.

The pressor response to angiotensin II (ANG II) is reduced in normal pregnancy but is unchanged to noradrenaline. The reduced sensitivity to ANG II presumably protects against the potentially pressor levels of ANG II found in normal pregnancy and is associated with lower receptor density; plasma noradrenaline is not increased in normal pregnancy. Pregnancy does not alter the response of intramyometrial arteries to a variety of vasoconstrictors. Nitric oxide may modulate myogenic tone and flow-mediated responses in the resistance vasculature of the uterine circulation in normal pregnancy.

The venous pressure in the lower circulation rises for both mechanical and hydrodynamic reasons. The pulmonary circulation is able to absorb high rates of flow without an increase in pressure; so pressure in the right

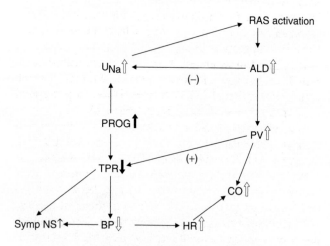

Fig. 2.1 Flow chart of the probable sequence of initial cardiovascular activation. ALD, aldosterone; BP, systemic arterial blood pressure; CO, cardiac output; HR, heart rate; PROG, progesterone; PV, plasma volume; RAS, renin-angiotensin system; Symp NS, sympathetic nervous system; TPR, total peripheral resistance; U_{Na}, urinary sodium excretion.

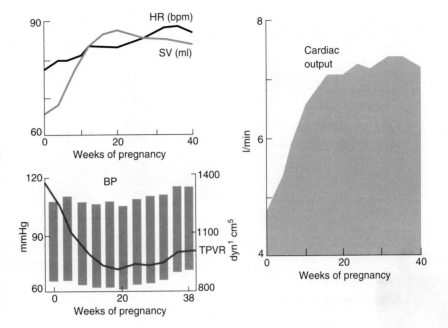

Fig. 2.2 Major haemodynamic changes associated with normal human pregnancy. The marked augmentation of cardiac output results from asynchronous increases in both heart rate (HR) and stroke volume (SV). Despite the increases in cardiac output, blood pressure (BP) decreases for most of pregnancy. This implies a very substantial reduction in total peripheral vascular resistance (TPVR).

Table 2.1 Percentage change in some cardiovascular variables during pregnancy

	First trimester	Second trimester	Third trimester
Heart rate (bpm)	+11	+13	+16
Stroke volume (ml)	+31	+29	+27
Cardiac output (l/min)	+45	+47	+48
Systolic BP (mmHg)	−1	+1	+6
Diastolic BP (mmHg)	−6	−3	+7
MPAP (mmHg)	+5	+5	+5
Total peripheral resistance (resistance units)	−27	−27	−29

BP, systemic blook pressure; MPAP, mean pulmonary artery pressure. Data are derived from studies in which pre-conception values were determined. The mean values shown are those at the end of each trimester, and are thus not necessarily the maxima. Note that most changes are near maximal by the end of the first trimester. (Data from Robson *et al.*, 1991.)

ventricle and the pulmonary arteries and capillaries does not change. Pulmonary resistance falls in early pregnancy and does not change thereafter. There is progressive venodilatation and rises in venous distensibility and capacitance throughout a normal pregnancy, possibly because of increased local nitric oxide synthesis.

The respiratory system

Tidal volume rises by ~30% in early pregnancy to 40–50% above non-pregnant values by term, with a fall in expiratory reserve and residual volume (Fig. 2.3) [6]. Neither FEV$_1$ nor peak expiratory flow rate are affected by pregnancy, even in women with asthma. The rise in tidal volume is largely driven by progesterone, which appears to decrease the threshold and increase the sensitivity of the medulla oblongata to carbon dioxide. Respiratory rate does not change, so the minute ventilation rises by a similar amount. This overbreathing also begins before conception; the P_{CO_2} is lowest in early gestation. Progesterone also increases erythrocyte [carbonic anhydrase], which will also lower P_{CO_2}. Carbon dioxide production rises sharply during the third trimester, as fetal metabolism increases. The fall in maternal P_{CO_2} allows more efficient placental transfer of carbon dioxide from the fetus, which has a P_{CO_2} of around 55 mmHg (7.3 kPa). The fall in P_{CO_2} results in a fall in plasma bicarbonate concentration (to ~18–22 mmol/l by comparison with 24–28 mmol/l) which contributes to the fall in plasma osmolality; the peripheral venous pH rises slightly (Table 2.2; Fig. 2.4).

The increased alveolar ventilation results in a much smaller proportional rise in P_{O_2}, from around 96.7 to 101.8 mmHg (12.9–13.6 kPa). This increase is offset by the rightward shift of the maternal oxyhaemoglobin dissociation curve caused by an increase in 2,3-diphosphoglycerate (2,3-DPG) in the erythrocytes. This facilitates oxygen unloading to the fetus, which has both a much lower P_{O_2} (25–30 mmHg; 3.3–4.0 kPa) and a marked leftwards shift of the oxyhaemoglobin dissociation curve, due to the lower sensitivity of fetal haemoglobin to 2,3-DPG.

There is an increase of ~16% in oxygen consumption by term, due to increasing maternal and fetal demands. Since the increase in oxygen-carrying capacity of the blood (see 'Haematology', p. 12) is ~18%, there is actually a

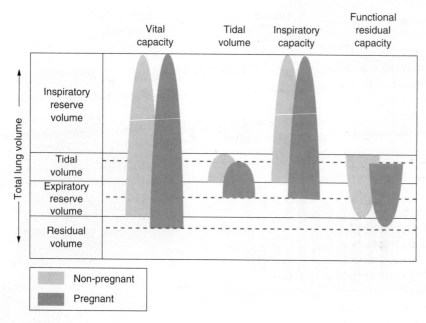

Fig. 2.3 Alterations in lung volumes associated with normal human pregnancy. In general terms, inspiratory reserve and tidal volumes increase at the expense of expiratory reserve and residual volumes.

Table 2.2 The influence of pregnancy on some respiratory variables

		Non-pregnant	Pregnant – term
P_{O_2}	mmHg (kPa)	93 (12.5)	102 (13.6)
O_2 consumption	ml/min	200	250
P_{CO_2}	mmHg (kPa)	35–40 (4.7–5.3)	30 (4.0)
Venous pH		7.35	7.38

Table 2.3 Although the increases in resting cardiac output and minute ventilation are of the same order of magnitude in pregnancy, there is less spare capacity for increases in cardiac output on moderate exercise than for increases in respiration

	Resting	Exercise
Cardiac output	+33% (4.5–6 l/min)	+167% (up to 12 l/min)
Minute ventilation	+40% 7.5–10.5 l/min	+1000% (up to ~80 l/min)

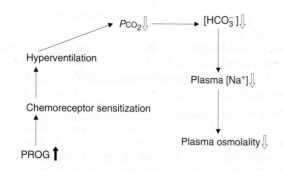

Fig. 2.4 Flow chart of the effects of over-breathing. HCO_3, bicarbonate; Na, sodium; P_{CO_2}, carbon dioxide tension; PROG, progesterone.

fall in arterio-venous oxygen difference. Pulmonary blood flow, of course, rises in parallel with cardiac output and enhances gas transfer.

Pregnancy places greater demands on the cardiovascular than the respiratory system [7]. This is shown in the response to moderate exercise (Table 2.3).

Haematology

The circulating red cell mass increases by 20–30% during pregnancy, with rises in both cell number and size. It rises more in women with multiple pregnancies, and substantially more with iron supplementation (~29% compared with 17%). Serum iron concentration falls, the absorption of iron from the gut rises and iron-binding capacity rises in a normal pregnancy, since there is increased synthesis of the β1-globulin, transferrin. Plasma folate concentration halves by term, because of greater renal clearance, although red cell folate concentrations fall less. Even now, only ~20% of fertile women in the UK have adequate iron reserves for a pregnancy and ~40% have virtually no iron stores. Even relatively mild maternal anaemia is associated with increased placental:birthweight ratios and decreased birthweight. However, inappropriate supplementation can itself be associated with pregnancy problems [8]. Erythropoietin rises in pregnancy, more if iron supplementation is not taken (55% compared with 25%) but the changes in red cell mass antedate this; human placental lactogen may stimulate haematopoiesis.

Pro rata, the plasma volume increases more than the red cell mass, which leads to a fall in the various concentration measures which include the plasma volume, such as the haematocrit, the haemoglobin concentration and the red cell count. The fall in packed cell volume from ~36% in early pregnancy to ~32% in the third trimester is a sign of normal plasma volume expansion.

The total white cell count rises, mainly because of increased polymorphonuclear leucocytes. Neutrophil numbers rise with oestrogen concentrations and peak at ~33 weeks stabilizing after that until labour and the early puerperium, when they rise sharply. Their phagocytic function increases during gestation. T and B lymphocyte counts do not change but their function is suppressed, making pregnant women more susceptible to viral infections, malaria and leprosy. The uterine natural killer cells express receptors that recognize the otherwise anomalous combination of human lymphocyte antigens (HLA-C, -E and -G) expressed by the invasive cytotrophoblasts. This is likely to be central to the maternal recognition of the conceptus [9].

Platelet count and platelet volume are largely unchanged in most pregnant women, although their survival is reduced. Platelet reactivity is increased in the second and third trimesters and does not return to normal until ~12 weeks after delivery.

Coagulation

Continuing low-grade coagulopathy is a feature of normal pregnancy [10]. Several of the potent procoagulatory factors rise from at least the end of the first trimester (Fig. 2.5). For example, Factors VII, VIII and X all rise and absolute plasma fibrinogen doubles, while antithrombin III, an inhibitor of coagulation, falls. The erythrocyte sedimentation rate rises early in pregnancy due to the increase in fibrinogen and other physiological changes. Protein C, which inactivates Factors V and VIII, is probably unchanged in pregnancy, but concentrations of Protein S, one of its co-factors, fall during the first two trimesters. An estimated 5–10% of the total circulating fibrinogen is consumed during placental separation, and thromboembolism is the main cause of maternal death in the UK. Plasma fibrinolytic activity is decreased during pregnancy and labour, but returns to non-pregnant values within an hour of delivery of the placenta, suggesting strongly that the control of fibrinolysis during pregnancy is significantly affected by placentally derived mediators. Table 2.4 summarizes changes in some coagulation and fibrinolytic variables during pregnancy.

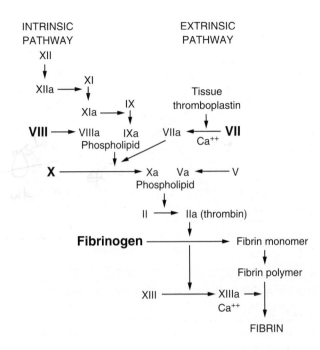

Fig. 2.5 Alterations in the coagulation pathways associated with human pregnancy. Factors which increase during normal pregnancy are printed in bold type.

Table 2.4 Percentage changes in some coagulation (upper) and fibrinolytic variables and fibronectin levels are expressed from postpartum data in the same women

	First trimester	Second trimester	Third trimester
PAI-1 (mg/ml)	−10	+68	+183
PAI-2 (mg/ml)	+732	+1804	+6554
t-PA (mg/ml)	−24	−19	+633
Protein C (% activity)	−12	+10	+9
AT III (% activity)	−21	−14	−10
TAT III	+362	+638	+785
Fibronection (mg/l)	+3	−12	+53

PAI-1 and PAI-2, plasminogen activator inhibitors 1 and 2; t-PA, tissue plasminogen activator antigen; AT III, antithrombin III; TAT III, thrombin-antithrombin III complex.
The mean values shown are those at the end of each trimester, and are thus not necessarily the maxima. Note the very large rises in PAI-2 (placental type PAI) and TAI III complexes in the first trimester. (Data from Halligan *et al.* 1994)

The renal system

The kidneys increase in size in pregnancy mainly because renal parenchymal volume rises by about 70% with marked dilatation of the calyces, renal pelvis and ureters in most women [11]. Ureteric tone does not decrease, but bladder tone does. The effective renal plasma flow (RPF) is increased by at least 6 weeks gestation and rises to some

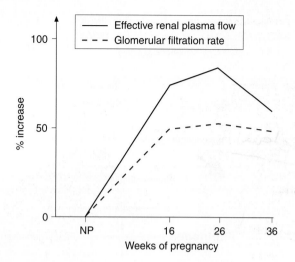

Fig. 2.6 The changes in renal function during pregnancy are largely complete by the end of the first trimester, and are thus pro-active, not reactive to the demands of pregnancy. The filtration fraction falls during the first trimester, but begins to return to non-pregnant levels during the third trimester. With permission from [11].

80% by mid-pregnancy falling thereafter to ~65% above non-pregnant values (Fig. 2.6). This increase is proportionally greater than the increase in cardiac output, presumably reflecting specific vasodilatation, probably via the increased renal prostacyclin synthesis. The glomerular filtration rate (GFR) also increases, by ~45% by the 9th week, only rising thereafter by another 5–10%, but this is largely maintained to term, so the filtration fraction falls during the first trimester, is stable during the second, and rises towards non-pregnant values thereafter. These major increments do not, however, exhaust the renal reserve. This differential changes in ERPF and GFR in late pregnancy suggest a mechanism acting preferentially at the efferent arterioles, possibly angiotensin II.

The filtered load of metabolites therefore increases markedly, and reabsorptive mechanisms frequently do not keep up (e.g. glucose and aminoacids; see below). These changes have profound effects on the concentration of certain plasma metabolites and electrolytes and 'Normal' laboratory reference ranges may thus be inappropriate in pregnancy. For example, plasma creatinine falls significantly by the 4th week of gestation and continues to fall to mid-pregnancy, to below 50 mmol/l, but creatinine clearance begins to fall during the last couple of months of pregnancy, so plasma creatinine rises again.

Total body water rises by about 20% during pregnancy (~8.5 l) with a very sharp fall in plasma osmolality between weeks 4–6 after conception, possibly through the actions of hCG. The volume-sensing arginine vasopressin (AVP) release mechanisms evidently adjust as pregnancy

progresses. As well as water present in the fetus, amniotic fluid, placenta and maternal tissues, there is also oedema fluid and increased hydration of the connective tissue ground substance with laxity and swelling of connective tissue.

The pregnant woman accumulates some 950 mmol sodium in the face of high circulating progesterone concentrations which competes with aldosterone at the distal tubule. The potentially natriuretic prostacyclin also rises markedly, with a small rise in atrial natriuretic peptide (ANP). This stimulates the renin-angiotensin system (RAS) with increased synthesis and release of aldosterone from the first trimester. The raised plasma prolactin concentration may also contribute to sodium retention. It is assumed that glomerulotubular balance must also change in pregnancy, to allow the sodium retention which actually occurs. There is a fall of some 4–5 mmol/l in plasma sodium by term, but plasma chloride does not change. Curiously, some 350 mmol potassium is also retained during pregnancy, in the face of the much-increased GFR, substantially raised aldosterone concentrations and a relatively alkaline urine. Renal tubular potassium reabsorption evidently adjusts appropriately to the increased filtered potassium load.

Serum uric acid concentration falls by about a quarter in early pregnancy, with an increase in its fractional excretion secondary to a decrease in net tubular reabsorption. The kidney excretes a progressively smaller proportion of the filtered uric acid, so a rise in serum uric acid concentration during the second half of pregnancy is normal. A similar pattern is seen in relation to urea, which is also partly reabsorbed in the nephron.

Glucose excretion may rise 10-fold as the greater filtered load exceeds the proximal tubular T_{max} for glucose (~1.6–1.9 mmol/min). If the urine of pregnant women is tested sufficiently often, glycosuria will be detected in 50% of them. The excretion of most amino acids increases, which is curious since these are used by the fetus as the building blocks from which it synthesises protein. The pattern of excretion is not constant and differs between individual amino acids. Excretion of the water-soluble vitamins is also increased. The mechanism for all these is inadequate tubular reabsorption in the face of a 50% rise in GFR.

Urinary calcium excretion is also two to threefold higher in normal pregnancy than in the non-pregnant woman, even though tubular reabsorption is enhanced, presumably under the influence of the increased concentrations of 1,25-dihydroxyvitamin D. To counter this, intestinal absorption doubles by 24 weeks, after which it stabilizes. Renal bicarbonate reabsorption and hydrogen ion excretion appear to be unaltered during pregnancy. Pregnant women can acidify their urine, but in pregnancy it is mildly alkaline.

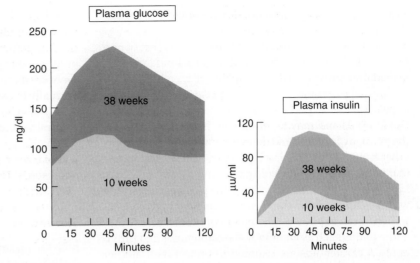

Fig. 2.7 Responses in normal pregnant women to a 50 g oral glucose load during early and late pregnancy. During early pregnancy there is a normal plasma insulin response with a relative reduction in plasma glucose concentrations compared to the non-pregnant state. In contrast, during late pregnancy plasma glucose concentrations reach higher levels after a delay, despite a considerably enhanced plasma insulin response, a pattern which could be explained by relative resistance to insulin.

Both total protein and albumin excretion rise during pregnancy, up to at least 36 weeks, due to the increased GFR and changes in both glomerular and tubular function. Thus in late pregnancy, an upper limit of normal of 200 mg total protein excretion/24 h collection is accepted. The assessment of proteinuria in pregnancy using dipsticks has been shown to give highly variable data.

The gastrointestinal system

Taste often alters very early in pregnancy. The whole intestinal tract has decreased motility during the first two trimesters, with increased absorption of water and salt, tending to increase constipation. Heartburn is common from the increased intragastric pressure. Hepatic synthesis of albumin, plasma globulin and fibrinogen increases, the latter two sufficiently to give increased plasma concentrations despite the increase in plasma volume. Total hepatic synthesis of globulin increases under oestrogen stimulation, so the hormone-binding globulins rise. There is decreased hepatic extraction of circulating amino acids.

The gallbladder increases in size and empties more slowly during pregnancy but the secretion of bile is unchanged. Cholestasis is almost physiological in pregnancy and may be associated with generalized pruritus but only rarely produces jaundice. The cholestasis can also occur in users of oral contraceptives and postmenopausal hormone replacement.

Carbohydrates/insulin resistance

Pregnancy is hyperlipidaemic and glucosuric. Although neither the absorption of glucose from the gut nor the half-life of insulin seems to change and the insulin response is well-maintained, by 6–12 weeks gestation, fasting plasma glucose concentrations fall by 0.11 mmol/l, and by the end of the first trimester the increase in blood glucose following a carbohydrate load is less than outside pregnancy [12]. This increased sensitivity stimulates glycogen synthesis and storage, deposition of fat and transport of amino acids into cells. The uptake of amino acids by the mother for gluconeogenesis may also be enhanced. After mid-pregnancy, resistance to the action of insulin develops progressively and plasma glucose concentrations rise, though remaining below non-pregnant levels (Fig. 2.7). Glucose crosses the placenta readily and the fetus uses glucose as its primary energy substrate, so this rise is presumably beneficial to the fetus. Fetal and maternal glucose concentrations are significantly correlated.

The insulin resistance is presumably largely endocrine-driven, possibly via increased cortisol or hPL. Leptin has been implicated in altered insulin sensitivity outside pregnancy, but appears not to play a role during gestation, while concentrations of glucagons and the catecholamines are unaltered.

Lipids

Total plasma cholesterol falls early in pregnancy, reaching its lowest point at 6–8 weeks, but then rises to term. There is a striking increase in circulating free fatty acids and complex lipids in pregnancy, with ~threefold increases in triglycerides and a 50% increase in very low density lipoprotein (VLDL) cholesterol by 36 weeks [13]. High density lipoprotein (HDL) cholesterol is also increased. Birthweight and placental weight are directly related to maternal VLDL triglyceride levels at term. The hyperlipidaemia of normal pregnancy is not atherogenic because the pattern of increase is not that of atherogenesis, although pregnancy can unmask pathological hyperlipidaemia.

Lipids undergo peroxidation in all tissues as part of normal cellular function. Excess production of lipid can result in oxidative stress with damage to the cell membrane. During normal pregnancy, increases in plasma lipid peroxides appear by the second trimester in step with the general rise in lipids and may taper off later in gestation [14]. As the peroxide levels rise so do those of vitamin E and some other antioxidants: this rise is proportionately greater than that of peroxides so physiological activities are protected. Lipid peroxidation is also active in the placenta, increasing with gestation. Since the placenta contains high concentrations of unsaturated fats under conditions of low P_{O_2}, antioxidants such as vitamin A, the carotenoids and provitamin A carotenoids are required to protect both mother and fetus from free radical activity Early in pregnancy fat is deposited but from mid-pregnancy it is used as a source of energy, mainly by the mother so that glucose is available for the growing fetus [15]. The absorption of fat from the intestine is not directly altered during pregnancy. The hormone leptin acts as a sensor alerting the brain to the extent of body fat stores and rises threefold during pregnancy. It may regulate maternal energy balance.

Endocrine systems

The placenta is a powerhouse of hormone production from the beginning of gestation and challenges the mother's autonomy.

Placental hormones

Human chorionic gonadotrophin is the signal for pregnancy, but indirect effects, such as oestrogen-driven increased hepatic synthesis of the binding globulins for hormones such as thyroxine, corticosteroids and the sex steroids also affect the mother's endocrinological function. The fetoplacental unit synthesizes very large amounts of oestrogens and progesterone, both probably being concerned with uterine growth and quiescence and with mammary gland development.

The hypothalamus and pituitary gland

The pituitary gland increases in weight by 30% in first pregnancies and by 50% subsequently. The number of lactotrophs is increased and plasma prolactin begins to rise within a few days of conception and by term may be 10–20 times as high as in the non-pregnant woman; the secretion of other anterior pituitary hormones is unchanged or reduced. Human chorionic gonadotrophin (hCG) and the gonadotrophins share a common α-subunit,

and the rapidly rising hCG suppresses secretion of both follicle-stimulating hormone and luteinizing hormone, thus inhibiting ovarian follicle development by a blunting of response to gonadotrophin-releasing hormone (GnRH). Thyroid-stimulating hormone (TSH) secretion responds normally to hypothalamic thyrotropin-releasing hormone (TRH; also synthesized in the placenta). Adrenocorticotropic hormone (ACTH) concentrations rise during pregnancy, partly because of placental synthesis of ACTH and of a corticotrophin-releasing hormone (CRH) and do not respond to normal control mechanisms.

The adrenal gland

Both the plasma total and the unbound cortisol and other corticosteroid concentrations rise in pregnancy from about the end of the first trimester. Concentrations of cortisol-binding globulin double. Excess glucocorticoid exposure *in utero* appears to inhibit fetal growth in both animals and humans. However, the normal placenta synthesizes a pregnancy-specific 11b-hydroxysteroid dehydrogenase, which inhibits transfer of maternal cortisol. The marked rise in secretion of the mineralocorticoid aldosterone in pregnancy has already been mentioned. Synthesis of the weaker mineralocorticoid 11-deoxycorticosterone is also increased by the 8th week of pregnancy, and actually increases proportionally more than any other cortical steroid, possibly due to placental synthesis.

The measurement of plasma catecholamines has inherent difficulties, but there is now broad consensus that plasma catecholamine concentrations fall from the first to the third trimesters. There is some blunting of the rise in noradrenaline (reflecting mainly sympathetic nerve activity) seen on standing and isometric exercise in pregnancy, but the adrenaline response (predominantly adrenal) is unaltered [16].

The thyroid gland

hCG may suppress thyroid-stimulating hormone (TSH) in early pregnancy because they share a common α-subunit. The thyroid remains normally responsive to stimulation by TSH and suppression by tri-iodothyronine (T3). There is a threefold rise in the thyroid's clearance of iodine, allowing the absolute iodine uptake to remain within the non-pregnant range. Thyroid-binding globulin concentrations double during pregnancy, but other thyroid-binding proteins do not increase. Overall, free plasma T3 and thyroxine (T4) concentrations remain at the same levels as outside pregnancy (although total levels are raised) and most pregnant women are euthyroid. Free T4 may fall in late gestation [17].

Calcitonin, another thyroid hormone, rises during the first trimester, peaks in the second and falls thereafter, although the changes are not large. It may contribute to the regulation of 1,25 dihydroxyvitamin D.

The parathyroid glands and calcium metabolism

Calcium homeostasis changes markedly [18,19]. Maternal total plasma calcium concentration falls, because albumin concentration falls, but unbound ionized calcium concentration is unchanged. Synthesis of 1,25 dihydroxycholecalciferol increases, promoting enhanced gastrointestinal calcium absorption. Parathyroid hormone (PTH) regulates the synthesis of 1,25 dihydroxyvitamin D in the proximal convoluted tubule. There is a fall in intact PTH during pregnancy but a doubling of 1,25 dihydroxyvitamin D; placentally synthesized PTH-related protein is also present in the maternal circulation.

Renal hormones

The RAS is activated from very early pregnancy (see 'The cardiovascular system', p. 10). Synthesis of erythropoietin appears to be stimulated by hCG; its concentration rises from the first trimester, peaking in mid-gestation and falling somewhat thereafter. Prostacyclin is a potent vasodilator, synthesized mainly in the kidney. Concentrations begin to rise rapidly by 8–10 weeks gestation, being fourfold higher than non-pregnant values by the end of the first trimester.

The pancreas

The size of the islets of Langerhans and the number of β-cells increase during pregnancy, as does the number of receptor sites for insulin. The functions of the pancreas in pregnancy were considered above.

Conclusion

This chapter attempts to outline the physiology of normal pregnancy. The changes mostly begin very early indeed, and it may be that two of the major problems of pregnancy, intrauterine growth retardation and pre-eclampsia, are initiated even before the woman knows that she is pregnant. Better understanding of the mechanisms of very early normal pregnancy adaptation may help us to understand the abnormal.

References

1. Chapman AB, Zamudio S, Woodmansee W *et al.* (1997) Systemic and renal hemodynamic changes in the luteal phase of the menstrual cycle mimic early pregnancy. *Am J Physiol* **273**(5 Pt 2), F777–82.
2. Chapman AB, Abraham WT, Zamudio S *et al.* (1998) Temporal relationships between hormonal and hemodynamic changes in early human pregnancy. *Kidney Int* **54**(6), 2056–63.
3. Ganzevoort W, Rep A, Bonsel GJ, de Vries JI & Wolf H (2004) Plasma volume and blood pressure regulation in hypertensive pregnancy. *J Hypertens* **22**(7), 1235–42.
4. Robson SC, Hunter S, Boys RJ & Dunlop W (1989) Serial study of factors influencing changes in cardiac output during human pregnancy. *Am J Physiol* **256**(4 Pt 2), H1060–5.
5. de Swiet M & Shennan A (1996) Blood pressure measurement in pregnancy. *Br J Obstet Gynaecol* **103**(9), 862–3.
6. de Swiet M (1998) The respiratory system. In: Chamberlain G & Broughton Pipkin F (eds) *Clinical Physiology in Obstetrics*, 3rd edn. Oxford: Blackwell Science Ltd., 111–28.
7. Bessinger RC, McMurray RG & Hackney AC (2002) Substrate utilization and hormonal responses to moderate intensity exercise during pregnancy and after delivery. *Am J Obstet Gynecol* **186**(4), 757–64.
8. Scholl TO (2005) Iron status during pregnancy: setting the stage for mother and infant. *Am J Clin Nutr* **81**(5), 1218S–22S.
9. Moffett A & Loke YW (2004) The immunological paradox of pregnancy: a reappraisal. *Placenta* **25**(1), 1–8.
10. Brenner B (2004) Haemostatic changes in pregnancy. *Thromb Res* **114**(5–6), 409–14.
11. Bayliss C & Davison JM (1998) The urinary system. In: Chamberlain G & Broughton Pipkin F (eds) *Clinical Physiology in Obstetrics*, 3rd edn. Oxford: Blackwell Science Ltd, 263–307.
12. Butte NF (2000) Carbohydrate and lipid metabolism in pregnancy: normal compared with gestational diabetes mellitus. *Am J Clin Nutr* **71**(5 Suppl), 1256S–61S.
13. Herrera E, Ortega H, Alvino G, Giovannini N, Amusquivar E & Cetin I (2004) Relationship between plasma fatty acid profile and antioxidant vitamins during normal pregnancy. *Eur J Clin Nutr* **58**(9), 1231–8.
14. Poston L & Raijmakers MT (2004) Trophoblast oxidative stress, antioxidants and pregnancy outcome – a review. *Placenta* **25**(Suppl A), S72–8.
15. Kopp-Hoolihan LE, van Loan MD, Wong WW & King JC (1999) Longitudinal assessment of energy balance in well-nourished, pregnant women. *Am J Clin Nutr* **69**(4), 697–704.
16. Barron WM, Mujais SK, Zinaman M, Bravo EL & Lindheimer MD (1986) Plasma catecholamine responses to physiologic stimuli in normal human pregnancy. *Am J Obstet Gynecol* **154**(1), 80–4.
17. Ramsay ID (1998) The thyroid gland. In: Chamberlain G & Broughton Pipkin F (eds) *Clinical Physiology in Obstetrics*,

3rd edn. Oxford: Blackwell Science Ltd, 374–84.

18. Prentice A (2000) Maternal calcium metabolism and bone mineral status. *Am J Clin Nutr* **71**(5 Suppl), 1312S–6S.

19. Haig D (2004) Evolutionary conflicts in pregnancy and calcium metabolism – a review. *Placenta* **25**(Suppl A), S10–5.

Further reading

Chamberlain G & Broughton Pipkin F (eds) (1998) *Clinical Physiology in Obstetrics*, 3rd edn. Oxford: Blackwell Science.

Broughton Pipkin F (2001) Maternal Physiology. In: Chamberlain, G & Steer P (eds) *Turnbull's Obstetrics*, 3rd edn. London: Churchill Livingstone.

Chapter 3: The placenta and fetal membranes

Berthold Huppertz and John C.P. Kingdom

The placenta

The placenta was already recognized and venerated by the early Egyptians, while it was the Greek physician Diogenes of Apollonia (ca. 480 BC) who first ascribed the function of fetal nutrition to the organ. Aristotle (384–322 BC) described that the fetus is fully enclosed within the chorion membranes; and it was only during the Renaissance that the term placenta, the word derived from the Latin root meaning a flat "cake", was introduced by Realdus Columbus in 1559.

Structural characteristic of the human placenta

Tissue interactions [1,2]

On the gross anatomic level, a placenta can be classified according to whether the physical interactions between fetal and maternal tissues are restricted to specific sites or are covering the whole surface of the chorionic sac and the inner uterine surface. On this level, the human placenta is classified to be a *discoidal* placenta, confining interactions to a more or less circular area (Fig. 3.1a).

Tissue interdigitations [1,2]

The next level of classification is based on the interdigitations between maternal and fetal tissues. In the human placenta, maternal and fetal tissues are arranged in such a way that there are three-dimensional tree-like structures called *villous* trees of fetal tissues that float in a lake of maternal blood. Like the knots and branches of a tree, the fetal tissues repeatedly branch into smaller and slender villi (Fig. 3.1b).

Tissue interactions [1,2]

On the level of interactions between uterine and fetal tissues, the human displays an invasive type of implantation and placentation. The uterine epithelium is penetrated and invasion of maternal tissues results in erosion into maternal vessels. This type of placentation is termed *hemochorial* and is characterized by the bathing of placental villi with covering trophoblast directly by the mother's blood (Fig. 3.1c).

Vascular arrangement [1,2]

It is not just the thickness and exact histological nature of the placental barrier that defines the rate of diffusional exchange. Another important determinant is the direction of the blood flows of mother and fetus in relation to each other. The vascular arrangement of the human placenta cannot be clearly defined due to the branching of the villous trees into all directions and a respective maternal blood flow somehow bypassing these branches. Therefore, this unpredictable and variable flow pattern has been termed *multivillous* flow (Fig. 3.1d).

Macroscopic features of the term placenta

Measures [1,2]

The placenta at term displays a round disc-like appearance with the insertion of the umbilical cord in a slightly eccentric position on the fetal side of the placenta. The average measures of a delivered placenta at term are a diameter of 22 cm, a central thickness of 2.5 cm, and a weight of 450–500 g. One has to keep in mind, though, that these data may vary considerably due to the mode of delivery, especially content versus loss of maternal and/or fetal blood.

Tissue arrangements [1,2]

On the fetal side of the placenta, the avascular *amnion* covers the *chorionic plate*. Underneath the amnion, chorionic vessels continue with those of the umbilical cord and are arranged in a star-like pattern. At the other end, these vessels continue with those of the villous

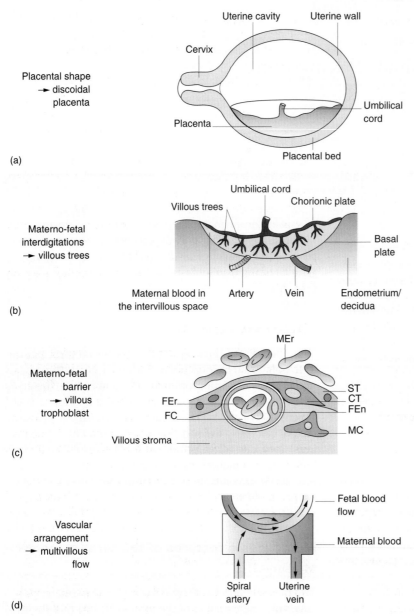

Fig. 3.1 Schematic representation of the structural characteristics of the human placenta. (a) The human placenta displays a discoidal shape. (b) The materno-fetal interdigitations are arranged in villous trees bathing in maternal blood that floats through the intervillous space. (c) The hemochorial type of placentation results in a materno-fetal barrier composed of villous trophoblast in direct contact with maternal blood. (d) Fetal and maternal blood flows are arranged in a multivillous flow. Abbreviations: CT, cytotrophoblast; FC, fetal capillary; FEn, fetal endothelium; FEr, fetal eryrocyte; MC, mesenchymal cells; MEr, maternal erythrocyte; ST, syncytiotrophoblast.

trees where the capillary system between arteries and veins is located. The *villous trees* originate from the chorionic plate and float in a lake of maternal blood. On the maternal side of the placenta, the *basal plate* is located (see Fig. 3.1b). It is an artificial surface generated by the separation of the placenta from the uterine wall during delivery. The basal plate is a colourful mixture of fetal trophoblast and maternal decidua cells, which are embedded in trophoblast-secreted matrix-type fibrinoid, decidual extracellular matrices, and fibrin-type fibrinoid. At the placental margin, chorionic plate and basal plate fuse with each other, thereby closing the intervillous space and generating the *fetal membranes* or *chorion laeve*.

Placental development
Trophoblast lineage [3,4]

At the transition between morula and blastocyst, the trophoblast lineage is the first to differentiate from the inner cell mass, the embryoblast (Fig. 3.2). Only after attachment of the blastocyst to the endometrial epithelium, further differentiation of the trophoblast occurs. Exact knowledge

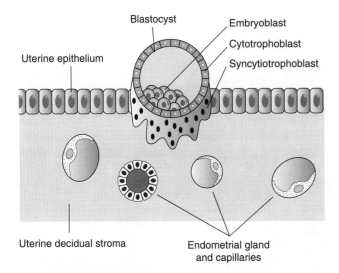

Fig. 3.2 During implantation of the blastocyst, trophoblast cells in direct contact with maternal tissues syncytially fuse and give rise to the syncytiotrophoblast. Only this multinucleated tissue is able to penetrate the uterine epithelium and implant the developing embryo.

of the processes in the human is still lacking, but it is anticipated that at this stage the first syncytial fusion of trophoblast cells takes place. Fusion of those trophoblast cells in direct contact with maternal tissues generates the very first syncytiotrophoblast and only this layer is able to penetrate the endometrial epithelium (Fig. 3.2).

Prelacunar stage [1,2]

At day 7–8 postconception, the blastocyst has completely crossed the epithelium and is embedded within the endometrium. The developing embryo is completely surrounded by the growing placenta, which at that stage consists of the two fundamental subtypes of the trophoblast. The multinucleated syncytiotrophoblast is in direct contact with maternal tissues, while the mononucleated cytotrophoblast as the stem cell layer of the trophoblast is directed towards the embryo.

All of the differentiation and developmental stages of the placenta described so far take place before fluid-filled spaces within the syncytiotrophoblast can be detected. This is why this stage is termed *prelacunar stage*.

Lacunar stage [1,2]

At day 8–9 postconception, the syncytiotrophoblast generates a number of fluid-filled spaces within its mass. These spaces flow together forming larger lacunae (*lacunar stage*) and are finally separated by parts of the syncytiotrophoblast (trabeculae) that cross the syncytial mass from the embryonic to the maternal side.

The development of the lacunar system leads to the subdivision of the placenta into its three compartments.
1 the embryonically oriented part of the trophoblast will develop into the *chorionic plate*,
2 the lacunae will become the *intervillous space*,
3 while the trabeculae will become the *anchoring villi*,
4 with the growing branches developing into *floating villi*,
5 finally, the maternally oriented part of the trophoblast will develop into the *basal plate*.
At the end of this stage, at day 12 postconception, the process of implantation is completed. The developing embryo with its surrounding extraembryonic tissues is totally embedded in the endometrium and the syncytiotrophoblast surrounds the whole surface of the conceptus. Mesenchymal cells derived from the embryo spread over the inner surface of the trophoblast, thus generating a new combination of trophoblast and mesoderm, termed *chorion*.

Early villous stage [1,2]

Starting on day 12 postconception, proliferation of cytotrophoblast pushes trophoblast cells to penetrate into the syncytial trabeculae, reaching the maternal side of the syncytiotrophoblast by day 14. Further proliferation of trophoblast cells inside the trabeculae (day 13) stretches the trabeculae resulting in the development of syncytial side branches filled with cytotrophoblast cells (*primary villi*).

Shortly after, the mesenchymal cells from the extraembryonic mesoderm too follow the cytotrophoblast and penetrate the trabeculae and the primary villi, thus generating *secondary villi*. At this stage there is always a complete cytotrophoblast layer between the penetrating mesenchyme and syncytiotrophoblast.

Around day 20–21, vascularization (development of new vessels from hemangioblastic precursor cells) within the villous mesenchyme gives rise to the formation of the first placental vessels (*tertiary villi*). Only later, the connection to the fetal vessel system will be established.

The villi are organized in villous trees that cluster together into a series of spherical units known as lobules or placentones. Each placentone originates from the chorionic plate by a thick villous trunk stemming from a trabecula. Continuous branching of the main trunk results in daughter villi mostly freely ending in the intervillous space [5,6].

Trophoblast cell columns [1,2]

During penetration of the syncytial trabeculae, the cytotrophoblast cells reach the maternal endometrial tissues while the following mesenchymal cells do not penetrate

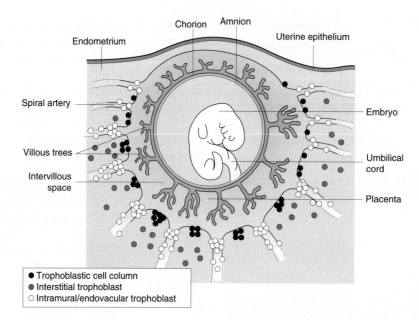

Chorion   Amnion

Endometrium   Uterine epithelium

Spiral artery   Embryo

Villous trees   Umbilical cord

Intervillous space   Placenta

- ● Trophoblastic cell column
- ● Interstitial trophoblast
- ○ Intramural/endovacular trophoblast

Fig. 3.3 Schematic representation of the developing embryo and its surrounding tissues at about 8–10 weeks of pregnancy. The amnionic cavity with the embryo inside is marked off by the amnion that has already contacted the chorion. From the chorion, villous trees protrude into the intervillous space where some villi have direct contact with the basal plate (anchoring villi). At these sites trophoblastic cell columns are the source for all extravillous trophoblast cells invading maternal tissues. Interstitial trophoblast cells derived from these columns invade the endometrium and myometrium, while a subset of these cells penetrates the spiral arteries first as intramural and then as endovascular trophoblast cells. Onset of maternal blood flow into the placenta starts in the upper regions of the placenta (the abembryonic pole) where development is slightly delayed. The local high concentrations of oxygen contribute to the regression of villi at the abembryonic pole.

to the tips of the trabeculae. At the tips multiple layers of cytotrophoblast cells are developing, referred to as trophoblastic *cell columns* (Fig. 3.3). Only those cytotrophoblast cells remain as proliferative stem cells that are in direct contact with the basement membrane separating trophoblast from mesenchyme of the anchoring villi.

Subtypes of extravillous trophoblast [1,2,7–9]

The formation of cell columns does not result in a complete trophoblastic shell but rather in separated columns from which extravillous trophoblast cells invade maternal uterine tissues (Fig. 3.3). These cells migrate as *interstitial trophoblast* into the endometrial stroma, while a subset of the interstitial trophoblast further penetrates the wall of the uterine spiral arteries (*intramural trophoblast*), finally reaching the vessels' lumen (*endovascular trophoblast*) (Fig. 3.3). Some of the interstitial trophoblast cells fuse and generate the *multinucleated trophoblast giant cells* (Fig. 3.4) at the boundary between the endometrium and myometrium.

Plugging of spiral arteries

The invasion of extravillous trophoblast cells is the ultimate means to transform maternal vessels into large-bore conduits to enable adequate supply of oxygen and nutrients to the placenta [1,2,10–12]. However, free transfer of maternal blood to the intervillous space is only established at the end of the first trimester of pregnancy [13,14]. Before the free transfer of maternal blood can occur, the extent of invasion and thus the number of endovascular trophoblast is so great that the trophoblast cells aggregate within the vessels' lumen and plug the distal segments of the spiral arteries (Fig. 3.3). Hence, before 10–12 weeks of gestation, the intervillous space contains mostly glandular secretion products together with a plasma filtrate that is free of maternal blood cells (Fig. 3.3) [13,14].

The reason for such a paradoxical plugging of already eroded and transformed arteries may be as follows: lack of blood cells keeps the placenta and the fetus in a low oxygen environment of less than 20 mmHg in the first trimester of pregnancy. This low oxygen environment may be necessary to prevent the formation of free radicals that affect the growing fetus in this critical stage of tissue and organ development [15–17].

Onset of maternal blood flow [13,14]

At the end of the first trimester the trophoblastic plugs become pervious and maternal blood cells enter the

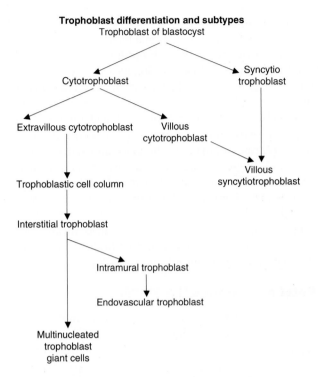

Trophoblast differentiation and subtypes

Fig. 3.4 Trophoblast differentiation and subtypes. The trophoblast lineage is the first to develop at the blastocyst stage. From this stage onwards, further differentiation leads to the generation of the syncytiotrophoblast and subsequently into the two main trophoblast types of placental villi, villous cytotrophoblast and villous syncytiotrophoblast. The trophoblast cells that start to invade maternal tissues are termed extravillous trophoblast with its respective subtypes.

intervillous space establishing the first arterial blood flow to the placenta. The inflow starts in those upper parts of the placenta that are closer to the endometrial epithelium (Fig. 3.3). These sites are characterized by a slight delay in development since the deeper parts have been the first to develop directly after implantation (Fig. 3.3). Therefore, at these upper sites the plugs inside the vessels contain fewer cells, enabling blood cells to penetrate the plugs earlier, and blood flow starts first at these sites. Here the placental villi degenerate in larger parts and the chorion becomes secondarily smooth. The regression leads to the formation of the fetal membrane or *chorion laeve*. The remaining part of the placenta develops into the *chorion frondosum*, the definitive disc-shaped placenta.

Basic structure of villi

Villous trophoblast [1,2]

The branches of the syncytial trabeculae are the forerunners of the placental villi. Throughout gestation the syncytial cover remains and forms the placental barrier between the maternal blood floating in the intervillous space and the fetal vessels within the mesenchymal villous core.

Cytotrophoblast [1,2]

The layer of the mononucleated *cytotrophoblast* cells is the basal layer of villous trophoblast and located underneath the multinucleated syncytiotrophoblast (see Fig. 3.1c). These stem cells rest on a basement membrane, maintaining their proliferative activity throughout gestation. Hence, the total number of villous cytotrophoblast cells continuously increases during pregnancy, from about 1×10^9 at 13–16 weeks to about 6×10^9 at 37–41 weeks of gestation.

During gestation, cytotrophoblast cells are prevented from coming into direct contact with maternal blood. Damaged areas of syncytiotrophoblast are filled with *fibrin-type fibrinoid* (a blood clot product) to cover the exposed cytotrophoblast cells and to separate them and to keep them from coming into direct contact with maternal blood [18].

Syncytiotrophoblast [1,2]

The *syncytiotrophoblast* is a multinucleated layer without lateral cell borders, hence there is a single syncytiotrophoblast covering all villi of a single placenta. Microvilli on its apical surface provide amplification of the surface (sevenfold) and are in direct contact to the maternal blood floating within the intervillous space (see Fig. 3.1c). Growth and maintenance of the syncytiotrophoblast is completely dependent on the fusion with the underlying cytotrophoblast, since syncytial nuclei do not display transcriptional activity.

Within the syncytiotrophoblast the incorporated nuclei first exhibit a large and ovoid shape, while during maturation they become smaller and denser. Finally, they display envelope convolution, increased packing density and increased heterochromatinization [19,20].

Syncytial fusion by far exceeds the needs for growth since the syncytiotrophoblast needs steady input for the maintenance of its functional and structural integrity. Consequently, the nuclei that are incorporated into the syncytium are accumulated and packed into protrusions of the apical membrane. These *syncytial knots* are then extruded into the maternal circulation [21].

Trophoblast turnover [1,2,21–23]

Like every epithelium, the villous trophoblast displays a continuous turnover comprising:
1 proliferation of cytotrophoblast stem cells,

2 differentiation of post-proliferative daughter cells (2–3 days),
3 syncytial fusion of these cells with the overlying syncytiotrophoblast,
4 further differentiation and maturation within the syncytiotrophoblast (3–4 weeks),
5 aging and late apoptosis at specific sites of the syncytiotrophoblast, and finally
6 packing of old material into syncytial knots and extrusion of membrane-sealed corpuscles into the maternal circulation.

Trophoblast release

Throughout gestation, syncytial knots are released into the maternal circulation [21–27] and are mostly lodged in the capillary bed of the lung. Hence, they can be found in uterine vein blood but not in arterial blood of a pregnant woman. It has been estimated that in late gestation up to 150,000 such corpuscles or 2–3 g of trophoblast material enter the maternal circulation each day [1,21].

Current knowledge places the multinucleated syncytial knots as products generated by apoptotic mechanisms [23]. As such, they are surrounded by a tightly sealed plasma membrane not releasing any content into the maternal blood. Hence, induction of an inflammatory response of the mother is not a normal feature of pregnancy. However, during placental pathologies with a disturbed trophoblast turnover such as pre-eclampsia the release of syncytiotrophoblast material is altered to a more non-apoptotic release. This necrotic or aponecrotic release of material could easily induce the endothelial damage typical of pre-eclampsia [21–23,25–27].

Villous stroma [1,2]

The stromal villous core comprises the population of fixed connective tissue cells including:
1 mesenchymal cells and fibroblasts in different stages of differentiation up to myofibroblasts [28,29],
2 placental macrophages (Hofbauer cells) and
3 placental vessels with smooth muscle cells and endothelial cells.

Oxygen as regulator of villous development

There is an increasing recognition of the role oxidative stress inside the placenta plays in the pathophysiology of pregnancy disorders ranging from miscarriage to pre-eclampsia [1,13,15–17,30–32]. During the first trimester, villous trophoblast is well adapted to low oxygen; and it appears that trophoblast is more susceptible to raised oxygen rather than low oxygen [23,30,32]. Hence, during

the first trimester if the upper side of the placenta is oxygenated by the onset of maternal blood flow, villi display increased evidence of oxidative stress, become avascular and finally regress. These physiological changes at the abembryonic pole result in the formation of the chorion laeve (Fig. 3.3).

If such early onset of maternal blood flow and consequently early onset of oxygenation occurs inside the whole placenta damage to the placenta itself will result. The most severe cases are missed miscarriages, while less severe cases may continue but may lead to pathologies such as pre-eclampsia and intrauterine growth restriction (IUGR) [13,17]. It becomes more and more clear that in pre-eclampsia increased oxidative stress is evident; and recent data point to hyperoxic changes or to the occurrence of fluctuating oxygen concentrations [23,30].

Fetal membranes [1,2,33–35]

Fluid accumulation within the amnionic cavity, that is, between embryo and chorionic sac leads to a complete separation of embryo and surrounding extraembryonic tissues, only leaving the developing umbilical cord as the connection between placenta and embryo. The amnionic mesenchyme comes into direct contact with the chorionic mesoderm lining the inner surface of the chorionic sac. Both tissue layers do not fuse, and it remains that amnion and chorion can easily slide against each other. As described above, it is only at the implantation pole that the definitive placenta develops. Due to regression of villi, most of the surface of the chorionic sac (about 70%) develops in such a way that the early chorionic plate, together with the amnion, remnants of villi and the early basal plate fuse and form a multilayered compact structure termed the chorion laeve or fetal membranes.

Layers of the chorion laeve

The layers of the chorion laeve from the fetal to the maternal side are as follows (Fig. 3.5):
1 *Amnionic epithelium.* It is a single cuboideal epithelium secreting and resorbing the amnionic fluid and involved in removal of carbon dioxide and pH regulation.
2 *Amnionic mesoderm.* It is a thin layer of connective tissue separated from the amnionic epithelium by a basement membrane.
3 *Chorionic mesoderm.* This second layer of connective tissue is separated from the amnionic mesoderm by slender, fluid-filled clefts. It is continuous with the connective tissue of the chorionic plate.
4 *Extravillous trophoblast of the fetal membranes.* This specific type of extravillous tropohblast does not display invasive properties and is separated from the chorionic mesoderm by another basement membrane.

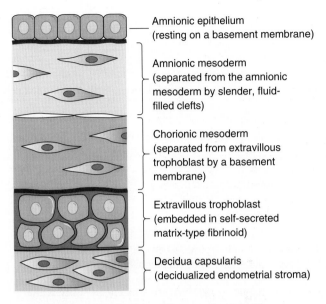

Amnionic epithelium
(resting on a basement membrane)

Amnionic mesoderm
(separated from the amnionic mesoderm by slender, fluid-filled clefts)

Chorionic mesoderm
(separated from extravillous trophoblast by a basement membrane)

Extravillous trophoblast
(embedded in self-secreted matrix-type fibrinoid)

Decidua capsularis
(decidualized endometrial stroma)

Fig. 3.5 Layers of the fetal membranes. The amnionic epithelium is a simple epithelium that secretes and resorbs the amnionic fluid. The two layers of connective tissues (amnionic and chorionic mesoderm) are separated by fluid-filled clefts. The extravillous trophoblast of the fetal membranes displays a non-invasive phenotype and is embedded in a self-secreted matrix, termed matrix-type fibrinoid. Finally, on the maternal side the fetal membranes are covered by capsular decidua of maternal origin.

5 *Capsular decidua.* This layer of maternal cells is directly attached to the extravillous trophoblast. At the end of the implantation process, the decidua closes again over the developing embryo, generating the capsular decidua. During the early second trimester, the capsular decidua fuses with the opposite wall of the uterus causing obliteration of the uterine cavity.

Characteristics [1,2]

After separation from the uterine wall, the fetal membranes have a mean thickness of about 200–300 μm at term. The presence of the decidua capsularis on the outer surface of the fetal membranes after delivery indicates that separation of the membranes takes place in between maternal tissues rather than along the materno-fetal interface. Due to the absence of vascular structures inside the chorionic as well as amnionic mesoderm, all paraplacental exchanges between fetal membranes and fetus have to pass the amnionic fluid.

Ultrasound [36–45]

Using ultrasound just a few days after the expected menstrual period a gestational sac with a diameter of 2–3 mm

can be detected within the uterine endometrium. Developmental changes in the structure and organization of the placenta and membranes can be seen by ultrasound [40]. Minor anatomical variations, such as cysts and lakes, can readily be distinguished from lesions that destroy functioning villous tissue, such as infarcts and intervillous thrombi. Small placentas typically have eccentric cords, due to chorionic regression, and can have progressive parenchymal lesions – these features are typical in early-onset IUGR [41]. Placental location and cord insertion are relevant to document. Pathological placental invasion (placenta acreta or percreta) may be suspected by ultrasound, and can be confirmed by magnetic resonance imaging (MRI).

Doppler ultrasound

Pulsed and colour Doppler ultrasound are valuable techniques for placental assessment. Umbilical cord flow can be seen at 7–8 weeks, though end-diastolic flow (EDF) is not established until 14 weeks. Early-onset IUGR pregnancies may be characterized by absent EDF in the umbilical arteries [41], associated with small malformed placentas, and defective angiogenesis in the gas-exchanging terminal placental villi [42]. A major role for Doppler ultrasound in placental assessment is to determine maternal flow in the uterine arteries. This screening test is performed either at the 18–20-week anatomical ultrasound or at a separate 22-week visit [43]. Integration of placental ultrasound, uterine artery Doppler and first + second trimester biochemistry screening tests (PAPP-A, hCG and AFP) is an effective way of screening for serious placental insufficiency syndromes before threatening fetal viability, thereby directing care to a high-risk pregnancy unit [44].

Colour power Doppler

Colour power angiography (CPA) is an extended application in Doppler ultrasound and velocimetry. CPA can be used to map out the vasculature within the placenta when combined with three-dimensional reconstruction (Fig. 3.6). This technique is able to identify red blood cells in small vessels with a diameter of more than 200 μm [45].

References

1. Benirschke K & Kaufmann P (2000) *Pathology of the Human Placenta.* New York: Springer.
2. Burton GJ, Kaufmann P & Huppertz B (2006) Anatomy and genesis of the placenta. In: Knobil E & Neil JD (eds) *Physiology of Reproduction*, 3rd ed. New York: Elsevier.
3. Cross JC (2000) Genetic insights into trophoblast differentiation and placental morphogenesis. *Semin Cell Dev Biol* **11**, 105–13.

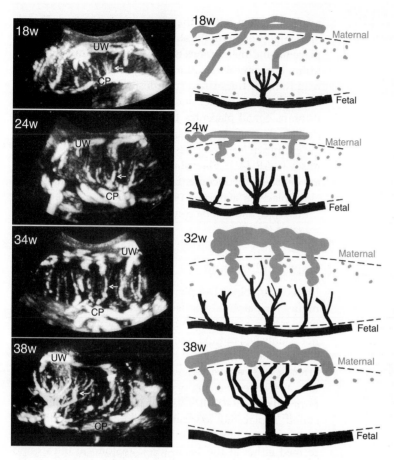

Fig. 3.6 Development of placental blood flow. Left column: Typical 3-D Power Doppler scans from placentas of normal pregnant women at weeks 18, 24, 34 and 38. The flow signals within placental villi (white arrows) increase in extent, intensity, width and height with advancing pregnancy. At term (38 weeks) tree like structures can be visualized. Since only anterior placentas have been used for these scans, the uterine wall (UW) is always at the top of the scan while the chorionic plate (CP) is always at the bottom of the scan. Courtesy of Justin Konje, Leicester, UK. Right column: Synoptic view of characteristic features of placental blood flow throughout pregnancy as depicted by 3-D Power Doppler. Adapted from drawings of Peter Kaufmann, Aachen, Germany.

4. Carter AM (2001) Evolution of the placenta and fetal membranes seen in the light of molecular phylogenetics. *Placenta* **22**, 800–07.

5. Castellucci M, Kosanke G, Verdenelli F, Huppertz B & Kaufmann P (2000) Villous sprouting: fundamental mechanisms of human placental development. *Hum Reprod Update* **6**, 485–94.

6. Kingdom J, Huppertz B, Seaward G & Kaufmann P (2000) Development of the placental villous tree and its consequences for fetal growth. *Eur J Obstet Gynecol Reprod Biol* **92**, 35–43.

7. Kaufmann P, Black S & Huppertz B (2003) Endovascular trophoblast invasion: implications for the pathogenesis of intrauterine growth retardation and preeclampsia. *Biol Reprod* **69**, 1–7.

8. Kemp B, Kertschanska S, Kadyrov M, Rath W, Kaufmann P & Huppertz B (2002) Invasive depth of extravillous trophoblast correlates with cellular phenotype: a comparison of intra- and extrauterine implantation sites. *Histochem Cell Biol* **117**, 401–14.

9. Kurman RJ, Main CS & Chen HC (1984) Intermediate trophoblast: a distinctive form of trophoblast with specific morphological, biochemical and functional features. *Placenta* **5**, 349–69.

10. Craven CM, Morgan T & Ward K (1998) Decidual spiral artery remodelling begins before cellular interaction with cytotrophoblasts. *Placenta* **19**, 241–52.

11. De Wolf F, De Wolf-Peeters C & Brosens I (1973) Ultrastructure of the spiral arteries in the human placental bed at the end of normal pregnancy. *Am J Obstet Gynecol* **117**, 833–48.

12. Pijnenborg R, Bland JM, Robertson WB & Brosens I (1983) Uteroplacental arterial changes related to interstitial trophoblast migration in early human pregnancy. *Placenta* **4**, 397–413.

13. Jauniaux E, Watson AL, Hempstock J, Bao YP, Skepper JN & Burton GJ (2000) Onset of maternal arterial bloodflow and placental oxidative stress; a possible factor in human early pregnancy failure. *Am J Pathol* **157**, 2111–22.

14. Rodesch F, Simon P, Donner C & Jauniaux E (1992) Oxygen measurements in endometrial and trophoblastic tissues during early pregnancy. *Obstet Gynecol* **80**, 283–85.

15. Burton GJ, Hempstock J & Jauniaux E (2003) Oxygen, early embryonic metabolism and free radical-mediated embryopathies. *Reprod BioMed Online* **6**, 84–96.

16. Burton GJ & Jauniaux E (2004) Placental oxidative stress: from miscarriage to preeclampsia. *J Soc Gynecol Investig* **11**, 342–52.

17. Jauniaux E, Hempstock J, Greenwold N & Burton GJ (2003) Trophoblastic oxidative stress in relation to temporal and regional differences in maternal placental blood flow in normal and abnormal early pregnancies. *Am J Pathol* **162**, 115–25.

18. Kaufmann P, Huppertz B & Frank HG (1996) The fibrinoids of the human placenta: origin, composition and functional relevance. *Annals Anat* **178**, 485–501.

19. Huppertz B, Frank HG, Kingdom JCP, Reister F & Kaufmann P (1998) Villous cytotrophoblastic regulation of the syncytial apoptotic cascade in the human placenta. *Histochem Cell Biol* **110**, 495–508.

20. Mayhew TM, Leach L, McGee R, Ismail WW, Myklebust R & Lammiman MJ (1999) Proliferation, differentiation and apoptosis in villous trophoblast at 13–41 weeks of gestation (including observations on annulate lamellae and nuclear pore complexes). *Placenta* **20**, 407–22.

21. Huppertz B, Kaufmann P & Kingdom J (2002) Trophoblast turnover in health and disease. *Fetal Matern Med Rev* **13**, 103–18.

22. Huppertz B, Tews DS & Kaufmann P (2001) Apoptosis and syncytial fusion in human placental trophoblast and skeletal muscle. *Int Rev Cytol* **205**, 215–53.

23. Huppertz B & Kingdom J (2004) Apoptosis in the trophoblast – role of apoptosis in placental morphogenesis. *J Soc Gynecol Investig* **11**, 353–62.

24. Iklé FA (1961) Trophoblastzellen im strömenden Blut. *Schweiz Med Wochenschr* **91**, 934–45.

25. Johansen M, Redman CW, Wilkins T & Sargent IL (1999) Trophoblast deportation in human pregnancy – its relevance for pre-eclampsia. *Placenta* **20**, 531–9.

26. Knight M, Redman CW, Linton EA & Sargent IL (1998) Shedding of syncytiotrophoblast microvilli into the maternal circulation in pre-eclamptic pregnancies. *Br J Obstet Gynaecol* **105**, 632–40.

27. Redman CWG & Sargent IL (2000) Placental debris, oxidative stress and pre-eclampsia. *Placenta* **21**, 597–602.

28. Graf R, Neudeck H, Gossrau R & Vetter K (1996) Elastic fibres are an essential component of human placental stem villous stroma and an integrated part of the perivascular contractile sheath. *Cell Tissue Res* **283**, 133–41.

29. Graf R, Matejevic D, Schuppan D, Neudeck H, Shakibaei M & Vetter K (1997) Molecular anatomy of the perivascular sheath in human placental stem villi: the contractile apparatus and its association to the extracellular matrix. *Cell Tissue Res* **290**, 601–7.

30. Burton GJ & Hung TH (2003) Hypoxia-reoxygenation; a potential source of placental oxidative stress in normal pregnancy and preeclampsia. *Fetal Matern Med Rev* **14**, 97–117.

31. Kingdom JCP & Kaufmann P (1997) Oxygen and placental villous development: origins of fetal hypoxia. *Placenta* **18**, 613–21.

32. Zamudio S (2003) The placenta at high altitude. *High Alt Med Biol* **4**, 171–91.

33. Bourne GL (1962) *The Human Amnion and Chorion*. London: Lloyd-Luke Ltd.

34. Menon R & Fortunato SJ (2004) The role of matrix degrading enzymes and apoptosis in rupture of membranes. *J Soc Gynecol Investig* **11**, 427–37.

35. Schmidt W (1992) The amniotic fluid compartment: the fetal habitat. *Adv Anat Embryol Cell Biol* **127**, 1–100.

36. Burton GJ & Jauniaux E (1995) Sonographic, stereological and Doppler flow velocimetric assessments of placental maturity. *Br J Obstet Gynaecol* **102**, 818–25.

37. Chaddha V, Viero S, Huppertz B & Kingdom J (2004) Developmental biology of the placenta and the origins of placental insufficiency. *Semin Fetal Neonat Med* **9**, 357–69.

38. Jauniaux E, Jurkovic D, Campbell S & Hustin J (1992) Doppler ultrasound features of the developing placental circulations: correlation with anatomic findings. *Am J Obstet Gynecol* **166**, 585–7.

39. Tabsh KMA (1983) Correlation of real-time ultrasonic placental grading with amniotic lecithin/sphingomyelin ratio. *Am J Obstet Gynecol* **145**, 504–8.

40. Alkazaleh F, Viero S, Kingdom JCP (2004). Doppler assessment in pregnancy. In: Rumack, Wilson, Charbonea, Johnson, eds., *Diagnostic Ultrasound*, Vol. 2, 3rd edition. Part V Obstetric and Fetal Sonography, Chapter 47, Elsevier Mosby, 1527–55.

41. Viero S, Chaddha V, Alkazaleh F *et al.* (2004) Prognostic value of placental ultrasound in pregnancies complicated by absent end-diastolic flow velocity in the umbilical arteries. *Placenta* **25**, 735–41.

42. Krebs C, Macara LM, Leiser R, Bowman AW, Greer IA & Kingdom JC (1996) Intrauterine growth restriction with absent end-diastolic flow velocity in the umbilical artery is associated with maldevelopment of the placental terminal villous tree. *Am J Obstet Gynecol* **175**, 1534–42.

43. Whittle W, Chaddha V, Wyatt P, Huppertz B, Kingdom J. Ultrasound detection of placental insufficiency in women with 'unexplained' abnormal maternal serum screening results. *Clin Genet* 2006; **69**: 97–104.

44. Chaddha V, Whittle WM & Kingdom JCP (2004) Improving the diagnosis and management of fetal growth restriction: the rationale for a placenta clinic. *Fetal Matern Med Rev* **15**, 205–30.

45. Konje JC, Huppertz B, Bell SC, Taylor DJ & Kaufmann P (2003) 3-dimensional colour power angiography for staging human placental development. *Lancet* **362**, 1199–201.

Further reading

For further reading on
structural characteristics of the placenta, see [1] or [2];
the definition of fibrinoid, see [18];
trophoblast and its changes during pre-eclampsia, see [23];
a detailed descriptions on pathologies of the macroscopic
   features of the placenta, see [1];
the classification of villi and the types of villi, see [1];
stereological parameters of the growing placenta, see [20];
syncytial fusion and the involvement of apoptosis, see [22]
   and [23];
the impact of oxygen on placental development and
   placental-related disorders of pregnancy, see [16];
the composition and characteristics of fetal membranes, see [35];
rupture of fetal membranes, see [34];
placental assessment by ultrasound, see [37];
placental Doppler, see [40,43,44];
developmental placental pathology, see [1,37].

Chapter 4: Normal fetal growth

Jason Gardosi

Developments in ultrasound imaging techniques and analysis of large databases have improved our understanding of normal fetal growth and maturation. Its understanding is of immediate relevance for the assessment of fetal well-being at any stage of pregnancy.

Length of pregnancy

In any large database, the distribution of the length of pregnancy is skewed because babies are more likely to be born preterm than post-term and at a wider range of gestations into the early preterm period. Thus neither the mean nor median, but the modal value is used to denote the typical length of pregnancy.

Starting from the time of conception, this typical length of gestation and the fetal age at the end of pregnancy is 266 days or 38 weeks (= conceptual age). In most (but by no means all) cases conception occurs in mid-cycle and thus 2 weeks are added to denote menstrual age. By convention, gestational age is also expressed in this manner: the formulae used for dating pregnancies by ultrasound, to determine the length of pregnancy at any point and the expected date of delivery (EDD), also add a standard 2 weeks to derive 'gestational age'. The typical length of pregnancy is 280 days or 40.0 weeks; term is conventionally denoted as 37–42 weeks, preterm as <37.0 weeks and post-term >42.0 weeks. However, these cut-offs may be varied for the purpose of looking at specific issues. For example, prematurity <34 weeks denotes babies that are more likely to require some form of special care; and limits of >290 days or even >287 days (41.0 weeks) have been used to study the effects of post-term pregnancy.

Determination of gestational age

Accurate dating of pregnancy is important for a number of reasons, each of them constituting milestones which are more important than the prediction of the actual EDD itself:

1 *Antenatal screening.* Values for serum tests for chromosomal abnormalities (e.g. Down's syndrome), PAPP-A, HCG or oestriol are strongly related to gestational age and may give false readings if the 'dates' are wrong. This can result in missing that a pregnancy is at risk, or in providing false positives and in unnecessary, invasive diagnostic procedures such as chorionic villous sampling or amniocentesis.

2 *Estimating fetal viability at extreme prematurity.* Between say 23 and 28 weeks, the chance of a baby's survival is heavily dependent on the gestational age [1] and inaccurate dates may lead to wrong advice to the parents and inappropriate management.

3 *Post-term pregnancy.* Prolonged gestation is associated with a rise in perinatal morbidity and mortality. The reasons for this are not well understood, but it has become established practice to offer mothers induction of labour in pregnancies that go beyond 290–294 days.

Before the advent of ultrasound, the menstrual age was used to determine gestational dates and the EDD. However, dating by menstrual history has several problems [2]. First the last menstrual period (LMP) may not be accurately remembered in a substantial proportion of cases. Second, dating by LMP assumes that conception occurred in mid-cycle, whereas it may have occurred earlier or (more likely) later. If the usual length of a woman's cycle tended to be longer, say 35 instead of 28 days, then an adjustment needs to be made by adding 7 days to the EDD. This is often not done, but even if it is, it represents an imprecise science as the actual length of the follicular phase at the beginning of that pregnancy is not known.

Dating by ultrasound has made the determination of gestational age more precise. The ultrasound scan dating can be done on the basis of the fetal crown rump length (CRL), which is reliable between 7 and 12 weeks, or in the second trimester, between say 15 and 22 weeks, by the bi-parietal diameter (BPD) or the head circumference (HC). There are few studies which have compared whether first or second trimester measurement is more accurate in routine practice. Between 13 and 15 weeks, dating by ultrasound can be less accurate, as the fetus flexes,

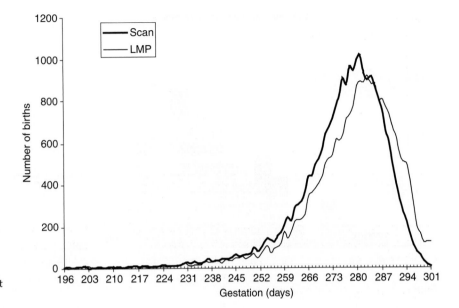

Fig. 4.1 Frequency distribution of gestational age at birth in $n = 24,524$ pregnancies in Nottingham 1988–1995, which had a record of the last menstrual period (LMP) and an ultrasound dating scan. The graph shows a general left shift associated with ultrasound dates.

making CRL difficult, while it may be too early for accurate measurements of the head (BPD or HC).

Ultrasound measurement can also have error, but this error is smaller than that of the LMP. Based on studies from pregnancies achieved with assisted reproduction techniques, that is, where the exact date of conception was known, the error of routine scan dating by ultrasound was normally distributed and had a standard deviation of ±4, which means a 95% confidence interval of −8 to +8 days [3]. In contrast, LMP dating error is heavily skewed towards overestimation of the true gestational age, with a 95% confidence interval of −9 to +27 days [4].

One manifestation of such a tendency of overestimation is that many pregnancies which are post-term by LMP dates and considered in need for induction of labour are in fact not post-term if ultrasound dates are used. About three-quarters of 'post-term' (>294 days) pregnancies by LMP are not post-term by ultrasound (11.3 to 3.6%) [5]. This would suggest that many 'post-term' pregnancies in clinical practice as well as in studies in the literature prior to routine dating by ultrasound were in fact not post-term but mis-dated (Fig. 4.1).

As an ultrasound scan is performed in most pregnancies in the UK at some stage in the first half of pregnancy, it is now recommended that gestation dates should preferentially be determined by ultrasound [2]. In many units, practices and protocols have sprung up whereby the LMP is used unless it has a discrepancy of greater than 7, 10 or 14 days from the dates by ultrasound. However, this is not based on any evidence; in fact, even within 14, 10 or even 7-day cut-offs, scan dates are known to be more accurate than LMP dates in predicting the actual date of delivery [5].

Small for gestational age and intrauterine growth restriction

The traditional method of denoting a small baby as being below 2500 g, or 1500 g, does not distinguish between smallness due to short gestation and smallness due to intrauterine growth restriction (IUGR).

The terms small for gestational age (SGA), average for gestational age (AGA) and large for gestational age (LGA) are therefore preferred, which adjust the limit for the average at the respective gestational age. Traditionally, the 10th and 90th centiles respectively are used, although the 5th and 95th, or the 3rd and 97th (equivalent to ±2 standard deviations) can also be applied. However, SGA is not synonymous with IUGR as it includes pathological as well as constitutional smallness.

Increasingly, it has become apparent that birthweight and fetal growth vary with a number of factors, apart from gestational age. These factors can be physiological (constitutional) or pathological.

Physiological factors include birth order (parity), maternal characteristics such as height, weight and ethnic origin and fetal gender [6]. Coefficients have been derived to allow for the normal birthweight ranges to be adjusted, from which then growth curves can be drawn (see below) [7].

Pathological factors affecting growth include smoking, alcohol, social class and deprivation, multiple pregnancy, and pregnancy complications such as placental failure and related underlying conditions associated with hypertensive diseases in pregnancy, antepartum haemorrhage and diabetes (see Chapter 27). However, such variables should

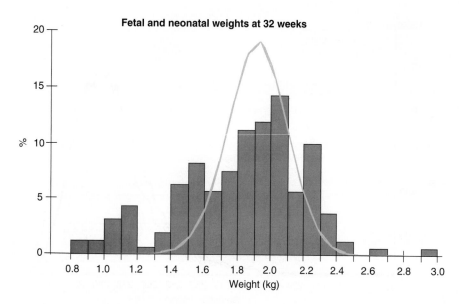

Fig. 4.2 Ultrasound versus birth weight standard at 32 weeks gestation. The line shows ultrasound weight estimations derived from pregnancies which have proceeded to normal term delivery. The curve is characterized by a relatively narrow, normal distribution. The histogram shows birth weights of babies born at this same, preterm gestation in dataset of approximately 40,000 cases in the Midlands. The distribution shows a lower median, a wider range and negative skewness.

not be adjusted for, as the standard should reflect the optimal growth potential of the fetus. For example, it is well established that maternal smoking adversely affects fetal growth; however, the standard or norm should not be adjusted downwards if a mother smokes, but it should be 'optimized' as if the mother did *not* smoke, to allow better detection of the fetus that is affected.

In practice, well-dated birthweight databases with sufficient details about maternal characteristics and pregnancy outcome are used to derive the coefficients needed to adjust for constitutional variation.

Fetal weight gain

In the first half of pregnancy, the fetus develops its organ systems and grows mainly by cell division. In the second half, most growth occurs by increase in cell size.

Determination of what is 'normal' is essential for the identification of abnormal growth in day-to-day clinical practice. Imaging techniques have allowed us to get a better understanding of normal fetal growth. They include two-dimensional and three-dimensional ultrasound as well as assessment of Doppler flow (see Chapter 19).

Previously, 'normal growth' was inferred from birthweight curves which showed wide ranges especially at early (preterm) gestations and flattening of the curve at term. A marked terminal flattening of birthweight curves is evident in some birthweight standards still in widespread use [8]. However, this is an artefact due to misdating, because LMP error is more likely to *over-* rather than *under*estimate true gestational age (Fig. 4.1). Many birthweights end up being plotted at later gestations than they should be, producing the erroneous impression of a flattening of fetal growth at term.

Birthweight curves also tend to show a depression or negative skewness at preterm gestations. This is associated with the known fact that many preterm births, including those following spontaneous onset of labour, are of babies whose growth was restricted *in utero* [9,10]. In contrast, ultrasound curves based on fetuses which continue growth until normal term delivery show no such skewness (Fig. 4.2).

In utero growth of the fetus is assessed by fetal biometry, including measurements of the head, abdomen and the femur. The results can be plotted on separate charts to check whether the growth is within normal limits. Alternatively, the measurements can be used to calculate and plot estimated fetal weight (EFW), which is now considered to be a more appropriate method to monitor fetal growth during pregnancy [11].

In fact, longitudinal ultrasound studies have shown that variation and the normal range of fetal weight is constant throughout pregnancy, at about 10–11%, and that growth continues until birth without any slowing [7,12,13] (Fig. 4.3).

The dynamics of growth in normal pregnancy can be studied by converting the weight-for-gestation curve into a 'proportionality' curve, where term weight in normal pregnancies is equated to 100%. As Fig. 4.4 shows, half of this weight should be expected to be reached at 31 weeks, and a third and two thirds should be reached by 28 and 31 weeks, respectively.

Such proportionality curves can be used to project backwards the predicted, individually adjusted birthweight endpoint. These constitutional variables can result in an infinite number of combinations, which require calculation by computer software (such as GROW – Gestation Related Optimal Weight software – www.gestation.net) to

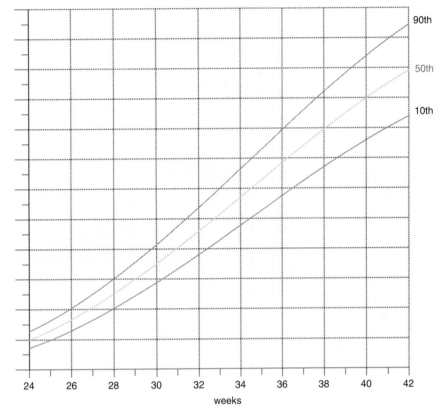

Fig. 4.3 Fetal growth curves derived from longitudinal ultrasound scans of normal pregnancies, showing a normal distribution and no flattening at term.

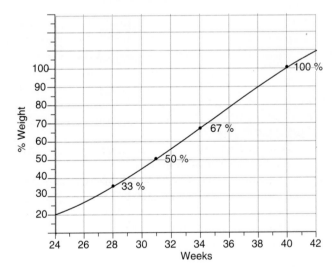

Fig. 4.4 'Proportionality' fetal growth curve. The line represents an equation derived from an *in utero* weight curve, transformed into a % term weight versus gestation curve for any predicted term (280 day) birthweight point.
% weight $= 299.1 - 31.85\,\text{GA} + 1.094\,\text{GA}^2 - 0.01055\,\text{GA}^3$.

produce individually adjusted or 'customized' norms for fetal growth in each pregnancy (Fig. 4.5).

Thus 'normal' growth is not an 'average' for the population, but one that defines the optimal growth that a fetus can achieve, that is, the 'growth potential' of each baby.

A number of studies have shown that standards for normal birthweight and growth adjusted for constitutional variation are better than local population norms to separate physiological and pathological smallness. Customized standards improve detection of pathologically small babies [14,15]. Smallness defined by customized standards were also more strongly associated with adverse pregnancy outcomes such as stillbirth, neonatal death or low Apgar scores [16] and were more closely linked with a number of pathological indicators such as abnormal antenatal Doppler, caesarean section for fetal distress, admission to the neonatal unit and prolonged hospital stay [17].

Significantly, each of these studies showed that babies that are considered small only by the (unadjusted) population method do *not* have an increased risk of adverse pregnancy outcome. In the general population, up to a third of babies are false positively small when general rather than individually adjusted norms for fetal growth are used, which can result in many unnecessary investigations and parental anxiety. Conversely, about a third of babies who should be suspected to be at risk are missed. In population subgroups such as minority ethnic groups, application of an unadjusted population standard results

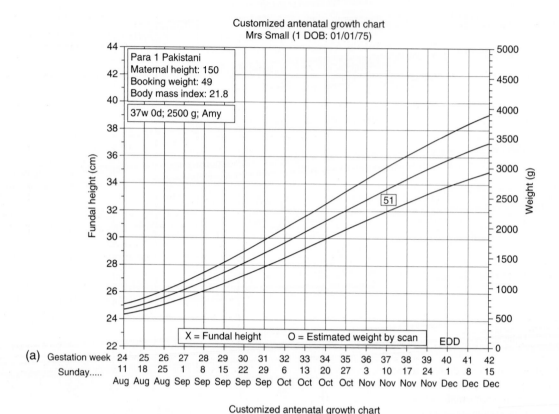

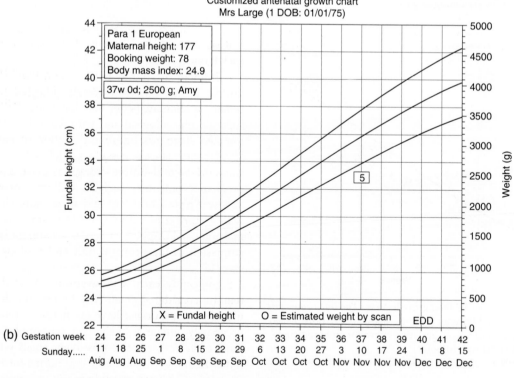

Fig. 4.5 Two examples of customized fetal growth curves, using GROW.exe version 5.11 (www.gestation.net). The charts can be used to calculate previous baby weights and ultrasound estimated fetal weight(s) in the current pregnancy. Serial fundal height measurements can also be plotted. The graphs are adjusted to predict the optimal curve for each pregnancy, based on the variables entered (maternal height and weight, parity and ethnic group). In the example, a baby born at 37.0 weeks weighing 2500 g was within normal limits for Mrs Small (51st centile) but FGR for Mrs Large (5th centile) as the latter's predicted optimal growth curve is steeper. The pregnancy details entered are shown on the top left, together with the (computer-) calculated body mass index (BMI). The horizontal axis shows the day and month of each gestation week, calculated by the software on the basis of the EDD.

in even more false positives and false negatives. The individual or customized method to determine normal fetal growth is recommended by guidelines of the Royal College of Obstetricians and Gynaecologists [18].

In summary, thanks to imaging techniques such as ultrasound, normal fetal maturation and growth can be better defined. Fetal growth is subject to constitutional variation which needs to be adjusted for. Such adjustment results in better definition of normal growth, and improved identification of the fetus whose growth is pathologically affected.

References

1. Draper ES, Manktelow B, Field DJ & James D (1999) Prediction of survival for preterm births by weight and gestational age: retrospective population based study. *Br Med J* **319**, 1093–7.
2. Gardosi J & Geirsson R (1998) Routine ultrasound is the method of choice for dating pregnancy. *Br J Obstet Gynaecol* **105**, 933–36.
3. Mul T, Mongelli M & Gardosi J (1996) A comparative analysis of second-trimester ultrasound dating formulae in pregnancies conceived with artificial reproductive techniques. *Ultrasound Obstet Gynecol* **8**, 397–402.
4. Gardosi J & Mongelli M (1993) Risk assessment adjusted for gestational age in maternal serum screening for Down's syndrome. *Br Med J* **306**, 1509.
5. Mongelli M, Wilcox M & Gardosi J (1996) Estimating the date of confinement: ultrasonographic biometry versus certain menstrual dates. *Am J Obstet Gynecol* **174**(1), 278–81.
6. Gardosi J, Chang A, Kalyan B, Sahota D & Symonds EM (1992) Customised antenatal growth charts. *Lancet* **339**, 283–7.
7. Gardosi J, Mongelli M, Wilcox M & Chang A (1995) An adjustable fetal weight standard. *Ultrasound Obstet Gynecol* **6**, 168–74.
8. Alexander GA, Himes JH, Kaufman RB, Mor J & Kogan M (1996) A United States National Reference for Fetal Growth. *Obstet Gynecol* **87**, 163–8.
9. Tamura RK, Sabbagha RE, Depp R *et al.* (1984) Diminished growth in fetuses born preterm after spontaneous labor or rupture of membranes. *Am J Obstet Gynecol* **148**, 1105–10.
10. Gardosi JO (2005) Prematurity and fetal growth restriction. *Early Hum Devt* **81**, 43–9.
11. Gardosi J (2002) Ultrasound biometry and fetal growth restriction. *Fetal Matern Med Rev* **13**, 249–59.
12. Gallivan S, Robson SC, Chang TC, Vaughan J & Spencer JAD (1993) An investigation of fetal growth using serial ultrasound data. *Ultrasound Obstet Gynecol* **3**, 109–14.
13. Marsal K, Persson P-H, Larsen T *et al.* (1996) Intrauterine growth curves based on ultrasonically estimated foetal weights. *Acta Paediatr* **85**, 843–8.
14. de Jong CLD, Gardosi J, Dekker GA, Colenbrander GJ & van Geijn HP (1998) Application of a customised birthweight standard in the assessment of perinatal outcome in a high risk population. *Br J Obstet Gynaecol* **105**, 531–5.
15. De Jong CLD, Francis A, Van Geijn HP & Gardosi J (2000) Customized fetal weight limits for antenatal detection of fetal growth restriction. *Ultrasound Obstet Gynecol* **15**, 36–40.
16. Clausson B, Gardosi J, Francis A & Cnattingius S (2001) Perinatal outcome in SGA births defined by customised versus population-based birthweight standards. *Br J Obstet Gynaecol* **108**, 830–4.
17. McCowan L, Harding JE & Stewart AW (2005) Customised birthweight centiles predict SGA pregnancies with perinatal morbidity. *Br J Obstet Gynaecol* **112**, 1026–33.
18. Royal College of Obstetricians and Gynaecologists (2002) *The Investigation and Management of the Small-For-Gestational Age Fetus*. RCOG Green Top Guideline 2002 (No.31). London: RCOG Press.

Chapter 5: Pre-conception counselling

Andrew McCarthy

Prepregnancy care

Traditionally obstetric care has been focused on ensuring a 'healthy' baby was delivered alive, free of the effects of hypoxic ischaemic damage and of perinatal infection. It is an intimidating prospect to consider that in the next few decades, obstetric care may have to assume greater responsibilities that can shape the lifelong risk of acquired disease for the individual neonate rather than simply immediate neonatal morbidity. It is in this context that prepregnancy care currently takes place.

Specific pre-conception counselling arises in a number of different environments. For doctors in primary care it will be dominated by the low-risk woman for whom advice on diet and access to care will be most important. The quality of this advice may have the potential to significantly affect public health. In a hospital setting, it will mostly involve women with specific complications seeking advice on the potential for successful pregnancy and implications for background medical conditions.

Age

Questions often arise as to the advisability of pregnancy at certain ages. Advanced maternal age is associated with increased risks of pre-eclampsia, gestational diabetes, incidental medical problems, aneuploidy and miscarriage. While this may sound overwhelming, and translates into increased maternal mortality [1], the vast majority of mothers in their forties will deliver satisfactorily and should not be deterred from conceiving unless there are specific issues for concern. Often concern about aneuploidy and miscarriage has a greater influence than maternal disease.

There are occasions when it is advisable to conceive at a younger age than planned, that is, in the presence of mild renal failure a satisfactory outcome may be anticipated, whereas a delay with consequent loss of renal function may result in a very-high-risk pregnancy. The natural history of background medical conditions must be considered when advising on optimal age for conception.

Diet and weight

There is little that the well-motivated woman can do to affect pregnancy outcome that is based on evidence, but weight has a clear impact on pregnancy outcome, that is, low body mass index (BMI) is associated with intrauterine growth retardation, high BMI with increased fetal weight, possibly greater risks of neural tube defects [2], gestational diabetes, risk of dystocia and shoulder dystocia, anaesthetic complications and other associated morbidity [3,4].

Maternal obesity is increasingly common, with increased calorie intake and increased fat intake. The potential implications of this change on developmental programming are huge, with subsequent increased risk of ischaemic heart disease, hypertension and type II diabetes in adult life [5,6]. There is also the potential for this to be amplified between generations specifically with reference to insulin resistance. The concept of functional deficit in response to adverse intrauterine stimuli must be extended to other stimuli such as medication or toxicology where structural deficits have attracted most attention in the past.

Folic acid is important in relation to risk of neural tube disorders. Some studies have suggested that a higher folic acid intake is associated with a lower risk of neural tube defect. This has been addressed in two ways. In the first instance some countries have fortified foods to increase folic acid content. These programmes have met with some success [7]. The alternative strategy is to advise women of childbearing age to take folic acid supplementation by way of tablets [8]. This clearly has the disadvantage that vulnerable women may never receive the message, compliance may be poor and offers no protection to unplanned pregnancies. There is also some evidence suggesting risk of other structural anomalies, that is, cardiac or craniofacial abnormalities, may also be reduced by folate supplementation [9].

Table 5.1 Issues that arise when counselling in a low-risk setting

Issue	Aims
Diet	Achieve normal BMI
	Balanced diet
Vitamin supplementation	Folic acid 400 mg daily (unless fortified food policy in place) 5 mg for high-risk mothers
Lifestyle factors	Avoid excessive caffeine intake [11]
	Reduce alcohol intake as much as possible
	Stop smoking
Review past medical history	Identify potential problems
	Achieve good control of chronic disease
	Review medications
Review family history	Identify potential problems, e.g. thrombosis and diabetes
Genetic disorders	Specialist genetic counselling
Review obstetric history	Previous pre-eclampsia or other preterm delivery: offer specialist advice
Check smear history	Ensure abnormal cytology appropriately treated
Reduce risk of viral disease	Check rubella immunity (varicella, hepatitis B and HIV are normally checked antenatally)

Infants of diabetic mothers are at increased risks of congenital abnormality, though it is not clear that all such abnormalities can be related to HbA1c levels [9,10]. This raises some doubt about the relationship to hyperglycaemia, though small elevations in HbA1c still increase risk of abnormality. It is known that infants of diabetic mothers are at increased risk of neural tube defects. There is concern that hyperglycaemia in non-diabetic women is predicted by high BMI, and that this is associated with increased risk of neural tube defects.

Excessive retinoic acid exposure in early pregnancy can also disrupt development, that is, craniofacial and CNS abnormalities have been described with isotretinoin which is used to treat acne [9]. Increased vitamin A intake in early pregnancy has been shown to increase risks of neural tube and heart defects. It is clear that there is a relationship between dietary intake and gene expression in the fetus which influences early development.

Pre-conceptual counselling in the low-risk setting

The issues that must be addressed in a pre-conceptual review in a low-risk setting are outlined in Table 5.1.

Rubella immunity must be checked. Most women in developed countries will be immune, and therefore particular care must be taken to screen immigrant groups. HIV and hepatitis are not normally checked other than in women undergoing fertility treatment or in immunocompromised groups, though a case can be made for such a check prior to conception. Hepatitis C and varicella may be checked selectively.

It is worth enquiring about the health of the male partner. Smoking cessation programmes are more available now and there has been concern about the smoking in male partner and miscarriage risk [12]. Regardless of this risk, it would be a clear advantage for the father to not smoke and the incentive of a healthy environment for the child may help smoking cessation. Occasionally fathers are on medication which may have implications for fertility and review of such medication may be worthwhile.

Counselling for women with medical disorders

Women with serious medical disorders require specific care and counselling prior to pregnancy. The aim is to provide seamless care from chronic disease state to early conception to delivery and back to long-term care. This has not been achieved within many traditional patterns of care. The aims of prepregnancy care in this context are outlined in Table 5.2.

It is important for women with certain medical problems that consideration is given to first trimester complications. Women with bleeding disorders will need admission plans in the event of miscarriage or ectopic pregnancy and clear plans for ultrasound assessment of pregnancy to try and prevent emergency admission. Hyperemesis can have more profound implications for women with diabetes making control at a critical time difficult to achieve and for women on maintenance medication such as steroids or other immunosuppressive treatment. Thromboembolic disorders can pose very specific risks in the first trimester as vomiting and hyperemesis can predispose to increased risks of thrombosis. Threshold for admission and assessment needs to be adjusted accordingly.

Medications should be prescribed pre-conceptually that are in general safe in the first trimester [13]. Some medications are important for long-term well-being and physicians may be reluctant to stop them to await conception.

Table 5.2 Issues that need to be considered when giving pre-conceptual advice to women with background medical conditions

Trimester	Plan
First	Clear contact arrangements with medical team
	Medications consistent with safe use in pregnancy
	Or clear plan to change treatment in first trimester
	Clear plan in the event of first trimester complications
Second	Appropriate medication
	High-quality anomaly scanning as appropriate
	Availability of perinatal care for late second trimester delivery, i.e. 25–28 weeks
Third	Appropriate medical and surgical backup
Puerperium	Clear plan for disease flares or incidental complications
	Smooth transition to optimal treatment to meet long-term healthcare needs

Table 5.3 Drugs known to be teratogenic [13]

Drug	Vulnerable period	Harm
Warfarin	First trimester	Warfarin embryopathy (abnormal cartilage and bone formation)
	Second and third	Fetal cerebral haemorrhage Warfarin microcephaly
ACE Inhibitors	Probably all trimesters	Fetal renal dysgenesis
Statins [15]	Uncertain (evidence mainly relates to first trimester)	CNS and limb defects
Antiepileptic drugs [13,16]	First trimester	Neural tube defects, oral clefts, cardiac defects
Valproate [17]	Probably second and third	Developmental delay
Tetracycline	Second and third	Staining of dentition
Retinoids	First +?	Multiple defects described

*This list is not exhaustive. Excellent reviews are available to guide clinicians and there are now many websites that offer continuously updated advice on risks of teratogenicity and the limitations of the advice that may be offered. www.uspharmacist.com

Conception may only be achieved after unpredictable periods of time and many will choose to leave women with hypertension or renal compromise on angiotensin converting enzyme (ACE) inhibitors, with a view to cessation of treatment as early as possible in the first trimester [14]. The same arguments may apply to warfarin treatment in women at high risk of thromboembolism. It is clear that seamless care with medical clinics is necessary for such treatment plans and well-informed patients.

The importance of good control in the diabetic mother has been covered in Chapter 27. Prior to pregnancy assessment of co-morbidities such as retinal disease, renal function and blood pressure control all aid a smooth transition into pregnancy. The cause of renal compromise is best addressed prior to pregnancy, and in the presence of nephrotic syndrome a plan for thromboprophylaxis needs to be instituted.

Phenylketonuria (PKU) is a specific genetic condition where appropriate dietary treatment can influence disease expression. This will have implications for an infant of an affected mother. Mothers with rare conditions of this nature tend to be well informed and to have ready access to specialist advice.

Conditions in which pregnancy is contraindicated

There are some medical conditions in which pregnancy is contraindicated. There is a general reluctance to instruct women not to get pregnant as ultimately it is their decision. In the presence of pulmonary hypertension with up to a 50% risk of mortality it is reasonable to give explicit advice against conception and advise on contraception

accordingly. Some other cardiac conditions may carry similar advice and contraception for this high-risk group may warrant specialist input. Respiratory compromise may mean that pregnancy is contraindicated. It will usually be clear that severe compromise is present in such patients as evidenced by their background medical condition such as cystic fibrosis or their limited exercise tolerance. A specialist opinion should always be sought before informing a patient that pregnancy is contraindicated. In the presence of certain cancers such as breast cancer, the focus will be more on ensuring a specific disease-free interval prior to conception. In the presence of renal compromise, the advice may be that pregnancy is better attempted sooner rather than later, that is, that conception occurs in mild to moderate renal failure rather than severe renal failure with advancing maternal age. Previous breakthrough thromboses in high-risk women may mean that pregnancy should not be considered. Clinical scenarios as described above are excellent opportunities to review contraceptive needs and to ensure that reliable methods, which are appropriate to the medical conditions involved, are being used.

Known teratogens

Most drugs are safe to use in pregnancy. When offering pre-conceptual care, medications must be reviewed to ensure that there are no inappropriate risks of teratogenicity. In certain clinical situations some risk must be taken, that is, with antiepileptic drugs (Table 5.3).

Table 5.4 Medications for which a washout period may be required

Medication	Clinical use	Concerns
Bisphosphanates	Osteoporosis	Very long tissue half-life Very limited data
Methotrexate [18]	Rheumatoid arthritis	Known potential teratogen But reassuring data available for certain treatment regimes Maintain high dose of folic acid
Leflunemide	Rheumatoid arthritis	Known teratogen

There have been major advances in drug therapy for women with rheumatic disease. This may result in patients presenting to obstetricians on medication which the obstetrician may not be familiar with. In such situations the doctor must seek expert advice. Some of these medications require a substantial washout period to minimize risk of teratogenicity. This can result in a recurrence of morbidity from the underlying disease, such that most patients would wish to be forewarned, and have a clear plan for assisted conception in the absence of spontaneous pregnancy (Table 5.4).

It is clear that there is a paucity of data in relation to the potential for functional deficits following treatment in pregnancy, that is, is there a renal deficit as a result of stopping ACE inhibitors at 6–7 weeks gestation? Or are there subtle immunological sequelae from the use of immunosuppressive treatment regimes in rheumatological disorders? Such putative functional deficits must be weighed against the need for long-term cardiovascular protection and protection against lupus flares. Nonetheless every effort must be made to gather long-term data on the offspring of mothers treated during pregnancy to gather this information. The duration of follow-up required makes this a difficult task, but one which is likely to become more important as healthcare improves, society becomes richer, more drug treatment becomes available and side effects of treatment become less well tolerated.

Psychiatric disease

Psychiatric disease also warrants good quality prepregnancy care and counselling. There are often concerns about transmission of mental illness to children, and risks of destabilizing mental illness. The estimate is that there is a 10–15% risk of schizophrenia or manic depressive illness in offspring. Risks of instability and potential plans for withdrawing medication must be discussed thoroughly with the professional most involved in long-term management of such patients, that is, commonly the psychiatrist and general practitioner.

Obstetric complications

Obstetric concerns may also lead to advice to avoid pregnancy, that is, previous recurrent post-partum haemorrhage or multiple uterine scars with risk of placenta accreta. Women with prior histories of early onset or severe pre-eclampsia or preterm delivery may warrant prepregnancy counselling. Recurrence risks and treatment plans have been addressed in Chapters 13 and 18. Women may come for counselling following a previous traumatic delivery. Such visits are usually very valuable in helping women come to terms with adverse events in previous pregnancies, offering explanations for previous management plans and making clear plans for subsequent pregnancies. It is not uncommon for women to choose not to conceive following particularly traumatic deliveries, as they perceive that they will necessarily be exposed to the same stress with subsequent pregnancies. The extent to which such situations arise has not been sufficiently formally studied. One visit for counselling in such circumstances can be very rewarding.

Organizational issues

The need for a smooth transition into pregnancy has been emphasized above. It is also clear that a similar smooth transition must take place after delivery. The puerperium is a very-high-risk time for cardiac patients and is also the time when considerable loss of renal function can occur in women with renal disease. Bleeding disorders can cause major morbidity in the puerperium and optimal control of insulin regimes can help the breastfeeding diabetic mother. Prompt treatment of flares of immunological problems can prevent major problems in the puerperium. It is frequently the case that traditional obstetric care becomes complacent once delivery has taken place. It is vitally important that good communication between specialist and obstetric teams takes place after delivery and that senior input continues for such patients. Plans for this transition must be put in place when care is handed over in early pregnancy.

References

1. Department of Health (2004) *Report on Confidential Enquiries into Maternal Deaths in the United Kingdom 2000–2002*. Lemanch, London.
2. Ray J, Wyatt P, Vermeulen M, Meier C & Cole D (2005) Greater maternal weight and the ongoing risk of neural tube defects after folic acid flour fortification. *Obstet Gynecol* **105**(2), 261–5.

3. Kristensen J, Vestergaard M, Wisborg K, Kesmodel U & Secher N (2005) Pre-pregnancy weight and the risk of stillbirth and neonatal death. *Br J Obstet Gynaecol* **112**(4), 403–8.

4. Sheiner E, Levy A, Menes T, Silverberg D, Katz M & Mazor M (2004) Maternal obesity as an independent risk factor for caesarean delivery. *Paediatr Perinat Epidemiol* **18**(3), 196–201.

5. Lau C & Rogers J (2004) Embryonic and fetal programming of physiological disorders in adulthood. *Birth Defects Res C Embryo Today* **72**(4), 300–12.

6. Armitage J, Taylor P & Poston L (2005) Experimental models of developmental programming: consequences of exposure to an energy rich diet during development. *J Physiol* **565**, 171–84.

7. Mills J & Signore C (2004) Neural tube defect rates before and after food fortification with folic acid. *Birth Defects Res A Clin Mol Teratol* **70**(11), 844–5.

8. Botto L, Lisi A, Robert-Gnansia E *et al.* (2005) International retrospective cohort study of neural tube defects in relation to folic acid recommendations: are the recommendations working? *Br Med J* **330**(7491), 571.

9. Finnell R, Shaw G, Lammer E *et al.* (2004) Gene-nutrient interactions: importance of folates and retinoids during early embryogenesis. *Toxicol Appl Pharmacol* **198**(2), 75–85.

10. Suhonen L, Hiilesmaa V & Teramo K (2000) Glycaemic control during early pregnancy and fetal malformations in women with type I diabetes mellitus. *Diabetologia* **43**(1), 79–82.

11. Tolstrup J, Kjaer S, Munk C *et al.* (2003) Does caffeine and alcohol intake before pregnancy predict the occurrence of spontaneous abortion? *Hum Reprod* **18**(12), 2704–10.

12. Venners S, Wang X, Chen C *et al.* (2004) Paternal smoking and pregnancy loss: a prospective study using a biomarker of pregnancy. *Am J Epidemiol* **159**(10), 993–1001.

13. Jacqz-Aigrain E & Koren G (2005) Effects of drugs on the fetus. *Semin Fetal Neonatal Med* **10**(2), 139–47.

14. Cooper WO, Hernandez-Dias S, Arbogast PG *et al.* (2006) *NEJM* **354**, 2443–51.

15. Edison R & Muenke M (2004) Mechanistic and epidemiologic considerations in the evaluation of adverse birth outcomes following gestational exposure to statins. *Am J Med Genet A* **131A**(3), 287–98.

16. Kaplan P (2004) Reproductive health effects and teratogenicity of antiepileptic drugs. *Neurology* **63**(10 Suppl 4) S13–23.

17. Adab N, Kini U, Vinten J *et al.* (2004) The longer term outcome of children born to mothers with epilepsy. *J Neurol Neurosurg Psychiatry* **75**(11), 1575–83.

18. Østensen M (2001) Drugs in pregnancy. Rheumatological disorders. *Best Pract Res Clin Obstet Gynaecol* **15**(6), 953–69.

Chapter 6: Antenatal care

Timothy G. Overton

Introduction

The care of pregnant women presents a unique challenge to modern medicine. Most women will progress through pregnancy in an uncomplicated fashion and deliver a healthy infant requiring little medical or midwifery intervention. Unfortunately, a significant number will have medical problems which will complicate their pregnancy or develop such serious conditions that the lives of both themselves and their unborn child will be threatened. In 1928, a pregnant woman faced a 1 in 290 chance of dying from an obstetric complication related to the pregnancy; the most recent Confidential Enquiry into Maternal and Child Health put this figure at 1 in 19,020 [1]. Undoubtedly, good antenatal care has made a significant contribution to this reduction. The current challenge of antenatal care is to identify those women who will require specialist support and help while allowing uncomplicated pregnancies to progress with minimal interference. The antenatal period also allows the opportunity for women, especially those in their first pregnancy, to receive information from a variety of health-care professionals regarding pregnancy, childbirth and parenthood.

Aims of antenatal care

Antenatal education

PROVISION OF INFORMATION

Women and their husbands/partners have the right to be involved in all decisions regarding their antenatal care. They need to be able to make informed decisions concerning where they will be seen, who will undertake their care, which screening tests to have and where they plan to give birth. Women must have access to evidence-based information in a format that they can understand. Current evidence suggests that insufficient written information is available especially at the beginning of pregnancy and that information provided can be misleading or inaccurate. 'The Pregnancy Book' [2] provides information on the developing fetus, antenatal care and classes, rights

and benefits as well as a list of useful organizations. Many leaflets have been produced by the Midwives Information and Resource Service (MIDIRS) helping women to make informed objective decisions during pregnancy. Written information is particularly important to help women understand the purpose of screening tests and the options that are available and to advise on lifestyle considerations including dietary recommendations. Available information needs to be provided at the first contact and must take into account cultural and language barriers. Local services should endeavour to provide information that is understandable to those whose first language is not English and to those with physical, cognitive and sensory disabilities. Translators will be required in clinics with an ethnic mix.

Couples should also be offered the opportunity to attend antenatal classes. Ideally such classes should discuss physiological and psychological changes during pregnancy, fetal development, labour and childbirth and how to care for the newborn baby. Evidence shows a greater acquisition of knowledge in women who have attended such classes compared with those that have not.

LIFESTYLE CONCERNS

At an early stage in the pregnancy women require lifestyle advice, including information on diet and food, work during pregnancy and social aspects, for example, smoking, alcohol, exercise and sexual activity.

Women should be advised of the benefits of eating a balanced diet such as plenty of fruit and vegetables, starchy foods such as pasta, bread, rice and potatoes, protein, fibre and dairy foods. They should be informed of foods that could put their fetus at risk. Listeriosis is caused by the bacterium *Listeria monocytogenes* which can present with a mild, flu-like illness but is associated with miscarriage, stillbirth and severe illness in the newborn. Contaminated food is the usual source including unpasteurized milk, ripened soft cheeses and pate. Toxoplasmosis contracted through contact with infected cat litter, or undercooked meat can lead to permanent neurological and visual problems in the newborn if the mother contracts the infection during pregnancy. (Salmonella food poisoning has not been shown to have adverse fetal effects.) To reduce the risk, pregnant women should be advised to thoroughly wash all fruits and vegetables before eating and to cook well all meats including ready-prepared chilled meats. Written information from the Food Standards Agency – 'Eating While you are Pregnant' can also be helpful. Women who have not had a baby with spina bifida, should be advised to take folic acid, 400 mg/day, from pre-conception until 12 weeks of gestation to reduce the chance of fetal neural tube defects (NTDs). A recent study has failed to show the efficacy of this strategy in analysing population incidence of NTD. This is suggested to relate to inadequate pre-conceptual taking of folate and/or poor compliance. Suggestions of adding folate to certain foods, for example, flour to ensure population compliance remain debatable. Current evidence does not support routine iron supplementation for all pregnant women and can be associated with some unpleasant side effects such as constipation. However, any woman who shows evidence of iron deficiency must be encouraged to take iron therapy prior to the onset of labour or any excess blood loss at delivery will increase maternal morbidity. The intake of vitamin A (liver and liver products) should be limited in pregnancy to approximately 700 mg/day because of fetal teratogenicity.

Because alcohol passes freely across the placenta, women should be advised not to drink excessively during pregnancy. Current evidence suggests that there is no harm in drinking 1–2 units of alcohol per week. Binge drinking and continuous heavy drinking causes the fetal alcohol syndrome, characterized by low birthweight, a specific facies, and intellectual and behavioural difficulties later in life.

Approximately 27% of women are smokers at the time of birth of their baby. Smoking is significantly associated with a number of adverse outcomes in pregnancy including an increased risk of perinatal mortality, placental abruption, preterm delivery, preterm premature rupture of the membranes, placenta praevia, low birthweight, etc. While there is evidence to suggest that smoking may decrease the incidence of pre-eclampsia this must be balanced against the far greater number of negative associations. Although there is mixed evidence for the effectiveness of smoking cessation programmes, women should be encouraged to partake. Pregnant women who are unable to stop smoking should be informed of the benefits of reducing the number of cigarettes they smoke. A 50% reduction can significantly reduce the fetal nicotine concentration and is associated with an increase in the birthweight.

Women who use recreational drugs must be advised to stop or be directed to rehabilitation programmes. Evidence shows adverse effects on the fetus and its subsequent development.

Continuing moderate exercise in pregnancy or regular sexual intercourse does not appear to be associated with any adverse outcomes. Certain physical activity should be avoided such as contact sports which may cause unexpected abdominal trauma. Scuba diving should also be avoided because of the risk of fetal decompression disease and an increased risk of birth defects.

Physically demanding work, particularly those jobs with prolonged periods of standing may be associated with poorer outcomes such as preterm birth, hypertension and pre-eclampsia and small-for-gestational-age babies but the evidence is weak and employment per se has not been associated with increased risks in pregnancy. Women require information regarding their employment rights in pregnancy and health-care professionals need to be aware of the current legislation.

Help for the socially disadvantaged and single mothers must be organized and ideally a one-to-one midwife allocated to support these women. The midwife should be able to liaise with other social services to ensure the best environment for the mother and her newborn child. Similar individual help is needed for pregnant teenagers and midwife programmes need to provide appropriate support for these vulnerable mothers.

Common symptoms in pregnancy

It is common for pregnant women to experience unpleasant symptoms in pregnancy caused by the normal physiological changes. However, these symptoms can be quite debilitating and lead to anxiety. It is important that health-care professionals are aware of such symptoms, can advise appropriate treatment and know when to initiate further investigations.

Extreme tiredness is one of the first symptoms of pregnancy and affects almost all women. It lasts for approximately 12–14 weeks then resolves in the majority.

Nausea and vomiting in pregnancy is one of the commonest early symptoms. While it is thought that this may be caused by rising levels of human chorionic gonalotropin (hCG) the evidence for this is conflicting. Hyperemesis gavidarum, where fluid and electrolyte imbalance and nutritional deficiency occur, is far less common complicating approximately 3.5/1000 deliveries. Nausea and vomiting in pregnancy varies in severity but usually presents within 8 weeks of the last menstrual period. Cessation of symptoms is reported by most by about 16 weeks. Various non-medical treatments have been advocated including ginger, vitamins B6 and B12, and P6 acupressure. There is evidence for the effectiveness of each of these but concerns about the safety of vitamin B6 (pyridoxine) remains and there is limited data on the safety of vitamin B12 (cyanocobalamin).

Constipation complicates approximately one-third of pregnancies usually decreasing in severity with advancing gestation. It is thought to be related in part to poor dietary fibre intake and reduction in gut motility caused by rising levels of progesterone. Diet modification with bran and wheat fibre supplementation helps, as well as increasing daily fluid intake.

Heartburn is also a common symptom in pregnancy, but unlike constipation, occurs more frequently as the pregnancy progresses. It is estimated to complicate one-fifth of pregnancies in the first trimester rising to three quarters by the third trimester. It is due to the increasing pressure caused by the enlarging uterus combined with the hormonal changes that lead to gastro-oesophageal reflux. It is important to distinguish this symptom from the epigastric pain associated with pre-eclampsia which will usually be associated with hypertension and proteinuria. Symptoms can be improved by simple lifestyle modifications such as maintaining an upright posture especially after meals, lying propped up in bed, eating small frequent meals and avoiding fatty foods. Antacids (especially Gaviscon®), H_2 receptor antagonists and proton-pump inhibitors are all effective, although it is recommended that the latter be used only when other treatments have failed because of its unproven safety in pregnancy.

Haemorrhoids are experienced by 1 in 10 women in the last trimester of pregnancy. There is little evidence for either the beneficial effects of topical creams in pregnancy or indeed their safety. Diet modification may help and in extreme circumstances surgical treatment considered although this is unusual since the haemorrhoids often resolve after delivery.

Varicose veins occur frequently in pregnancy. They do not cause harm and while compression stockings may help symptoms they unfortunately do not prevent varicose veins from appearing.

The nature of physiological vaginal discharge changes in pregnancy. If, however, it becomes itchy, malodorous or is associated with pain on micturition, it may be due to an underlying infection such as trichomoniasis, bacterial vaginosis or candidiasis. Appropriate investigations and treatment should be instigated.

Screening for maternal complications

ANAEMIA

Maternal iron requirements increase in pregnancy because of the demands of the developing fetus, the formation of the placenta and the increase in the maternal red cell mass. With an increase in the maternal plasma volume of up to 50% there is a physiological drop in the haemoglobin (Hb) concentration during pregnancy. It is generally recommended that an Hb level below 11 g/dl up to 12 weeks' gestation or less than 10.5 g/dl at 28 weeks signifies anaemia and warrants further investigation. A low Hb (8.5–10.5 g/dl) may be associated with preterm labour and low birthweight. Routine screening should be performed at the booking visit and at 28 weeks gestation. While there are many causes of anaemia including thalassaemia and sickle cell disease, iron deficiency remains the commonest. Serum ferritin is the best way of assessing maternal iron stores and if found to be low iron supplementation should be considered. Routine iron supplementation in women with a normal Hb in pregnancy has not been shown to improve maternal or fetal outcome and is currently not recommended.

BLOOD GROUPS

Identifying the maternal blood group and screening for the presence of atypical antibodies is important in the prevention of haemolytic disease, particularly from rhesus alloimmunization. Routine antibody screening should take place at booking in all women and again at 28 weeks' gestation in those who did not have antibodies at booking. Detection of atypical antibodies should prompt referral to a specialist fetal medicine unit. In the UK, 15% of women are RhD negative and should be offered anti-D prophylaxis after potentially sensitizing events (such as amniocentesis or antepartum haemorrhage) and routinely at 28 and 34 weeks' gestation [3].

INFECTION

Maternal blood should be taken early in pregnancy and with consent screened for hepatitis B, HIV, rubella and syphilis. Identification of women who are hepatitis B carriers can lead to a 95% reduction in mother to infant transmission following postnatal administration of vaccine and immunoglobulin to the baby. Women who are HIV positive can be offered treatment with antiretroviral drugs which, when combined with delivery by Caesarean section and avoidance of breast feeding, can reduce the maternal transmission rates from approximately 25 to 1% [4]. Such women need to be managed by appropriate specialist teams. Rubella screening aims to detect those women who are susceptible to the virus allowing postnatal vaccination to protect future pregnancies. All women who are rubella non-immune must be counselled to avoid contact with any infected person and if inadvertently she does, she must report the event to her midwife or doctor. Serial antibody levels will determine whether infection has occurred. Vaccination during pregnancy is contraindicated because the vaccine may be teratogenic. Although the incidence of infectious syphilis is low, there have been a number of recent outbreaks in England and Wales. Untreated syphilis is associated with congenital syphilis, neonatal death, stillbirth and preterm delivery. Following positive screening for syphilis, testing of a second specimen is required for confirmation. Interpretation of results can be difficult and referral to specialist genitourinary medicine clinics is recommended. Current evidence does not support the routine screening for cytomegalovirus, hepatitis C or toxoplasmosis.

Asymptomatic bacteriuria occurs in approximately 2–5% of pregnant women and when untreated is associated with pyelonephritis and preterm labour. Appropriate treatment will reduce the risk of preterm birth. Screening should be offered early in pregnancy by midstream urine culture.

HYPERTENSIVE DISEASE

Chronic hypertension pre-dates pregnancy or appears in the first 20 weeks whereas pregnancy-induced hypertension develops in the pregnancy, resolves after delivery and is not associated with proteinuria. Pre-eclampsia defines hypertension that is associated with proteinuria occurring after 20 weeks and resolving after birth. Pre-eclampsia occurs in 2–10% of pregnancies and is associated with both maternal and neonatal morbidity and mortality [5]. Risk factors include nulliparity, age of 40 years and above, family history of pre-eclampsia, history of pre-eclampsia in a prior pregnancy, a body mass index greater than 35, multiple pregnancy and pre-existing diabetes or hypertension. Hypertension is often an early sign that pre-dates the development of serious maternal and fetal disease and should be assessed regularly in pregnancy. There is little evidence as to how frequently blood pressure should be checked and so it is important to identify risk factors for pre-eclampsia early in pregnancy. In the absence of these, blood pressure and urine analysis for protein should be measured at each routine antenatal visit and mothers should be warned of the advanced symptoms of pre-eclampsia (frontal headache, epigastric pain, vomiting and visual disturbances).

GESTATIONAL DIABETES

Currently there is little agreement as to the definition of gestational diabetes, whether we should routinely screen for it and how to diagnose and manage it. Accordingly, the National Institute for Clinical Excellence (NICE) recently recommended that routine screening for gestational diabetes should not be offered [3].

PSYCHIATRIC ILLNESS

The importance of psychiatric conditions related to pregnancy was highlighted in the most recent Confidential Enquiry into Maternal and Child Health [1]. At booking, details of a significant history of psychiatric illness should be established and at-risk women referred for specialist psychiatric assessment during the pregnancy.

PLACENTA PRAEVIA

In approximately 1.5% of women the placenta will cover the os on the 20-week scan but by delivery, only 0.14% will have placenta praevia. Only those women whose placenta covers the os in the second trimester should be offered a scan at 36 weeks to check the position. If this is not clear on transabdominal scan, a transvaginal scan should be performed.

Screening for fetal complications

CONFIRMATION OF FETAL VIABILITY

All women should be offered a 'dating' scan. This is best performed between 10 and 13 weeks' gestation and the crown–rump length measured when the fetus is in a neutral position (i.e. not curled up or hyperextended). Current evidence shows that the estimated day of delivery predicted by ultrasound at this gestation will reduce the need for induction of labour at 41 weeks when compared with the due date predicted by the last menstrual period. In addition, a dating scan will improve the reliability of serum screening for Down's syndrome, diagnose multiple pregnancy and allow accurate determination of chorionicity and diagnose up to 80% of major fetal abnormalities. Women who present after 14 weeks' gestation should be offered a dating scan by ultrasound assessment of the biparietal diameter or head circumference.

SCREENING FOR DOWN'S SYNDROME

Current recommendations from the National Screening Committee and the National Institute for Clinical Excellence advocate that Down's screening programmes should detect 60% of affected cases for a 5% false positive rate. By 2007 the detection rate should be 75% for a 3% false positive rate. These performance measures should be age standardized and based on a cut-off of 1/250 at term. There are numerous screening strategies operational in the UK at the present time using either first trimester ultrasound markers (nuchal translucency) or maternal serum markers (alpha-fetoprotein, oestriol, free-beta hCG, inhibin-A and pregnancy associated plasma protein A) in either the first or second trimester. Some programmes use a combination of both serum and ultrasound markers. To achieve the 2007 targets, it is likely that combination screening will be required. Because screening for Down's syndrome is a complex issue, health-care professionals must have a clear understanding of the options available to their patients. Unbiased, evidence-based information must be given to the woman at the beginning of the pregnancy so that she has time to consider whether to opt for screening and the opportunity to clarify any areas of confusion before the deadline for the test passes. Following a 'screen positive' result the woman needs careful counselling to explain the test result does not mean the fetus has Down's syndrome and to explain the options for further testing by either chorion villus sampling or amniocentesis. A positive screen test does not mean further testing is mandatory. Likewise, a woman with a 'screen negative' result must understand the fetus may still have Down's syndrome (see 'Fetal medicine in clinical practice').

SCREENING FOR STRUCTURAL ABNORMALITIES

The identification of fetal structural abnormalities allows the opportunity for *in utero* therapy, planning for delivery, for example, when the fetus has major congenital heart disease, parental preparation and the option of termination of pregnancy should a severe problem be diagnosed. Major structural anomalies are present in about 3% of fetuses screened at 20 weeks' gestation. Detection rates vary depending on the system examined, skill of the operator, time allowed for the scan and quality of the ultrasound equipment. Follow-up data is important to audit the quality of the service. Women must appreciate the limitations of such scans. Local detection rates of various anomalies such as spina bifida, heart disease, facial clefting and the like should be made available. Written information should be given to women early in pregnancy explaining the nature and purpose of such scans highlighting conditions that are not detected such as cerebral palsy and many genetic conditions. It is important to appreciate that the fetal anomaly scan is a screening test which women should opt for rather than have as a routine part of antenatal care without appropriate counselling (see 'Fetal medicine in clinical practice').

SCREENING FOR FETAL WELL-BEING

Each antenatal clinic attendance allows the opportunity to screen for fetal well-being. Auscultation for the fetal heart will confirm that the fetus is alive and can usually be detected from about 14 weeks of gestation. While hearing the fetal heart may be reassuring there is no evidence of a clinical or predictive value. Likewise there is no evidence to support the use of routine cardiotocography in uncomplicated pregnancies. Physical examination of the abdomen by inspection and palpation will identify approximately 30% of small-for-gestational-age fetuses [6]. Measurement of the symphysio-fundal height in centimetres starting at the uterine fundus and ending on the fixed point of the symphysis pubis has a sensitivity and specificity of approximately 27 and 88%, respectively, although serial measurements may improve accuracy. Customized growth charts make adjustments for maternal height, weight, ethnicity and parity. Their use increases the antenatal detection of small-for-gestational-age fetuses and result in fewer unnecessary hospital admissions. While the evidence for the benefits of plotting serial symphysio-fundal height measurements is limited, it is recommended that women are offered estimation of fetal size at each antenatal visit and when there is concern, referred for formal ultrasound assessment. Traditionally, women have been advised to note the frequency of fetal movements in the third trimester. Although the evidence does not support formal counting of fetal movements to reduce the incidence of late fetal death, women who notice a reduction of fetal movements should contact their local hospital for further advice.

Organization of antenatal care

Antenatal care has been traditionally provided by a combination of general practitioners, community midwives and hospital midwives and obstetricians. The balance has depended on the perceived normality of the pregnancy at booking. However, pregnancy and childbirth is to a certain extent an unpredictable process. The frequency of antenatal visits and appropriate carer must be planned carefully allowing the opportunity for early detection of problems without becoming over-intrusive.

Who should provide the antenatal care?

A meta-analysis comparing pregnancy outcome in two groups of low-risk women, one with community-led antenatal care (midwife and general practitioner) and the other with hospital-led care did not show any differences in terms of preterm birth, Caesarean section, anaemia, antepartum haemorrhage, urinary tract infections and perinatal mortality. The first group had a lower rate of pregnancy-induced hypertension and pre-eclampsia which could reflect a lower incidence or lower detection [7]. Clear referral pathways need to be developed, however, that allow appropriate referral to specialists when either fetal or maternal problems are detected.

There is little evidence regarding women's views on who should provide antenatal care. Unfortunately, care is usually provided by a number of different professionals often in different settings. Studies evaluating the impact of continuity of care do not generally separate the antenatal period from labour. The studies consistently show that with fewer caregivers women are better informed and prepared for labour, attend more antenatal classes, have fewer antenatal admissions to hospital and have higher satisfaction rates. Differences in clinical end-points such as Caesarean section rates, post-partum haemorrhage, admission to the neonatal unit and perinatal mortality are generally insignificant [3]. While it would appear advantageous for women to be seen by the same midwife throughout pregnancy and childbirth there are practical and economic considerations that need to be taken into account. Nevertheless, where possible, care should be provided by a small group of professionals.

Documentation of antenatal care

The antenatal record needs to document clearly the care the woman has received from all those involved. It will also serve as a legal document, a source of useful information for the woman and a mechanism of communication between different health-care professionals. There is now good evidence that women should be allowed to carry their own notes. Women feel more in control of their pregnancy and do not lose the notes any more often than the hospital! In addition, useful information will be available to clinicians should the women require emergency care while away from home. Many areas of the UK are endeavouring to work towards a standard format for the records. This would be of benefit to those women who move between hospitals so that the caregivers would automatically be familiar with the style of the notes. If we are to move to an electronic patient record, there must be general agreement in a minimum data set and a standard antenatal record would be a step in this direction.

Frequency and timing of antenatal visits

There had been little change in how frequently women are seen in pregnancy for the last 50 years. In 2003, the National Institute for Clinical Excellence produced a clinical guideline entitled 'Antenatal care; routine care for the healthy pregnant woman' [3]. This document recognized the large amount of information that needs to be discussed at the beginning of pregnancy particularly with regard to screening tests. The first appointment needs to be early in pregnancy, certainly before 12 weeks if possible. This initial appointment should be regarded as an opportunity for imparting general information about the

Table 6.1 Factors indicating the need for additional specialist care in pregnancy

---

Conditions such as hypertension, cardiac or renal disease, endocrine, psychiatric or haematological disorders, epilepsy, diabetes, autoimmune disease, cancer or HIV
Factors that make the woman vulnerable such as those who lack social support
Age 40 years and older or 18 years and younger
BMI greater than or equal to 35 or less than 18
Previous Caesarean section
Severe pre-eclampsia or eclampsia
Previous pre-eclampsia or eclampsia
Three or more miscarriages
Previous preterm birth or midtrimester loss
Previous psychiatric illness or puerperal psychosis
Previous neonatal or stillbirth
Previous baby with congenital anomaly
Previous small-for-gestational or large-for-gestation aged baby
Family history of genetic disorder

(By kind permission of the National Collaborating Centre for Women's and Children's Health)

pregnancy such as diet, smoking, folic acid supplementation etc. A crucial aim is to identify those women who will require additional care in the pregnancy (Table 6.1). A urine test should be sent for bacteriological screen and a booking for ultrasound arranged. Sufficient time should be set aside for an impartial discussion of the screening tests available including those for anaemia, red-cell antibodies, syphilis, HIV hepatitis and rubella. Because of the complexity of Down's syndrome, this too should be discussed in detail and supplemented with written information. Ideally another follow-up appointment should be arranged before the screening tests need to be performed to allow further questions and arrange a time for the tests following maternal consent.

The next appointment needs to be around 16 weeks gestation to discuss the results of the screening tests. In addition, information about antenatal classes should be given and a plan of action made for the timing and frequency of future antenatal visits including who should see the woman. As with each antenatal visit, the blood pressure should be measured and the urine tested for protein. The 20-week anomaly scan should also be discussed and arranged and women should understand its limitations.

At each visit the symphysio-fundal height is plotted, the blood pressure measured and the urine tested for protein. At 28 weeks' gestation, blood should be taken for haemoglobin estimation and atypical red-cell antibodies. Anti-D prophylaxis should be offered to women who are rhesus negative. A follow-up appointment at 32 weeks will allow the opportunity to discuss these results. A second dose of anti-D should be offered at 34 weeks. At 36 weeks, the position of the baby needs to be checked and if there is uncertainty, an ultrasound scan arranged to exclude breech presentation. If a breech is confirmed, external-cephalic version should be considered. If placenta praevia had been noted at 20 weeks a follow-up scan at 36 weeks is needed. For women who have not given birth by 41 weeks, both a membrane sweep and induction of labour should be discussed and offered.

References

1. Confidential Enquiry into Maternal and Child Health (2004) *Why Mothers Die; 2000–2002*. London: RCOG Press.
2. National Health Service (2001) *The Pregnancy Book*. London: Health Promotion England.
3. National Collaborating Centre for Women's and Children's Health (2003) *Antenatal Care: Routine Care for the Healthy Pregnant Woman*. London: RCOG Press.
4. Mandelbrot L, Le Chenadec J, Berrebi A *et al.* (1998) Perinatal HIV-1 transmission. Interaction between zidovudine prophylaxis and mode of delivery in the French perinatal cohort. *J AM Med Assoc* **280**, 55–60.
5. Sibai B, Dekker G & Kupferminc M (2005) Pre-eclampsia. *Lancet* **365**, 785–99.
6. Royal College of Obstetricians and Gynaecologists (2002) *The Investigation and Management of the Small-For-Gestational-Age Fetus*. RCOG Guideline (No. 31) London: RCOG Press.
7. Villar J, Carroli G, Khan-Neelofur D *et al.* (2003) Patterns of routine antenatal care for low-risk pregnancy. Cochrane Database Syst Rev **1**, 000934.

Chapter 7: Normal labour

A.A. Calder

Of all the experiences of the human condition, birth surely represents the most important. Human society places great importance upon it: for social, not to mention legal, reasons knowledge of our birth date is a lifelong requirement. Much more important than its timing is the need for our birth to release us towards independent existence with the fullest possible endowment for physical and intellectual development. Despite its enormous importance it is doubtful if any of us can recollect any of this experience.

In contrast, few, if any, women can forget their birth-giving experiences; yet the imperative that the offspring should complete the birth process unscathed applies almost equally to the mother. The spectrum of maternal experiences of childbirth extends from exhilarated, fulfilled and enriched mothers, to those women who are permanently crippled physically or emotionally and even, still all too commonly, those who pay for the experience with their lives. Safe motherhood is a wholly reasonable expectation but one which still ranks too low in the priorities of male-dominated political arenas.

Amidst the complexity and sophistication that is modern obstetrics it is important to remind ourselves of the simple objective of every pregnancy, namely the delivery of a healthy baby to a healthy mother. The fullest possible understanding of the birth process, its perturbations and appropriate management policies is central to that objective.

Physiology of the birth process

Traditional teaching of the mechanisms of labour has focused on the three participants:
1 The powers.
2 The passages.
3 The passenger.

It would be difficult to improve on this approach but before addressing these in detail it is first necessary to consider the pregnancy phase. The labour phase represents a fraction (perhaps only 1/1000th) of the total time between conception and birth. For the preceding 999 parts it is imperative that the mother is not in labour, thus ensuring that the offspring grows and develops to the appropriate

extent before birth. The fetus then undergoes a complex process of maturation. Hitherto dependent almost entirely on the placenta via its umbilical lifeline for nutritional, respiratory and excretory functions, not to mention a host of other regulatory processes, the fetus must be prepared for its adaptation to extrauterine life by maturational changes in several key organ systems, notably the lungs. These processes probably occupy several weeks at the end of pregnancy.

For successful reproduction the uterus must display two fundamental qualities. It must first receive and nurture the pregnancy, and it must then launch the finished product into the world. In these two roles it must display diametrically opposite properties and to do so it has two components, very different in both structure and function – the corpus uteri and the cervix uteri. The corpus is almost entirely composed of smooth muscle – the myometrium. This must remain quiescent through almost the entire course of pregnancy before performing its contractile heroics during labour. In contrast, the cervix contains little muscle, consisting largely of connective tissue whose principal component is collagen. The collagen in the cervical stroma must retain the cervix in a firmly closed condition throughout pregnancy and then be capable of yielding during labour to allow passage of the fetus to delivery. Just as fetal maturation is a gradual process, so too is the 'maturation' which concerns the corpus and the cervix, and it seems clear that the complex endocrine and other changes which 'mature' both the fetus and the uterus are, in normal conditions, intimately linked.

While labour proper is generally a process lasting a few hours, its onset, far from being sudden, is the culmination of a gradual process which has been evolving over several weeks. This development phase of preparation for parturition has been suitably entitled prelabour [1].

Prelabour and labour: hormonal and immunological mechanisms

The multitude of biological substances which interact in the control of the human birth process seem to increase almost daily. To catalogue more than 60 such factors might

Table 7.1 A far from comprehensive list of substances and categories of substances which are known to participate in the birth process

Actin	Lipocortin
Adenylate cyclase	Lipopolysaccharide
Adhesion molecules	Lipoxygenase
(ICAM, VCAM, etc.)	Magnesium
Adrenaline	Matrix metalloproteinases
Bradykinin	*Monocyte chemotactic protein-1*
Calcium	*Myosin*
Calmodulin	Myosin light chain kinase
Chemokines	Neutrophil elastase
Chondroitin sulphate	Nitric oxide
Collagen	Noradrenaline
Collagenases	Oestrogens
Connexin 43	*Oxytocin*
Corticotrophin (ACTH)	Oxytocinase
Corticotrophin-releasing factor	Phosphatases
Cortisol	Phosphodiesterase
cAMP	Phospholipases
cGMP	Platelet-activating factor
Cyclo-oxygenase-1	Potassium
Cyclo-oxygenase-2	*Progesterone*
Cytokines	Prostacyclin
Dehydroepiandrosterone sulphate	*Prostaglandin dehydrogenase*
Dermatan sulphate	*Prostaglandin E$_2$*
Endothelins	*Prostaglandin F$_{2\alpha}$*
Glycosaminoglycans	Proteoglycans
G proteins	Relaxin
Gravidin	Sodium
Inositol trisphosphate	Substance P
IL-8	Sulphatase
Leukotrienes	Surfactant
	Vasopressin

Those shown in italic are discussed in detail in the text

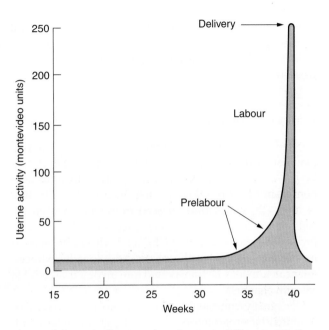

Fig. 7.1 Schematic diagram of uterine contractility quantitation through the course of labour and delivery (from [2]).

cyclic adenosine monophosphate (AMP), prostacyclin, the prostaglandin-degrading enzyme prostaglandin dehydrogenase, and various cytokines and chemokines, notably interleukin 8 (IL-8, the neutrophil attractant and activating peptide) and monocyte chemotactic peptide (MCP-1).

TRANSITION FROM PREGNANCY TO LABOUR

The classical studies of Caldeyro-Barcia [2] demonstrate the gradual 'coming to the boil' of myometrial contractility during 'prelabour' which occupies the last seventh or so of pregnancy (Fig. 7.1). Although the parameter shown on the vertical axis is Caldeyro's Montevideo unit whereby he quantifies uterine contractility as the product of the frequency and amplitude of contractions, the same figure pattern could be used, simply by altering the labelling, to illustrate a host of other events. These include the concentrations of myometrial gap junctions, those elements consisting of the protein connexin 43 which allow the spread of action potentials between smooth muscle cells by intercellular transmission of ions thereby allowing individual myometrial fibres to change from a disorganized rabble into a disciplined regiment marching to the same drum beat in labour. Equally the factor in question might be the myometrial sensitivity to oxytocin or the concentration of various receptors in the myometrium. Nor does the recipe for this broth contain only myometrial ingredients. To these can be added fetal endocrine changes (which may carry responsibility for initiating the process)

seem extravagant, yet such a list can readily be made (Table 7.1). A detailed description of the precise interactive roles of these factors is beyond the scope of this chapter. Discussion is mainly restricted to the roles of those shown in italic type in Table 7.1, since these are of special importance, both to the natural process and to its clinical manipulations. This description is inevitably a gross oversimplification of a hugely complex process, but one which may afford the clinician the appropriate insights with which to manage the problems of labour and delivery.

KEY SUBSTANCES

Everyday clinical experience, not least from the effective use of natural substances or drugs which interfere with their function, suggests that the following may deserve special prominence: progesterone, calcium, oxytocin and prostaglandins (especially PGE$_2$ and PGF$_{2\alpha}$). Less obviously, to these may be added: connexin 43, cortisol, as well as a contribution from the cervix. The numerical expression of cervical ripening, the Bishop score, also fits Caldeyro's diagram during prelabour and labour almost perfectly.

ACTIVATION OF THE MYOMETRIUM

The individual myometrial fibre contracts when the two filaments actin and myosin combine by phosphorylation by the enzyme myosin light chain kinase to form actinomyosin. This reaction requires increased availability of intracellular calcium, released from stores within the cell (mainly in the sarcoplasmic reticulum) which may be provoked by oxytocin or $PGF_{2\alpha}$ or both via the second messenger inositol trisphosphate. Additionally, extracellular calcium may be transported into myometrial cells via calcium channels.

Conversely, contractility of the myometrial cell may be inhibited by progesterone and by the intracellular availability of cAMP, a mechanism which the use of β mimetic agents as tocolytics seeks to exploit.

RIPENING OF THE CERVIX

The substance most closely associated by clinicians with cervical ripening is PGE_2 and this probably reflects a key biological role for this compound. Softening of the cervix entails not only degradation of stromal collagen, but also changes in the proteoglycan complexes and water content of the ground substance, which may be likened to glue or cement binding individual collagen fibrils into the rigid bundles which confer on the tissue its tensile strength. The process of cervical ripening remains improperly understood, but recent studies of a number of inflammatory mediators, notably IL-8 and MCP-1 have focused attention on neutrophils and monocytes recruited from the circulation as likely factors in the process. Neutrophils are a rich source of collagenases and neutrophil elastase as well as matrix metalloproteinase enzymes which play a crucial role in the breakdown of cervical collagen. One attractive hypothesis [3] implicates PGE_2 as mainly responsible for vasodilatation of cervical capillaries and increasing their permeability to circulating neutrophils which are captured by surface adhesion molecules and drawn into the cervical stroma under the chemoattractant influence of IL-8. This chemokine is also responsible for stimulating their degranulation within the tissues to release these collagenolytic enzymes. Monocytes are also recruited into the cervix by MCP-1 and might potentially play a unifying role as a source of both PGE_2 and IL-8. Both IL-8 and MCP-1 may prove in time to be effective agents in the pharmacological orchestration of cervical ripening.

INTEGRATION OF CONTROL PATHWAYS

Studies in humans, subhuman primates, domestic species (notably sheep), rodents, and especially guinea pigs have allowed concepts to be elaborated to explain the biological control of human parturition. As emphasized above, the transition from pregnancy maintenance to birth develops gradually during a month or more of 'prelabour'. From early naïve concepts which credited the mother as responsible for initiating labour by producing oxytocin from her posterior pituitary, the hypothesis has gradually been developed whereby the control is initiated and largely vested within the fetoplacental unit (Fig. 7.2). The key component appears to be the fetal brain whose influence is exerted on fetoplacental endocrinology via the hypothalamopituitary-adrenoplacental axis. Activation of corticotrophin (adrenocorticotrophic hormone or ACTH) stimulates adrenal production of (1) cortisol which brings about maturation of the fetal lungs with the generation of pulmonary surfactant; and (2) dehydroepiandrosterone sulphate. The latter, a key precursor of placental oestradiol production, ordains a shift in the oestrogen to progesterone ratio in favour of oestrogen and provokes an endocrine dialogue between fetus, placenta, membranes and uterus (Fig. 7.3). Cortisol promotes maturation of the fetal lungs and this, together with similar events in the fetal kidneys, may modify the content of the amniotic fluid and thereby activate the fetal membranes (amnion and chorion), particularly in respect of prostaglandin synthesis. By means of such biological changes in the fetal components – fetus, placenta, amniotic fluid and the membranes – a new dialogue is created with the uterine (maternal) tissues which envelop them – the

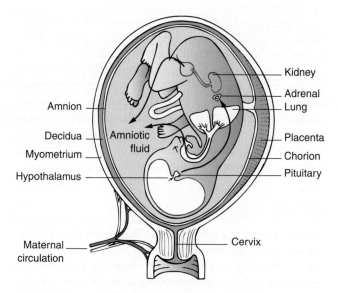

Fig. 7.2 The fetoplacental unit and the intrauterine and uterine structures with which it interacts.

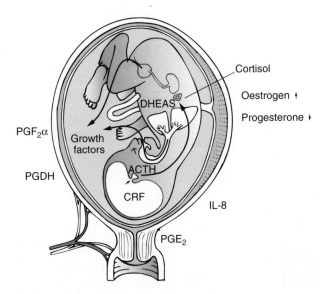

Fig. 7.3 Scheme of the principal biochemical factors participating in the control of human labour.

decidua, myometrium and cervix – producing a positive cascade of interactions among prostaglandins, cytokines and oxytocin.

PROSTAGLANDINS – ESSENTIAL REGULATORS OF PARTURITION

Only one small group of compounds involved in labour, the prostaglandins, appear to play an essential command role. It is probably no exaggeration to state that without prostaglandins labour is impossible, whereas when they appear in abundance labour is irresistible. $PGF_{2\alpha}$ appears to be the principal prostaglandin generating contractility of the myometrium, while PGE_2 is more important in the process of cervical ripening. The main sources of these prostanoids within the uterus are, respectively, the decidua and the amnion. Conveniently placed in intimate contact between these structures lies the chorion, a rich source of the prostaglandin-degrading enzyme 15-hydroxyprostaglandin dehydrogenase (PGDH). Activation of uterine prostaglandins in labour is vested in the inducible isoform of cyclo-oxygenase, COX-2, and it seems likely that the high capacity of the chorion to metabolize prostaglandins represents a defence mechanism against the early and inappropriate production of prostaglandins before the scheduled time. The influences which may bring about this precocious production of prostaglandins include trauma, haemorrhage and (most importantly) infection, now recognized as a major factor in initiating many premature deliveries. The chorion may thus be regarded as a biological metabolic barrier rather like blotting paper designed to mop up unwelcome prostaglandins.

CERVICAL EFFACEMENT – THE KEY TO SUCCESSFUL DELIVERY

As is emphasized below, effacement of the cervix is an essential prerequisite to its dilatation and one which depends on the softening and ripening of its connective tissue. Attention has focused on the apparent obstacle presented by the chorion to PGE_2 derived from the amnion. It must be conceded that the PGE_2 required in cervical ripening might be synthesized within the cervical stroma itself, but an alternative and attractive hypothesis lies in the possibility that a selective loss of PGDH activity in that area of chorion overlying the cervix might afford access of PGE_2 from the amnion and amniotic fluid to the precise part of the cervix where it is most required, namely the internal cervical os. Support for such a concept comes from the clinical observation that loss of the fetal membranes from that key site following either their spontaneous or their artificial rupture adversely prejudices the prospects of successful delivery. Recently we have provided evidence that the area of fetal membranes overlying the cervix changes from exhibiting the highest activity of PGDH during pregnancy to the lowest during labour ([4]; Fig. 7.4). Nature may thus have provided a mechanism whereby the long firm cervix is progressively softened and shortened from the top downwards during the process of 'taking up' or effacement. Beginning just below the fibromuscular junction (Fig. 7.5) the softened tissue at the internal os is progressively transported outwards around the fetal presenting part and the 'fore-waters' thereby bringing the lower portions of the cervix into intimate contact with that fetal membrane source of PGE_2.

SUBSEQUENT COURSE OF CLINICAL LABOUR

Clinical labour, as opposed to prelabour, is considered to begin with the onset of regular painful uterine contractions. The events of prelabour should have set everything in place for a comparatively short birth process, but not all labours will follow a straightforward course. In its simplest terms, labour consists of the muscle of the uterine corpus progressively stretching the cervix over the fetal head by means of rhythmic contraction and retraction. This process is usefully compared to pulling on a woollen jumper with a tight polo neck, where the action of the arms represent the contractions of the myometrium, while the changes in the neck of the garment replicate effacement and dilatation of the cervix. This analogy can be carried further with the observation that just as the first attempt at pulling on the garment is generally the most difficult, so too is the first labour. Furthermore, appropriate flexion of the head to present the cranial vertex to the neck of the garment, or the womb, is just as important for the wearer as it is for the fetus.

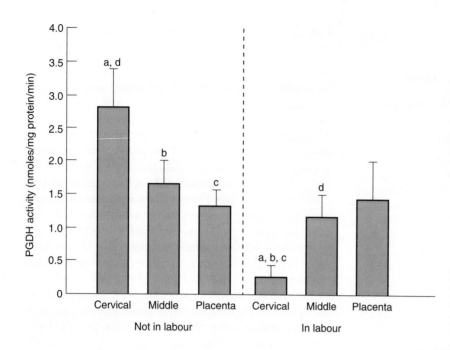

Fig. 7.4 Changes in the activity of prostaglandin dehydrogenase in different areas of the fetal membranes between late pregnancy and established labour (from [4]).

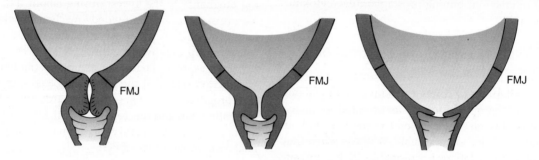

Fig. 7.5 Shape change in the cervix with the approach of labour (FMJ = fibromuscular junction).

Effacement is thus a vital forerunner to dilatation. The uneffaced cervix cannot dilate although this is less absolute in parous women than in nulliparous. Early stages of dilatation appear before the parous cervix is fully effaced.

PARTOGRAPHY

The simplest partogram plots dilatation of the cervix in centimetres against time in hours. This concept was introduced by Friedman in New York in 1954. 'The graphic analysis of labour' [5] was the first of a series of classical contributions whereby the science of partography was established, to become the cornerstone of clinical evaluation of progress in labour. Figure 7.6 shows the Friedman curve of cervimetric progress in normal labour. The sigmoid nature of Friedman's curve is a source of some interest. The gradual rise in the latent phase (0–3 cm dilatation) is followed by the steep slope of the active phase

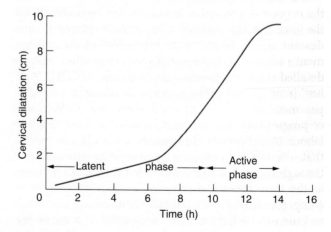

Fig. 7.6 The classic 'sigmoid' curve of progress of cervical dilatation during labour (after [5]).

(4–9 cm) and then a short less steep curve to full dilatation. Although the intensity of uterine contractions may rise during the course of labour, there is no evidence of any significant surge coinciding with the change from the latent to the active phase. Rather the slow rate of cervimetric progress in latent labour has more to do with the evolution of effective uterine contractility and the completion of cervical effacement. The steepening of the rate of progress after 3 cm dilatation is also partly explained by improved alignment of the traction force of the myometrium on the cervix as the latter begins to turn around the contours of the advancing presenting part which also begins to 'wedge' its way into the dilating os. By the same token the final deceleration phase reflects mechanical factors, the slowing rate of the final centimetre of dilatation being explained on the basis that the dilating head has farther to travel down the birth canal to stretch the cervix to full dilation as the widest part of the fetal head passes through; in addition, the cervical tissue has to be moved further by the myometrium to reach that configuration.

The duration of the phases of Friedman's original curve is now viewed with some scepticism: a latent phase of more than 10 h seems as excessive as an active phase of less than 2 h seems unduly short. Later studies have modified these initial estimates such that the latent phase might be expected to last between 3 and 8 h and the active between 2 and 6 h depending on parity and other factors including the distinction between spontaneous and induced labours. Of special importance in respect of the latent phase, however, is the almost insurmountable difficulty of defining when it starts. As has already been emphasized, labour evolves as the culmination of weeks of prelabour and the borderline between the two is impossible to define precisely.

The second sentence of Friedman's first paper reads: 'Of the major observable events that occur during labour, i.e. the force, frequency and duration of uterine contractility, descent of the presenting fetal part, and cervical effacement and dilatation, only the last named was selected for detailed study because *it seemed to parallel overall progress best*' [emphasis added]. While one might argue that this parameter is in some circumstances not the best mirror of progress (e.g. when cervical dilatation continues in a labour obstructed by cephalopelvic disproportion) and that ultimately the best measure is descent of the fetus through the birth canal, cervimetry has become accepted as the first measure of progress because it is simple to comprehend, easy to measure, reproducible and subject to little observer error. Later partograms have in some aspects been simplified, while in others they have become more sophisticated (Figs 7.7 and 7.8). The issue of rate of cervimetric progress can be reduced to a target of 1 cm/h (always recognizing that first labours may be expected to

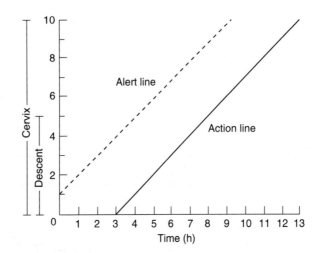

Fig. 7.7 The partogram with 'alert' and 'action' lines proposed by Philpott and Castle [6,7].

take longer). Conversely, a useful additional component to the partogram is a record of descent of the presenting part, since that represents the ultimate measure of labour progress.

The refinements of partography suggested by Philpott and Castle [6,7] some 25 years ago not only added alert lines and action lines to the graph with material advantages for clinical management, they also displayed the descent of the presenting part (see Fig. 7.7). The measure of descent is usually made at the same time as that of dilatation during a vaginal examination and is based on recording the level of the presenting part relative to the level of the ischial spines (the station). It should not be forgotten, however, that in circumstances of caput formation and moulding of the fetal head such an observation may exaggerate progress. The simple and often neglected assessment of how much fetal head (usually expressed as fifths) can be felt above the pelvic brim by abdominal examination may in the final analysis represent a more valid and reliable measure of progress.

PROGRESS IN LABOUR

The modern approach to labour, and the clinical imperative of ensuring its adequacy, has been influenced by the work of O'Driscoll and colleagues at the National Maternity Hospital in Dublin. Much of this issue is addressed in Chapter 22 of O'Driscoll and Meagher [8] which in its entirety represents one of the most significant milestones in modern obstetrics.

Poor progress in labour can be attributed to faults in the powers, the passages or the passenger (P). Faults in the powers should be considered first. Uterine contractions may be hypotonic or incoordinate. Clinical assessment of

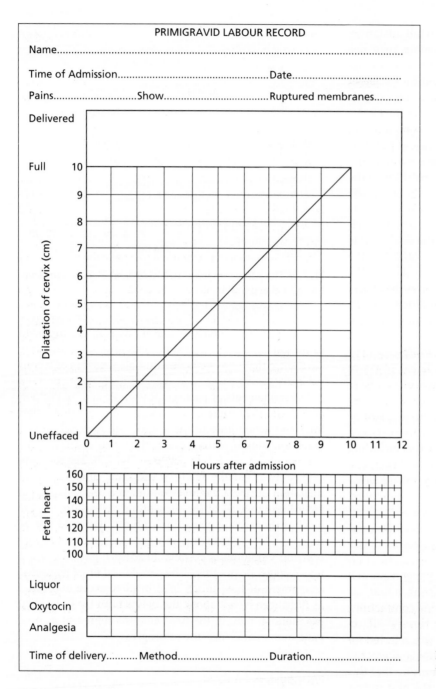

PRIMIGRAVID LABOUR RECORD

Name..

Time of Admission...Date..................................

Pains..........................Show..............................Ruptured membranes..........

Delivered

Full   10
        9
        8
        7
        6
Dilatation of cervix (cm)   5
        4
        3
        2
        1
Uneffaced   0   1   2   3   4   5   6   7   8   9   10   11   12

Hours after admission

Fetal heart   160
        150
        140
        130
        120
        110
        100

Liquor

Oxytocin

Analgesia

Time of delivery...........Method..............................Duration............................

Fig. 7.8 The simple partogram favoured by the National Maternity Hospital, Dublin.

this is subjective and unreliable; external tocography may assist somewhat; internal tocography using an intrauterine pressure sensor may be best but has never really progressed beyond a research tool. In general, if poor uterine action is suspected steps should be taken to improve it. If the fetal membranes are still intact they should be ruptured, but ideally only if the cervix is fully effaced and at least 3 cm dilated. Intravenous oxytocin is the cornerstone of therapy and this issue is addressed in the next chapter.

There is evidence that primary dysfunctional labour may be associated with deficient production of $PGF_{2\alpha}$ [9] but to date no studies have supported the clinical use of this agent to correct such problems, perhaps because it causes unpleasant side effects.

Faults in the passages may come from distortion in the maternal bony pelvis by disease, damage or deformity. There is little that can be done to overcome these, and unless they present only marginal difficulty, delivery by

Caesarean section is usually required. The soft tissues of the birth canal – cervix, vagina, perineum, and so on – may, if rigid, obstruct progress.

The passenger may be uncooperative by being excessively large, in the wrong position or presentation, or in the wrong attitude, notably with a deflexed head.

If these problems prove insurmountable then Caesarean section is necessary, but in most labours where progress is slow it is appropriate to take steps to maximize the quality of uterine contractility, an expedient which may often overcome minor problems of the passages or the passenger or both.

MANAGEMENT AND SUPERVISION OF NORMAL LABOUR

The first imperative in the conduct of labour is to determine whether labour has in fact started. The accurate diagnosis of labour is essential because so much depends on defining starting points. The diagnosis is often difficult, notably when preterm (see Chapter 21) and reliance on observing contractions is not enough by itself. A progressive change in the cervix over a few hours will confirm established labour, and so a vaginal examination at the time of admission to the labour ward is important to establish a baseline.

The partogram should be started 'provisionally' unless the initial assessment indicates that labour is unlikely. The mother's vital signs should be recorded and this should be repeated at intervals, pulse and blood pressure at least every hour and temperature every 3 h. Abnormal recordings require that the frequency of these observations be increased. The mother should be encouraged to empty her bladder regularly and her urine should be tested on each occasion for the presence of ketones, sugar, protein and blood.

It is important to establish when painful regular contractions began and what their frequency has been since. A graphic record should thus be made of the apparent strength, frequency and, if possible, the duration of the contractions.

FETAL MEMBRANES

Particular attention should be paid to the condition of the fetal membranes. If the history suggests that they have ruptured before admission it is important to look for confirmatory evidence of this especially during the initial vaginal examination. Adequate clear liquor draining is generally a reassuring sign that the fetus is in good condition to withstand the rigours of labour. In contrast scanty or absent liquor when it is fairly certain that the membranes have ruptured or have been ruptured should

occasion concern and prompt steps to establish more clearly the condition of the fetus, such as cardiotocography and, if feasible, blood gas estimation.

It is important to note the presence of blood or meconium in the liquor. The possibility that the blood may be fetal in origin should always be considered and appropriate diagnostic steps taken. The presence of meconium staining should lead to similar responses in clarifying the fetal condition as should the apparent absence of liquor.

The timing of amniotomy is critical. Some mothers resent the assumption that the membranes should always be ruptured when it becomes feasible to do so, a practice of which many obstetricians and midwives can be guilty. Mothers who crave 'natural childbirth' may see this as clinical interference and their wish to have the membranes left intact should be respected unless there is a clear benefit to be argued in favour of their rupture. Although Theobald is remembered for his dictum 'intact membranes are the biggest single hindrance to progress in labour', if the labour is progressing well, and the mother and offspring seem well, there is no compelling requirement for amniotomy. Nevertheless there would seem to be an optimum time for amniotomy during the course of spontaneous labour. This lies at the point of transition from latent to active labour when the contractions are well in train and the cervix is fully effaced and dilated 3–4 cm. Earlier amniotomy may be counterproductive, but if performed around this point then the subsequent labour is likely to be more efficient. Furthermore, fetal surveillance is enhanced by the opportunity to examine the amniotic fluid directly for meconium or blood staining and by applying a fetal scalp electrode if desired. In addition, although the quality and strength of contractions may be improved there is no persuasive evidence that labour is any more painful. Indeed requirements for analgesia are likely to be reduced partly because the increased efficiency of labour is reflected in its shorter duration.

PAIN RELIEF

We have come a long way in the century and a half since James Young Simpson discovered the analgesic effects of chloroform and applied them in the first significant attempts to relieve the anguish of labouring women in 1847. A wide variety of analgesic options have been provided for labouring women; a detailed account of their advantages and disadvantages will not be offered here. The benefits of pain relief in labour, however, extend far beyond mere humanitarian ones, and it should be clearly recognized that appropriate pain relief may improve the general course and success of labour. Obstetricians may still argue about whether epidural analgesia can on occasion lead to increased need for other interventions such as operative delivery, or may even adversely influence the progress of labour, but there seems little doubt concerning its overall benefits.

A THREE-POINT SCHEME FOR LABOUR SUPERVISION

Failure to reach the simple objective of intrapartum care – ensuring the delivery of a healthy baby to a healthy fulfilled mother – results in unhappiness, complaints and litigation, and may even lead to death or damage of mothers or babies. Opportunities for failure are numerous and varied.

The proposals with which this chapter concludes are designed to avoid these problems and are based on the following concerns:

1 Problems when they arise often do so from the neglect of simple basic principles.

2 Lines of communication, responsibility and authority need to be clearly defined.

3 Meticulous record keeping is essential, including the need for the author of the record to be easily identified.

With this in mind, the three fundamental requirements in labour are to ensure that: (1) the mother is well; (2) the fetus is in good condition; and (3) the labour is progressing. It is imperative to identify who is the lead professional in the care of each and every labour. This is likely to be a qualified midwife in most normal labours, but might be an obstetrician depending on the particular circumstances. In tune with the broad philosophy which has evolved in the latter half of the twentieth century that labour is a journey whose duration and progress should be carefully observed and managed, the three issues listed above should be addressed at regular intervals and recorded in a disciplined fashion, perhaps every hour. Thus at these intervals (and perhaps at longer intervals by a more senior midwife or obstetrician if indicated) the lead carer should formally pose the questions: (1) Is the mother well? (2) Is the fetus in good condition? (3) Is the labour progressing? The answer to each will be either 'yes', 'no' or 'unclear'. If the answer to all three is 'yes', no special investigation is called for. If the answer to any is unclear, steps must be taken to clarify it. Where the answer to a question is 'no', steps are required to rectify the problem.

Examples of problems for the mother include distress from pain, ketosis, hypertension or bleeding. Possible trouble for the fetus would most commonly be fetal heart abnormalities, meconium staining or bleeding. Finally, failure to progress in labour demands early recognition and, where possible, correction.

TIME	06.00	07.00	08.00	09.00	10.00	11.00
	M ✓	M ✓	M ✓	M ✓	M ✓	M ✓
Observation ✓/u/p	F ✓	F ✓	F ✓	F ✓	F ✓	F u
	P ✓	P ✓	P u	P p	P ✓	P ✓
Problem/Action	/	/	①	②	/	③
Name	A Smith (Sister)	A Smith (Sister)	A Smith (Sister)	C. Jones (Registrar)	A Smith (Sister)	P White (SHO)

Fig. 7.9 Scheme for expanded partogram. For each of Mother (M), Fetus (F) and Progress (P) the observer records Satisfactory (s) or Unclear (u) or Poor (p) at each recording interval. Whenever an entry is either u or p a number is entered against PROBLEM/ACTION which relates to an entry in the expanded text, e.g. (**1**) Progress in labour seems poor, head still 4/5 palpable contractions irregular. Registrar review requested. Signed: A Smith, midwifery sister. (**2**) V.E. shows cervix 3 cm dilated vertex at 0–3, some caput. Amniotomy performed, moderate clear liquor. Signed: C Jones, obstetric registrar. (**3**) Slight meconium staining of liquor. Continuous fetal monitoring begun. Signed: P White, SHO in obstetrics.

The record of answers to these three recurring questions could readily be entered on the partogram. Most hospital partograms contain a large section on which to plot the blood pressure and pulse, most of which is largely wasted space. A simple redesign of the partogram to include a requirement to record the above scheme of answers (Fig. 7.9) could constitute a significant advance in intrapartum care.

References

1. Demelin L (1927) *La Contraction Uterine et les Discinesies Correlative*. Paris: Dupont.
2. Caldeyro-Barcia R (1959) Uterine contractility in obstetrics. *Proceedings of the 2nd International Congress of Gynecology and Obstetrics*, vol. 1. Montreal, 65–78.
3. Kelly RW (1994) Pregnancy maintenance and parturition: the role of prostaglandin in manipulating the immune and inflammatory response. *Endocr Rev* **15**, 684–706.
4. Van Meir CA, Ramirez MM, Matthews SG, Calder AA, Keirse MJNC & Challis JRG (1997) Chorionic prostaglandin catabolism is decreased in the lower uterine segment with term labour. *Placenta* **18**, 109–14.
5. Friedman EA (1954) The graphic analysis of labour. *Am J Obstet Gynecol* **68**, 1568.
6. Philpott RM & Castle WM (1972) Cervicographs in the management of labour in the primigravida. 1. The Alert line

for detecting abnormal labour. *J Obstet Gynaecol Br Cmmw* **79**, 592.

7. Philpott RH & Castle WM (1972) Cervicographs in the management of labour in the primigravida. 2. The Action line and treatment of abnormal labour. *J Obstet Gynaecol Br Cmmw* **75**, 599.

8. O'Driscoll K & Meagher D (1980) *The Active Management of Labour*. London: Saunders.

9. Johnson TA, Greer IA, Kelly RW & Calder AA (1993) Plasma prostaglandin metabolite concentrations in normal and dysfunctional labour. *Br J Obstet Gynaecol* **93**, 483–8.

Chapter 8: Fetal monitoring during labour

James A. Low

What is the problem?

The objective of fetal monitoring during labour is the prediction and diagnosis of fetal asphyxia before fetal/newborn morbidity with particular reference to brain damage has occurred.

Fetal asphyxia is defined as 'a condition of impaired blood gas exchange leading, if it persists, to progressive hypoxemia and hypercapnia' [1]. The operative term in this definition is 'progressive'. Hypoxemia and hypercapnia as an event during labour may occur in a transient fashion with physiological but no pathological significance. Fetal asphyxia of pathological significance during labour requires progressive hypoxemia with a significant metabolic acidosis.

Thus the diagnosis of fetal asphyxia requires a blood gas and acid–base assessment. In respect to intrapartum fetal asphyxia, the threshold at delivery beyond which cerebral dysfunction or brain damage may occur is an umbilical artery base deficit greater than 12 mmol/l.

Relationship of fetal asphyxia to brain damage

During the last 50 years, asphyxia has been examined in the research laboratory using a number of different animal models. These studies have confirmed that fetal asphyxia of a particular degree and duration may cause brain damage. However, the striking feature of all these studies is that in spite of a uniform single exposure to asphyxia many fetuses have no brain damage, some will have brain damage and a few fetal deaths will occur. The outcome is influenced by the fetal response to asphyxia. Fetal cardiovascular compensation with an increase of arterial pressure, centralization of cardiac output and increased cerebral blood flow will maintain cerebral oxygen consumption in spite of the hypoxemia. However if the asphyxia continues, a point will be reached when fetal cardiovascular decompensation reverses this process leading to cerebral hypoxia and, if sustained, brain damage. Variability of this fetal cardiovascular response is an important

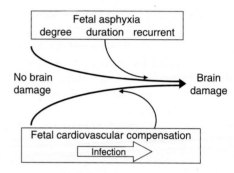

Fig. 8.1 The outcome, i.e. no brain damage/brain damage is a result of the characteristics of the fetal asphyxia and the quality of the fetal cardiovascular compensation.

factor in the differing outcome in these laboratory studies.

Our understanding of the relationship between fetal asphyxia and brain damage has been based on these studies in the research laboratory. It has become evident that the relationship between fetal asphyxia and brain damage is complex and may be influenced by a number of factors including: maturity of the fetus; degree, duration and nature of the asphyxia and the quality of the fetal cardiovascular response (Fig. 8.1).

The clinical introduction of microelectrode blood gas systems provided the opportunity to examine these measures in all pregnancies at delivery without risk to the fetus and newborn. Umbilical vein and artery blood gas and acid–base measures at delivery represent valuable reference points of asphyxia during labour. The umbilical vein reflects the effectiveness of maternal fetal blood gas exchange while the umbilical artery reflects the acid–base status of the fetus. Reference data for these measures in the umbilical vein and artery for 21,744 deliveries in our centre are presented in Table 8.1.

Recognizing the importance of these measures, recent studies have emphasized the need for quality data to provide the basis for interpretation [2]. Several procedural and technical errors may occur during umbilical cord blood sampling and subsequent blood gas analysis. Optimal

Table 8.1 Mean blood gas and acid–base measures for 21,744 deliveries

	Umbilical vein		Umbilical artery	
	Mean	SD	Mean	SD
pH	7.340	0.07	7.248	0.069
pCO_2	40.4	7.7	54.5	9.7
pO_2	27.2	6.1	15.1	5.1
BD	3.0	2.7	6.8	3.2

BD, base deficit.

Table 8.2 Prevalence of intrapartum fetal asphyxia

Fetal asphyxia	Rate per 1000 live births	
	Preterm	Term
Prevalence	73	25
Mild	38	21
Moderate/severe	35	4

interpretation requires a paired sample from both umbilical vein and artery. A single sample from the umbilical vein will define venous metabolic state but cannot rule out an arterial metabolic acidosis. During sampling, two aliquots may be drawn from the umbilical vein. Such a procedural error is implied when the vein–artery pH difference is less than 0.02. The accuracy of the calculated measures of metabolic acidosis is dependent upon the quality of the pH and pCO_2 estimations. The accuracy of the pCO_2 estimation should be questioned when the pCO_2 value is outside the physiological range or the pCO_2 artery–vein difference is a negative value or less than 4 mgHg. In these circumstances, the interpretation should be limited to pH alone.

An umbilical artery blood measure of metabolic acidosis is the best indicator of tissue oxygen debt experienced by the fetus. Recent studies have suggested an increased risk to the fetus begins when the umbilical artery base deficit exceeds the mean [3]. In a study to determine the threshold for significant morbidity, moderate and severe newborn complications occurred only in the fetuses with an umbilical artery base deficit >12 mmol/l. The incidence of moderate and severe complications with an umbilical artery base deficit 12–16 mmol/l was 10% [4]. There is a progression of frequency of such complications with increasing metabolic acidosis with a 40% incidence of moderate and severe complications when the umbilical artery base deficit was >16 mmol/l.

The objective of clinical studies since the introduction of microelectrode blood gas systems has been to determine if the concepts emerging from the research laboratory are relevant to the human fetus. The findings are consistent with the contention that a fetus may experience asphyxia without morbidity; however, the occurrence of fetal asphyxia of a particular degree and duration may cause cerebral dysfunction in the newborn [5,6] and in some cases brain damage accounting for handicap in surviving children [7,8].

Prevalence of intrapartum fetal asphyxia

The classification of fetal asphyxia in the research laboratory is based upon continuous measures of the degree and duration of the asphyxia and the quality of the fetal cardiovascular response. Since most measures obtained in the laboratory are not available in the clinical setting, the clinical classification of asphyxia as mild, moderate or severe is based on the presence of metabolic acidosis to confirm the occurrence of asphyxia with measures of neonatal encephalopathy and other organ system complications to express the severity of the asphyxia [9].

Clinical studies in recent years have provided insight into the prevalence of mild, moderate and severe fetal asphyxia during the intrapartum period. The prevalence and severity of fetal asphyxia at delivery in preterm and term pregnancies at delivery is outlined in Table 8.2.

There is no evidence of an association between mild fetal asphyxia and major deficits while long-term follow-up has demonstrated no association with minor disabilities later in childhood [10]. These findings suggest that mild fetal asphyxia represents a window of opportunity in clinical management when a diagnosis of fetal asphyxia can be confirmed and if necessary intervention initiated to prevent cerebral dysfunction and deficits in these children.

Although the prevalence of intrapartum fetal asphyxia as determined at delivery has been established the duration and nature of the asphyxia in most cases is not known. Since the duration and nature of the asphyxia cannot be determined it is not known when the asphyxia identified at delivery began before the onset of labour and how often the asphyxia identified at delivery represents the last in a series of asphyxial exposures that may have begun before the onset of labour.

Prediction and diagnosis of fetal asphyxia

The diagnosis of fetal asphyxia requires a blood gas and acid–base assessment. A reliable method to provide a continuous recording of fetal acid–base status in the clinical setting is not yet available. At the present time a diagnosis can be confirmed by means of periodic fetal blood sampling during labour or at delivery for a blood gas and acid–base assessment. Thus, the requirements are criteria to identify the fetus at risk for fetal asphyxia to justify the intervention for fetal blood sampling particularly during labour for a fetal blood gas and acid–base assessment.

The clinical paradigm that has been widely used to identify the fetus at risk of asphyxia combines clinical risk scoring with fetal heart rate surveillance. This has not resolved the problem due to shortfalls of each element of the paradigm that have become evident with increasing clinical experience.

CLINICAL RISK SCORING

The limitations of clinical risk scoring have been demonstrated in several studies. In our experience, 23–40% of fetal asphyxia occurred in pregnancies with no clinical risk factors [11,12]. The term 'low risk' based on clinical markers cannot be applied in regard to fetal asphyxia during labour.

In those cases in which clinical risk factors were present, a wide range of clinical complications determined risk with no single risk factor demonstrating a strong association with intrapartum fetal asphyxia. The positive predictive value for both antepartum and intrapartum risk factors for intrapartum fetal asphyxia was 3%. Thus clinical risk scoring has a major problem with false positive prediction of intrapartum fetal asphyxia.

Electronic fetal heart rate monitoring

The publication by Edward Hon in 1958 [13] reflects the beginning of the expectation that electronic fetal heart rate monitoring (EFM) would be useful in the prediction of intrapartum fetal asphyxia.

Observations during the 1960s and 1970s supported the contention that EFM could be a useful screening test for the prediction of intrapartum fetal asphyxia. Our clinical experience paralleled that of other investigators in this field with anecdotal examples of an association between abnormal fetal heart rate patterns and fetal asphyxia with a range of outcomes. Laboratory studies demonstrated a relationship between fetal heart rate behaviour and fetal hypoxemia and metabolic acidosis. Late decelerations have been shown to occur when fetal oxygen tension decreases below a critical level. The interval between the onset of the contraction and the onset of the deceleration reflects the time necessary for fetal oxygen tension to fall below this threshold [14,15]. Late decelerations due to fetal hypoxemia in a previously normoxic fetus are due to chemoreceptor initiated reflex bradycardia which can be blocked by atropine, while in previously hypoxic fetuses the bradycardia is presumably due to a direct effect upon the myocardium [16]. Based on such reports the use of EFM expanded rapidly in the 1970s.

The evaluation of EFM as a screening test

There are two requirements for a screening test. The clinical problem must justify intervention. Intrapartum fetal asphyxia is important and in selected circumstances justifies intervention. The benefits of the test must outweigh the harm. It was recognized in the late 1970s that this had not been determined.

The introduction of EFM was associated with a reduction in the number of intrapartum fetal deaths [17]. However, intrapartum fetal deaths continue to be reported in studies of perinatal mortality. In the UK Confidential Enquiry into stillbirths and death in infancy, 9% of all deaths between 20 and 44 weeks of gestation were related to labour and, of the normally formed babies weighing at least 2500 g, 4.3% could be linked to intrapartum events [18].

Well-designed, randomized, controlled trials are proposed as a means of providing a measure of the true risks and benefits of a medical intervention. There have been no randomized clinical trials to compare no fetal heart rate surveillance with intermittent fetal heart rate auscultation. Nine randomized clinical trials, three with electronic fetal monitoring alone and six with electronic fetal monitoring with scalp sampling, have been analysed in the Cochrane Pregnancy and Child Birth Data Base [19,20]. The randomized clinical trials comparing intermittent auscultation and continuous EFM have not provided consistent evidence that EFM was associated with a decrease of fetal and newborn morbidity. The randomized clinical trials have made an important contribution, confirming the occurrence of false positive interpretation of electronic fetal heart rate recording with unnecessary interventions. These studies have demonstrated that electronic fetal heart rate monitoring in relation to intermittent auscultation has been associated with increased incidence of Caesarean section for fetal distress and dystocia, increased operative delivery and general anaesthesia. It must be recognized that these outcomes are not due to the method of fetal heart rate surveillance but are a result of inappropriate interpretation of the fetal heart rate data.

Clinical management guidelines for EFM

Faced with the available evidence, national organizations began to prepare consensus papers in regard to fetal surveillance during labour. Examples of the most recent clinical guidelines include: ACOG Technical Bulletin Number 207, 1995 in United States [21]; SOGC Clinical Practice Guideline Number 112, 2001 in Canada [22]; and RCOG Evidence-based Clinical Guideline Number 8, 2001 in the United Kingdom [23]. These guidelines prepared by recognized experts in the field endeavoured to reflect the best evidence available at that time.

What is missing from all the current guidelines is a specific algorithm for the interpretation of fetal heart rate patterns. The ACOG and the SOGC guidelines classify fetal heart rate patterns as reassuring and non-reassuring. Detailed criteria and time are not noted. The Royal College Evidence-based Guidelines have defined traces as normal, suspicious and pathological. No guidelines have provided data as to the sensitivity, specificity and predictive value of the patterns as defined.

This issue was addressed by an NIH research-planning workshop in 1997 [24]. The specific purpose of the workshop was to develop standardized and unambiguous definitions of fetal heart rate tracings for future research. Although all members of the workshop were of the opinion that EFM was of value, there was no consensus regarding strict guidelines for clinical management using fetal heart rate (FHR) patterns. The position expressed was that many fetuses have FHR tracings that are intermediate between two extremes, that is, normal and patterns so severe that the fetus is at risk of morbidity or mortality. The workshop concluded that evidence-based algorithms for management awaits further research. This view has been recently expressed again [25].

An FHR algorithm to predict fetal asphyxia

Interpretation of the FHR record

Two issues important in the interpretation of an FHR record are the classification of FHR variables and inter-observer reliability in the visual interpretation of these variables.

Many definitions of the individual FHR variables, baseline FHR, baseline FHR variability, accelerations and decelerations have been provided. A good example is provided in the RCOG Evidence-based Clinical Guideline Number 8. However differences of classification criteria remain, particularly for decelerations. In the classification of late decelerations, some clinicians have given first priority to the timing of the nadir of the deceleration, whereas others have emphasized the waveform. In the interpretation of the waveform, both the onset to the nadir [26] and the residual component of the waveform have been examined [27]. Until a consensus is developed, criteria should be clearly defined and consistently used.

Although progress is being made in the computer-based interpretation of FHR records, with few exceptions, clinical records are read visually. The limited inter-observer reliability for the interpretation of FHR variables has been well documented [28]. Our experience has demonstrated the following good-to-fair inter-observer Kappa values: baseline FHR, 0.70; baseline FHR variability, 0.55; FHR accelerations, 0.57; variable decelerations, 0.46 and late and prolonged decelerations, 0.57. Scoring FHR patterns over time can offset this limited inter-observer reliability of individual FHR variables. The record should be scored in 10 min epochs (cycles). Determination of the pattern requires careful scoring of a number of cycles that in most cases can be achieved with six cycles representing 1 h of the FHR record. Our experience has been a high degree

of inter-observer reliability in the classification of FHR patterns in 1 h of recording [29].

An FHR algorithm to predict fetal asphyxia

We have addressed this question. A matched case control study was conducted in term pregnancies to demonstrate that a threshold of FHR patterns can be defined and that intermediate patterns of FHR can be determined for intrapartum fetal asphyxia [29]. The FHR records were scored for each FHR variable for six 10-min cycles in each hour.

FHR variables with an independent association with fetal asphyxia (i.e. umbilical artery base deficit greater than 16 mmol/l at delivery) in this study were absent as well as minimal baseline variability and late and prolonged decelerations. Three FHR patterns were defined based on the presence of these four FHR variables in six 10-min cycles in 1 h. The patterns proposed as an algorithm for the interpretation of electronic FHR records are outlined in Table 8.3.

A number of relevant observations emerged from this study. The sensitivity of predictive and potentially predictive FHR patterns was good identifying 75% of the cases with fetal asphyxia. In the 25% of cases not identified, the fetal asphyxia was mild. The positive predictive value of a predictive FHR pattern that occurred in 17% of the cases was very good. However, in these cases the fetal asphyxia was already moderate or severe. The positive predictive value of potentially predictive FHR patterns, 10 and 5% respectively, was very poor. These potentially predictive patterns accounted for over 50% of the fetal asphyxia ranging from mild to moderate in degree.

The potentially predictive patterns unless clarified by supplementary tests represent a dilemma for the clinician. The pattern can be ignored and in ten cases, fetal asphyxia will not be present in nine; however, in one case, fetal asphyxia accounting for at least 50% of asphyxia will be present and continue. On the other hand, the pattern can serve as an indication for intervention leading to an unnecessary intervention in nine out of ten cases.

Table 8.3 Predictive and potentially predictive fetal heart rate patterns for intrapartum fetal asphyxia

	Baseline variability (cycles/h)		Decelerations late/prolonged (cycles/h)
Predictive	Absent ≥ 1	+	≥ 2
Potentially predictive			
#1	Minimal ≥ 2	+	≥2
#2	Minimal ≥ 2	or	≥2

Can an algorithm of predictive FHR patterns prevent moderate/severe fetal asphyxia

Although there is no Grade 1 definitive evidence that the benefits of EFM outweigh the harm, our experience would support the contention that this EFM algorithm used as a screening test can make a difference in the outcome of some cases.

The benefits of EFM as a screening test in the prediction and prevention of intrapartum fetal asphyxia derived from a decade of experience was examined in term and preterm pregnancies [30,31]. A predictive or potentially predictive FHR pattern was present in most cases. Intervention and delivery occurred in 98 of the 166 term pregnancies and 21 of the 24 preterm pregnancies. A predictive or potentially predictive FHR pattern was the indication for intervention in most cases.

This assessment paradigm did not prevent all cases of moderate or severe fetal asphyxia. However in some cases, prediction and diagnosis leading to intervention during the first or second stage of labour likely prevented the progression of mild to moderate or severe asphyxia and limited the severity of moderate asphyxia.

Supplementary assessments

The predictive value of vibroacoustic stimulation with an acceleration response as a means of ruling out fetal acidosis has been equivocal [32,33]. A number of trials of amnioinfusion, particularly in the presence of oligohydramnios, have demonstrated a beneficial effect, reducing variable decelerations and the rate of Caesarean section for fetal distress [34,35].

The assessment of the fetal electrocardiographic (ECG) waveform is an attractive option since the signal can be obtained from the same fetal scalp electrode used for recording the FHR. Laboratory studies have examined the effect of hypoxemia and acidosis on the ST segment. In studies of acute hypoxemia, the ratio of the T-wave height to QRS height increased [36], although this association has not been a consistent finding [37]. Preliminary clinical observations suggested caution in the interpretation of ST waveforms [38]. The recent development of higher order FHR analysis has provided monitoring systems that can add automated fetal electrocardiographic ST segment analysis to the standard FHR and uterine contraction information which have been applied in a number of clinical trials. Meta-analysis of two randomized clinical trials of FHR assessment with the support of ST waveform analysis has shown that the number of babies born with metabolic acidosis at delivery could be reduced in conjunction with a reduction of operative deliveries for fetal distress [39]. Subsequent reports indicate some limitations of the sensitivity of ST waveform analysis in the identification of fetal asphyxia with a significant metabolic acidosis [40,41].

Fetal pulse oximetry was introduced to provide a non-invasive measure of oxygen saturation to improve intrapartum assessment during labour. However, the randomized clinical trials have not provided convincing evidence that this supplementary test will reduce unnecessary intervention [42,43].

Near-infrared spectroscopy (NIRS) has been developed as a means of continuous, non-invasive real time measurement of change in fetal cerebral oxygenation and hemodynamics during labour. Preliminary reports of the application of this technology for fetal assessment during labour have been published [44,45].

Although these supplementary tests provide additional information, further research remains to be done before the role of these tests in clinical practice can be determined.

Current challenges in fetal monitoring

There are a number of issues that must be considered if the current paradigms are to be effective in the prediction and diagnosis of intrapartum fetal asphyxia.

The first issue is to acknowledge the diversity of fetal asphyxia. Fetal asphyxia is not either on or off but rather simulates a dimmer switch that may vary in duration and degree. This may range from mild hypoxemia beginning in the antepartum period as demonstrated in cordocentesis studies to acute near total fetal asphyxia associated with a sentinel event such as a uterine rupture or prolapsed cord. Fetal asphyxia may occur in either a continuous or intermittent fashion, features that may relate to the effect of uterine contractions during labour on utero-placental blood flow. On the other hand, there is a corresponding range in the effectiveness of the fetal cardiovascular compensation that serves as the defence mechanism protecting the fetal brain, a response that may be confounded by the concurrent presence of intrauterine infection and cytokines.

In the development of clinical management protocols, it is important to remember that fetal surveillance cannot prevent fetal asphyxia or brain damage due to fetal asphyxia that occurs before fetal surveillance begins. The objective of fetal monitoring is the prediction of mild fetal asphyxia and prevention of progression to moderate or severe fetal asphyxia with newborn cerebral dysfunction and brain damage. The window of opportunity for the prediction and diagnosis of mild fetal asphyxia will vary widely in relation to the diversity of fetal asphyxia. The determination of the duration of this window in the individual clinical situation is difficult because of the limited information available in respect to the duration, degree and nature of the asphyxia and the quality of the fetal cardiovascular response. This makes the definition of a 'decision-delivery time' in clinical management protocols difficult.

At present the primary screening test available for the prediction of the fetus at risk for fetal asphyxia is EFM. The second and most important issue is the lack of a detailed algorithm for the interpretation of FHR patterns with appropriate recommendations for management. Although the FHR algorithm outlined in this presentation requires further testing in clinical trials it highlights the difficulties facing the clinician at the present time.

If an algorithm such as this is to be used the FHR record must be continuously scored to identify predictive and particularly potentially predictive patterns. A predictive pattern is an indication for intervention. If the objective to prevent moderate and severe asphyxia is to be achieved, the clinician cannot wait for a predictive FHR pattern at which point the fetal asphyxia is usually already moderate or severe. The key to the problem is the intermediate patterns expressed by the potentially predictive patterns in this algorithm that accounts for 50% of the fetal asphyxia. Potentially predictive patterns require supplementary assessments because of the associated high false positive rate. A blood gas and acid–base assessment is required to confirm the diagnosis.

The final issue is a fetal surveillance protocol for 'low-risk obstetric patients' who account for approximately 25% of fetal asphyxia. Current guidelines advocate the use of intermittent auscultation in the surveillance of the 'low-risk obstetric patient' even though there are no randomized clinical trials to support the benefit of this procedure. If the goal of prevention of fetal asphyxia is to be achieved, the intermediate potentially predictive patterns must be identified. This requires the early recognition of minimal baseline variability and late or prolonged decelerations by auscultation. Even in a continuously recorded FHR record, the inter-observer reliability for the discrimination between moderate and minimal baseline FHR variability and between variable and late decelerations is low. It is not realistic to anticipate that intermittent auscultation can effectively determine FHR patterns in six 10-min cycles over 1 h to identify the onset of potentially predictive patterns. It is counter intuitive to anticipate that current fetal assessment protocols for 'low-risk obstetric patients' are effective.

References

1. Bax M & Nelson KB (1993) Birth asphyxia: a statement. World Federation of Neurology Group. *Dev Med Child Neurol* **35**, 1022–4.
2. Westgate J, Garibaldi JM & Greene KR (1994) Umbilical cord blood gas analysis at delivery: a time for quality data. *Br J Obstet Gynaecol* **101**, 1054–63.
3. Victory R, Penava D, da Silva O, Natale R & Richardson B (2004) Umbilical cord pH and base excess values in relation to adverse outcome events for infants delivering at term. *Am J Obstet Gynecol* **191**, 2021–8.
4. Low JA, Lindsay BG & Derrick EJ (1997) Threshold of metabolic acidosis associated with newborn complications. *Am J Obstet Gynecol* **177**, 1391–4.
5. Low JA, Panagiotopoulos C & Derrick EJ (1994) Newborn complications after intrapartum asphyxia with metabolic acidosis in the term fetus. *Am J Obstet Gynecol* **170**, 1081–7.
6. Low JA, Panagiotopoulos C & Derrick EJ (1995) Newborn complications after intrapartum asphyxia with metabolic acidosis in the preterm fetus. *Am J Obstet Gynecol* **172**, 805–10.
7. Low JA, Galbraith, RS, Muir DW, Killen HL, Pater EA & Karchmar EJ (1988) Motor and cognitive deficits after intrapartum fetal asphyxia in the mature infant. *Am J Obstet Gynecol* **158**, 356–61.
8. Low JA, Galbraith RS, Muir DW, Killen HL, Pater EA & Karchmar EJ (1992) Mortality and morbidity after intrapartum asphyxia in the preterm fetus. *Obstet Gynecol* **80**, 57–61.
9. Low JA (1997) Intrapartum fetal asphyxia: definition, diagnosis, and classification. *Am J Obstet Gynecol* **176**, 957–9.
10. Handley-Derry M, Low JA, Burke SO, Waurick M, Killen H & Derrick EJ (1997) Intrapartum fetal asphyxia and the occurrence of minor deficits in 4- to 8-year-old children. *Dev Med Child Neurol* **39**, 508–14.
11. Low JA, Simpson LL, Tonni G & Chamberlain S (1995) Limitations in the clinical prediction of intrapartum fetal asphyxia. *Am J Obstet Gynecol* **172**, 801–4.
12. Low JA, Simpson LL & Ramsey DA (1992) The clinical diagnosis of asphyxia responsible for brain damage in the human fetus. *Am J Obstet Gynecol* **167**, 11–15.
13. Hon EH (1958) The electronic evaluation of the fetal heart rate. *Am J Obstet Gynecol* **75**, 1215–30.
14. James LS, Morishimo HO, Daniel SS, Bowe ET, Cohen H & Niemann WH (1972) Mechanism of late decelerations of the fetal heart rate. *Am J Obstet Gynecol* **113**, 578.
15. Murata Y, Martin CB, Ikenoue T, Hashimoto T, Sagawa T & Sakata H (1982) Fetal heart rate accelerations and late decelerations during the course of intrauterine death in chronically catheterized rhesus monkeys. *Am J Obstet Gynecol* **144**, 218–23.
16. Harris JL, Krueger TR & Parer JT (1982) Mechanisms of late decelerations of the fetal heart rate during hypoxia. *Am J Obstet Gynecol* **144**, 491–6.
17. Quilligan EJ & Paul RH (1975) Fetal monitoring: is it worth it? *Obstet Gynecol* **45**, 96–100.
18. Gardosi J (1996) Monitoring technology and the clinical perspective. *Baillieres Clin Obstet Gynaecol* **10**, 325–39.
19. Neilson JP (1995) EFM alone vs. intermittent auscultation in labor (revised 04 May 1994). In: Keirse MJNC, Renfrew MJ, Neilson JP & Crowther C (eds) *Pregnancy and Childbirth Module. The Cochrane Pregnancy and Childbirth Database.* The Cochrane Collaborative Issue 2. Oxford: Update Software.

20. Neilson JP (1995) EFM + scalp sampling vs. intermittent auscultation in labor (revised 04 May 1994). In: Keirse MJNC, Renfrew MJ, Neilson JP & Crowther C (eds) *Pregnancy and Childbirth Module. The Cochrane Pregnancy and Childbirth Database.* The Cochrane Collaboration Issue 2. Oxford:Update Software.

21. American College of Obstetrics and Gynecology (1995) ACOG Technical Bulletin. Fetal heart rate patterns: monitoring, interpretation, and management. Number 207–July 1995. *Int J Gynaecol Obstet* **51**, 65–74.

22. Society of Obstetricians and Gynaecologists of Canada. Clinical Practice Guidelines. Fetal health surveillance in labour. Clinical Practice Guideline No 112, March 2001.

23. Royal College of Obstetricians and Gynaecologists (2001) *The Use of Electronic Fetal Monitoring.* Evidence-based Clinical Guideline May 2001 (No. 8). London: RCOG Press.

24. National Institute of Child Health and Human Development Research Planning Workshop (1997). Electronic fetal heart rate monitoring research guidelines for interpretation. *Am J Obstet Gynecol* **177**, 1385–90.

25. Freeman R (2002) Problems with intrapartum fetal heart rate monitoring interpretation and patient management. *Obstet Gynecol* **100**, 813–26.

26. Hon EH & Quilligan EJ (1968) Electronic evaluation of fetal heart rate. Further observations on pathologic fetal bradycardia. *Clin Obstet Gynecol* **11**, 145–67.

27. Uzan S, Fouillot JP & Sureau C (1989) Computer analysis of FHR patterns in labour. In: Spencer JAD (ed) *Fetal Monitoring.* Tunbridge Wells: CHP 159–64.

28. Paneth N, Bommarito M & Stricker J (1993) Electronic fetal monitoring and later outcome. *Clin Invest Med* **16**, 159–65.

29. Low JA, Victory R & Derrick EJ (1999) Predictive value of electronic fetal monitoring for intrapartum fetal asphyxia with metabolic acidosis. *Obstet Gynecol* **93**, 285–91.

30. Low JA, Pickersgill H, Killen HL & Derrick EJ (2001) The prediction and prevention of intrapartum fetal asphyxia in term pregnancies. *Am J Obstet Gynecol* **184**, 724–30.

31. Low JA, Killen HL & Derrick EJ (2002) The prediction and prevention of intrapartum fetal asphyxia in preterm pregnancies. *Am J Obstet Gynecol* **186**, 279–82.

32. Elimian A, Figueroa R & Tejani N (1997) Intrapartum assessment of fetal well being: a comparison of scalp stimulation with scalp blood ph sampling. *Obstet Gynecol* **89**, 373–6.

33. Skupski DW, Rosenberg CR & Eglington GS (2002) Intrapartum fetal stimulation tests: a meta-analysis. *Obstet Gynecol* **99**, 129–34.

34. Perrson-Kjerstadius N, Forsgen H & Westgren M (1999) Intrapartum amnioinfusion in women with oligohydramnios. A prospective randomized trial. *Acta Obstet Gynaecol Scand* **78**, 116–9.

35. Hofmeyr GJ (2000) Prophylactic versus therapeutic amnioinfusion for oligohydramnios in labour. *Cochrane Database Syst Rev* **2**, CD000176.

36. Widmark C, Lindecrantz K, Murray H & Rosen KG (1992) Changes in the PR, RR intervals and the ST waveforms of the fetal lamb electrocardiogram with acute hypoxemia. *J Dev Physiol* **18**, 99–103.

37. deHaan HH, Ijzermans ACM, deHaan J & Hasaart THM (1995) The T/QRS ratio of the electrocardiogram does not reliably reflect well-being in fetal lambs. *Am J Obstet Gynecol* **172**, 35–43.

38. MacLachlan NA, Spencer JAD, Harding K & Arulkumaran S (1992) Fetal acidemia, the cardiotocograph and the T/QRS ratio of the fetal ECG in labour. *Br J Obstet Gynaecol* **9**, 26–31.

39. Amer-Wahlin I, Hellsten C, Noren H *et al.* (2001) Cardiotocography only versus cardiotocography plus ST analysis of fetal electrocardiogram for intrapartum fetal monitoring: a Swedish randomized controlled trial. *Lancet* **358**, 534–38.

40. Dervaitis KI, Poole M, Schmidt G, Penava D, Natale R & Gagnon R (2004) St segment analysis of the fetal electrocardiogram plus electronic fetal heart rate monitoring in labor and its relationship to umbilical cord arterial blood gases. *Am J Obstet Gynecol* **191**, 879–84.

41. Kwee A, van der Hoorn-van den Beld CW, Veerman J, Dekkers AH & Visser GH (2004) Stan S21 fetal heart monitor for fetal surveillance during labor: an observational study in 637 patients. *J Matern Fetal Neonatal Med* **15**, 400–7.

42. Garite TJ, Dildy GA, McNamara H *et al.* (2000) A multicenter controlled trial of fetal pulse oximetry in the intrapartum management of nonreassuring fetal heart rate patterns. *Am J Obstet Gynecol* **183**, 1049–58.

43. Kuhnert M & Schmidt S (2004) Intrapartum management of nonreassuring fetal heart rate patterns: a randomized controlled trial of fetal pulse oximetry. *Am J Obstet Gynecol* **191**, 1989–95.

44. Peebles DM, Edwards AD & Wyatt JS (1992) Changes in human fetal cerebral hemoglobin concentration and oxygenation during labor measured by near-infrared spectroscopy. *Am J Obstet Gynecol* **166**, 1369–73.

45. Aldrich CJ, D'Antona D, Wyatt JS, Spencer JA, Peebles DM & Reynolds EO (1994) Fetal cerebral oxygenation measured by near-infrared spectroscopy shortly before birth and acid–base status at birth. *Obstet Gynecol* **84**, 861–6.

Chapter 9: Analgesia and anaesthesia

John A. Crowhurst

Pain

The distress and pain women often endure while they are struggling through a difficult labour are beyond description, and seem to be more than human nature would be able to bear under any other circumstances.

Medical men may oppose for a time the superinduction of anaesthesia in parturition, but our patients will force the use of it upon the profession. The whole question is, even now, one merely of time.

These statements by James Young Simpson in 1847 [1] are still most pertinent, as they encapsulate today's widely held view of both parturients and most perinatal care-providers. Firstly because most of today's labouring women do not want to suffer severe pain, and more importantly they know that it is no longer necessary to do so.

Pain is defined by the International Association for the Study of Pain as: 'An unpleasant, subjective, sensory & emotional experience associated with real or potential tissue damage, or described in terms of such damage.' In colloquial terms, 'Pain is what hurts', and is an unnecessary accompaniment to most labours. *Severe* pain is common, affecting some 60–70% of nulliparous and 35–40% of multiparous labours. So many factors may contribute to pain in labour that a specific aetiological diagnosis of the causes of such pain is difficult, but ALL causes of pain must be considered, and investigated, before analgesia is administered. While contraction pain, cervical dilatation and second stage labour pain have obvious physiological causes, the basis of severe pain in any individual may be due to obstructed labour; fetal position; extreme anxiety; uterine hyperstimulation; uterine rupture or extant pathology, such as fibromyata or other tumours; haemorrhoids, adhesions or scarring from previous surgery, and so on.

The effects of severe pain are principally a sympathetic autonomic response and include exhaustion, dehydration, misery, raised heart rate, blood pressure, oxygen and glucose consumption, decreased blood flow and oxygen to placenta and fetus, hyperventilation and cramps.

Obviously in many individuals such effects are undesirable and in some may even be life-threatening.

While many authors distinguish between physiological and pathological pain of any kind, in the individual, if severe enough to exceed that person's threshold of tolerance, it results in the sympathetically mediated responses listed above. In such circumstances, pain relief should be readily available. Most women desire to be in control when they are in labour, but many cannot achieve this if/when they cannot cope with severe pain. For most women, the duration, nature and severity of pain in labour is unpredictable. Thus it is prudent to advise all expectant mothers to keep an open mind about pain and its relief, and to understand the advantages and disadvantages, benefits and risks of all techniques of analgesia available. In at-risk pregnancies, be they due to fetal, obstetric or maternal factors, analgesia or anaesthesia is almost always required, and frequently recommended. If such risk factors increase the hazards of any anaesthetic procedure, consultation with an anaesthetist during the pregnancy is prudent.

Obstetric analgesia and anaesthesia

The ideal analgesic technique in labour should:
1 Provide rapid, effective and safe pain relief for all stages.
2 Not compromise maternal vital physiology or normal activity.
3 Not compromise fetal vital physiology or well-being.
4 Not hamper the normal processes of labour.
5 Be flexible enough to convert to anaesthesia for urgent operative delivery or other intervention, e.g. manual removal of placenta.

Meeting such an ideal would leave the mother awake, alert, comfortable and able to void, bear down, and, if desired, even ambulate throughout labour. Unfortunately such ideals are rarely met in medicine, but for the past twenty or so years the development of low-dose neuraxial anaesthesia and analgesia (epidural and combined spinal-epidural (CSE)) has all but achieved these.

There are two *strategies* for obstetric analgesia:

1 Reduction of the **perception** of pain, i.e. reduction of the brain's perception of, and the body's and mind's response to, pain – i.e. reduce the effects of pain.

2 Reduction of the **transmission** of pain, i.e. reduction of the ability of the nerves to conduct pain.

Three *methods* of implementing these strategies are possible:

1 *Psychological techniques*, such as a positive attitude, pre-natal education, conditioning (physical and mental relaxation) and hypnosis are helpful to many women for mild and moderately severe pain.

2 *Physical methods* include massage, relaxation techniques and transcutaneous electrical nerve stimulation (TENS), but like the psychological techniques listed above, they often fail when pain exceeds one's threshold of tolerance.

3 *Pharmacological techniques* may be systemic or regional/local.

Systemic drugs are as effective as they are for trauma, post-operative or other severe pain situations, but in the parturient they may have the disadvantage of affecting uteroplacental blood flow and the fetus, either directly or indirectly. Nevertheless, some gaseous drugs such as nitrous oxide and sevoflurane have extremely rapid action, elimination and minimal metabolism and accumulation, which properties make them ideal for intermittent use, 'with contractions'. As with all systemic, centrally-acting drugs, however, side effects such as vertigo, nausea and drowsiness limit their efficacy.

Parenterally administered analgesics have been popular in obstetrics for many decades, but the same caveats apply. Older opiates such as morphine and pethidine (meperidine) are difficult to titrate to effect; are usually given intramuscularly, resulting in variable absorption and efficacy, and with prolonged, or poorly timed use, accumulate in the fetus and affect fetal well-being and neonatal cardiorespiratory physiology. This is particularly true of pethidine and its primary metabolite, norpethidine, when pethidine is used throughout a long labour. However, two opioids – Fentanyl and Remifentanil – which are potent, short acting and rapidly redistributed and metabolized are most efficacious and safe if given in accordance with approved guidelines and monitoring. Small intravenous boluses of fentanyl (20–25 mcg) may be given in the second stage of labour to alleviate pain and assist the mother to cooperate. This is particularly useful when a spontaneous delivery is imminent and there is no indication for epidural or other anaesthesia. Neonatal depression is uncommon, but if it does occur it is readily reversed with a single dose of naloxone into the umbilical cord vein.

Ketamine is a potent non-opioid analgesic, which, in small intermittent intravenous doses (3–5 mg), is useful too for short-term, late-second-stage analgesia in selected patients.

Both fentanyl and remifentanil can be self-administered by patient-controlled analgesia (PCA) devices. Remifentanil in particular holds much promise in this context, but there have been few controlled trials to date. Most anaesthetists would recommend a PCA regime with either of these agents when neuraxial analgesia is contraindicated, provided that attending midwives have been trained in supervising this type of analgesia.

Regional, most commonly neuraxial, analgesia has dramatically changed medical and public attitudes to obstetric anaesthesia and pain relief since the 1980s. Although lumbar epidurals have been the benchmark neuraxial technique since the late 1960s, the classic observations of Wang [2] and Behar [3], that demonstrated the spinal actions of neuraxial opioids, opened a remarkable chapter of development of epidural and spinal blockade. When intraspinal opioids are combined with local anaesthetics (LAs), their action is synergistic, enabling lower dose of both drugs to be used to provide neural blockade of varying intensity [4]. These techniques, still widely referred to as 'epidurals', include continuous subarachnoid (spinal) anaesthesia (CSA), epidurals, and particularly low-dose CSE are most suitable for labour analgesia in the vast majority of parturients and are quickly and reliably convertible to anaesthesia for operative delivery or other obstetric or surgical interventions [4]. CSE, and less commonly CSA, have largely replaced the use of 'single-shot' spinal anaesthesia for operative delivery in most obstetric units in the UK [5,6]. Similarly, low-dose CSE is rapidly becoming the preferred choice of neuraxial analgesia for labour [7].

Caudal epidural block, while useful for some gynaecological procedures, is now rarely used in obstetrics, and is not recommended. Trans-vaginal pudendal block is occasionally used for a 'lift-out' forceps or ventouse delivery, but the failure rate is high (30%), LA dose is high, which may cause acute toxicity and there is a risk of injection into the fetal head.

In the rare situations when the obstetrician is the sole operator or does not have expert anaesthesia services available, a low-dose single shot spinal anaesthetic at L3–4 or L4–5 is arguably the best anaesthesia for operative vaginal delivery or repair of vaginal/perineal trauma.

The most common type of CSE used for analgesia is the needle-through-needle technique illustrated in Fig. 9.1. The procedure comprises a low-dose intrathecal injection of LA, usually bupivacaine (2–2.5 mg) plus fentanyl (15–25 mcg), followed by insertion of an epidural catheter which is used for ongoing analgesia or anaesthesia if required. For anaesthesia the subarachnoid dose is increased appropriately. Compared with single-shot

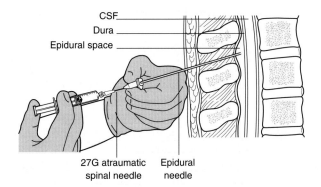

CSF
Dura
Epidural space

27G atraumatic spinal needle Epidural needle

Fig. 9.1 Needle-through-needle CSE technique.

Table 9.1 Low-dose CSE compared with epidural and S-S spinal

	S-S spinal*	Epidural	CSE
Onset of action (min)	Fast (1–5)	Slow (10–20)	Fast (1–5)
Median pain score 60–90 min	0	0–3	0
Total drugs dose	Low	High	Low
Observable leg weakness (%)[†]	100	5–50	0–40
Postdural puncture headache (%)	1–2	0.3–1.0	0.2–0.7
Hypotension (%)[†]	20–80	5–10	5–10
Failure (i.e. GA is required) (%)[†]	1.7–6.0	2–6	0.3–0.7
Pruritus (%)[†]	50–80	20–80	20–80
Duration (min)	60–240	∞	∞

Source: Modified from Paech M (2003) *Anesth Clin North Am* **21**, 1–17.
* Single-shot spinal *anaesthesia* dose = 2 − 3x subarachnoid dose of CSE.
[†] These side effects are dose dependent with epidural and CSE. High ranges associated with full *anaesthesia* doses.

spinal anaesthesia, a subarachnoid dose of 50% or less will provide surgical anaesthesia for Caesarean delivery in >70% cases [6,7]. In the remainder, the epidural is 'topped-up' to establish the required level of block.

The advantages of this CSE technique compared with epidural injection alone are listed in Table 9.1. Foremost are the rapidity of onset, the markedly reduced failure rate and the reduced density of motor block in the legs, which, with low dose, can be fine-tuned to permit normal ambulation in >90% of labouring women [8,9].

Ambulation in labour has not been shown to significantly affect the mode of delivery, but the 'lighter' degree of blockade and the ability to ambulate have been shown to provide much greater satisfaction and 'control' [9–11]. To permit safe ambulation, all delivery unit staff must be appropriately trained and certain conditions must be met (Table 9.2). Despite many studies, the only definitive test

Table 9.2 Requirements for safe 'walking epidurals' in labour

Cooperative, understanding parturient
Presenting part of fetus engaged and well applied to cervix
Minimal or no motor and proprioceptive block
No postural hypotension
Continuous fetal monitoring (CTG), when indicated
Suitable conditions: good epidural catheter fixation; attending midwife; disconnect (bung) IV line; no shoes; safe, even floor without cables, steps, mats, etc.

to assess a mother's ability to ambulate is to allow her to judge her own ability. This should be done in stages, firstly monitoring blood pressure and vital signs, including Cardiotocograph (CTG) when sitting on the bedside, then standing. When walking or moving about her room, no mother should be left unattended.

Disadvantages of CSE include a slightly more complex technique, but this is easily mastered, and the dural puncture made by the fine gauge, atraumatic spinal needle, which is not significantly different from when epidurals alone are used. Hypotension is uncommon with low-dose epidural or CSE and is easily monitored and corrected [12]. The fact remains, however, that neuraxial blockade is an invasive technique with the potential for serious, though fortunately rare, morbidity.

The true incidence of traumatic neuropathy, infections, such as epidural abscess and meningitis is unknown with estimates between 1 in 5000 to 1 in 15,000 [13,14]. These complications can be minimized, if not prevented entirely, with careful attention to skilled technique. Peripheral nerve injuries due to labour and delivery are far more common and have been reported as frequently as almost 1% (96 in 10,000) in a population of women receiving all kinds of analgesia [15]. Such neuropraxias almost always recover within a year.

Spinal epidural haematoma (SEH) is a very significant risk in patients with a coagulopathy or who are receiving thromboprophylactic therapy. Following the introduction of low molecular weight heparins (LMWHs), many cases of SEH were reported, especially in the United States, where LMWH doses were 1.5 times that used in Europe and elsewhere. Clear communication between anaesthetist and obstetrician, and strict guidelines must be observed when neuraxial block and anticoagulant therapy are used together.

While neuraxial anaesthesia is the most commonly used procedure for operative delivery, it is not appropriate for all women. There are several important contraindications, see Table 9.3.

Apart from pain, there are many obstetric indications for neuraxial block in labour. In these cases – breech and other malpresentations; previous operative delivery; large fetus; multiple pregnancy – it is generally agreed that such

Table 9.3 Contraindications to neuraxial blockade

Absolute	Patient refusal
	Raised intracranial pressure
	Infection: systemic and localized
	Uncorrected hypovolaemia
Relative	Coagulopathy, anticoagulant therapy
	Spinal/neurological pathology, abnormality
	Some complex cardiovascular and other conditions
	Inadequately skilled management team
	Urgency (Degree of urgency)

mothers should have a neuraxial block administered during labour, so that if the need for intervention arises, the epidural catheter can be quickly 'topped-up' to provide appropriate anaesthesia.

For instrumental delivery, where maternal 'powers' are required, the top-up block can be tailored to provide sensory blockade of sacral dermatomes and up to the T10 level, while retaining motor power in the abdominal muscles. Bearing down can then be instituted in time with contractions.

For abdominal delivery, the epidural is topped-up with dosage sufficient to provide relaxation of abdominal muscles, and a sensory block of dermatomes to T4.

One disadvantage of neuraxial anaesthesia for operative delivery is that the anaesthesia does not provide tocolysis, although this can be achieved with intravenous glyceryl trinitrate or other drugs, (see 'Acute tocolysis', p. 67) Because severe pain increases sympathetic tone with a resultant rise in blood pressure, oxygen consumption and redistribution of cardiac output resulting in reduced utero-placental perfusion, many at-risk parturients can benefit from optimal analgesia during labour. Pre-eclampsia and other hypertensive states, and other cardio-respiratory disorders are therefore good indications for neuraxial analgesia in labour, even if severe pain is absent. In high-risk patients, neuraxial anaesthesia for surgery or operative delivery is often the technique of choice. Low-dose CSE can provide marked haemodynamic stability in parturients with severe aortic or mitral stenosis; obstructive cardiomyopathy and pulmonary hypertension delivered by elective Caesarean section [16]. Such patients require expert team management, beginning early in the pregnancy. Because maternal and fetal morbidity and mortality is high in such cases, early consultation with a cardiologist and an anaesthetist is imperative so that management plans can be agreed to, both for ongoing monitoring and care, and for elective or emergency delivery. Any anaesthesia in such patients is potentially hazardous, and because neuraxial techniques may fail, a back-up strategy must be planned for, with all appropriate facilities and carers.

Informed consent for anaesthetic procedures

Through the 1990s, in developed countries, the number of women receiving an anaesthetic procedure in association with a pregnancy increased to more than 60% [17] in line with the increasing popularity of, and demand for, neuraxial analgesia – older mothers, obesity, increased Caesarean delivery rates, *in vitro* fertilization procedures and the like.

Because ALL expectant mothers *may* require analgesia or anaesthesia it is imperative that appropriate information on all aspects of pain, analgesia and anaesthesia is given to all women in the antenatal period. When anxiety, fear or refusal is expressed, a consultation with an obstetric anaesthetist should be arranged during the pregnancy. Such pre-education is mandatory to prevent difficulties in obtaining informed consent when the analgesia or anaesthesia is required or requested, especially in urgent or emergency situations and when the mother is experiencing severe pain [18].

General anaesthesia

'If we could induce anaesthesia without loss of consciousness, most would regard it as a even greater advance', remarked James Young Simpson soon after a maternal anaesthetic death in the early days of chloroform anaesthesia in 1847 [1]. In 2000, The National Sentinel Caesarean Section Audit reported that general anaesthesia (GA) was used in less than 30% of Caesarean deliveries, and most of these were emergencies [19]. At Queen Charlotte's Hospital, London, GA is used for only 5% of all Caesarean deliveries. Moreover GA remains the anaesthesia of choice for failed neuraxial blocks; situations when regional anaesthesia is contraindicated and other surgery in pregnancy and the puerperium – see also below. Indeed the 'greater advance' prophesied by Simpson can be seen in the marked reduction in maternal mortality as neuraxial anaesthesia has superceded GA during the past 50 years. GA in pregnancy is considered far more hazardous than for the normal population, with airway difficulties, failed intubation, pulmonary aspiration of gastric contents and their sequelae accounting for the majority of deaths. However, the triennial Confidential Maternal Mortality Reports since 1952 repeatedly suggested that most of the direct anaesthetic deaths attributed to GA, whatever the cause, could have been prevented with better communication between obstetricians and anaesthetists. As stated above, ALL gravidae are potential candidates for anaesthesia, and this is often required in an emergency. As expectant mothers are a 'captive' population attending for regular antenatal care and review, it is imperative that anaesthetic risk factors be identified, and an appropriate anaesthetic

Table 9.4 Principal anaesthetic risk factors

Patient refusal of analgesic/anaesthetic procedures
Previous complications or adverse reactions to anaesthesia
Proven sensitivity or allergy to anaesthetic drugs
Severe medical disorders
Anticoagulant therapy or risk of coagulopathy
Thrombocytopaenia
Airway abnormalities
Obesity
Spinal abnormalities or previous spinal surgery
Intervertebral disc prolapse
Neurological disease
(Some) complex obstetric and/or fetal situations
Planned operative delivery or other surgery in pregnancy

consultation arranged early in the pregnancy. 'At-risk' gravidae should include all those with such risk factors, even though there may be no perceived obstetric, fetal or medical complications. Major anaesthetic risk factors are listed in Table 9.4, but this list is not comprehensive. Clinical judgement should always govern the need for antenatal anaesthesia consultation in many cases.

Because ALL parturients are at risk of pulmonary aspiration of gastric contents, prophylactic antacid and/or H-2 blocking premedication is standard practice before both regional and GA.

General anaesthesia is usually used for emergencies and for surgery when neuraxial block is contraindicated. However, in many labours, the likelihood for operative or assisted delivery can be anticipated, and an urgent GA avoided by having neuraxial analgesia already *in situ*, which can be used to induce anaesthesia quickly when required.

Many anaesthetists will recommend a combination of general and neuraxial anaesthesia for Caesarean hysterectomy and other complicated surgery, enabling the mother to be awake for the delivery, and then receive GA for the remainder of the operation. The epidural catheter is then used for post-operative analgesia. Similarly for fetal surgery, or other surgery during pregnancy, combined GA and block is frequently used. Such combination provides optimal tocolysis with volatile anaesthetic agents such as isoflurane.

Modern GA drugs do not increase the risk of uterine atony post-delivery, but uterine tone should be monitored closely and appropriate oxytocics administered as needed.

Acute tocolysis

Tocolytic drugs are discussed elsewhere, but during operative delivery and fetal surgery the anaesthetist may be required to provide acute tocolysis. Arguably, volatile anaesthetic drugs are the most effective acute tocolytics,

but by definition they induce unconsciousness and thus general anaesthesia. Intravenous alternatives are available, and can be used with regional anaesthesia, but they must be used with caution and appropriate monitoring lest cardiovascular collapse occur. As outlined above, GA, and optimal tocolysis are often preferred for complex surgery involving uterine manipulations, and some multiple pregnancy deliveries, for example, conjoined or monoamniotic twins.

In summary, modern obstetrics includes anaesthetic procedures for most parturients. Close cooperation, consultation and planning, minimal use of general anaesthesia, especially in emergency situations have markedly reduced maternal and perinatal mortality and morbidity, and will continue to do so. All expectant mothers may require analgesia or anaesthesia, so risk factors must be sought and acted upon antenatally to maintain the impressive record of safety of anaesthesia in obstetrics.

References

1. Simpson JY (1847) Notes on Chloroform.
2. Wang JK, Nauss LA & Thomas JE (1979) Pain relief by intrathecally applied morphine in man. *Anesthesiology* **50**, 149–51.
3. Behar M, Magora F, Olshwang D & Davidson JT (1979) Epidural morphine in treatment of pain. *Lancet* **1**, 527–9.
4. Campbell DC, Camann WC & Datta S (1995) The addition of bupivacaine to sufentanil for labor analgesia. *Anesth Analg* **81**, 305–9.
5. Crowhurst JA & Birnbach D (2000) Low-dose neuraxial block: heading towards the new millennium. (Editorial). *Anesth Analg* **90**, 24.
6. Rawal N, Van Zundert A, Holmström B & Crowhurst J (1997) Combined spinal-epidural technique. *Reg Anesth* **22**, 406–23.
7. Ranasinghe JS, Steadman J, Toyama T, Lai M. (2003) Combined spinal epidural anaesthesia is better than spinal or epidural alone for Caesarean delivery. Br J Anaesth 91, 299–300.
8. Plaat F, Alsaud S, Crowhurst JA *et al.* (1996) Selective sensory blockade with low-dose combined spinal/epidural (CSE) allows safe ambulation in labour. A pilot study. *Int J Obstet Anaesth* **5**(3), 220.
9. Collis RE, Baxandall ML, Srikantharajah ID *et al.* (1993) Combined spinal epidural analgesia with ability to walk throughout labour. *Lancet* **341** 767–8.
10. Rawal N (1995) European trends in the use of combined spinal epidural technique – a 17-nation survey. *Reg Anesth* **20**(2S), 162.
11. 'COMET' study group UK (2001) Effect of low-dose mobile versus traditional epidural techniques on mode of delivery: a randomised controlled trial. *Lancet* **358**, 19–23.
12. Vercauteren MP, Coppejans HC, Hoffman VH *et al.* (2000) Prevention of hypotension by a single 5-mg dose of ephedrine during small-dose spinal anesthesia in prehydrated caesarean delivery patients. *Anesth Analg* **90**, 324–7.

13. Ong BY, Cohen MM, Esmail A *et al.* (1987) Paresthesias and motor dysfunction after labor and delivery. *Anesth Analg* **66**, 18–22.

14. Holdcroft A, Gibberd FB, Hargrove RL *et al.* (1995) Neurological complications associated with pregnancy. *Br J Anaesth* **75**, 522–6.

15. Wong CA, Scavone BM, Dugan S *et al.* (2003) Incidence of postpartum lumbosacral spine and lower extremity nerve injuries. *Obstet Gynecol* **101**, 279–98.

16. Hamlyn L, Plaat F, Stocks G & Crowhurst JA (2005) Low-dose combined spinal-epidural anaesthesia for caesarean delivery of high-risk cardiac disease parturients. *Int J Obstet Anesth* **14**, 355–61.

17. Crowhurst JA (1992) Epidurals in obstetrics – how safe? (Editorial). *Med J Aust* **157**(4), 220–22.

18. Crowhurst JA & Plaat F (2001) Pain relief in labour and the anaesthetist. In: MacLean AB, Stones RW & Thornton S (eds) *Pain in Obstetrics and Gynaecology*. London: RCOG Press, 356–7.

19. Thomas J & Paranjothy S (2001) *The National Sentinel Caesarean Section Audit Report*. London: RCOG Press.

Chapter 10: Puerperium and lactation

D. Keith Edmonds

The puerperium is a period that lasts from delivery of the placenta till 6–12 weeks after delivery. It is a time of enormous importance to the mother and her baby and yet it is an aspect of maternity care that has received relatively less attention than pregnancy and delivery. During the puerperium the pelvic organs return to the non-gravid state, the metabolic changes of pregnancy are reversed and lactation is established. In the absence of breastfeeding, the reproductive cycle may start again within a few weeks. The puerperium is a time which is steeped in cultural customs and rituals in many different countries and indeed many of the medical recommendations about the puerperium have developed as adaptations of socially acceptable traditions rather than science.

The puerperium is also a time of psychological adjustment and while most mothers' enjoyment of the arrival of a newborn baby is obvious the transition to becoming a responsible parent and the anxiety about a child's welfare will influence the mothers' ability to cope. These anxieties may be compounded if she is tired after her labour or if she has any medical complications. However, the majority of women are subjected to another problem that new mothers find very difficult to cope with and this is the plethora of well-meaning but conflicting advice from doctors, midwives, relatives and friends. Here again, the cultural influences may be at conflict with the mother's own beliefs. It is extremely important that an atmosphere be created whereby a mother can learn to handle her baby with confidence, and here the influence of midwifery and obstetric staff plays an important role in trying to establish what will be an important part of their lives. In caring for a woman during the early puerperium, the role of the obstetrician and midwife is to monitor the physiological changes of the puerperium, to diagnose and treat any postnatal complications, to establish infant feeding, to give the mother emotional support and to advise about contraception and other measures which will contribute to continuing health. It is important to bear in mind that maternal death may still occur in the puerperium and hence its importance cannot be understated.

Physiology of the puerperium

There are two major physiological events that occur during the puerperium. The first is the establishment of lactation and the second is the return of the physiological changes of pregnancy to the non-pregnant state. During the first 2 weeks after childbirth, the changes in the organs are quite rapid but some take 6–12 weeks to complete.

The uterus

The crude weight of the pregnant uterus at term is approximately 1000 g and the weight of the non-pregnant uterus is between 50 and 100 g. By 6 weeks post-partum, the uterus has returned to its normal size and from a clinical perspective, the uterine fundus is no longer palpable abdominally by 10 days post-partum. The cervix itself is very flaccid after delivery but within a few days returns to its original state. The placental site in the first 3 days after delivery is infiltrated with granulocytes and mononuclear cells and this reaction extends into the endometrium and the superficial myometrium. By the seventh day there is evidence of the regeneration of endometrial glands and by day 16 post-partum the endometrium is fully restored. Decidual necrosis begins on the first day and by the seventh day a well-demarcated zone exists between necrotic and viable tissue. The presence of mononuclear cells and lymphocytes persists for about 10 days and it is presumed that this acts as some form of antibacterial barrier. Haemostasis immediately after a birth is accomplished by arterial smooth muscle contraction and compression of vessels by the uterine muscle. The vessels in the placental site are characterized during the first 8 days by thrombosis, hyalinization and obliterative fibrinoid endarteritis. Immediately post delivery, bleeding lasts for several hours and then rapidly diminishes to a red-brown discharge by the third or fourth day post-partum. This vaginal discharge is known as lochia and after the third or fourth day the discharge becomes mucopurulent and sometimes malodorous. This is known as the lochia serosa and it

69

has a mean duration of 22–27 days. However, 10–15% of women will have lochia serosa for at least 6 weeks [1]. Not infrequently, there is a sudden but transient increase in uterine bleeding between 7 and 14 days post-partum. This corresponds to the shedding of the slough over the placental site and as myometrial vessels are still at this stage larger than normal it accounts for the dramatic bleeding that can occur with this phenomenon. However, it is self-limiting and subsides within 1–2 h. A new endometrium will grow from the basal layers of the decidua but this is influenced by the method of infant feeding. If lactation is suppressed, the uterine cavity may be covered by new endometrium within 3–4 weeks, but if lactation is established, endometrial growth may be suppressed for many months.

Ovarian function

Women who breastfeed their infants will be amenorrhoeic for long periods of time, often until the child is weaned. However, in non-lactating women, ovulation may occur as early as 27 days after delivery although the mean time is approximately 70–75 days. Among those women who are breastfeeding, the mean time to ovulation is 6 months. Menstruation resumes by 12 weeks post-partum in 70% of women who are not lactating and the mean time to the first menstruation is 7–9 weeks. The risk of ovulation within the first 6 months post-partum in women exclusively breastfeeding is between 1 and 5% [2]. The hormonal basis of puerperal ovulation suppression in lactating women appears to be the persistence of elevated serum prolactin levels. Prolactin levels fall to the normal range by the third week post-partum in non-lactating women but remain elevated to the sixth week post-partum in lactating women.

Cardiovascular and coagulation system

Changes take place in the cardiovascular and coagulation systems which have practical and clinical implications and these are summarized in Table 10.1. Although both heart rate and cardiac output fall in the early puerperium there may be an early rise in stroke volume and together with the rise in blood pressure due to increased peripheral resistance it is a time of high risk for mothers with cardiac disease. Such mothers require extra supervision at this time (see Chapter 26). Although it is assumed that by 6 weeks the woman's body has changed physiologically back to the non-pregnant state, it can be seen from Table 10.1 that cardiac output may remain elevated for up to 24 weeks post-natally. During the immediate post-natal period, fibrinolytic activity is increased for 1–4 days before it returns to normal by 1 week. Platelet counts are normal

Table 10.1 Changes in the cardiovascular and coagulation systems during the puerperium

	Early puerperium	Late puerperium
Cardiovascular		
Heart rate	Fall – 14% by 48 h	Normal by 2 weeks
Stroke volume	Rise over 48 h	Normal by 2 weeks
Cardiac output	Remains elevated and then falls over 48 h	Normal by 24 weeks
Blood pressure	Rises over 4 days	Normal by 6 weeks
Plasma volume	Initial increase and then fall	Progressive decline in first week
Coagulation		
Fibrinogen	Rise in first week	Normal by 6 weeks
Clotting factors	Most remain elevated	Normal by 3 weeks
Platelet count	Fall and then rise	Normal by 6 weeks
Fibrinolysis	Rapid reversal of pregnancy inhibition of tissue plasminogen activator	Normal by 3 weeks

Adapted from Dunlop [29].

during pregnancy but there is a sharp rise in platelets after delivery, making it a time of high risk for thromboembolic disease [3].

Urinary tract

During the first few days the bladder and urethra may show evidence of mild trauma sustained at delivery although these changes are usually associated with localized oedema. These are transient and do not remain in evidence for long. The changes that occur in the urinary tract during pregnancy disappear in a similar manner to other involutional changes and within 2–3 weeks the hydroureter and pelvic dilatation in the kidney are almost eliminated and completely return to normal by 6–8 weeks post-partum.

Weight loss

There is an immediate loss of 4.5–6 kg following birth due to the placenta, amniotic fluid and blood loss that occurs at delivery. By 6 weeks post-partum, 28% of women will have returned to their pre-pregnancy weight and in those women who did not have excessive weight gain in pregnancy, they should have returned to their normal pre-pregnancy weight by 6 months post-partum. Women with excessive weight gain in pregnancy (>15 kg) are likely to find that at 6 months they still have net gain of 5 kg, which may persist indefinitely [4]. Breastfeeding has no effect on post-partum weight loss unless lactation continues for 6 months [5] and diet and exercise have no effect on the growth of infants who are being breastfed and women can therefore be encouraged to return to normal activity and to regain their weight even though they are lactating [6].

Thyroid function

Thyroid volume increases by approximately 30% during pregnancy and this returns to normal over a 12-week period. Thyroxine and triiodothyronine return to normal within 4 weeks post-partum.

Hair loss

Hair growth slows in the puerperium and women will often experience hair loss as temporarily more hair is lost than regrown. This is a transient phenomenon but it is important for women to realize that this may take between 6 months and a year to return to normal.

Management of puerperium

The morbidity associated with the puerperium is underestimated and an important review (Table 10.2) shows that after childbirth mothers have high levels of post-partum problems. Thirty-one per cent of women felt that they had major problems for up to 8 weeks post-partum. In trying to reduce the impact of this morbidity there are a number of principles which need to be applied in planning post-natal care. These include:

1 *Continuity of care*. An ideal pattern of care is one that offers continuity from the antenatal period through childbirth and into the puerperium involving the smallest team of health professionals with which the mother can identify.
2 *Mother/infant bonding*. It is now well established that mothers and their partners should be able to hold and touch their babies as soon as possible after delivery. Good

post-natal facilities which allow rooming in, privacy and the opportunity for close contact play an important part in helping parents to have a good experience of childbirth.
3 *Flexible discharge policies*. The optimum duration of post-natal stay varies with the needs of the individual mother and her baby. Some mothers will elect to have a home confinement, some will elect to have early discharge at 6 h post-natally and others may have greater needs, particularly those who have had complicated deliveries and those who wish to establish breastfeeding before going home. The current pressure on maternity services in the Western world means that any length of stay in hospital to respond to maternal needs as opposed to medical necessity has meant that this flexibility has been curtailed. While this has not had an impact on successful breastfeeding, the psychological morbidity may have increased.
4 *Emotional and physical support*. Mothers require help and support after childbirth and this may come from her partner, relatives and friends. Good professional support is also important and good communication between hospital staff, community midwives, the general practitioner and health visitor is essential.

Routine observations

During the patient's stay in hospital, she will be asked if she has any complaints and regular checks are made of her pulse, temperature, blood pressure, fundal height and lochia. The perineum should be inspected daily if there has been any trauma and the episiotomy or other wounds checked for signs of infection. It is also important that urinary output is satisfactory and that the bladder is being emptied completely. These observations are necessary to give the earliest warning of any possible complications.

Ambulation in the puerperium

It is now well established that early mobilization after childbirth is extremely important. Once the mother has recovered from the physical rigours of her labour, she should be encouraged to mobilize as soon as possible. The physiotherapist has an important role to play in returning the patient to normal health during the puerperium and limb exercises will be particularly important to encourage venous flow in the leg veins of any mother who has been immobilized in bed for any reason. Exercises to the abdominal and pelvic floor muscles are most valuable in restoring normal tone which may have been lost during pregnancy.

Complications of the puerperium

Serious and sometimes fatal complications may arise during the puerperium. The most serious complications are

Table 10.2 Proportion of mothers having major, intermediate and minor morbidity after childbirth

	In hospital (0–5 days) $n = 1249$ Percentage of women	95% CI	At home (up to 8 weeks) $n = 1116$ Percentage of women	95% CI
Minor	67	64–69	74	71–77
Intermediate	60	58–63	48	46–57
Major	25	22–27	31	29–34

From Glazener *et al.* [15].
Minor problems: tiredness, backache, constipation, piles, headache. Intermediate: perineal pain, breast problems, tearfulness/depression. Major: hypertension, vaginal discharge, abnormal bleeding, stitch breakdown, voiding difficulties/incontinence, urinary infection, side effects of epidural.

Table 10.3 Deaths from pulmonary embolism reported by Confidential Enquiry into Maternal and Child Health

Triennium	Total deaths	Rate/100,000	Post-natal	Rate/100,000
1985–87	30	1.3	13	0.6
1988–90	24	1.0	11	0.5
1991–93	30	1.3	17	0.7
1994–96	46	2.1	25	1.1
1997–99	31	1.5	13	0.6
2000–02	25	1.3	16	0.8

Table 10.4 Deaths from puerperal sepsis as reported in Confidential Enquiry into Maternal and Child Health

Triennium	Total deaths	Rate/million	Post-natal	Rate/million
1985–87	9	4	2	0.9
1988–90	17	7.2	4	1.7
1991–93	15	6.5	4	1.7
1994–96	16	7.3	11	5.0
1997–99	18	8.5	4	1.9
2000–02	13	6.5	5	2.5

thromboembolism, infection and haemorrhage, as well as mental disorders and breast problems.

Thrombosis and embolism

The Confidential Enquiry into Maternal and Child Health 2000–2002 [7] shows that pulmonary embolism is still a major cause of death in the puerperium. Of a total of 25 deaths that occurred in the triennium, 16 occurred in the post-natal period. Table 10.3 illustrates how the rate of pulmonary embolism as a cause of death has remained static since 1985. The report identifies that there are three major areas that give rise to this increased risk of pulmonary embolism. These were increased maternal age, a family history of thromboembolism and obesity with its associated lack of mobility. Of the 16 deaths that occurred, 7 occurred within 7 days of delivery and 6 in the subsequent 2 weeks. The other 3 deaths occurred after this time. Currently, the use of prophylactic, subcutaneous, low molecular weight heparin as prophylaxis in the puerperium is given only to women who are having Caesarean sections but attention should be given to this increased risk group for prophylactic heparin in the puerperium following vaginal delivery.

Puerperal infection

Puerperal pyrexia may have several causes but it is an important clinical sign which merits careful investigation. Infection may occur in several sites and each needs to be investigated in the presence of elevated temperature.

Genital tract infection

Genital tract infection continues to present a life-threatening problem to women and Table 10.4 shows the risk of puerperal sepsis and maternal death over the last 17 years. The most virulent organism is beta-haemolytic streptococcus but more commonly Chalmydia, *Escherichia coli* and other gram negative bacteria will be the infective agents. Table 10.5 summarizes the main causes of post-natal pyrexia. Early diagnosis and treatment are

Table 10.5 Risk factors for post-natal depression

Unmarried
Under age 20
Brought up by single parent
Poor parental support in childhood
Poor relationship with partner
Socially disadvantaged
Poor achievement educationally
Low self-esteem
Previous emotional problems
Previous depressive illness

imperative if the long-term sequelae are to be avoided. Of importance in the five deaths that occurred between 2000 and 2002, four out of the five became ill in the community and it is important that healthcare professionals who are caring for women after discharge from hospital should be aware of the dangers of puerperal sepsis and the need for early treatment.

Urinary tract infection

This is a common infection in the puerperium following the not infrequent use of catheterization during labour. Some women will also develop urinary retention and require indwelling catheters. *E. coli* is the commonest pathogen and again early treatment is advised.

Respiratory infection

These are now seen less commonly during the puerperium as fewer women have a general anaesthetic for delivery. However, chest symptoms may be a sign of pulmonary embolism and in all women who present with any chest problems a possible diagnosis of pulmonary embolism should be considered.

Other causes

Any surgical wound should be examined for evidence of infection and this is obviously important following

Caesarean section. Wound infection may manifest itself as a reddened, tender area, deep to the incision, which may be surrounded by induration. Treatment will depend on the extent and severity of the infection. If the infection is well localized it may discharge spontaneously or if an abscess has formed this may require incision and drainage. The use of broad spectrum antibiotics will be required and bacteriological specimens should be sent for examination. It is occasionally necessary to re-suture wounds after infection but often wounds will granulate from the base and heal spontaneously. The legs should always be inspected if a puerperal pyrexia is present because of the risk of thrombophlebitis and it may also be a sign of deep venous thrombosis. The breasts should be examined for signs of breast infection; breast abscess formation is very unusual until after the fourteenth post-natal day.

Urinary complications

Other than infection, urinary retention is the commonest complication following delivery especially if there has been any trauma to the urethra or oedema round the bladder neck. A painful episiotomy may make it very difficult for women to spontaneously micturate and retention of urine may occur. Following epidural anaesthesia, there may be temporary interruption of the normal sensory stimuli for bladder function and over-distension of the bladder may occur. It is extremely important that, in the immediate post-natal period, urinary retention is avoided as over-distension may lead to an atonic bladder, which is then unable to empty spontaneously. If the bladder is distended, it is usually palpable abdominally but if this is not the case or the clinician is uncertain of the abdominal findings, an ultrasound scan should be performed to determine the volume of urine retained in the bladder. The treatment of urinary retention is to leave an indwelling catheter on continuous drainage for 48 h. The patient can be ambulant during this time and after the bladder has been continuously emptied, the catheter can be removed and then the volumes of urine passed can be monitored. If there is any suspicion that further retention is occurring, then a suprapubic catheter should be inserted so that the bladder can undergo a further period of continuous drainage and then intermittent clamping of the catheter can be instituted until normal bladder function returns.

Incontinence of urine

Urinary incontinence will occur in many women immediately following delivery and approximately 15% of women will have urinary incontinence which persists for 3 months after birth [8]. However, a recent study by Glazener *et al.* [9] showed that three quarters of

women with urinary incontinence 3 months after childbirth still have this 6 years later. Urinary incontinence is more frequently seen following instrumental delivery and least frequently seen after elective Caesarean section. Urinary fistulae are uncommon in obstetric practice today although direct injury from the obstetric forceps may occasionally occur. Complications to the ureter are most commonly seen at a complicated Caesarean section when ureteric injury may either result in a ureteric fistula or ureteric occlusion. Women with this type of urinary problem should not be managed by obstetricians but should be referred to a urological colleague for surgical management.

Incontinence of faeces

It is now recognized that 35% of women undergoing their first vaginal delivery develop anal sphincter injury [10,11]. Approximately 10% will still have anal symptoms of urgency or incontinence at 3 months post-natal. Again, in the 6-year follow-up study by Glazener *et al.* [9], there was no improvement in this anal incontinence rate over time and at 6 years the faecal incontinence rate actually increased to 13%. The aetiology of this type of anal sphincter trauma is complex in the same way as the mechanisms that maintain continence are complex. Instrumental delivery is a recognized cause of trauma and randomized trials suggest that the use of the vacuum extractor is associated with less perineal trauma than forceps delivery [12,13]. In looking at the incidence of anal incontinence, forceps delivery gave a 32% incidence versus 16% for vacuum extraction. The incidence of third and fourth degree tears varies enormously from centre to centre suggesting the clinical ability to recognize this type of trauma may vary. In those women who have a recognized anal sphincter rupture, 37% continue to have anal incontinence despite primary sphincter repair [14].

Secondary post-partum haemorrhage

Delayed post-partum bleeding occurs in 1–2% of patients. It occurs most frequently between 8 and 14 days post-partum and in the majority of these cases it is due to sloughing of the placental site. However, if this bleeding is not self-limiting, further investigation will be required. Ultrasound examination of the uterine cavity will usually determine whether there is a significant amount of retained products although it can be at times difficult to distinguish between blood clot and retained placental tissue. Suction evacuation of the uterus is the treatment of choice and if this is required, it is imperative that antibiotic cover is given. If curettage is not required immediately to arrest bleeding, it is best to start antibiotics at least 12 h beforehand. This will reduce the risk of endometritis leading to uterine synechae. A combination of metronidazole and augmentin can be used in those patients who have endometritis without retained products of conception. In those that do have retained products who require curettage, intravenous antibiotics in the form of metronidazole and a cephalosporin or clindomycin are the antibiotics of choice. Great care must be taken at the time of curettage as the infected uterus is soft and easy to perforate. Rarely, these measures do not result in cessation of the bleeding and in life-threatening circumstances embolization of the uterine arteries may be effective in controlling the bleeding, as may the use of uterine tamponade using a Foley catheter balloon.

Puerperal psychological disorders

Mild pyschological and transient depression is extremely common in the few days post-partum. This transient state of tearfulness, anxiety, irritation and restlessness has been variously described as 'the blues' and it may occur in up to 70% of women. It is usually resolved by day 10 post-natally and is probably associated with disruptive sleep patterns and the adaptation and anxiety of having a newborn baby. The changes in steroid hormone levels that occur immediately following delivery are not correlated with this transient depressive state and because it is transient no therapy is needed. Post-partum depression occurs in approximately 8–15% of women and this disorder may vary in severity from mild to suicidal depression [15]. The signs and symptoms of post-natal depression are not different from those of depression in non-pregnant women and there are a number of antenatal factors that increase the risk of major post-partum depression. These are outlined in Table 10.5. There is a high incidence of recurrence of post-partum depression in subsequent pregnancies (around 50%). Mode of delivery has not been associated with an increased risk of post-partum depression but early recognition of this condition is extremely important. When diagnosed early and treated the prognosis is extremely good, although symptoms may persist for up to a year. Unfortunately, there may be delays in the diagnosis as this type of depression occurs most commonly when the mother has returned home and is in the community. A worrying trend over the last few years has been that suicide is now the leading cause of maternal mortality. In the Confidential Enquiry into Maternal and Child Health 2000–2002 [7], there were a total of 30 deaths in the post-natal period in relation to psychiatric disorders. These 30 deaths were the result of suicide by hanging, jumping from a height, cutting of the throat or overdose. It is therefore obvious that patients at risk must be identified in the antenatal period and communication between the hospital, obstetrician, midwife, GP, healthcare worker and the psychiatric liaison services must be improved if we are to reduce the level of suicide.

Post-natal psychosis

Approximately 0.1% of women post-partum may exhibit some signs of psychosis. Post-partum psychosis is usually characterized by an increased degree of anxiety, a combination of mania and depression, suicidal thoughts, an expression of delusion and a wish to self-harm or to harm the baby. Women manifesting signs of post-partum psychosis should be referred immediately to a psychiatrist and transferred to a mother and baby unit where they can be appropriately cared for as 5% of these women may commit suicide and the infanticide rate is also 5% if they are not treated.

Counselling of patients after perinatal death

When a woman and her family experience a loss associated with pregnancy, special attention must be given to the grieving that they are going to undergo. Mourning is an extremely important part of coping and the clinical signs and symptoms of grief are important to recognize so that the healthcare workers can be sympathetic to this grieving process. These symptoms include sleeplessness, fatigue, poor eating habits, preoccupation with pictures of the baby, feelings of guilt, hostility and anger and a general disruption in the normal pattern of daily life. Unless the clinicians are aware of these changes, misunderstanding may occur and the ability to help the process of grieving will be lost. These families require a sympathetic person so that they have the opportunity to express and discuss their feelings in an open way. The establishment of identified individuals who are trained to deal with perinatal death is extremely important and centres should have doctors, midwives and counsellors available to help the grieving families. It is also extremely important that trained individuals are able to help the family with the legal and administrative processes that are needed in association with the death so that they are not overburdened with these which will then interfere with their ability to grieve. Counselling and support for these families may need to go on for many weeks or months after the event and appropriate staff must be available to help them.

Drugs during lactation

Drugs which are taken by a breastfeeding mother may pass to the child and it is important to consider whether particular drugs will have any effect on the fetus. This

Table 10.6 Comparison of the constituents of human and cow's milk

Constituent	Human milk	Cow's milk
Energy (kcal/100 ml)	75	66
Protein (g/100 ml)	1.1	3.5
Fat (g/100 ml)	4.5	3.7
Lactose (g/100 ml)	6.8	4.9
Sodium (mmol/l)	7	2.2

is often a difficult problem and the reader is referred to Shehata *et al.* [16] on Drugs in Pregnancy.

Infant feeding

The major physiological event of the puerperium is the establishment of lactation. Some mothers in developed countries still reject breastfeeding in favour of artificial feeding but there is increasing evidence of the important short-and long-term benefits of breastfeeding.

Advantages of breastfeeding

NUTRITIONAL ASPECTS OF BREAST MILK

Human milk is not a constant substance because colostrum differs from mature milk and the milk of the early puerperium differs from the milk of late lactation. Indeed, the content of milk varies at differing stages of the same feed. Nevertheless, the approximate concentrations of human milk and cow's milk show substantial differences (Table 10.6) with human milk having less protein but more fat and lactose. A number of specific components also differ between human milk and formulae, such as the long-chain polyunsaturated fatty acids, which have important neurodevelopmental consequences for the baby [17]. There is no doubt that breast milk is the ideal nutrition for the human baby.

PROTECTION AGAINST INFECTION

One of the most important secondary functions of breastfeeding is to protect the infant against infection. This is particularly important in developing countries where it has been estimated that in each year there are 500 million cases of diarrhoea in infants and children and about 20 million of these are fatal. The extent to which breastfeeding protects against infection in infants in developed countries, however, has been a matter of dispute. In a study from Dundee, Scotland, it was found that babies who had been breastfed for at least 3 months had greatly reduced incidences of vomiting and diarrhoea compared with babies who were either bottlefed from birth or completely weaned within a short time of delivery [18]. This study also found that the protection against gastrointestinal illness in breastfed babies persisted beyond the period of breastfeeding itself and, in the developed country setting at least, was not undermined by the early introduction of at least some supplements. There was a smaller protection against respiratory tract infections but not against other illnesses.

A number of mechanisms contribute to the anti-infective properties of breast milk. Breast milk contains lactoferrin which binds iron, and because *E. coli* requires iron for growth, the multiplication of this organism is inhibited. Breastfeeding also encourages colonization of the gut by non-pathogenic flora which will competitively inhibit pathogenic strains. In addition, there are bacteriocidal enzymes, such as lysozyme, present in breast milk, which will contribute to its protective effect.

The most specific anti-infective mechanism, however, is an immunological one. If a mother ingests a pathogen which she has previously encountered, the gut-associated lymphoid tissue situated in the Peyer's patches of the small intestine will respond by producing specific immunoglobulin A, which is transferred to the breast milk via the thoracic duct (Fig. 10.1). This immunoglobulin, which is present in large amounts in breast milk, is not absorbed from the infant's gastrointestinal tract but remains in the gut to attach to the specific offending pathogen against which it is directed. In this way the breastfed infant is given protection from the endemic infections in the environment against which the mother will already have immunity. Breast milk contains living cells, such as polymorphs, lymphocytes and plasma cells and although their functions are not yet fully understood they may also be active against invading pathogens.

BREASTFEEDING AND NEUROLOGICAL DEVELOPMENT

A number of studies have shown positive associations between breastfeeding and improved childhood cognitive functions, such as increased intelligence quotient, which persist even after allowing for potential confounding variables. For example, one study found that, at 2 years of age, babies who had been breastfed for more than 4 months had a 9.1 point advantage in the Bayley score [19]. Other studies have shown similar but smaller benefits and preterm babies also have improved neurological development if exposed to breast milk [20,21].

The mechanism for the improved neurological development is not fully understood but the presence of long-chain ω-3 fatty acids in breast milk, particularly docosohexanoic acid, may be important; the composition of the infant brain is sensitive to dietary intake but the relationship between the biochemical composition of brain lipid and cognitive function is not yet known. Nevertheless, the possible

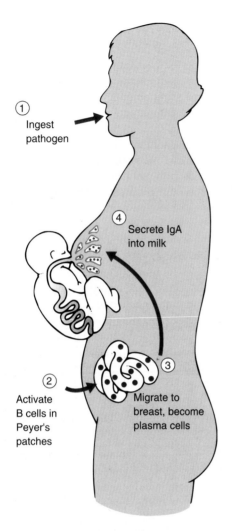

① Ingest pathogen

④ Secrete IgA into milk

② Activate B cells in Peyer's patches

③ Migrate to breast, become plasma cells

Fig. 10.1 Pathways involved in the secretion of immunoglobulin A in breast milk by the enteromammary circulation. (Courtesy of Professor R.V. Short, Melbourne, Australia.)

beneficial effect of breastfeeding on cognitive function is a topic of great potential importance.

BREASTFEEDING AND ATOPIC ILLNESS

There are a number of reports that show lower incidences of atopic illness such as eczema and asthma in breastfed babies. This effect is particularly important when there is a family history of atopic illnesses [22]. When the atopic illness is present, it is commonly associated with raised levels of immunoglobulin E, especially cow's milk protein.

Oddy *et al.* [22] suggest that, apart from a positive family history, the most important predisposing factor for atopic illness is the early introduction of weaning foods. The protective effect of breastfeeding against atopic illness, therefore, may be secondary, rather than primary,

because breastfeeding mothers tend to introduce supplements at a later stage. Nevertheless, mothers with a family history of atopic illness should be informed of the advantages of breastfeeding and of the dangers of introducing supplements too quickly.

BREASTFEEDING AND DISEASE IN LATER LIFE

Breastfeeding may be associated with reduced juvenile-onset diabetes mellitus [23] and neoplastic disease in childhood [24]. It is possible that some of these benefits are related to the avoidance of cow's milk during early life rather than to breastfeeding *per se*, for example, it is possible that early exposure to bovine serum albumin could trigger an autoimmune process leading to juvenile-onset diabetes. Breast milk is a particularly important ingredient in the diet of preterm infants as it appears to help in the prevention of necrotizing enterocolitis among these particularly vulnerable babies.

BREASTFEEDING AND BREAST CANCER

There is an epidemic of breast cancer among women of developed countries in the Western world. A number of recent studies have shown a reduced risk of breast cancer among women who have breastfed their babies [25]. Because breastfeeding appears to have no effect on the incidence of postmenopausal breast cancer, its overall protective effect will be relatively small but the protection offered by lactation still represents an important advantage against a much feared and common disease.

BREASTFEEDING AND FERTILITY

The natural contraceptive effect of breastfeeding has received scant attention in the Western world because it is not a reliable method of family planning in all cases. Nevertheless, on a population basis, the antifertility effect of breastfeeding is large and of major importance in the developing world. It has to be remembered that the majority of women in the developing world do not use artificial contraception and rely on natural checks to their fertility. By far the most important of these natural checks is the inhibition of fertility by breastfeeding. In many developing countries mothers breastfeed for 2 years or more, with the effect that their babies are spaced at about 3-yearly intervals. In the developing world, more pregnancies are still prevented by breastfeeding than by all other methods of family planning combined. The current decline in breastfeeding in the developing world is a cause for great concern because, without a sharp rise in contraceptive usage, the loss of its antifertility effect will aggravate the population increase in these countries.

BREASTFEEDING AND OBESITY

Artificially fed children have twice the risk of childhood obesity in comparison to breastfed children [26]. Breastfed children have a significantly reduced blood pressure [27]. These children have a significantly reduced chance of being obese as adults and dying prematurely from cardiovascular disease.

MECHANISMS OF LACTATIONAL AMENORRHOEA

The mechanisms of lactational amenorrhoea are complex and incompletely understood. The key event is a suckling-induced change in the hypothalamic sensitivity to the feedback effects of ovarian steroids. During lactation, the hypothalamus becomes more sensitive to the negative feedback effects and less sensitive to the positive feedback effects of oestrogen. This means that if the pituitary secretes enough follicle-stimulating hormone and luteinizing hormone to initiate the development of an ovarian follicle, the consequent oestrogen secretion will inhibit gonadotrophin production and the follicle will fail to mature. During lactation there is inhibition of the normal pulsatile release of luteinizing hormone from the anterior pituitary gland which is consistent with this explanation.

From a clinical standpoint, the major factor is the frequency and duration of the suckling stimulus although other factors such as maternal weight and diet may be important confounding factors. If supplementary food is introduced rapidly at an early stage, the suckling stimulus will fall and early ovulation and a return to fertility will be the consequence.

Trends in infant feeding in the UK

Because of the many advantages of breastfeeding, it is important that mothers are given accurate information and encouraged to breastfeed successfully whenever possible. Conversely, mothers who choose to bottle feed should be given proper instructions on best practice and to be supported in their decision.

In the UK, about 69% of mothers overall start to breastfeed but many discontinue after a short time. The prevalence of breastfeeding in the UK in 2002 is shown in Table 10.7 and the figures have shown no significant change over the previous 10 years, although a small increase in breastfeeding at birth is noted. Factors which are associated with higher breastfeeding prevalence are higher social class, primiparity, older age of mother and place of residence (mothers in the south of the country have a higher prevalence).

In attempting to improve these disappointing low rates of successful breastfeeding, it is important that

Table 10.7 Prevalence of breastfeeding from birth until 9 months from 1985–2000

	1985	1990	1995	2000
Birth	63	62	66	69
6 weeks	41	42	42	42
4 months	26	28	27	28
6 months	23	22	21	21
9 months	14	14	14	13

health professionals should understand the physiology of lactation.

Physiology of lactation

At puberty, the milk ducts which lead from the nipple to the secretory alveoli are stimulated by oestrogen to sprout, branch and form glandular tissue buds from which milk-secreting glands will develop (Fig. 10.2). During pregnancy, this breast tissue is further stimulated so that pre-existing alveolar-lobular structures hypertrophy and new ones are formed. At the same time milk-collecting ducts also undergo branching and proliferation. Both oestrogen and progesterone are necessary for mammary development in pregnancy but prolactin, growth hormone and adrenal steroids may also be involved. During pregnancy only minimal amounts of milk are formed in the breast despite high levels of the lactogenic hormones, prolactin and placental lactogen. This is because the actions of these lactogenic hormones are inhibited by the secretion of high levels of oestrogen and progesterone from the placenta and it is not until after delivery that copious milk production is induced.

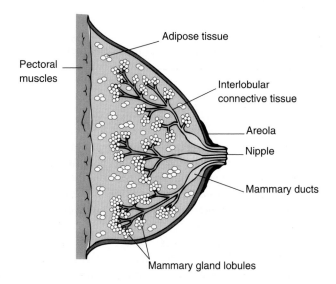

Fig. 10.2 Structure of the lactating breast.

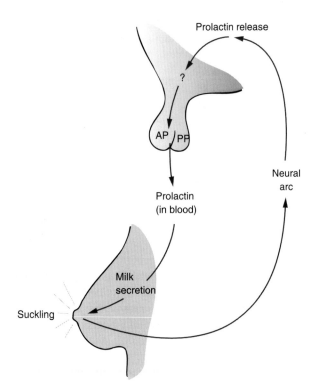

Fig. 10.3 Pathway of prolactin release from the anterior pituitary gland.

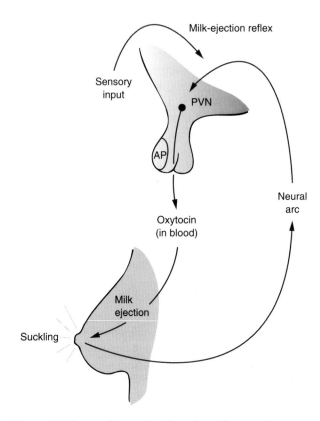

Fig. 10.4 Pathway of oxytocin release from the posterior pituitary gland.

Milk production

Two similar, but independent, mechanisms are involved in the establishment of successful lactation (lactogenesis); the first mechanism causes the release of prolactin which acts upon the glandular cells of the breast to stimulate milk secretion (Fig. 10.3) and the second induces the release of oxytocin which acts upon the myoepithelial cells of the breast to induce the milk ejection reflex (Fig. 10.4). Although these two mechanisms are similar, in that they can both be activated by suckling, they are mediated through two entirely different neuroendocrinological pathways. As can be seen in Figs 10.3 and 10.4, the key event in lactogenesis is suckling and the sensitivity of the breast accommodates itself to this important activity. During pregnancy the skin of the areola is relatively insensitive to tactile stimuli but becomes much more sensitive immediately after delivery. This is an ingenious physiological adaptation which ensures that there is an adequate stream of afferent neurological stimuli from the nipple to the hypothalamus to initiate and maintain the release of prolactin and oxytocin, both of which are required for successful lactation.

Milk-ejection reflex

Successful breastfeeding depends as much upon effective milk transfer from the breast to the baby as upon adequate milk secretion. The milk-ejection reflex is mediated by the release of oxytocin from the posterior pituitary gland (see Fig. 10.4). Oxytocin causes contraction of the sensitive myoepithelial cells which are situated around the milk-secreting glands and also dilates the ducts by acting upon the muscle cells which lie longitudinally in the duct walls. Contraction of these cells, therefore, has the dual effect of expelling milk from the glands and of encouraging free flow of milk along dilated ducts. This is recognized by the mother as the milk 'let-down' and she may be aware of milk being ejected from the opposite breast from which the baby is suckling. In contrast to prolactin, which is secreted only in response to suckling, oxytocin can be released in response to sensory inputs such as the mother seeing the baby or hearing its cry. Oxytocin has a very short half-life in the circulation and is released from the posterior pituitary in a pulsatile manner. As shown in Fig. 10.5 the highest levels of oxytocin may be released prior to suckling in response to the baby's cry, while prolactin is released only after suckling commences. The milk-ejection reflex is readily inhibited by emotional stress and this may explain why maternal anxiety frequently leads to a failure of lactation. Successful breastfeeding depends upon engendering confidence in the mother and ensuring correct fixing and suckling at the breast.

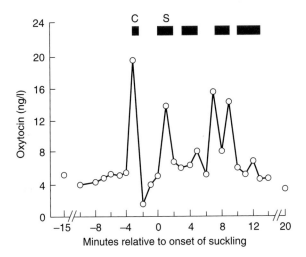

Fig. 10.5 Pattern of oxytocin release in response to the infant's cry (C) and to suckling (S). Redrawn from McNeilly *et al.* (1982) with permission.

Another factor is of potential physiological importance as an inhibitor of breast milk. If the milk is not effectively stripped from the breast at each feed this will inhibit lactopoiesis and lead to a fall in milk production.

Volumes of breast milk

During the first 24 h of the puerperium, the human breast usually secretes small volumes of milk but with regular suckling, milk volumes steadily increase and, by the sixth day of the puerperium, an average volume of 500 ml will be taken by the baby. Once lactation is fully established, an average daily milk volume is about 800 ml. In well-established lactation, it is possible to sustain a baby on breast milk alone for 4–6 months.

Management of breastfeeding

Despite the fact that it is a physiological event, many women experience difficulties in establishing breastfeeding. The greatest asset that a nursing mother can have is the support of an experienced and sympathetic counsellor. This counsellor may be a midwife, a health visitor or a lay person but the creation of a relaxed and confident environment is vital for successful breastfeeding. Babies are individuals, so there is no simple strategy that works in every case; mothers should be encouraged to learn to respond to their own babies but all too often well-meaning but dogmatic and conflicting advice is given. The best approach is to give mothers all of the options and let them make their own decisions; they will soon learn by trial and error what is best for their own babies. As an important stimulus to the promotion of effective breastfeeding, the

Table 10.8 Ten steps to successful breastfeeding

1. Have a written breastfeeding policy
2. Train all staff
3. Inform all pregnant women about the benefits and management of breastfeeding
4. Help mothers to initiate breastfeeding within 30 min of birth
5. Show mothers how to breastfeed
6. Foster the establishment of breastfeeding support groups
7. Practice 24 h rooming in
8. Encourage breastfeeding on demand
9. Give newborn infants no other food or drink, unless medically indicated
10. Use no artificial teats

From UNICEF UK Baby Friendly Initiative 2004 [30].

concept of 'baby-friendly hospitals' has been developed with breastfeeding being an important part of that assessment. The 'baby-friendly' initiative has adopted the 10 successful steps to breastfeeding as its central strategy and these are outlined in Table 10.8. Support for the breastfeeding mother is both an art and a science and the reader is referred to some of the detailed texts on the subject (e.g. [28]).

References

1. Oppenheimer LW, Sherriff EA, Goodman JD *et al.* (1986) The duration of lochia. *Br J Obstet Gynaecol* **93**, 754–7.
2. Kovacs GT (1985) Post partum fertility – a review. *Clin Reprod Fertil* **3**, 107–14.
3. Greer IA (2003) Prevention of venous thromboembolism in pregnancy. *Best Pract Res Clin Haematol* **16**, 261–78.
4. Rooney BL & Schauberger CW (2002) Excess pregnancy weight gain and long-term obesity: one decade later. *Obstet Gynecol* **100**, 245–52.
5. Dewey KG (2004) Impact of breast feeding on maternal nutritional status. *Adv Exp Med Biol* **554**, 91–100.
6. Larson-Meyer DE (2002) Effect of post partum exercise on mothers and their offspring. *Obes Res* **10**, 841–53.
7. Confidential Enquiry into Maternal and Child Health (2004) *Why Mothers Die 2000–2002*. London: RCOG Press.
8. Chaliha C & Stanton SL (2002) Urological problems in pregnancy. *BJU International* **89**, 469–76.
9. Glazener CM, Herbison GP, Macarthur C *et al.* (2004) Randomised controlled trial of conservative management of post natal urinary incontinence and faecal incontinence: six year follow up. *Br Med J* **12** (Dec), doi:10.1136/bmj.38320.613461.82.
10. Donnelly VS, Fynes M & Campbell D (1998) Obstetric events leading to anal sphincter damage. *Obstet Gynecol* **92**, 955–61.
11. Sultan AH, Kamm MA, Hudson CN *et al.* (1993) Anal-sphincter disruption during vaginal delivery. *N Eng J Med* **329**, 1905–11.
12. Bofill JA, Rust OA, Schorr SJ *et al.* (1996) A randomized prospective trial of the obstetric forceps versus the M-cup vacuum extractor. *Am J Obstet Gynecol* **175**, 1325–30.

13. Johansson RB, Rice C & Doyle MA (1993) A randomised prospective study comparing the new vacuum extractor policy with forceps delivery. *Br J Obstet Gynaecol* **100**, 524–30.

14. Sultan AH (2002) Third degree tear repair. In: McJean AB (ed.) *Incontinence in Women*. London: RCOG Press, 379–90.

15. Glazener CM, MacArthur C & Garcia J (1993) Post natal care: time for a change. *Contemp Rev Obstet Gynaecol* **5**, 130–6.

16. Shehata HA & Nelson Piercy C (2001) Drugs in pregnancy. *Best Pract Clin Obstet Gynaecol* **15**, 971–86.

17. Anderson JW, Johnstone BM & Remley DT (1999) breastfeeding and cognitive development: a meta-analysis. *Am J Clin Nutri* **70**, 525–35.

18. Howie PW, Forsyth JS, Ogston SA *et al.* (1990) Protective effect of breast feeding against infection. *Br Med J* **300**, 11–16.

19. Morrow-Tlucak M, Haude RH & Ernhart CB (1988) Breastfeeding and cognitive development in the first 2 years of life. *Soc Sci Med* **26**, 635–9.

20. Lucas, A, Morley R, Cole TJ *et al.* (1992) Breast milk and subsequent intelligence quotient in children born preterm. *Lancet* **339**, 261–4.

21. Vestergaard M, Obel C, Henriksen TB *et al.* (1999) Duration of breastfeeding and developmental milestones during the latter half of infancy. *Acta Paediatr* **88**, 1327–32.

22. Oddy WH, Peat JK & de Klerk NH (2002) Maternal asthma, infant feeding, and the risk of asthma in childhood. *J Allergy Clin Immunol* **110**, 65–67.

23. Gerstein HC (1994) Cow's milk exposure and type I diabetes mellitus. A critical overview of the clinical literature. *Diabetes Care* **17**, 13–19.

24. Davis MK (1998) Review of the evidence for an association between infant feeding and childhood cancer. *Int J Cancer Suppl* **11**, 29–33.

25. Colloborative group on breast cancer and breastfeeding: collaborative reanalysis of individual data from 47 epidemiological studies in 30 countries, including 50302 women with breast cancer and 96973 women without the disease. (2002) *Lancet* **360**, 187–95.

26. von Kries R, Koletzko B, Sauerwald T *et al.* (1999) Breast feeding and obesity: cross sectional study. *Br Med J* **319**, 147–50.

27. Martin RM, Ness AR, Gunnell D *et al.* (2004) Does breastfeeding in infancy lower blood pressure in childhood? The Avon Longitudinal Study of Parents and Children (ALSPAC). *Circulation* **109**, 1259–66.

28. Renfrew M Fisher C & Arms S (1990) *Breast Feeding: Getting Breastfeeding Right for You*. Berkeley, CA: Celestial Arts.

29. Dunlop W (1989) The puerperium. *Fetal Med Rev* **1**, 43–60.

30. UNICEF Baby Friendly Initiative (2005) @ www.babyfriendly.org.uk

Chapter 11: Neonatal care for obstetricians

M.A. Thomson and A.D. Edwards

The transition to the extrauterine life

Lungs

Expansion of the lungs at birth presents a considerable challenge to the newborn infant. In fetal life, lung liquid is actively secreted into the alveolar space and the lung is a fluid-filled organ. During term labour lung liquid production ceases, high fetal blood concentrations of thyroid hormone, adrenaline and corticosteroids cause the direction of fluid flow to be permanently reversed, preparing the air spaces for air breathing. The majority of lung liquid is absorbed into the pulmonary lymphatics and capillaries with a small amount squeezed out of the lungs as a result of high vaginal pressure during the second stage of labour.

In response to a number of stimuli following birth which include the change in environmental temperature, audiovisual, proprioceptive changes, touch and physiological hypoxia which occurs when the umbilical cord is clamped a healthy term baby usually takes the first breath within 60 s. The first breaths must generate high pressure within the lungs to overcome several factors, such as the surface tension at the air–liquid interface of collapsed alveoli, the high flow resistance and inertia of fluid in the airways and the elastic recoil and compliance of the lungs and chest wall. Therefore initial respiratory effort results in both large inspiratory breaths which create high negative pressures (20 cmH$_2$0) within the lungs and forced active expiration producing pressure ranging from 20–100 cmH$_2$O. Replacement of lung liquid by air is largely accomplished within a few minutes of birth although this may be delayed if the delivery occurs before the onset of labour or the respiratory drive is compromised by such factors as prematurity, surfactant deficiency, perinatal hypoxia and general anaesthesia.

Once expanded, lung compliance is much improved and the pressure required for normal tidal breathing is only about 5 cmH$_2$O. Failure to reabsorb lung liquid may produce transient tachypnoea in a term baby.

Expanded alveoli must be prevented from collapsing again and this depends on the surfactant system. Surfactant, a complex mixture of mainly phospholipids, with smaller amounts of neutral lipids and proteins is produced by type II alveolar cells. These cells can be identified from about 24 weeks gestation. However, surfactant production is limited until much later in gestation. It is the phospholipids notably dipalmitoyl phosphatidylcholine (DPPC) which forms a monolayer at the alveolar air–tissue interface thereby significantly reducing surface tension and preventing alveolar collapse. The four surfactant-associated proteins SP-A, SP-B, SP-C, and SP-D each have essential roles; SP-B and C aid spreading, adsorption and recycling of the phospholipids, SP-A has a dual role in improving surfactant function and with SP-D is part of the innate host defence mechanism against infection.

Surfactant production and release increases during the latter part of pregnancy under control of hormones such as corticosteroids and thyroid hormone. Maturation of the surfactant system can be stimulated by numerous agents including maternal glucocorticoids. Babies born preterm may fail to clear lung liquid or produce surfactant so that pulmonary compliance remains low and the high negative intrathoracic pressures required for lung inflation during the first breath persist. These infants develop respiratory distress and may require ventilation and surfactant replacement.

The heart and circulation

In the fetus, oxygenated blood from the placenta is preferentially streamed through the ductus venosus to the right atrium and across the foramen ovale into the left atrium. Here it mixes with the small quantity of pulmonary venous blood, then passes to the left ventricle from where it is pumped into the aortic root and to the cerebral and coronary circulations.

A small proportion of inferior vena cava blood enters the right atrium and mixes with the poorly oxygenated blood returning through the superior vena cava, passing to the right ventricle and pulmonary artery. In the fetus, pulmonary vascular resistance is extremely high and very little blood passes from the pulmonary artery into the lungs. Most blood passes though the patent ductus arteriosus to the aorta and supplies the lower body and placenta.

The fetal pattern of circulation is dependent on high pulmonary vascular resistance, the presence of the patent ductus arteriosus and the low-resistance placental component of the systemic circulation. At birth, expansion of the lung and the onset of air breathing increase the local oxygen concentration within the lungs which causes a dramatic fall in pulmonary vascular resistance, effected by a complex series of vasoactive mediators which include prostaglandins and nitric oxide.

The fall in pulmonary resistance allows pulmonary artery pressure to decrease, and thus right atrial pressure falls below left atrial pressure, so stopping the flow of blood from right to left atrium, and promoting mechanical closure of the foramen ovale. This process is aided by the increase in systemic vascular resistance (and thus left heart pressures) caused by clamping of the umbilical cord with the sudden loss of the low-resistance placental circulation.

Increased oxygenation of arterial blood induces closure of the arterial and venous ducts, largely by inhibition of the dilator prostaglandins PGE_2 and PGI_2. This system may be immature in the preterm infant and the ductus arteriosus may not close.

Lung expansion and oxygenation are thus essential to the circulatory changes at birth, allowing both a fall in pulmonary vascular resistance and the closure of the ductus arteriosus. Situations of impaired respiratory function are frequently associated with pulmonary hypertension leading to a physiological right to left shunt and exacerbation of hypoxaemia. This is evident in respiratory distress syndrome when the pulmonary artery pressure is high, and in conditions such as meconium aspiration or diaphragmatic hernia persistence of the fetal circulatory pattern is the major clinical problem.

Haemoglobin

In the term infant, the haemoglobin concentration is high, between 16 and 18 g/dl. Of this 80% is fetal haemoglobin (HbF). HbF has a lower affinity for 2,3-diphosphoglycerite which shifts the haemoglobin–oxygen dissociation curve to the left, leading to maximum oxygen transfer at lower pO_2 levels. The proportion of HbF falls gradually during the months after birth and by six months only 5% haemoglobin is HbF.

The relatively high total haemoglobin concentration also declines after birth. Haemoglobin is removed through the formation of bilirubin which is removed by the liver; hepatic immaturity frequently leads to jaundice in the normal newborn infant. Excessive haemolysis or liver impairment can lead to levels of unconjugated bilirubin sufficiently high to cause neurological damage.

Feeding and nutrition

Human breast milk is the preferred nutrition source for both term and preterm babies; it is associated with a significant reduction in both morbidity and mortality. Every effort should be made to encourage a mother to breastfeed. There are few genuine contraindications to breastfeeding; these include some rare inborn errors of metabolism in the baby such as galactosaemia. It is not the practice in the UK to encourage HIV-positive mothers to breastfeed; however, this is not the case in developing countries. Breastfeeding is generally safe for the baby if the mother requires medication; rarely breastfeeding is absolutely contraindicated. Examples of drugs which require caution are given in Table 11.1. When prescribing for a breastfeeding mother it is wise to check that the drug prescribed is safe. Information can be found in the British National Formulary; if a contraindication, caution or a potential problem is identified, the advice of the local paediatric pharmacist or local drug information centre should be sought. Often alternative drugs can be prescribed and breastfeeding continued. Information is also available via websites such as www.ukmi.nhs.uk.

Human breast milk is a complex bioactive fluid that alters in composition over time. Colostrum has a greater concentration of protein and minerals than mature milk and provides a large number of active substances and cells. Term colostrums contains approximately 3 million cells per ml, of which about 50% are polymorpholeucocytes, 40% macrophages, 5% lymphocytes and the remainder epithelial cells. Colostrum also contains antibodies, humoral factors, growth factors and interleukins.

Table 11.1 Drugs and breastfeeding

Breastfeeding contraindicated	
Cytotoxics, ergotamine, immunosuppressants, lithium, phenindione, chloramphenicol, tetracyclines	
Example of drugs to be used with caution during breastfeeding	
Antiarrhythmic	Amiodarone
Antibiotic	Metronidazole
Anticonvulsant	Gabapentin, levetiracetam, oxcarbazepine, phenobarbital, phenytoin, pregabalin, primidone, topiramate, vigabatrin
Antidepressant	Doxepin, selective serotonin re-uptake inhibitors (SSRI)
Antihypertensive	Betablockers
Anxiolytic	Benzodiazepines, buspirone
Radioisotopes	

The majority of the immunoglobin (Ig) in milk is secretory IgA, with specific antibodies against antigens recognized by the mothers' intestinal mucosa which protect against the extrauterine environment. However, most circulating immunoglobulin in the human infant is acquired transplacentally.

Healthy term infants feeding on demand usually suckle 2 to 4 hourly. On the first day of life they require about 40 ml/kg of milk, and some 20–30 ml/kg more each day until they take approximately 150 ml/kg per day by the end of the first week. Infants weighing 1.5–2.0 kg need approximately 60 ml/kg, again increasing to 150 ml/kg per day after 1 week. Feeding infants smaller than 1.5 kg often requires specialized practices such as gavage or parenteral feeds.

Body composition, fluids and electrolyte metabolism

Table 11.2 shows the average body composition of appropriately grown infants at different gestational ages. During pregnancy total body water declines from 94% in the first trimester to about 70% at term. Extracellular fluid decreases from 65% body weight at 26 weeks to 40% at term. Administration of intravenous fluids to a mother or Caesarean section increases the infant's body water after birth.

Following birth, an abrupt contraction of the extracellular compartment occurs; term infants lose about 5% and preterm infants 10–15% of body weight by diuresis during the first 5 days. This important adjustment to extrauterine life is interrupted by stress which causes secretion of anti-diuretic hormone; infants with respiratory problems show little weight loss until the lung condition improves. However, infants who are sick from many causes may also show excessive weight loss and loss of more than 10% in a term infant is cause for concern.

The glomerular filtration rate is low in newborn infants and only reaches mature levels by the end of the first year. Thus infants initially require little water, and 40–60 ml/kg per 24 h is adequate. Infants have a concomitant obligatory sodium loss and do not require dietary sodium until weight loss is complete. In a sick or preterm infant, fluid and electrolyte administration must be carried out with great care as well as frequent measuring of weight and blood electrolyte concentrations.

Table 11.2 Infantile body compositions

Gestational age (weeks)	22	26	29	40
Weight (g)	500	1000	1500	3500
Water (g)	433	850	1240	2380
Fat (g)	6	23	60	525

Temperature control

The placenta is a heat exchanger which transfers heat generated by metabolism from fetus to mother. After birth the newborn infant functions as a homeotherm, maintaining deep body temperature at 37°C. Heat control places a large demand on neonatal metabolism and physiology because a large surface area to volume ratio and wet skin make the newborn baby vulnerable to excessive heat loss.

Newborn infants have a specialized organ for heat production: brown adipose tissue, which allows non-shivering thermogenesis. Catecholamines are released in response to cold, stimulating oxidative phosphorylation in these cells, where uncoupling energy metabolism from ATP generation allows chemical energy to be converted into heat. Non-shivering thermogenesis is impaired in the first few hours of life in sick infants and after maternal sedative administration.

Despite this, the newborn infant has a limited capacity to maintain core temperature. At environmental temperatures below 32°C non-shivering thermogenesis increases oxygen consumption and maintains core temperature. However, at environmental temperatures below 24°C heat production is inadequate and the body temperature will fall. It is therefore important to ensure the environmental temperature in delivery rooms and theatre is 20°C for a term baby and at least 23°C if a preterm delivery is expected to prevent initial hypothermia.

Preterm infants are at particular risk of hypothermia because of lack of brown fat, small energy reserves, high evaporative heat loss through immature skin and a higher surface area to volume ratio. Sickness places extreme demands on the infant's homeothermic capacity and an unstable core temperature frequently accompanies severe illness. While a healthy term infant can be adequately cared for by dressing and wrapping in warm blankets, sick or preterm infants require incubators or radiant heaters to maintain a normal core temperature.

Resuscitation of the newborn

Assessment and simple resuscitation at birth

Most infants born at term and without specific indicators of high risk during pregnancy do not need resuscitation. Almost all those who do can be resuscitated by simple methods using bag and mask ventilation. A small number of term infants and the many extremely preterm infants require resuscitation involving endotracheal intubation. Thus, while having equipment for resuscitation ready, the first task of the attendant is to decide whether resuscitation is required or not.

Assignment of American Pediatric Gross Assessment Record (APGAR) scores as described in Table 11.3 can

Table 11.3 Clinical evaluation of the newborn infant (Apgar scoring method)

Sign	0	1	2
Heart rate	Absent	Slow (below 100 beats/min)	Over 100 beats/min
Respiratory effort	Absent	Weak	Good; strong cry
Muscle tone	Limp	Some flexion of extremities	Active motion; extremities well flexed
Reflex irritability (response to stimulation of sole of foot)	No response	Grimace	Cry
Colour	Blue; pale	Body pink; extremities blue	Completely pink

The Apgar score is obtained by assigning the value of 0, 1 or 2 to each of five signs and summing the result.

be helpful. These scores are conventionally determined at 1 and 5 min and describe cardiorespiratory and neurological depression. There are many causes of depression at birth, and low Apgar scores are neither evidence of birth asphyxia, nor, except in extreme circumstances, a guide to neurological prognosis. Nevertheless, a low Apgar score signifies a problem that needs explanation and management.

It is helpful to commence a time clock at the moment of delivery and some attendants aspirate the nasal passages immediately after delivery to remove fluid and debris from the pharynx and exclude choanal atresia, although many believed this to be excessive for low-risk births.

In an infant who breathes immediately on delivery, it takes minutes for the cerebral oxygenation concentration to reach normal extrauterine levels and there is no reason to believe that a short period of apnoea at birth causes significant injury. At least three quarters of normal term infants breathe within a minute of delivery and most of the rest have breathed before 3 min. The low-risk newborn can thus be safely given immediately to the mother, while drying with a warm towel, which should then be discarded, and the baby then covered in dry warm towels to allow skin-to-skin contact with the mother. The infant can then be observed, and failure to breath by 30 s should persuade the attendant that resuscitation might be needed. Initially drying, or blowing cold air or oxygen over the face may stimulate respiration. If this fails then resuscitation is appropriate. In many units preterm babies are placed directly in plastic bags without drying. If the bag covers the whole baby except the face better thermal control is achieved and hypothermia, which is known to significantly increase mortality and morbidity, can be prevented.

In infants who have taken a first breath, mask ventilation is highly effective provided the right equipment is used. The mask must be soft so as to form a seal around the airway. Pressurized air or oxygen is provided either by a compressible bag or an interruptible pressurized gas source; both should have a valve which releases pressure at 30 cm of water. After the airway has been adequately cleared by suction, the mask is positioned over the nose and mouth with the baby lying prone and the bag squeezed (or gas provided) to deliver several long inspiratory breaths followed by regular ventilation at a rate of 30–40 breaths/min. In many cases ventilating with air is as effective as using oxygen. This technique requires practice and obstetricians and midwives should maintain their skills, if necessary, using an appropriate resuscitation dummy.

The best guide to successful resuscitation is the baby's heartbeat. This can be determined in most cases by feeling the umbilical cord or the femoral pulsation, or can be heard through a stethoscope over the chest. A heart rate above 120 usually signifies adequate oxygenation, but a heart rate below this implies a need for more effective therapy. The heart rate provides a more immediate and accurate guide to the baby's state than respiratory effort or skin colour and, especially for the occasional or inexperienced resuscitator, is the best short-term measure of success or failure.

The Resuscitation Council UK course in Neonatal Life Support (NLS) teaches and assesses basic neonatal resuscitation practice (www.resus.org.uk).

Advanced life support

If mask ventilation fails to produce an adequate heart rate check again for evidence of upper airway obstruction and aspirate the nasal passages and nasopharynx. Meconium present in the trachea should have been aspirated under direct vision using a laryngoscope before ventilation, but this may need repeating. If clearing of the airway and reventilation fails to produce a normal heart rate, endotracheal intubation is required. This technique is not difficult but requires practice and carries a considerable danger in inexperienced hands: the endotracheal tube will enter the oesophagus easily and significantly inhibit ventilation. If an infant does not rapidly improve after attempted endotracheal intubation, there is presumptive evidence of the tube being in the oesophagus. It should be removed and intubation repeated. If there is doubt it may be safer to concentrate on bag and mask ventilation while awaiting skilled assistance.

Once the endotracheal tube is placed, auscultate the chest over both lungs to ascertain that breath sounds are equal. Inequality implies that the tube has been inserted too far and entered one lung, but could also suggest major problems such as pneumothorax or congenital diaphragmatic hernia.

Endotracheal intubation secures access for mechanical ventilation. Initial ventilation should include an inspiratory time of approximately 1 s to distend collapsed alveoli, and peak pressures sufficient to visibly move the chest. Once the alveoli are expanded less pressure is required. Thus the first breaths may require peak pressures of 30 cm of water or more in term babies, whereas after this it is usually possible to ventilate the lungs with pressures of approximately half this, and a respiratory time of 0.5 s at a rate of 40 breaths/min. If there is evidence or presumption of surfactant deficiency, exogenous surfactant should be administered early.

Effective ventilation is enough to resuscitate most infants and only rarely is cardiac massage or the administration of blood because of bleeding required. On very rare occasions, endotracheal adrenaline may need to be administered for persistent bradycardia and if this fails intravenous adrenaline may be given. It is no longer good practice to administer sodium bicarbonate intravenously to infants unless blood gases are measured or circulatory failure is very prolonged.

Most low-risk infants who require resuscitation can be extubated within a few minutes and can usually be nursed by their mothers as long as (1) there is no specific problem such as meconium aspiration, prematurity or a history of infection and (2) adequate observation can be maintained. Infants who cannot be extubated successfully in this time or who continue to have respiratory problems require admission to a neonatal unit.

Admission to neonatal units

Approximately 8–10% of births require admission to a neonatal unit; however, a much small number (2–3%) require neonatal intensive care. The criteria for admission vary between units but should include the following: (1) birth weight less than 1.8 kg or gestational age below 34 weeks, as these infants rarely feed from the nipple and have difficulty controlling their temperature or (2) proven or suspected illness, such as respiratory distress, cardiac disease, fits or sepsis.

Unnecessary admission of infants to neonatal units can strain resources and put the infant at risk of nosocomial disease, as well as interrupting bonding and frightening parents. Adequate transitional care facilities are essential to avoid misuse of neonatal care.

Examination of the newborn infant

A preliminary examination is made in the delivery room to establish that the baby does not have a major abnormality such as spina bifida and the full examination at a later time. In this way bonding and the initiation of breastfeeding are not interrupted.

A full examination should be carried out on every baby in the presence of the mother before discharge from hospital. Ideally it should take place 24–48 h after birth; however, if discharged before this the examination should still be undertaken. It is then advisable to examine the baby again during the first week of life. Any trained practitioner can carry out the newborn examination. A history should be taken including maternal obstetric and family history to identify problems in the baby that will require further management or follow up.

During examination one relies heavily on observational skills. Note abnormalities of posture and asymmetry of facial or limb movements. Evidence of jaundice, polycythaemia, anaemia or rashes is noted and choanal atresia excluded.

A systematic search for congenital abnormalities can be rapidly performed by examining along the midline and then passing to the limbs. Starting with the head, the facial features should be noted and thought given to dysmorphic syndromes. The palate needs to be examined visually to exclude a clef palate or bifid uvula which signifies a sub-mucus cleft. The eyes must be examined by ophthalmoscopy to exclude cataracts: in a normal eye the red reflex is immediately obvious. Eye movements may not be fully coordinated in the first week of life and momentary strabismus is common.

Examination should be made of (1) the back of the neck and the spine for skin lesions suggesting spinal dysraphism; (2) the anus; (3) the genitalia; (4) the femoral pulses; (5) hips; (6) the abdomen; and (7) the chest for examination of the cardiovascular and respiratory system (chest). Then the limbs are examined: digits need to be counted and palmar and planter creases examined; the ankles should be examined for talipes.

Examination of the cardiovascular system includes not only auscultation of the heart but also palpation of all pulses and the liver. Murmurs are not necessarily evidence of cardiac abnormalities, whereas major heart disease can occur in infants with normal heart sounds. Important signs of cardiac disease include cyanosis, tachypnoea, recession and absent or high-volume pulses.

Respiratory problems also present with cyanosis, recession or tachypnoea, but these two problems can be separated by echocardiography. If this is unavailable a hyperoxia test may be used in which an infant is given 100% oxygen to breathe for 10–20 min and a sample of arterial blood taken from the right arm. Assuming ventilation is adequate, a baby with lung disease will normally have an oxygen tension exceeding 20 kPa whereas in a baby with cyanotic heart disease it normally remains below 15 kPa. The test is now more frequently undertaken with pulse oximetry substituted for arterial blood gas measurement; however, this is prone to error. As the hyperoxia test is not infallible echocardiography is preferred.

Examination of the hip is mandatory to exclude congenital dislocation. The infant lies supine, a femur is held in either hand and the hips fully abducted until the femurs lie parallel to the bed. If this cannot be achieved by gentle pressure, the hip is probably dislocated and ultrasound examination is required. The pelvis is then held firmly by one hand while the other grasps the femur in a vertical position, applying pressure downwards and outwards. If the hip is unstable, this will allow the head of the femur to leave the acetabulum. The examiner then abducts the femur, which rides forwards and inwards as it re-enters the acetabular cup producing a low pitched clunk: this signifies a dislocatable hip. High-pitched clicks can also occur because of ligamental laxity. It is wise to obtain ultrasound examinations of all suspect hips, in infants born after breech delivery and in those with a family history of congenital dislocation.

A great deal can be learnt about an infant's neurological status by observation and assessing posture and tone. A normal term infant when left supine will adopt a position in which the limbs are flexed and adducted. If lifted and held prone the baby will momentary hold its head extended before dropping it forward, with the spine adopting a smooth curvature. Reflexes can also be helpful signs of normality. To elicit the Moro reflex gentle but abrupt neck extension is allowed by moving the head, and this results in sudden extension and abduction of the limbs followed by slower adduction and flexion. Slow rotational movement of the head will also elicit dolls eye movement in which the point of gaze remains relatively fixed despite the movement. If the cheek is touched gently, a rooting response will be elicited in which the baby turns his head slightly towards the stimulus and gives a unilateral grimace. Sucking is a valuable neurological sign, and babies who suck well and effectively rarely have a severe encephalopathy.

A complete examination includes measurement and plotting on standard charts of weight and head circumference; this forms the basis of developmental surveillance in following years. It should also be ascertained that the infant has passed meconium and urine within 24 h of birth.

The examiner should be prepared to answer maternal questions and discuss the merits of BCG and hepatitis B vaccination, and routine screening tests if appropriate. Universal newborn hearing screening has recently been introduced in the United Kingdom. Universal biochemical screening for phenylketonuria and hypothyroidism during the newborn period is well established. In addition, galactosaemia, cystic fibrosis, haemoglobinopathies and various aminoacidopathies are screened for in some parts of the United Kingdom.

Disorders in the newborn period

Preterm birth

Infants born significantly before term usually require neonatal care until around the expected date of delivery. Following the introduction of surfactant coupled with the widespread use of antenatal corticosteroids in the mid-90s mortality rates for these infants fell significantly although in the smallest the risks of death remained high (Fig. 11.1). Rates in the twenty-first century remain similar to those shown. Mortality in extremely preterm babies can be significantly reduced if hypothermia is prevented at birth; this is only possible if the delivery room is maintained at an appropriate temperature. Most survivors do not suffer long-term disability, but in infants of less than 28 weeks gestation some 20% suffer neurodevelopmental impairment.

The stress on parents and family of having a baby who undergoes intensive care can be immense. They have to suffer prolonged uncertainly about the infant's survival as well as a loss of control over their baby's and their own

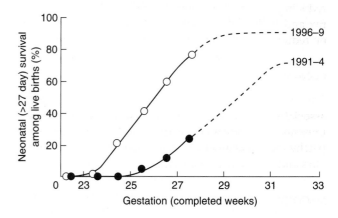

Fig. 11.1 Neonatal survival among registered live births. Redrawn from Tin *et al.* (1997) *Br Med J* **314**, 107–10.

lives. Careful preparation of parents, with visits to the intensive care unit and meetings with unit staff may help, but the difficulties for families in this situation should not be underestimated.

Respiratory disorders

Abnormal breathing is a common presentation of many illnesses in the newborn period. Intermittent or periodic breathing is common and not usually significant. However, a respiratory rate persistently above 60 breaths/min needs further investigation, as do periods of apnoea lasting more than a few seconds, especially if associated with cyanosis and bradycardia.

Tachypnoea with recession and nasal flaring is frequently the presentation of respiratory or cardiac disorders, while apnoea may be the presentation of a great many disorders such as septicaemia, meningitis, gastrointestinal obstruction or heart disease.

SURFACTANT DEFICIENCY

The respiratory distress syndrome caused by inadequate surfactant production is mainly a disease of the preterm infant. However, it can occur in term infants, particularly those of diabetic mothers or after caesarean section without labour.

Affected infants may require mechanical ventilation and intensive care. The classical clinical presentation is an infant with tachypnoea, subcostal and intercostal recession and nasal flaring which becomes progressively worse over the first 60 h after birth, and a chest X-ray showing a ground glass appearance with air bronchograms. It can be associated with pneumothorax, bronchopulmonary dysplasia (BPD) and intracerebral haemorrhage although in more mature infants it normally resolves without sequelae. The combined use of antenatal corticosteroids and surfactant modify the illness, improving survival and reducing the rates of complication such as pneumothorax and intracerebral haemorrhage but have little effect on reducing the incidence of BPD.

CONGENITAL PNEUMONIA

Congenital pneumonia is a relatively common problem associated with a variety of microorganisms. The infant presents with respiratory distress and a chest X-ray shows patchy inconsistent shadowing. Treatment is with antibiotics and intensive care as required.

MECONIUM ASPIRATION

Inhalation of meconium before or during delivery can be an extremely severe problem if pulmonary hypertension with reduced lung perfusion and severe hypoxaemia develop. Meconium may block large and/or small airways and lead to a ventilatory deficit. Although meconium aspiration may be apparent at birth, severe disease may present an hour or more later and it is important that babies suspected of having aspirated are carefully observed.

Treatment of meconium aspiration complicated pulmonary hypertension requires expert intensive care. Early surfactant administration may be beneficial, high-frequency oscillatory ventilation and the administration of nitric oxide reduce mortality. When other measures fail extracorporeal membrane oxygenation should be considered.

TRANSIENT TACHYPNOEA OF THE NEWBORN

Transient tachypnoea of the newborn is due to delayed reabsorption of lung liquid which leads to a moderate degree of intracostal recession and tachypnoea. In the preterm infant this can lead to marked respiratory distress, but in a term baby needing high inspired oxygen concentrations other causes of respiratory distress should be excluded.

BRONCHOPULMONARY DYSPLASIA

This is a chronic condition affecting up to 50% of infants born at 26 weeks or less. Premature delivery, pre- and postnatal inflammation and infection, ventilation, oxygen and poor nutrition are among the many factors contributing to the development and persistence of BPD. The underlying problem is an arrest in alveolar and peripheral vascular development. The severity is variable ranging from the need for supplementary oxygen for several weeks to prolonged respiratory support with a ventilator or continuous positive airways pressure and death. A small proportion of babies are discharged home on supplementary oxygen; most outgrow the need by 12 months of age. All babies born prematurely have an increased risk of respiratory illness within the first few years of life. This is increased in the group with BPD and respiratory problems may persist into adult life.

Cardiac disorders

Some form of congenital heart disease affects between 7 and 9 per 1000 live births of whom approximately one quarter will present in the newborn period. Fetal anomaly ultrasound can detect many lesions; antenatally, however, some are more difficult to diagnose (see Chapter 17).

Cardiac disease in the newborn baby presents in five main ways:

CYANOSIS DUE TO REDUCED PULMONARY BLOOD FLOW

The commonest causes are transposition of the great arteries (TGA), right to left shunts such as Tetralogy of Fallot and pulmonary or tricuspid atresia. Administration of 100% oxygen fails to increase arterial saturation and a chest X-ray may show oligaemia. Tachypneoa may occur; however, respiratory distress is often not a prominent feature of the presentation whereas cyanosis may be profound. A measurement of blood gases is mandatory both to the diagnosis and as a measure of the baby's condition: metabolic acidosis is an ominous sign. For those presenting in the neonatal period immediate treatment is required to prevent the ductus arterious from closing with transfer to a specialist paediatric cardiac centre.

CARDIORESPIRATORY DISTRESS DUE TO INCREASED PULMONARY BLOOD FLOW

Left to right shunting though septal defects with a consequent increase in pulmonary blood flow decreases the compliance of the lung leading to chest recession and tachypnoea. The homeostatic response to this shunt is fluid retention, leading to congestive cardiac failure with a large liver and oedema. Infants with large left to right shunts are not particularly hypoxaemic except when cardiac failure is severe. The commonest cause of large left to right shunts are large ventricular septal defect, atrioventricular septal defects and patent ductus arteriosus.

CYANOSIS AND CARDIORESPIRATORY DISTRESS

Infants in whom mixing between systemic and pulmonary circulations is impaired can present with breathlessness and cyanosis. Complex conditions such as transposition of the great arteries may lead to this presentation.

SHOCK SYNDROME DUE TO LOW CARDIAC OUTPUT

The clinical picture of shock is a desperately ill infant with generalized pallor, cyanosis, cool peripheries and weak or absent pulses. Breathing is laboured or gasping, and the infant is hypotonic. Neonatal shock is usually due to major sepsis, significant blood loss or major interruption to the circulation such as hypoplastic left heart syndrome, severe coarctation of the aorta or complex cardiac defects. Shock can also be part of the later natural history of other cardiac defects. Causes of significant blood loss in the newborn baby are given in Table 11.4.

Table 11.4 Blood loss in newborn infants

Before and during delivery	Fetomaternal transfusion
	Fetofetal transfusion in twins
	Rupture of umbilical cord vessels
	Abnormal vessels – varices, aneurysm or vasa praevia
	Normal vessels – precipitate delivery
	Rupture of placental vessels
	Placenta praevia (abruptio placenta)
After delivery	External blood loss
	Cord stump
	Gastrointestinal – haematemesis and melaena
	Skin injury – bruising and incisions
	Internal blood loss
	Cephalohaematoma
	Suboponeurotic haemorrhage
	Intraventricular, subarachnoid and subdural
	Liver or spleen – rupture and subcapsular

THE ASYMPTOMATIC MURMUR

Murmurs are common in newborn infants and are frequently innocent. A low-amplitude-ejection systolic murmur is audible in some 60% of normal newborn infants. It is normally best heard over the pulmonary area and may be due to a ductus arterious that has not fully closed or a pulmonary artery branch flow murmur which disappears before 6 months of age. Innocent murmurs are systolic, short, localized and may change. Infants may develop murmurs when unwell, because of increased cardiac output or reopening of the ductus arterious. Other causes of asymptomatic murmurs in the newborn period include septal defects, aortic or pulmonary stenosis and Tetralogy of Fallot. A thorough search for other signs of cardiac disease should be made and an expert opinion arranged where appropriate. It is important to remember that the mention of a heart murmur can strike panic into even the calmest of parents and the situation needs to be handled with great tact. Rapid definitive diagnosis by echocardiography is the mainstay of successful management.

Neurological disorders

NEONATAL ENCEPHALOPATHY

Neonatal encephalopathy can be caused by hypoxia ischaemia due to birth asphyxia but also by other conditions including metabolic disorders and infections. These conditions should be excluded before a confident diagnosis of hypoxic ischaemic encephalopathy due to birth asphyxia can be accepted.

Table 11.5 Classification of severity of hypoxic ischaemic encephalopathy in the term newborn

Clinical features	Severity of encephalopathy		
	Mild	Moderate	Severe
Level of consciousness	Hyperalert	Lethargic	Stuporous, comatose
Muscle tone	Normal	Mild hypotonia	Flaccid
Seizures	None	Common	Interactable
Intracranial pressure	Normal	Normal	Elevated
Primitive reflexes			
Suck	Weak	Weak or absent	Absent
Moro	Strong	Weak	Absent
Autonomic function	Generalized sympathetic activity	Generalized parasympathetic activity	Both systems depressed
EEG findings	Normal (awake)	Early: low-voltage delta and theta Later: periodic pattern, seizures	Early: periodic pattern and suppression Later: generalized suppression
Duration	<24 h	2–14 days	Weeks

Data from Sarnat and Sarnat (1976), source from Roberton's Textbook of Neonatology 2005.

Hypoxia-ischaemia followed by resuscitation may lead to apparent recovery followed by inexorable deterioration beginning 6–8 h later and ending in severe cerebral injury. Consequently, it is frequently difficult to determine the prognosis soon after birth on clinical grounds alone. However, if asphyxia is severe or happened some time before delivery the infant will not develop spontaneous breathing; therefore, if despite advance life support there is no sign of spontaneous breathing 20 min after birth the outcome is extremely poor.

Hypoxic ischaemic encephalopathy is graded clinically using clinical signs. A frequently used grading system – that of Sarnat and Sarnat – is given in Table 11.5. Infants with grade 1 encephalopathy have a very good prognosis whereas infants with Grade 3 almost all die or are severely impaired. About half the infants with Grade 2 have severe neurodevelopmental impairment. Unfortunately a large number of infants at risk fall into Grade 2, limiting the utility of the system.

If asphyxia is suspected, further investigation is required, preferably by paediatricians specialized in neonatal neurology and with access to sophisticated equipment such as electrophysiology, magnetic resonance imaging or magnetic resonance spectroscopy. Diagnosis and an accurate guide to prognosis can then be obtained.

CEREBRAL PALSY

Cerebral palsy is a non-progressive brain syndrome which may not be apparent until after the first year of life and which cannot be confidently diagnosed at birth. Population based studies have shown that about 20% of all cases of cerebral palsy are due to birth asphyxia in the term infant, approximately one third are associated with preterm birth, and the remainder have no obvious fetal or perinatal antecedent.

CONVULSIONS

Convulsions occurring just after delivery in term infants may be due to hypoxic ischaemic encephalopathy, metabolic disorders, infections, hypoglycaemia, hypocalcaemia, hypomagnesaemia or pyridoxine deficiency. Many otherwise idiopathic fits are caused by focal cerebral infarction, which have a much better prognosis than generalized hypoxic ischaemic injury but are difficult to diagnose without magnetic resonance imaging.

BRAIN INJURY IN PRETERM INFANTS

Preterm infants are at high risk of cerebral injury and approximately 10% of infants born preterm develop significant neurodevelopmental impairment and another 10% have minor neurological lesions: two classical lesions which occur in preterm infants.

First, intracerebral haemorrhage may affect only the germinal layers or ventricles in which case the prognosis is good; however, haemorrhage into the brain parenchyma is caused by haemorrhagic infarction and this is associated with neurodevelopmental impairment.

Second, in periventricular leucomalacia there is a general loss of white matter, sometimes with cavitation. Whereas haemorrhagic parenchymal infarctions can be usually seen by cerebral ultrasonography, periventricular leucomalacia is difficult to see and is probably under diagnosed. Both these conditions seem to be becoming less common than a more subtle loss of cerebral matter; this may present as dilated cerebral ventricles on cerebral ultrasonography but is often only apparent with magnetic resonance imaging. The aetiology of this condition is poorly understood, the extremely preterm infant seems to be most at risk. The usefulness of cerebral ultrasonography alone to predict neurological prognosis in extremely preterm infants is therefore limited.

The more mature preterm infants with normal ultrasound scans at discharge from intensive care have a very low risk of neurodevelopmental impairment whereas those with definable loss of brain tissue from whatever cause have a greater than 50% chance of long-term impairment.

BRACHIAL PLEXUS INJURY

Brachial plexus injury occurs in 0.4–2.5 per 1000 live births. The commonest type, Erb's palsy, involves C5 and 6 nerve roots. The incidence has not declined over the past few decades; however, the prognosis for recovery, has improved with full recovery expected in the majority of babies with Erb's palsy. Injury to the brachial plexus results in the characteristic waiters tip position, a fracture to the clavical may also be present. Careful neurological examination is needed to determine the level of the lesion as this affects the prognosis for recovery of function; an associated Horner's syndrome is a bad prognostic sign.

Effects of maternal drug ingestion

Infants of mothers who take drugs such as opiates, cocaine, amphetamines, barbiturates, benzodiazepines and some other medical drugs may develop a withdrawal syndrome with irritability, poor feeding, apnoea and fits. The babies of mothers who have high alcohol or nicotine intake may also exhibit withdrawal. Wherever possible the mother and baby should be kept together; in many cases breastfeeding in not contraindicated. If a history of maternal drug abuse was known antenatally a plan of management can be agreed before birth and a referral to the social work team may be appropriate. Management of a baby at risk of drug withdrawal involves careful observation and skilled nursing. If withdrawal is severe treatment with opiates may be required. Naloxone should never be given to infants at risk of opiate withdrawal as it can provoke convulsions. Many labour wards no longer stock naloxone for fear it will be given inadvertently to an infant of a substance-abusing mother.

Jaundice

Jaundice beginning in the first 24 h after birth is pathological. It is usually unconjugated and the commonest causes are haemolytic anaemia or infection. Jaundice beginning on days 2–5 is commonly physiological, but unconjugated hyperbilirubinaemia may have many causes including haemolytic disease, ABO incompatability and G-6-PD deficiency.

Guidelines for the management of neonatal jaundice are derived from the belief that bilirubin levels greater than 340 mmol/l in term infants can cause deafness and kernicterus. This is based on data established when kernicterus due to severe rhesus disease was common but it has not been demonstrated that 340 mmol/l is the critical level for nervous system injury in other conditions. It is generally believed that in preterm infants critical levels are lower than this, especially if the infants have intercurrent illness, while at term higher concentrations may be tolerated without neurological deficit provided the infant does not have additional pathology such as infection or acidosis. Many authorities now advocate a more relaxed view of neonatal jaundice in a well, term infant, but haemolytic jaundice and jaundice in the sick or preterm infant should always be treated aggressively. Failure to control bilirubin levels by phototherapy should lead to urgent exchange transfusion.

Conjugated hyperbilirubinaemia signifies liver disease and requires urgent specialist investigation. These infants may be at risk of complications such as significant bleeding and neurological damage.

Hypoglycaemia

Blood glucose concentration is only one measure available of metabolic fuel and in term infants who are able to produce and utilize ketones, it is not easy to define an unequivocal level at which the baby is at risk of the neurological sequelae of hypoglycaemia. Authorities differ, but a pragmatic solution is to consider term infants with two consecutive blood glucose levels below 2 mmol/l or a single blood glucose level below 1 mmol/l in need of intervention. The blood glucose must be measured using an accurate device as commercial test strips are not adequate for making the diagnosis of hypoglycaemia.

Conditions commonly associated with transient low blood glucose are hypothermia, infection, prematurity, intrauterine growth retardation and maternal diabetes. Some infants develop transient hyperinsulinaemia, particularly infants of diabetic mothers with poor antenatal control or those with severe rhesus disease. Rare causes include the Beckwith-Wiedemann syndrome and metabolic defects such as cortisol deficiency, galactosaemia and other enzyme defects of glycogenolysis, gluconeogenesis or fatty acid β oxidation. Preterm infants are much less able to mount a ketotic response and hypoglycaemia should be treated promptly.

Treatment is initially to give calories in the form of milk or as intravenous glucose infusion. Rapid bolus injections of concentrated glucose solutions (20–50%) are not recommended. If hypoglycaemia persists investigations, including insulin measurements, are required.

Infections

Newborn infants are particularly prone to perinatal infection; risk factors include low-birthweight infants, prolonged ruptured membranes, maternal fever or chorioamnionitis. Iatrogenic infection is problematic for those undergoing intensive care; the presence of indwelling cannulae, central venous lines and invasive mechanical ventilation increase the risk. Organisms responsible for later neonatal infection frequently come from the skin or gut. Breastfeeding helps promote normal gut flora and reduces the risk of acquired neonatal infections. Adherence to good hand-washing practices by all staff, parents and visitors can significantly reduce the risk of acquired infection.

SEPTICAEMIA

The signs of systemic sepsis are non-specific. Infants may present with apnoea, bradycardia or cyanotic episodes; poor feeding is a common association. They may be lethargic and hypotonic and they are hyper or hypothermic. Sepsis frequently presents as a metabolic acidosis or shock and occasionally causes petechial skin rash or severe jaundice.

Organisms which commonly cause infection in the newborn period are group B streptococci, and gram-negatives such as *Escherichia coli* or Klebsiella. The prolonged use or multiple changes of antibiotics in the antenatal period may increase the risk of infection with resistant organisms. Rapid treatment with antibiotics, immediate resuscitation and, frequently, mechanical ventilation is required. Investigations include chest X-ray, blood cultures, urine culture, and examination and culture of the placenta. A lumbar puncture is performed once the baby is stable and will tolerate the procedure. The mortality of infants who develop septicaemia in the neonatal period is high with a significant number of survivors developing subsequent impairment.

GROUP B STREPTOCOCCUS INFECTION

Mortality due to maternal colonization by Group B streptococcus (GBS) is reduced by antibiotic therapy to the mother during labour and early treatment of infants with evidence of infection. About 2% of infants of colonized mothers develop infections, and 70% of these manifest risk factors at birth such as preterm labour, prolonged rupture of the membranes or meconium stained liquor. Urgent antibiotic therapy is indicated for these infants. Well infants shown by surface cultures to be colonized, do not require treatment. Recurrent GBS infection can occur but more commonly GBS infection can occur later in infancy when meningitis is the presenting problem.

MENINGITIS

Signs of meningitis in newborn infants are non-specific with a bulging fontanelle; opisthotonos and seizures occur late in the disease. Meningitis usually presents as septicaemia and can be complicated by cerebral oedema, cerebral infarction, brain abscess or deafness. Common causal organisms are GBS and *E. coli*. *Listeria monocytogenes* is a rare cause of perinatal infection in the United Kingdom.

URINARY TRACT INFECTION

Urinary tract infections may present as jaundice, vomiting, poor feeding or septicaemia. The main cause is believed to be spread of blood-borne organisms to the kidney during septicaemia. Further investigation is essential as 35–50% are associated with urinary tract abnormalities such as vesico-ureteric reflux or ureterocele. Breastfeeding offers a significant degree of protection.

EYE INFECTION

The majority of sticky eyes are not infected but are due to a blocked nasolacrimal duct. In the absence of conjunctival redness or swelling investigation for infection and treatment with topical antibiotics is not required. Simple measures such as cleaning with boiled water and lacrimal duct massage suffice with symptoms usually resolving in 3–6 months. Neonatal conjunctivitis can be caused by such organisms as *Staphylococcus aureus*, *Chlamydia trachomatis*, *Haemophlus influenzae*, *Streptococcus pneumoniae* and *Neisseria gonorrhoeae*. Gonococcal ophthalmia usually presents within 24 h of delivery with profuse purulent conjunctival discharge and immediate diagnosis and treatment (systemic and topical) is required to prevent damage to the cornea.

Chlamydial ophthalmia which is now among the commonest causes of neonatal conjunctivitis presents between 5 and 12 days postnatal age; some babies infected as neonates will develop chlamydial pneumonia later in infancy. Corneal scarring is rare; 14 days systemic and topical treatment is required. The identification of either

N. gonorrhoeae or chlamydia in the baby requires referral of mother and her sexual partner for investigation and treatment.

SKIN INFECTION

Simple hygienic methods such as bathing, hand washing and routine umbilical cord care can prevent many skin infections. The infant's skin is vulnerable to infection by Staphylococci, which usually leads to small pustules or lesions but can also cause scalded skin syndrome with severe exfoliation. Staphylococcal infections should therefore be treated with antibiotics after appropriate cultures have been taken. Streptococci can also cause skin infection and both may cause systemic illness.

Infection of the umbilical cord is commonly limited to periumbilical redness with a small amount of discharge. The presence of oedema indicating cellulitis can occasionally lead to complications such as spreading cellulites of the abdominal wall, fasciitis and septicaemia and requires treatment with systemic antibiotics.

Candidiasis usually presents after the first week of life with napkin dermatitis with or without oral thrush. Topical and oral treatment is required to prevent the candidiasis returning as the gut is colonized with candidia. Maternal nipple candidial infection can occur in breastfeeding mothers.

TUBERCULOSIS

Tuberculosis is a re-emergent disease and many hospitals now offer Bacille Calmette-Guérin (BCG) immunization to newborn infants. Infants born to mothers infected with active tuberculosis should be vaccinated with isoniazid-resistant BCG vaccine and kept with the mother while both receive treatment with appropriate drugs. Breastfeeding should be encouraged. Expert advice on drug therapy is advisable as patterns of antibiotic susceptibility change over time.

TETANUS

Neonatal tetanus due to infection of the umbilical stump by *Clostridium tetanii* is the result of poor hygiene and is a distressing and severe condition with extremely high mortality. Opisthotonus and muscle spasms of the jaw and limbs are presenting features and can appear very rapidly after birth. Prevention centres on maternal vaccination during pregnancy and education to improve hygiene and change of local cultural practices.

Gastrointestinal disorders

OESOPHAGEAL ATRESIA OR TRACHEO-OESOPHAGEAL FISTULA

These conditions should be suspected when there is polyhydramnios or excessive mucous from the mouth at birth. The baby may show rapid onset of respiratory stress and cyanosis particularly after the first feed. X-ray confirms the diagnosis, the naso- or orogastric tube does not pass into the stomach. A large bore nasogastric tube should be placed in the oesophageal pouch, constant suction and regular aspiration help prevent aspiration pneumonia. Associated congenital anomalies occur in 50% or more of infants. Surgery involves division of the fistula and oesophageal repair; if primary anastomosis is not possible lengthened procedures are required before later oesophageal repair. Common long-term complications are gastro-oesophageal reflux and anastomotic stricture formation both of which may require further surgical treatment and long-term medication. Survival is usually determined by the severity of associated congenital anomalies and not the defect itself.

DIAPHRAGMATIC HERNIA

Herniation of the abdominal contents into the hemithorax leads to severe respiratory difficulties with persistent pulmonary hypertension. Most cases present with respiratory distress and cyanosis at birth. Essential early management is the passage of a large bore nasogastric tube into the stomach to prevent gaseous distension, ventilation and rapid transfer to intensive care. All these infants require tertiary level intensive care, with access to sophisticated mechanical ventilation and modern vasodilator therapy such as nitric oxide. Surgery is delayed until the infant's respiratory status has been stabilized. Survival depends on the degree of underlying pulmonary hypoplasia and the presence of associated congenital anomalies such as cardiac defects. Long-term complications include persistent gastro-oesophageal reflux and respiratory problem; neurodevelopmental problems can develop if neonatal hypoxia was severe.

ABDOMINAL WALL DEFECTS

Exopmhalos, in which part or all of the intestine and abdominal organs are in a peritoneal sack outside the abdomen, should be differentiated from gastroschisis where a congenital defect of the abdominal wall allows herniation of the abdominal contents without a peritoneal sac. The former is frequently associated with other congenital defects, while the latter is not. Urgent surgery is

Table 11.6 Frequently asked questions

	Answers
Is milk from the newborn infant's breast normal?	Normal in boys and girls
Is vaginal bleeding in girls normal?	Normal
What causes persistent sticky eye after culture and treatment of infection?	Blocked nasolacrimal duct. Will recanulate spontaneously – does not need probing
How often should a baby feed 'on demand'?	Usually about 2–4 h, but 6 h is not uncommon in healthy infants
My baby is squinting. Is this normal?	Yes, in the first week after birth
Is my breastfed baby getting enough milk?	If the baby is gaining weight properly, yes

required if the amniotic sac has broken and for gastroschisis; immediate management is to wrap the abdominal contents in a plastic wrapper taking care not to twist the bowel and disrupt its vascular supply. This should help prevent hypovalaemia due to fluid loss from the exposed bowel. A large bore nasogastric tube is passed and the baby's circulatory status constantly assessed. Hypovalaemia or excessive nasogastric output should be treated with 20 ml/kg 0.9% sodium chloride bolus intravenous infusions. The risk of hypothermia is high unless good thermal management is present from birth. Primary repair is not always possible if the abdominal cavity is not large enough to accommodate all the contents; a silo made of sterile prosthetic material is attached to the abdominal wall and the contents gradually reduced over 7–10 days. Outcomes are worse for those requiring silo treatment as infected complications are high. The long-term outcome for most with exopmhalos is determined by the presence of associated congenital anomalies. In gastroschisis 90% or more now survive. However, their postnatal course is often protracted and parenteral nutrition may be required for several weeks with its risks and complications. In addition bowel atresias and necrotizing enterocolitis may develop.

INTESTINAL OBSTRUCTION

High intestinal obstructions usually present with vomiting which may be bile stained, and this ominous sign demands urgent investigation. Plain X-ray film of the abdomen can confirm the presence of obstruction by showing a lack of air in the lower gut or a sign such as the 'double bubble' of duodenal atresia. Hypertropic pyloric stenosis does not usually present until 2–6 weeks of age.

Lower intestinal obstruction usually presents as failure to pass meconium within 24 h followed by abdominal distension with or without vomiting. Causes include Hirshprung's disease, meconium ileus due to cystic fibrosis, low bowel atresia or hypoplasia and imperforate anus. A meconium plug can sometimes mimic obstruction especially in preterm infants.

NEONATAL NECROTIZING ENTEROCOLITIS

This poorly understood inflammatory condition is primarily a condition of preterm infants and those with congenital heart disease. It presents as an acute abdomen in the days or weeks after birth and varies in severity from mild to fatal. Diagnosis is clinical, aided by characteristic X-ray changes such as air in the bowel wall or biliary tree. Treatment is conservative with cessation of enteral feeding and with antibiotics or surgery.

Common queries from parents

Many minor alterations to physiology cause alarm to parents. Some common questions and responses to them are outlined in Table 11.6 and in the absence of disease, reassurance is all that is required. It is wise to read your unit's breastfeeding policy so as not to contradict the advice given by midwives and lactation consultants.

Further reading

Rennie JM (ed) (2005) *Roberton's Textbook of Neonatology*, 4th ed. Elsevier: Philadelphia. ISBN 0443073554.

Abman SH, Fox WW & Polin RA (eds) (2003) *Fetal and Neonatal Physiology*, 3rd edn. Saunders: London. ISBN 0721696546.

Brindley S & Richmond S (2001) *Resuscitation at Birth. The Newborn Life Support Provider Manual*. UK: Resuscitation Council, ISBN 1903812011.

Levene M & Evans DJ (2005) Hypoxic-ischaenic brain injury. In: Rennie J (ed) Roberton's text of Neonatology. Elsevier: Philadelphia. 1128–48.

Lissauer T, Fanaroff AA & Weindling AM (2006) *Neonatology at a Glance*. UK: Blackwell Publishing. ISBN 0632055979.

Chapter 12: Spontaneous miscarriage

Joanne Topping and Roy G. Farquarson

Definition

The commonest early pregnancy complication of spontaneous miscarriage occurs in approximately 15–20% of all pregnancies, as recorded by hospital episode statistics. The actual figure, from community based assessment, may be up to 30%, as many cases remain unreported to hospital [1]. The great majority occur early before 12 weeks gestation, while mid trimester loss, between 12 and 24 weeks, occurs less frequently and constitutes <3% of all pregnancy outcomes.

The clinical assessment of every pregnancy loss history demands clarification of pregnancy loss type and accurate classification, whenever possible. The traditional grouping of all pregnancy losses prior to 24 weeks as 'abortion' may have had pragmatic origins, but it is poor in terms of definition and makes little sense. Increasing knowledge about early pregnancy development, with the more widespread availability of serum Beta HCG (human chorionic gonadotrophin) measurement, the advent of high resolution ultrasound and a clearer description of gestational age at pregnancy loss make for a more sophisticated assessment of miscarriage history. The advent of these important information milestones has neither been fully realized nor incorporated into clinical event description for mainstream article publication.

The emergence of the Early Pregnancy Unit (EPU) in many hospitals has addressed the need for a dedicated clinical area for the diagnosis of miscarriage and patient support at a distressing time [2]. With the establishment of an EPU network, it becomes more important that a standardized diagnostic classification system be employed for accurate and reproducible reporting of ultrasound findings and clinical outcomes so that direct comparisons between units can be readily made and understood for both research and audit purposes.

The most recent Confidential Enquiry into Maternal Deaths conclusively demonstrates that mortality from ectopic pregnancy has not declined and is still on the increase compared to rates described 10 years ago [3]. As the EPU represents the most likely point of ectopic pregnancy diagnosis, the importance of standardized reporting of very early pregnancy changes requires a robust approach following recent recommendations [4].

Diagnosis

Role of ultrasound

The first demonstration of an intrauterine pregnancy by means of transvaginal ultrasound was reported in 1967 [5]. Major improvements in ultrasound resolution since then have revolutionized the assessment and management of early pregnancy problems. For instance, longitudinal study of early pregnancy development can be made in terms of viability and growth in the same patient (Table 12.1).

Ultrasound plays a major role in maternal reassurance, where fetal cardiac activity is seen and is pivotal in the assessment of early pregnancy complications, such as vaginal bleeding [6]. However, there are limits to ultrasound resolution of normal early pregnancy development. Expert advice concludes that the diagnosis of an empty gestation sac can only be made when the mean gestation sac diameter is greater than 20 mm (Fig. 12.1), and that the crown–rump length must be 6 mm or greater before one can say for certain that fetal heart activity is absent (Fig. 12.2). If measurements are below these thresholds a repeat transvaginal ultrasound examination after at least a week should be offered [7]. Ultrasound features such as a sac that is much smaller than expected from a certain last menstrual period; a sac that is low in the uterus or the presence of fetal bradycardia are strongly suggestive but not diagnostic of impending miscarriage [8]. In addition, the possibility of incorrect dates should always be remembered by the alert clinician. Wherever possible, the term 'missed abortion' should be replaced by 'delayed miscarriage' [9].

As ultrasound findings are not diagnostic in a significant number of women with early pregnancy failure,

Table 12.1 Ultrasound features in early pregnancy

Gestational age	Anatomical landmarks	Comments
4 weeks 2 days	Eccentrically placed gestational sac GSD 2–3 mm	
5th week	Double decidual sign (DDS)	Results from approximation of d.capsularis and d.vera
5th week	GSD 5 mm Yolk sac (YS)	Confirms intrauterine pregnancy (IUP)
6th week	GSD 10 mm Embryo 2–3 mm Cardiac activity	
7th week	GSD 20 mm Head and trunk distinguishable	GSD > 20 mm If no yolk sac poor prognosis
8th week	GSD 25 mm Limb buds Midgut herniation Rhomboncephalon	
9th week	Choroid plexus, spine limbs	
10th week	Cardiac chambers, Stomach, bladder Skeletal ossification	
11th week	Gut returning Most structures identified	

Association of Early Pregnancy Units Guidelines (www.earlypregnancy.org.uk).

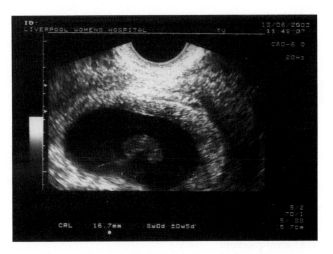

Fig. 12.2 This fetus was inert when scanned, it is very flexed and has a maximum crown–rump length of 16.7 mm. No fetal heart activity could be demonstrated. The findings are in keeping with a silent miscarriage.

many units now measure various biochemical parameters, which are used within the context of diagnostic models to predict pregnancy outcome [10]. Similar models have been designed to predict the success of expectant management of failing pregnancies both intrauterine and ectopic. To use this approach effectively one requires access to the results of biochemical parameters within 24–48 h. This is feasible for HCG and in some cases progesterone, but not at present for inhibin A and insulin growth factor binding protein 1, which at present can only be recommended within a research setting.

The impact of a diagnosis of a miscarriage should not be underestimated. The RCOG recommends 'Early intrauterine death should be regarded as of equal significance to fetal death occurring at a later stage.' It is therefore important that within an area where early pregnancy scans are performed, there is a quiet room for counselling, and staff working within this setting should have training in the emotional aspects of early pregnancy loss.

Classification

There has been a plea to classify pregnancy losses according to the gestation at which they occur and detail the event, for example, intrauterine fetal death at 8 weeks gestation (Table 12.2). In this way, possible pathophysiological mechanisms may be postulated and studied. Historically, clinicians have grouped all pregnancy losses that occur at a gestation prior to theoretical viability under the umbrella of 'abortion'.

Between 1 and 2% of fertile women will experience recurring miscarriage (RM) [11]. Recently, among researchers in the field of RM, it has been recognized that

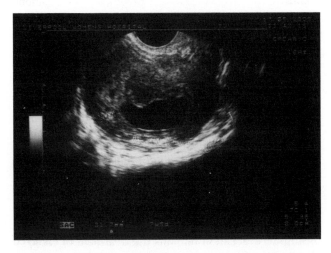

Fig. 12.1 An empty gestations sac with mean sac diameter 31.7 mm. The sac has an irregular contour and internal structures are seen within the sac.

Table 12.2 Revised nomenclature of early pregnancy events

Avoid	Prefer
Egg	Oocyte
Fetus	Ultrasound based definition to include fetal heart activity and/or crown–rump length >10 mm
Embryo	Absence of fetus definition
Spontaneous abortion	Spontaneous miscarriage
Early pregnancy loss	Pregnancy loss of <12 weeks gestation
Recurrent abortion/ Habitual abortion	Recurrent miscarriage consisting of three early consecutive losses or two late pregnancy losses
Medical abortion	Termination of pregnancy
Menstrual abortion	Biochemical pregnancy loss
Preclinical abortion	
Early embryonic demise	Empty sac
Anembryonic pregnancy	
Missed abortion	Delayed pregnancy loss
Embryonic death	Fetal loss
Late abortion	Late pregnancy loss between 12 and 24 weeks gestation
Hydatidiform mole/ partial mole/ molar pregnancy	Gestational trophoblastic disease (complete or partial)
Preclinical embryo loss	Biochemical pregnancy loss
Heterotopic pregnancy	Intrauterine plus Ectopic pregnancy (e.g. tubal, cervical, ovarian, abdominal)
Trophoblast regression	Biochemical pregnancy loss
Threatened abortion	Bleeding in early pregnancy
Pregnancy test	Serum/urine level of human chorionic gonadotrophin (HCG)
No identifiable pregnancy on ultrasound with positive blood/urine HCG	Pregnancy of unknown location (PUL)

Words NEVER used: Abortion, habitual, preclinical.

the classification of pregnancy loss is more complex as the developing pregnancy undergoes various important stages, and different pathology at the time of pregnancy loss is exhibited at these different stages. As the majority of RM cases following investigation are classified as idiopathic, it is generally accepted that within the idiopathic group there is considerable heterogeneity and it is unlikely that one single pathological mechanism can be attributed to their RM history. Furthermore, there is considerable debate about cause and association as the exact pathophysiological mechanisms have not been elucidated. Current research is directed at theories related to implantation, trophoblast invasion and placentation, as well as factors which may be embryopathic.

Modern classification of pregnancy loss type

The revision of early pregnancy nomenclature is both desirable and essential in raising the standard of reporting. To improve the accuracy of observational studies it is desirable to present a clear and consistent description of the pregnancy event that is universally understood by the clinician. It is essential to have a clear classification of pregnancy loss type to differentiate between fetal (late) or empty sac (early) loss events (Table 12.3). For randomized controlled treatment trial reports, there is a strong argument for mandatory karyotyping of all pregnancy losses where supportive pharmacologic intervention is employed. This is because a false treatment 'failure' may be ascribed to a lethal trisomy or triploid karyotype. Recent data testify to significant observations that are observed when these karyotype outcome measures are included [12–16].

It is understandable that a modernized classification system cannot answer every clinical scenario but the adoption of revised terminology is a better way forward than persisting with an antiquated description that precedes the universal use of transvaginal ultrasound findings or serum HCG levels.

Management of miscarriage
Surgical evacuation

If a woman in the earlier months is labouring under aflooding, no obvious danger attending, the less you actively interfere the better. If the womans life is in jeopardy practice more vigorous may be required

Since the nineteenth century, surgical evacuation of the uterus has been the standard treatment offered by gynaecologists to those requiring treatment following first-trimester miscarriage. This approach was based on an assumption that retained tissue increase the risk of infection and haemorrhage. However, surgical evacuation was introduced at a time when high rates of retained products and infection with ensuing morbidity and mortality were likely to be due to the high numbers of illegal terminations of pregnancy and the absence of any antibiotic medication.

The incidence of septic miscarriage has dramatically fallen in the United Kingdom following the introduction of the 1967 abortion act.

Surgical evacuation remains the treatment of choice if bleeding is excessive; vital signs are unstable or infected tissue is retained. Fewer than 10% of women experiencing a miscarriage fall within these categories [17]. However,

Table 12.3 Pregnancy loss classification

Type of loss	Typical gestation (weeks)	Fetal heart activity	Principal ultrasound finding	Beta HCG level
Biochemical loss	<6	Never	Unknown location	Low then fall
Early pregnancy loss	6–8	Never	Empty sac	Initial rise then fall
Late pregnancy loss	>10	Lost	Crown–rump length and fetal heart activity identified	Rise then static or fall

many women when offered treatment options will still choose surgical evacuation as it offers an immediate termination of the pregnancy and allows women to schedule treatment around work and childcare commitments.

If surgical evacuation is to be used, suction curettage is the method of choice as this is associated with fewer complications [18]. Serious complications including uterine perforation, cervical tears, intrauterine adhesions and haemorrhage should be included on all patient information leaflets and clearly stated on all surgical consent forms prior to operation. In all cases where surgical evacuation is the treatment option consideration should be given to the use of a cervical priming agent.

Over the past decade alternative management options (expectant and medical) have been developed and many women prefer the option of a treatment without the attendant risks associated with a surgical procedure.

EXPECTANT MANAGEMENT

Expectant management often results in absorption of retained tissue with little associated bleeding. For those women managed in general practice expectant management has long been the treatment of choice.

It is likely that at least 74% of non-viable pregnancies would miscarry successfully without intervention [19]. Observational and controlled trials of expectant management of miscarriage show wide variations in reported efficacy. Factors affecting the success rate were the type of miscarriage, duration of follow-up and whether clinical or ultrasound features were used for review. The clinical dilemma is therefore which patients are suitable for expectant management.

When ultrasound assessment of the uterine cavity is suggestive of retained products with an antero-posterior diameter of 15 mm or less genuine retained products are less likely to be confirmed histologically, hence such cases are best managed expectantly. These women are said to have suffered a complete miscarriage. One study showed that 98% of women treated expectantly following a scan report of complete miscarriage had an uneventful recovery [20].

A non-randomized study [21] provided detailed information about short-term complications. Women with complete miscarriage were managed expectantly, whereas those showing retained products of conception on ultrasonography were treated surgically. Short-term complications occurred in 3% of those managed expectantly and 6% after surgery. The latter group suffered complications of uterine perforation, cervical laceration and in one case hysterectomy.

Nielsen and Hahlin [22] published the first randomized controlled trial which compared expectant management with surgical evacuation. The inclusion criteria were women with either inevitable or incomplete abortion and they reported similar success rates and complications in both groups. Further large-scale observational data demonstrated spontaneous resolution in 91% for incomplete miscarriage, 76% for fetal loss and 66% for empty sac pregnancy loss among 1096 consecutive patients treated conservatively [23]. A similar outcome was confirmed in a patient choice study of 545 women using continued ultrasound surveillance [24] Completed miscarriage rates are higher in those patients who have bleeding at the time of diagnosis [25] and those who have detectable intervillous pulsatile blood flow on scan [26].

This data suggests that expectant management is the treatment of choice for complete miscarriage and a valid option for the management of incomplete miscarriage. Success rates for silent miscarriages are lower.

MEDICAL MANAGEMENT

Several pharmacologic agents, capable of inducing abortion, have become available in the last 20 years. Medical termination of pregnancy is now well recognized as an effective treatment option. It was thus a logical progression to use these drugs in the management of miscarriage.

Mifepristone blocks the progesterone receptors, reversing the influence of progesterone during pregnancy. As a result, there is an influx of leukocyte and red cells into the decidua followed by the release of prostaglandins and cytokines [27]. Addition of a synthetic prostaglandin E1 analogue results in powerful contractions, which supplement those induced by the withdrawal of progesterone. This process closely mimics events in a spontaneous miscarriage.

The use of medical management in cases of incomplete miscarriage may show no great benefit over conservative management [28]. However, in the management of silent miscarriage there is a significant advantage. One randomized clinical trial demonstrated 80% success with vaginal misoprostol compared to 16% in the placebo arm [29].

The two commonly used prostaglandin analogues are gemeprost and misoprostol. As misoprostol is cheaper, does not require refrigeration and can be given in different dosages by different routes, it is the most commonly used in recent published studies. Research seems to indicate that although oral or sublingual misoprostol is effective, the vaginal route of administration appears to give maximum efficacy with least side effects. An increase in misoprostol dosage appears to achieve a slightly higher success rate but with an increased risk of side effects (mainly gastrointestinal).

Mifepristone may be used to induce cervical change and is usually given orally, followed 36–48 h later by one of the prostaglandin analogues. Mifepristone has been given in doses ranging from 200 mg to 600 mg; however, studies have demonstrated that the lower dosage has similar efficacy but with a significant reduction in side effects, mainly nausea and vomiting [30].

The selection of women with silent miscarriage based on gestation and initial B-HCG level may increase the success of medical treatment [31]. Although some centres offer medical management as an outpatient procedure, in most studies a significant number of women require parenteral analgesia [32].

The treatment option should take into account the patient's symptoms, type of miscarriage, volume of retained tissue and patient choice. A patient choice study reported treatment preferences for future miscarriage in women with a miscarriage randomized to either expectant or surgical management [33]. Women who were managed according to their own treatment choice held onto their initial treatment preference (expectant versus surgical 84 and 88%, respectively). In patients who have no strong preference impartial advice on success rates and potential risks should be given and the patient allowed to make her own decision.

At present we do not have any specific investigation which will help predict which miscarriages can be successfully treated by either the medical or expectant route.

It is very important whichever treatment option is chosen that the psychological impact of miscarriage on the patient is not overlooked. It is impossible to provide all women who miscarry with counselling appointments due to the high frequency with which pregnancy loss occurs. It is, however, important that they have contact details for the hospital and also information on local or national support groups such as the 'Miscarriage Association'. The development of EPUs has helped address some of the patient's needs and it is essential that they are staffed by personnel who are knowledgeable and dedicated to the field of early pregnancy care.

References

1. Everett C (1997) Incidence and outcome of bleeding before the 20th week of pregnancy: prospective study from general practice. *Br Med J* **315**, 32–4.
2. Twigg J, Moshy R, Walker JJ & Evans J (2002) Early pregnancy assessment units in the United Kingdom: an audit of current clinical practice. *J Clin Excell* **4**, 391–402.
3. Early Pregnancy Confidential Enquiry into Maternal and Child Health (2004) *Why Mothers Die: 2000–2002*. Executive summary, p. 13. London: RCOG Press.
4. Kirk E, Condous G & Bourne T (2004) Ectopic pregnancy deaths: what should we be doing? Hosp Med **65**, 657–60.
5. Kratochwill A & Eisenhut L (1967) Der fruheste nachweis der fatalen herzaction durch ultrscall. Gerburtsh Frauenheilk **27**, 176–80.
6. Jauniaux E, Kaminopetros P & El-Rafaey H (1999) Early pregnancy loss. In: Rodeck CH & Whittle MJ (eds) *Fetal Medicine*. Edinburgh: Churchill Livingstone, 835–47.
7. Royal College of Obstetricians and Gynaecologists (1995) *Guidance and Ultrasound Procedures in Early Pregnancy*. London: RCOG Press.
8. Chittacharoen A & Herabutya Y (2004) Slow fetal heart rate may predict pregnancy outcome in first-trimester threatened abortion. *Fertil Steril* **82**, 227–9.
9. Hutchon DJ & Cooper S (1997) Missed abortion versus delayed miscarriage. *Br J Obstet Gynaecol* **104**, 73.
10. Elson J & Jurkovic D (2004) Biochemistry in diagnosis and management of abnormal early pregnancy. *Curr Opin Obstet Gynecol* **16**, 339–44.
11. Stirrat GM (1990) Recurrent miscarriage: definition and epidemiology. *Lancet* **336**, 673–5.
12. Morikawa M, Yamada H, Kato EH, Shimada S, Yamada T & Minakami H (2004) Embryo loss pattern is predominant in miscarriages with normal chromosome karyotype among women with repeated miscarriage. *Hum Reprod* **19**, 2644–7.
13. Philipp T, Philipp K, Reiner A, Beer F & Kalousek DK (2003) Embryoscopic and cytogenetic analysis of 233 missed abortions: factors involved in the pathogenesis of developmental defects of early failed pregnancies. *Hum Reprod* **18**, 1724–32.
14. Stephenson MD, Awartini KA & Robinson WP (2002) Cytogenetic analysis of miscarriages from couples with recurring miscarriage: a case-control study. *Hum Reprod* **17**, 446–51.
15. Levine JS, Branch DW & Rauch J (2002) The antiphospholipid syndrome. *N Engl J Med* **346**, 752–63.
16. Bricker L & Farquharson RG (2002) Types of pregnancy loss in recurrent miscarriage: implications for research and clinical practice. *Hum Reprod* **17**, 1345–50.
17. Ballagh SA, Harris HA & Demasio K (1998) Is curettage needed for an uncomplicated incomplete abortion? *Am J Obstet Gynecol* **179**, 1279–82.

18. Verkuyl DA (1993) Suction versus conventional curettage in incomplete abortion: a randomised controlled trial. *S Afr Med J* **83**, 13–5.
19. Schauberger CW, Mathiason MA & Rooney BL (2005) Ultrasound assessment of first-trimester bleeding. *Obstet Gynecol* **105**(2), 333–8.
20. Rulin MC, BornsteinSG & Campbell JD (1993) The reliability of ultrasonography in the management of spontaneous abortion, clinically thought to be complete: a prospective study. *Am J Obstet Gynecol* **168**, 12–5.
21. Cheung LP, Sahota DS, Haines CJ & Chang AMZ (1998) Spontaneous abortion: short term complications following either conservative or surgical management. *Aust N Z J Obstet Gynaecol* **38**, 61–4.
22. Nielsen S & Hahlin M (1995) Expectant management of first-trimester spontaneous abortions. *Lancet* **345**, 84–6.
23. Luise C, Jermy K, May C *et al.* (2002) Outcome of expectant management of spontaneous first trimester miscarriage: observational study. *Br Med J* **324**, 873–5.
24. Sairam S, Khare M, Michailidis *et al.* (2001) The role of ultrasound in the expectant management of early pregnancy loss. *Ultrasound Obstet Gynecol* **17**, 506–9.
25. Wieringa-de Waard M, Bindels PJ, Vos J, Bonsel GS, Stalmeier PF (2004) *J Clin Epidemiol* **57**, 167–73.
26. Schwarzler P, Holden D, Neilsen S, Hahlin M, Sladkevicus P & Bourne TH (1999) The conservative management of first trimester miscarriages and the use of colour Doppler sonography for patient selection. *Hum Reprod* **14**, 1341–5.
27. Baird DT (2000) Mode of action of medical methods of abortion. *J Am Med Womens Assoc* **55**(3 Suppl), 121–6.
28. Shelley JM, Healy D & Grover S (2005) A randomised trial of surgical, medical and expectant management of first trimester spontaneous miscarriage. *Aust N Z J Obstet Gynaecol* **45**(2), 122–7.
29. Wood SL & Brain PH (2002) Medical management of missed abortion : a randomised clinical trial. *Obstet Gynecol* **99**(4), 563–6.
30. Coughlin LB, Roberts D, Haddad NG & Long A (2004) Medical management of first trimester miscarriage (blighted ovum and missed abortion): is it effective? *J Obstet Gynaecol* **24**(1), 69–72.
31. Gronlund A, Gronlund L, Clevin L, Andersen B, Palmgren N & Lidegaard O (2002) Managementof missed abortion: comparison of medical treatment with either mifepristone + misoprostol 0r misoprostol alone with surgical evacuation. A multi-center trial in Copenhagen county, Denmark. *Acta Obstet Gynecol Scand* **81**(11), 1060–5.
32. El–Refaey H, Hinshaw K, Henshaw R, Smith N & Templeton A (1992) Medical management of missed abortion and anembryonic pregnancy. *Br Med J* **305**(6866), 1399.
33. Wieringa-de Waard M, Bindels PJ, Vos J, Bonsel GS, Stalmeier PF & Ankum WM (2004) Patient preferences for expectant management vs. surgical evacuation in first-trimester uncomplicated miscarriage. *J Clin Epidemiol* **57**, 167–73.

Further reading

Royal College of Obstetricians and Gynaecologists (www.rcog.org.uk).
Miscarriage Association (www.miscarriageassociation.org.uk).
Association of Early Pregnancy Units (www.earlypregnancy.org.uk).
European Society of Human Reproduction and Embryology Early Pregnancy Group (www.earlypregnancy.com).
Ectopic Pregnancy Trust (www.ectopic.org).
Confidential Enquiries into Maternal and Child Health 2004 (www.cemach.org.uk).

Chapter 13: Recurrent miscarriage

Raj Rai

Recurrent miscarriage (RM), the accepted definition of which is three or more consecutive miscarriages, is relatively uncommon – affecting about 1 to 2% of couples who conceive. Three strands of evidence support the contention that RM is a distinct clinical entity rather than one which occurs purely by chance alone. First, the observed incidence of RM is significantly higher than that expected by chance alone (0.4%); second, a woman's risk of miscarriage is directly related to the outcome of her previous pregnancies [1]; and third, in contrast to sporadic miscarriage, women with RM tend to lose pregnancies with a normal chromosome complement, suggesting the presence of a persistent underlying cause for pregnancy loss among these women [2,3].

Despite major advances in our understanding of the aetiology of RM over the last 20 years, even after comprehensive investigation, no cause for pregnancy failure is identified in approximately 50% of couples. This has led to the situation where women with RM have been, and continue to be, subjected to investigations and treatments based on anecdotal evidence, historical beliefs and the personal prejudices of their clinicians [4]. This chapter aims to provide a comprehensive, evidence-based approach to the investigation and treatment of RM while at the same time highlighting new avenues of research.

Aetiology

Genetic

PARENTAL CHROMOSOME ABNORMALITIES

On the basis of conventional Geisma banding techniques, a parental structural chromosome abnormality is identified in between 3 and 5% of couples with RM. The most common abnormality is a balanced or reciprocal translocation. While carriers of a balanced reciprocal translocation are phenotypically normal, abnormal segregation at meiosis leads to between 50 and 70% of their gametes and hence embryos being unbalanced. Twice as many females compared with males are identified as carrying a structural chromosome abnormality. This is most likely due

Table 13.1 Contemporary investigative screen for recurrent miscarriage

Male and female parental blood karyotypes
Lupus anticoagulant
IgG and IgM anticardiolipin antibodies
Factor V genotype
Factor II genotype
Activated protein C resistance
Pelvic ultrasound to determine ovarian morphology and uterine anatomy
Early follicular phase FSH
Insulin resistance status

to structural abnormalities among males being associated with sterility. While translocations have been reported for all chromosomes in a variety of combinations, the clinical miscarriage rates and subsequent pregnancy outcome for different abnormalities have not been reported.

Until recently, little active treatment could be offered to those with a parental karyotype abnormality other than referral to a genetic counsellor for informed advice regarding the prognosis for a future pregnancy. This has changed with the introduction of *in vitro* fertilization (IVF) and pre-implantation genetic diagnosis (PGD), in which fluorescent in situ hybridization (FISH) is used to infer the genetic status of an embryo from a single cell biopsied three days after fertilization. However, before embarking on this treatment avenue it should be recognized that the live birth rate/cycle for those with a reciprocal translocation undergoing PGD is lower than would be hoped – between 29%/oocyte retrieval rising to 38%/embryo transfer [5]. This has to be compared to the live birth rate among those with a reciprocal translocation who persevere with spontaneous conception where the chance of a successful pregnancy, even after three miscarriages, is between 50 and 65% [6] (Table 13.1).

FETAL ANEUPLOIDY

Aneuploidy (trisomy or monosomy) is the most commonly identified chromosome abnormality in humans and fetal aneuploidy is the single most common cause of miscarriage. Approximately 30% of all miscarriages are trisomic and a further 10% are due to either sex-chromosome monosomy or polyploidy.

The incidence of fetal trisomy rises with increasing age of the mother, whereas sex-chromosome monosomy and polyploidy do not. The hypothesis of a 'limited oocyte pool' in which the effect of age is due to a relative scarcity of oocytes at optimal stages of maturation has been advanced [7]. In support of this hypothesis, women who have lost at least one trisomic fetus have been reported to have a diminished ovarian reserve and to enter the menopause at an earlier age compared to those with no such history [8].

It is possible that some women with RM are more prone to hetero-trisomy (recurrence of a different trisomy subsequent to a trisomic pregnancy). Rubio *et al.* [9], using FISH to screen the embryos of couples with RM undergoing IVF, reported a significantly higher incidence of abnormal embryos (70%) compared with an age matched control group with no history of RM.

ENDOCRINOPATHIES

Many cases of RM have been thought to be secondary to an underlying endocrine defect. However, the search for such a defect has proven elusive.

Interest has traditionally centred on the concept of deficient secretion of progesterone by the corpus luteum leading to early miscarriage. This has come to be termed the luteal phase defect which has been reported to be present in between 23 and 60% of women with RM. The diagnosis of a luteal phase defect is based on luteal phase progesterone levels and endometrial biopsies in non-fertile cycles. This is not reliable as there is low concordance between endocrine and histological variables in consecutive cycles. Moreover, pre-conceptual hormone profiles are similar among pregnancies that are successful and those that end in miscarriage [10].

Historically, progestational agents have been used from early post-conception in an attempt to prevent miscarriage. This practice is not supported by the results of two meta-analyses of the use of progesterone to reduce the miscarriage rate among women with sporadic miscarriage [11,12]. It should be noted, however, that a subgroup analysis among women with unexplained first trimester RM suggests that progesterone use in the first trimester may be of benefit.

Well-controlled diabetes is not a risk factor for RM. While the prevalence of thyroid auto-antibodies are increased among women with RM, the prospective live-birth rate among women with RM who have thyroid antibodies is similar to that of those who do not have these antibodies [13].

Of more interest is the relationship between polycystic ovaries (PCO), the various endocrinopathies associated with the polycystic ovarian syndrome (PCOS) and RM.

The prevalence of PCO, using established ultrasound criteria, is significantly higher among women with RM (40%) compared to those with an uncomplicated reproductive history. It has previously been thought that hypersecretion of luteinizing hormone (LH) is causal of pregnancy loss both among women undergoing assisted conception and those conceiving spontaneously. This is no longer held to be the case. A prospective randomized study reported that suppression of endogenous LH followed by ovulation induction did not decrease the miscarriage rate [14]. As important, women who hypersecreted LH and who did not have their endogenous LH suppressed had an excellent live birth rate in later untreated pregnancies.

Attention is now focused on the relationship between PCOS, insulin resistance and pregnancy loss. Impairment of insulin metabolism is a prominent feature of the syndrome and appears to play a key pathogenetic role precipitating the cascade of other disorders associated with PCOS. Insulin resistance has been reported to be associated with a higher rate of miscarriage among women with PCOS undergoing ovulation induction compared to those not insulin resistant. Recent studies report that the insulin-sensitizing agents, such as metformin, reduce hyperinsulinemia, reverse the endocrinopathy of PCOS and normalize endocrine, metabolic and reproductive function. Retrospective studies report that metformin use during pregnancy is associated with a significant reduction in the miscarriage rate among women with PCOS [15]. This effect of metformin, however, remains to be tested in a large prospective placebo-controlled study of a well-defined cohort of women with RM.

ANTIPHOSPHOLIPID SYNDROME

Over the last decade the antiphospholipid syndrome (APS), also known more recently as Hughes Syndrome, has emerged as the most important treatable cause of RM.

Antiphospholipid antibodies (aPL) are a family of approximately 20 auto-antibodies directed against negatively charged phospholipids-binding proteins. Of this family of antibodies, only the lupus anticoagulant (LA) and the anticardiolipin antibodies (aCL) have been shown to be of reproductive significance. The reproductive criteria for the diagnosis of APS are shown in Table 13.2 [16].

Prevalence studies have reported that 15% of women with RM have persistently positive tests for either LA and/or aCL and hence have a diagnosis of APS [17]. In

Table 13.2 Contemporary reproductive criteria for the diagnosis of antiphospholipid syndrome

One or more unexplained deaths of a morphologically normal fetus at or after the 10th week of gestation
One or more premature births of a morphologically normal fetus before 34 weeks gestation
Three or more consecutive unexplained miscarriages before the 10th week of gestation

After Wilson *et al.* (1999) *Arthritis Rheum.* **42**, 1309–11.
Together with persistently positive tests for either lupus anticoagulant and/or IgG/IgM anticardiolipin antibodies.

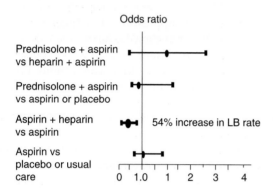

Fig. 13.1 Meta-analysis of treatments for aPL-associated pregnancy loss. After [21].

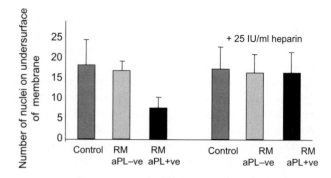

Fig. 13.2 Antiphospholipid antibodies impair extra-villous trophoblast invasion. This is restored by unfractionated heparin. RM, recurrent miscarriage; aPL, antiphospholipid antibodies.

future untreated pregnancies, women with APS have a miscarriage rate as high as 90% [18]. The majority of miscarriages occur in the first trimester of pregnancy after the establishment of fetal cardiac activity.

Pregnancy failure associated with APS has traditionally been ascribed to thrombosis of the uteroplacental vasculature. Indeed, placental thrombosis and infarction are seen in phospholipid pregnancies but these findings are neither universal nor specific to aPL pregnancy losses. Not withstanding this, two randomized studies which used aspirin in combination with heparin as thromboprophylactic agents reported a significant increase in the live birth rate from 40% with aspirin alone to 70% with aspirin together with heparin [19,20]. These results have been confirmed in a meta-analysis (Fig. 13.1) [21].

More recently, advances in our understanding of early pregnancy development and of aPL biology have challenged the primacy of thrombosis as the underlying pathology of pregnancy loss in APS. *In vitro* studies report that aPL (1) impair signal transduction mechanisms controlling endometrial cell decidualization; (2) increase trophoblast apoptosis; (3) decrease trophoblast fusion and (4) impair trophoblast invasion (Fig. 13.2) [22]. Interestingly, the effects of aPL on trophoblast function are reversed, at least *in vitro*, by low molecular weight heparin.

THROMBOPHILIC DEFECTS

Pregnancy is a hypercoaguable state secondary to both an increase in the levels of certain coagulation factors and a simultaneous decrease in both the levels of anticoagulant proteins and fibrinolysis. The evolutionary advantage of this response is to counteract the inherent instability associated with haemochorial placentation. The hypothesis has been advanced that some cases of recurrent miscarriage and later pregnancy complications are due to an exaggerated haemostatic response during pregnancy leading to thrombosis of the uteroplacental vasculature and subsequent fetal demise. This hypothesis is supported by both histological data reporting that microthrombi are a common finding in the placental vasculature of women with recurrent miscarriage and by prospective studies reporting an increased prevalence of thrombophilic abnormalities among women with recurrent miscarriage.

The first prevalence studies of coagulation abnormalities among women with a history of adverse pregnancy outcome appeared in the mid-1990s. Since this time, numerous publications have reported the prevalence of individual coagulation defects among women with recurrent miscarriage to be either similar to or increased when compared with controls. As far as the genetic thrombophilic defects are concerned, two meta-analyses report that only maternal carriage of either the Factor V (Leiden) G1691A or the Factor II (prothrombin) G20210A mutations are associated with RM (Fig. 13.3) [23,24].

Analagous to concepts on aPL-associated pregnancy failure, we have escaped from the restrictive concept of pregnancy loss associated with thrombophilic defects being due to thrombosis to now emphasizing the non-coagulant actions of thrombin. Thrombin has an important role in cell signalling (acting via protease activating receptors). Excess thrombin generation, as seen in hypercoaguable states, impairs decidualization of the endometrium and increases trophoblast apoptosis.

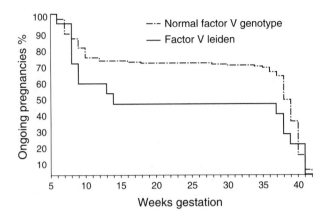

Fig. 13.3 Survival plot of the outcome of untreated pregnancies among women with recurrent miscarriage who carry the Factor V Leiden mutation and those with a Normal Factor V genotype.

Immune dysfunction

IMMUNE RESPONSE IN PREGNANCY

Traditionally, pregnancy from an immunological perspective, has been viewed as a conflict between the semi-allogenic fetus and the mother in which fetal survival is dependent on suppression of the maternal immune response. However, it is clear that while lymphocyte function does indeed change during pregnancy, there is no generalized suppression of the maternal immune response. Indeed, the concept of immunization of the mother, for example with paternal white blood cells, in order that she may mount a protective immune response to prevent rejection of the genetically dissimilar fetus has been refuted by randomized therapeutic studies [25].

Contemporary concepts in reproductive immunology now emphasize the co-operative nature of the interaction between individual cells and molecules of the immune system and the fetus in governing pregnancy outcome. In particular, interest is currently focused on the relationship between Natural Killer (NK) cells and reproductive failure.

Natural Killer cells are lymphocytes which are part of the innate immune system. The NK cells may be divided into those found in peripheral blood and those present in the uterine decidua. There are important phenotypic and functional differences between NK cells present at the two sites. Unlike peripheral blood NK cells, uterine NK cells have little killing ability. Micro-array analysis combined with flow cytometric and RT-PCR studies have demonstrated that the phenotype of uNK cells is different from that of NK cells in peripheral blood [26]. Hence, it may be erroneous to extrapolate data examining peripheral blood NK cells to implantation failure and RM.

While some have advocated the use of glucocoritcoids as adjuvant therapy in women with raised peripheral NK cell levels, there is no evidence base to support this.

Indeed, glucocorticoids themselves during pregnancy are associated with an increased risk of preterm delivery secondary to rupture of membranes and the development of pre-eclampsia and gestational diabetes [27]. Importantly, glucocorticoid receptors are present in the stromal compartment of the endometrium thus suggesting they play an important role in decidualization. The effect of exogenous glucocorticoid therapy on the endometrial gene expression profile during decidualization has not been examined.

The cytokine response at the maternal–fetal interface is also the subject of current investigation. This response may be broadly divided into being either a predominantly Th-1 type response (characterized by the production of interleukin 2, interferon-γ and tumour necrosis factor-β) or a Th-2 type response (characterized by the production of interleukins -4, -6 and -10). It has been suggested that normal pregnancy is the result of a Th-2 type cytokine response which allows the production of blocking antibodies to mask fetal trophoblast antigens from immunological recognition by a maternal Th-1 cell-mediated cytotoxic response [28]. In contrast, women who recurrently miscarry tend to produce a predominantly Th-1 type response both in the period of embryonic implantation and during pregnancy [29]. Immuno-modulation of the cytokine response during early pregnancy represents an important future avenue of research for therapeutic trials.

Structural uterine abnormalities

The prevalence and reproductive implications of uterine anomalies in the general population have not been clearly established. Hence, it is difficult to assess the contribution that congenital uterine anomalies make to RM. The prevalence of uterine anomalies among women with RM has been reported to range between 1.8% and 37.6% [30]. This wide range reflects the differences in criteria and techniques used for diagnosis and the fact that available studies have included women with two, three or more miscarriages at both early and late stages of pregnancy. A recent retrospective review of reproductive performance in patients with untreated uterine anomalies has suggested that these women experience high rates of miscarriage and preterm delivery [31]. Open uterine surgery is associated with post-operative infertility and carries a significant risk of uterine scar rupture during pregnancy. These complications are less likely to occur after hysteroscopic surgery but no randomized trial assessing the benefits of surgical correction of

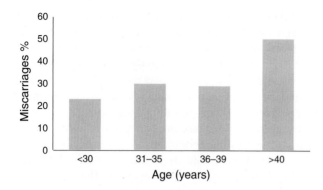

Fig. 13.4 Outcome of index pregnancy is related to maternal age.

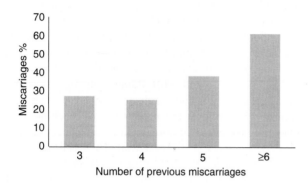

Fig. 13.5 Outcome of index pregnancy is related to number of previous miscarriages.

uterine abnormalities on pregnancy outcome has been performed.

Management of unexplained recurrent miscarriage

A significant number of couples investigated for recurrent miscarriage will have no cause identified to account for their pregnancy losses. While this is a frustrating situation for both patient and clinician, the prospective live-birth rate of women who are aPL negative is good [32]. The main determinants of future pregnancy outcome are the maternal age and the number of previous miscarriages she has had (Figs 13.4 and 13.5). A woman less than 38 years of age who has had less than five consecutive first trimester miscarriages and who is aPL negative has a 65% chance of her next pregnancy being successful with supportive care alone. While the scientific basis for the benefit of supportive care in early pregnancy remains to be elucidated, it is possible that elevated stress hormones (e.g. catecholamines and cortisol) may be able to reduce fetal vascularization and oxygen supply and thereby induce miscarriage.

References

1. Regan L, Braude PR & Trembath PL (1989) Influence of past reproductive performance on risk of spontaneous abortion. *Br Med J* **299**(6698), 541–5.
2. Sullivan AE, Silver RM, LaCoursiere DY, Porter TF & Branch DW (2004) Recurrent fetal aneuploidy and recurrent miscarriage. *Obstet Gynecol* **104**(4), 784–8.
3. Stephenson MD, Awartani KA & Robinson WP (2002) Cytogenetic analysis of miscarriages from couples with recurrent miscarriage: a case-control study. *Hum Reprod* **17**(2), 446–51.
4. Rai R, Clifford K & Regan L (1996) The modern preventative treatment of recurrent miscarriage. *Br J Obstet Gynaecol* **103**(2), 106–10.
5. Braude P, Pickering S, Flinter F & Ogilvie CM (2002) Preimplantation genetic diagnosis. *Nat Rev Genet* **3**(12), 941–53.
6. Carp H, Feldman B, Oelsner G & Schiff E (2004) Parental karyotype and subsequent live births in recurrent miscarriage. *Fertil Steril* **81**(5), 1296–301.
7. Warburton D (1989) The effect of maternal age on the frequency of trisomy: change in meiosis or in utero selection? *Prog Clin Biol Res* **311**, 165–81.
8. Kline J, Kinney A, Levin B & Warburton D (2000) Trisomic pregnancy and earlier age at menopause. *Am J Hum Genet* **67**(2), 395–404.
9. Rubio C, Simon C, Vidal F *et al.* (2003) Chromosomal abnormalities and embryo development in recurrent miscarriage couples. *Hum Reprod* **18**(1), 182–8.
10. Wilcox AJ, Weinberg CR, O'Connor JF *et al.* (1998) Incidence of early loss of pregnancy. *N Engl J Med* **319**(4), 189–94.
11. Goldstein P, Berrier J, Rosen S, Sacks HS & Chalmers TC (1989) A meta-analysis of randomized control trials of progestational agents in pregnancy. *Br J Obstet Gynaecol* **96**(3), 265–74.
12. Oates-Whitehead RM, Haas DM & Carrier JA (2003) Progestogen for preventing miscarriage. *Cochrane Database Syst Rev* **4**, CD003511.
13. Rushworth FH, Backos M, Rai R, Chilcott IT, Baxter N & Regan L (2003) Prospective pregnancy outcome in untreated recurrent miscarriers with thyroid autoantibodies. *Hum Reprod* **15**(7), 1637–9.
14. Clifford K, Rai R, Watson H, Franks S & Regan L (1996) Does suppressing luteinising hormone secretion reduce the miscarriage rate? Results of a randomised controlled trial. *Br Med J* **312**(7045), 1508–11.
15. Glueck CJ, Wang P, Goldenberg N & Sieve-Smith L (2002) Pregnancy outcomes among women with polycystic ovary syndrome treated with metformin. *Hum Reprod* **17**(11), 2858–64.
16. Rai RS, Clifford K, Cohen H & Regan L (1995) High prospective fetal loss rate in untreated pregnancies of women with recurrent miscarriage and antiphospholipid antibodies. *Hum Reprod* **10**(12), 3301–4.
17. Rai RS, Regan L, Clifford *et al.* (1995) Antiphospholipid antibodies and beta 2-glycoprotein-I in 500 women with recurrent miscarriage: results of a comprehensive screening approach. *Hum Reprod* **10**(8), 2001–5.

18. Wilson WA, Gharavi AE & Piette JC (2001) International classification criteria for antiphospholipid syndrome: synopsis of a post-conference workshop held at the Ninth International (Tours) aPL Symposium. *Lupus* **10**(7), 457–60.

19. Rai R, Cohen H, Dave M & Regan L (1997) Randomised controlled trial of aspirin and aspirin plus heparin in pregnant women with recurrent miscarriage associated with phospholipid antibodies (or antiphospholipid antibodies). *Br Med J* **314**(7076), 253–7.

20. Kutteh WH (1996) Antiphospholipid antibody-associated recurrent pregnancy loss: treatment with heparin and low-dose aspirin is superior to low-dose aspirin alone. *Am J Obstet Gynecol* **174**(5), 1584–9.

21. Empson M, Lassere M, Craig JC & Scott JR (2002) Recurrent pregnancy loss with antiphospholipid antibody: a systematic review of therapeutic trials. *Obstet Gynecol* **99**(1), 135–44.

22. Bose P, Black S, Kadyrov M *et al.* (2005) Heparin and aspirin attenuate placental apoptosis *in vitro*: implications for early pregnancy failure. *Am J Obstet Gynecol* **192**(1), 23–30.

23. Rey E, Kahn SR, David M & Shrier I (2003) Thrombophilic disorders and fetal loss: a meta-analysis. *Lancet* **361**(9361), 901–8.

24. Kovalevsky G, Gracia CR, Berlin JA, Sammel MD & Barnhart KT (2004) Evaluation of the association between hereditary thrombophilias and recurrent pregnancy loss: a meta-analysis. *Arch Intern Med* **164**(5), 558–63.

25. Scott JR (2003) Immunotherapy for recurrent miscarriage. *Cochrane Database Syst Rev* **1**, CD000112.

26. Koopman LA, Kopcow HD, Rybalov B *et al.* (2003) Human decidual natural killer cells are a unique NK cell subset with immunomodulatory potential. *J Exp Med* **198**(8), 1201–12.

27. Laskin CA, Bombardier C, Hannah ME *et al.* (1997) Prednisone and aspirin in women with autoantibodies and unexplained recurrent fetal loss. *N Engl J Med* **337**(3), 148–53.

28. Wegmann TG, Lin H, Guilbert L & Mosmann TR (1993) Bidirectional cytokine interactions in the maternal-fetal relationship: is successful pregnancy a TH2 phenomenon? *Immunol Today* **14**(7), 353–6.

29. Raghupathy R, Makhseed M, Azizieh F, Omu A, Gupta M & Farhat R (2000) Cytokine production by maternal lymphocytes during normal human pregnancy and in unexplained recurrent spontaneous abortion. *Hum Reprod* **15**(3), 713–8.

30. Salim R, Regan L, Woelfer B, Backos M & Jurkovic D (2003) A comparative study of the morphology of congenital uterine anomalies in women with and without a history of recurrent first trimester miscarriage. *Hum Reprod* **18**(1), 162–6.

31. Grimbizis GF, Camus M, Tarlatzis BC, Bontis JN & Devroey P (2001) Clinical implications of uterine malformations and hysteroscopic treatment results. *Hum Reprod Update* **7**(2), 161–74.

32. Clifford K, Rai R & Regan L (1997) Future pregnancy outcome in unexplained recurrent first trimester miscarriage. *Hum Reprod* **12**(2), 387–9.

Chapter 14: Ectopic pregnancy

Davor Jurkovic

Introduction

First descriptions of ectopic pregnancy in England date back to 1731 when Gifford described implantation of a pregnancy outside the uterine cavity. Charles Meigs provided particularly vivid descriptions of severe cases of ectopic pregnancy in the mid-nineteenth century, when ectopic pregnancy was considered to be a rare, but universally fatal condition. With the improvements in surgical techniques at the turn of the twentieth century ectopic pregnancy became curable [1]. However, it was still considered a very serious problem with high mortality rates. This perception has changed only recently with the increased ability to establish the diagnosis of ectopic pregnancy non-invasively in women with minimal clinical symptoms. Although there has been a massive increase in the incidence of ectopic pregnancy in recent years, the mortality of the disease has been static [2]. Therefore the main challenge in modern clinical practice is to identify and treat as early as possible cases of ectopic pregnancy with the potential to cause serious morbidity and death, and at the same time to minimize interventions in those destined to be resolved without causing any harm.

Epidemiology and aetiology

Over the past 30 years the incidence of ectopic pregnancy has dramatically increased in most industrialized countries. The incidence of ectopic pregnancy may be expressed in various ways, for example, number of births, number of pregnancies or number of women of reproductive age may be used as a denominator. Due to difficulties in registering all pregnancies, the number of women aged 15–44 is often used as the denominator when comparing the figures from different populations. The reported annual incidence rates vary between 100 and 175 per 100,000 women aged between 15 and 44 [3]. In recent years a stabilization or even decline of ectopic rates has been noted in some countries such as Sweden and Finland [4]. The incidence in the United Kingdom has changed little in the last decade with 9.6 ectopics per 1000 pregnancies in 1991–1993 and 11.0 per 1000 pregnancies in 2000–2002 [2].

The perceived increase in the incidence of ectopic pregnancy may be due to a number of factors. The increase may be a true reflection of the larger number of cases in the population or a result of the improved sensitivity of diagnostic tests for ectopic pregnancy. In the past a significant number of ectopic pregnancies may have resolved spontaneously without being detected, which is less likely to occur in modern clinical practice. Therefore the increased incidence of ectopic pregnancy rate may be partly explained by the increased effectiveness of screening.

A number of factors have been identified, which increase individual risk of ectopic implantation. An association between increased maternal age and ectopic pregnancy has been well documented in the past. The incidence of ectopic pregnancy is three times higher in women aged 35–44 in comparison to those in the age group 15–24 [5,6]. In recent years the age at first conception has increased, which may have contributed to the increased incidence.

The observed increase in incidence of ectopic pregnancy could also be attributed to an increase in risk factors such as sexually transmitted infections. A recent meta-analysis showed that the odds of having an ectopic pregnancy are significantly higher in women with history of pelvic infection, multiple partners and early age of intercourse. Odds were particularly high in women with history of chlamydia infection [7]. Another study from Sweden also supports an association between ectopic pregnancy and preceding infection by chlamydia. These data showed that a surge in the incidence of ectopic pregnancy was preceded by a similar peak in the incidence of acute salpingitis 15 years earlier [8]. It has also been found that the reduction in the rate of chlamydia infection due to screening and treatment leads to concomitant decline in the incidence of ectopic pregnancy [4]. However, the findings from epidemiological studies may have been confounded by other factors and they should be interpreted with caution. It is possible that the temporal association between the incidence of chlamydia infection and ectopic pregnancy may actually be due to the changes in screening policies for chlamydia and continuous improvement of diagnostic methods for the detection of ectopic pregnancy.

Table 14.1 Risk factors for ectopic pregnancy

History of previous ectopic pregnancy
(IUCD) or sterilization failure
Pelvic inflammatory disease
Chlamydia infection
Early age of intercourse and multiple partners
History of infertility
Previous pelvic surgery
Increased maternal age
Cigarette smoking
Strenuous physical exercise
In utero DES exposure

All methods of contraception are effective in reducing both the number of intrauterine and extrauterine pregnancies. However, when pregnancies occur as a result of contraceptive failure the risk of ectopic pregnancy is significantly increased in women who fall pregnant after tubal sterilization or while using the intrauterine contraceptive device (IUCD), but not in women conceiving due to the failure of oral hormonal contraception or barrier methods [9].

Other factors associated with an increased risk of ectopic pregnancy are previous pelvic surgery, history of infertility, *in utero* diethylstilbestrol (DES) exposure, strenuous physical exercise and cigarette smoking. The risk of ectopic pregnancy among black women and other ethnic minorities is 1.6 times higher than the risk among white women in the United States [5].

In women with previous ectopic pregnancy the risk of recurrent ectopic pregnancy is 12–18%. The future risk increases further with every successive occurrence [10,11] (Table 14.1).

Mortality

Ectopic pregnancy remains an important cause of maternal mortality worldwide. Figures from the United States show that the incidence of ectopic pregnancy increased fourfold between 1972 and 1987. At the same time the mortality has decreased nearly sixfold from 19.6/10000 to 3.4/10000 cases. However, the absolute number of deaths has decreased by less than half from 47 to 30 cases per year [12]. In the United Kingdom both the number of ectopics and the number of deaths have been static in the last 12 years with the mortality rate at 0.4/1000 pregnancies [2]. This trend has been maintained despite a massive expansion in the services available to women with suspected early pregnancy complications over the last decade. A possible explanation is that women with the most serious forms of ectopic pregnancies, such as interstitial ectopics, are typically asymptomatic until sudden rupture accompanied by a massive internal bleeding

occurs. The lack of early warning signs prevents women seeking the semi-elective services available to them.

Pathophysiology

Any abnormality in tubal morphology or function may lead to ectopic pregnancy. In normal pregnancy the egg is fertilized in the Fallopian tube, and then it is transported into the uterus. It is believed that the most important cause of ectopic pregnancy is damage to the tubal mucosa, which could obstruct the embryo transport due to scarring. The other possibility is that a small defect in the mucosa attracts implantation in the Fallopian tube [13]. The mucosal damage may be caused by infection or surgical trauma. However, evidence of tubal damage is lacking in many cases of ectopic pregnancy. In these women the cause of ectopic pregnancy may be a dysfunction in the tubal smooth muscle activity. In general, oestrogens stimulate tubal myoelectrical activity and progesterone has an inhibitory effect. An altered oestrogen/progesterone ratio may affect tubal motility in different ways. Abnormally high oestrogen levels may cause tubal spasm, which could block transport of the embryo towards the uterine cavity. This may be an explanation for increased rates of ectopics following ovarian hyperstimulation and post-coital oral contraception. Conversely, pharmacological doses of progesterone in women using progesterone-only contraception could cause complete tubal relaxation leading to retention of the fertilized egg within the tube [14].

Embryonic abnormalities have also been studied in an attempt to explain occurrence of ectopics in the absence of tubal pathology and although the majority of tubal pregnancies are non-viable, the incidence of chromosomal defects is no higher than in samples obtained from intrauterine pregnancies [15].

Clinical presentation

The clinical presentation of ectopic pregnancy is very variable and reflects the biological potential of pregnancy to develop beyond a very early stage. This in turn is largely determined by the location of pregnancy within the tube. In general, more proximal implantation to the uterine cavity shows more advanced development. Ampullary ectopics, which represent 70% of all tubal ectopics, rarely develop beyond a very early stage and clinical symptoms of tubal abortion may be present as early as 5 weeks gestation. On the other hand one third of interstitial tubal ectopics develop in a similar way to healthy intrauterine pregnancies with evidence of a live embryo on ultrasound examination. These pregnancies tend to be clinically silent until sudden rupture occurs [16].

Most ectopic pregnancies represent a form of early pregnancy failure and the first symptom is usually brown vaginal discharge, which starts soon after the missed menstrual period. However, the amount of bleeding varies and in some women it can be quite heavy. Passage of a decidual cast may sometimes lead to an erroneous diagnosis of miscarriage. Abdominal pain is usually a late feature in the clinical presentation of ectopic pregnancy. The localization of pain is not specific and it is not unusual for women to complain of pain on the side contralateral to the ectopic. Some women may complain of period-like pain or upper abdominal discomfort. The pain is usually caused by tubal miscarriage and bleeding through the fimbrial end of the tube into the peritoneal cavity. The pain varies in intensity and does not necessarily reflect the volume of blood lost inside the abdominal cavity.

About 10–20% of ectopic pregnancies present without bleeding [17]. In a significant proportion of these cases a viable embryo is detected on ultrasound scan, which increases the risk of rupture. Pain associated with rupture tends to be more intense, with signs of peritonism on abdominal palpation. Severe rupture sometimes presents with nausea, vomiting and diarrhoea, which may resemble a gastrointestinal disorder. This confusing picture may cause a delay in the diagnosis of ectopic pregnancies. Indeed this misdiagnosis was made in more than a third of women who have died from ectopic pregnancy in the United Kingdom since 1998 [2]. Significant intra-abdominal bleeding, however, can be recognized by the typical signs of haemorrhagic shock, which include pallor, tachycardia, hypotension and oliguria.

Women with suspected early pregnancy complications have traditionally been subjected to vaginal examination including speculum and bimanual palpation. Speculum examination has very little value in the detection of ectopic pregnancy. It may help to diagnose miscarriage by the visualization of the products of conception within the cervix or vagina. Although this reduces the chance of an ectopic, it does not eliminate the possibility of a heterotopic pregnancy.

Palpation of pelvic organs is also of limited diagnostic value. Most ectopic pregnancies are very small and they cannot be felt on palpation. The assessment of the uterine size is rarely helpful and cervical excitation is not a specific sign of an ectopic [18]. Internal examination is unpleasant for pregnant woman and is often uncomfortable even in those with normal intrauterine pregnancies. One could also argue that the application of significant pressure on a tube swollen with an ectopic pregnancy during such an examination could facilitate tubal rupture and complicate the further management of ectopic pregnancy.

In modern clinical practice where ultrasound diagnostic facilities are readily available, vaginal examination in women with suspected ectopic pregnancy is of little value and it should not be routinely employed.

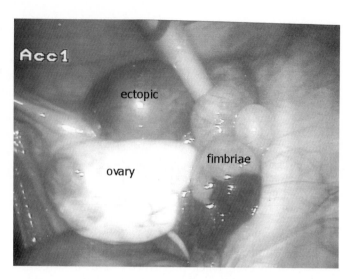

Fig. 14.1 A laproscopic view of an isthmic tubal ectopic pregnancy with bleeding from the fimbrial end of the tube. (Courtesy of Dr E. Saridogan, University College Hospital, London)

Diagnosis

Surgery

Traditionally the diagnosis of ectopic pregnancy was made at surgery and then confirmed on histological examination following salpingectomy. At laparoscopy an unruptured ectopic pregnancy typically presents as a well-defined swelling in the Fallopian tube [19] (Fig. 14.1). The diagnosis may be difficult in the presence of extensive pelvic adhesions, which impair the visualization of the tubes. Anecdotal cases of false positive and false negative laparoscopic findings have been reported, but no formal assessment of the accuracy of laparoscopy in the diagnosis of ectopic pregnancy has been published so far. Some authors have advocated the use of dilatation and curettage in the diagnosis of ectopic pregnancy. The presence of chorionic villi helps to provide some reassurance since the incidence of heterotopic pregnancy is relatively low, but as mentioned previously it does not exclude an ectopic. However, the majority of women with absent villi on curettage do not have ectopic pregnancies on subsequent laparoscopies and therefore the diagnostic value of curettage is very limited [20].

Ultrasound

With the advent of diagnostic ultrasound and the increasing use of conservative treatment, the diagnosis of ectopic pregnancy is increasingly made without the help of surgery. The sensitivity of ultrasound examination in the diagnosis of ectopic pregnancy depends on the quality

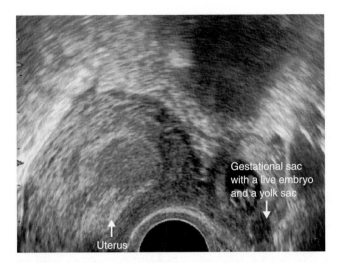

Fig. 14.2 An ultrasound image of a tubal ectopic gestational sac left of the uterus, which contained a live embryo and a yolk sac.

Table 14.2 Differential diagnosis between early intrauterine gestational sac and pseudosac

	Early gestational sac	Pseudosac
Location	Below the midline echo buried into the endometrium	Along the cavity line, between endometrial layers
Shape	Steady, usually round	May change during scan, usually ovoid
Borders	Double ring	Single layer
Colour flow pattern	High peripheral flow	Avascular

of ultrasound equipment and the experience and skill of the operator. With the use of transabdominal ultrasound, direct visualization of ectopic pregnancy is rarely possible. The only value of transabdominal ultrasound is therefore the detection of an intrauterine pregnancy in women with a clinical suspicion of ectopic. Even the diagnosis of intrauterine pregnancy is difficult to make with confidence until 6 to 7 weeks' gestation. In addition, it is almost impossible to differentiate between interstitial ectopics and intrauterine pregnancies on transabdominal scan. For these reasons transabdominal ultrasound should not be routinely used in women with a clinical suspicion of ectopic pregnancy.

Transvaginal scanning provides much clearer images of pelvic structures in comparison to transabdominal scanning. By using the transvaginal approach it is possible to palpate pelvic organs under visual control, which enables assessment of their mobility and helps to establish the source of pelvic pain. Gentle pressure applied with the tip of the probe may be used to see whether the suspected tubal ectopic moves separately from the ovary. This 'sliding organs sign' helps to avoid false positive diagnosis of ectopic pregnancy in women with a prominent corpus luteum on ultrasound scan [21]. In experienced hands, transvaginal ultrasound will detect 75–80% of clinically significant tubal ectopic at the initial examination [22]. The remaining 20–25% can be detected on follow-up visits and ultrasound should rarely fail to visualize an ectopic pre-operatively.

The morphology of ectopic pregnancy can be classified into five categories: gestational sac with a live embryo (Fig. 14.2), sac with an embryo but no heart rate, sac containing a yolk sac, an empty gestational sac and solid tubal swelling. The first three morphological types are very specific and enable a conclusive diagnosis of an ectopic to be made. The potential for false positive diagnosis is higher when the sac is empty or in cases with an inhomogeneous tubal swelling [23].

The presence of free fluid in the pouch of Douglas is a frequent finding in women with normal intrauterine pregnancies and it should not be used to diagnose an ectopic. However, the presence of blood clots is important and is a common finding in ruptured ectopics. Blood clots appear hyperechoic and irregular on the scan and they may be mistaken for bowel loops. Checking for the presence of peristalsis helps in the differential diagnosis.

In women with ectopic pregnancies bleeding within the uterine cavity may resemble an early intrauterine pregnancy ('pseudosac'). The distinction between a pseudosac and a true gestational sac may be difficult on transabdominal scan. Therefore in all women at risk of ectopic pregnancy and an empty sac on transabdominal scan a transvaginal scan should be performed in order to differentiate between the two using the criteria listed in Table 14.2 (Figs 14.3 and 14.4).

In women with intrauterine pregnancy on the scan a possibility of heterotopic pregnancy should be excluded. This is particularly the case in women who conceived after stimulation of ovulation or IVF (*in vitro* fertilization). In symptomatic women with spontaneous pregnancies it is helpful to examine the number of corpora lutea. If more than one corpus is present, a concomitant ectopic needs to be excluded.

Biochemical measurements

SERUM HUMAN CHORIONIC GONADOTROPIN

Serum human chorionic gonadotropin (hCG) measurements have traditionally been used as a secondary investigation in women with suspected ectopic pregnancy in whom ultrasound examination has failed to identify an

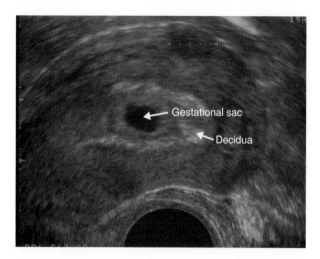

Fig. 14.3 A longitudinal section through the uterus showing a normal early intrauterine pregnancy at 5 weeks' gestation. The sac is surrounded by a well-defined layer of trophoblast tissue and thick decidua.

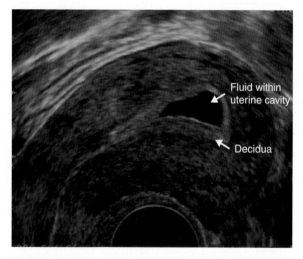

Fig. 14.4 Uterine cavity distended with fluid resembling an intrauterine pregnancy ('pseudosac') in a woman with a tubal ectopic pregnancy.

intrauterine or ectopic pregnancy. With the use of transabdominal ultrasound, a normal pregnancy could be seen in most cases when serum hCG exceeded 6500 IU/l (Third International Reference 75/537, World Health Organization) [24]. With the transvaginal ultrasound this threshold can be lowered to 1000 IU/l [25]. These observations have helped to introduce the concept of 'discriminatory hCG zone' above which a normal intrauterine pregnancy should be detectable on ultrasound scan. However, the concept of discriminatory zone is often misinterpreted in clinical practice. There are many clinicians who assume that in the absence of a visible intrauterine pregnancy on

ultrasound scan, serum hCG reading below a predefined level equals normal intrauterine pregnancy and that the reading above that level is diagnostic of an ectopic [26]. This is clearly not the case as hCG levels are often high in the aftermath of a complete miscarriage because of its long clearance half time of 24–36 h. It has also been shown that more than 50% of ectopics, which are detectable on the scan, present with hCG levels <1000 IU/l [27]. In view of this, the concept of discriminatory zone is of limited value in clinical practice and it is only useful in assessing asymptomatic women with uncertain menstrual dates.

Abnormally slow rise in serum hCG has also been used to diagnose ectopic pregnancy. In normal early pregnancy the hCG doubling time is 1.4 days before 5 weeks' gestation and 2.4 days from then until the seventh week of gestation. A prolonged hCG doubling time is an indicator of an abnormal pregnancy. However, it cannot discriminate between intrauterine miscarriages and ectopics. It has also been shown that in about 10% of ectopic pregnancies serum hCG increases at a normal rate [28].

The use of hCG to select patients for expectant, medical and surgical management of ectopic pregnancy and to assess the efficacy of treatment at follow-up visits will be discussed later.

PROGESTERONE

The progesterone production from corpus luteum is dependent on the slope of hCG increase in early pregnancy. The half-life of progesterone clearance is only 2 h compared to 24–36 h for serum hCG [29]. As a result serum progesterone levels will respond quickly to any decrease in hCG production. The progesterone measurement can therefore be used as a bioassay of early pregnancy viability. Serum progesterone <20 nmol/l reflects fast decreasing hCG levels and can be used to diagnose spontaneously resolving pregnancies with a sensitivity of 94% and specificity of 91% [27]. Progesterone levels >60 nmol/ indicate a normal increase in hCG levels, but those between 20 and 60 are strongly associated with abnormal pregnancies. In clinical practice serum progesterone measurements are particularly useful in women with a non-diagnostic ultrasound scan. Although the majority of these women have failed intrauterine pregnancies, they are usually followed up with serial hCG measurement because of the fear of missing potentially significant ectopic pregnancies. The routine measurement of serum progesterone can reliably diagnose pregnancies in regression and can reduce by 50–60% the need for follow-up scans and serial hCG measurements in pregnant women with non-diagnostic scan findings [27,29].

Management

Surgery

Surgery has been traditionally used both for the diagnosis and treatment of ectopic pregnancy. In the second half of the twentieth century laparoscopy was mostly used as a diagnostic tool and open surgery was used to treat ectopic pregnancy. With recent advances in operative laparoscopy, the minimally invasive approach has also become accepted as the method of choice to treat most tubal ectopic pregnancies. There are important advantages of laparoscopic over open surgery which include less post-operative pain, shorter hospital stay and faster resumption of social activity [30]. However, the future reproductive outcomes following laparoscopic or open surgery are not significantly different. Although the rate of recurrent ectopic is slightly lower following laparoscopic surgery, the rates of subsequent intrauterine pregnancies appear to be similar [31].

It remains unclear whether laparoscopic salpingotomy with tubal conservation offers any advantage over salpingectomy. Laparoscopic salpingotomy is usually a longer operation, with a higher risk of intraoperative and post-operative bleeding. In addition there is a 10–15% risk of persistent trophoblast following salpingotomy, which may require further surgical or medical treatment. However, data from observational studies indicate that tubal conservation results in slightly higher rates of subsequent intrauterine pregnancies [32]. Until this finding is tested in a prospective randomized trail the choice between removal of the tube and tubal conservation should be made depending on the circumstances in each individual case. At present there is a consensus that tubal conservation should be attempted if a woman desires further pregnancies and there is evidence of contralateral tubal damage at laparoscopy. In the presence of a healthy contralateral tube salpingectomy may be performed with the patient's consent [31].

Medical management

Medical management of ectopic pregnancy has grown in popularity in recent years following several observational studies which reported success rates with a single dose systemic methotrexate in excess of 90% [33]. However, the diagnosis of ectopic pregnancy was based in many cases on monitoring the dynamics of serum hCG and progesterone, rather than on direct visualization of ectopic on ultrasound scan or at laparoscopy. It is therefore possible that in a significant number of cases intrauterine miscarriages were misdiagnosed as ectopics, contributing to the high success rates. Nevertheless there are some obvious attractions of medical treatment such as the possibility

Table 14.3 Selection criteria for conservative management of ectopic pregnancy

Minimal clinical symptoms
Certain ultrasound diagnosis of ectopic
No evidence of embryonic cardiac activity
Size <5 cm
No evidence of haematoperitoneum on ultrasound scan
Low serum hCG (methotrexate <3000 IU/l; expectant <1500 IU/l)

to manage patients on an outpatient basis and avoidance of surgery. However, due to the need for prolonged follow up and increased failure rate in women presenting with higher initial hCG measurements, medical treatment is only cost effective in ectopics with serum hCG <1500 IU [34].

Selection criteria for treatment with methotrexate are usually strict and they are listed in Table 14.3. Two randomized trials which compared methotrexate to surgery showed that only one third of all tubal ectopics satisfied these criteria and were suitable for medical treatment with the success rates between 65 and 82% [35,36]. The overall contribution of methotrexate to successful treatment of tubal ectopic was between 23 and 30% while all other women required surgery. The other problem with methotrexate is the risk of tubal rupture and blood transfusion, which occurred significantly more often in women receiving methotrexate compared to those who had surgery, this emphasizes the need for a very close follow up [35]. There is also a risk of side effects such as gastritis, stomatitis, alopecia, headaches, nausea and vomiting. Disturbances in hepatic and renal function and leukopenia or thrombocytopaenia may also occur.

In view of this, the overall role of methotrexate in the management of ectopic pregnancy is limited, but it may be offered on an individual basis to highly motivated women with small unruptured ectopics and a serum hCG level of 1500–3000 IU/l, who are likely to comply with well-organized follow-up.

Expectant management

Expectant management has important advantages over medical treatment as it follows the natural history of the disease and is free from serious side effects of methotrexate. The progress of ectopic pregnancy is easier to monitor as serum hCG measurements accurately reflect trophoblastic activity of the ectopic pregnancy, with rising levels indicating an increased risk of rupture. This is different from medical treatment, which is characterized by an initial rise in serum hCG following administration of methotrexate in cases with both successful and unsuccessful outcomes. Therefore with medical treatment it is often impossible to be confident about the probability of successful treatment for up to a week following injection, which increases the risk of adverse outcomes in comparison to expectant management.

Expectant management requires prolonged follow-up and it may cause anxiety to both women and their carers. However, the main limiting factor in the use of expectant management is the relatively high failure rate and the inability to identify with accuracy the cases that are likely to fail expectant management. To minimize the risk of failure many authors have used very strict selection criteria for expectant management such as the initial hCG <250 IU [37]. The use of strict selection criteria has resulted in relatively high success rates of expectant management sometimes reaching 70–80% [38,39]. However, only a small minority of ectopics was considered suitable for expectant management resulting in a low overall contribution to successful management of tubal ectopic of only between 7 and 25%. Recent studies showed that by using more liberal selection criteria for expectant management up to 40% of all tubal ectopics may resolve spontaneously on expectant treatment [40]. This observation also reflects the increased sensitivity of modern ultrasound equipment, which enables detection of very small ectopics (Fig. 14.5). It is very likely that a large proportion of these small ectopics were undiagnosed in the

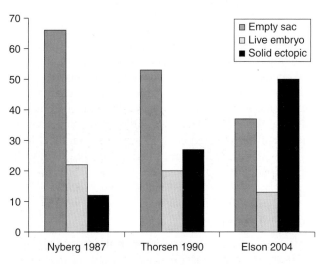

Fig. 14.5 Relative frequencies of different morphological types of ectopic pregnancies detected on ultrasound scan in the last two decades. The proportion of more severe forms such as live ectopics and well-formed gestational sacs is decreasing, while the proportion of mild forms such as small solid ectopics is increasing. This finding reflects the ability of modern equipment to detect tubal ectopics, rather than the change in the nature of the condition.

past and treated as early intrauterine miscarriages. However, the sensitivity of equipment will probably improve further in the future and it is imperative for modern practice to continue efforts to refine the selection criteria for expectant management of tubal ectopics.

According to the current literature the success of expectant management may be determined by the serum hCG levels at the initial presentation. In general, if hCG is less than 1500 IU and the ectopic pregnancy is clearly visible on ultrasound scan the success of expectant management is 60–70% [40]. The addition of the serum progesterone and morphological features of ectopics on ultrasound scan enable further refinement in the prediction of the likely success of expectant management.

Long-term fertility outcomes in women treated expectantly are similar to those treated by conservative surgery or medically. Several authors examined reproductive outcomes in women with ectopic pregnancies following successful expectant management compared to those who required surgery. They found no significant differences in the ipsilateral tubal patency rates and the rates of subsequent intrauterine and extrauterine pregnancies [41]. Therefore the main advantage of expectant management is avoidance of any intervention, rather than an improvement in the reproductive outcomes.

Fertility after ectopic pregnancy

Intrauterine pregnancy rates following ectopic pregnancy range between 50 and 70% [41]. Recurrent ectopic pregnancies occur in 6–16% of women with previous history of ectopics [42] and these women should be offered early scans in all future pregnancies to detect recurrent ectopics before complications can occur.

Non-tubal ectopics
Interstitial ectopics

The implantation of the conceptus in the proximal portion of the Fallopian tube, which is within the muscular wall of the uterus, is called an interstitial pregnancy. The incidence of interstitial ectopic is 1 in 2500–5000 live births and it accounts for 2–6% of all ectopic pregnancies [43]. Risk factors predisposing to an interstitial pregnancy are the same as those for tubal ectopics and include previous ectopic pregnancy (40.6%), assisted reproduction treatment (37.5%) and sexually transmitted infections (25%) [44]. A unique predisposing factor to interstitial pregnancy is previous ipsilateral salpingectomy.

The maternal morbidity associated with interstitial pregnancy is still high, and the maternal mortality rate of this form of ectopic pregnancy is about 2–2.5% [2].

Interstitial pregnancy remains the most difficult type of ectopic pregnancies to diagnose pre-operatively. This is partly due to lack of any symptoms prior to sudden rupture. In modern clinical practice the diagnosis of interstitial pregnancy should be made non-invasively using transvaginal ultrasound. The diagnosis is based on the visualization of the interstitial tube adjoining the lateral aspect of the uterine cavity and the gestational sac, and the presence of a continuous myometrial layer surrounding the chorionic sac [45] (Figs 14.6 and 14.7).

Ruptured interstitial pregnancy usually presents dramatically with severe intra-abdominal bleeding, which requires urgent surgery. Haemostasis can usually be achieved by removing the pregnancy tissue and suturing the rupture site. However, in cases of extreme bleeding a cornual resection or in rare cases a hysterectomy may be necessary to arrest the bleeding.

Unruptured interstitial pregnancy <12 weeks in size can be managed conservatively. Medical treatment with methotrexate should be given to all women with rising serum hCG on follow-up visit. Good results have been reported with both systemic and local methotrexate [46,47]. However, in viable interstitial pregnancies local injection under ultrasound guidance is preferable as it enables fetocide to be carried out at the same time, which increases the success rate of medical treatment. Small interstitial pregnancies with declining serum hCG levels can be managed expectantly without any intervention.

Apart from the side effects of methotrexate, the main disadvantage of conservative treatment is the time taken for the pregnancy to be fully absorbed and in larger pregnancies this may take up to a year.

Pregnancies located below the internal os – cervical and Caesarean scar ectopics

Cervical pregnancy is defined as the implantation of the conceptus within the cervix, below the level of the internal os. Caesarean scar pregnancy is a novel entity, which refers to a pregnancy implanted into a deficient uterine scar following previous lower segment Caesarean section [48]. Prior to the introduction of high resolution transvaginal scanning, the distinction between cervical and Caesarean section scar pregnancies was not possible. In older literature 33% of 'cervical' pregnancies occurred in women with a history of previous Caesarean section, which indicates that scar pregnancies probably account for a significant number of ectopics below the level of the internal os [49].

The common characteristic of both cervical and Caesarean scar pregnancies is their implantation into myometrial defects following previous intrauterine surgery (Fig. 14.8). In case of cervical pregnancy the implantation

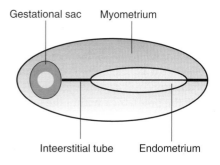

Fig. 14.6 Schematic illustration of interstitial pregnancy.

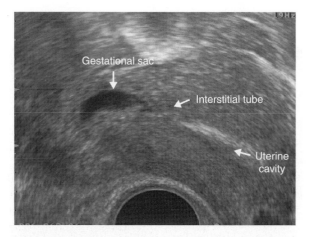

Fig. 14.7 An oblique section through the uterus showing an empty uterine cavity and the interstitial portion of the tube adjoining the cavity and an ectopic sac. The sac is completely surrounded by a myometrial mantle, which is typical of interstitial pregnancy.

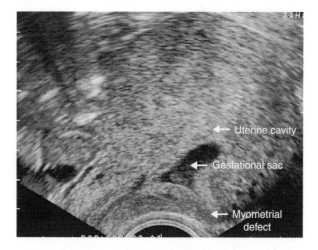

Fig. 14.8 A 7 weeks' Caesarean scar pregnancy with the gestational sac herniating into the myometrial defect.

is usually into the false passage which occurred during previous attempts at cervical dilatation. As a result of myometrial involvement surgical evacuation of cervical or Caesarean ectopics often results in serious haemorrhage. The bleeding tends to be more severe with increasing gestation. Pregnancies below the internal os are often viable and it is not unusual for Caesarean ectopics to progress to full term. In these cases women usually develop placenta praevia/accreta, which is often complicated by severe post-partum haemorrhage and peri-partum hysterectomy [50].

An attempt to remove cervical or Caesarean section pregnancy is likely to cause severe vaginal bleeding and hysterectomy rates of 40% have been described when a D&C was attempted without pre-operative diagnosis of cervical pregnancy [51]. Various additional methods directed at reducing the bleeding from the implantation site have been used in conjunction with D&C. They include: insertion of a Foley catheter into the cervix, intracervical vasopressin injection, cervical Shirodkar cerclage, transvaginal ligation of the cervical branches of uterine arteries or angiographic uterine artery embolization. The use of any of these methods in adjunction with D&C reduces the risk of hysterectomy to <5% (Fig. 14.9).

Similar to other types of ectopic pregnancy medical treatment with methotrexate or expectant management can be used in smaller non-viable cervical pregnancies. Although conservative management is successful in some cases, it is associated with prolonged vaginal bleeding which may last for many months and there is also a risk of infection and sepsis. For these reasons surgery should be used in preference for cervical/Caesarean scar ectopic except in very small cases on non-viable pregnancies which can be managed expectantly [52].

The risk of recurrence of cervical/Caesarean ectopic is low, and provided the next pregnancy is located normally within the uterine cavity, it is likely to be uncomplicated.

Ovarian pregnancy

Ovarian pregnancy is defined as the implantation of the conceptus on the surface of the ovary or inside the ovary, away from the fallopian tubes. There are no direct risk factors associated with primary ovarian pregnancy. The role of IUCD as a direct risk factor for ovarian pregnancy is unclear [53]. The role of pelvic inflammatory disease and assisted reproduction as predisposing factors is also not clear. Chance might also have played a role in some cases, as recurrent cases of ovarian pregnancy have rarely been reported.

The diagnosis of ovarian pregnancy is rarely achieved pre-operatively; hence most women are treated surgically as the diagnosis is reached only at operation [54]. On ultrasound scan a small ovarian pregnancy can be seen implanted into the ovary next to the corpus luteum Fig. 14.10.

Laparoscopy has emerged as the gold standard method for the management of most ovarian pregnancies. The technique of laparoscopic removal depends on the size and location of the pregnancy within the ovary, as well as the patients' haemodynamic status. Conservative laparoscopic surgery involves ovarian resection or aspiration of the pregnancy combined with coagulation of the implantation site using a thermocoagulator [55]. However, in cases with profuse intraoperative bleeding an oophorectomy or salpingo-oophorectomy may be necessary to achieve haemostasis.

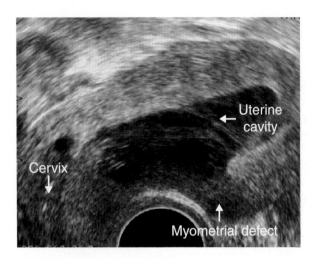

Fig. 14.9 An anterior myometrial defect is clearly visible following evacuation of a Caesarean pregnancy.

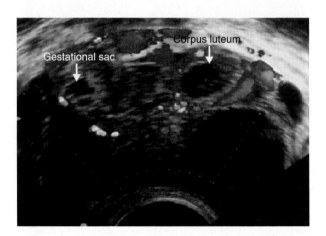

Fig. 14.10 A case of ovarian pregnancy diagnosed on ultrasound scan. The gestational sac with a distinctive trophoblastic ring is seen lateral to a cystic corpus luteum.

Abdominal pregnancy

Abdominal pregnancy is a rarity that only a few gynaecologists will encounter during their professional career. Most abdominal pregnancies are the result of re-implantation of ruptured undiagnosed tubal ectopic pregnancies. With the increasing accuracy of first-trimester transvaginal scanning it is likely the prevalence of advanced abdominal pregnancy will decrease even further in the future. The clinical and ultrasound features of an early abdominal pregnancy are very similar to tubal ectopic pregnancies. However, viable abdominal pregnancies, which progress beyond the first trimester, are typically missed on routine transabdominal scanning. Abdominal pregnancy should be suspected in women with persistent abdominal pain later in pregnancy and in those who complain of painful fetal movements. In abdominal pregnancy it is often difficult to obtain clear images of the fetus due to overlying bowel loops, there is often evidence of oligohydramnios and early intrauterine growth resriction (IUGR). Perinatal mortality is high (>40%) and the incidence of fetal malformations is also increased [56].

In women with a clinical suspicion of abdominal pregnancy a transvaginal scan should be performed to assess the uterus and establish the continuity between the cervical canal, uterine cavity and gestational sac. If pregnancy is clearly outside the uterine cavity the differential diagnosis includes abdominal pregnancy and pregnancy in an atretic non-communicating cornu of a unicornuate uterus. The visualization of both interstitial portions of the tubes favours the diagnosis of abdominal pregnancy.

Treatment of abdominal pregnancy is surgical. The timing of the intervention depends on clinical signs and patient's symptoms. In advanced abdominal pregnancies accompanied by normal fetal development diagnosed in the late second trimester termination of pregnancy may be delayed for a few weeks until the fetus reaches viability. At surgery the gestational sac should be opened carefully avoiding disruption of the placenta. The fetus should be removed, the cord cut short and the placenta should be left in situ [57]. Any attempt to remove the placenta may result in massive uncontrollable haemorrhage. Adjuvant treatment with methotrexate is not necessary and the residual placental tissue will absorb slowly over a period of many months, sometimes a few years. The placental tissue left in situ may become infected leading to the formation of a pelvic abscess, which may require drainage.

References

1. Tait RL (1884) Five cases of extrauterine pregnancy operated upon at the time of rupture. *Br Med J* 1, 1250.
2. RCOG (2004) Why mothers die 2000–2002. The Sixth Report of the Confidential Enquiries into Maternal Deaths in the United Kingdom 2000–2002. London: RCOG Press.
3. Coste J, Bouyer J, Ughetto S et al. (2004) Ectopic pregnancy is again on the increase. Recent trends in the incidence of ectopic pregnancies in France (1992–2002). Hum Reprod **19**(9), 2014–8.
4. Egger M, Low N, Davey Smith G, Lindblom B & Herrmann B (1998) Screening for chlamydial infections and the risk of ectopic pregnancy in a county in Sweden: ecological analysis. *Br Med J* **316**, 1776–80.
5. Goldner T, Lawson H, Xia Z & Atrash H (1993) Surveillance for Ectopic Pregnancy – United States, 1970–1989. CDC Surveillance summaries **42**, 73–85.
6. Westrom L, Bengtsson LPH & Mardh PA (1981) Incidence, trends and risks of ectopic pregnancy in a population of women. *Br Med J* **282**, 15–18.
7. Ankum WM, Mol BWJ, Van der Veen F & Bossuyt PMM (1996) Risk-factors for ectopic pregnancy – a meta-analysis. *Fertil Steril* **65**, 1093–9.
8. Bjartling C, Osser S & Persson K (2000) The frequency of salpingitis and ectopic pregnancy as epidemiologic markers of *Chlamydia trachomatis*. *Acta Obstet Gynecol Scand* **79**, 123–8.
9. Mol BW, Ankum WM, Bossuyt PM & Vand Derveen F (1995) Contraception and the risk of ectopic pregnancy: a meta-analysis. *Contraception* **52**, 337–41.
10. Bouyer J, Job-Spira N & Pouly JL et al. (1996) Fertility after ectopic pregnancy – results of the first three years of the *Auvergne registre*. *Contracept Fertil Sex* **24**, 475–81.
11. Maymon R, Shulman A, Halperin R, Michell A & Bukovsky I (1995) Ectopic pregnancy and laparoscopy – review of 197 patients treated by salpingectomy or salpingotomy. *Eur J Obstet Gynecol Reprod Biol* **62**, 61–7.
12. Cartwright PS (1993) Incidence, epidemiology, risk factors and etiology. In: Stovall TG, Ling FW (eds) *Extrauterine pregnancy. Clinical Diagnosis and Management*. New York: McGraw-Hill, 27–64.
13. Vasquez G, Winston RML & Brosens IA (1983) Tubal mucosa and ectopic pregnancy. *Br J Obstet Gynaecol* **90**, 468.
14. Pulkkinen MO & Talo A (1987) Tubal physiologic consideration in ectopic pregnancy. *Clin Obstet Gynecol* **30**, 164.
15. Coste J, Fernandez H & Joye N (2000) Role of chromosome abnormalities in ectopic pregnancy. *Fertil Steril* **74**, 1259–60.
16. Hafner T, Aslam N, Ross JA, Zosmer N & Jurkovic D (1999) The effectiveness of non-surgical management of early interstitial pregnancy: a report of ten cases and review of the literature. *Ultrasound Obstet Gynecol* **13**, 131–6.
17. Elson J, Tailor A, Banerjee S, Salim R, Hillaby K & Jurkovic D (2004) Expectant management of tubal ectopic pregnancy: prediction of successful outcome using decision tree analysis. *Ultrasound Obstet Gynecol* **23**, 552–6.
18. Kitchin JD, Wein RM & Nunley WC (1979) Ectopic pregnancy – current clinical trends. *Am J Obstet Gynecol* **134**, 870.
19. Beck P, Broslovsky L, GaI D & Tancer ML. (1984) The role of laproscopy in the diagnosis of ectopic pregnancy. Int J Gynaecal Obstet **22**, 307–9.
20. Lindahl B & Ahlgren M (1986) Identification of chorion vili in abortion specimens. *Obstet Gynecol* **67**, 79–81.

21. Timor-Tritsch IE & Rottem S (1987) Transvaginal ultrasonographic study of the Fallopian tube. *Obstet Gynecol* **70**, 424–8.

22. Condous G, Okaro E, Khalid A *et al.* (2005) The accuracy of transvaginal sonography for the diagnosis of ectopic pregnancy prior to surgery. *Hum Reprod* **20**, 1404–9.

23. Brown DL & Doubilet PM (1994) Transvaginal sonography for diagnosing ectopic pregnancy. *J Ultrasound Med* **13**, 259–66.

24. Kadar N, DeVore G & Romero R (1981) Discriminatory hCG zone: its use in the sonographic evaluation for ectopic pregnancy. *Obstet Gynecol* **58**, 156–61.

25. Cacciatore B, Stenman U-H & Ylostalo P (1990) Diagnosis of ectopic pregnancy by vaginal ultrasonography in combination with a discriminatory serum hCG level of 1000 IU/L (IRP). *Br J Obstet Gynecol* **97**, 904–8.

26. Pisarska MD, Carson SA & Buster JE (1998) Ectopic pregnancy. *Lancet* **351**, 1115–20.

27. Banerjee S, Aslam N, Woelfer B, Lawrence A, Elson J & Jurkovic D (2001) Expectant management of early pregnancies of unknown location: a prospective evaluation of methods to predict spontaneous resolution of pregnancy. *BJOG* **108**, 158–63.

28. Fridstrom M, Garoff L, Sjoblom P & Hillens T (1995) Human chorionic gonadotropin patterns in early pregnancy after assisted conception. *Acta Obstet Gynecol Scand* **74**, 534–38.

29. Hahlin M, Thorburn J & Bryman I (1995) The expectant management of early pregnancies of uncertain site. *Hum Reprod* **10**, 1223–27.

30. Gray D, Thorburn J, Lundorff P, Strandell A & Lindblom B (1995) A cost-effectiveness study of a randomised trial of laparoscopy versus laparotomy for ectopic pregnancy. *Lancet* **345**, 1139–43.

31. Royal College of Obstetricians and Gynaecologists (2004) The management of tubal pregnancy. Guideline 21. London: RCOG Press.

32. Bangsgaard N, Lund C, Ottensen B & Nillas I (2003) Improved fertility following conservative surgical treatment of ectopic pregnancy. *BJOG* **110**, 765–70.

33. Stovall TG & Ling FW (1993) Single-dose methotrexate: an expanded clinical trial. *Am J Obstet Gynecol* **168**, 1759–65.

34. Sowter M, Farquhar C & Gudex G (2001) An economic evaluation of single dose methotrexate and laparoscopic surgery for the treatment of unruptured ectopic pregnancy. *BJOG* **108**, 204–12.

35. Hajenius PJ, Engelsbel S, Mol BW *et al.* (1997) Randomised trial of systemic methotrexate versus laparoscopic salpingostomy in tubal pregnancy. *Lancet* **350**, 774–9.

36. Sowter MC, Farquhar CM, Petrie KJ & Gudex G (2001) A randomised trial comparing single dose systemic methotrexate and laparoscopic surgery for the treatment of unruptured tubal pregnancy. *BJOG* **108**, 192–203.

37. Cacciatore B, Korhonen J, Stenman U-H & Ylostalo P (1995) Transvaginal sonography and serum hCG in monitoring of presumed ectopic pregnancies selected for expectant management. *Ultrasound Obstet Gynecol* **5**, 297–3.

38. Ylostalo P, Cacciatore B, Sjoberg J, Kaaraianen M, Tenhunen A & Stenman U-H (1992) Expectant management of ectopic pregnancy. *Obstet Gynecol* **80**, 345–8.

39. Makinen JI, Kivijarvi AK & Irjala KMA (1990) Success of non-surgical management of ectopic pregnancy. *Lancet* **335**, 1099.

40. Elson J, Tailor A, Banerjee S, Salim R, Hillaby K & Jurkovic D (2004) Expectant management of tubal ectopic pregnancy: prediction of successful outcome using decision tree analysis. *Ultrasound Obstet Gynecol* **23**, 552–6.

41. Strobelt N, Mariani E, Ferrari L, Trio D, Tiezzi A & Ghidini A (2000) Fertility after ectopic pregnancy. *J Reprod Med* **45**, 803–7.

42. Dubuisson JB, Aubriot FX & Foulot H (1990) Reproductive outcome after laparoscopic salpingectomy for tubal ectopic pregnancy. *Fertil Steril* **53**, 1004–7.

43. Bouyer J, Coste J, Fernandez H, Pouly JL & Job-Spira N (2002) Sites of ectopic pregnancy: a 10 year population-based study of 1800 cases. *Hum Reprod* **17**, 3224–30.

44. Tulandi T & Al-Jaroudi D (2004) Interstitial pregnancy: results generated from the society of reproductive surgeons registry. *Obstet Gynecol* **103**, 47–50.

45. Ackerman TE, Levi CS, Dashefsky SM, Holt SC & Lindsay DJ (1993) Interstitial line: sonographic finding in interstitial (cornual) ectopic pregnancy. *Radiology* **189**, 83–7.

46. Hafner T, Aslam N, Ross JA, Zosmer N & Jurkovic D (1999) The effectiveness of non-surgical management of early interstitial pregnancy: a report of ten cases and review of the literature. *Ultrasound Obstet Gynecol* **13**, 131–6.

47. Jermy K, Thomas J, Doo A & Bourne T (2004) The conservative management of interstitial pregnancy. *Br J Obstet Gynaecol* **111**, 1283–8.

48. Vial Y, Petignat P & Hohlfeld P (2000) Pregnancy in a cesarean scar. *Ultrasound Obstet Gynecol* **16**, 592–3.

49. Ushakov FB, Elchalal U, Aceman PJ & Schenker JG (1996) Cervical pregnancy: past and future. *Obstet Gynecol Surv* **52**, 45–57.

50. Herman A, Weinraub Z, Avrech O, Maymon R, Ron-El R & Bukovsky Y (1995) Follow up and outcome of isthmic pregnancy located in a previous caesarean section scar. *Br J Obstet Gynaecol* **102**, 839–41.

51. Jurkovic D, Hacket E & Campbell S (1996) Diagnosis and treatment of early cervical pregnancy: a review and a report of two cases treated conservatively. *Ultrasound Obstet Gynecol* **8**, 373–80.

52. Jurkovic D, Hillaby K, Woelfer B, Lawrence A, Salim R & Elson CJ (2003) First-trimester diagnosis and management of pregnancies implanted into the lower uterine segment Cesarean section scar. *Ultrasound Obstet Gynecol* **21**, 220–7.

53. Raziel A, Golan A, Pansky M, Ron-El R, Bukovsky I & Caspi E (1990) Ovarian pregnancy: a report of twenty cases in one institution. *Am J Obstet Gynecol* **163**, 1182–5.

54. Seinera P, Di Gregorio A, Arisio R, Decko A & Crana F (1997) Ovarian pregnancy and operative laparoscopy: a report of eight cases. *Hum Reprod* **12**, 608–10.

55. Morice P, Dubuisson JB, Chapron C, De Gayffier A & Mouelhi T (1996) Laparoscopic treatment of ovarian pregnancy. *Gynecol Endo* **5**, 247–9.

56. Attapattu JAF & Menon S (1993) Abdominal pregnancy. *Int J Gynecol Obstet* **43**, 51–5.

57. Martin JN Jr, Sessums JK, Martin RW, Pryor JA & Morrison JC (1988) Abdominal pregnancy: current concepts of management. *Obstet Gynecol* **71**, 549–57.

Chapter 15: Trophoblast disease

Philip Savage and Michael Seckl

Introduction

The abnormal proliferation of gestational trophoblast tissue forms a spectrum of diseases from the usually benign partial hydatidiform mole through to the highly malignant choriocarcinoma and placental site trophoblast tumours. The biology, diagnosis and therapy of these diseases, combined with their psychological impact, makes trophoblast disease an extremely important and interesting area of gynaecological and oncology care. Despite the rarity of these illnesses, patients generally have very successful outcomes with overall cure rates in excess of 95%. Using the treatments that have been established for over 20 years, the majority of trophoblast patients including those with advanced metastatic disease can be treated with a high expectation of cure with minimal long-term toxicity.

With the effectiveness of the current medical therapies, the main developments in trophoblast disease management in the UK are now aimed at improving the supportive care. These areas include strategies for ensuring human chorionic gonadotrophin (hCG) monitoring after molar pregnancies, improvements in pathology reporting and maintaining clinical awareness for the early diagnosis of choriocarcinoma and placental site tumours.

Since 1973 the UK has had centralized surveillance, follow-up and treatment facilities and much of the content of this chapter is based on the experience from the National Trophoblast Tumour Centre at Charing Cross Hospital (CXH) in London.

Classification

The World Health Organization classification divides trophoblast disease into the premalignant partial and complete hydatidiform moles and the malignant disorders of invasive mole, choriocarcinoma and placental site tumours.

While there are some geographical and racial variations, with perhaps a higher incidence in Africa and Asia, the widely varying standards in the frequency and accuracy of pathology reporting makes comparisons difficult. However, the reported incidence of molar pregnancies in Europe and North America is in the order of 0.2–1.5 per 1000 live births although these figures are also of limited accuracy [1].

The relative risk of hydatidiform mole is highest in pregnancies at the extremes of the reproductive age group with a modestly increased incidence in teenagers (1.3-fold) but a 10-fold increased relative risk in those aged 40 and over [2].

Historically the incidence of partial and complete molar pregnancies have been reported as approximately 3:1000 and 1:1000, respectively; however, this situation may well represent an over diagnosis of partial mole (PM). Nearly 40% of partial moles referred for expert review are reclassified as either complete moles (CMs) or non-molar pathologies [3].

Premalignant pathology and presentation

Partial mole

The genetic origins of the different types of molar pregnancies are demonstrated in Fig. 15.1. PMs are triploid with two sets of paternal and one set of maternal chromosomes. Macroscopically PM often resembles the normal products of conception with an embryo initially present which usually dies by week 8–9. The histology shows less swelling of the chorionic villi than in complete mole and there are usually only focal changes. As a result the diagnosis of PM can often be missed after a miscarriage or termination.

The clinical presentation of PM is most frequently via irregular bleeding or by detection on routine ultrasound. The obstetric management is by suction evacuation and these patients should all be followed up by serial hCG measurement.

Fortunately PM rarely moves onto malignant disease with generally only one or two cases of malignant disease seen per year at CXH with an overall risk of 0.5% requiring chemotherapy after a PM [4].

Complete mole

In the majority of CMs all of the genetic material is male in origin and results from the fertilization of an 'empty'

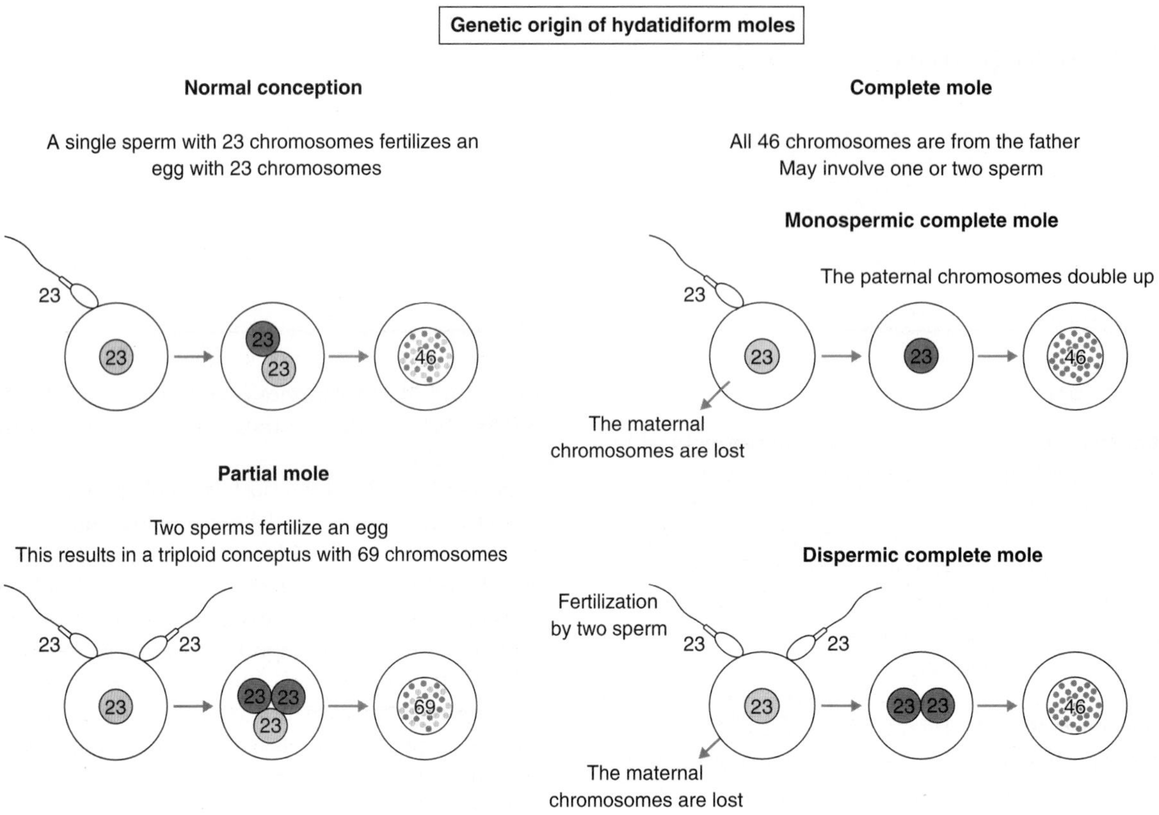

Genetic origin of hydatidiform moles

Normal conception

A single sperm with 23 chromosomes fertilizes an
egg with 23 chromosomes

Complete mole

All 46 chromosomes are from the father
May involve one or two sperm

Monospermic complete mole

The paternal chromosomes double up

The maternal
chromosomes are lost

Partial mole

Two sperms fertilize an egg
This results in a triploid conceptus with 69 chromosomes

Dispermic complete mole

Fertilization
by two sperm

The maternal
chromosomes are lost

Fig. 15.1 Genetic formation of hydatidiform moles.

oocyte lacking maternal DNA. The chromosome count is most commonly 46XX, which results from one sperm that duplicates its DNA, or less frequently 46XX or 46XY from the presence of two different sperms. On rare occasions CM can be biparental in origin and this type is associated with a high risk of further molar pregnancies.

The clinical diagnosis of CM is most often as a result of bleeding, a large for date uterus or an abnormal ultrasound. Macroscopically there is no visible foetal material although microscopically some embryonic cells can be present. The histology shows the characteristic oedematous villous stroma; however, the textbook 'bunch of grapes' appearance is only seen in the second trimester and as most cases are diagnosed earlier, this is now rarely seen. In Plate 15.1 (*facing p. 562*) the typical macroscopic appearances of a CM are shown. The obstetric management is by suction evacuation followed by serial hCG measurement and surveillance registration. In contrast to PM, CM more frequently proceeds to invasive disease with 8–20% of patients requiring chemotherapy.

REGISTRATION AND SURVEILLANCE

The majority of patients with molar pregancies will prove to have no requirement for further treatment beyond evacuation. The residual trophoblast tissue will fail to proliferate and as the cells stop growing and their numbers reduce the hCG levels fall back to normal. However, at present there is no effective prognostic system that allows distinction between the patients who after evacuation will develop invasive disease and the majority who will not. As a result all molar pregnancy patients should be registered for an hCG follow-up system. The use of this system allows the early identification of patients whose disease is continuing to proliferate, while also allowing the careful watch of patients with more slowly falling hCG, so producing minimization of unneccessary chemotherapy.

Analysis of the natural history of the illness in this surveillance phase has allowed the development of a set of guidelines that are employed to select out the patients most at risk of developing malignant disease. As shown in Table 15.1, these rules help to distinguish patients whose disease is either clearly progressing, destined to fail to remit spontaneously or those who are getting significant symptoms and so would benefit from early treatment.

The post molar pregnancy patients from the surveillance service who go on to require treatment have a cure rate approaching 100% and nearly always fall into the low-risk treatment group. Overall from the 1400 patients registered annually we give chemotherapy to approximately 8%.

Table 15.1 Post molar pregnancy surveillance patients

Indications for chemotherapy
1 Raised hCG level 6 months after evacuation (even if falling)
2 hCG plateau in three consecutive serum samples
3 hCG >20,000 IU/l more than 4 weeks after evacuation
4 Rising hCG in two consecutive serum samples
5 Pulmonary, vulval or vaginal mets unless the hCG level is falling
6 Heavy PV bleeding or GI/intraperitoneal bleeding
7 Histological evidence of choriocarcinoma
8 Brain, liver, GI mets or lung metastases >2 cm on CXR

Malignant pathology and presentation

Invasive mole (chorioadenoma destruens)

Invasive mole nearly always arises from a CM and is characterized by invasion of the myometrium, which can lead to perforation of the uterus. Microscopically invasive mole has a similarly benign histological appearance as CM but is characterized by the ability to invade in to the myometrium and local structures if untreated. Fortunately the incidence of invasive mole has fallen substantially with the introduction of routine ultrasound, the early evacuation of CMs and effective hCG surveillance.

Choriocarcinoma

Choriocarcinoma is histologically and clinically overtly malignant and presents the most frequent emergency medical problems in the management of trophoblast disease. The diagnosis most frequently follows a CM [50%], when the patients are usually in a surveillance programme but can also arise in unsupervised patients after a non-molar abortion [25%] or term pregnancy [25%]. The clinical presentation of choriocarcinoma can be from the disease locally in the uterus leading to bleeding, or from distant metastases that can cause a wide variety of symptoms with the lungs, central nervous system and liver the most frequent sites of distant disease.

The cases of choriocarcinoma presenting with symptoms from distant metastases can be diagnostically challenging. However, the combination of the gynaecology history and elevated serum hCG usually makes the diagnosis clear and so avoid biopsy which can be hazardous due to the risk of haemorrhage.

On the occasions that pathology is available the characteristic findings show the structure of the villous trophoblast but sheets of syncytiotrophoblast or cytotrophoblast cells, haemorrhage, necrosis and intravascular growth are common. The genetic profile of choriocarcinoma is a range of gross abnormalities without any specific characteristic patterns.

Placental site trophoblast tumour

Placental site trophoblast tumours (PSTTs) were originally described in 1976 [5] and are the least common type of gestational trophoblast disease forming less than 2% of all cases. PSTT most commonly follows a normal pregnancy but can also occur after a non-molar abortion or a complete molar pregnancy, and very rarely following a PM.

In contrast to the more common types of trophoblast disease which characteristically present fairly soon after the index pregnancy, in PSTT the average interval between the prior pregnancy and presentation is 3.4 years. The most frequent presentation is bleeding following amenorrhea and the hCG level, while elevated, is characteristically lower for the volume of disease than in the other types of gestational trophoblastic tumour (GTT). The tumour is diploid and arises from the non-villous trophoblast and the pathology is characterized by intermediate trophoblastic cells with vacuolated cytoplasm, the expression of placental alkaline phosphotase (PLAP) rather than hCG and the absence of cytotrophoblast and villi.

The clinical presentation of PSTT can range from slow growing disease limited to the uterus to more rapidly growing metastatic disease that is similar in behaviour to choriocarcinoma.

The role of hCG in trophoblast disease diagnosis and management

Produced predominantly by the syncytiotrophoblast cells, hCG is a glycosylated heterodimer protein consisting of the alpha and beta units held together non-covalently. However, in malignant disease a number of variants can occur including hyperglycosylated hCG, nicked hCG, hCG missing the beta subunit C terminal peptide and the free beta subunit. With the exception of a few atypical cases of PSTT, hCG is constitutively expressed by malignant trophoblast cells. The measurement of hCG allows an estimation of the tumour bulk, forms an important part of the assessment of the patient's disease risk and provides a simple method to follow the response to treatment. The hCG level can be measured by a variety of immunoassays but at present there is no internationally standardized assay and the various commercially available kits used in different hospitals can vary in their ability to detect different portions of partially degraded hCG molecules and so can give divergent results and occasional false negatives [6]. Fortunately the hCG assay used at CXH has been demonstrated to recognize all forms of hCG and can be used as reference test in difficult cases.

In the absence of tumour hCG production the serum half-life of hCG is 24–36 h; however, in the clinical situation total hCG levels characteristically show slower falls

Table 15.2 FIGO scoring system

Scores	0	1	2	4
Age	<40	≥40	–	–
Antecedent pregnancy	Mole	Abortion	Term	–
Months from index pregnancy	<4	4–6	7–13	≥13
Pre-treatment hCG	<1000	1000–10,000	1000–100,000	>100,000
Largest tumour size	<3 cm	3–5 cm	≥5 cm	–
Site of mets	Lung	Spleen, kidney	Gastro-intestinal	Brain, liver
Number of mets	–	1–4	5–8	>8
Previous chemotherapy	–	–	Single agent	Two or more drugs

as the tumour cells continue to produce some hCG as their number decreases with treatment.

Hyperglycosylated hCG

There is increasing evidence that the hyperglycosylated form of hCG, also known as invasive trophoblast antigen (ITA) may be an early and powerful indicator of the risk of disease progression. At present this test is not routinely available but when available assessment of hyperglycosylated hCG could be a helpful assay particularly in determining the course and potential need for treatment of patients with persistent low levels of hCG [7].

Prognostic factors and treatment groups

Data from the early days of chemotherapy treatment for trophoblast disease show clearly that there is a relationship between the level of elevation of hCG at presentation, the presence of distant metastases and the reducing chances of cure with single-agent chemotherapy. This relationship and the impact on treatment choice and cure rate were first codified by the Bagshawe scoring system published in 1976 [8]. Subsequently there have been a number of revisions and parallel systems introduced that are broadly similar to this original. In Table 15.2 the revised 2000 FIGO prognostic score table is shown. From assessment of these parameters, an estimate of the risk category can be obtained and patients offered initial treatment either with single-agent chemotherapy if their score is 6 or less or multiagent combination chemotherapy for scores of seven and over [9].

Low-risk disease management

Our standard treatment and the most widely used for patients with low-risk trophoblast disease is methotrexate given intramuscularly with oral folinic acid rescue following the schedule shown in Table 15.3a. The first course of treatment is administered in hospital with the subsequent

Table 15.3a Methotrexate/folinic acid treatment schedule

Day 1	Methotrexate 50 mg im at noon
Day 2	Folinic acid 30 mg po at 6 p.m.
Day 3	Methotrexate 50 mg im at noon
Day 4	Folinic acid 30 mg po at 6 p.m.
Day 5	Methotrexate 50 mg im at noon
Day 6	Folinic acid 30 mg po at 6 p.m.
Day 7	Methotrexate 50 mg im at noon
Day 8	Folinic acid 30 mg po at 6 p.m.

courses administered at home. However, patients with an hCG of >10,000 iµ/ml often stay in for 3 weeks as they have a higher risk of bleeding, particularly as the tumour shrinks rapidly with the initial chemotherapy. Bleeding usually responds well to bed rest and less than 1% of our low-risk patients have required emergency interventions such as vaginal packing, embolization or hysterectomy.

The low-risk chemotherapy treatment is usually well tolerated without much major toxicity. Methotrexate does not cause alopecia or significant nausea and myelosuppression is extremely rare. Of the side effects that do occur, the most frequent problems are from pleural inflammation, mucositis and mild elevation of liver function tests. For the low-risk patients with lung metastases visible on their chest X-rays, our policy is to add CNS prophylaxis with intrathecal methotrexate administration to minimize the risk of development of CNS disease.

The data shows that 67% of the low-risk group patients will be successfully treated with methotrexate and we monitor their disease response by twice weekly serum hCG measurement. Following normalization of the serum hCG level it is usual to continue treatment for another 3 cycles (6 weeks) to ensure eradication of any residual disease that is below the level of serological detection [10].

Patients who have an inadequate response to methotrexate therapy as shown by an hCG plateau or rise have their treatment changed to second line therapy. For this we have used either single-agent actinomycin-D, given

Table 15.3b EMA/CO chemotherapy

Week 1	
Day 1	Actinomycin-D 0.5 mg iv
	Etoposide 100 mg/m^2 iv
	Methotrexate 300 mg/m^2 iv
Day 2	Actinomycin-D 0.5 mg iv
	Etoposide 100 mg/m^2 iv
	Folinic acid 15 mg po 12 hourly × 4 doses
	Starting 24 h after commencing methotrexate
Week 2	
Day 8	Vincristine 1.4 mg/m^2 (max 2 mg)
	Cyclophosphamide 600 mg/m^2

at 0.5 mg for days 1–5 every 2 weeks if their hCG is below 100 iμ/l, or etoposide, methotrexate, actinomycind, cyclophoshamide, vincristine (EMA/CO) combination chemotherapy (Table 15.3b) if the hCG is above 100 iμ/l. More recently, with the aim of minimizing exposure to combination cytotoxicity, we have revised our hCG cut-off point from 100 iμ/l to 300 iμ/l. An individual example of the pattern of hCG levels during the course of management is shown in Fig. 15.2. This demonstrates the rise in hCG that lead to the introduction of methotrexate chemotherapy; following this the hCG initially fell rapidly but after two cycles appeared to plateau. The introduction of second line treatment with EMA/CO chemotherapy lead to a rapid fall in the hCG to normal and the discontinuation of chemotherapy after 6 weeks further treatment. Overall the survival in this group is nearly 100% and the sequential introduction of additional chemotherapy as necessary minimizes the potential long-term carcinogenic risks of excess treatment.

High-risk disease management

Historical data from before the introduction of multiagent chemotherapy schedules demonstrated that only 31% of the high-risk patients would be cured with single-agent therapy [11]. The introduction of combination chemotherapy treatments in the 1970s transformed this situation and our recent series shows a cure rate for high risk patients of 86% using EMA/CO chemotherapy [12,13]. This combination delivers a dose intense treatment with the five chemotherapy agents, delivered in two groups 1 week apart as shown in Table 15.3b. This approach to chemotherapy, rather than the more usual 3 or 4 weekly cycles used in other malignancies, appears to be the most effective approach to this rapidly proliferating malignancy. However, these drugs are fairly myelosuppressive and G-CSF (granulocyte stimulating factor) support is frequently helpful. Fortunately serious or life-threatening toxicity is rare and the majority of patients tolerate treatment without any major problems. As in the low-risk situation, treatment is continued for 6 weeks after the normalization of the hCG. In selected patients the dose of etoposide can be reduced after the hCG falls to normal, to contain the total dose exposure and so minimize the potential risk of developing secondary malignancies.

Of the high-risk patients treated with EMA/CO, approximately 17% develop resistance to this combination and require a change to second line drug treatment. In this situation we generally use the etoposide, cisplatin (EP)/EMA regimen as shown in Table 15.3c which incorporates cisplatin and a further dose of etoposide replacing the vincristine and cyclophosphamide. This treatment combined with surgery mostly to the uterus for defined areas of drug resistant disease, produces a cure rate approaching 90% in this relatively small group of patients [14].

With the aim of minimizing short-term infective risks and that of long-term bone toxicity we avoid the routine use of dexamethasone in the antiemetics, as this can be associated with both pneumocystis infection and avascular necrosis of the femoral head.

Approximately 4% of patients presenting with trophoblast disease have cerebral metastases at the time of diagnosis. In contrast to most other malignancies where cerebral metastases are associated with a very poor prognosis, trophoblast patients with CNS disease can routinely be cured of their disease. Treatment may include an initial surgical resection if the disease is superficial and then chemotherapy with modified EMA/CO containing a higher dose of methotrexate which enhances penetration into the CNS. This treatment, combined with intrathecal methotrexate administration, has produced a cure rate of 86% for patients with CNS disease who were fit enough at presentation to commence effective treatment [15].

The management of placental site trophoblast disease

The original description of placental site trophoblast disease suggested a relatively benign malignancy. However, further data demonstrated that this is a malignancy that can often metastasize but can be cured with effective therapy.

The management depends on careful staging. When the disease is limited to the uterus curative treatment can be achieved with hysterectomy alone. For patients with disseminated disease we recommend treatment with EP/EMA chemotherapy, which is continued for 6–8 weeks after the normalization of the hCG level. Following successful chemotherapy treatment we usually recommend hysterectomy. Our data for patients with PSTT treated

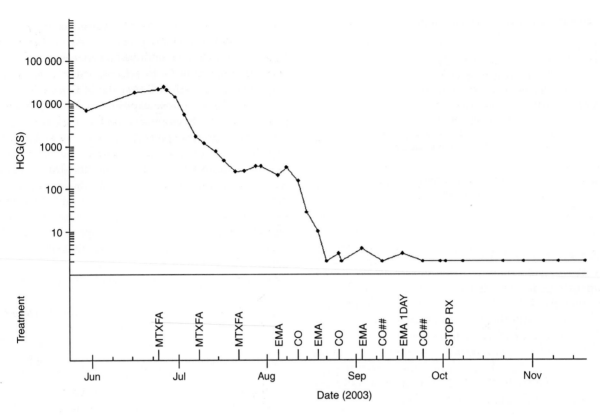

Fig. 15.2 An individual example of the pattern of hCG levels during the course of management.

Table 15.3c EP/EMA chemotherapy

Week 1
Day 1   Actinomycin-D 0.5 mg iv
         Etoposide 100 mg/m^2 iv
         Methotrexate 300 mg/m^2 iv
Day 2   Folinic acid 15 mg po 12 hourly × 4 doses
         Starting 24 h after commencing methotrexate

Week 2
Day 8   Etoposide 150 mg/m^2 iv
         Cisplatin 75 mg/m^2 iv

between 1975 and 2001 demonstrates a 100% cure rate for those presenting within 4 years of the antecedent pregnancy, but a poorer prognosis for those presenting after a longer interval [16].

RISK OF RELAPSE AND LATE TREATMENT
COMPLICATIONS

For the majority of patients with trophoblast disease who achieve a serological remission the outlook is very bright in terms of future risks of relapse, the possibility of further pregnancy and only modest long-term health risks from the chemotherapy exposure. Once the hCG has fallen to normal, the risk of relapse is less than 5% for patients treated with the low-risk protocols and only 3% for patients treated with the high-risk EMA/CO regimen. Generally these recurrences occur within the first 12 months after treatment but may occur many years later. Even in this situation trophoblast disease retains the possibility of cure, with further chemotherapy and on occasion surgery to sites of disease often providing satisfactory outcomes.

Subsequent fertility

Following either low- or high-risk chemotherapy treatment, fertility is usually maintained and regular menstruation restarts 2–6 months after the end of chemotherapy. However chemotherapy treatment does bring the average age of the menopause forward, by approximately 1 year for those treated with methotrexate and 3 years for those treated with EMA/CO [17].

We normally recommend that for 12 months after treatment further pregnancy is avoided to minimize any teratogenic effects on developing oocytes and to minimize the possible confusion from the rising hCG between a new pregnancy and disease relapse. The modest impact on future fertility is reflected in the data demonstrating that 83% of women wishing to conceive after chemotherapy treatment have been able to have at least one live birth. Despite the frequent long exposure to cytotoxic chemotherapy in the high-risk group there does not appear to be any significant increase in fetal abnormalities.

Many patients after experiencing one molar pregnancy and particularly those who require chemotherapy are anxious of the problem occurring again in any subsequent pregnancy. While the data suggest that the risk of a further molar pregnancy is about 10-fold higher than in the normal population this only equates to an approximate 1 in 70 risk [18]. This risk appears to be independent of chemotherapy exposure, being similar for those patients who required chemotherapy and those where the molar pregnancy was cured by evacuation alone.

Long-term toxicities

With the prolonged follow-up data available from trophoblast disease patients treated from the 1970s onwards, it is clear that the exposure to combination chemotherapy carries some long-term health risks. Data from a study of 1377 patients treated at CXH show that those receiving combination chemotherapy have enhanced risks of developing a second malignancy. From our series of patients the overall relative risk (rr) was increased 1.5-fold and is particularly marked for myeloid leukaemia (rr 16.6), colon cancer (rr 4.6), breast cancer (rr 5.8) and melanoma (rr 3.41) malignancies [19]. This database is being updated and as the cohorts of treated patients get older, these risks may further increase. In contrast the patients treated with single-agent methotrexate do not appear to have increased risks of second malignancies.

This long-term health concern from the use of combination chemotherapy reinforces the benefits from surveillance, allowing treatment to be commenced with single-agent methotrexate while the patient falls within the low-risk group.

Personal and psychological issues

Despite the very high cure rates and the low long-term toxicity from chemotherapy treatment, it is perhaps unsurprising that the diagnosis of a molar pregnancy and particularly treatment with chemotherapy can result in a number of psychological sequelae. The areas that lead to stress in the short term are the loss of the pregnancy, the impact of the 'cancer' diagnosis, the treatment process and the delay of future pregnancy. During chemotherapy treatment issues regarding potential side effects, emotional problems and fertility concerns are frequent. Other studies have shown that the concerns can remain for many years, with feelings regarding the wish for more children, a lack of control of fertility and an ongoing mourning for the lost pregnancy still frequently reported 5–10 years after treatment [20]. Additionally issues regarding self-esteem, and loss of sexual desire can be troublesome for many years after treatment; however, overall marital happiness does not seem to be impaired for trophoblast patients and their partners [21]. A number of surveys have demonstrated the wish of many patients to have more support through counselling and support at diagnosis and continuing even after treatment, and the recognition of this need must be addressed at centres and in the community subsequently.

References

1. Smith HO & Kim SJ (2003) In: Epidemiology. Hancock BW, Newlands ES, Berkowitz RS & Cole, LA (eds) *Gestational Trophoblastic Diseases*, 2nd edn. Sheffield: International Society for the Study of Trophoblastic Diseases.
2. Sebire NJ, Foskett M, Fisher RA, Rees H, Seckl M & Newlands E (2002) Risk of partial and complete hydatidiform molar pregnancy in relation to maternal age. *BJOG* **109**, 99–102.
3. Paradinas FJ (1998) The diagnosis and prognosis of molar pregnancy. the experience of the National Referral Centre in London. *Int J Gynaecol Obstet* **60**, S57–64.
4. Seckl MJ, Fisher RA, Salerno G *et al.* (2000) Choriocarcinoma and partial hydatidiform moles. *Lancet* **356**, 36–9.
5. Kurman RJ, Scully RE & Norris HJ (1976) Trophoblastic pseudotumor of the uterus. an exaggerated form of 'syncytial endometritis' simulating a malignant tumor. *Cancer* **38**, 1214–26.
6. Cole LA, Shahabi S, Butler SA *et al.* (2000) Utility of commonly used commercial human chorionic gonadotropin immunoassays in the diagnosis and management of trophoblastic diseases. *Clin Chem* **47**, 308–15.
7. Cole LA & Khanlian SA (2004) Inappropriate management of women with persistent low hCG results. *J Reprod Medical* **49**, 423–32.
8. Bagshawe KD (1976) Risk and prognostic factors in trophoblastic neoplasia. *Cancer* **38**, 1373–85.
9. FIGO Oncology Committee (2002) FIGO staging for gestational trophoblastic neoplasia. *Int J Gynaecol Obstet* **77**, 285–7.
10. McNeish IA, Strickland S, Holden L *et al.* (2002) Low-risk persistent gestational trophoblastic disease: outcome after initial treatment with low-dose methotrexate and folinic acid from 1992 to 2000. *J Clin Oncol* **20**, 1838–44.
11. Bagshawe KD, Dent J, Newlands ES, Begent RH & Rustin GJ (1989) The role of low-dose methotrexate and folinic acid in gestational trophoblastic tumours (GTT). *Br J Obstet Gynaecol* **96**, 795–802.
12. Newlands ES, Bagshawe KD, Begent RH, Rustin GJ & Holden L (1991) Results with the EMA/CO (etoposide, methotrexate, actinomycin D, cyclophosphamide, vincristine) regimen in high risk gestational trophoblastic tumours, 1979 to 1989. *Br J Obstet Gynaecol* **98**, 550–7.
13. Bower M, Newlands ES, Holden L Bagshawe KD (1997) EMA/CO. for high-risk gestational trophoblastic

tumors: results from a cohort of 272 patients. *J Clin Oncol* **15**, 2636–43.

14. Newlands ES, Mulholland PJ, Holden L, Seckl MJ & Rustin GJ (2000) Etoposide and cisplatin/etoposide, methotrexate, and actinomycin D (EMA) chemotherapy for patients with high-risk gestational trophoblastic tumors refractory to EMA/cyclophosphamide and vincristine chemotherapy and patients presenting with metastatic placental site trophoblastic tumors. *J Clin Oncol* **18**, 854–9.

15. Newlands ES, Holden L, Seckl MJ, McNeish I, Strickland S & Rustin GJ (2002) Management of brain metastases in patients with high-risk gestational trophoblastic tumors. *J Reprod Med* **47**, 465–71.

16. Papadopoulos AJ, Foskett M, Seckl MJ *et al.* Twenty-five years' clinical experience with placental site trophoblastic tumors. *J Reprod Med* **47**, 460–4.

17. Bower M, Rustin GJ, Newlands ES *et al.* (1998) Chemotherapy for gestational trophoblastic tumours hastens menopause by 3 years. *Eur J Cancer* **34**, 1204–7.

18. Bagshawe KD, Dent J & Webb J (1986) Hydatidiform mole in England and Wales 1973–83. *Lancet* **2**, 673–7.

19. Rustin GJ, Newlands ES, Lutz JM *et al.* (1996) Combination but not single-agent methotrexate chemotherapy for gestational trophoblastic tumors increases the incidence of second tumors. *J Clin Oncol* **14**, 2769–73.

20. Wenzel L, Berkowitz RS, Newlands E *et al.* (2002) Quality of life after gestational trophoblastic disease. *J Reprod Med* **47**, 387–94.

21. Wenzel L, Berkowitz R, Robinson S, Bernstein M & Goldstein D (1992) The psychological, social, and sexual consequences of gestational trophoblastic disease. *Gynecol Oncol* **46**, 74–81.

Further reading

Hancock BW, Newlands ES, Berkowitz RS & Cole LA (eds) (2003) *Gestational Trophoblastic Disease*, 2nd edn. Sheffield: International Society for the Study of Trophoblastic Diseases.

The management of gestational trophoblastic neoplasia RCOG Guideline No. 38.

Soper JJ, Mutch DG, Schink JC (2004) American College of Obstetricians and Gynecologists, Diagnosis and treatment of gestational trophoblastic disease: ACOG, Practice Bulletin No.53, *Gynecal. Oncol.* **93**, 575–85.

Soper JT, Mutch DG and Schink JC () *Gynecol Oncol* **93**, 575–85.

International Society for the Study of Trophoblastic Diseases (ISSTD). http://www.isstd.org/index.html

USA hCG reference service. Website http://www.hcglab.com/

UK Hydatidiform mole and Choriocarcinoma Information and support service. http://www.hmole-chorio.org.uk/

Chapter 16: Prenatal diagnosis and genetics

Sailesh Kumar

Introduction

The main purpose of any prenatal screening or diagnostic test is, first, the identification of fetuses at risk of serious structural, genetic, metabolic or haematologic abnormalities before the application of a confirmatory diagnostic test. The difference between screening and diagnostic tests is that the former are designed to have high sensitivity but may also have a high false positive rate. In contrast, diagnostic tests are highly accurate on which management and clinical decisions can be made. Screening tests are safe and applicable either universally or to low risk populations whereas diagnostic tests may involve invasive procedures and only applicable to a high risk group or those with a positive screen result.

It is now possible to diagnose a range of conditions antenatally that previously could only be detectable after birth. This has allowed parents the ability to make much more informed choices about the pregnancy than was hitherto possible. Parents have a myriad of reasons as to why they want prenatal diagnosis. In some instances, it is because of a previously affected child or a family history of a serious genetic condition, in others a raised risk on a screening test may be the impetus to seek a definite result. Whatever their reason, prenatal diagnosis for the vast majority of conditions will require a fetal sample and hence carry a risk of fetal loss. This chapter will concentrate on some of the developments and techniques currently available for prenatal diagnosis and the implications of these advances on clinical practice.

Advances in molecular genetics

There are three methods for finding genes contributing to complex diseases: candidate gene screening, linkage mapping, and association (case-control) studies. Candidate gene screening relies on selecting potential disease-causing genes, for example, genes causing inherited forms of disease and sequencing these genes in patients with complex diseases. Linkage mapping follows the segregation of chromosomal regions marked by random genetic

variants in families with complex diseases, in search of regions that co-segregate with the disease trait. Finally, case-control association studies look for differences in the frequencies of common genetic variants between ethnically matched cases and controls to find variants that are strongly associated with the disease. The eventual goal of each method is to identify either definite mutations with a strong causal relation to the disease or polymorphic variants which have a weak causal link to the disease.

An extremely wide range of techniques is now available for the diagnosis of genetic disorders, a review of which is beyond the scope of this chapter. The Human Genome Project showed that the current genome sequence contains approximately 2.85 billion nucleotides interrupted by only 341 gaps and seems to encode only 20,000–25,000 protein-coding genes [1]. If only 5% of these genes have diagnostic significance, approximately 1200 gene-based tests should be available. No single laboratory will be able to offer the breadth of these testing requirements and close liaison with a clinical genetics unit is imperative to ensure that samples are sent to the appropriate laboratory.

Invasive fetal tests

In the majority of instances, amniocentesis and chorionic villous sampling (CVS) are performed to obtain a fetal sample for analysis. It is estimated that around 5% of the pregnant population (approximately 30,000 women per year in the UK) could be offered a choice of invasive prenatal diagnostic tests. Amniocentesis is the most common invasive prenatal diagnostic procedure undertaken in the UK. Most amniocenteses are performed to obtain amniotic fluid for karyotyping and the majority are undertaken from 15 completed weeks (15 + 0) onwards. Amniocentesis prior to 15 completed weeks of gestation is referred to as 'early'. Chorionic villus sampling (CVS) is usually performed between 10 and 13 weeks of gestation and involves aspiration of placental tissue rather than amniotic fluid. CVS can be performed either transabdominally or the transcervically. It is usually performed after

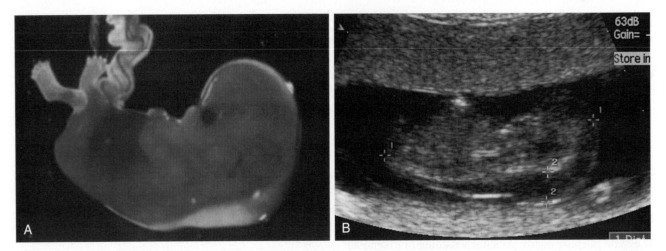

Fig. 16.1 1st trimester fetas with increased nuchal edema.

nuchal translucency screening (Fig. 16.1) which identifies fetus at risk for Down syndrome.

The best estimate of miscarriage risk associated with amniocentesis comes from the study by Tabor *et al* in 1986 [2]. This study randomised 4606 low-risk women and showed that the amniocentesis group had a loss rate which exceeded the control group by 1%; a figure which is often quoted in pretest counseling. Several more recent studies suggest that procedure related loss rates of around 0.5% are achievable [3,4]. There are no studies that compare CVS with no testing but randomised trials comparing CVS (by any route) with second trimester amniocentesis showed an excess pregnancy loss rate of 3% [5]. Other forms of invasive fetal testing include fetal blood sampling, fetal skin and muscle biopsy. The risk of an uncomplicated fetal blood sampling is between 1–3%, however, if the fetus is hydropic, the risk may be as high as 20% [6]. Once a fetal sample is obtained, chromosomal or non-chromosomal testing can begin.

Cytogenetics

Although karyotyping remains the gold standard of chromosome analysis and is still the most frequently used genetic method in prenatal diagnosis, the most important advance in cytogenetics has been the development of fluorescent in situ hybridization (FISH) technology and quantitative fluorescent polymerase chain reaction techniques (QF-PCR).

Full karyotype analysis takes approximately two weeks from amniotic fluid or chorionic villi (Fig. 16.2). Samples are cultured until sufficient dividing cells are harvested and the metaphase chromosomes spread onto microscope slides. These chromosomes are then banded by enzyme digestion and finally analysed under the microscope. In addition to detecting numerical chromosomal abnormalities (aneuploidies), this method also detects structural rearrangements and abnormalities where the size of the aberration is greater than 3Mb. A similar technique is used for fetal blood although a much more rapid result can be obtained (within 48 hours) as cultured lymphocytes divide much more quickly than amniocytes.

Fluorescent in situ hybridization (FISH)

The FISH technique is based on the discovery that labelled ribosomal ribonucleic acid (RNA) hybridises to acrocentric chromosomes (i.e. chromosomes that have a non-centrally located centromere, and therefore unequal chromosome arms) [7,8]. It involves a fluorescently labelled deoxyribonucleic acid (DNA) probe being hybridised to genomic DNA sequences and can be used to study a specific site on a chromosome. These specific probes can be hybridized not only to metaphase chromosomes but also incorporated directly onto fixed interphase nuclei of non-mitotic cells [9] (Fig. 16.3). Four main classes of FISH probes are now available: repetitive-sequence probes, whole genomic DNA probes, locus specific probes and chromosome specific painting probes [9]. FISH signals are visualised by fluorescence microscopy using a light source that illuminates the fluorescently labelled specimens.

Conventional high-resolution chromosome banding techniques can result in up to 1000 bands per genome; however, even at such high resolution, deletions, duplications or translocations are difficult to detect. FISH, however, can be used to determine the origin of marker chromosomes and to confirm numerical and structural anomalies. FISH probes can detect regions as small as 0.5 kb on metaphase chromosomes in contrast to only much larger regions (2–3 Mb) using conventional banding

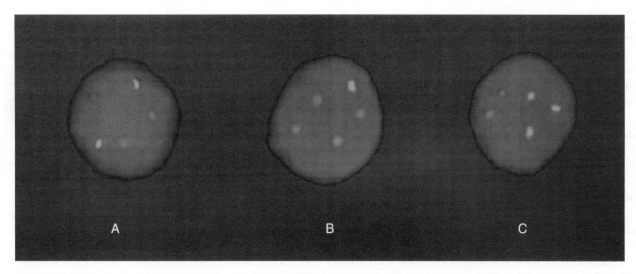

Fig. 16.2 Aneuploidy screening using FISH.

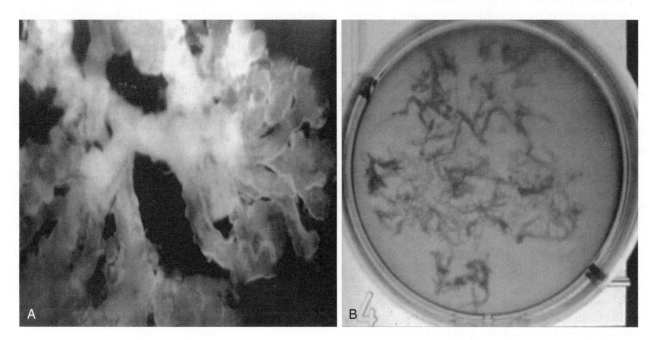

Fig. 16.3 Chorionic villi obtained after CVS.

techniques. The increased resolution provided by FISH is particularly suited to the study of microdeletion syndromes (e.g. Prader-Willi and Miller-Dieker) because the size of the DNA region that has been deleted is often very small.

Quantitative fluorescent polymerase chain reaction (QF-PCR)

Polymerase chain reaction is a rapid and reliable method for the detection of chromosome copy number by the amplification of highly polymorphic chromosome specific short tandem repeats (STR). A fluorochrome incorporated into the products of amplification permits visualization and quantification using an automated DNA scanner. Two fluorescence peaks with a ratio of 1:1 will be produced for each chromosome specific STR from normal euploid fetuses. Samples from trisomic fetuses will usually demonstrate either three peaks with a ratio of 1:1:1 (trisomic triallelic) or two peaks with a ratio of 2:1 (trisomic diallelic). The advantage of QF-PCR over FISH is its cost effectiveness especially when large numbers are processed. In addition, less material is required, bloody specimens may be successfully analysed and it is less time-consuming and less labour-intensive. The introduction of both techniques now enable rapid exclusion of the common trisomies (13, 18 and 21) giving reassurance to the majority of patients and allowing earlier management decisions to be made in the case of abnormal results [10].

The introduction of rapid testing of all prenatal samples has raised the issue of necessity for full karyotype analysis and reporting of these samples. The majority of women who undergo invasive testing do so because they have been identified as high risk by a particular screening method. Full karyotype analysis may detect abnormalities of unknown significance (small 'marker' chromosomes, balanced chromosome rearrangements, or regions of variability) which may be inherited and thus of minimal, if any, significance. These findings often cause counselling difficulties and raise ethical issues for patients both in how to interpret and choose between termination of pregnancy or ongoing anxiety for the rest of the pregnancy. Overall, around 0.07–0.14% of pregnancies karyotyped will have a clinically significant chromosome abnormality that would not be detected by rapid testing [11,12] and this needs to be considered by those performing prenatal testing in their pre-test counselling of patients.

Non-invasive prenatal diagnosis: fetal cells and cell-free fetal DNA

This remains the holy grail of prenatal diagnosis. Because invasive fetal testing carries risks to both mother and fetus alternative non-invasive methods are being actively explored. It is now abundantly clear that intact fetal cells and cell-free nucleic acid are present in the maternal circulation and are ideal targets for diagnosis.

One approach is the isolation of intact fetal cells from the maternal circulation. Several cell types have been isolated – nucleated red blood cells (NRBC), CD34 positive hematopoietic progenitors and trophoblasts. Although these cell types have been unequivocally proven to be present in the maternal circulation, each bears a significant disadvantage, rendering their application in clinical testing currently very problematic: NRBCs cannot be expanded in culture, thereby ruling out metaphase chromosome analysis, an essential component of prenatal diagnosis. CD34 positive cells do posses the potential for in vitro proliferation, however, they have been found to persist in the maternal circulation after delivery, thereby complicating diagnosis in consecutive pregnancies. Trophoblasts are not consistently detected in the maternal circulation. Moreover, due to the lack of a definitive fetal cell marker and a reliable sorting method, consistent and reliable fetal cell identification of any of these cell types is at the present time challenging.

Once fetal cells are isolated from maternal blood, there are sensitive new techniques that can be applied for genetic analysis. The major limitation in applying these techniques clinically (in addition to the specific problems detailed above) is the generally low number of fetal cells found in the maternal circulation (approximately one fetal cell per ml of maternal blood) [13]. The sensitivity of aneuploidy detection through analysis of intact fetal cells in maternal blood approaches 75% in some reports, with a false-positive rate estimated between 0.6 and 4.1% [14,15].

In 1997, Lo *et al.* [16] demonstrated the presence of large amounts of *cell-free* fetal DNA in plasma and serum from pregnant women. This same group also showed that there was rapid drop in fetal DNA levels in the maternal circulation after delivery with undetectable levels of circulating DNA two hours post partum [17]. Considerably more fetal DNA is present in the cell-free fraction of maternal plasma and serum compared with fetal DNA extracted from the cellular fraction of maternal blood [18]. The predominant source of fetal DNA in the maternal circulation appears to be the placenta [19]. Levels of fetal DNA increase with gestation with a significant rise in the last 8 weeks of pregnancy [20].

Unlike nucleated fetal cells in maternal blood, which usually requires the use of sophisticated cell enrichment techniques, fetal DNA analysis has the advantage of being reliably processed and easily performed for a large number of samples. The main problem precluding its more widespread application at present appears to be the lack of availability of uniquely fetal gene sequences that identify and/or measure the presence of fetal DNA in both male and female fetuses.

In general, the clinical applications of fetal DNA measurement in maternal plasma and serum have focused on the *measurement* of fetal DNA sequences and the *detection* (presence or absence) of uniquely fetal gene sequences [21].

Gender detection

In one study [22], fetal gender was correctly predicted by fetal DNA from maternal plasma samples taken between 10 and 13 weeks with 100% sensitivity. As the identification of male fetal DNA sequences is relatively easy, one potential application is the non-invasive identification of male fetuses at risk for an X-linked condition. Fetal sexing in early pregnancy therefore could be the first step to identify fetuses that are at risk and would require invasive testing for confirmation of the diagnosis [23] or in cases where the fetal sex affects clinical management such as in the use of corticosteroid therapy for congenital adrenal hyperplasia in those carrying female but not male fetuses [24].

Non-invasive diagnosis of aneuploidy

Using real-time PCR, one group [25] demonstrated a 2-fold increase in fetal DNA levels for trisomy 21, compared with euploid cases. Subsequent studies have supported these observations on confirmed trisomy 21, but not on trisomy 18 [26], suggesting that different fetal growth and placental abnormalities result in different levels of fetal DNA in the maternal circulation. Analysis of stored maternal serum samples has also shown a 1.8-fold increase in the amount of fetal DNA levels in trisomy positive pregnancies as compared with gestational age-matched controls. Taken together, these findings suggest the possible use of fetal DNA as an additional screening analyte. Another novel application of fetal DNA analysis is in the investigation of pregnancies at risk for aneuploidy due to a parental balanced translocation [27].

Pre-eclampsia

In pre-eclampsia, there is an almost five fold increase in fetal DNA in the maternal circulation compared with controls [28,29]. In women destined to develop pre-eclampsia, fetal DNA is noted to be elevated before the disease becomes symptomatic [30]. A two stage rise is noted in these patients. Raised levels of fetal DNA were detected as early as 17 weeks gestation followed by a second rise approximately 3 weeks before the onset of symptoms [31]. This phenomenon may allow both screening for the disease, as well as indicating impending pre-eclampsia. However, this test is not yet in routine clinical practice as it requires further validation.

Monogenic disorders

Perhaps one of the most important application of fetal DNA in maternal plasma is the non-invasive genotyping of the fetus in pregnancies complicated by red cell alloimmunisation. Non-invasive fetal Rh-D genotyping was first reported in 1998 [20] and since 2001, the International Blood Group Reference Laboratory (IBGRL) in Bristol has offered fetal Rh-D typing using cell free fetal DNA in maternal plasma, to obstetricians caring for alloimmunised women. This has significantly reduced the number of invasive procedures carried out in the UK for fetal Rh-D genotyping [32]. More recently, the IBGRL has also started offering fetal Rh-c and Kell genotyping using the same technique.

Other genetic disorders such as myotonic dystrophy [33], achondroplasia [34] and cystic fibrosis [35] have all been diagnosed using fetal DNA in maternal plasma. In addition, Hong Kong investigators [36], using fetal DNA to exclude or confirm the presence of the paternally inherited mutant allele in beta-thalassaemia major, have been able to identify at-risk fetuses who then need invasive testing.

A major limitation of using DNA in maternal blood is the fact that the mother and fetus share, on average, half of their genomic DNA sequences. Thus, it is only possible to detect uniquely fetal DNA sequences that are paternally inherited. Novel approaches, such as using gender-independent polymorphisms, epigenetic markers, or circulating mRNA sequences, will eventually allow this technology to be applied to female fetuses. Comparative genome hybridization and microchip assays may make it possible that amplified fetal nucleic acids will ultimately permit a non-invasive fetal genome scan as part of routine prenatal screening.

Preimplantation genetic diagnosis

The first reports of preimplantation genetic diagnosis (PGD) were published almost 15 years ago [37,38]. The main purpose of PGD is to perform genetic testing before pregnancy and in order to avoid the termination of pregnancy which is a major limitation of conventional prenatal diagnosis. To date more than 7000 PGD have been performed with the birth of almost 1000 healthy children. The list of disorders to which PGD has been applied now number more than 100 with the most frequent ones being cystic fibrosis and haemoglobin disorders (see review by Kuliev and Verlinsky) [39]. PGD is an attractive option for couples carrying translocations because of their poor reproductive outcome. There is a four fold reduction of spontaneous abortions in women undergoing PGD compared to those not undertaking PGD [40,41].

PGD is currently performed either by testing oocytes for maternally derived genetic abnormalities, or by genetic analysis of single cells removed from preimplantation embryos, so only unaffected embryos may be transferred back to the uterus ensuring the establishment of an unaffected pregnancy [42]. Each of these approaches has advantages and disadvantages and is applied depending on the clinical circumstances.

Embryo biopsy is performed as early as the 6–8-cell stage, or at blastocyst, allowing testing for both maternally and paternally derived genetic abnormalities. Despite reduction in embryo cell number, which may have an influence on the embryo viability, embryo biopsy is the method of choice for paternally derived dominant conditions and translocations, as well as for gender determination and HLA typing. In contrast, oocyte testing is used for maternally derived genetic abnormalities and is performed by removing the first and second polar bodies (PB1 and PB2) from oocytes, representing the by-products of meiosis I (PB1) and meiosis II (PB2), respectively. Whilst oocyte testing does not give information on gender or paternal mutations, it may be the method of choice for PGD of recessive conditions and maternally derived dominant mutations and translocations. Because over 90% of chromosomal errors originate from maternal meiosis, this approach is of special value for PGD of age-related aneuploidies. It is also of particular importance due to the relatively high rate of mosaicism at the cleavage stage, which is the major limitation of blastomere based tests for chromosomal disorders.

PGD may now be applied to any genetic disease presently diagnosed by prenatal diagnosis and also for those not conventionally tested prenatally, such as late onset and complex disorders and the pre-selection of unaffected and HLA matched embryos. However, PGD is not an option that is applicable to most couples contemplating assisted reproduction and like any other technique has its place in a select group of patients.

Conclusion

Much of the advance in prenatal diagnosis has come from major breakthroughs in molecular techniques which have greatly enhanced our knowledge of many genetic diseases and thus allowed the development of precise diagnostic tests for these conditions. However, hand in hand with the immense possibilities these new techniques offer, come problems that are not so easily resolved. For example, quality assurance and standards have to be rigorously set and consistently achieved in every laboratory involved in genetic testing. Often this is difficult to achieve because of the lack of universally accepted quality assurance programmes.

Ethical dilemmas have arisen surrounding the screening and identification of genetic markers responsible with late onset conditions. Is it appropriate to offer or perform prenatal diagnosis when it is known that the condition only develops late in life (e.g. Huntington's disease)? The abuse of prenatal tests is a very real issue that will challenge society both ethically and legally in a multitude of ways. The practising obstetrician will have to be aware of some of the issues in order to manage affected patients appropriately. In the future, current arguments about the best Down syndrome screening test will seem very simplistic and probably very naïve indeed.

References

1. Consortium IHGS (2004) Finishing the euchromatic sequence of the human genome. *Nature* **431**(7011), 931–45.
2. Tabor A, Philip J, Madsen M, Bang J, Obel EB, Norgaard-Pedersen B. Randomised controlled trial of genetic amniocentesis in 4606 low-risk women. *Lancet* 1986;**1**(8493):1287–93.
3. Horger EO, 3rd, Finch H and Vincent VA (2001) A single physician's experience with four thousand six hundred genetic amniocenteses. *Am J Obstet Gynecol* **185**(2), 279–88.
4. Scott F, Peters H, Boogert T, Robertson R, Anderson J, McLennan A, et al. The loss rates for invasive prenatal testing in a specialised obstetric ultrasound practice. *Aust N Z J Obstet Gynaecol* 2002;**42**(1):55–8.
5. Alfirevic Z Sundberg K and BS (2004) Amniocentesis and chorionic villous sampling for prenatal diagnosis. *Cochrane Database Syst Rev* (CD003252).
6. Maxwell DJ, Johnson P, Hurley P, Neales K, Allan L, Knott P. Fetal blood sampling and pregnancy loss in relation to indication. *Br J Obstet Gynaecol* 1991;**98**(9):892–7.
7. Schrock E, Veldman T, Padilla-Nash H, Ning Y, Spurbeck J, Jalal S, et al. Spectral karyotyping refines cytogenetic diagnostics of constitutional chromosomal abnormalities. *Hum Genet* 1997;**101**(3):255–62.
8. Bayani J and Squire JA (2001) Advances in the detection of chromosomal aberrations using spectral karyotyping. *Clin Genet* **59**(2), 65–73.
9. McNeil N and Ried T (2000) Novel molecular cytogenetic techniques for identifying complex chromosomal rearrangements: technology and applications in molecular medicine. *Expert Rev Mol Med* **2000**, 1–14.
10. Nicolini U, Lalatta F, Natacci F, Curcio C, Bui TH. The introduction of QF-PCR in prenatal diagnosis of fetal aneuploidies: time for reconsideration. *Hum Reprod Update* 2004;**10**(6):541–8.
11. Thein AT, Abdel–Fattah SA, Kyle PM, Soothill PW. An assessment of the use of interphase FISH with chromosome specific probes as an alternative to cytogenetics in prenatal diagnosis. *Prenat Diagn* 2000;**20**(4):275–80.
12. Ryall RG, Callen D, Cocciolone R, Duvnjak A, Esca R, Frantzis N, alGjerde E. M, Haan E. A, Hocking T, Sutherland G, Thomas D. W, Webb F. Karyotypes found in the population declared at increased risk of Down syndrome following maternal serum screening. *Prenat Diagn* 2001;**21**(7):553–7.
13. Bianchi DW (1997) Progress in the genetic analysis of fetal cells circulating in maternal blood. *Curr Opin Obstet Gynecol* **9**(2), 121–5.
14. Bianchi DW, Simpson JL, Jackson LG, Elias S, Holzgreve W, Evans MI et al. Fetal gender and aneuploidy detection using fetal cells in maternal blood: analysis of NIFTY I data. National Institute of Child Health and Development Fetal Cell Isolation Study. *Prenat Diagn* 2002;**22**(7): 609–15.
15. de la Cruz F, Shifrin H, Elias S, Bianchi DW, Jackson L, Evans MI, et al. Low false-positive rate of aneuploidy detection using fetal cells isolated from maternal blood. *Fetal Diagn Ther* 1998;**13**(6):380.
16. Lo YM, Corbetta N, Chamberlain PF, Rai V, Sargent IL, Redman CW, et al. Presence of fetal DNA in maternal plasma and serum. *Lancet* 1997;**350**(9076):485–7.
17. Lo YM, Zhang J, Leung TN, Lau TK, Chang AM, Hjelm NM. Rapid clearance of fetal DNA from maternal plasma. *Am J Hum Genet* 1999;**64**(1):218–24.
18. Lo YM, Hjelm NM, Fidler C, Sargent IL, Murphy MF, Chamberlain PF, Poon P. M, Redman, C. W, Wainscoat, J. S.

Prenatal diagnosis of fetal RhD status by molecular analysis of maternal plasma. *N Engl J Med* 1998;**339**(24): 1734–8.

19. Bianchi DW (2004) Circulating fetal DNA: its origin and diagnostic potential-a review. *Placenta* **25 (Suppl A)**, S93–S101.

20. Lo YM *et al.* (1998) Prenatal diagnosis of fetal RhD status by molecular analysis of maternal plasma. *N Engl J Med* **339**(24), 1734–8.

21. Pertl B and Bianchi DW (2001) Fetal DNA in maternal plasma: emerging clinical applications. *Obstet Gynecol* **98**(3), 483–90.

22. Costa JM *et al.* (2002) [First trimester fetal sex determination in maternal serum using real-time PCR]. *Gynecol Obstet Fertil* **30**(12), 953–7.

23. Honda H, Miharu N, Ohashi Y, Samura O,Kinutani M, Hara T, Kinutani M. Hara T, Ohama K. Fetal gender determination in early pregnancy through qualitative and quantitative analysis of fetal DNA in material serum. *Hum Genet* 2002;**110**(1):75–9.

24. Bartha JL, Finning K and Soothill PW (2003) Fetal sex determination from maternal blood at 6 weeks of gestation when at risk for 21-hydroxylase deficiency. *Obstet Gynecol* **101**(5 Pt 2), 1135–6.

25. Lo YM, Lau TK, Zhang J, Leung TN, Chang AM, Hjelm NM, Elmes R. S, Bianchi DW. Increased fetal DNA concentrations in the plasma of pregnant women carrying fetuses with trisomy 21. *Clin Chem* 1999;**45**(10):1747–51.

26. Zhong XY, Burk MR, Troeger C, Jackson LR, Holzgreve W, Hahn S. Fetal DNA in maternal plasma is elevated in pregnancies with aneuploid fetuses. *Prenat Diagn* 2000;**20**(10):795–8.

27. Chen CP, Chern SR and Wang W (2001) Fetal DNA analyzed in plasma from a mother's three consecutive pregnancies to detect paternally inherited aneuploidy. *Clin Chem* **47**(5), 937–9.

28. Lo YM, Leung TN, Tein MS, Sargent IL, Zhang J, Lau TK, Haines C. J, Redman C. W. Quantitative abnormalities of fetal DNA in maternal serum in preeclampsia. *Clin Chem* 1999;**45**(2):184–8.

29. Zhong XY, Laivuori H, Livingston JC, Ylikorkala O, Sibai BM, Holzgreve W, Hahn S. Elevation of both maternal and fetal extracellular circulating deoxyribonucleic acid concentrations in the plasma of pregnant women with preeclampsia. *Am J Obstet Gynecol* 2001;**184**(3):414–9.

30. Leung TN, Zhang J, Lau TK, Chan LY, Lo YM. Increased maternal plasma fetal DNA concentrations in women who eventually develop preeclampsia. *Clin Chem* 2001;**47**(1): 137–9.

31. Levine RJ, Qian C, Leshane ES, Yu KF, England LJ, Schisterman EF, Wataganara T, Romero R, Bianchi D. W. Two-stage elevation of cell-free fetal DNA in maternal sera before onset of preeclampsia. *Am J Obstet Gynecol* 2004;**190**(3):707–13.

32. Finning K, Martin P and Daniels G (2004) A clinical service in the UK to predict fetal Rh (Rhesus) D blood group using free fetal DNA in maternal plasma. *Ann N Y Acad Sci* **1022**, 119–23.

33. Amicucci P, Gennarelli M, Novelli G, Dallapiccola B. Prenatal diagnosis of myotonic dystrophy using fetal DNA obtained from maternal plasma. *Clin Chem* 2000;**46**(2): 301–2.

34. Saito H, Sekizawa A, Morimoto T, Suzuki M, Yanaihara T. Prenatal DNA diagnosis of a single-gene disorder from maternal plasma. *Lancet* 2000;**356**(9236):1170.

35. Gonzalez-Gonzalez MC, Garcia-Hoyos M, Trujillo MJ, Rodriguez de Alba M, Lorda-Sanchez I, Diaz-Recasens J, Gallardo E, Ayuso C, Ramos C. Prenatal detection of a cystic fibrosis mutation in fetal DNA from maternal plasma. *Prenat Diagn* 2002;**22**(10):946–8.

36. Chiu RW, Lau TK, Leung TN, Chow KC, Chui DH, Lo YM. Prenatal exclusion of beta thalassaemia major by examination of maternal plasma. *Lancet* 2002;**360**(9338):998–1000.

37. Handyside AH, Kontogianni EH, Hardy K, Winston RM. Pregnancies from biopsied human preimplantation embryos sexed by Y-specific DNA amplification. *Nature* 1990;**344**(6268):768–70.

38. Verlinsky Y, Ginsberg N, Lifchez A, Valle J, Moise J, Strom CM. Analysis of the first polar body: preconception genetic diagnosis. *Hum Reprod* 1990;**5**(7):826–9.

39. Kuliev A and Verlinsky Y (2005) Place of preimplantation diagnosis in genetic practice. *Am J Med Genet A* **134**(1), 105–10.

40. Munne S, Sandalinas M, Escudero T, Fung J, Gianaroli L, Cohen J. Outcome of preimplantation genetic diagnosis of translocations. *Fertil Steril* 2000;**73**(6):1209–18.

41. Verlinsky Y, Cieslak J, Evsikov S, Galat V, Kuliev A. Nuclear transfer for full karyotyping and preimplantation diagnosis for translocations. *Reprod Biomed Online* 2002;**5**(3):300–5.

42. Verlinsky Y and Kuliev A (Editors) (2000) Atlas of preimplantation genetic diagnosis. Panthern Publishing Group.

Chapter 17: Fetal medicine in clinical practice

R.C. Wimalasundera

Introduction

Historically, fetal medicine has been limited by the inaccessibility of the human fetus in the uterus. Advances in the last three decades in imaging techniques such as ultrasound and MRI as well as cytogenetics and intrauterine surgical techniques mean that we can now accurately diagnose and offer curative or ameliorative treatments for many conditions that were previously only treatable in the neonatal period.

Referrals for specialist fetal medical assessments are usually based on women falling into a high-risk category either on routine antenatal screening for Down's syndrome or a structural anomaly or on her own medical or family history such as a known genetic syndrome or because of a previously affected pregnancy/child. Once a referral has been made then the underlying principles of fetal medicine are broadly categorized into either preventing 'wrongful birth' or prevention of perinatal mortality and post-natal disability. These are achieved by accurate diagnosis of the fetal anomaly, a multidisciplinary approach to decisions on management and counselling of parents. Management options would include conservative management, offering a termination of pregnancy where appropriate, antenatal therapeutic interventions and decisions on timing, mode and place of delivery.

However, the practical aspects of fetal medicine are far from the simplistic pathway outlined earlier. Although in some cases the diagnosis may be clear from the initial detailed imaging or invasive karyotyping, in many cases the diagnosis is uncertain either because of poor images, fetal position or the complex nature of an anomaly. Even if a diagnosis is made the detailed natural history of many fetal conditions are unknown or the lesions may evolve during the pregnancy such that the prognosis will change as the pregnancy progresses.

The aim of this chapter is to discuss some of the practical aspects of fetal medicine in terms of being able to make accurate diagnosis and deciding on management options such as which pregnancies should be offered a termination of pregnancy and which should be offered therapeutic interventions *in utero* or simply monitored until delivery when post-natal intervention would be most appropriate and finally decisions on the timing, mode and place of delivery.

Diagnosis of fetal anomaly

The impact of fetal medicine practice is obviously directly influenced by the detection of fetal anomalies in the general population and therefore referred for an opinion. Women who are at high risk of a fetal anomaly are usually referred directly to a fetal medicine unit, but within a low-risk population detection of an anomaly is based on antenatal screening programmes. These are primarily based on screening for Down's syndrome, blood group antibody screening and second trimester anomaly scan screening.

The National Institute of Clinical Excellence (NICE[1]) guidelines on antenatal care in the UK stipulate that all women should be offered a dating scan between 10 and 16 weeks as well as some form of screening for Down's syndrome either based on first or second trimester screening or a combination of both.

Down's syndrome screening

The screening procedures offered currently in the UK are listed here. Each consists of a risk assessment based on maternal age and a scan performed in the first trimester or a blood test in the first or second trimester or a combination of scans and blood test.

Triple test

Early second trimester (14–20 completed weeks) test is based on the measurement of α-fetoprotein, unconjugated oestriol (uE3) and hCG (either total hCG or free β-hCG) together with maternal age.

Nuchal translucency scan

A first trimester (11–13 weeks) test is based on the measurement of the fold of skin on the back of the fetal neck (Nuchal translucency (NT)) together with the maternal age.

Quadruple test

Early second trimester (14–21 weeks) test is based on the measurement of α-fetoprotein, uE3, free β-hCG (or total hCG) and inhibin-A together with maternal age.

Combined test

Late first trimester (10–13 weeks) test is based on combining NT measurement with free β-hCG, pregnancy associated plasma protein-A (PAPP-A) and maternal age.

Integrated test

This is the integration of different screening markers measured at different stages of pregnancy into a single test result. Unless otherwise qualified, 'Integrated test' refers to the integration of NT measurement and PAPP-A in the first trimester with serum α-fetoprotein, β-hCG and uE3 in the second.

The NICE Guideline – Antenatal Care, Routine Care for the Healthy Pregnant Woman [1] stated that by April 2007, pregnant women should be offered screening for Down's Syndrome with a test which provides a detection rate of >75% and a false-positive rate of <3%. These performance measures should be age-standardized and based on cut-off of 1 in 250 at term. These guidelines were based on the SURUSS report [2], which was a multicentre study of nearly 50,000 singleton pregnancies in women where the most effective, safe and cost-effective method of screening for Down's syndrome using NT, maternal serum and urine markers in the first and second trimester of pregnancy and maternal age in various combinations were analysed. The authors concluded that the Integrated test was the best performing with the highest detection and lowest false-positive rates at any given risk cut-off (Table 17.1). Subsequently the National Screening Committee Model of Best Practice in the UK also concluded that the Integrated test resulted in the lowest loss rate of unaffected fetuses (Table 17.2).

Table 17.1 Data from the SURUSS [2] study of screening performance with a constant early second trimester risk cut-off of 1:250

Screening test	Detection rate (%)	False-positive rate (%)
Triple test	81	6.9
Quadruple test	84	5.7
Combined test	83	5
Integrated test	90	2.8

Ultrasound screening for fetal anomalies

Routine first trimester dating scanning has a number of benefits – (1) it is more accurate at assessing gestational age than menstrual periods, and therefore reduces the rates of induction of labour for post-term pregnancies (2) detects multiple pregnancies early in pregnancy and (3) can detect some major structural anomalies such as anencephaly. However a more detailed, although limited, anomaly scan is incorporated into a NT scan such as the shape of the fetal skull, presence of nose, hands and feet and presence of stomach and bladder. Therefore, instigation of Down's syndrome screening strategies such as the Combined or Integrated test which involve an NT scan are likely to not only increase the detection of aneuploidy but also major structural anomalies and particularly cardiac defects earlier in gestation.

In the UK there is a policy of routine second trimester ultrasound screening for fetal anomalies [1]. However, detection of fetal anomalies varies considerably depending on the anomaly being screened for as well as the gestation at screening, the skill of the operator and the quality of the equipment used. A systematic review of routine ultrasound [3] screening for fetal anomalies included 96,633 babies between 1996 and 1998. The overall detection rate was 44.7% with detection being considerably higher <24 weeks (41.3%) than >24 weeks (18.6%) (Table 17.3). In the UK although the detection rates appear to be higher there is a considerable geographic variation. Chitty *et al.* [4] reported an overall detection rate of 74% in an inner London unit, whereas Boyd *et al.* [5] reported a detection rate of 50% in Oxford.

The detection of cardiac anomalies is of particular interest. Early prenatal detection of congenital heart disease (CHD) has increased due to advances in ultrasound resolution and the incorporation of at least a 4-chamber cardiac view in the routine anomaly scan, which is now accepted as standard in the UK. There is, however, regional variation in antenatal detection of CHD, with those obstetric centres close to cardiac units faring better than those situated in more remote areas. There also appears to be a discrepancy between countries, which reflect different obstetric practice; for example, the policy of universal anomaly scanning between 20 and 22 weeks in the UK compared with targeted anomaly scanning in the USA.

The risk of aneuploidy varies as to the structural anomaly detected and it would be outside the scope of this chapter to detail the risk for each structural anomaly. However, cardiac anomalies are the commonest type of structural anomalies detected in fetal life and at birth with a frequency of 8:1000 and Table 17.4 illustrates the variation in risk of aneuploidy with the various cardiac defects [6].

Table 17.2 Outcome in 100,000 women screened with a constant detection rate of 75% (derived from SURUSS report [2])

Test	Unaffected women referred for CVS or amnio	No. of Down's syndrome diagnosed	No. of unaffected fetuses lost	No. of Down's syndrome diagnosed per unaffected fetuses lost
Triple	4200	152	30	5.1
Quadruple	2500	152	18	8.5
Combined	2300	152	17	9
Integrated	300	152	2	76.3

Assuming an 80% acceptance rate of amnio/CVS and 0.9% loss rate from the procedure.

Table 17.3 Percentage of fetal anomalies detected by routine second trimester ultrasound screening according to anatomical systems (Bricker *et al.* [3])

Anatomical systems	Detected (%)
Central nervous system	76
Urinary tract	67
Pulmonary	50
Gastrointestinal	42
Skeletal	24
Cardiac	17

Mid-trimester ultrasound markers

Soft-tissue markers are signs that can be detected on a second trimester anomaly scan that in themselves are not structural defects but have an association with aneuploidy, and therefore their presence increases the risk of aneuploidy. Markers include nuchal skin oedema, short femoral or humeral length measurements, choroid plexus cysts, bilateral renal pelvic dilatation, echogenic fetal bowel and hyperechogenic foci ('golf balls') in the fetal heart. Early publications reporting increased prevalence of these markers in Down fetuses compared to euploid fetuses were used to derive increased risks for trisomy 21. However, a meta-analysis of 56 studies by Smith-Bindmen *et al.* [7] found sensitivities for individual markers in isolation of only 1–16% (Table 17.5), whereas the sensitivity of multiple markers in association with structural anomalies was 69%. Most of the markers in isolation had low relative risks (positive predictive values or likelihood ratios of 3–7 only). Indeed, it is now known that choroid plexus cysts in isolation, which are found in 0.65% of normal fetuses, do not increase the risk of Down's syndrome [7].

Based on this meta-analysis only the presence of a thickened nuchal fold or echogenic bowel in isolation would significantly increase the risk of aneuploidy. However,

the presence of any of the other soft markers would alert the person performing the scan to perform a thorough check for other features of aneuploidy. If indeed more than one soft marker or any structural anomaly is detected this would significantly increase the risk of aneuploidy and warrant further counselling regarding invasive karyotyping.

However, Nicolaides *et al.* [8] suggested that based on the analysis of two of the largest published studies on soft markers and trisomy 21, each soft marker has a positive likelihood ratio (PLR) that its presence is associated with trisomy 21 and a negative likelihood ratio (NLR) that its absence is associated with a normal karyotype. Therefore an individual's risk of trisomy 21 before a second trimester scan, based on age or Down's syndrome screening, can be adjusted more accurately by multiplying by the PLR of an individual soft marker if it were detected on the scan and by the NLR of the soft makers not detected on the scan (Table 17.6). For example, a woman with a serum triple test risk of trisomy 21 of 1:1000 has an anomaly scan which shows the presence of an echogenic intracardiac foci (PLR: 6.41) and a short femur (PLR: 7.94), but no major structural defects (NLR: 0.79), no nuchal fold thickening (NLR: 0.67), no short humerus (NLR: 0.68), no hydronephrosis (NLR: 0.85) and no echogenic bowel (NLR: 0.87). The combined likelihood ratio is $6.41 \times 7.94 \times 0.79 \times 0.67 \times 0.68 \times 0.85 \times 0.87 = 13.5$. Therefore based on this calculation the woman would be counselled that her risk of trisomy 21 would be increased from 1:1000 to 1:74 ($13.5 \times 1/1000$) and offered invasive karyotyping.

Invasive prenatal diagnosis

Once a woman has been given a high risk of aneuploidy based on a Down screening, a structural anomaly detected on scan or because of her previous history an obstetrician would normally counsel the women on the options of invasive karyotyping. This counselling should be based on the

Table 17.4 Meta-analysis performed by Wimalasundera *et al.* [6]

Cardiac anomaly	Overall aneuploidy rate (%)	T 21 (%)	T18 (%)	T 13 (%)	45XO (%)	Other (%)	22q11 deletion
AVSD	46	79	13			8	
VSD	46	43	45	2	4	6	10–17
TOF	31	43	29	7		21	6–30
CoA	33	18	24	24	12	22	
CAT	19				25	75	10
IAAb							17–50
APVS	20						
HLHS	7		56	22	11	11	
DORV	21	10	40	20	30		1
Mitral atresia	18						
UVH	15						
PS/PA + IVS	5						
Tricuspid atresia	7				50	50	
TVD	4						
Aortic stenosis	5						
ASD	17						
TGA	0						
cTGA	0						
Tumours	0						
Cardiomyopathy	0						
Cardiosplenic syndromes	0						
DIV	0						

Data expressed as overall rate of aneuploidy (%) for individual congenital cardiac defects.
AVSD, atrioventricular septal defect; VSD, ventricular septal defect; TOF, Tetralogy of Fallot; CoA, Coarctation of the aorta; CAT, common arterial trunk; APVS, absent pulmonary valve syndrome; HLHS, hypoplastic left heart syndrome; DORV, double outlet right ventricle; UVH, univentricular heart; PS/PA + IVS, pulmonary stenosis/pulmonary atresia with intact ventricular septum; TVD, tricuspid valve dysplasia; ASD, atrial septal defect; TGA, transposition of the great arteries; cTGA, corrected transposition of the great arteries; DIV, double inlet ventricle; IAAb, interrupted aortic arch type B.

Table 17.5 Test performance for mid-trimester ultrasonic markers as isolated findings to predict trisomy 21, based on a meta-analysis of 56 studies [20]

Marker	Sensitivity (%)	Positive likelihood ratio (%)
Thickened nuchal fold	4	17
Choroid plexus cyst	1	1
Short femur length	16	2.7
Short humeral length	9	7.5
Echogenic bowel	4	6.1
Echogenic intracardiac focus	11	2.8
Renal pyelectasis	2	1.9

Table 17.6 Data published by Nicolaides [8] on the positive and negative likelihood ratios for trisomy 21 when isolated soft-tissue markers and major defects are detected in the second trimester

Soft marker	Positive LR	Negative LR	LR isolated
Nuchal fold	53	0.67	9.8
Major defect	33	0.79	5.2
Echogenic bowel	21	0.87	3.0
Short femur	8	0.62	1.6
Short humerus	23	0.68	4.1
Hydronephrosis	6.8	0.85	1.0
Echogenic foci	6.4	0.75	1.1

risk of aneuploidy, the voluntary nature of the test, the option of no testing, the technique of the proposed test, the procedure-related loss rate and other common complications associated with the test, the timing of the result and the possible management options depending on the result of the test. This decision to balance the potential risk of the loss of an unaffected fetus against that of having an affected child is a very difficult and traumatic one and it is important that the parents are not rushed into a premature decision.

Amniocentesis

Amniocentesis should be performed after 15 weeks when the uterus is an abdominal organ and the proportion of fluid needed to be removed (15–10 ml) is relatively small compared to the overall liquor volume at this gestation (150–250 ml).

The procedure is performed under aseptic conditions under continuous ultrasound guidance. Best practice is for the operator to introduce a gauge 22–20 needle percutaneously while he or she is continuously scanning using the free hand. The needle is preferably introduced into a cord free pool of liquor avoiding the placenta. Once in place the inner stylet of the needle is withdrawn and an initial 2 ml of amniotic fluid is withdrawn by an assistant and discarded to avoid maternal contamination. Then a further 15–20 ml is removed using a 10–20 ml syringe. A few operators use a needle guide attached to the transducer, but this has the disadvantage of being less flexible if the needle needs to be realigned.

There is clearly a learning curve with any invasive procedure. Studies have demonstrated the significance of operator experience in terms of both failed attempts and miscarriage rates. Earlier studies had suggested that the difference in miscarriage rates in operators performing over 50 cases per year (0.3%) was considerably lower than ones performing less than 10 cases per year (3.7%) [9]. Amniocentesis is therefore not a routine procedure and it is recommended by the Royal College of Obstetricians and Gynaecologists (RGOG) that it is only performed by adequately trained individuals with at least 50–100 supervised procedures and 50 procedures per annum to maintain their skills. In general only two needle insertions should be attempted and if these fail then the woman should be referred to a tertiary level fetal medicine unit for repeat attempts.

The miscarriage rate for amniocentesis is generally quoted as 1:100 (1%) and is based on the single randomized controlled trial of second trimester amniocentesis by Tabor *et al.* [10] in Denmark in 1986. He demonstrated that the women randomized to not have amniocentesis had a miscarriage rate of 0.7% compared to 1.7% in the group who had an amniocentesis and therefore suggested that amniocentesis increased the background miscarriage rate by 1%. More recent uncontrolled series suggest lower miscarriage rates of 0.5%, but it is important that each tertiary level fetal medicine unit should audit their own amniocentesis and chorionic villus sampling (CVS) outcomes and be able to quote an individual miscarriage rate for the unit.

Leakage of amniotic fluid vaginally following an amniocentesis is relatively common occurring in up to 2% but is almost always self-limiting and associated with a normal outcome. Post-amniocentesis chorioamnionitis is also rare occurring in <1.5/1000. However, if signs of chorioamnionitis should be apparent following a recent amniocentesis a repeat amniocentesis with gram staining and culture of the amniotic fluid should be undertaken. If infection is confirmed immediate emptying of the uterine cavity is needed to prevent maternal septicaemia.

Cytogenetic analysis

Amniotic fluid will contain fetal skin, urogenital and pulmonary epithelial cells and cells from the extra-embryonic membranes. The cells are first concentrated by centrifuging and are cultured for 7–10 days with the result of the karyotype being available in 14–15 days. Culture failure occurs in about 0.5% and can be minimized by taking an adequate volume of fluid and limiting the delay from the sample being taken and sent to the laboratory. There is also the possibility of *in vitro* mitotic abnormalities occurring as a result of the culture process and therefore multiple cultures are performed for each amniocentesis. Only if a mosaicism or karyotypic anomaly occurs in more than one culture is it likely to be of clinical significance and will need further investigation. This occurs in 0.1–0.2% of samples and may require confirmation on fetal blood sampling.

More recently chromosome-specific probes and fluorescence in situ hybridization (FISH) techniques have been developed to detect numerical aberrations in interphase as well as, non-dividing cells, eliminating the need for prolonged cell culture. Most cytogenetic laboratories will now offer rapid prenatal diagnosis of amniotic fluid using either, fluorescence-based probes for short-tandem-repeat (STR) markers on chromosomes 21, 13 and 18 and polymerase chain reaction (PCR) amplification of these STRs [11], or FISH and fluorescence-labelled DNA probes for chromosomes 21, 18 and 13 [12]. This allows identification of the three commonest chromosomal anomalies within 3 working days.

Chorionic villus sampling

CVS involves sampling of placental tissue rather than amniotic fluid and can be performed between 11 and 14 weeks. There are two routes used for CVS either transabdominal which is now the preferred option or the transcervical route if the former is not possible.

The transabdominal route was developed in the late 1980s and involves a similar technique to that of second trimester amniocentesis. There are various techniques for performing CVS and as there are no studies comparing techniques, the operators should use one that they are most familiar with. Nevertheless, the technique preferred by the author is as follows. It is an aseptic single operator technique, under continuous ultrasound guidance where the operator performs the ultrasound scan and the needling. A 20-gauge needle is inserted percutaneously directly into the placenta being careful not to enter the amniotic sac. The stylet of the needle is removed by an assistant and a 20-ml syringe with 5 ml of heparinized saline is attached to the needle. Negative pressure is then applied to the syringe and the needle moved backwards and forwards in the placenta a few times to suction placental tissue within the needle. While the negative pressure is maintained the needle is then withdrawn and the contents syringed into a sterile container.

The older transcervical approach was developed in the early 1980s. This is now used rarely when the placenta is low and posterior and is not approachable directly by the transabdominal route. This is a 2-operator technique with the patient in the lithotomy position. While one operator scans transabdominally with the transducer in the midline, the other operator attaches a tenaculum to the cervix and inserts a 2-mm CVS forceps through the cervix into the placenta under ultrasound guidance and takes a sample.

Meta-analysis of the randomized trials of transcervical CVS yields an excess loss rate in the CVS group of 3.7% compared to mid-trimester amniocentesis [13]. One study reported a significantly lower miscarriage of transabdominal CVS compared to the transcervical [14], which is then comparable to that after amniocentesis. The transabdominal approach is preferred, not just because it may be associated with a lower miscarriage risk, but also because it avoids putting the women through an uncomfortable procedure in the lithotomy position.

It is now recommended that CVS is not performed before 10 weeks because of the reported association of early CVS and isolated fetal limb disruption and oromandibular hypoplasia. However, large series of CVS performed after 10 weeks do not show any increase in the rate of limb defects [15].

Cytogenetic analysis of the CVS sample is similar to that of amniocentesis. However, placental karyotype may not be exactly the same as the fetus, especially if there has been a post-zygotic non-disjunctive event after cells destined to become the placenta have separated off from those giving rise to the fetus. Confined placental mosaicism occurs in around 1% of chorionic villus samples and will require reanalysis with a second trimester amniocentesis. Mosaicism is only confirmed in the fetus in about 10% of cases.

Multiple pregnancies

Invasive prenatal diagnosis should only be performed in multiple pregnancies by a specialist in a tertiary level fetal medicine unit who has experience in performing selective termination of pregnancy if required. The uterine contents need to be mapped thoroughly before the procedure is undertaken to ensure that separate samples are taken from each fetus and that each twin can be identified accurately at a later stage. Detailed mapping involves identification of chorionicity, location of individual placental sites and cord insertions, plane of the dividing septum in three dimensions and identifying fetal sex.

Amniocentesis is the preferred option in most units because of the relatively high risk of cross contamination of chorionic tissue with CVS in dichorionic twins (2–6%), leading to false-positive or false-negative results. However, CVS is appropriate in a monochorionic pregnancy if the operator is sure of the chorionicity. Most clinicians use two separate puncture sites when performing amniocentesis again to limit the risk of cross contamination although there are series with single entry techniques traversing the placental membranes and low complication rates.

There are no randomized trials to indicate procedure-related loss rates in twins. Background loss rates, however, are appreciably higher. Recent series suggest that total fetal loss rates in twins after amniocentesis (3.5–4.0%) or CVS (2–4%) may not be much higher than background rates. A case-control study of 202 twins undergoing mid-trimester amniocentesis reported a loss rate only 0.3% higher than in control twins [16].

Fetal blood sampling

The availability of rapid karyotypic diagnosis with both CVS and amniocentesis and their considerably easier utility has resulted in fetal blood sampling (FBS) now rarely being used to assess karyotype. It is now almost exclusively used for the assessment of fetal anaemia or infection. It is performed under sterile conditions with continuous ultrasound guidance. Again a single operator usually performs the ultrasound and needle insertion. A 20-gauge needle is inserted into the placental cord insertion or intrafetally into the intrahepatic vein, with colour Doppler mapping of the vessels. There are significantly greater risks of FBS than with amniocentesis or CVS. These include fetal bradycardia, haemorrhage, cord haematoma or tamponade and fetal death. Sampling from the intrahepatic cord appears to be safer than the placental cord insertion or free loops of cord. There needs to be immediate access to laboratory facilities for analysis of the fetal blood. Because of the significantly higher density of nucleated cells in an FBS a full karyotype culture of lymphocytes should be available within 48 h.

Management options

Following a diagnosis of fetal abnormality, the women should be referred for appropriate counselling regarding the nature of the abnormality, the possibility of therapy, and the probable outcome for the child. Further consultation with the relevant paediatric specialist may be indicated, especially where post-natal interventions are contemplated or where there is a major risk of serious handicap. Counselling should address the certainty of the diagnosis, the possible association with other anomalies and the associated risk of aneuploidy or other serious undiagnosed genetic syndromes. They also need to be advised of the prognosis for the fetus including perinatal morbidity including the risk of intrauterine death, the post-natal morbidity associated with the findings and the life expectancy for the child. Finally, they need to be counselled as to whether any curative or ameliorating procedures can be offered in the neonatal period, whether early delivery and what mode of delivery may be required and if any procedure could be offered while the fetus is *in utero*.

Termination of pregnancy

Although some conditions are amenable to fetal treatment, neonatal correction or surgery in infancy, for chromosomal anomalies and many structural abnormalities there is no treatment and the management issues are essentially limited to termination versus continuation of pregnancy. Unless the abnormality is trivial, termination of pregnancy is a management option that should be discussed in parental counselling. The RCOG Report on Termination of Pregnancy for Fetal Abnormality [17] advises that where abortion falls within the grounds specified in the Abortion Act of 1967, doctors 'must advise the woman that she has this option. They must ensure she understands the nature of the fetal abnormality, and the probable outcome of the pregnancy, whether it continues to term or is aborted. The woman is then able to decide whether she wishes to have an abortion and to give her informed consent.'

In England and Wales, termination of pregnancy is allowed under Clause E of the 1967 Abortion Act where two medical practitioners acting in good faith certify that 'there is a substantial risk that if the child were born it would suffer from such physical or mental abnormalities as to be seriously handicapped'. This has been the main Clause under which termination is offered in most fetal medicine centres. Termination can also be offered under Clause C of the Act where 'the pregnancy has not exceeded its 24th week and the continuance of the pregnancy would involve risk, greater than if the pregnancy were terminated, of injury to the physical or mental health of the pregnant woman or any existing children of her family.' This is the clause under which more than 90% of terminations in England and Wales are performed. Where practitioners have difficulty justifying termination prior

to 24 weeks for fetal abnormality, which they do not necessarily consider 'severe' (Clause E), termination is instead then frequently offered under Clause C.

Termination of pregnancy in later pregnancy is largely confined to referral centres both because of the need for an expert opinion on fetal diagnosis and prognosis and because of the need for feticide before it is born. This is usually achieved by ultrasound-guided intracardiac injection of potassium chloride, which is recommended for all terminations after 21 weeks and 6 days' gestation. These are skilled procedures usually restricted to fetal medicine specialists and fetal asystole must be confirmed at least 5 min post-procedure and then checked again on ultrasound half an hour later.

It must be stressed that as Clause E is relatively vague and *'substantial'* and *'significantly'* are not clearly defined, the decision to offer a termination of pregnancy for a fetal anomaly is usually based on a consensus decision of a multidisciplinary team and not by the fetal medicine specialist alone.

Continuation of pregnancy

Once aneuploidy has been excluded, many isolated structural anomalies are best corrected in the term neonate or indeed later in life. These include conditions such as duodenal/jejunal atresia, omphalocele, gastroschisis, unilateral renal problems, ovarian cysts, cleft lip and palate and most cardiac anomalies. This list is by no means exhaustive. Under these circumstances the parents need to be counselled on the morbidity and mortality for corrective surgery. Detection of these anomalies, however, allows for appropriate perinatal management of the pregnancy to be undertaken. This will involve antenatal review and counselling with the appropriate paediatric specialist such as the surgeon, urologist, cardiologist and cardiac surgeons. It also allows for the timing and mode of delivery to be discussed as well as the location such as delivery in a tertiary level unit where the neonatal surgery is to be performed. Indeed these same principles apply even when the fetus has a non-lethal chromosomal anomaly such as trisomy 21 and the parents wish to continue the pregnancy. However, conditions such as trisomy 18 and 13 which have almost no chance of long-term survival are usually not offered surgical correction as this would not influence survival and the parents need to be counselled of this.

Parents who decide to continue with a pregnancy where the prognosis is universally fatal such as anencephaly or trisomy 18 need to be supported in their decision by all staff concerned in their care. However, they need to be counselled regarding the high risk of intrauterine death and if they should reach term, management of the labour needs to be discussed. The parents should be given the option of no monitoring in labour to avoid delivery by Caesarean section, which would not improve neonatal survival and would significantly increase maternal morbidity. Neonatal resuscitation with an option of no active resuscitation also needs to be discussed by the neonatologist and carefully detailed in the notes.

With most structural anomalies Caesarean section does not improve outcome compared with a vaginal delivery. Nonetheless there are some conditions preferably delivered by Caesarean section. This primarily applies to conditions where the neonate is likely to need immediate surgery such as duodenal atresia or gastroschisis and organization of neonatologist, paediatric surgeons and paediatric anaesthetist is easier when the delivery is planned. With some conditions a Caesarean section may be the only option because of unstable lie or dystocia as with a large sacrococcygeal teratoma, massive intra-abdominal masses and severe macrocephaly.

Fetal therapy *in utero*

However, there are now a number of conditions where *in utero* therapy may be offered in specialist fetal medicine units. This has only been possible due to recent advances in imaging as well as ultrasound-guided or fetoscopic techniques. The goal of fetal surgery is to interrupt the *in utero* progression of an otherwise treatable condition and improve perinatal outcome in the neonate. However, it must be stated that many of the techniques of fetal surgery have not been tested in randomized control studies and until they have been, the ability to treat *in utero* may not necessarily be the best option for the mother or fetus. It is also important that these new techniques are tested against current conservative management and not historical data, as neonatal care and post-natal outcomes have improved dramatically over the last two decades as demonstrated by the data on management of congenital diaphragmatic hernias [18]. Below are detailed some of the conditions that have been treated *in utero* and a summary of the evidence for treatment.

Red cell and platelet alloimmunization

Intrauterine therapy for fetal anaemia and thrombocytopaenia by intravascular fetal transfusion was probably the first major success story in fetal medicine. There have been two recent advances which have revolutionized the management of fetal anaemia. First, the development of PCR techniques to identify fetal Rh genotype from free-fetal DNA in the maternal serum [19]. Rh D status of the fetus can now be accurately determined non-invasively in Rh D negative women and is now a routine test offered by the International Blood Group Reference Laboratory (IBGRL) to alloimmunized women in the UK. This has significantly reduced the number of invasive procedures required for genotyping for Rh D in the UK. In the study by Finning *et al.* [20] only 7 out of 230 cases could not have their Rh status confirmed using this technique. Currently the IBGRL are also offering genotyping for Rhc and Kell using a similar technique as these can both cause fetal haemolytic anaemia.

The second major advance is in the abandonment of invasive amniocentesis for detecting ODΔ450 in amniotic fluid as a surrogate for fetal haemolysis, in favour of non-invasive monitoring for fetal anaemia by using fetal middle cerebral artery Doppler velocimetry. Mari *et al.* [21] demonstrated using a cut of 1.5 multiples of the median (MOM) that the middle cerebral artery Doppler peak systolic velocity (MCA PSV) could be used with a sensitivity of 100% and false positive rate of 12% to detect fetal anaemia (Plate 17.1, *facing p. 562*).

Current practice is to perform maternal sera fetal Rh D genotyping in all Rh D negative alloimmunized women. In women who have a Rh D positive fetus maternal serum titres of Rh D antibodies are monitored and the patient referred for weekly MCA PSV monitoring using ultrasound once maternal serum levels reach 4 IU/ml or if there has been a previously affected child. If the MCA PSV is above 1.5 [21] a FBS under continuous ultrasound guidance is performed with immediate access to fetal blood analysis. If the fetus is anaemic it is transfused using maternally cross-matched O Rh negative, cytomegalovirus negative, irradiated, concentrated (haematocrit 70–90%) blood. Weekly MCA PSV monitoring is continued and further FBS is performed if indicated on MCA PSV or at a 3–5 week interval to assess the rate of fall of haemoglobin. Women who have been transfused are usually delivered electively at 37–38 weeks and the neonate should go onto double phototherapy post-natally.

Fetal alloimmune thrombocytopaenia is caused by maternal sensitization to the human platelet antigens (HPA) and can lead to devastating intracranial haemorrhage in 10–20% of affected pregnancies. The diagnosis is usually made following the birth of a previously affected child. Previous management was based on frequent FBS and platelet transfusion, with the timing based on the gestation and severity of a previously affected pregnancy. However, the risk to the fetus of repeated FBS are considerable with a procedure-related loss rate per procedure of 1.2% and up to 8.4% per pregnancy. More recently a European collaborative study concluded that the start of treatment can be stratified on the basis of sibling history and that maternal intravenous immunoglobulin (IVIG) treatment should be the first-line treatment of choice thereby delaying and limiting the number of invasive procedures as the procedure-related complication rate was high [22].

Twin–twin transfusion syndrome

Twin–twin transfusion syndrome (TTTS) is discussed in more detail elsewhere. It affects 15% of monochorionic pregnancies and historically has perinatal mortalities of up to 80% if untreated. Recent advances in management such as amnioreduction, septostomy, laser ablation of placental vessels or selective reduction using bipolar cord occlusion has significantly improved perinatal survival such that between 60 and 79% of affected pregnancies have at least one fetus surviving with the various techniques. However, a recent randomized control trial of placental laser ablation versus amnioreduction/septostomy demonstrated that as compared with the amnioreduction group, the laser group had a higher likelihood of survival of at least one twin to 28 days of age (76 versus 56%; relative risk of the death of both fetuses, 0.63; 95% confidence interval, 0.25–0.93; $p = 0.009$) and 6 months of age ($p = 0.002$). Infants in the laser group also had a lower incidence of cystic periventricular leukomalacia (6 versus 14%, $p = 0.02$) and were more likely to be free of neurologic complications at 6 months of age (52 versus 31%, $p = 0.003$) [23]. The authors suggested that endoscopic laser coagulation of anastomoses is a more effective first-line treatment than serial amnioreduction for severe twin-to-twin transfusion syndrome diagnosed before 26 weeks of gestation. However, it remains unclear what the most appropriate management for early stage disease should be and randomized trial in this group is awaited.

Multifetal pregnancy reduction

Multifetal pregnancy reduction (MFPR) has been used over the last 15–20 years to reduce high-order multiple pregnancies in the late first trimester, usually to twins, with the perinatal outcome of reduced twins approaching that of spontaneous twins. A finishing number of 2 has become standard practice, as the perinatal outcome of twin pregnancies is considered acceptable and as two fetuses still leave an option of selective feticide if discordant fetal abnormalities manifest later on ultrasound scan.

Expansion of the technique has been associated with a progressive fall in miscarriage rates due to a combination of better resolution ultrasound and the learning curve of fetal medicine specialists performing the technique. The procedure is performed by an intracardiac injection of strong potassium chloride solution (1.5 g in 10 ml) into the targeted fetus under ultrasound guidance using a 20-gauge needle. Because of a lower miscarriage rate (5.4 versus 12%) the transabdominal approach has almost entirely replaced the transvaginal technique.

MFPR is performed between 11 and 14 weeks for three reasons. First, the risk of spontaneous reduction or 'vanishing twin' has by then passed and second, a limited anomaly scan can be performed to detect gross structural anomalies and features of aneuploidy to guide selection of the fetus(es) for reduction. Finally, screening for aneuploidy using NT can also be performed prior to MFPR again to guide selection if the NT measurements are discordant. To minimize the risk of ascending infection, if there are no structural anomalies and the NT risk of aneuploidy is low, the fetus furthest away from the cervix is normally selected for reduction.

The literature remains relatively evenly divided as to whether MFPR in triplets improves outcome compared with unreduced triplets. A meta-analysis of studies of triplets reduced to twins and expectantly managed [24] show that the pregnancy loss rate <24 weeks for triplets reduced to twins appeared lower than that of unreduced triplets but was not statistically significant (5.7 versus 7.5% respectively, Odds Ratio (OR) 0.74 [0.54–1.03]; $p = 0.09$). However, the extreme preterm delivery rate <28 weeks was significantly lower for the reduced group (4 versus 10%, OR 0.37 [0.2–0.5]; $p < 0.0001$) as was the rate of preterm delivery <32 weeks (9 versus 24%; OR 0.32 [0.25–0.42]; $p < 0.0001$) and the perinatal mortality (43/1000 live births versus 110/1000; OR 0.37 [0.3–0.5]; $p < 0.0001$) compared with unreduced triplets, although there was no difference in the take-home baby rate (92 versus 87%; OR 0.7 [0.4–1.2]; $p = 0.23$).

Although expectant management of trichorionic triplets has improved significantly in the last two decades the evidence suggests that reduction to dichorionic twins significantly reduces the risk of preterm delivery and low birthweight infants without a significant increase in the risk of miscarriage. Therefore, parents of trichorionic triplets need to have balanced counselling early in pregnancy where clear facts are presented and time given for them to make an informed decision based on their individual moral and religious values and fully supported in any decision they make.

Fetal *in utero* surgical interventions

In utero fetal surgery for structural anomalies that can interfere with organ development may allow normal development to take place and therefore improve perinatal outcome. However, there are a number of major factors that need to be considered before fetal surgery can be offered. First, appropriate patient selection is essential, the condition needs to have been detected early enough to intervene before irreversible damage has already occurred and the maternal risks of anaesthesia and surgery which may involve hysterotomy needs to be considered as well as the risks of preterm labour and fetal demise during the procedure. Finally, the evidence that the intervention is of benefit to the fetus needs to be discussed with the parents.

Spina bifida

Open neural tube defects are characterized by exposure of the meninges and neural tissue to the amniotic fluid. Although it had previously been assumed that the spinal cord was intrinsically defective, it is becoming more evident that secondary destruction of the spinal tissue occurs due to exposure to the amniotic fluid or direct trauma from fetal movements. This led to the development of techniques for open hysterotomy repair of myleomeningoceles. Bruner *et al.* [25] published outcome on the first 178 cases of intrauterine surgery for spina bifida performed in their centre since 1997, with post-natal follow-up data on 116 cases. This data suggest that among fetuses who underwent operation *in utero* for spina bifida, fetuses with a ventricular size of <14 mm at the time of surgery, fetuses who had surgery at ≤25 weeks of gestation and fetuses with defects that were located at ≤ L4 were less likely to require ventriculoperitoneal shunting for hydrocephalus during the first year of life.

Notwithstanding this, there is still considerable maternal and fetal morbidity and mortality associated with the procedure. This is primarily due to the general anaesthesia and hysterotomy required for the procedure with its inherently high risk of preterm labour. Currently the National Institute of Health (NIH) in the USA are undertaking a multicentre prospective randomized controlled study on *in utero* repair called the Management of Myelomeningocele Study (MOMS: www.spinabifidamoms.com). The study plans to recruit 200 patients between 19 and 25 weeks gestation, who will be randomized into conservative management with post-natal repair or fetal surgery at three tertiary fetal surgical units in the USA. The primary outcome measures will be death and need for ventriculoperitoneal shunts by 1 year of age. This study began in 2003 and has as yet not completed recruitment. Until this study has been published there is an informal embargo on other centres outside the NIH study performing intrauterine surgery for spina bifida and until this study is published *in utero* repair cannot be recommended.

Congenital diaphragmatic hernia

Although congenital diaphragmatic hernia (CDH) is a simple anatomical defect to correct post-natally, the perinatal mortality has historically been high (58%) because of the pulmonary hypoplasia and the resulting pulmonary hypertension already established in fetal life. Open hysterotomy and surgical repair of the CDH proved to be very unsuccessful and was abandoned early. A number of techniques have been developed for the *in utero* management of CDH. These were primarily based on animal studies that showed that occlusion of the fetal trachea could improve pulmonary development by accumulation of pulmonary secretions. This led to the development and clinical use of reversible techniques for fetal tracheal occlusion. This could be achieved either by open hysterotomy and direct application of a removable external metal clip on the trachea or endoscopic neck dissection and tracheal clip application and more recently by the use of endoscopic bronchoscopy and placement of a tracheal balloon, which can be deflated *in utero* or at the time of delivery.

However, a randomized trial performed by Harrison *et al.* [18] whose group had previously published most of the data on *in utero* therapy, comparing standard post-natal management with that of endoscopic tracheal occlusion demonstrated that there was no benefit in either neonatal morbidity or mortality of *in utero* surgery. Probably the most significant finding of this study was that the conservatively managed group had a surprising high survival rate (75% compared with an expected 37% from historical data) and reflected the improvement in neonatal management of pulmonary hypoplasia and pulmonary hypertension. Following the publication of this study, *in utero* fetal therapy for CDH cannot currently be recommended.

Sacrococcygeal teratoma

Sacrococcygeal teratomas (SCT) are teratomas which arise from the presacral space and can grow to massive proportions leading to high-output cardiac failure with perinatal mortality in nearly 50%. The Rationale for *in utero* therapy was to occlude the vascular flow to the teratoma and therefore reverse the vascular steal and high-output cardiac failure. Although intrauterine surgical procedures such as cyst aspiration, amnioreduction and open debulking have been tried the perinatal mortality and obstetric complication rates remain high [26]. Other minimally invasive techniques such as ultrasound-guided radio frequency ablation of the SCT vasculature appear promising but require further evaluation.

Congenital cystic adenomatous malformation

Congenital cystic adenomatous malformation (CCAM) is a space occupying cystic lesion of the lungs that can lead to cardiac failure by causing mediastinal shift leading to cardiac and vascular compression. Fetuses that develop hydrops with CCAM have a very poor prognosis which can be improved by *in utero* open hysterotomy and resection of the CCAM with improved survival (60%) [27]. However, less invasive procedures such as cyst aspiration or cyst shunting may also be considered before open hysterotomy.

Stenosis of semilumnar valves

Congenital heart disease with pulmonary or aortic stenosis/atresia can lead to progressive hypoplasia of the affected ventricle and a functional univentricular heart. *In utero* valvuloplasty can allow forward flow across the valve, therefore permitting growth of the affected ventricle and the potential for biventricular repair post-natally. Once again although the few case series published are promising [28,29] further studies are awaited to support its use.

Lower urinary tract obstruction

Lower urinary tract obstruction (LUTO) is a heterogenous condition that affects 1:5000–8000 newborns. The aetiology can vary depending on the fetal sex with posterior urethral valves being most common in male infants and urethral atresia being more common in females. Complete obstruction of the lower urinary tract can lead to massive distension of the bladder and back pressure on the kidneys leading to destruction of the renal cortex as well as the resultant oligo/anhydramnios causing pulmonary hypoplasia and limb deformities. The rationale for *in utero* therapy is to alleviate the obstruction and therefore prevent bladder and renal damage and restore liquor volume to allow pulmonary development. Careful patient selection is crucial and involves serial bladder aspiration and analysis of urinary electrolytes to confirm normal renal function, as well as confirmation of karyotype and exclusion of other major structural anomalies on detailed ultrasound scan.

Current management options include vesico-ureteric shunting or fetal cystoscopy. Vesico-ureteric shunting involves ultrasound-guided insertion of a pig-tail shunt between the fetal bladder and the amniotic cavity. However, there appears to be considerable complications related to shunting and survival remains poor with considerable post-natal morbidity with the majority requiring bladder augmentation post-natally. Fetal cystoscopy seems to be more promising. Direct visualization and exploration of the fetal bladder allows the presence of posterior urethral valves to be identified and even disrupted using laser or gentle saline pressure injections. Once again the data for its use is based on small case series and further studies are needed to support its use.

Medical interventions and stem cell therapy

Medical intervention *in utero* for certain fetal conditions have been successful. Treatment of fetal congenital adrenal hypoplasia (CAH) with maternal dexamethasone was the first inborn error of metabolism to be successfully treated *in utero*. Currently CVS and the use of molecular markers can be used to diagnose CAH in at-risk fetuses and steroid treatment started as early as possible to prevent masculinization of female fetuses [30].

Fetal heart block due to maternal anti-Ro and anti-La antibodies have also been treated antenatally. Maternal anti-Ro and anti-La antibodies can lead to varying degrees of fetal heart block. If a complete heart block should occur with a fetal ventricular rate of <55 bpm this usually leads to hydrops and a very poor prognosis. As the damage to the fetal cardiac conduction tissue is immune mediated, maternal administration of high-dose steroids have been tried with varying degrees of success in a number of case reports [31]. However, there are considerable maternal and fetal complications of using such high-dose steroids such as maternal diabetes, intrauterine growth restriction and fetal and maternal Cushing's disease. More recent studies on the use of IVIG as a blocking antibody have shown more promising results but again larger controlled studies are needed [32].

The use of stem cells for *in utero* therapy is purely experimental at this stage but the results are encouraging. Gene therapy has been developed for use in osteogenesis imperfecta [33] and in theory at least could be used *in utero* in an affected fetus; although this is as yet to be reported on. Another promising area is in the use of gene therapy for cystic fibrosis which has already been successful in animal models [34]. It is likely that the major advances in the next two decades will be in the field of stem cell *in utero* therapy.

Conclusion

The basic principles of practice in fetal medicine are based around the identification of high-risk pregnancies, accurate diagnosis of fetal anomalies using invasive prenatal diagnostic techniques and detailed imaging and a multidisciplinary approach to counselling of parents. This counselling will be centred on the accuracy of the diagnosis, prognosis for the fetus and neonate and the possibility of *in utero* therapy. Many conditions such as aneuploidy are not amenable to treatment and many others are best managed in the neonatal period. However, recent advances in *in utero* therapy have made *in utero* treatment for some conditions possible. Nevertheless, despite the great strides forward and initial euphoria, many fetal therapeutic interventions have not be shown to improve outcome and cannot now be recommended. Others have yet to be tested in controlled trials and remain anecdotal case series.

Notwithstanding this, continued advances in minimally invasive techniques, *in utero* imaging and suppression of preterm labour may allow development of therapeutic techniques for a wider range of conditions. This will likely be coupled with advances in stem cell research and *in utero* gene therapy. However, it must be accepted that any new technique as well as older established techniques need to be exposed first to the rigors of good quality research before they can be accepted as standard practice.

References

1. National Institute of Clinical Excellence (2003) *Antenatal Care: Routine Care for the Healthy Pregnant Women*. Clinical Guideline October 2003.
2. Wald NJ, Rodeck C, Hackshaw AK, Walters J, Chitty L, Mackinson AM (2003) First and second trimester antenatal screening for Down's syndrome: the results of the Serum, Urine and Ultrasound Screening Study (SURUSS). *Health Technol Assess* **7**(11), 1–77.
3. Bricker L, Garcia J, Henderson J, Mugford M, Neilson J, Roberts T *et al.* (2000) Ultrasound screening in pregnancy: a systematic review of the clinical effectiveness, cost-effectiveness and women's views. *Health Technol Assess* **4**(16), i–193.
4. Chitty LS, Hunt GH, Moore J & Lobb MO (1991) Effectiveness of routine ultrasonography in detecting fetal structural abnormalities in a low risk population. *Br Med J* **303**(6811), 1165—9.
5. Boyd PA, Chamberlain P & Hicks NR (1998) 6-year experience of prenatal diagnosis in an unselected population in Oxford, UK. *Lancet* **352**(9140), 1577–81.
6. Wimalasundera RC & Gardiner HM (2004) Congenital heart disease and aneuploidy. *Prenat Diagn* **24**(13), 1116–22.
7. Smith-Bindman R, Hosmer W, Feldstein VA, Deeks JJ & Goldberg JD (2001) Second-trimester ultrasound to detect fetuses with Down syndrome: a meta-analysis. *J Am Med Assoc* **285**(8), 1044–55.
8. Nicolaides KH (2003) Screening for chromosomal defects. *Ultrasound Obstet Gynecol* **21**(4), 313–21.
9. Wiener JJ, Farrow A & Farrow SC (1990) Audit of amniocentesis from a district general hospital: is it worth it? *Br Med J* **300**(6734), 1243–5.
10. Tabor A, Philip J, Madsen M, Bang J, Obel EB & Norgaard-Pedersen B (1986) Randomised controlled trial of genetic amniocentesis in 4606 low-risk women. *Lancet* **1**(8493), 1287–93.
11. Verma L, Macdonald F, Leedham P, McConachie M, Dhanjal S & Hulten M (1998) Rapid and simple prenatal DNA diagnosis of Down's syndrome. *Lancet* **352**(9121), 9–12.
12. Morris A, Boyd E, Dhanjal S *et al.* (1999) Two years' prospective experience using fluorescence in situ hybridization on uncultured amniotic fluid cells for rapid prenatal diagnosis of common chromosomal aneuploidies. *Prenat Diagn* **19**(6), 546–51.
13. Medical Research Council European trial of chorion villus sampling (1991) MRC working party on the evaluation pf chorion villus sampling. *Lancet* **337**(8756), 1491–9.
14. Smidt-Jensen S, Permin M *et al.* (1992) Randomised comparison of amniocentesis and transabdominal and transcervical chorionic villus sampling. *Lancet* **340**(8830), 1237–44.
15. Froster UG & Jackson L (1996) Limb defects and chorionic villus sampling: results from an international registry, 1992–94. *Lancet* **347**(9000), 489–94.
16. Ghidini A, Lynch L, Hicks C, Alvarez M & Lockwood CJ (1993) The risk of second-trimester amniocentesis in twin gestations: a case-control study. *Am J Obstet Gynecol* **169**(4), 1013–6.
17. Royal College of Obstetricians and Gynaecologist (1996) *Termination of Pregnancy for Fetal Abnormality in England, Wale and Scotland*. London: RCOG Press.
18. Harrison MR, Keller RL, Hawgood SB *et al.* (2003) A randomized trial of fetal endoscopic tracheal occlusion for severe fetal congenital diaphragmatic hernia. *N Engl J Med* **349**(20), 1916–24.
19. Lo YM, Bowell PJ, Selinger M *et al.* (1994) Prenatal determination of fetal rhesus D status by DNA amplification of peripheral blood of rhesus-negative mothers. *Ann N Y Acad Sci* **731**, 229–36.
20. Finning K, Martin P & Daniels G (2004) A clinical service in the UK to predict fetal Rh (Rhesus) D blood group using free fetal DNA in maternal plasma. *Ann N Y Acad Sci* **1022**, 119–23.
21. Mari G, Deter RL, Carpenter RL *et al.* (2000) Noninvasive diagnosis by Doppler ultrasonography of fetal anemia due to maternal red-cell alloimmunization. Collaborative Group for Doppler Assessment of the Blood Velocity in Anemic Fetuses. *N Engl J Med* **342**(1), 9–14.
22. Birchall JE, Murphy MF, Kaplan C & Kroll H (2003) European collaborative study of the antenatal management of feto-maternal alloimmune thrombocytopenia. *Br J Haematol* **122**(2), 275–88.
23. Senat MV, Deprest J, Boulvain M, Paupe A, Winer N & Ville Y (2004) Endoscopic laser surgery versus serial amnioreduction for severe twin-to-twin transfusion syndrome. *N Engl J Med* **351**(2), 136–44.
24. Wimalasundera RC (2006) *Recommendations arising from the Royal College of Obstetricians and Gynaecologist 50th Study Group: Multiple Pregnancy*. London: RCOG Press.
25. Bruner JP, Tulipan N, Reed G *et al.* (2004) Intrauterine repair of spina bifida: preoperative predictors of shunt-dependent hydrocephalus. *Am J Obstet Gynecol* **190**(5), 1305–12.
26. Hedrick HL, Flake AW, Crombleholme TM *et al.* (2004) Sacrococcygeal teratoma: prenatal assessment, fetal intervention, and outcome. *J Pediatr Surg* **39**(3), 430–8.
27. Adzick NS, Harrison MR, Flake AW, Howell LJ, Golbus MS & Filly RA (1993) Fetal surgery for cystic adenomatoid malformation of the lung. *J Pediatr Surg* **28**(6), 806–12.
28. Kohl T, Sharland G, Allan LD *et al.* (2000) World experience of percutaneous ultrasound-guided balloon valvuloplasty in human fetuses with severe aortic valve obstruction. *Am J Cardiol* **85**(10), 1230–3.
29. Tulzer G, Arzt W, Franklin RC, Loughna PV, Mair R & Gardiner HM (2002) Fetal pulmonary valvuloplasty for

critical pulmonary stenosis or atresia with intact septum. *Lancet* **360**(9345), 1567–8.

30. Evans MI, Harrison MR, Flake AW & Johnson MP (2002) Fetal therapy. *Best Pract Res Clin Obstet Gynaecol* **16**(5), 671–83.

31. Jaeggi ET, Fouron JC, Silverman ED, Ryan G, Smallhorn J & Hornberger LK (2004) Transplacental fetal treatment improves the outcome of prenatally diagnosed complete atrioventricular block without structural heart disease. *Circulation* **110**(12), 1542–8.

32. Wong JP, Kwek KY, Tan JY & Yeo GS (2001) Fetal congenital complete heart block: prophylaxis with intravenous gammaglobulin and treatment with dexamethasone. *Aust N Z J Obstet Gynaecol* **41**(3), 339–41.

33. Chamberlain JR, Schwarze U, Wang PR *et al.* (2004) Gene targeting in stem cells from individuals with osteogenesis imperfecta. *Science* **303**(5661), 1198–201.

34. Boyle MP, Enke RA, Adams RJ, Guggino WB & Zeitlin PL (2001) In utero AAV-mediated gene transfer to rabbit pulmonary epithelium. *Mol Ther* **4**(2), 115–21.

Further reading

Diana W Bianchi (ed.) (2000) *Fetology: Diagnosis and Management of the Fetal Patient*. Columbus: McGraw-Hill Education.

Michael R Harrison (ed.) (2001) *The Unborn Patient Prenatal Diagnosis and Treatment*. Philadelphia: Saunders (W.B.) Co Ltd.

Chapter 18: Obstetric emergencies

Sara Paterson-Brown

Introduction

The variety of emergencies which can present to the obstetrician is vast and includes acute medical and surgical as well as obstetric conditions. Many such emergencies can be preceded by warning signs in women with risk factors and rapid recognition and response is crucial in optimizing outcome. A sound understanding of the pathologies involved and the principles of their treatment should help the obstetrician to build up a reliable, reproducible and robust systematic approach to recognizing and managing these life-threatening conditions. This chapter will address how to minimize the risks and consequences of such emergencies as well as how to manage them in the acute situation.

General principles for minimizing the risk of an emergency occurring

Promote good antenatal health

Good general health and a supportive home environment promote good health during pregnancy. The Confidential Enquiry into Maternal and Child Health (CEMACH): Why Mothers Die 2000–2002 [1] reminds us of the increased risks not only of those with pre-existing disease, but also of the socially excluded, the obese, and those abusing substances. Good antenatal care is paramount in promoting health: women should be screened for a variety of risk factors and any problem that is identified should be acted upon [2]. We know from the confidential enquiries over the years that we sometimes fail to recognize, communicate or act on risk factors which are apparent in the antenatal period. This makes it imperative, when considering intrapartum care, to review a woman's antenatal health to identify any such risks, and pay heed to any instructions made in the antenatal period.

Organized intrapartum care

The senior sister in charge and the senior obstetrician on the delivery suite should work together as a team to co-ordinate clinical activity. The skills required to coordinate workload and staffing are multiple and often acquired over years; but if you recognize calm and control in those you work with, take a moment or two to try to define what they are doing differently and try to emulate these features:

- Keep your mind open to all the activity going on.
- Try to coordinate activity so that things happen in sequence and not all at the same time.
- Listen to your midwives' and doctors' concerns and address them;
- Prioritize according to risk (triage – see below).
- Get simple things done quickly, as once resolved they relieve staff.
- Do not defer decisions unnecessarily (work just builds up).
- Give each woman a carer with the appropriate skills to match the complexity of the clinical problem.
- Recognize if a doctor or midwife is out of their depth support them and encourage them to call for help.
- Regularly revisit women with risk factors to check the situation is not deteriorating (do not assume you will be called).

Triage

The principles behind effective triage have hinged on the ABC approach to prioritizing casualties according to whether they have an airway (A) problem (which can lead to death within minutes if left untreated), through difficulties with breathing (B) to circulatory disorders (C). Although this can also be useful in obstetrics it doesn't always address the fact that there are two patients, the mother and the baby which may sometimes be a dilemma. Indeed there is little written about obstetric triage [3,4] and how to fit the fetus (F) into the equation. Clearly it is not as easy as ABCF and emergency care to save a baby may take priority over a less than life-threatening maternal condition. However, in most societies, a mother's life is given priority over that of an unborn baby and most importantly the fetus is best treated by adequate, rapid and effective resuscitation or stabilization of the mother anyway [5].

General principles for minimizing adverse consequences resulting from an emergency

If risk factors have been identified preparations can be made to deal with the anticipated problem and staff should be informed, briefed and their roles defined. It is not uncommon that when such problems are anticipated, everything goes smoothly; this does not mean that staff are overcautious; it means they did their job well. Sadly, events do not always turn out well or an unexpected emergency occurs, and in such situations there are some features of general care which are important.

Communication and teamworking

In any emergency multiple workers will become involved which can produce problems in itself:
- some staff may not know each other;
- no one knows what anyone else is doing;
- activity can become disordered and inefficient;
- basic important treatment can be forgotten.
Therefore
- someone needs to take the lead role and coordinate activity in a systematic way such that staff work together as a team;
- the skills of any unknown staff need to be clarified;
- roles need to be allocated which match the skills of the staff concerned;
- specific tasks need to be given to designated people to avoid duplications and omissions;
- when someone is asked to do something it is worth checking that they understand and are happy with what is being asked of them;
- someone needs to document timings and actions;
- someone needs to talk to the patient (and her partner) even if only briefly to keep them calm and informed and help them feel confident and supported.
Although the most senior obstetrician present is likely to become the team leader, this is not always either necessary or appropriate and an anaesthetist or senior midwife may take the lead in some emergencies. Senior personnel need to talk to each other and interchange roles as is dictated by the needs of the clinical scenario. In all situations the team leader should keep a cool head and deal with problems logically and efficiently as this will help keep others calm and will promote a cohesive team.

Documentation

This has been mentioned briefly above, but in all emergencies it helps to have someone looking at the clock, holding paper and pen. They can and should be spoken to as things are happening so that they document the important facts – otherwise if, as is often the case, this person is fairly junior, they may not know or understand exactly what is going on and therefore fail to document key activity. Once the emergency is over notes should be written carefully and comprehensively and signed legibly: this is the best time to account for what has happened and any relevant diagnosis, follow-up care plan and prognosis for future pregnancies should be spelt out clearly at this stage whenever possible.

Risk management

After the emergency is over, recounting and analysing events with staff is hugely appreciated and very important: this is usually multidisciplinary but will sometimes be in small groups. Health-care assistants and porters may need this support too and should not be forgotten. If things went well everyone should be congratulated, and if some things were less than perfect, discussing why the difficulties were encountered and what might make things easier/work better another time is often helpful. This is a time for positive critical reflection: any negative feedback can wait.

Emergency training

With the reduced duration of junior doctors' training combined with the dramatic cuts in their working hours, it is unsurprising that their clinical experience of obstetric emergencies is much less than that of their predecessors. They rely increasingly on formal training which can be gained locally to an extent but tends to be supplemented by regional or national courses, a few of which are listed below:

ALSO – Advanced life support in obstetrics – This course is aimed at midwives, obstetric senior house officers (SHOs) and junior specialist registrars (SpRs) and deals with the main obstetric emergencies in a structured systematic fashion. Candidates should gain a sound understanding of the problems and the structured approaches in how to manage them (http://www.also.org.uk).

MOET – Managing obstetric emergencies and trauma – This course is organized for a more senior and multidisciplinary groups, for example, obstetric consultant and senior SpRs (Post-Membership of Royal College of Obstetricians and Gynaecologists (MRCOG) and at least year 3), anaesthetic consultant and senior SpRs, and senior accident and emergency doctors. These courses also include midwives (as 'observers' as they are not formally assessed) who receive the same training during the course and their presence emphasizes and promotes the team approach, which is so important in the obstetric emergency. This course deals with more advanced and complex aspects of emergency obstetrics (http://www.moet.org.uk).

MOSES – Multidisciplinary Obstetric Simulated Emergency Scenarios – This course focuses on emergency behaviour and teamworking dynamics as they apply to the obstetric patient, rather than training on knowledge or techniques. It involves midwives, anaesthetists and obstetricians who often attend together from the same department. This course is very different from, but complements MOET or ALSO (blsimcentre@bartsandthelondon.nhs.uk).

Although acute obstetric emergency training courses are now well established, their formal evaluation is limited [6] and they are certainly no substitute for clinical exposure or indeed for ongoing local training. Most units are now incorporating multidisciplinary emergency drills and scenarios within their teaching programmes. These serve not only to improve knowledge and teamwork, but can also be invaluable aids to identifying problems within the system [7,8].

Collapse

Collapse as it presents to the obstetrician can be due to a variety of causes, including innocent vasovagal faint through to cardiac arrest, but the initial assessment and management of the patient is remarkably similar and requires a systematic disciplined ABC approach (airway, breathing, circulation) combined with lateral tilting of the pregnant patient to minimize aortocaval compression. The essential steps of how to approach the apparently lifeless patient are summarized in Fig. 18.1 and aim to make the crucial diagnosis of cardiac arrest (as opposed to reduced consciousness due to another cause) so that cardiopulmonary resuscitation can be commenced early. Most other conditions require basic resuscitation with attention to the airway and breathing combined with intravenous access and circulatory support while the cause of the problem is diagnosed and then treated (Table 18.1).

Cardiac arrest (Fig. 18.1)

Cardiopulmonary resuscitation (CPR) is not only difficult to administer but is particularly inefficient in the pregnant patient due to:
- difficulties in performing CPR on a tilted patient;
- increased oxygen requirement in pregnancy (20% increase in resting oxygen consumption);

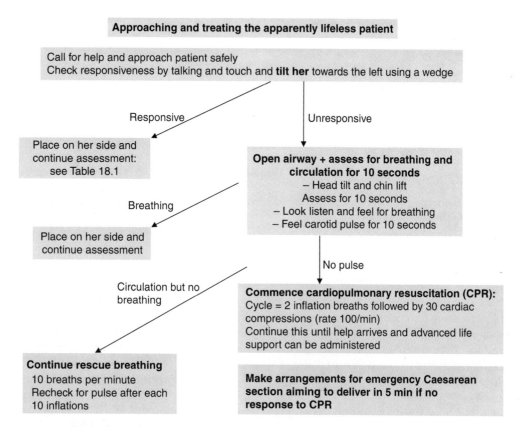

Fig. 18.1 Basic life support [9].

Table 18.1 Causes, features and initial treatment of collapse in the obstetric patient (distinguishing features in bold)

(alphabetical order)	Cause/risk factors	Specific clinical features	Specific treatment points: all need ABC + lateral tilt if undelivered
Adrenal insufficiency	Inadequate or absent steroid cover in someone previously taking steroids	Drug history Hypotensive collapse Metabolic imbalance	Supportive with IV fluids (check electrolytes especially sodium may be low) Hydrocortisone (200 mg IV stat) check BM – may need glucose
Amniotic fluid embolism [13]	Uterine tachysystole Syntocinon hyperstimulation Previous uterine surgery Multiparity Polyhydramnios	Restless, shortness of breath and cyanosis **Vaginal bleeding follows within 30 min due to disseminated intravascular coagulation [15]**	O₂ + ventilate Deliver the baby ASAP Hydrocortisone (200 mg IV stat) *(aminophylline, diuretics, adrenaline morphine)
Anaphylaxis [12,14]	Drug administration, e.g. antibiotics, voltarol, anaesthetic agents, haemocell Latex	History of drugs/latex Rash Stridor Oedema	Adrenaline* (1 ml of 1 in 10,000 IV repeated as needed) with IV fluids Hydrocortisone (200 mg IV stat) Chlorpheniramine (20 mg IV)
Aspiration (Mendelson's syndrome)	Inhalation after vomiting/passive regurgitation (reduced consciousness with unprotected airway)	Shortness of breath, restlessness cyanosis **Bronchospasm**	O₂ + ventilate *(aminophylline, steroids, diuretics and antibiotics)
Bacteraemic shock	Overwhelming sepsis due to esp. Gram negative rods or strep. B	Hypotensive **Warm/fever/blotchy**	Replenish circulation, systems support Antibiotics IV (e.g. Imipenem)
Cardiogenic shock	Congenital or acquired disease Cardiomyopathy	History Restless **SOB/chest pain**	**Sit up** O₂ + frusemide
Eclampsia	Associated with cerebrovascular events or pulmonary oedema or Mg toxicity	Hypertensive Proteinuria	Magnesium sulphate (antidote = calcium gluconate) Control blood pressure with hypotensives
Hyperglycaemia	Diabetes	Hyperventilation and ketosis	IV fluids, Insulin (and potassium)
Hypoglycaemia	Diabetes, Addison's hypopituitary, hypothyroid	**Sweating/clammy** loss of consciousness	IV glucose
Intracerebral bleed	a-v malformation	Fits, CNS signs and **neck stiffness**	Supportive
Massive PE	Usually deep pelvic thrombosis	Restless/cyanosis **elevated JVP**	**Lie down** + O₂ IV fluids + anticoagulate
Neurogenic	Vasovagal (uterine inversion)	**Vaginal examination**	IV fluids ± atropine/reduce uterine inversion
Oligaemic [16]	Haemorrhage (can be concealed) Previous history of labour/pushing	**Tachycardia, pale and cold** Chest pain SOB	Restore circulation and treat Aspirate/drain
Pneumo: thorax/mediastinum			

*These treatments should be undertaken under anaesthetic supervision on high dependancy unit (HDU)/intensive care unit (ITU).

• decreased chest compliance due to splinting of the diaphragm (20% decrease in functional residual capacity);
• reduced venous return due to caval compression limiting cardiac output from chest compressions (stroke volume 30% at term compared to non-pregnant state);
• risk of gastric regurgitation and aspiration (relaxation of cardiac sphincter).

For these reasons it is considered appropriate to empty the uterus to aid maternal survival by performing a *perimortem* Caesarean section if CPR performed with lateral tilt is ineffective after 5 min [5,10]. To achieve this the obstetrician at such an arrest should therefore be preparing for Caesarean section almost immediately. It is reiterated that the point of emptying the uterus is to aid in the resuscitation of the mother and is not for fetal reasons. Fetal viability issues should not delay this procedure which is worthwhile when the pregnancy is of sufficient size to compromise resuscitation: as a guide, if the uterus has reached the level of the umbilicus it should be considered.

To perform a perimortem Caesarean section rapidly the skin incision should be that with which the operator is most familiar, and the uterine incision will be influenced by the gestation of the pregnancy. These details matter little compared to the pressing need to evacuate the uterus and render the mother more receptive to life-saving resuscitation techniques. A large Caesarean section pack is unnecessary and in extremis all the obstetrician needs is a scalpel to commence the procedure while other instruments are being collected.

It is stressed again that this is not done for fetal reasons but there is no doubt that fetal viability is more likely the more quickly the baby is delivered: 70% survive intact if delivered within 5 min, falling to 13% after 10 min [11].

To detail the management of each possible condition which can cause maternal collapse is beyond the scope of this chapter, but Table 18.1 summarizes the different possibilities and those features specific to them in terms of risk factors, clinically distinguishing features and specific points of treatment. More detailed accounts are referenced for further reading [12–16], but a few summary points are highlighted here.

Airway problems

The airway of an obstetric patient is more vulnerable than in the non-pregnant state: not only is there more likely to be swelling and oedema, but the progestogenic effects which reduce gastric emptying and relax the cardiac sphincter increase the chance of regurgitation and subsequent aspiration of gastric contents. For these reasons the management of any obstetric patient with reduced consciousness requires careful attention to maintaining and protecting the airway and this should involve an anaesthetist. In simple circumstances she should at the very least be nursed on her side, and a jaw thrust and chin lift can aid in bringing the tongue forward to open the airway. Severe laryngeal oedema due to pre-eclampsia or anaphylaxis are examples of situations which can critically compromise the airway in the obstetric patient, and in these circumstances an anaesthetist is needed extremely urgently to establish and maintain a protected airway (usually by a cuffed endotracheal tube).

Breathing problems

If the airway is patent but breathing is laboured or consciousness impaired then supplementary oxygen is vital. This should be given by face mask with a reservoir bag, and the oxygen should be turned up to maximum at the wall in the emergency situation. Restlessness and confusion are signs of hypoxaemia and can precede collapse and therefore should be taken extremely seriously. Oxygen saturation should be measured in air by a pulse oximeter and arterial blood taken for gas analysis if there is any concern, and results of these should be reviewed with the anaesthetist on duty.

Circulatory problems

Circulatory problems can be due to cardiac disease (where the resulting pathology is usually pulmonary oedema and low output failure), inadequate venous return with resultant low output failure (massive pulmonary embolus) or an under-filled circulation (hypovolaemia – due to haemorrhage or sepsis). Early intravenous access with large bore cannulae is vital, but then treatment needs to be specific to the cause. Cardiac failure patients do not require (and indeed may be killed by) volume expansion, but are helped by sitting up and diuretics. On the other hand, a woman with a pulmonary embolus or who is hypovolaemic needs volume expansion and to be laid flat. Distinguishing between these conditions is vital as the management of each would clearly be dangerous to the other. Fluid replacement strategies remain controversial [17] but crystalloids and colloids both have a place in obstetric resuscitation, with crystalloids being the first line therapy. The use of albumen in the critically ill is controversial [18] and is currently the subject of a large double blind randomized controlled trial [19].

Haemorrhage

Obstetric haemorrhage is one of the most common causes of major maternal morbidity and mortality [1,20,21] and the most recent triennial report raises the unhappy truth that these deaths have increased (from 7 in 1997–1999 to 17 in 2000–2002) due to a rise in post-partum haemorrhages (CEMACH). The confidential enquiries into maternal deaths in the UK have highlighted repeatedly the importance of clear local procedures and policies to trigger rapid and appropriate responses which should be rehearsed regularly. Furthermore there should be senior input in high-risk cases and women at high risk of bleeding should be delivered in centres equipped for blood transfusion [1].

Clinical care should concentrate on identifying risk factors for haemorrhage to enable preparations and avoiding action to be taken: but, once massive haemorrhage occurs management should follow a logical sequence of diagnos-

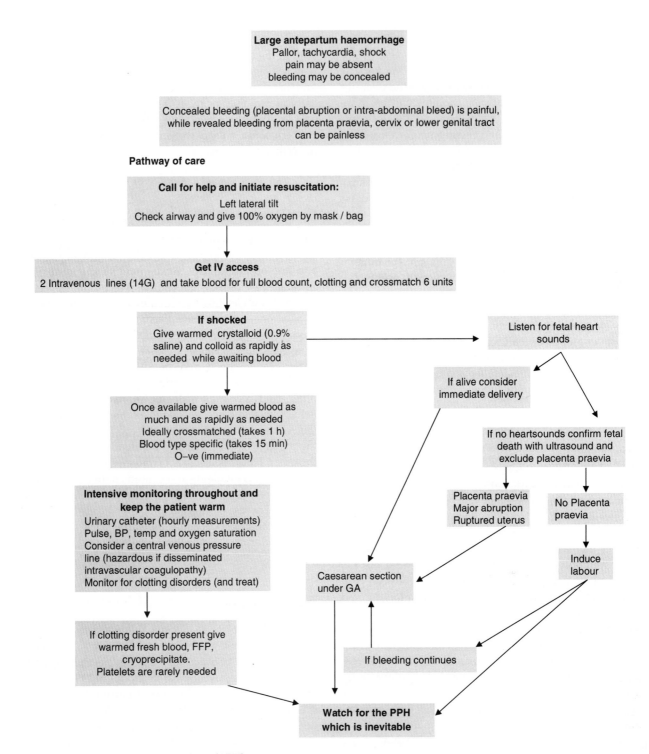

Fig. 18.2 Large antepartum haemorrhage (APH).

tic and therapeutic options as illustrated in Figs 18.2 and 18.3. A few additional points are made below as warning hints:

• In the case of antepartum haemorrhage: if it is due to severe abruption with an accompanying bradycardia

the urgency of delivery is clear, and a decision to delivery interval of 20 min or less is associated with reduced neonatal adverse outcome [22].

• 'Heavy lochia' or 'she's trickling' descriptions are misleading and should be avoided. If the loss is considered

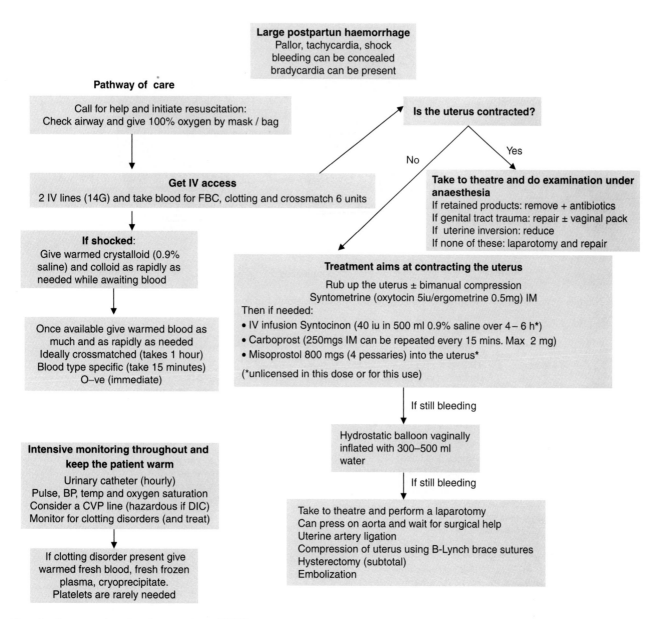

Fig. 18.3 Large post-partum haemorrhage (PPH).

above the norm the woman should be reviewed and the problem addressed.

• Continued vaginal bleeding with a contracted uterus is either due to retained placenta/membrane/clot or due to trauma and needs to be managed actively while the patient is stable.

• Hypotension is a very late sign and tachycardia, peripheral perfusion, skin colour and urine output should be noted.

• If the lower segment of the uterus or the cervix fills up with blood or clot it can cause vagal stimulation producing a bradycardia – this can mislead when there is no visible vaginal bleeding and a vaginal examination should be done.

• Bleeding can be concealed.
  – A rising uterine fundus indicates increasing clot in the uterus due to uterine atony.
  – intra-abdominal bleeding–massive volumes of blood can be accommodated within the peritoneal cavity without affecting girth measurements which are unhelpful and can be falsely reassuring.
  – the uterus which is not central but shifted to one side may suggest a broad ligament haematoma

• Petichiae suggest DIC [15].

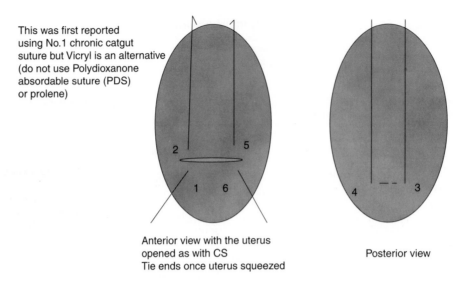

This was first reported using No.1 chronic catgut suture but Vicryl is an alternative (do not use Polydioxanone absorbable suture (PDS) or prolene)

Anterior view with the uterus opened as with CS
Tie ends once uterus squeezed

Posterior view

Fig. 18.4 B-Lynch 'brace' suture for treatment of bleeding due to uterine atony, but some uterine tone is needed.

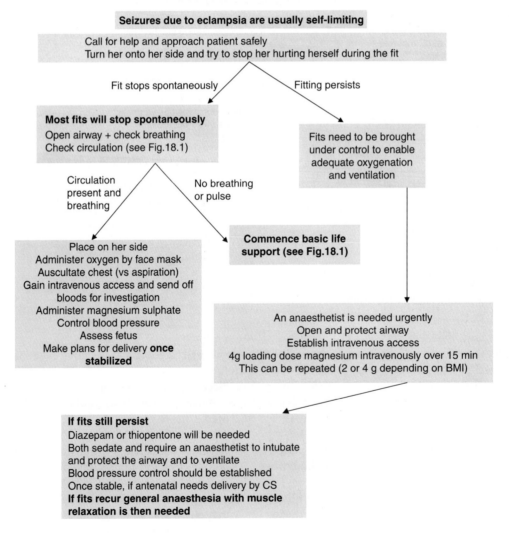

Seizures due to eclampsia are usually self-limiting

Call for help and approach patient safely
Turn her onto her side and try to stop her hurting herself during the fit

Fit stops spontaneously   Fitting persists

Most fits will stop spontaneously
Open airway + check breathing
Check circulation (see Fig.18.1)

Fits need to be brought under control to enable adequate oxygenation and ventilation

Circulation present and breathing   No breathing or pulse

Place on her side
Administer oxygen by face mask
Auscultate chest (vs aspiration)
Gain intravenous access and send off bloods for investigation
Administer magnesium sulphate
Control blood pressure
Assess fetus
Make plans for delivery **once stabilized**

Commence basic life support (see Fig.18.1)

An anaesthetist is needed urgently
Open and protect airway
Establish intravenous access
4g loading dose magnesium intravenously over 15 min
This can be repeated (2 or 4 g depending on BMI)

If fits still persist
Diazepam or thiopentone will be needed
Both sedate and require an anaesthetist to intubate and protect the airway and to ventilate
Blood pressure control should be established
Once stable, if antenatal needs delivery by CS
If fits recur general anaesthesia with muscle relaxation is then needed

Fig. 18.5 Eclampsia.

Life-saving measures and advanced techniques for massive postpartum haemorrhage

Aortic compression

If bleeding is out of control and the anaesthetist needs to stabilize the patient, it is worth trying aortic compression while waiting for senior or specialist help to arrive. In the woman who has delivered vaginally tilt the uterus forward and press a closed fist down onto the abdomen just below the umbilicus. If the abdomen is already open, sweep the small bowel mesentery up towards the liver and compress the aorta. The effect is dramatic and can be life-saving.

Uterine packing

This is useful for placental bed bleeding but can also be used with uterine atony when there is an element of uterine tone present. The technique is not new, but rather than using a gauze pack an inflatable balloon has the advantage of being quick and expandable. Various balloon catheters have been reported for this technique including the Sengstaken-Blakemore, but the urological Rusch balloon catheter is cheaper and effective [23]. The balloon of a normal urinary catheter itself is not suitable as its capacity is far too small. The volume needed is very individually dependent and the key is to insert the balloon catheter and gently fill it up while keeping the uterus as

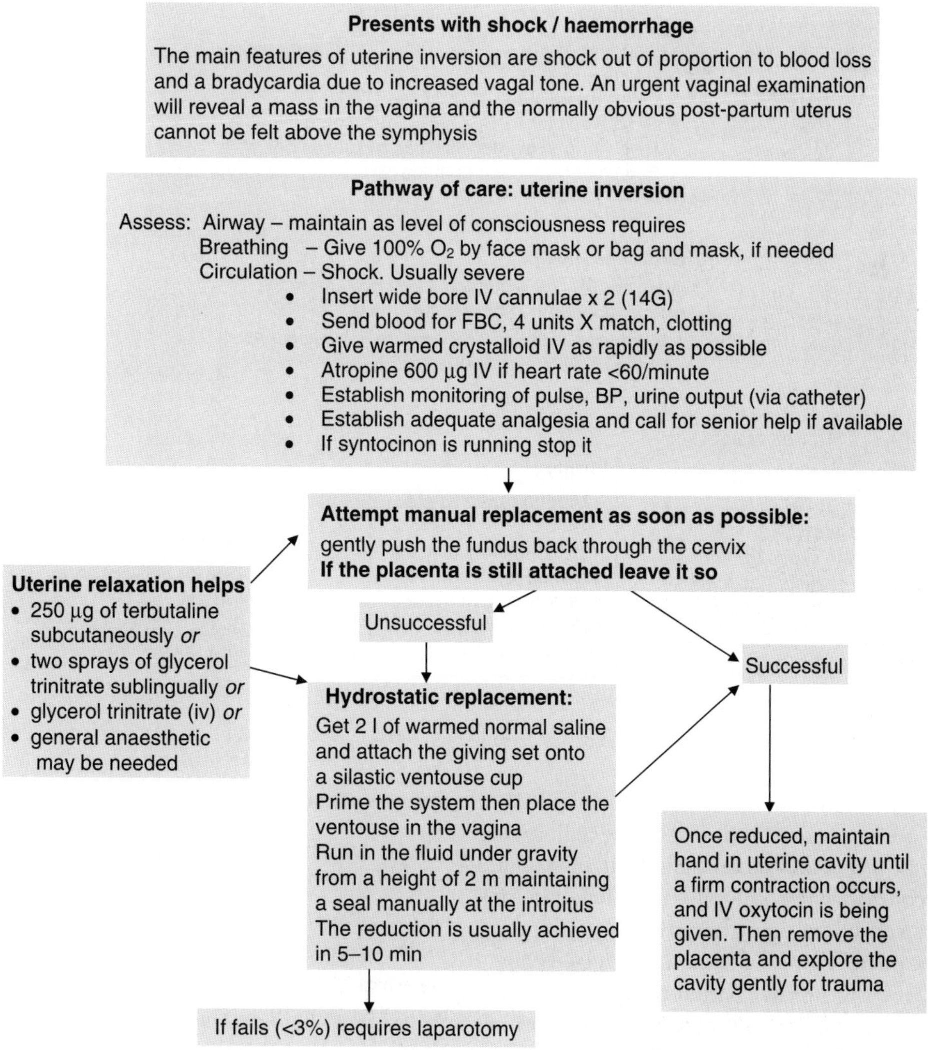

Presents with shock / haemorrhage

The main features of uterine inversion are shock out of proportion to blood loss and a bradycardia due to increased vagal tone. An urgent vaginal examination will reveal a mass in the vagina and the normally obvious post-partum uterus cannot be felt above the symphysis

Pathway of care: uterine inversion

Assess: Airway – maintain as level of consciousness requires
Breathing – Give 100% O_2 by face mask or bag and mask, if needed
Circulation – Shock. Usually severe
- Insert wide bore IV cannulae x 2 (14G)
- Send blood for FBC, 4 units X match, clotting
- Give warmed crystalloid IV as rapidly as possible
- Atropine 600 µg IV if heart rate <60/minute
- Establish monitoring of pulse, BP, urine output (via catheter)
- Establish adequate analgesia and call for senior help if available
- If syntocinon is running stop it

Attempt manual replacement as soon as possible:
gently push the fundus back through the cervix
If the placenta is still attached leave it so

Uterine relaxation helps
- 250 µg of terbutaline subcutaneously *or*
- two sprays of glycerol trinitrate sublingually *or*
- glycerol trinitrate (iv) *or*
- general anaesthetic may be needed

Unsuccessful

Successful

Hydrostatic replacement:
Get 2 l of warmed normal saline and attach the giving set onto a silastic ventouse cup
Prime the system then place the ventouse in the vagina
Run in the fluid under gravity from a height of 2 m maintaining a seal manually at the introitus
The reduction is usually achieved in 5–10 min

Once reduced, maintain hand in uterine cavity until a firm contraction occurs, and IV oxytocin is being given. Then remove the placenta and explore the cavity gently for trauma

If fails (<3%) requires laparotomy

Fig. 18.6 Uterine inversion.

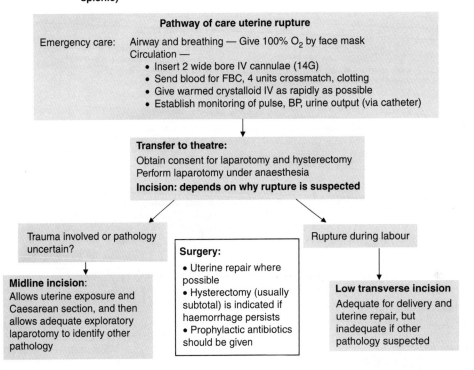

Fig. 18.7 Uterine rupture.

contracted as possible. As a rough guide approximately 300–500 ml or so is usually required, and as the balloon is blown up resistance is met and bleeding is seen to reduce. Once bleeding is controlled the balloon is usually left in for approximately 24 h and then, again an advantage over the traditional uterine pack, it can be deflated in stages. Whatever is used to pack the uterus, antibiotic cover should be given for the procedure and until the pack/balloon is removed; and similarly the bladder should be catheterized until the pack is removed.

Brace suture

The B-Lynch brace suture, first described in 1997 [24] can avoid hysterectomy in cases of bleeding from uterine atony. It aims to exert longitudinal lateral compression to the uterus combined with a tamponade effect and is performed by means of one long suture placed as illustrated in Fig. 18.4. The key to this technique is to check the theory that it might work by exteriorizing the uterus and compressing it (bleeding should be controlled) before

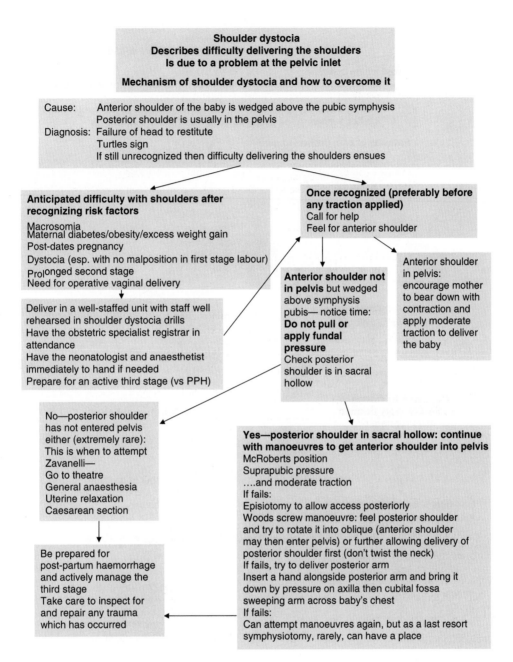

Shoulder dystocia
Describes difficulty delivering the shoulders
Is due to a problem at the pelvic inlet

Mechanism of shoulder dystocia and how to overcome it

Cause: Anterior shoulder of the baby is wedged above the pubic symphysis
          Posterior shoulder is usually in the pelvis
Diagnosis: Failure of head to restitute
          Turtles sign
          If still unrecognized then difficulty delivering the shoulders ensues

Anticipated difficulty with shoulders after recognizing risk factors

Macrosomia
Maternal diabetes/obesity/excess weight gain
Post-dates pregnancy
Dystocia (esp. with no malposition in first stage labour)
Prolonged second stage
Need for operative vaginal delivery

Deliver in a well-staffed unit with staff well rehearsed in shoulder dystocia drills
Have the obstetric specialist registrar in attendance
Have the neonatologist and anaesthetist immediately to hand if needed
Prepare for an active third stage (vs PPH)

Once recognized (preferably before any traction applied)
Call for help
Feel for anterior shoulder

Anterior shoulder not in pelvis but wedged above symphysis pubis— notice time:
Do not pull or apply fundal pressure
Check posterior shoulder is in sacral hollow

Anterior shoulder in pelvis: encourage mother to bear down with contraction and apply moderate traction to deliver the baby

No—posterior shoulder has not entered pelvis either (extremely rare):
This is when to attempt Zavanelli—
Go to theatre
General anaesthesia
Uterine relaxation
Caesarean section

Yes—posterior shoulder in sacral hollow: continue with manoeuvres to get anterior shoulder into pelvis
McRoberts position
Suprapubic pressure
....and moderate traction
If fails:
Episiotomy to allow access posteriorly
Woods screw manoeuvre: feel posterior shoulder and try to rotate it into oblique (anterior shoulder may then enter pelvis) or further allowing delivery of posterior shoulder first (don't twist the neck)
If fails, try to deliver posterior arm
Insert a hand alongside posterior arm and bring it down by pressure on axilla then cubital fossa sweeping arm across baby's chest
If fails:
Can attempt manoeuvres again, but as a last resort symphysiotomy, rarely, can have a place

Be prepared for post-partum haemorrhage and actively manage the third stage
Take care to inspect for and repair any trauma which has occurred

Fig. 18.8 Shoulder dystocia.

continuing. Since its first description there have been many reports of its successful use [25] but there have been modifications suggested [26] which have confused the understanding of the principles behind it, and some of these have been associated with problems [27–29].

Intervention radiology

Arterial embolization is increasingly reported in the management of post-partum haemorrhage [30–32]. It is especially effective in achieving haemostasis in cases of genital tract trauma where surgical control has failed or is inaccessible. It can, however, also help in more non-specific haemorrhage such as uterine atony, when the internal iliacs or their tributaries can be embolized. Developing links with, and knowing contact details of, an intervention radiology department in advance of the emergency scenario makes the urgent referral easier. It has been suggested that morbidity is better if embolization is carried out before rather than after hysterectomy [33],

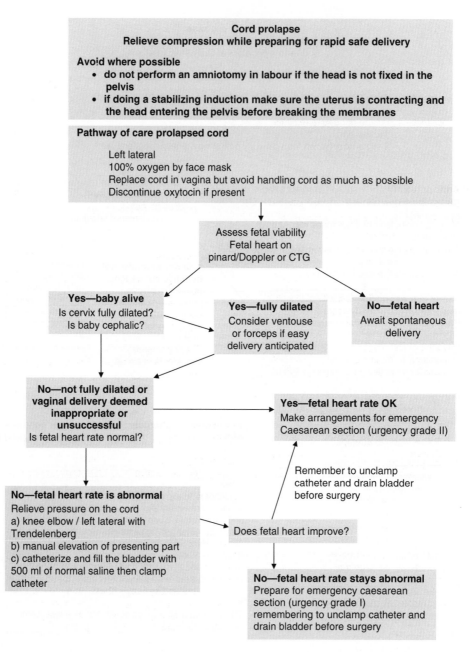

Fig. 18.9 Cord prolapse.

but this will clearly depend on local facilities and arrangements and the stability of the patient. Embolization cannot be carried out if the internal iliac arteries have been tied off; and this technique, which so threatens trauma to the internal iliac vein, should rarely be attempted by the obstetrician.

Cell salvage

This technique of contemporary peri-operative autologous blood salvage and retransfusion for use in obstetrics

has recenty been approved by NICE [34]. It has an excellent safety record, is acceptable to Jehovah's witnesses and avoids the risks associated with homologous blood transfusion [35,36]. With the impending blood shortages and the risk of post-transfusion infection, it is likely to be adopted in an increasing number of obstetric units.

Activated factor VIIa

The use of this novel, prohaemostatic agent has potential for treating severe obstetric haemorrhage [37]. Its use is limited to patients with complicated coagulation disorders and should only be considered in life-threatening bleeding.

Obstetric causes of collapse

Eclampsia can present with collapse due to the fitting and post-ictal phase of the disease, an intracerebral catastrophe, magnesium toxicity or pulmonary oedema. The principles of treatment are as for any collapse but, in addition, blood pressure control, magnesium sulphate and strict fluid balance to avoid fluid overload provide the basis of good care. If the patient is antenatal, then the mother must be stabilized before delivery – this is dealt with in the chapter on hypertensive disorders of pregnancy – but a summary flow chart of acute management of this condition is shown in Fig. 18.5.

Uterine inversion and uterine rupture can both contribute to maternal collapse as listed in Table 18.1 and their management is illustrated in Fig. 18.6 and 18.7. It is worth noting that 18 of the 42 cases of uterine rupture in the confidential inquiry into still births and deaths in infancy (CESDI) report had a laparotomy before a diagnosis was made [38]. Signs can be subtle and fetal heart abnormalities in the presence of a uterine scar should be taken extremely seriously and rarely, if ever, justify fetal blood sampling. Similarly, a multiparous patient with secondary arrest should arouse suspicion and syntocinon augmentation should only be decided after careful clinical assessment of the patient by a senior obstetrician.

Emergency obstetric deliveries

Most emergency operative deliveries (Caesarean section, instrumental delivery, breech and twin deliveries and interventions for fetal distress) together with neonatal resuscitation are mentioned in the relevant chapters, but the management of shoulder dystocia and cord prolapse are indicated in Fig. 18.8 and 18.9 and mentioned here.

Shoulder dystocia is a very serious obstetric emergency. The flow chart in Fig. 18.8 highlights the processes and sequences of its management, but additional points to add are:

- Stay calm – do not panic – think logically.
- Always remember that the problem is at the pelvic brim and pulling on the baby or pushing down on the fundus are both unhelpful and dangerous.
- Time is deceptive (try to glance at a clock or get someone to note timings).
- There remains a place for symphysiotomy which can be life-saving [39,40].
- Careful and precise documentation is essential after the event.

Cord prolapse

Figure 18.9 highlights the main features of this emergency: the principles of treatment are as follows:

- Handle the cord as little as possible.
- If an operative vaginal delivery is proposed it should be simple and achieved quickly – if it is not it should not be attempted.
- If there is no fetal bradycardia, there is time to administer a regional block with the patient lying on her side and this may be appropriate.
- If the bladder has been filled up with saline remember to **empty** it before surgery.

Summary

Good antenatal care, anticipating possible problems and preparing for them, and running a well-coordinated delivery suite are the mainstays of coping with obstetric emergencies. Training and drills helps to focus on teamwork and a supportive system to reduce adverse consequences from them. Keep things simple and focus on the problem to hand. The ABC principle is a good one for dealing with any ill patient, but is particularly useful in the apparently lifeless patient and those who require resuscitation, although it is crucial to remember to apply lateral tilt in anyone still pregnant. In any obstetric emergency keep the basic pathology in your mind: why has this happened, where is the problem, and what can be done about it?

References

1. Confidential Enquiry into Maternal and Child Health (2004) *Why Mothers Die 2000–2002.* London: RCOG Press.
2. NICE Guideline (2003) *Antenatal care. Routine care for the healthy pregnant woman.* NO309. London: National Institute for Health and Clinical Excellence.
3. Grady K & Cox C (2003) Triage. In: Johanson R, Cox C, Grady K & Howell C (eds) *Managing Obstetric Emergencies and Trauma: The MOET Course Manual.* London: RCOG Press, 275–7.
4. Sen R & Paterson-Brown S (2005) Prioritisation on the labour ward. *Curr Obstet Gynaecol.* **15**, 228–36.
5. Grady K, Prasad BGR & Howell C (2003) Cardiopulmonary resuscitation in the non-pregnant and pregnant patient. In: Johanson R, Cox C, Grady K & Howell C (eds) *Managing Obstetric Emergencies and Trauma: the MOET Course Manual.* London: RCOG Press, 17–26.
6. Black RS & Brocklehurst P (2003) A systematic review of training in acute obstetric emergencies. *Br J Obstet Gynaecol,* **110**, 837–41.
7. Rizvi F, Mackey R, Barrett T *et al.* (2004) Successful reduction of massive postpartum haemorrhage by use of guidelines and staff education. *Br J Obstet Gynaecol,* **111**, 495–8.

8. Thompson S, Neal S & Clark V (2004) Clinical risk management in obstetrics: eclampsia drills. *Br Med J*, **328**, 269–71.

9. Resuscitation Council (UK). *Adult advanced life support algorithm*. In: Resuscitation Guidelines, 2005. London: www.resus.org.uk.

10. Morris S & Stacey M (2003) Resuscitation in pregnancy. *Br Med J*, **327**, 1277–9.

11. Katz VL, Dotters DJ & Droegemueller W (1986) Perimortem cesarean delivery. *Obstet Gynecol*, **68**, 571–6.

12. Ewan PW (1998) Anaphylaxis. *Br Med J*, **316**, 1442–5.

13. Goswami K, Young P, Grady K & Cox C (2003) Amniotic fluid embolism. In: Johanson R, Cox C, Grady K & Howell C (eds) *Managing Obstetric Emergencies and Trauma: The MOET Course Manual*. London: RCOG Press, 29–34.

14. Stannard L & Bellis A (2001) Maternal anaphylactic reaction to a general anaesthetic at emergency caesarean section for fetal bradycardia. *Br J Obstet Gynaecol*, **108**, 539–40.

15. Baglin T (1996) Disseminated intravascular coagulation: diagnosis and treatment. *Br Med J*, **312**, 683–7.

16. Penna L & Clarke J (2003) Post-partum collapse. *Curr Obstet Gynaecol*, **13**, 67–73.

17. Schierhout G & Roberts I (1998) Fluid resuscitation with colloid or crystalloid solutions in critically ill patients: a systematic review of randomised trials. *Br Med J*, **316**, 961–4.

18. Cochrane Injuries Group Albumin Reviewers (1998) Human albumin administration in critically ill patients: systematic review of randomised controlled trials. *Br Med J*, **317**, 235–40.

19. Finfer S, Bellomo R, Myburgh J et al. (2003) Efficacy of albumin in critically ill patients. *Br Med J*, **326**, 559–60.

20. Brace V, Penney G & Hall M (2004) Quantifying severe maternal morbidity: a Scottish population study. *Br J Obstet Gynaecol*, **111**, 481–4.

21. Pattinson RC, Buchmann E, Mantel G et al. (2003) Can enquiries into severe acute maternal morbidity act as a surrogate for maternal death enquiries? *Br J Obstet Gynaecol*, **110**, 889–93.

22. Kayani SI, Walkinshaw SA & Preston C (2003) Pregnancy outcome in severe placental abruption. *Br J Obstet Gynaecol*, **110**, 679–83.

23. Johanson R, Kumar M, Obhrai M et al. (2001) Management of massive postpartum haemorrhage: use of a hydrostatic balloon catheter to avoid laparotomy. *Br J Obstet Gynaecol*, **108**, 420–2.

24. B-Lynch C, Coker A, Lawal AH et al. (1997) The B-Lynch surgical technique for the control of massive postpartum haemorrhage: an alternative to hysterectomy? Five cases reported. *Br J Obstet Gynaecol*, **104**, 372–5.

25. Ferguson JE, Bourgeois FJ & Underwood PB (2000) B-Lynch suture for postpartum hemorrhage. *Obstet Gynecol*, **95**, 1020–2.

26. Hayman RG, Arulkumaran S & Steer PJ (2002) Uterine compression sutures: surgical management of postpartum hemorrhage. *Obstet Gynecol*, **99**, 502–6.

27. B-Lynch C (2005) Partial ischemic necrosis of the uterus following a uterine brace compression suture. *Br J Obstet Gynaecol*, **112**, 126–7.

28. El Hamamy E (2005) Partial ischemic necrosis of the uterus following a uterine brace compression suture. *Br J Obstet Gynaecol*, **112**, 126.

29. Joshi VM & Shrivastava M (2004) Partial ischemic necrosis of the uterus following a uterine brace compression suture. *Br J Obstet Gynaecol*, **111**, 279–80.

30. Duggan PM, Jamieson MG & Wattie WJ (1991) Intractable postpartum haemorrhage managed by angiographic embolization: case report and review. *Aust NZ J Obstet Gynaecol*, **31**, 229–34.

31. Hansch E, Chitkara U, McAlpine J et al. (1999) Pelvic arterial embolization for control of obstetric hemorrhage: a five-year experience. *Am J Obstet Gynecol* **180**, 1454–60.

32. Jackson N & Paterson-Brown S (1999) Postpartum haemorrhage. *Hosp Med*, **60**, 868–72.

33. Bloom AI, Verstandig A, Gielchinsky Y et al. (2004) Arterial embolisation for persistent primary postpartum haemorrhage: before or after hysterectomy? *Br J Obstet Gynaecol*, **111**, 880–4.

34. NICE Guideline (2005) Intraoperative blood ell salvage in obstetrics. N0935. London: National Institute for Health and Clinical Excellence.

35. Catling S & Joels L (2005) Cell salvage in obstetrics: the time has come. *Br J Obstet Gynaecol*, **112**, 131–2.

36. de Souza A, Permezel M, Anderson M et al. (2003) Antenatal erythropoietin and intra-operative cell salvage in a Jehovah's Witness with placenta praevia. *Br J Obstet Gynaecol*, **110**, 524–6.

37. Boehlen F, Morales MA, Fontana P et al. (2004) Prolonged treatment of massive postpartum haemorrhage with recombinant factor VIIa: case report and review of the literature. *Br J Obstet Gynaecol*, **111**, 284–7.

38. Confidential Enquiry into Stillbirths and Deaths in Infancy (1998) *5th Annual Report. Focus Group on Ruptured Uterus*. London: Maternal and Child Health Consortium.

39. Johanson R & Wykes CB (2003) Symphysiotomy. In: Johanson R, Cox C, Grady K & Howell C (eds) *Managing Obstetric Emergencies and Trauma: The MOET Course Manual*. London: RCOG Press, 237–9.

40. Wykes CB, Johnston TA, Paterson-Brown S et al. (2003) Symphysiotomy: a lifesaving procedure. *Br J Obstet Gynaecol*, **110**, 219–21.

Further reading

Johanson R, Cox C, Grady K & Howell C (eds) (2003) *Managing Obstetric Emergencies and Trauma: The MOET Course Manual*. London: RCOG Press.

Baskett TF (2004) *Essential Management of Obstetric Emergencies* 4th edn. Bristol: Clinical Press Ltd.

Cox C & Grady K (2004) *Managing obstetric emergencies*. Oxford: BIOS Sc Pub Ltd.

Myerscough PR (1982) *Munro Kerr's Operative Obstetrics* 10 edn. London: B-T.

Chapter 19: Disorders of fetal growth and assessment of fetal well-being

G.C.S. Smith and C.C. Lees

Introduction

Defining disorders of growth requires relating a given achieved growth to an expected growth. In the case of fetal growth, three further levels of complexity arise. First, growth is determined in part by gestational age and an apparent growth disorder may reflect an inaccurate assessment of gestational age. Second, even if gestational age is known accurately, the size of the fetus can only be assessed indirectly by ultrasound. Third, even accepting these limitations, fetal measurements are typically related to a population-based norm. Deviation from normal may arise from parental determinants of growth, such as race and stature. The primary interest in assessing fetal growth is to avoid the complications associated with a fetus that is poorly grown due to uteroplacental insufficiency. The most important consequence of fetal compromise is perinatal death, principally antepartum stillbirth.

Endocrine regulation of fetal growth

Fetal growth is critically regulated by the insulin-like growth factors (IGFs). There are two IGFs, numbered I and II. There are two main receptors for the IGFs, numbered 1 and 2. The type-1 IGF receptor mediates most of the major biological effects of IGF-I and IGF-II and it binds the two growth factors with similar affinity. The type-2 IGF receptor appears mainly to be involved in clearance of IGF-II. Mice lacking IGF-I, IGF-II or the type-1 IGF receptor are growth restricted at birth. Mice lacking the type-2 receptor are large at birth. Following birth, IGF levels are stimulated by growth hormone (GH). However, in fetal life, levels of the IGFs appear largely independent of GH and are stimulated by human placental lactogen. The effects of IGFs are influenced by six distinct IGF binding proteins (IGFBP). Binding of IGF to an IGFBP may decrease or enhance its physiological effect. A number of IGFBP proteases exist, such as pregnancy associated plasma protein A (PAPP-A), a protease for IGFBP-4 and IGFBP-5. Many associations have been described between cord blood, amniotic fluid and maternal serum levels of components of the IGF system and fetal growth.

Placental regulation of fetal growth

The placenta is clearly crucial for fetal growth as it provides all the substrates for fetal growth and performs gaseous exchange in fetal life. Some of the associations between IGF system proteins and eventual birth weight are placentally derived components, such as PAPP-A, as IGFs are also important in controlling placentation. A number of tests of placental function demonstrate associations with eventual fetal growth (see p. 162). A view emerged that many complications of pregnancy associated with poor placental function may be due to failure of the so-called 'second wave' of trophoblast invasion in the second trimester. However, more recent studies have suggested that trophoblast invasion takes place as a continuous process during the first half of pregnancy. The process of implantation and early placentation may be crucial in determining fetal growth disorder and there are associations between both the size of the fetus in the first trimester of pregnancy and maternal levels of PAPP-A and the eventual birth weight of the baby (Fig. 19.1).

Genomic imprinting and fetal growth

Key genes of the IGF system are imprinted. Genomic imprinting is the selective inactivation of a gene in the conceptus in relation to whether it is the maternal or paternal copy. This is referred to as an epigenetic process as it alters the code for expression of genes without changing the actual genome. Genomic imprinting is primarily a feature of placental mammals and is thought to be important in controlling the conflict of the paternal interest in fathering large offspring and the maternal interest of dividing resources equally among all her offspring. Imprinted genes may act in balancing these conflicting interests at all stages of development. In fetal life, this is primarily manifested in the control of fetal growth. The

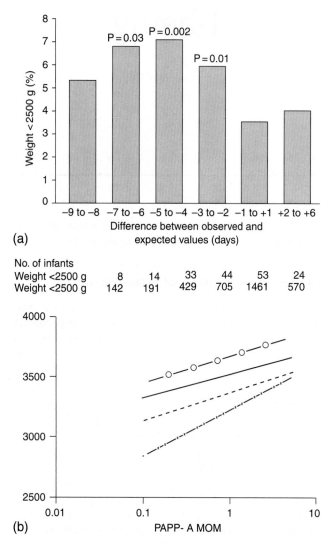

No. of infants
| Weight <2500 g | 8 | 14 | 33 | 44 | 53 | 24 |
| Weight <2500 g | 142 | 191 | 429 | 705 | 1461 | 570 |

Fig. 19.1 First trimester measurements and eventual birthweight. (a) Relationship between observed and expected crown–rump length and the incidence of low birthweight. From Smith GCS *et al*. 1998 *NEJM* **339**, 1817–22. (b) Relationship between first trimester levels of PAPP-A and eventual birthweight at term. Line with circles 41 weeks, straight line 40 weeks, broken line 39 weeks and line with stars 38 weeks. From Smith GCS *et al*. (2002) *Nature* **417**, 916.

key role of the placental IGF system is underlined by the fact that IGF-II, a stimulator of placental invasion, is paternally imprinted and the type-2 IGF receptor, which degrades IGF-II, is maternally imprinted. The importance of imprinting in the regulation of human fetal growth is illustrated by a number of genetic conditions which are manifestations of aberrant expression of imprinted genes. These can result in fetal overgrowth (e.g. Beckwith-Wiedemann syndrome) or intrauterine growth restriction (e.g. Silver-Russell syndrome).

Table 19.1 Epidemiological associations with intrauterine growth restriction

Primarily genetic	Primarily environmental	Mixed/genetic environmental
Infant sex	Parity	Maternal height
Paternal height	Gestational weight gain	Maternal pre-pregnancy weight
Race	Illness	Paternal weight
Maternal birth weight	Drug use (alcohol, tobacco, other)	Previous IUGR

Definition of fetal growth disorder

Fetal growth disorder is strictly defined as the failure of a fetus to grow according to its genetic potential. In practice this is never known and fetal growth is defined on the basis of the expected dimensions of the infant in relation to its gestational age. At birth, these measurements can be made directly. In fetal life, ultrasound is employed (see p. 164). Defining whether a given value of a continuous variable is normal, whether weight or an ultrasonic measurement, involves identifying a value which is thought to be the limit of the normal range. Often, measurements which are within two standard deviations of the mean are regarded as normal: this includes approximately 95% of the population. It follows that approximately 2.5% of the population will be regarded as small and 2.5% large, assuming a normal distribution. In practice, due to error in estimating gestational age, inaccuracy in weight estimation, and variation in true genetic potential, there will be no cut off that correctly separates normal and abnormal. In practice, if the threshold is set at an extremly low value, most of the fetuses less than that level will be growth restricted. As the threshold increases, the proportion which is truly growth restricted will decrease. The converse follows for identifying large infants. In practice, three percentile thresholds are commonly employed: less than the 3rd, less than the 5th, and less than the 10th percentile and the equivalent upper limits used for large infants. Fetuses outside the given threshold are called small for gestational age (SGA) or large for gestational age (LGA), as appropriate, and those within the range are called appropriate for gestational age (AGA). The terms SGA and intrauterine growth restriction (IUGR) are often used interchangeably although they are clearly not synonymous.

Epidemiology of fetal growth disorder

The epidemiological associations with delivering an SGA infant are tabulated (Table 19.1). These can be classified as primarily genetic, environmental or mixed genetic and environmental, although clearly the distinctions are not absolute. Similar factors will be involved in determining a large fetus, although the associations will clearly be reversed. Fetal growth may also be affected by pathological processes. These in turn can be classified as maternal disease, abnormalities of the placenta and fetal disease. Maternal cardiovascular and connective tissue disease are particularly associated with poor growth. Conversely maternal diabetes and obesity are common causes of a large infant. Placental causes of growth restriction include confined placental mosaicism but more commonly poor growth is associated with biochemical and ultrasonic tests which suggest poor placental function but do not establish the cause of the dysfunction. Intrinsic fetal causes of poor growth include chromosomal abnormalities (in particular aneuploidy) non-chromosomal syndromes (such as Cornelia de Lange syndrome) and congenital infection. Careful elucidation of history, structural and Doppler assessment of the placenta and fetus and other appropriate investigations will help clarify whether a growth abnormality is pathological.

Physiological fetal response to adverse intrauterine environment

In cases where a fetus is poorly grown due to an adverse intrauterine environment, it adapts to survive the challenge. The primary purpose of these adaptations is to maintain oxygen supply to the key organs, namely, the brain, heart and adrenals. These reflexes are stimulated by the peripheral arterial chemoreceptors. Unlike the child or adult, chemoreceptor stimulation inhibits breathing movements in the fetus. These adaptive responses underlie many of the biophysical assessments of fetal well-being. The responses and the biophysical measurements are listed in Table 19.2.

Consequences of fetal growth disorder

The most common single cause of perinatal death is unexplained antepartum stillbirth. Analysis of these events suggests that poor fetal growth is the major single determinant of these deaths. Moreover, antepartum stillbirth

Table 19.2 Physiological basis for biophysical assessment of the poorly grown fetus

Organ	Normal state	Association with adverse environment	Biophysical measurement
Fetal placenta	Low resistance circulation	Poor placental development results in high resistance	Doppler velocimetry of umbilical arteries demonstrates increased resistance
Fetal body	Moderately high resistance circulation	Peripheral arterial chemoreceptors stimulate vasoconstriction in non-vital organs	Doppler velocimetry of descending aorta demonstrates high resistance. The descending aorta also supplies the umbilical arteries and increased resistance in the fetal side of the placenta also contributes
Maternal placenta	Low resistance circulation	Poor placental development results in high resistance	Doppler velocimetry of the uterine artery demonstrates high resistance flow and notching: predictive of IUGR, abruption and stillbirth
Cerebro-vascular circulation	High resistance	Peripheral arterial chemoreceptors stimulate vasodilation to maintain brain oxygen supply	Doppler velocimetry of middle cerebral artery demonstrates reduced resistance
Kidney	Adequate blood flow and urine output	Increased vasopressin and reduced blood flow reduces urine output	Decreased liquor volume
Thorax	Breathing movements prepare for birth	Peripheral arterial chemoreceptors inhibit breathing movements	Decreased fetal breathing movements
Heart	Low central venous pressure	Central venous pressure rises as heart fails when fetus fails to compensate for adverse intrauterine environment	High resistance flow in the ductus venosus, absent or reversed flow during atrial systole, pulsatile flow in umbilical vein
CNS	Stimulation of fetal movement in cycles of activity	Fetal movements inhibited to reduce oxygen consumption by non-vital organs	Decreased or absent fetal movements

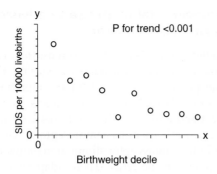

Fig. 19.2 Association between birthweight percentile and the risk of sudden infant death syndrome. Redrawn from Smith GCS *et al.* (2004) *NEJM* **351**, 978–86.

of structurally normal fetuses is also associated with abruption and pre-eclampsia. Both these outcomes are associated with IUGR. Poor growth is also associated with perinatal death due to prematurity. It has been shown that growth restriction in early pregnancy is associated with an increased risk of spontaneous preterm birth. Labour appears to be initiated by the activation of the fetal hypothalamo-pituitary adrenal axis. In sheep, the effector hormone from the adrenal is cortisol, whereas in primates and – it is assumed – in the human, it is likely to be androgenic precursors of oestrogen. The effect in both species is stimulation of labour. Therefore, spontaneous preterm delivery may be a physiologically indicated response to a poor environment. Poor growth is also directly related to prematurity in the context of elective delivery for suspected fetal compromise. Poor fetal growth is also associated with increased morbidity and mortality in infancy. For example, the risk of sudden infant death syndrome (SIDS) varies inversely with the birth weight percentile (Fig. 19.2). It is thought that the susceptibility of the adult to a range of diseases may also be affected by IUGR (the Barker hypothesis). The basis for this is associations between birth weight and birth proportions and the rates of disease in later life. These associations are not particularly strong, however, with a relative risk of death from ischaemic heart disease (IHD) of approximately 1.7 across the range of birth weights. Interestingly, the mother who delivers a low birth weight infant has a much higher relative risk of IHD, suggesting a genetic component. Nevertheless, animal models appear to confirm associations between intrauterine stress and later cardiovascular and metabolic function.

Investigation and management of fetal growth disorder

The challenge of perinatal care is to distinguish those fetuses that are small but healthy ('constitutionally small')

from those with pathologically reduced growth. In practice, fetal growth disorders are rare as an isolated finding before 24 weeks and routine assessment of fetal growth is therefore normally performed only after 24 weeks. While fetal size may be assessed both clinically and by ultrasound, fetal growth may only be ascertained by serial assessments.

The concept of symmetric and asymmetric IUGR have been taken to describe early onset (chromosomal/genetic) and later onset (uteroplacental) IUGR respectively. Thus poor fetal growth before 24 weeks is more commonly associated with genetic and chromosomal abnormalities or fetal infection whereas after 24 weeks fetal growth is determined to a far greater extent by maternal influences and uteroplacental function. As ultrasound techniques have advanced, it has become clear that the symmetric/asymmetric IUGR is somewhat of an oversimplification. The growth restriction thought to be inherent to chromosomal and genetic conditions may in fact be mediated by uteroplacental insufficiency; hence severely growth restricted trisomy 18 babies in the third trimester frequently exhibit asymmetrical growth restriction with abnormal uteroplacental and fetal Doppler. Conversely, ultrasound assessment of fetuses with severe early onset uteroplacental insufficiency often reveals symmetrically reduced abdominal and head measurements.

Prediction of fetal growth restriction

The epidemiological factors described above might be used to identify fetuses which are likely to have growth abnormalities allowing an increased level of surveillance. However, although many statistical associations are described, few of these are particularly strong. Therefore, although a study may show that a woman with a body mass index of 17 has an increased risk of delivering an SGA infant, the majority of these women would deliver an AGA infant. Most adverse pregnancy outcomes occur to women with no identified risk factors. These statements can be expressed in terms of screening: maternal history has low sensitivity and low positive predictive value in detecting fetal growth disorder. Biochemical prediction of IUGR has been investigated primarily using analytes measured in the first or second trimesters in the context of Down's screening programmes. While low first trimester PAPP-A levels are associated with low birthweight, studies of first and second trimester AFP, hCG and inhibin-A have shown a less consistent picture. None of these biochemical analytes has sufficient predictive value to be useful in a clinical context.

Uterine artery Doppler allows indirect assessment of downstream resistance in the arteries, arterioles and capillaries of the maternal side of the placenta. It is a quick,

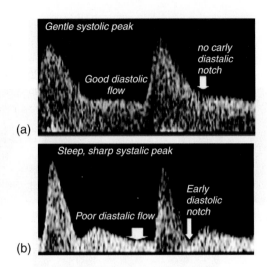

Fig. 19.3 Assessment of uterine artery Doppler. (a) Normal uterine artery Doppler flow velocity waveform. (b) Abnormal uterine artery Doppler flow velocity waveform.

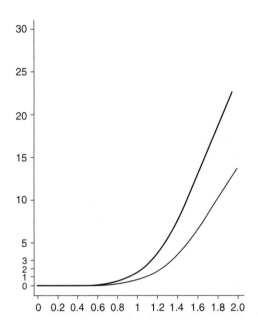

Fig. 19.4 Likelihood ratio for severe adverse outcome (vertical axis) relating to mean pulsatility index (horizontal axis). Smokers are represented by a thick black line (to left), non-smokers by a thin line. From Lees *et al.* (2001) *Obstet Gynecol* **98**(3), 369–73.

simple and non-invasive technique which involves the placement, using colour Doppler ultrasound, of a sample gate over the uterine artery just distal to its origin from the internal iliac artery. Pulsed wave (PW) Doppler is then applied, and a flow velocity waveform is obtained from which resistance indices such as resistance index, pulsatility index (PI) and A/B or S/D ratios can be derived. Low-resistance waveforms indicate good trophoblast invasion to the spiral arterioles, whereas high-resistance waveforms (characterized by low levels of end-diastolic flow and notches) indicate abnormal placentation (Fig. 19.3). The higher the uterine artery PI, the higher the risk of severe adverse outcome due to abnormal placentation (Fig. 19.4). Large studies with good reproducibility reported since the late 1990s have suggested its potential utility as a screening tool from as early as 12 weeks to, optimally, 24 weeks in predicting both pre-eclampsia and fetal growth restriction.

Although the sensitivity of uterine Doppler is poor for growth restriction at any gestation, it becomes better for the more severe and early onset forms. For example, its sensitivity in predicting IUGR<10th centile requiring delivery before 34 weeks is around 80%, for a 5% screen positive rate in an unselected population. It is, however, less reliable at predicting IUGR in twins and if performed earlier in gestation. It has not become a feature of routine antenatal care as controversy still exists over its utility in screening low risk populations, although concerns over reproducibility have now been largely overcome.

Clinical assessment of fetal growth

Clinical examination is most commonly by symphysis–fundal height (SFH) measurement, and SFH assessment has traditionally been performed from 24 weeks gestation onwards by measuring the distance from the mother's pubic symphysis to the uterine fundus, and successive measurements recorded in the woman's notes or on a chart. The SFH measurement after 24 weeks has been taken to be equal in centimetres to the week of gestation ± 2 cm to 36 weeks, and 3 cms from 36–42 weeks. The problems associated with SFH measurement are poor intra and inter observer reproducibility and those inherent to the technique. As it relies on assessment of the height of the uterine fundus as a proxy measure of fetal growth, it can, therefore, take no account of confounding maternal factors such as height, weight and physical build, and uterine–fetal factors such as fibroids, poly or oligohydramnios, multiple pregnancy and fetal lie. Two large retrospective studies in the 1980s suggested that reduced SFH measurements correctly identified only 25–50% of fetuses whose birthweight was <10th centile.

Ultrasound biometry

Ultrasound is the most sensitive method of assessing fetal growth. It is important to note that while a single ultrasound measurement may give an indication of whether the fetal abdominal circumference or estimated fetal weight is above or below a pre-defined centile, this does not in itself diagnose a fetal growth abnormality. Abnormal fetal growth can only be ascertained by successive measurements, usually of the abdominal circumference, plotted either manually or by specialized software on a centile chart.

Growth parameters, primarily biparietal diameter (BPD), head circumference (HC), femur length (FL) and abdominal circumference (AC), are plotted on charts which delineate the normal range of growth within a population. In an attempt to refine identification of true IUGR, ultrasound growth charts that adjust for baseline maternal and fetal characteristics have been devised. They also allow the differentiation between fetuses that are small, but have normal growth rate (hence might have been mis-labelled 'growth restricted' using normal population centile charts) from those whose growth was originally within the normal range but has fallen below a given centile.

Fetal arterial and venous Doppler

The decision to deliver a small for gestational age infant is based on a combination of investigations. Fetal arterial and venous Doppler assessment has shown itself to be useful and reproducible in tracking the cardiovascular responses to hypoxia and acidaemia in the fetuses compromised through uteroplacental insufficiency. Fetal vessels most commonly assessed are the umbilical and middle cerebral arteries, thoracic aorta and the ductus venosus. Meta-analysis of randomized controlled trials has shown that in high-risk pregnancies, umbilical artery Doppler improves perinatal outcome. It remains unclear why this should be as on this study no consistent management plan was followed.

As the feto-placental unit becomes more hypoxic, the umbilical artery Doppler resistance increases as does that of the thoracic aorta (Fig. 19.5); there is a concomitant fall in middle cerebral artery resistance known as centralization or 'brain sparing'. Later venous changes can be observed with PW Doppler of the ductus venosus; as acidaemia and impaired contractility of the heart supervene the biphasic waveform becomes abnormal with an exaggerated 'a' wave – sometimes reaching or falling below the baseline, indicating 'back pressure' during atrial contraction (diastole) (Fig. 19.6). This finding in the ductus venosus, often mirrored by increased pulsatility in the umbilical vein, is an ominous and usually pre-terminal event.

Cardiotocography and biophysical assessment

The most reproducible method of assessing the fetal heart rate (FHR) is by computerized FHR analysis; several software packages exist which allow storage, comparison

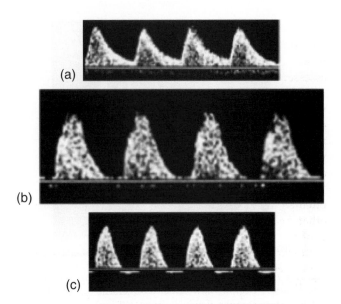

Fig. 19.5 Assessment of umbilical artery Doppler. (a) Normal umbilical artery Doppler flow velocity waveform, (b) absent end-diastolic flow, (c) reversed end-diastolic flow.

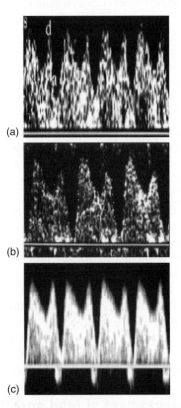

Fig. 19.6 Assessment of ductus venosus Doppler. (a) Normal waveform, (b) reduced 'a' wave to baseline, (c) reversed 'a' wave.

and print out of successive traces. Chronic uteroplacental insufficiency may lead to hypoxia and in severe cases to acidaemia. The short-term variation (STV) in FHR, assessed by computerized analysis, is the best indicator of fetal compromise in this context. STV increases with gestational age; the 2.5th centile is approximately 4.4 ms at 26 weeks and 6 ms at 34 weeks. It is very rare for there to be fetal acidaemia at values above these whereas reduced STV correlates well with fetal hypoxia and metabolic acidaemia. Successive recordings of an 'at risk' growth restricted fetus over days or weeks will often show a gradual reduction in STV in parallel with other findings such as reduced amniotic fluid, reduced fetal movements and raised umbilical artery resistance with centralization of blood flow. Spontaneous decelerations seen on cardiotocography (CTG) are a relatively late finding and usually coincide with reduced STV on computerized recordings. Unprovoked CTG decelerations are related to the occurrence of fetal hypoxemia and acidaemia.

Other elements of the biophysical profile (BPP) such as fetal tone, movements and amniotic fluid should be reported on alongside fetal growth, Doppler findings, maternal condition and CTG at every ultrasound scan of a potentially compromised fetus. In UK and European practice, a formal biophysical score is however rarely used to dictate management and delivery timing.

Timing of delivery

The optimal timing of delivery in hypoxic, growth restricted fetuses is simply not known. There have been no randomized studies that give an indication as to which method of fetal assessment to use and when to deliver. The Growth Restriction Intervention Trial (GRIT) reported on over 500 compromised babies where the timing of delivery was in doubt. This demonstrated a *non-significant* trend towards better long-term outcome when delivery was delayed among infants recruited between 24 and 30 weeks, but not at later gestations. The risk of fetal hypoxaemia and acidaemia (hence possible intrauterine death) must be weighed against the complications arising from prematurity. There is considerable geographical variation in practice: in North America the biophysical profile usually determines delivery timing whereas in Europe this decision is usually made on a combination of CTG and Doppler findings. The inconsistency reflects the lack of very strong evidence favouring one method over another.

There is a general consensus that reversed umbilical artery Doppler end-diastolic flow (EDF) after 32 weeks of gestation, and absent EDF after 34 weeks is an indication for immediate delivery. However, reversed umbilical EDF at 26, or even 28 weeks is not necessarily an indication for delivery as in earlier gestation these Doppler findings may follow a more chronic course. An assessment of all Doppler and biophysical parameters is most informative before making a decision for delivery.

Further reading

Baschat A (2004) Fetal responses to placental insufficiency: an update. *BJOG* **111**, 1031–41.

Baschat A (2004) Pathophysiology of fetal growth restriction: implications for diagnosis and surveillance. *Obstet Gynecol Surv* **23**, 617–27.

Das UG & Sysyn G (2004) Abnormal fetal growth: intrauterine growth retardation, small for gestational age, large for gestational age. *Pediatr Clin N Am* **51**, 639–54.

Smith GCS (2004) First trimester origins of fetal growth impairment. *Semin Perinatol* **28**, 41–50.

Lees C & Baumgartner H (2005) The TRUFFLE study – a collaborative publicly funded project from concept to reality: how to negotiate an ethical, administrative and funding obstacle course in the European Union. *Ultrasound Obstet Gynecol* **25** 105–7.

Chapter 20: Multiple pregnancy

Nicholas M. Fisk

With the decline in perinatal morbidity and mortality from other causes, multiple pregnancy now warrants special attention from obstetricians. First, they are common, having increased in incidence by 50% in developed countries over the last two decades. Second, they make a disproportionate contribution to perinatal morbidity and mortality, well in excess of that due to multiplication of singleton risks by fetal number. Next, almost every maternal and obstetric problem occurs more frequently in multiples. Finally, there are a number of intrapartum considerations, including manipulations no longer practised in singletons. Whereas previously maternal management was stressed, the modern approach to managing multiple pregnancy focuses on recognizing fetal risk as stratified by chorionicity, monitoring fetal growth and well-being by ultrasound and reducing risks of preterm delivery. Recognizing the specialized nature of multiple pregnancy management, the RCOG Study Group on Multiple Pregnancy has recommended that, like for diabetes, multiple pregnancies be managed within any one hospital by a single consultant-led multidisciplinary team [1].

Incidence

The considerable geographical and temporal variation in twinning incidence reflects factors influencing dizygotic or non-identical twinning, which results from multiple ovulation. Twinning occurs in from 4/1000 births in Japan to 54/1000 in Nigeria, and is common in older mothers, presumably due to their rising follicle-stimulating harmone (FSH) levels. Familial predisposition to multiple ovulation can be demonstrated ultrasonically [2], although a gene has yet to be identified. In contrast, monozygous or identical twinning, which results from early cleavage division of a single blastocyst, occurs with a constant incidence of 3.9/1000.

Since 1980, the twinning rate in the UK has risen from 9.8 to 14.7/1000 maternities while the triplet rate increased from 0.14 to 0.45 in 1998, before falling to 0.2/1000 last year

(Fig. 20.1). The increase has been largely due to assisted reproductive technologies (ART), both ovulation induction by anti-oestrogens or gonadotrophins and assisted conception by *in vitro* fertilization (IVF). Avoidance of iatrogenic multiple pregnancy is a clinical and societal priority. Thus the recent fall in triplet incidence is welcome, reflecting both judicious monitoring of induced ovulation and proscription of three embryo transfers, which has reduced the triplet, but not the take-home baby, rate [3]. Attention is now turning to the prevention of twins, with single embryo transfer and a subsequent cryopreservation cycle achieving the same pregnancy rate as two embryo transfers [4]. It is increasingly recognized that ART increases the incidence of monozygous (MZ) twinning 2–6 fold, particularly two blastocyst transfer.

Perinatal wastage

Perinatal mortality in twins is nearly four times higher and in triplets six times higher than in singletons. Cerebral palsy is nearly three times more common in twins, and more than 10 times as common in triplets as in singletons. These figures are per baby, whereas the more relevant figure in counselling parents is the chance of their multiple pregnancy producing any one baby with these complications. Thus a twin pregnancy has eight times and a triplet pregnancy nearly 50 times the chance of a singleton of producing a baby with cerebral palsy [5–7]. This high perinatal wastage is largely attributable to the increased chance overall of prematurity and intrauterine growth restriction and of complications specific to monochorionic twins.

Chorionicity and zygosity

Two thirds of twins are dizygous (DZ) and one third MZ. However, chorionicity, not zygosity, mediates the degree of perinatal risk in any individual multiple pregnancy. Perinatal mortality is 2–3 times higher in monochorionic

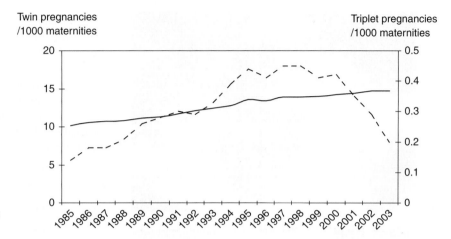

Fig. 20.1 UK data showing temporal trend since 1985 in incidence of twin (solid line, left *y* axis) and triplet pregnancies (dashed line, right *y* axis)/1000 maternities (Source: UK Office National Statistics).

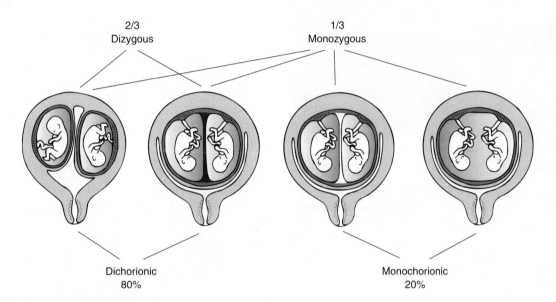

Fig. 20.2 Relationship between zygosity and chorionicity, with relative frequencies.

(MC) compared to dichorionic (DC) twins [8,9]. Morbidity seems similarly related, with MC twins having an increased chance of antenatally acquired cerebral lesions and of long-term handicap [10,11]. This excess morbidity and mortality is attributed to transfusional complications mediated via placental vascular anastomoses connecting the circulations in almost all MC twins.

The relationship between zygosity and chorionicity is shown in Fig. 20.2. Whereas all DZ pregnancies are DC, MZ pregnancies assume one of three placental configurations. Splitting within three days of fertilization results in separate DC placentae, which as with dizygous DC placentae may or may not come to lie adjacent to each other to appear fused. Splitting after formation of the inner cell mass at four days results in a single MC diamniotic pla-

centa and splitting after 7 days in MC monoamniotic twins. About 20% of all twins are MC.

Ultrasonic determination of chorionicity

Chorionicity can be determined on ultrasound with 100% accuracy in the first trimester, by counting the constituent layers of the dividing membranes. Thick chorion is obvious in a DC intertwin septum, while the tissue paper thin amnion is normally resolved separately from the chorion in the first trimester (Fig. 20.3). A simple method involves inspecting the placental base of the membrane which has a thick 'lambda' shape if DC, or a thin 'T' shape if MC. Finally, a single extra-embryonic coelom with two yolk sacs confirms MC diamniotic placentation,

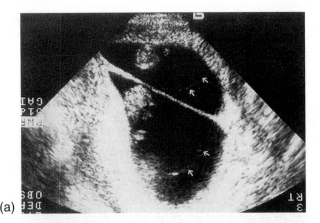

(a)

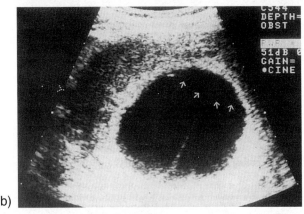

(b)

Fig. 20.3 First trimester chorionicity determination. (a) A thick intertwin septum, with each twin's amnion (arrows) identified separately from the chorion, indicating dichorionicity. (b) A thin intertwin septum, which diverges (arrows) into a single extra-embryonic coelom, indicating the absence of intervening chorion and thus monochorionicity (reproduced with permission from [1]).

whereas a single coelom with a single yolk sac and no dividing septum indicates monoamnionicity. In the midtrimester, after the thinned chorion leave has fused with the amnion, chorionicity determination is only 80–90% accurate. Qualitative interpretation as thick (DC) or thin (MC) appears as accurate as septal measurement [12]. Discordant external genitalia indicate dizygosity and thus dichorionicity and separate placentae dichorionicity, as does demonstration of a tongue of placental tissue within the base of the septum known as the 'twin peak' sign. In contrast a thin septum in concordant-sex twins with a single placental mass suggests MC. Demonstration by colour Doppler of a functional artery-to-artery anastomosis is more challenging but provides definitive proof of monochorionicity.

Chorionicity should be determined on ultrasound in all multiple pregnancies [13]. This is because chorionicity is relevant to: (1) counselling parents about perinatal risks; (2) counselling parents about their risk of genetic and structural abnormality; (3) invasive testing and management of discordant abnormality; (4) feasibility of multifetal pregnancy reduction; (5) risk of sequelae in the presence of fetal compromise; (6) early detection and management of twin–twin transfusion syndrome. It should be done at the first ultrasound, as it is most accurate in the first trimester; fortunately all ART pregnancies have an early scan, as do the increasing number undergoing nuchal screening.

Zygosity determination

MC twins by definition are MZ, while discordant sex twins are DZ. In the remaining 50%, zygosity cannot be determined without DNA fingerprinting, which is rarely indicated *in utero*. Zygosity studies on cord blood are no longer offered routinely, as the babies can be tested any time in childhood. Not only are parents often curious, but knowledge of zygosity influences the twins rearing, sense of identity, genetic risk and their transplantation compatibility. Rarely there may be indications for zygosity testing *in utero* on invasively collected fetal tissue, such as deducing genetic risk or excluding contamination at prenatal diagnosis or demonstrating dichorionicity in the presence of fetal compromise.

Miscarriage

Twins have a high incidence of spontaneous early pregnancy loss, one study suggesting 12% of human conceptions start off as twins [14]. Studies of ultrasound or abortal pathology indicate that twins are found twice as commonly in the first trimester as at birth. First trimester resorption of one previously ultrasonically viable twin known as the 'vanishing twin' phenomenon is estimated to occur in over 20% of twins [15]. Spontaneous first trimester loss of one or more fetuses in high-order multiple pregnancies is common, with nearly 40% of pregnancies in which three sacs are seen in early pregnancy delivering twins. When one twin dies *in utero* in the mid-trimester, a *fetus papyraceus*, its squashed paper-like remains may be found among the placenta after delivery.

Prenatal diagnosis
Structural anomalies

Zygosity determines the risk of abnormality and chorionicity what can be done if one is present. Zygosity can be deduced definitively in cases of monochorionicity (=MZ) or discordant external genitalia (=DZ) while in DC concordant-sex twins, the chance of dizygosity is 75–80%. MZ twins have a 50% increase in structural abnormalities per baby, which are sought at the routine anomaly scan at 20 weeks. In particular they have twice the frequency of congenital heart disease, and thus a fourfold increase per pregnancy, so that fetal echocardiography is recommended [16].

Aneuploidy

Women with DZ twins can be counselled that the chance of their pregnancy producing a child with Down's syndrome is theoretically double their age-related risk, whereas women with MZ twins simply have their age-related risk that both twins will be aneuploid. Nevertheless, there is some evidence that Down's syndrome may occur less frequently in twins [17,18]. Serum screening is inapplicable in multiple pregnancy, because aberrant placental or fetal hepatic hormone production in an affected twin is masked by normal levels from the unaffected co-twin. In contrast, nuchal translucency, although rarely used in isolation any more in singletons because of its high false positive rate, is readily applicable as a fetally-specific marker. Because the background rate of increased neckfolds is doubled in MC twins, the average of the twins' measurements is used to avoid high false positive rates [19].

Invasive procedures

Invasive procedures in twins are complex and should only be performed in fetal medicine centres. Great care is taken to avoid mislabelling and misidentification of an affected twin. While this may be facilitated in the presence of discordant gender or structural abnormality, it is good practice always to map the topography in terms of location within the uterus, placental site, cord insertion and plane of the dividing septum. This is a prerequisite for interpretation of discordant results and for selective feticide. Ideally the operator doing the diagnostic procedure should also undertake any selective feticide to minimize uncertainty and obviate any need for confirmatory invasive testing. In structurally concordant MC twins, only one needs sampling for prenatal diagnosis, but the operator should be certain of this on first trimester scanning. With this exception, it is important to ensure that both fetuses are sampled separately. With amniocentesis this is best achieved by two separate ultrasound-guided procedures as far away as possible from the dividing septum, although there are series using single-entry techniques with low rates of complications. With fetal blood sampling, the intrahepatic vein can be sampled to avoid confusing the cord origins. Most operators consider chronic villus sample (CVS) contraindicated in DC twins, because of a 1–5% rate of contamination [20,21], and thus potential for false positive and negative results through inadvertently sampling the same twin twice. Otherwise DNA fingerprinting

and/or confirmatory amniocentesis may be necessary in DC twins with concordant-sex karyotypes at CVS.

Miscarriage rates after amniocentesis in twins seem higher than in singletons [22], although the lack of randomized trials or large cohorts preclude estimation of the procedure-related risk.

Selective feticide in DC twins discordant for fetal abnormality by injection of intracardiac KCL is associated with a 7% loss rate in the international registry, with marginally lower rates if the procedure is done before than after 13 weeks [23]. The same technique in MC twins leads to death of the healthy twin due to agonal exsanguination along vascular anastomoses. To obviate this, a variety of cord occlusion techniques have recently been developed to render selective termination in MC twins now feasible.

Maternal responses

All the normal physiological adaptations such as increased cardiac output, glomerular filtration rate and renal blood flow are increased in multiple pregnancy. Red cell mass increases approximately 300 ml more than in singletons, but because this is disproportionately less than the one third increase in plasma volume, haemoglobin values fall. Iron stores are diminished in 40% of women with twins, so that routine haematinic supplementation is recommended, particularly given the increased risk of post-partum haemorrhage and Caesarean section.

Hyperemesis gravidarum is more likely and severe cases may respond to steroid therapy or odansetron. All the minor complications of pregnancy such as backache, oedema, varicose veins, reflux, haemorrhoids etc. are also increased, both as a result of the physical effects of greater uterine size and also of greater placental hormone production. Gestational diabetes is increased in most studies.

Pre-eclampsia is two to three times more common in multiple than singleton pregnancies and likely to be more severe [24]. There is no good evidence that it is increased in MC compared to DC pregnancies. Unlike other high-risk groups, uterine artery Doppler screening has low sensitivity. Management is based on standard principles, save that the risks of iatrogenic prematurity with delivery apply to two fetuses.

After delivery, the difficulties coping with the demand of two or more babies are considerable, with depression, stress and relationship difficulties more common in mothers of multiples than singletons [25]. Given the high perinatal wastage in multiple pregnancy, there is often the added burden in the post-natal period of coping with bereavement. Antenatal classes dedicated to multiples have a role in preparing parents not just for differences in antenatal care and delivery, but also for the extra demands of breast feeding and coping.

Intrauterine growth restriction

Ultrasound is the primary tool for monitoring growth in multiple pregnancies for two reasons. First, they are at high risk of intrauterine growth restriction (IUGR), with 25% of twins being small for gestational age at birth. In most cases IUGR will be discordant affecting one twin only. Second, abdominal palpation and symphysis–fundal height measurement are unreliable as indices of individual fetal growth as, instead, they reflect total intrauterine growth.

There is no agreement on the ideal frequency of ultrasound examinations in twins, but a conservative policy for detecting IUGR in DC twins is four weekly scanning from 24 weeks, with further scans and/or Doppler measurements as indicated. MC twins should be scanned at fortnightly intervals from 16 weeks, both to allow early diagnosis and thus treatment of twin–twin transfusion syndrome, and to pre-empt intrauterine death from IUGR through timely delivery (or pre-emptive cord occlusion prior to viability) to protect the healthy co-twin.

There is controversy as to whether singleton or twin biometric charts should be used. The former seems the more logical, as twins are at high risk of IUGR with attendant morbidity, and separate charts are not used for other high-risk groups, such as pre-eclamptics or diabetics. Further, increasing emphasis is placed on growth profile and fetal condition (liquor volume, umbilical Doppler). Many use percentage discordancy in estimated fetal weight (=100* [EFWlarger − EFWsmaller] EFWlarger) as an index of discordant IUGR. Discordancy >25–30% has some predictive value in MC twins for poor outcome in twin–twin transfusion syndrome (TTTS) and for fetal death [26], whereas in DC twins, it is controversial whether or not it denotes poorer outcome independent of the degree of IUGR [27,28].

The standard principle of management in IUGR (i.e. deliver when the risks of continued intrauterine outweigh those of extra-uterine existence) needs modification in twin pregnancy to account for the risks to both fetuses. Thus whereas cessation in fetal growth with preterminal Doppler studies might warrant delivery at 25 weeks with a singleton fetus, discordant IUGR with this picture in DC twins might better be managed by allowing the IUGR fetus to die *in utero*, sparing the healthy fetus the risks of iatrogenic prematurity.

In MC twins the decision-making is more complex. On the one hand, latency (absent end diastolic frequencies in the umbilical artery) may persist weeks longer without decompensation than in DC twins [29]. On the other hand,

delivery or pre-emptive cord occlusion must be instituted before any intrauterine death to protect the co-twin from acute transfusional sequelae. Such balancing of risks is always difficult and decision making should occur in concert with the parents and neonatal paediatricians.

Preterm labour

This is the major cause of neonatal death in multiple pregnancy. The median gestational ages at delivery in twins and triplets of 37 and 34 weeks, respectively, are not so much a concern in terms of survival, as the proportion delivering less than <30 weeks (c. 7 and 15%, respectively). Although plurality substantially increases the chance of preterm delivery, once in the neonatal unit an individual baby's prognosis is the same or better than gestational age- and weight-matched singletons [28]. Parents should be informed of the symptoms and signs of threatened preterm labour and the advisability of early presentation. Management of preterm labour in multiple pregnancies differs little from that of singletons, other than the consequences of prematurity affecting a greater number of babies. The following discussion concentrates on those aspects, which pertain especially to multiple pregnancy.

Prevention

Preterm labour in multiple pregnancy, as with polyhydramnios, is attributed to uterine over-distension. Accordingly, there are no specific preventative measures aside from fetal reduction in high-order multiples, as discussed pp. 173–174.

Although hospitalization for bed rest has been practised in the past, there is little evidence to support its use. Indeed, meta-analysis of six randomized controlled trials suggests that bed rest in twins increases the chance of preterm delivery [30]. With the exception of progesterone, prophylactic tocolytics are of no benefit in singletons, and thus it is not surprising that randomized trials similarly report no clear benefit in twins [31]. There was no reduction in preterm birth or related outcomes in the only trial of 17-hydroxyprogesterone caproate in twins [32].

Prediction

Cervical length on transvaginal ultrasound is shorter and the risk of preterm labour higher than in singletons, so the cut off for identifying those at risk or preterm delivery before 32–34 weeks is set higher at 20–25 mm [33]. Cervical length of 20 mm is found in 8% of twins at 23 weeks but 40% of those delivering spontaneously <32 weeks. Meta-analysis of studies in asymptomatic twin pregnancies shows that a cervical length of <25 mm at 20–24 weeks increases the pre-test probability of delivery before

34 weeks from 19 to 48%, whereas a negative test reduces it only slightly to 14% [34]. Although useful for identifying those at risk, screening remains controversial because of the lack of evidence that cerclage improves outcome in twin pregnancies with a short cervix [35]; indeed, the only randomized trial showed a doubling in preterm birth.

Management

β2 mimetics are no longer used for tocolysis, given their cardiovascular side effects and in particular pulmonary oedema for which multiple pregnancy was a risk factor.

Although atosiban and nifedipine seem equally effective in delaying preterm labour [36], there is increasing concern in twin pregnancies about the adverse cardiovascular effects of nifedipine. Nine of the 14 reported cases of pulmonary oedema associated with tocolytic calcium channel blockers were in twins; therefore nifedipine should not be used in multiple pregnancies [37].

Glucocorticoids should be used in multiple pregnancies at risk of delivery < 34–36 weeks in the next 7–14 days. Meta-analysis of randomized trials in multiple pregnancies suggests a trend towards reduced respiratory distress syndrome, although as with other subgroups this falls short of significance (OR 0.72, 95% CI 0.35–1.68) [38]. This could be due to small numbers or to sub-therapeutic drug levels in twin pregnancies. Consistent with this, retrospective studies suggest that multiple pregnancy attenuates the beneficial effect of antenatal steroids. The possibility that a larger dose is required remains to be tested. Repeated prophylactic steroids are not recommended. First, retrospective data show that fortnightly steroids from 24 weeks did not reduce the incidence of respiratory problems in twins [39]. Second, there is concern that these may impair fetal growth and/or brain development. Finally, they may prevent indicated courses working, as only the first course has been shown to be beneficial.

Complications of monochorionic twinning

MC twinning is a congenital abnormality of the placenta whereby the twins' circulations communicate via placental vascular anastomoses. These occur in almost all MC placentae. Large bidirectional superficial artery–artery or vein–vein anastomoses compensate for any haemodynamic imbalance set up by smaller deep uni-directional arteriovenous anastomoses. Intertwin transfusion is thus a normal event but, when unbalanced, may result in a number of complications.

Acute transfusion

When one MC twin dies *in utero*, there is an empiric 25% risk of ischaemic, neurological or renal lesions in the survivor [40]. The mechanism is now known to be acute transfusion from the healthy twin's circulation into the hypotensive dying twin's circulation. There is also a comparable risk of the initially healthy twin exsanguinating into the dying twin's circulation, resulting in double intrauterine death. These risks appear greater in the presence of an arterio-arterial anastomosis [41,42].

Unlike DC twins discordant for fetal compromise, where the risks of intrauterine demise in one are balanced against those of iatrogenic prematurity in the other, delivery needs to be expedited in MC twins discordant for fetal compromise, not only to prevent intrauterine death in the compromised twin but also to prevent sequelae in the co-twin. Where this occurs prior to viability ultrasound-guided bipolar cord occlusion is an alternative to expectant management, whereby the dying twin's cord is intentionally blocked prior to its demise to protect the co-twin from acute transfusional sequelae.

If one twin is found dead *in utero*, delivery is rarely indicated except near term. Instead middle cerebral artery Doppler helps identify surviving fetuses with anaemia [43], and they should all undergo neuro-imaging by MR or ultrasound to exclude transfusional brain injury. If abnormal, handicap is likely and termination of pregnancy maybe offered where allowed, even in late pregnancy.

Twin–twin transfusion syndrome

Chronic TTTS occurs in 15% of MC twins and is responsible for 15–20% of perinatal death in twins. The pathophysiology involves chronic net shunting of blood from the donor to recipient twin. The donor becomes growth restricted, oliguric and develops anhydramnios ('stuck twin') and the recipient becomes polyuric with polyhydramnios and can go on to develop cardiac sequelae and hydrops. TTTS usually presents in the mid- but sometimes the third trimester, with gross discordance in amniotic fluid volume, with polyhydramnios in the recipient's and oligohydramnios in the donor's sac. The usual placental configuration comprises unbalanced deep artery to vein anastomoses with absent or inadequate compensation along superficial anastomoses [44]. Thus Doppler detection of a compensatory artery-to-artery anastomosis antenatally substantially reduces the chance of developing TTTS, and where it does develop, predicts better prognosis [42,45].

Untreated, perinatal loss rates in the mid-trimester exceed 80%, with survivors at risk both of neurological morbidity acquired *in utero* or at birth and of cerebral palsy. Perinatal mortality rates have fallen to around 50% over the last decade due to a range of treatments comprising serial amnioreduction, septostomy, fetoscopic laser ablation of placental anastomoses (Plate 20.1, *facing p. 562*) and cord occlusion. The recent randomized trial of endoscopic laser versus serial amnioreduction demonstrated that laser therapy as first line treatment was associated with better outcome, more pregnancies having at least one survivor to 6 months of age (76 versus 51%) along with fewer short-term neurological sequelae [46]. These results are confirmed in a systematic view that included observational studies [47]. Notwithstanding this, overall outcomes are far from perfect, in that two thirds of affected pregnancies still result in a dead or brain injured baby [48]. The current management dilemma concerns early stage disease [47], of which there were few patients in the randomized trial. Because TTTS resolves in 20–30% of stage I–II cases treated with a single amnioreduction, because perinatal survivals in the randomized amnioreduction/septostomy trial and the amnioreduction registry [49] were empirically better than in the laser trial [50], and because laser could still be used in those that progress, there remains a role for test amnioreduction in early stage disease. This requires evaluation as amnioreduction may rarely lead to septal detachment, which can impede the technical success of a subsequent laser procedure.

Twin reversed arterial perfusion sequence

This rare condition (1:35,000 pregnancies) arises in MC twins with two cords linked by a large arterio-arterial anastomosis such that flow from one, the 'pump twin,' supplies the other, the 'perfused' twin, in a retrograde fashion. The term 'twin reversed arterial perfusion' (TRAP) sequence is preferred to the older 'acardiac monster', so named as reversed deoxygenated arterial supply is associated with only rudimentary development of upper body structures such as the heart, face and arms. Perinatal mortality in the pump twin is up to 55%, due to polyhydramnios and cardiac failure [51]. Although polyhydramnios may be alleviated by amnioreduction or sulindac therapy, definitive treatment requires occlusion of the perfused twin's cord, which can now be achieved by a variety of fetoscopic or ultrasound-guided techniques. Techniques such as radiofrequency ablation and interstitial laser which occlude intrafetal rather than cord vessels give the best results, with a pump twin survival rate of > 80% [52].

Monoamniotic twins

One per cent of identical twins lie in the same sac, so that they almost all develop cord entanglement in the first trimester [53]. Their high perinatal mortality rate of up to 30–50% is attributed to cord accidents both at delivery and in the last half of pregnancy [54]. Perinatal mortality has fallen in recent series to 10–25% due to elective preterm delivery, mandatory Caesarean section and intensive fetal monitoring [55,56]. Prophylactic maternal sulindac therapy to reduce fetal urine output and thus amniotic fluid volume has been successfully used in over 20 cases in our centre to split the twins' excessive movements through relative oligohydramnios and thus reduce the risk of cord tautening [57].

Monoamniotic placenta are characterized by a high frequency of large artery to artery anastomoses, which explains why they rarely get TTTS and also why single intrauterine death frequently progresses to double fetal death.

Delivery

Timing

The antepartum stillbirth rate in twins exceeds that of singletons, both per fetus and, in particular, per pregnancy. Thus while awaiting the results of a randomized trial in progress [58], it seems prudent to recommend elective delivery at 37–38 weeks when neonatal morbidity is lowest. The large rise in stillbirths seen in population data at 38 weeks is artifactual, reflecting gestational age at delivery not at intrauterine death. There is an argument for delivering MC twins earlier, based on their high rate of unexplained death rate *in utero* and the desire to avoid the consequences of fetal death to its co-twin. Twins are not a contraindication to induction [59].

Vaginal delivery

Mode of delivery has traditionally been decided on the presentation of the first twin (cephalic in 70%, breech in 30%), and fetal growth and well-being. Caesarean section has been advised where the first twin is breech, based on extrapolation from the term breech trial, and the desire to avoid the rare interlocking with head entrapment of a presenting breech above a second cephalic twin. The presentation of the second twin is of little relevance until after the birth of the first. Parturients with a previous Caesarean section are probably best delivered by repeat Caesarean, because of greater risks of scar dehiscence/rupture due both to uterine distension and to intrauterine manipulation of the second twin.

For vaginal delivery, continuous cardiotocography (CTG) of both twins is facilitated by use of a dual channel recorder and/or a combination of internal and external electrodes. An intravenous line is sited, antacids given and blood drawn for cross matching, in view of the increased incidence of Caesarean section and post-partum haemorrhage. Augmentation may be used as in singletons. An epidural is strongly advised in case internal manipulation of the second twin is needed; if one is not sited, an

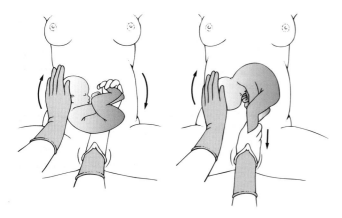

Fig. 20.4 Internal podalic version. Left: cephalic presentation; grasping both feet. Right: Downward traction on feet. Upward pressure on head. Cephalic presentation converted to footling breech.

Table 20.1 Comparison of external cephalic version with internal podalic version in pooled data from four observational studies

	External cephalic version N = 118	Internal podalic version N = 164	p value
Successful vaginal delivery	45%	97%	<0.001
Caesarean section for second twin	38%	3%	<0.001
Fetal distress	18%	1%	<0.001

After [61].

anaesthetist will be required at delivery in case general anaesthesia is required.

The delivery of the first twin proceeds as for a singleton. Its cord is clamped to prevent haemorrhage from the second twin along any placental anastomoses. An experienced obstetrician discerns the presentation of the second twin, either by abdominal and vaginal examination or increasingly by transabdominal ultrasound. Oblique or transverse lies are then converted to longitudinal. The membranes should be left intact to facilitate version. External cephalic version may be used to manipulate the fetal head over the pelvic inlet. However, internal podalic version (Fig. 20.4) and breech extraction is preferred as the primary procedure as observational studies (Table 20.1) show that it is associated with a higher chance of success and lower rate of fetal distress. One or preferably both feet are grasped and brought down into the vagina followed by assisted breech delivery with contractions and maternal effort.

Although historical series suggested that the risk to the second twin increased the greater the delay until its delivery, intervals of >30 min are acceptable providing the CTG is satisfactory and the presenting part is descending. Uterine inertia with a longitudinal-lying second twin is corrected by oxytocin infusion. Fetal distress can be managed by ventouse delivery even if the head is high or breech extraction if podalic. The already stretched vaginal tissues after birth of the first twin allow these procedures in circumstances where they are normally contraindicated. Caesarean section for a second twin is rarely indicated for disproportion, usually only where the second twin is unexpectedly much bigger than the first, and is associated with an increased complication rate compounding the complications of vaginal and abdominal delivery [60]. An oxytocin infusion is given prophylactically in the third stage.

Caesarean section

There is an increasing trend to Caesarean section with 59% of twins now delivered abdominally in the UK. Essentially the risks of vaginal delivery are increased in twins compared to singletons, as are the risks of Caesarean section [61]. A large international randomized trial is underway to resolve the optimal mode of delivery in twins. In the interim, it seems reasonable to offer women Caesarean section where otherwise suitable for vaginal delivery. This is based on (1) a high intrapartum section rate in twins, with evidence from other trials suggesting that maternal morbidity from elective section is comparable where the emergency rate exceeds one in three and (2) increasing recognition that the second twin has a chance of intrapartum-related death some five-fold higher than first twin or singletons [62]. Because the latter risk is not seen after Caesarean delivery, Smith *et al.* used Scottish national data to estimate that one death would be prevented every 264 Caesarean sections [63].

High order multiples

Perinatal risk increases exponentially with increasing fetal number. Most high-order multiple pregnancies are the result of ART and thus should be preventable with closer monitoring of follicular response and stricter controls on IVF. Although triplet rates have fallen in several Northern European countries including the UK, there is still much work to be done in proscribing three embryo transfers in other settings.

Every woman with a high-order multiple pregnancy should be counselled about the risk of continuing the pregnancy, the likely management and the offer of multifetal pregnancy reduction (MFPR). In addition to mortality rates, parents are informed of the mean gestational age at

Table 20.2 Principles of management of multiple pregnancy

Twins	High-order multiples
Routine chorionicity determination	As for twins
	Offer multifetal pregnancy reduction
	Manage in comprehensive tertiary perinatal centre with fetal medicine service
Down screening based on nuchal translucency & chorionicity	As for twins
Counselling regarding perinatal risks, agree management plan	As for twins
Haematinic supplementation	As for twins
Refer to fetal medicine centre for invasive procedures	As for twins
Anomaly scan and, if MC, fetal echocardiography	As for twins
Consider screening for cervical length	Cervical length scan 20–24 weeks
	Consider prophylactic progesterone
Ultrasound for growth/well-being (2 weekly if MC, 4 weekly DC)	2 weekly scans
Refer to fetal medicine centre if complications in MC	As for twins
Hospitalization for clinical indications	As for twins
Early detection and management of preterm labour	As for twins
Offer vaginal if presenting twin cephalic and fetal condition adequate	Deliver by Caesarean section
Continuous dual CTG monitoring, and epidural in labour	
Internal podalic version for non-longitudinal second twin	
Prophylactic oxytocin infusion in 3rd stage	As for twins

delivery of 33–34 and 31 weeks for triplets and quadruplets, respectively, and more importantly of the chance of delivering <28 weeks (5–10%, and 20–25% respectively) with attendant gestation-specific risks of long-term handicap. MFPR is done by intrathoracic KCl injection under ultrasound guidance. It is usually done at 11–13 weeks to allow prior nuchal translucency screening. Fetal number is reduced usually to two, because the outcome of twins is considered acceptable, and in case a structural malformation is shown on later scans. International registry data and meta-analysis of observational series suggest that the outcome after reduction approaches but never quite reaches that of spontaneous twins [64–66]. There is now general consensus that MFPR should be recommended for quadruplets and higher multiples. The situation with triplets has been more controversial with many considering this a social issue for parents. However, pooling of the available series suggests that the overall miscarriage rate is no higher and may even be lower in triplets reduced to twins compared to those left intact, with the chance of taking home at least one healthy baby higher in reduced compared to non-reduced triplets [64].

High-order multiple pregnancies should be managed in tertiary perinatal centres with a fetal medicine service. Management is along standard lines for twins, but with greater emphasis on preventing preterm delivery and on monitoring fetal growth and condition (Table 20.2). Prophylactic progesterone should be considered. Although there have been successful reports of triplets and even quadruplets being delivered vaginally, it is safer to deliver high-order multiples abdominally. This obviates difficulties with electronic fetal monitoring, avoids unrecognized hypoxia especially given the high incidence of IUGR, and prevents birth trauma from manipulative delivery of very preterm non-presenting fetuses. Given the high incidence of preterm labour in the mid-trimester, the option after delivery of the presenting fetus of conservative management with passive retention of residual fetuses to prolong their gestational age at delivery should be considered [67].

References

1. Ward RH, & Whittle M (eds) (1995) *Multiple Pregnancy.* London: RCOG Press.
2. Martin NG, Shanley S, Butt K *et al.* (1991) Excessive follicular recruitment and growth in mothers of spontaneous dizygotic twins. *Acta Genet Med Gemellol Roma* **40**, 291–301.
3. Fisk NM, Trew G (1999) Two's company, three's a crowd for embryo transfer. *Lancet* **354**, 1572–3.
4. Pandian Z, Templeton A, & Serour G *et al.* (2005) Number of embryos for transfer after IVF and ICSI: a Cochrane review. *Hum Reprod* **20**, 2681–7.
5. Petterson B, Nelson KB, Watson L *et al.* (1993) Twins, triplets, and cerebral palsy in births in Western Australia in the 1980s. *Br Med J* **307**, 1239–43.
6. Yokoyama Y, Shimizu T & Hayakawa K (1995) Prevalence of cerebral palsy in twins, triplets and quadruplets. *Int J Epidemiol* **24**, 943–8.
7. Pharoah PO & Cooke T (1996) Cerebral palsy and multiple births. *Arch Dis Child Fetal Neonatal Ed* **75**, F174–7.

8. Dube J, Dodds L & Armson BA (2002) Does chorionicity or zygosity predict adverse perinatal outcomes in twins? *Am J Obstet Gynecol* **186**, 579–83.

9. Sebire NJ, Snijders RJ, Hughes K *et al.* (2997) The hidden mortality of monochorionic twin pregnancies. *Br J Obstet Gynaecol* **104**, 1203–7.

10. Minakami H, Honma Y, Matsubara S *et al.* (1999) Effects of placental chorionicity on outcome in twin pregnancies. A cohort study. *J Reprod Med* **44**, 595–600.

11. Adegbite AL, Castille S, Ward S. *et al.* (2004) Neuromorbidity in preterm twins in relation to chorionicity and discordant birth weight. *Am J Obstet Gynecol* **190**, 156–63.

12. Stagiannis KD, Sepulveda W, Southwell D *et al.* (1995) Ultrasonographic measurement of the dividing membrane in twin pregnancy during the second and third trimesters: a reproducibility study. *Am J Obstet Gynecol* **173**, 1546–50.

13. Fisk NM, Bryan E (1993) Routine prenatal determination of chorionicity in multiple gestation: a plea to the obstetrician. *Br J Obstet Gynaecol* **100**, 975–7.

14. Boklage CE (1990) Survival probability of human conceptions from fertilization to term. *Int J Fertil* **35 75**, 79–80, 81–94.

15. Landy HJ, Keith LG (1998) The vanishing twin: a review. *Hum Reprod Update* **4**, 177–83.

16. Karatza AA, Wolfenden JL, Taylor MJ *et al.* (2002) Influence of twin–twin transfusion syndrome on fetal cardiovascular structure and function: prospective case-control study of 136 monochorionic twin pregnancies. *Heart* **88**, 271–7.

17. Jamar M, Lemarchal C, Lemaire V *et al.* (2003) A low rate of trisomy 21 in twin-pregnancies: a cytogenetics retrospective study of 278 cases. *Genet Couns* **14**, 395–400.

18. Cuckle H (1998) Down's syndrome screening in twins. *J Med Screen* **5**, 3–4.

19. Vandecruys H, Faiola S, Auer M *et al.* Screening for trisomy 21 in monochorionic twins by measurement of fetal nuchal translucency thickness. *Ultrasound Obstet Gynecol* **25**, 551–3.

20. Taylor M & Fisk NM (2000) Prenatal diagnosis in multiple pregnancy. In: Rodeck C (ed.) *Bailliere's Best Practice & Research: Diagnosis of Genetic Defects in the Fetus*. London: Bailliere Tindall, 663–76.

21. De Catte L, Liebaers I & Foulon W (2000) Outcome of twin gestations after first trimester chorionic villus sampling. *Obstet Gynecol* **96**, 714–20.

22. Yukobowich E, Anteby EY, Cohen SM (2001) Risk of fetal loss in twin pregnancies undergoing second trimester amniocentesis. *Obstet Gynecol* **98**, 231–4.

23. Evans MI, Goldberg JD, Horenstein J *et al.* (1999) Selective termination for structural, chromosomal, and mendelian anomalies: international experience. *Am J Obstet Gynecol* **181**, 893–7.

24. Day MC, Barton JR, O'Brien JM *et al.* (2005) The effect of fetal number on the development of hypertensive conditions of pregnancy. *Obstet Gynecol* **106**, 927–31.

25. Ellison MA, Hotamisligil S, Lee H *et al.* (2005) Psychosocial risks associated with multiple births resulting from assisted reproduction. *Fertil Steril* **83**, 1422–8.

26. Rydhstrom H (1994) Discordant birthweight and late fetal death in like-sexed and unlike-sexed twin pairs: a population-based study. *Br J Obstet Gynaecol* **101**, 765–9.

27. Hollier LM, McIntire DD, Leveno KJ (1999) Outcome of twin pregnancies according to intrapair birth weight differences. *Obstet Gynecol* **94**, 1006–10.

28. Garite TJ, Clark RH, Elliott JP *et al.* (2004) Twins and triplets: the effect of plurality and growth on neonatal outcome compared with singleton infants. *Am J Obstet Gynecol* **191**, 700–7.

29. Vanderheyden TM, Fichera A, Pasquini L *et al.* (2005) Increased latency of absent end-diastolic flow in the umbilical artery of monochorionic twin fetuses. *Ultrasound Obstet Gynecol* **26**, 44–9.

30. Crowther CA (2001) Hospitalisation and bed rest for multiple pregnancy. *Cochrane Database Syst Rev* CD000110.

31. Yamasmit W, Chaithongwongwatthana S, Tolosa JE *et al.* (2005) Prophylactic oral betamimetics for reducing preterm birth in women with a twin pregnancy. *Cochrane Database Syst Rev* CD004733.

32. Hartikainen-Sorri AL, Kauppila A, Tuimala R (1980) Inefficacy of 17 alphahydroxyprogesterone caproate in the prevention of prematurity in twin pregnancy. *Obstet Gynecol* **56**, 692–5.

33. Skentou C, Souka AP, To MS *et al.* (2001) Prediction of preterm delivery in twins by cervical assessment at 23 weeks. *Ultrasound Obstet Gynecol* **17**, 7–10.

34. Honest H, Bachmann LM, Coomarasamy A *et al.* (2003) Accuracy of cervical transvaginal sonography in predicting preterm birth: a systematic review. *Ultrasound Obstet Gynecol* **22**, 305–22.

35. Berghella V, Odibo AO, To MS *et al.* (2005) Cerclage for short cervix on ultrasonography: meta-analysis of trials using individual patient-level data. *Obstet Gynecol* **106**, 181–9.

36. Kashanian M, Akbarian AR & Soltanzadeh M (2005) Atosiban and nifedipine for the treatment of preterm labor. *Int J Gynaecol Obstet* **91**, 10–4.

37. Oei S (2006) Calcium channel blockers: a review of their efficacy and safety of tocolysis following reports of serious adverse events. *Eur J Obstet Gynecol Reprod Biol* **126**, 137–45.

38. Crowley P (2004) Prophylactic corticosteroids for preterm birth (Cochrane Review). The Cochrane Library, **4**, CD000065.

39. Murphy DJ, Caukwell S, Joels LA *et al.* (2002) Cohort study of the neonatal outcome of twin pregnancies that were treated with prophylactic or rescue antenatal corticosteroids. *Am J Obstet Gynecol* **187**, 483–8.

40. Nicolini U & Poblete A (1999) Single intrauterine death in monochorionic twin pregnancies. *Ultrasound Obstet Gynecol* **14**, 297–301.

41. Bajoria R, Wee LY, Anwar S *et al.* (1999) Outcome of twin pregnancies complicated by single intrauterine death in relation to vascular anatomy of the monochorionic placenta. *Hum Reprod* **14**, 2124–30.

42. Taylor MJ, Denbow ML, Tanawattanacharoen S *et al.* (2000) Doppler detection of arterio-arterial anastomoses in monochorionic twins: feasibility and clinical application. *Hum Reprod* **15**, 1632–6.

43. Senat MV, Loizeau S, Couderc S *et al.* (2003) The value of middle cerebral artery peak systolic velocity in the diagnosis of fetal anemia after intrauterine death of one monochorionic twin. *Am J Obstet Gynecol* **189**, 1320–4.

44. Galea P, Jain V & Fisk NM (2005) Insights into the pathophysiology of twintwin transfusion syndrome. *Prenat Diagn* **25**, 777–85.

45. Tan TY, Taylor MJ, Wee LY *et al.* (2004) Doppler for artery-artery anastomosis and stage-independent survival in twin-twin transfusion. *Obstet Gynecol* **103**, 1174–80.

46. Senat MV, Deprest J, Boulvain M *et al.* (2004) Endoscopic laser surgery versus serial amnioreduction for severe twin-to-twin transfusion syndrome. *N Engl J Med* **351**, 136–44.

47. Fox C, Kilby MD, Khan KS (2005) Contemporary treatments for twin-twin transfusion syndrome. *Obstet Gynecol* **105**, 1469–77.

48. Fisk NM & Galea P (2004) Twin–twin transfusion - as good as it gets? *N Engl J Med* **351**,182–4.

49. Mari G, Roberts A, Detti L *et al.* (2001) Perinatal morbidity and mortality rates in severe twin-twin transfusion syndrome: results of the International Amnioreduction Registry. *Am J Obstet Gynecol* **185**, 708–15.

50. Moise KJ Jr, Dorman K, Lamvu G *et al.* (2005) A randomized trial of amnioreduction versus septostomy in the treatment of twin-twin transfusion syndrome. *Am J Obstet Gynecol* **193**, 701–7.

51. Moore TR, Gale S & Benirschke K (1990) Perinatal outcome of forty-nine pregnancies complicated by acardiac twinning. *Am J Obstet Gynecol* **163**, 907–12.

52. Tan TY & Sepulveda W (2003) Acardiac twin: a systematic review of minimally invasive treatment modalities. *Ultrasound Obstet Gynecol* **22**, 409–19.

53. Overton TG, Denbow ML, Duncan KR *et al.* (1999) First-trimester cord entanglement in monoamniotic twins. *Ultrasound Obstet Gynecol* **13**,140–2.

54. Roque H, Gillen-Goldstein J, Funai E *et al.* (2003) Perinatal outcomes in monoamniotic gestations. *J Matern Fetal Neonatal Med* **13**, 414–21.

55. Allen VM, Windrim R, Barrett J *et al.* (2001) Management of monoamniotic twin pregnancies: a case series and systematic review of the literature. *Br J Obstet Gynaecol* **108**, 931–6.

56. Heyborne KD, Porreco RP, Garite TJ *et al.* (2005) Improved perinatal survival of monoamniotic twins with intensive inpatient monitoring. *Am J Obstet Gynecol* **192**, 96–101.

57. Pasquini L, Wimalasundera R, Fichera A, *et al.* (in press) High perinatal survival in monoamniotics twins managed by prophylactic sulindac, intensive surreillance, and caesarean delivery at 32 weeks. *Ultrasound Obset Gynecol.*

58. Dodd JM, Crowther CA (2003) Elective delivery of women with a twin pregnancy from 37 weeks' gestation. *Cochrane Database Syst Rev* CD003582.

59. Barigye O, Pasquini L, Galea P *et al.* (2005) High risk of unexpected late fetal death in monochorionic twins despite intensive ultrasound surveillance: a cohort study. *PLoS Med* **2**, 521–7.

60. Crowther CA (2002) Caesarean delivery for the second twin. *Cochrane Database Syst Rev* CD000047.

61. Barrett JF, Ritchie WK (2002) Twin delivery. *Best Pract Res Clin Obstet Gynaecol* **6**, 43–56.

62. Smith GC, Pell JP & Dobbie R (2002) Birth order, gestational age, and risk of delivery related perinatal death in twins: retrospective cohort study. *Br Med J* **325**, 1004.

63. Smith GC, Shah I, White IR (2005) Mode of delivery and the risk of delivery-related perinatal death among twins at term: a retrospective cohort study of 8073 births. *Br J Obstet Gynaecol* **112**, 1139–44.

64. Wimalasundera RC, Trew G, Fisk NM (2003) Reducing the incidence of twins and triplets. *Best Pract Res Clin Obstet Gynaecol* **17**(2), 309–29.

65. Dodd J & Crowther C (2004) Multifetal pregnancy reduction of triplet and higher-order multiple pregnancies to twins. *Fertil Steril* **81**, 1420–2.

66. Evans M, Wapner R, Carpenter R *et al.* (1999) International collaboration on multifetal, pregnancy reduction (MFPR): dramatically improved outcomes with increased experience. *Am J Obstet Gynecol* **190**, S28.

67. Trivedi AN, Gillett WR (1998) The retained twin/triplet following a preterm delivery – an analysis of the literature. *Aust NZ J Obstet Gynaecol* **38**, 461–5.

Further reading

Blickstein I & Keith LG (eds) (2005) *Multiple Pregnancy: Epidemiology, Gestation & Perinatal Outcome.* Oxford: Taylor & Francis.

Dodd JM & Crowther CA (2005) Evidence-based care of women with a multiple pregnancy. In: Neilson J (ed.) *Best Practice & Research Clinical Obstetrics and Gynaecology: Evidence-based Obstetrics.* Amsterdam: Elsevier, 131–54.

Jain V & Fisk NM (2004) The twin-twin transfusion syndrome. *Clin Obstet Gynecol* **47**, 181–202.

Kilby MD, Baker P, Critchley H, Field D (eds) (2006) Multiple Pregnancy: Proceedings of the RCOG study Group. London: RCOG Press.

Pasquini L, Wimalasundera R & Fisk NM (2004) Management of other complications specific to monochorionic twin pregnancies. In: Keith L & Penna L (eds) *Best Practice & Research Clinical Obstetrics and Gynaecology: Multiple Pregnancy.* Amsterdam: Elsevier, 577–99.

Chapter 21: Preterm labour

Phillip Bennett

Epidemiology

Definitions

Preterm birth is defined as delivery of a baby before 37 completed weeks of pregnancy. Legally, in the United Kingdom, the 1992 Amendment to the Infant Life Preservation Act, defined the limit of viability as 24 weeks. A small number of infants born at 23 weeks will, however, survive. Mortality and morbidity in preterm babies born after 32 weeks gestation is similar to that of babies born at term. The risk of neonatal mortality of survival with handicap becomes significant in 'Very Preterm Infants' defined as those born between 28 and 32 weeks but is most significant in 'Extremely Preterm Infants' defined as those born before 28 weeks. In modern obstetric practice assessment of gestational age is based both upon the date of the last menstrual period and ultrasound fetal biometry. In the past, however, assessment of gestational age was not always accurate and paediatric statistics may be based upon birthweight rather than gestational age data. 'Low Birthweight' is defined as less than 2.25 kg, 'Very Low Birthweight' as less than 1.5 kg and 'Extremely Low Birthweight' as less than 1 kg. Using these definitions to describe outcome data leads to blurring of the distinction between preterm babies and small for gestational age babies, particularly in the low birthweight category and also fails to differentiate the normally grown preterm neonate from the neonate who is both preterm and small for gestational age (Table 21.1).

Incidence

The incidence of preterm birth in the developed world is between 7 and 12%. There has been a small gradual rise in the incidence of preterm birth associated with assisted reproduction causing multiple pregnancy and an increased tendency to obstetric intervention. The rate of preterm birth prior to 32 weeks has remained relatively stable at 1–2%. About one quarter of preterm births are elective deliveries, usually for pre-eclampsia, intrauterine growth restriction, or maternal disease. The remainder are due to preterm labour and delivery. The incidence of spontaneous preterm labour is at its lowest in women in their 20s. The risk is increased in teenagers and in women over 30. There is a higher incidence of preterm labour in first pregnancies. Higher parity alone is not a risk factor for preterm labour. Indeed there is a progressively lower risk with each successive term birth. Marital status, cigarette smoking, environmental stress, poor nutrition and use of alcohol, coffee and street drugs (especially cocaine) have all been linked to an increased risk of preterm birth. Many of these factors are, however, interlinked and are all factors associated with social disadvantage.

There does appear to be an association between race and a risk of preterm delivery. In the United Kingdom the risk of preterm birth is 6% in white Europeans but 10% in Africans or Afro-Caribbeans but it is also difficult to differentiate genetic variation from social deprivation. In studies of populations where black and white women have similar life styles, levels of income and access to medical care (for example in US Army personnel) preterm delivery rates show a less marked ethnic variation. The recent identification of specific genetic polymorphisms which increase the risk of preterm labour does suggest, however, that there may be genetic as well as environmental factors, which explains the increased risk of preterm labour in certain ethnic populations. Intervention studies have shown that antenatal smoking cessation programmes reduce the risk of preterm birth but there is no evidence currently that other interventions such as increased frequency of antenatal care, dietary advice or an increase in social support reduce the risk.

Neonatal outcomes after preterm birth

Survival rates for preterm babies have improved steadily over the past two decades due to the introduction of surfactant therapy, improvements in neonatal respiratory management and more widespread use of antenatal steroids. While the number of babies above 24 weeks who

Table 21.1

Gestational age	Weight: 50th centile	Weight: 10th centile	Weight: 90th centile	Survival (%)	Survival percent without major morbidity
23	600	450	970	6	2
24	700	550	1180	15	5
25	790	620	1250	45	15
26	880	700	1350	60	20
27	960	780	1450	75	50
28	1080	820	1600	85	60
29	1220	940	1720	90	80
30	1400	1050	1900	93	85
31	1600	1180	2100	96	90
32	1760	1300	2300	97	92
33	1980	1480	2500	97	95
34	2200	1650	2700	98	97

survive has increased there has been no improvement in survival at the lower limits of viability below 23 weeks. The Epicure study [1] reported mortality rates of 100, 90 and 80% for preterm infants admitted to the Neonatal Unit at 21, 22 and 23 weeks gestation, respectively. Improved survival for very preterm infants has been associated with an increase in the proportion of children with cerebral palsy who were born preterm. Neonatal mortality rises gradually between 32 and 28 weeks from 2 to 8% and then more dramatically and exponentially to 80% at 23 weeks.

In the past surfactant deficiency leading to neonatal respiratory distress syndrome was the major cause of morbidity and mortality in preterm infants. Alveolar surfactant production begins at 30–32 weeks gestation. Therefore preterm infants born prior to 30 weeks are at highest risk. The impact of respiratory distress syndrome upon neonatal morbidity and mortality has been dramatically reduced in the past two decades through use of antenatal corticosteroids and exogenous surfactant replacement. The risk of chronic lung disease, defined as a need for ventilation or oxygen supplementation at 36 weeks after conception, has continued to rise, however, because of the increased survival of extremely preterm infants. The fetal and neonatal brain is especially susceptible to injury between 20 and 32 weeks post-conception. The greatest risk of long-term neural developmental problems is in infants born before 28 weeks or at birth weights of less than 1 kg. The Epicure study showed that in infants born before 26 weeks gestation approximately half had some disability at 30 months and approximately one quarter had severe disability (Figs 21.1 and 21.2). Cerebral palsy may be related to periventricular haemorrhage, post-haemorrhagic hydrocephalus and periventricular leukomalacia. Hypoxic ischaemia is a major risk factor for neonatal cerebral damage. However, there is

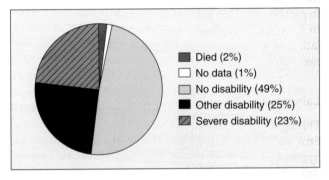

Fig. 21.1 Outcomes for surviving infants born before 26 weeks' gestation when assessed at 30 months. Adapted from Wood NS *et al.* N *Engl J Med.* (2000) 10; 343(6): 378–4 and Colvin M *et al.* (2004) *Br Med J* **329**, 1390–3.

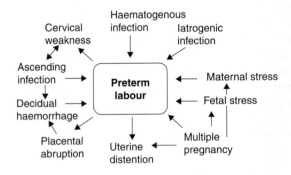

Fig. 21.2 The innerplay of causes of the 'preterm labour syndrome'.

growing evidence for a strong link between chorionamnionitis, fetal inflammation and the risk of periventricular leukomalacia.

The risk of visual impairment due to retinopathy of prematurity is inversely related to gestational age and directly related to the concentration and duration of oxygen treatment. Despite improvements in the management of oxygen therapy, most infants born before 28 weeks gestation will develop some form of retinopathy. The risk of retinopathy of prematurity rises dramatically from less than 10% at 26 weeks to above 50% in infants born at 24 weeks. About 3% infants born before 28 weeks gestation will require a hearing aid and 50% will be found to have learning difficulties at school requiring additional educational support.

The endocrinology and biochemistry of labour

To effectively predict and prevent labour requires a good understanding of the endocrinology and biochemistry underlying the onset of labour in humans, both at term and preterm. Unfortunately our understanding of the mechanisms leading to the onset of human labour is incomplete, in part because the mechanisms in different species appear to have evolved differently making the direct extrapolation of data from animal models to the human not necessarily valid.

Labour as an inflammatory process

Throughout pregnancy the uterine cervix needs to remain firm and closed while the body of the uterus grows by hypertrophy and hyperplasia but without significant fundally dominant contractions. For labour to be successful the cervix is converted into a soft and pliable structure that can efface and dilate and the uterus becomes a powerful contractile organ. There is no single endocrinological or biochemical switch in the human which changes the uterus from its no-labour state to its labour state. The onset of labour is a gradual process which begins several weeks before delivery itself with changes in the lower pole of the uterus which cause cervical ripening and effacement. The onset of clinically identifiable contractions is a relatively late event in this process. Cervical ripening occurs through breakdown of collagen, changes in proteoglycan concentrations and an increase in water content. The lower segment of the uterus also stretches and relaxes and behaves physiologically more like the cervix than the contractile upper segment of the uterus. These changes in the lower segment of the uterus are associated with an increase in the production of inflammatory cytokines, particularly interleukins-1, -6 and -8 and prostaglandins from the overlying fetal membranes and decidua and from the cervix itself. Cervical ripening is associated with an influx of inflammatory cells into the cervix which release matrix metalloproteins which contribute to the anatomical changes associated with ripening. The later increase in fundally dominant contractility in the upper segment of the uterus is associated with an increase in the expression of receptors for oxytocin and prostaglandins, in gap-junction proteins which mediate electrical connectivity between myocytes, and in more complex changes in the intracellular signalling pathways which increase the contractility of the myocytes.

The roles of progesterone, corticotrophin releasing hormone and oxytocin

In many species progesterone is thought to play an important role in suppressing the onset of labour. Progesterone has a generally anti-inflammatory action within the uterus. The biochemical events associated with cervical ripening and the onset of labour are similar to those seen at sites of inflammation. In some species the onset of labour is heralded by withdrawal of progesterone. So, for example, in the rodent prostaglandin mediated regression of the corpus luteum leads to a fall in progesterone concentrations immediately prior to the onset of labour. In the sheep increased production of cortisol from the fetal adrenal signals fetal maturation and induces placental 17-alpha hydroxylase which increases synthesis of oestrogen at the expense of progesterone, again leading to progesterone withdrawal prior to the onset of labour. There is no systemic withdrawal of progesterone in the human prior to labour although there is an increase in the expression of genes formerly repressed by progesterone, which has led to the hypothesis of a 'functional progesterone withdrawal' mediated by changes in the expression of progesterone receptors or of cofactors needed for the function of the progesterone receptor. Another hypothesis is that inflammatory events seen within the uterus at the time of labour are associated with increased activity of the transcription factor nuclear factor-kappa B (NF-kappa B) (which is a transcription factor strongly associated with inflammation in other contexts such as asthma, inflammatory bowel disease or arthritis). NF-kappa B is known to repress the function of the progesterone receptor and so could mediate 'functional progesterone withdrawal'. Although in the mouse progesterone concentrations fall due to luteolysis just prior to labour, there is still sufficient circulating progesterone to activate progesterone receptors. In the mouse it appears that the final event leading to parturition is the increased production of surfactant protein A from the fetal lung which stimulates the activity of NF-kappa B within the uterus leading to an influx of inflammatory cells, an increase in inflammatory cytokine synthesis and depression of the residual function of the progesterone receptor. It is an attractive hypothesis that pulmonary maturation in the human may also signal the final phase of the onset of labour but there is at present no direct evidence that this mechanism applies in the human.

Circulating levels of corticotrophin releasing hormone (CRH), synthesized in the placenta, increase progressively throughout pregnancy and especially during the weeks prior to the onset of labour. CRH binding protein concentrations fall with advancing gestational age such that, approximately 3 weeks prior to the onset of labour the concentration of CRH exceeds that of its binding protein. Unlike CRH in the hypothalamus, placental CRH is up regulated by cortisol. Several studies have linked placental production of CRH with the timing of birth and have demonstrated that a premature rise in CRH is associated with preterm delivery.

In the monkey uterine contractions occur only at night. In the days preceding labour and delivery there are nocturnal non-fundally dominant contractions which have been termed 'contractures'. The conversion from contractures to contractions is mediated by an increase in the production of oxytocin from the maternal posterior pituitary gland. In the monkey, therefore, while the fetus might signal its general readiness to be born through increased cortisol production from the adrenal, the precise timing of birth is signalled by the mother. This may be a mechanism of defence against predators which ensures that delivery is always at night. Contrary to the experience of many obstetricians, this phenomenon does not apply to the human. There is no increase in the production of oxytocin associated with the onset or progression of either preterm or term labour. There is, however, an increase in the expression of oxytocin receptors within the uterus and there is local production of oxytocin in the uterus, decidua and fetal membranes. Although oxytocin probably does not play an important role in the precise timing of parturition in the human, an increase in the density of oxytocin receptors suggests that oxytocin does play a role in mediating contractility.

The causes of preterm labour

Preterm labour is not a single disease entity but is a symptom or a syndrome which may have one or more of a number of causes (Fig. 21.3). Preterm labour has been linked to cervical incompetence, abnormalities of haemostasis, infection within the uterus, placental abruption or decidual haemorrhage, fetal or maternal stress and multiple pregnancy. In some cases several of these factors may act together to increase the likelihood of preterm delivery or to affect the gestational age at which preterm delivery occurs. So, for example, twin pregnancies deliver at 36 weeks. Multiple pregnancy probably leads to preterm delivery through at least two mechanisms. Over-distension of the uterus leads to premature up regulation of contraction associated proteins and of factors which mediate cervical ripening, all of which have been

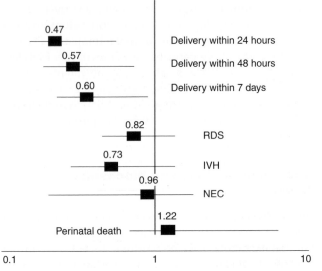

Fig. 21.3 Meta-analysis of the effect of tocolytic administration upon preterm delivery and neonatal outcomes. Adapted from Gyetvai K *et al*. Obstet Gynecol. 1999 94(5 Pt 2): 869–77.

shown to be sensitive to mechanical stretch. Multiple pregnancy is associated with multiple placentas and therefore with an earlier rise in placental CRH concentrations in the circulation. A preterm delivery in twins at 28 weeks will not be due simply to the multiple pregnancy and must have another aetiology associated with it, for example, infection or cervical weakness. Had the same pregnancy been a singleton pregnancy it is probable that the preterm delivery would have occurred at a later gestational age.

Cervical function

With improved survival at early gestational ages, there is now overlap between second trimester pregnancy loss and early preterm delivery. Historically cervical incompetence was diagnosed in women who experienced persistent, often rapid and painless, late second trimester pregnancy loss. More recently the concept of cervical competence as a continuum has evolved. It is probable that cervical length (Table 21.2) and strength together with the quality of the cervical mucus contribute towards the cervix's function, both to retain the pregnancy within the uterus and to exclude potential bacterial pathogens from ascending from the vagina. Numerous studies have demonstrated a strong relationship between cervical length and the risk of preterm delivery. The cervix may be damaged (or completely removed) by surgery in the treatment of cervical cancer or rarely, during a difficult instrumental vaginal delivery or Caesarean section at full dilatation. There are also associations between diethylstilbestrol exposure *in utero* and developmental anomalies in the genital tract and

Table 21.2 Survival rates and birth centiles at gestational ages between 23 and 34 weeks

Cervical length	Risk of PTL	
	Before 20 weeks (mm)	Between 20 and 24 weeks (mm)
15	62	56
20	28	30
22	20	15
25	12	9
27	10	6
30	6	4.6

cervical weakness. A short or partially dilated cervix may allow bacteria to ascend into the lower pole of the uterus where, acting through the toll-like receptors of the innate immune system, they stimulate activation of NF-kappa B, the production of inflammatory cytokines, prostaglandins and inflammatory response. This then leads to cervical ripening and shortening which in turn decreases the ability of the cervix to act as either a mechanical or a microbiological barrier and so, ultimately, the development of either localized or generalized chorionamnionitis and to preterm delivery. A short or weak cervix may therefore contribute to preterm delivery not only by leading to simple second trimester miscarriage but also by contributing to a risk of ascending infection leading to a more classical spontaneous preterm labour.

Genital tract infection

There is a strong correlation between infection within the uterus and the onset of spontaneous preterm labour. As discussed above, infection within the uterus has the potential to activate all of the biochemical pathways ultimately leading to cervical ripening and uterine contractions. A scenario has been described above where it is cervical weakness or shortness which is the primary factor leading to a risk of ascending bacterial infection. However, it is also possible that with a high number of virulent pathogens in the vagina, bacteria may gain access to the lower pole of the uterus through a normally functioning cervix, where they activate inflammatory mediators leading to cervical ripening and shortening. Bacteria may also gain access to the amniotic cavity through haematogenous spread or by introduction at the time of invasive procedures. Following preterm delivery histological chorionamnionitis is usually more common and severe at the site of membrane rupture than elsewhere. In virtually all cases of congenital pneumonia, inflammation of the fetal membranes is also

Table 21.3 Identification of bacterial vaginosis (BV)

Nugent's criteria
Scoring system. BV diagnosed if Score >7
Zero = No morphotypes per oil-immersion field
1+ = Less than one morphotype per oil-immersion field
2+ = One to four morphotypes per oil-immersion field
3+ = Five to 30 morphotypes per oil-immersion field
4+ = More than 30 morphotypes per oil-immersion field

Score	Large gram-positive rods*	Small gram-variable or gram-negative rods[†]	Curved gram-variable rods[‡]
0	4+	0+	0
1	3+	1+	1–2+
2	2+	2+	3–4+
3	1+	3+	
4	0+	4+	

* *Lactobacillus acidophilus*
[†] *Gardnerella vaginalis* and bacteroides species (small gram-variable or gram-negative rods)
[‡] Mobiluncus species (curved gram-variable rods)

Spiegel's criteria
Normal: Gram stain shows a predominance of *Lactobacillus acidophilus* (3+ or 4+), with or without *Gardnerella vaginalis*
Bacterial vaginosis: Gram stain shows mixed flora (gram-positive, gram-negative or gram-variable bacteria) and absent or decreased *L. acidophilus* (zero to 2+)
  L. acidophilus (large gram-positive bacilli)
  G. vaginalis (small gram-variable rods)
Scoring for each of the above bacterial morphotypes
0 = No morphotypes per oil-immersion field
1+ = Less than one morphotype per oil-immersion field
2+ = One to five morphotypes per oil-immersion field
3+ = Six to 30 morphotypes per oil-immersion field
4+ = More than 30 morphotypes per oil-immersion field

Amsel's diagnostic criteria
Thin, homogeneous discharge
Positive "whiff" test
"Clue cells" present on microscopy (highly significant criterion)
Vaginal pH > 4.5
Three of four criteria must be met

Gas-liquid chromatography
Succinate to lactate ratio >4

present. The bacterial species identified in the majority of cases of congenital infections is usually also found in the maternal lower genital tract. Following twin preterm delivery, chorionamnionitis is more common and severe in the presenting twin than in the second twin. These factors all suggest that ascending infection from the lower genital tract is the commonest mechanism for chorionamnionitis (Table 21.3).

Romero, Mazor *et al.* [2] have proposed a four stage sequence in chorionamnionitis which consists of
1 overgrowth of potential pathogens in the vagina or cervix possibly associated with bacterial vaginosis;
2 presence of the organisms in the uterine cavity, particularly in the decidua of the lower segment;
3 a localized inflammatory reaction leading to deciduitis, chorionitis and the extension through the amnion into the amniotic cavity;
4 infection of the fetus itself by aspiration and swallowing of infected amniotic fluid. The most common microbial isolates from the amniotic cavity of women in preterm labour are ureaplasma, urealiticum, fusibacteria and micoplasma hominis.

More than 50% of patients in preterm labour will have more than one microorganism isolated from the amniotic cavity. Microorganisms can be identified in the fetal membranes of the majority of women delivering both preterm and at term. It is probable that some cases of spontaneous preterm delivery are due to the generation of an excessive inflammatory response and to a lesser degree, of bacterial invasion of the amniotic cavity. So, for example, it has recently been demonstrated that bacterial vaginosis (see below) may be a greater risk factor for preterm labour in women who carry a high secretory form of the tumour necrosis factor alpha gene.

Haemorrhage

Placental abruption may lead to the onset of preterm labour. This is thought to be through release of thrombin which stimulates myometrial contractions by protease activated receptors but independently of prostaglandin synthesis. This may explain the clinical impression that preterm labour associated with chorionamnionitis is often rapid whereas that associated with placental abruption is less so because in placental abruption there is no periripening of the uterine cervix. Generation of thrombin may also play a role in preterm labour associated with chorionamnionitis when it is released as a consequence of decidual haemorrhage.

Fetal and maternal stress

There is evidence that both fetal and maternal stress may be risk factors for preterm labour. Fetal stress may arise in association with abnormal placentation and growth restriction. Maternal stress could be due to environmental factors. In both cases it is postulated that over secretion of cortisol leads to upregulation of CRH production in the placenta.

Prediction of preterm labour

In many cases of preterm labour obstetric management consists principally of attempting to suppress contractions in women who are already in established labour. As will be discussed in greater detail, this strategy is essentially ineffective. It is probable that in the future obstetric strategies to reduce perinatal morbidity and mortality associated with preterm labour will involve the early identification of women at risk and the use of prophylactic therapies. Attempts have been made to devise risk scoring systems based on socio-demographic characteristics, anthropomorphic characteristics, past history, patient behaviour and habits and factors in the current pregnancy. None of these systems has been found to have positive predictive values or sensitivities which make them clinically useful. Most systems rely heavily on past obstetric history and are therefore irrelevant to women having their first baby. At the present time there are no screening tests which are routinely applied to gravid women who are not at high risk for preterm labour.

Past obstetric history

Women at high risk of preterm labour will initially be detected based upon past obstetric history. (Table 21.4) Having had a single previous preterm delivery increases the risk of preterm delivery in a subsequent pregnancy four times when compared to a woman whose previous delivery was at term. Interestingly a past obstetric history which consists of a term delivery followed by a preterm delivery confers a higher risk of preterm delivery in the third pregnancy than a past obstetric history that consists of a preterm delivery followed by a term delivery. This may be because the latter group contains a disproportionate number of women whose preterm delivery was for 'non-recurring' causes such as placental abruption, whereas in the former group some cases of preterm delivery following the term delivery may be

Table 21.4 Effect of past obstetric history upon relative risk of preterm delivery. Adapted from Hoffman HJ and Bakketeig LS. Clin Obstet Gynecol. (1984) 27(3): 539–52

First delivery	Second delivery	RR of PTL
Term		1
Preterm		4
Term	Term	0.5
Preterm	Term	1.3
Term	Preterm	2.5
Preterm	Preterm	6.5

due to damage to the cervix during the original term delivery.

Bacterial vaginosis

The principle organism in normal vaginal flora is lactic bacillus, a bacterium which produces lactic acid from glycogen and leads to an acid pH in vaginal secretions. The combination of large numbers of lactobacilli and the low pH is a protective mechanism against colonization with potential pathogens. Many important potential pathogens can be found in the vagina of healthy women. However, in normal healthy pregnancies the numbers of lactobacilli increase as pregnancy progresses. Bacterial vaginosis is an abnormality of the normal vaginal flora characterized by a reduced number of lactobacilli, a higher pH and increased numbers of potential pathogens including *Gardenerella vaginalis*, bacteroides, *Escherichia coli*, group B streptococcus and the anaerobes peptostreptococcus, bacteroides and Mycoplasma hominis. Since the presence of large numbers of lactobacilli and a low vaginal pH are important mechanisms to protect against the growth of potential pathogenic organisms, bacterial vaginosis represents a risk factor for preterm delivery. Diagnosis of bacterial vaginosis can be made on gram staining of vaginal fluid, by gas–liquid chromatography of vaginal fluid or on clinical grounds based upon a high vaginal pH, a fishy odour in a thin homogenous vaginal discharge and the presence of clue cells in the discharge on a wet mount. There is no significant difference in the ability of each of these diagnostic tests to predict preterm birth. Studies of the risk of preterm labour associated with bacterial vaginosis have reported widely varying results. However, it appears that, overall, bacterial vaginosis approximately doubles the risk of preterm delivery.

Although there is evidence that bacterial vaginosis is a risk factor for preterm delivery, it is less clear that treating bacterial vaginosis with antibiotics is beneficial. This may in part be because various studies of bacterial vaginosis have used different antibiotics in different regimens and at different times. However, it may also reflect the fact that antibiotics may not necessarily result in the re-establishment of normal bacterial flora. The two antibiotics commonly used in the treatment of bacterial vaginosis are metronidazole administered orally or clindamycin which may be given either orally or vaginally. Clindamycin may have advantages over metronidazole since it has better activity against anaerobic bacteria, Mycoplasma hominis and Urea urealyticum which are often associated with bacterial vaginosis. The current evidence is that screening of pregnant women who are at high risk for preterm delivery based upon their past obstetric history or other factors and treatment of bacterial vaginosis (BV) can be justified but there is not currently strong evidence to recommend the routine screening and treatment of the general obstetric population.

Ultrasound measurement of cervical length

There is now good evidence that transvaginal sonographic measurement of cervical length can be used to predict the risk of preterm labour in both low- and high-risk pregnancies and in women who are symptomatic. Transabdominal measurement of cervical length is unreliable because of the need for a full bladder which may compress the cervix leading to an overestimate of its length and because it is more difficult to obtain adequate views of the cervix with this technique. Two strategies are currently in common use – either serial measurement of cervical length throughout the second and early third trimester of pregnancy or a single measurement of cervical length usually at the time of the routine ultrasound between 18 and 22 weeks. At any given gestational age there is a direct relationship between cervical length and the risk of preterm delivery. So, for example, a cervical length of 15 mm or less at 20–24 weeks predicts a 50% risk of preterm delivery prior to 34 weeks in a low-risk population. In multiple pregnancies the risk of preterm labour is higher, at any given cervical length than in a singleton pregnancy with the same cervical length. A large number of studies have examined the relationship between gestational age, cervical length and the risk of preterm delivery (see table and review by Honest *et al.* 2002). It appears that it is absolute cervical length rather than the presence or absence of funnelling which is the principle predictor of spontaneous preterm birth. If a screening strategy using a single ultrasound measurement of cervical length is used, then assessment between 21 and 24 weeks gestation appears to be better than assessment prior to 20 weeks gestation in predicting the risk of preterm labour. It is arguable, however, that identification of a risk of preterm labour as late as 23 weeks may be too late for any potential prophylactic therapies to be effective. Serial measurement of cervical length is more costly but appears to be superior to a single measurement in assessing the risk of preterm delivery.

On the continent of Europe it is common practice to perform a vaginal assessment of cervical length at each antenatal consultation. However, multicentre trials have shown that this policy is of no benefit in predicting the risk of preterm delivery.

Prevention of preterm delivery

In primigravid women with no other significant risk factors for preterm delivery there is no effective method for the prediction of preterm labour and therefore management can only be instituted at the time of acute presentation with contractions. It is possible, however, to identify a subgroup of women as being at risk of preterm delivery based upon their past obstetric history, the presence of abnormalities of the genital tract and the use of screening tests such as measurement of cervical length and detection of fetal fibronectin in vaginal secretions. At the present time there is no prophylactic therapy which has been demonstrated to be unequivocally beneficial in preventing the onset of preterm labour in a high-risk population. There is no evidence that oral beta-sympathomimetic drugs reduce the risk of preterm delivery and their use has generally been abandoned in UK obstetric practice. Commonly used therapies include cervical cerclage, non-steroidal anti-inflammatory drugs and more recently progesterone.

Cervical cerclage

As discussed earlier, cervical competence is not a discreet entity but should be considered to be a continuum. Abnormalities of cervical function may be a major factor or a minor contributor to the biochemical and mechanical events that lead to preterm delivery. There is probably considerable overlap between the mechanisms of second trimester pregnancy loss and early preterm delivery. It is clear that in women whose history strongly suggests cervical weakness, for example, those with a past history of cervical surgery or those with recurrent episodes of rapid relatively painless second trimester fetal loss, cervical cerclage will significantly improve the prospects for success in subsequent pregnancies. Where the aetiology of previous second trimester pregnancy losses or preterm deliveries points less clearly to an obvious role for cervical weakness, then whether to insert a cervical cerclage is largely a matter for individual clinical judgement. A short cervix prior to pregnancy or in early pregnancy, relatively rapid or painless early preterm deliveries, an absence of symptoms of dysmenorrhoea, all point to the possibility that cervical dysfunction may contribute to preterm delivery. An association between preterm delivery and chorionamnionitis does not necessarily discount a cervical problem since, as discussed earlier, there is an interplay between cervical function and genital tract microbiology which means that, even in cases where cervical function is undoubtedly abnormal, there is likely to be a degree of chorionamnionitis associated with preterm delivery. Preterm deliveries which are beyond 32 weeks or which are associated with major placental abruption, fetal growth restriction or pre-eclampsia are less likely to have a cervical element in their aetiology.

There have been few studies of the benefit of cervical cerclage in reducing the risk of preterm delivery partly because the views of obstetricians in this area are polarized and it has been difficult to persuade clinicians to randomize their patients into trials. The Royal College of Obstetricians and Gynaecologists/Medical Research Council (RCOG/MRC) trial showed that cervical cerclage does reduce the risk of preterm delivery but that 25 patients would need to receive a cerclage for it to benefit one patient. Although it was previously widely believed that cervical cerclage increased the risk of genital tract infection, there is not good evidence for this. Nevertheless there are clearly risks associated with the actual insertion of cervical cerclage and there has, therefore, been interest in trying to more precisely target cervical cerclage. There have been several studies in which women previously defined as at high risk of preterm delivery have had serial ultrasound measurements of cervical length performed with cerclage being performed when cervical length reaches a predetermined cut off. The Cipract study randomized women found to have a cervical length of 25 mm or less before 27 weeks to either cervical cerclage and bed rest or bed rest alone. This study showed a significant benefit of cerclage in reducing the preterm delivery rate and improving neonatal morbidity. Rust *et al.* (2005) randomly assigned 138 women whose cervical length was less than 25 mm between 16 and 24 weeks to cerclage or no cerclage and showed no benefit of cerclage. However, in this study there was a delay in the introduction of cerclage to allow the results of amniocentesis to be obtained and a higher incidence of placental abruption.

More recently To *et al.* (2004) randomized 255 women from a low-risk population whose cervical length was found to be 15 mm or less at a single ultrasound examination at 22–24 weeks to either cerclage or no cerclage and found that although strategy identified a group of women who were at high risk of early preterm birth, cervical cerclage did not reduce that risk. The screening event in this study was, however, relatively late in pregnancy. The study therefore inevitably excluded any women having a late second trimester pregnancy loss or very early preterm delivery and the failure of cervical cerclage to be beneficial may have been due to the fact that those women who had the potential to benefit from cerclage had already developed biochemical and mechanical changes in the lower pole of the uterus which made their preterm delivery inevitable.

If ultrasound indicated cervical cerclage is to be used the appropriate threshold has not yet been established. Groom *et al.* have shown that the presence of visible fetal membranes at the time of cervical cerclage is a strong prognostic indicator for the risk of preterm delivery. Visible fetal membranes are never seen at a cervical length greater than 15 mm. The threshold for cervical cerclage should therefore probably be greater than 15 mm which may also explain the lack of positive findings in the large study of To *et al*. Given the fact that the data on ultrasound indicated cervical cerclage is currently limited and variable in its conclusions further evaluation of this strategy is required before it is used widely in routine clinical practice.

Emergency 'rescue' cerclage

Rescue cervical cerclage may be performed when a woman is admitted with silent cervical dilatation and bulging of the membranes into the vagina but without the onset of uterine contractions. Characteristically such women present with slight vaginal bleeding, a watery vaginal discharge, or vague pelvic or vaginal pain. One small prospective-non-randomized study has suggested that rescue cervical cerclage improves birth weight and is not associated with a significant increase in the frequency of chorionamnionitis, maternal morbidity or perinatal mortality. The median pregnancy prolongation following emergency cervical cerclage is approximately 7 weeks. Whether antibiotics are beneficial in such cases has not been established.

Non-steroidal anti-inflammatory drugs

The central role for prostaglandins and inflammatory cytokines in the aetiology of preterm labour suggests that non-steroidal anti-inflammatory drugs (NSAIDs) may be beneficial in preventing preterm delivery. NSAIDs work largely by inhibition of the cyclo-oxygenase enzymes which catalyse the synthesis of prostaglandins. However, various NSAIDs also have other mechanisms of action including effects on intracellular signalling pathways and on transcription factors including NF-kappa B. There are two major isoforms at the cyclo-oxygenase enzyme termed COX-1 and COX-2. COX-1 is constitutively expressed in the majority of cells whereas COX-2 is inducible and catalyses the synthesis of prostaglandins at the sites of inflammation. COX-2 is the principle cyclo-oxygenase associated with the increased prostaglandin synthesis that occurs at the time of labour. NSAIDs may be divided into three classes. Those that are non-selective, those that are selective for COX-2 but still have some action against COX-1 and those that are specific for COX-2.

While there are several studies of the use of NSAIDs in the acute management of preterm labour, there are few good randomized trials of their use as prophylaxis. NSAIDs are associated with significant fetal side effects, in particular oligohydramnios and constriction of the ductus arteriosus. Oligohydramnios occurs in up to 30% of fetuses exposed to indomethacin. The effect is dose dependent and may occur with both short-term and long-term exposure. Discontinuation of therapy usually results in a rapid turn of normal fetal urine output and resolution of the oligohydramnios.

Constriction of the ductus arteriosus occurs in up to 50% of fetuses exposed to indomethacin at gestational ages greater than 32 weeks. There is a relationship between dose and duration of therapy and gestational age. Ductal constriction is seen less commonly below 32 weeks and rarely below 28 weeks. Long-term indomethacin therapy, particularly after 32 weeks is therefore associated with a significant risk of neonatal pulmonary hypertension.

It has been suggested that the use of NSAIDs which are selective or specific for COX-2 might be associated with a lower risk of fetal side effects. However, Nimesulide which is approximately 100-fold more effective in inhibition of COX-2 than COX-1 is nevertheless associated with an incidence of fetal oligohydramnios similar to that seen in fetuses exposed to indomethacin and there have been isolated case reports of fetal renal failure. Recently Groom *et al*. (2005) reported a study of the use of the COX-2 specific NSAID Rofecoxib used prophylactically in a cohort of women at high-risk of preterm delivery, although Rofecoxib was also associated with less effect on fetal renal function and the ductus arteriosus than is seen with indomethacin or Nimesulide. Unfortunately the risk of preterm delivery prior to 32 weeks was not reduced by Rofecoxib therapy and, once Rofecoxib was discontinued at 32 weeks, the rate of preterm delivery then increased in the Rofecoxib exposed patients. At the present time therefore there is no good evidence that NSAID confer benefit when used as prophylaxis for preterm labour. They are associated with a significant risk of potentially life-threatening side effects. If NSAIDs such as indomethacin are to be used, for example, as short-term therapies in association with cervical cerclage, then it is essential that there should be ultrasound surveillance of fetal urine production or amniotic fluid index and of the ductus arteriosus and that therapy should be stopped when fetal side effects become evident.

Progesterone

Progesterone is thought to inhibit the production of proinflammatory cytokines and prostaglandins within the uterus and to inhibit myometrial contractility. Although a meta-analysis by Kierse *et al*. in 1990 suggested that progesterone may be beneficial in reducing the risk of preterm delivery, it was not until the publication of two trials in 2003 that there was more widespread interest in the possibility that progesterone may be used as a prophylactic treatment in women at high risk of preterm delivery. In 2003, Da Fonseca *et al.* reported that women who were at high risk of preterm delivery and were randomized to receive a 100-mg vaginal suppository daily between 24 and 33 weeks had a lower rate of preterm delivery (13.8% at 37 weeks, 2.8% before 34 weeks) versus the placebo group (28% before 37 weeks, 18.6% before 34 weeks). In a similar study Mies *et al.* used weekly injections of 17 α hydroxyprogesterone capruate (250 mg) between 16 and 36 weeks which reduced the preterm delivery rate from 55 to 36% before 37 weeks and 19 to 11% before 32 weeks. In this study the neonates of mothers treated with progesterone also had lower rates of necrotizing enterocolitis, intraventricular haemorrhage and the need for supplemental oxygen. There are now a number of randomized controlled trials being conducted in various countries and, ideally, patients at high risk of preterm labour should be enrolled in one of these studies. However, the weight of both basic science and clinical evidence currently points towards progesterone being potentially beneficial in women at high risk of preterm delivery and there appear to be few, if any side effects.

Management of acute preterm labour

Diagnosis

There is little evidence to suggest that use of tocolytic drugs, intended to suppress uterine contractions, confers any real benefit in cases of preterm labour. There is, however, good evidence that the antenatal administration of corticosteroids, Olexa- or betamethazonem, to the mother and *in utero* transfer from a peripheral unit to a hospital with neonatal intensive care facilities significantly improves the outcome for the preterm neonate. It is therefore essential that a diagnosis of preterm labour should not be overlooked. It is usual to define the onset of labour at term as being when regular uterine contractions lead to cervical change or dilatation. To leave a woman with preterm contractions without either administering steroids or arranging an *in utero* transfer until there is cervical dilatation may be disadvantageous to the neonate. Preterm labour is therefore generally diagnosed solely on the basis of the presence of uncomfortable or painful regular uterine contractions. All of the placebo-controlled trials of tocolytic drugs show a very high placebo response rate. From these it can be concluded that of women who attract a diagnosis of preterm labour sufficient to lead to them being treated with tocolytic drugs, some 60% will remain undelivered after 48 h and close to 50% will deliver at term. Tocolytic drugs may be potentially harmful or expensive. Unnecessary *in utero* transfer consumes healthcare resources and there is growing concern about the possible long-term side effects of exposure of the fetus to high-dose corticosteroid therapy. It is therefore highly desirable that

obstetricians should have some form of test which can differentiate the woman genuinely in preterm labour from the woman with preterm contractions who will not go on to deliver preterm. Tests based upon the spectrum of electrical activity in the uterus currently are in development and are yielding encouraging results. At present, however, the two tests best able to differentiate true from false preterm labour are transvaginal measurement of cervical length and detection of fetal fibronectin in the vagina. In the United Kingdom the lack of availability of a transvaginal ultrasound machine on the Labour Ward and of an appropriately qualified or experienced clinician to perform the ultrasound together with the ready availability of bedside testing for fetal fibronectin means that fetal fibronectin testing is probably the optimal diagnostic test.

Fetal fibronectin testing

Fetal fibronectin is a glycoprotein present in amniotic fluid, placenta and the extra cellular substance of the decidua. Its synthesis and release is increased by the mechanical and inflammatory events which occur prior to the onset of labour. Fetal fibronectin may normally be detected in vaginal secretions up to 20 weeks gestation (at which time the amnion and chorion become fused) and is then normally undetectable until about 36 weeks gestation.

The presence of fibronectin in vaginal secretions between 20 and 36 weeks may be used to predict a risk of preterm labour. Fibronectin testing may be used to assess risk in asymptomatic women at high risk of preterm labour. However, it is in distinguishing 'true' from 'false' preterm labour in symptomatic women that fibronectin testing is probably of most value. While a positive fibronectin test in a symptomatic woman only predicts a risk of preterm delivery within the next 7 days for approximately 40%, a negative fetal fibronectin test reduces the risk to less than 1%. This is a level of risk at which it would be reasonable to withhold *in utero* transfer and treatment.

Acute tocolysis: sympathomimetics

The maximum benefit to the preterm neonate from antenatal corticosteroid administration is from 24 h to 7 days after the first dose of the course (Fig. 21.5). *In utero* transfer has also been shown to improve neonatal morbidity and mortality and clearly time would be required to move a mother in preterm labour from one hospital to another. Suppression of uterine contractions may therefore be an obvious solution to the problem of preterm labour. With the introduction of beta-sympethomitotics into obstetric practice in the 1970s accompanied by small clinical trials which suggested great efficacy in inhibiting preterm contractions, most obstetricians developed the impression that tocolysis with ritodrine or salbutamol was an effective therapy for acute preterm labour. This impression was strengthened because of the very high placebo response rate. More modern studies have shown that ritodrine will delay preterm delivery in a minority of patients for 24 and 48 h but that its use is not associated with any improvement of any marker of neonatal morbidity or in neonatal mortality rates. Ritodrine and salbutamol are associated with significant, potentially life-threatening maternal side effects (particularly if given in combination with corticosteroids) which include fluid overload, pulmonary oedema, myocardial ischaemia, hyperglycaemia and hypocalcaemia. Numerous maternal deaths have been reported in which tocolysis using sympathomimetic drugs has played a role. Sympathomimetic as tocolytics are now rarely used in the United Kingdom and, since safer, although not necessarily more effective tocolytic drugs are now available, their use should now be completely abandoned.

Non-steroidal anti-inflammatory drugs

The NSAID most widely studied as an acute tocolytic is indomethacin. Randomized placebo-controlled studies suggest that indomethacin may significantly delay preterm delivery for 24 and 48 h and for 7 days. However, the total number of women enrolled in all of the three randomized placebo-controlled trials is only 90. As discussed above, indomethacin has a major effect upon fetal renal function and upon the fetal cardiovascular system, in particular on the fetal ductus arteriosus. Use of indomethacin for tocolysis has also been associated with higher incidences of necrotizing enterocolitis, intraventricular haemorrhage and abnormalities in neonatal haemostasis. In experimental animals the combination of a COX-2 specific NSAID and a tocolytic (either a calcium channel blocker or an oxytocin antagonist) appears to be superior to the use of a tocolytic alone. However, this type of combination therapy has not yet been properly evaluated in the human. At present there is no evidence that indomethacin or any other NSAID has any advantage as a first line tocolytic over calcium channel blockers or oxytocin antagonists, each of which has a much better maternal and fetal side-effect profile.

Magnesium sulphate

Prior to the 1980s magnesium sulphate was widely used in the United States in the intrapartum management of pre-eclampsia and eclampsia and the clinical impression that magnesium sulphate made induction of labour more difficult led to its evaluation as a tocolytic agent. With the withdrawal of sympathomimetic drugs from the American market and the failure of atosiban, an oxytocin antagonist, to obtain FDA approval, there are no licensed tocolytic drugs available for the American obstetrician to use and magnesium sulphate is therefore in common use (Fig. 21.6). However, randomized placebo-controlled trials of magnesium sulphate show no significant short-term delay of delivery, increase in birthweight or difference in perinatal mortality when compared to placebo. Studies where magnesium has been compared to sympathomimetics have suggested equal efficacy. These two apparently contradictory findings can probably be explained by the lack of power of the studies to detect a significance difference between drugs with little or no efficacy but a high placebo response rate.

Oxytocin antagonists

Although there is no good evidence for an increase in circulating concentrations of oxytocin in either term or preterm labour, both term and preterm labour are associated with an increase in the expression of the oxytocin receptor in the myometrium and oxytocin is synthesized within the uterus itself, in both the myometrium and the decidua. This has led to the exploration of drugs which antagonize the oxytocin receptor as tocolytics. At the time of writing no specific oxytocin antagonist is available for clinical use. However atosiban, which is principally an Arginine vasopressin (AVP) receptor antagonists but also binds the oxytocin receptor at appropriate therapeutic concentrations, has a European licence for the treatment of preterm labour. Atosiban has been the subject of both placebo comparison trials and comparisons with sympathomimetic drugs. The placebo-controlled trials undertaken in the USA were, to a certain extent, flawed in that randomization at early gestational ages was skewed resulting in an increase in neonatal deaths among very preterm babies whose mothers were treated with atosiban. The primary outcome of the placebo-controlled trial (which was the time between the initiation of treatment and therapeutic failure defined as either preterm delivery or the need for an alternate tocolytic) showed that atosiban was no better than placebo. There were, however, statistically significant differences in the number of women who remained undelivered and did not require an alternative tocolytic at the specific 24 and 48 h and 7 day time points. As with all previous trials of tocolytic drugs, this trial was complicated by a very high placebo response rate. Analysis of the data shows that at, for example, 48 h, although 70% of women randomized to receive atosiban appeared to respond to it, in reality the majority of these represent placebo responses and that in fact only 11% had a genuine clinical response. This represents one quarter of those women who were

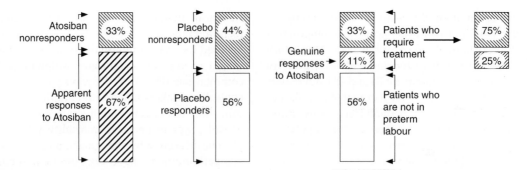

Fig. 21.4 Analysis of the 48 hours outcome data from the placebo controlled trial of atosiban (Romero et al, Am J Obstet Gynecol (2000) 182(5): 1173–83). Of all patients allocated to atosiban treatment only 11% showed a genuine clinical response, which represents one quarter of those with the potential to benefit.

genuinely in preterm labour and had a potential to have a genuine clinical response (Fig. 21.4).

Trials comparing atosiban with sympathomimetic drugs showed equal clinical efficacy to beta-sympathomimetics but with atosiban having a dramatically improved maternal side-effect profile. The clinical response rate to either atosiban or sympathomimetic drugs in those trials was, however, so high (over 90%) that it is probable that the majority of patients enrolled in the study were not genuinely in preterm labour. Neither the placebo-controlled trial nor the sympathomimetic comparison trials demonstrated any improvement in any aspect of neonatal morbidity or in neonatal mortality associated with the use of atosiban.

Calcium channel blockers

The central role of calcium in the biochemistry of myometrial contractions led to the exploration of the use of calcium channel blockers, specifically nifedipine, as a tocolytic drug. Because there has been no interest from the pharmaceutical industry in promoting nifedipine for this indication, there have only been small, locally funded comparison trials of nifedipine versus sympathomimetics. There are no placebo-controlled trials of nifedipine as a tocolytic. Meta-analysis of the sympathomimetic comparison trials suggest that nifedipine may be superior in its ability to delay delivery and is associated with a reduction in the rate of respiratory distress syndrome and intraventricular haemorrhage in preterm neonates, although not with any improvement in perinatal mortality. It is unlikely that there will ever be any large-scale placebo-controlled trials of nifedipine or any large trials comparing nifedipine with atosiban. There has been one study which indirectly compared atosiban with nifedipine by taking advantage of the fact that each had been compared with sympathomimetic drugs. This study suggested that nifedipine is superior to atosiban in delaying delivery and, unlike

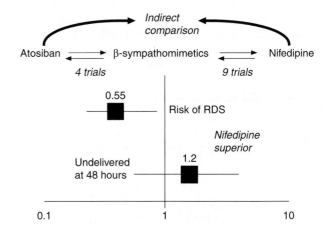

Fig. 21.5 Indirect comparison for Atbosiban with Nifedipine in the acute management of preterm labour. Adapted from Coomarasamy A et al. BJOG. 2003 110(12): 1045–9.

atosiban, is associated with a reduction in the risk of respiratory distress syndrome (Fig. 21.5).

At the present time the obstetrician has a choice between atosiban and nifedipine and it is probably reasonable, in our current state of knowledge, not to use tocolytic therapy at all. More specific oxytocin antagonists are in development, as are drugs which target other receptors, such as prostaglandin receptors. It is probable that the disappointing results of tocolytics in trials to date may be because of poor trial design and, in particular, the high placebo response rates. In future trials which are able to target tocolytic drugs more specifically at women genuinely in preterm labour, for example, by taking advantage of fetal fibronectin testing, may more properly define the potential value of tocolytic therapy.

Corticosteroid therapy

The potential for antenatally administered corticosteroids to accelerate lung maturity was discovered by Liggens

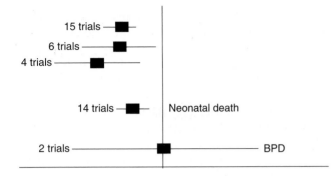

Fig. 21.6 Meta-analysis of the effect of antenatal corticosteroid administration upon neonatal outcomes, Adapted from Roberts D and Dalziel S. Cochrane Database Syst Rev. 2006 CD004454.

by experiments in which preterm labour was induced in sheep by injection of corticosteroids (Fig. 21.6). A large number of randomized trials took place during the 1970s and 1980s which, taken together, have shown that a single course of either betamethasone or dexamethasone administered to pregnant women between 24 and 34 weeks gestation up to 7 days before preterm delivery has a significant effect upon neonatal morbidity and mortality. Although the paediatric use of surfactant has had a major impact upon the incidence and consequence of respiratory distress syndrome, nevertheless antenatal corticosteroid therapy is still associated with a reduction in neonatal mortality principally due to a significant reduction in RDS and intraventricular haemorrhage rates. Antenatal corticosteroids have a receptor mediator effect on all of the components of the surfactant system in type-2 pneumocytes. They also, however, have effects on structural development of the lungs and lead to accelerated maturation of the fetal intestine and have effects upon the myocardium and on catecholamine responsiveness which may explain the reduced incidences of necrotizing entocolitis and intraventricular haemorrhage seen in extremely preterm infants that appear to be independent of the effect upon RDS.

The dramatic effects of a single course of corticosteroids unfortunately led in the past to the routine prescription of multiple courses of steroids, often at weekly intervals, in women deemed to be at risk of preterm delivery, especially those with multiple pregnancies. Recent concern about the long-term consequences of recurrent exposure to high dose steroids suggesting adverse effects on development and behaviour has generally led to an abandonment of this policy. Both dexamethasone and betamethasone have been explored in randomized trials with each having similar effects on RDS rates. Studies in France suggested that betamethasone reduced the incidence of periventricular leukomalacia whereas dexamethasone had no such protective effect. However this may be explained by the presence of sulphating agents used as preservatives in French preparations of dexamethasone. It is probably the case that either steroid will be suitable, provided that the preparation is non-sulphated.

Antibiotics

Meta-analysis of the use of antibiotics in symptomatic preterm labour is dominated by the ORACLE trials. These show that administration of antibiotics to the mother do not delay delivery or improve any aspect of neonatal morbidity or mortality. The only positive health benefit is a reduction in maternal infection rates.

Conduct of preterm delivery

Rates of neonatal morbidity and mortality are higher in babies transferred *ex utero* to neonatal intensive care units when compared to those born in the tertiary referral centre. Every effort should therefore be made to transfer a woman to an obstetric unit linked to a neonatal intensive care unit prior to a preterm delivery. The introduction of fetal fibronectin testing may reduce the numbers of unnecessary *in utero* transfers which currently take place. Except at the extremes of prematurity there should be continuous electronic fetal heart rate monitoring once preterm labour is clearly established. There is no evidence for a benefit of routine delivery by Caesarean section where the presentation is cephalic. However, hypoxia is a major risk factor for the development of periventricular leukomalacia and there should therefore be a relatively low threshold for delivery by Caesarean section in the presence of abnormal fetal heart rate patterns. The preterm delivery of a breech continues to be an obstetric dilemma. Although it is now established that elective Caesarean section is preferable for the term breech, it has proved impossible to undertake randomized trials of Caesarean section for the preterm breech. One potential disadvantage of planning to deliver the preterm breech (or indeed the cephalic presentation preterm) by 'elective' Caesarean section is the high incidence of 'threatened' preterm labour which does not lead to preterm delivery. An aggressive policy of delivering preterm babies by Caesarean section has the potential to lead to iatrogenic preterm deliveries. At the other end of the spectrum, Caesarean section preterm where the breech is already in the vagina, may be more traumatic than a vaginal delivery. At the present time, until further evidence becomes available, the mode of delivery of the preterm breech will need to be made on a case by case basis by the obstetrician at the time. There is no evidence for the old practice of elective forceps delivery to protect the fetal head during preterm delivery and episiotomy is rarely required.

Preterm prelabour rupture of membranes

Preterm prelabour rupture of membranes (PPROM) occurs in approximately 2% of all pregnancies and accounts for up to one third of preterm deliveries. The most frequent consequence of PPROM is preterm delivery with some 50% cases delivering within a week, 75% within 2 weeks and 85% within a month. There appears to be an inverse relationship between gestational age and latency with a shorter interval between membrane rupture and preterm labour at later gestational ages. As with preterm labour, postnatal survival following PPROM is directly related to gestational age at delivery and birthweight. However, there is the additional complication that where PPROM occurs prior to 23 weeks gestation there may be neonatal pulmonary hyperplasia leading to an increased risk of neonatal death, even if delivery occurs at gestational ages at which the outcome would usually be good. The risk of pulmonary hyperplasia following PPROM is approximately 50% at 19 weeks falling to about 10% at 25 weeks. The retention of amniotic fluid within the uterus is associated with better outcome. A pool of amniotic fluid greater than 2 cm is associated with a low incidence of pulmonary hypoplasia.

Once PPROM has been confirmed, through history, identification of the pool of liquor in the vagina and of oligohydramnios on ultrasonography, the management is a balance between the risks of prematurity if delivery is encouraged versus the risks of maternal and fetal infection if there is conservative management. The ORACLE study showed that the use of erythromycin improves neonatal morbidity and is associated with a longer latency period while coamoxiclav increased the risk of necrotizing enterocolitis and should therefore be avoided. Management of PPROM continues to be controversial. However, many obstetricians will institute conservative management in preterm premature rupture of membranes before 34 weeks and would induce labour relatively early in women whose membrane rupture occurs subsequent to 37 weeks. There is currently no good evidence as to what ideal management should be between 34 and 37 weeks.

Conservative management should include clinical surveillance for signs of chorionamnionitis including regular recording of maternal temperature and heart rate and cardiotocography. A rising white cell count or a rising C-reactive protein (CRP) level may indicate the development of chorionamnionitis. Neither of these are highly specific, however, and many cases of histologically proven chorionamnionitis are associated with normal white cell counts and CRP concentrations. Lower genital tract swabs are routinely taken in women with PPROM. Positive cultures for potential pathogens do not correlate well with the risk of chorionamnionitis. However, they are useful in determining the causative organisms once chorionamnionitis develops and in directing antibiotic therapy for both the mother and the preterm neonate.

Experiments have been performed in which amnioinfusion has been used in PPROM in an attempt to reduce the risk of pulmonary hyperplasia and/or orthopaedic abnormalities. Unfortunately the literature contains only a few case reports. In the majority of cases it is likely that fluid infused into the amniotic cavity will simply leak out. If it is retained then it is probable that the amniotic fluid would reaccumulate in any case because of fetal urine production. The onset of regular contractions and the establishment of preterm labour in cases of PPROM may be the first evidence of chorionaminonitis. The potential benefits of tocolytic drugs do not apply in the majority of cases of PPROM since there is usually time for administration of corticosteroids and *in utero* transfer before the onset of preterm labour itself. The few studies of the use of tocolysis in pregnancies complicated by PPROM show no improvement in perinatal outcome and suggest that long-term tocolysis may be associated with an increase in the risk of maternal and fetal infection.

References

1. Astle S, Slater DM & Thornton S (2003) The involvement of progesterone in the onset of human labour. *Eur J Obstet Gynecol Reprod Biol* **108**(2), 177–81. Review.
2. Blanks AM & Thornton S (2003) The role of oxytocin in parturition. *Br J Obstet Gynaecol* **110**(Suppl 20), 46–51. Review.
3. Challis JR & Lye S (2000) Endocrine and paracrine regulation of birth at term and preterm. *Endocr Rev* **21**(5), 514–50. Review.
4. Challis JR, Lye SJ, Gibb W, Whittle W, Patel F & Alfaidy N (2001) Understanding preterm labor. *Ann N Y Acad Sci* **943**, 225–34. Review.
5. Critchley H, Bennett PR & Thornton S (2004) *Preterm Birth*. London: RCOG Press.
6. Crowley P (2003) Antenatal corticosteroids-current thinking. *Br J Obstet Gynaecol* **110**(Suppl 20), 77–8.
7. Honest H, Bachmann LM, Coomarasamy A, Gupta JK, Kleijnen J & Khan KS (2002) Accuracy of cervical transvaginal sonography in predicting preterm birth: a systematic review. *Ultrasound Obstet Gynecol* **22**(3), 305–22. Review.
8. Honest H, Bachmann LM, Gupta JK, Kleijnen J & Khan KS (2002) Accuracy of cervicovaginal fetal fibronectin test in predicting risk of spontaneous preterm birth: systematic review. *Br Med J* **325**(7359), 301. Review.
9. Kenyon S, Boulvain M & Neilson J (2003) Antibiotics for preterm rupture of membranes. *Cochrane Database Syst Rev* **2**, CD001058. Review.
10. King J & Flenady V (2002) Prophylactic antibiotics for inhibiting preterm labour with intact membranes. *Cochrane Database Syst Rev* **4**, CD000246. Review.

11. McDonald H, Brocklehurst P & Parsons J (2005) Antibiotics for treating bacterial vaginosis in pregnancy. *Cochrane Database Syst Rev* **25**(1), CD000262.

12. Mendelson CR & Condon JC (2005) New insights into the molecular endocrinology of parturition. *J Steroid Biochem Mol Biol* **93**(2–5), 113–9.

13. Terzidou V & Bennett PR (2002) Preterm labour. *Curr Opin Obstet Gynecol* **14**(2), 105–13. Review.

14. To MS, Alfirevic Z, Heath V, Cicero S, Cacho A, Williamson PR & Nicolaides KH (2004) Cervical cerclage for the prevention of preterm delivery in women with short cervix—randomized controlled trial. *Lancet* **363**, 1849–53.

15. Rust OA, Roberts WE (2005) Does cerclage prevent preterm birth. Obstet Gynecol Clin North Am **32**, 441–56.

16. Groom KM, Shennan AH, Bennett PR (2002) Ultrasound indicated cervical cerclage: outcomes depend on preoperative cervical length and presence of visible membranes at time of cerclage. *Am J Obstet Gynecol* **187**, 445–9.

17. Wood NS, Costeloe K, Gibson AT, Hennessy EM, Marlow N, Wilkinson AR, EPI, Cure Study Group (2005) The EPICure study: associations and antecedents of neurological and developmental disability at 30 months of age following extremely preterm birth. *Arch Dis Child Fetal Neonatal Ed* **90**(2), F134–40.

Further reading

Costeloe K, Hennessy E, Gibson AT, Marlow N & Wilkinson AR (2000) The EPICure study: outcomes to discharge from hospital for infants born at the threshold of viability. *Pediatrics* **106**(4), 659–71.

Romero R, Mazor M, Munoz H, Gomez R, Galasso M & Sherer DM (1994) The preterm labor syndrome. *Ann N Y Acad Sci* **734**, 414–29. Review.

Chapter 22: Prolonged pregnancy

Patricia Crowley

Pregnancies of 294 days duration or more are defined as 'prolonged', 'post-dates', or 'post-term' [1]. Prolonged pregnancy is associated with an increase in perinatal mortality and morbidity in pregnancies which appear to be otherwise low risk. This chapter will show that many of the perinatal risks previously attributed to prolonged pregnancy increase in a continuous rather than a 'threshold' manner. Discussions about issues relating to prolonged pregnancy and interventions to prevent it often take place at 41 weeks' gestation. To cater for these clinical and epidemiological realities, the scope of this chapter has been expanded beyond the strict definition of prolonged pregnancy.

Epidemiology of prolonged pregnancy

An accurate estimation of the 'natural' incidence of prolonged pregnancy would require meticulous early pregnancy dating, universal follow-up of all pregnancies and an absence of obstetric intervention.

The 14% prolonged pregnancy rate quoted for the Hawaiian island Kauai [2] may be regarded as informative because of low rates of obstetric intervention and full follow-up, but lacks correction for dates errors. Boyce *et al.* [3] showed that reliance on menstrual dates gave an incidence of prolonged pregnancy of 10.7%, whereas the use of basal body temperature charts gave a much lower rate of 4.7%. In Britain, the fall in incidence of prolonged pregnancy from 11.5% in 1958 [4] to 4.4% in 1970 [5] illustrates the effect of the rise in rates of induction of labour from 13 to 26% over the same period.

Smith [6] studied 1514 healthy pregnant women in whom the discrepancy between the menstrual dates and those based on first trimester crown–rump length (CRL) was less than −1 to +1 days. The duration of pregnancy was estimated, using time-to-event analysis; non-elective delivery was taken to be the event while elective delivery was taken to be censoring. The median time to non-elective delivery was 283 days from the last menstrual period. The life-table graph published in this study gives an incidence of prolonged pregnancy of about 6%.

The use of ultrasound to establish gestational age lowers the incidence of prolonged pregnancy. Eik-Nes *et al.* [7] showed that adjustment of dates following measurement of the biparietal diameter at 17 weeks' gestation led to an incidence of prolonged pregnancy to 3.9%. Subsequently, several randomized trials of routine versus selective second trimester ultrasound have shown that routine second trimester biometry reduces the number of pregnancies that are classified as prolonged [8]. Bukowski *et al.* [9] studied 3588 women undergoing first trimester ultrasound as part of the multicentre First and Second Trimester Evaluation for Aneuploidy Trial (The FASTER Trial). Gestational age determination using the CRL as opposed to last menstrual period (LMP) reduced the apparent incidence of pregnancies greater than 41 weeks' gestation from 22.1 to 8.2%, $P < 0.001$).

An analysis of 171,527 births in residents of the Northeast Thames in 1989–1991 gave an incidence of 6.2% for prolonged pregnancy [10].

Prolonged pregnancy is increased in first pregnancies, but is not related to maternal age and the median duration of pregnancy is 2 days longer in nulliparae compared with multiparae. Women with a body mass index of greater than 30 are at increased risk of prolonged pregnancy (odds ratio 1.4 (1.2–1.7)).

Aetiology of prolonged pregnancy

It is likely that the majority of prolonged pregnancies represent the upper range of a normal distribution. The effects of anencephaly and of placental sulphatase deficiency on the duration are interesting examples of extreme post-term pregnancy but are unhelpful in elucidating the aetiology of the majority of cases of prolonged pregnancy.

There may be a genetic factor regulating the onset of labour. Prolonged pregnancy tends to repeat itself. Analysis of data from the Norwegian Birth Registry showed that a woman delivering post-term in her first pregnancy had a relative risk of a second post-term pregnancy of 2.2 and a woman with two post-term pregnancies had a 3.2-fold relative risk of a third post-term pregnancy [11]. Swedish

Medical Birth Registry data confirm these results and also indicate a tendency for daughters of mothers who deliver post-term to have prolonged pregnancies [12] but overall these factors account for only a small proportion of the overall population attributable risk for post-term pregnancy. Male fetuses may be associated with a higher risk of prolonged pregnancy.

Low vaginal levels of fetal fibronectin at 39 weeks are predictive of an increased likelihood of post-term pregnancy [13]. Ramanathan *et al.* [14] showed how transvaginal measurement of cervical length at 37 weeks predicts both prolonged pregnancy and failed induction. These observations suggest that a defect or delay in the remodelling of the cervix that takes place prior to successful initiation of labour, may cause prolonged pregnancy and may also be associated with some of the apparent increase in dystocia associated with prolonged pregnancy.

Prolonged pregnancy could result from variations in the corticotrophin releasing hormone (CRH) system during pregnancy, such as an alteration in the number or expression of myometrial receptor subtypes, altered signal-transduction mechanisms or increase in the capacity of CRH binding hormone protein to bind and inactivate CRH. Prospective, longitudinal studies have shown that women destined to deliver preterm tend to have a more rapid exponential rise in CRH in mid-pregnancy while women who go on to deliver post-term babies have a slower rate of rise [15]. Efforts currently directed towards researching the initiation of labour preterm may lead to greater understanding of the aetiology of post-term pregnancy.

Risks associated with prolonged pregnancy

Perinatal mortality

Tables 22.1 and 22.2 summarize some of the epidemiological studies that attempt to compare perinatal mortality rates of babies delivered at 42 weeks or over with those delivered between 37 weeks and 41 weeks and 6 days.

The methodological problems are considerable. There may be errors or biases in recording of information relating to gestational age. Women with uncertain dates have been repeatedly shown to be at increased risk of perinatal mortality [16,17]. Their inclusion may inflate the apparent perinatal risks of prolonged pregnancy. Older studies of perinatal outcome in post-term pregnancy showed that about 25% of the excess mortality risk in post-term pregnancy relates to congenital malformations [18]. Of the studies quoted in Tables 22.1 and 22.2 only that by Smith [19] specifies that cases of lethal congenital malformation have been excluded from the analysis. Hilder *et al.* [20] re-analysed the data presented in their 1998 [10] study after correcting for congenital malformation, showing that the outcomes presented were not biased by fetuses with congenital malformation being preferentially represented among post-term pregnancies. Another potential bias is the interval between intrauterine death and delivery. A fetus that dies in utero at 41 weeks and is delivered at 42 weeks will be counted as a perinatal death at 42 weeks' gestation.

Yudkin *et al.* [21] questioned the validity of using perinatal mortality rates as a means of relating outcome to gestational age, arguing that the population at risk of intrauterine fetal death at a given gestational age is the population of fetuses *in utero* at that gestational week and not those delivered at that week. However, the population at risk of intrapartum and neonatal complications such as cord prolapse or meconium aspiration syndrome is clearly the population of babies delivered at that week of pregnancy [19]. These issues are clearly explained by Smith [19], who related the perinatal risks at each gestational week to the appropriate denominators. Antepartum deaths were related to the number of ongoing pregnancies, intrapartum deaths to all births at that gestational age, excluding antepartum stillbirths and neonatal deaths were related to the number of live births. Yudkin *et al.* [21] expressed the prospective risk of stillbirth for the next fortnight of the pregnancy; Hilder *et al.* [10] expressed the risk as a rate over the next week; Cotzias *et al.* [22] generated considerable controversy [20,23], by expressing the risk of

Table 22.1 Perinatal mortality rates term versus post-term pregnancies

Authors	Source	Outcome	37–41 [86]	42 Weeks and over
Campbell *et al.* [25]	444,241 births Norway 1978–87	Relative risk of perinatal death	1	1.30 (1.13–1.50)
Fabre *et al.* [86]	547,923 births Spain 1980–92	Stillbirth rate	3.3	3.6
		Early neonatal mortality rate	1.7	2.8
		Perinatal mortality rate	4.9	6.4
Olesen *et al.* [87]	78,033 prolonged pregnancies	Adjusted odds ratio – stillbirth	1	1.24 (0.93–1.66)
	Danish birth register 1978–93	Adjusted odds ratio – neonatal death	1	1.60 (1.07–2.37)
	5% sample of deliveries at term	Adjusted odds ratio – perinatal death	1	1.36 (1.08–1.72)

Table 22.2 Perinatal outcomes by week of gestation, 37–43 weeks

Author	Source	Outcome	38–39	39–40	40–41	41–42	42–43	43 and more
Bakketeig & Bergsjo [11]	157,577 births Sweden 1977–78	Perinatal mortality rate	7.2	3.1	2.3	2.4	3	4
Ingemarsson & Kallen [24]	914,702 births Sweden 1982–91	Stillbirth rate in nulliparae	2.72	1.53	1.23	1.86	2.26	
		Neonatal mortality rate nulliparae	0.62	0.54	0.54	0.9	1.03	
		Stillbirth rate in multiparae	2.1	1.42	1.35	1.4	1.51	
		Neonatal mortality rate multiparae	0.55	0.45	0.53	0.5	0.86	
Divon *et al.* [88]	181,524 singleton pregnancies. Reliable dates, 40 weeks or more Sweden 1987–92	Odds ratio for fetal death			1	1.5	1.8	2.9
Hilder *et al.* [10]	171,527 births London 1989–91	Stillbirth rate	3.8	2.2	1.5	1.7	1.9	2.1
		Infant mortality rate	4.7	3.2	2.7	2	4.1	3.7
		Stillbirth rate per 1000 OP*	0.56	0.57	0.86	1.27	1.55	2.12
		Infant mortality rate per 1000 OP	0.7	0.83	1.57	1.48	3.29	3.71
Caughey & Musci [89]	Hospital based California 1992–2002 45 673 births after 37 weeks	fetal death rate per 1000 OP	0.36	0.4	0.26	0.92	3.47	
Smith [19]	700, 878 births in Scotland 1985–96	Cumulative probability of antepartum Stillbirth	0.0008	0.0013	0.0022	0.0034	0.0053	0.0115
	Multiple births and congenital anomalies excluded	Estimated probability of intrapartum & neonatal death	0.0006	0.0005	0.0006	0.0006	0.0006	0.0008

* Ongoing pregnancies

prospective stillbirth for the remainder of the pregnancy. This is a counter-intuitive concept for most obstetricians, whereas many find the concept of the prospective risk of stillbirth over the coming week an accessible concept, particularly in pregnancies of 40–42 weeks' gestation. ('If this woman remains undelivered in the next seven days, what is the chance of a fetal death occurring *in utero*?').

The outcomes presented in Table 22.1 compare pregnancies fulfilling the epidemiological definition of prolonged pregnancy with those delivered at 'term'. In modern obstetric practice, women with epidemiological and obstetric risk factors are more likely to be delivered before 42 weeks. Women with twin pregnancies, pre-eclampsia, diagnosed intrauterine growth restriction, antepartum haemorrhage, previous perinatal death are likely to be over-represented in the 37–41 week population

and under-represented among those delivered at 42 weeks and later.

Table 22.2 addresses the argument that the duration of pregnancy is a continuum and that perinatal risks are unlikely to alter abruptly on day 294 of a pregnancy. Outcomes are presented by week of gestational age from 37 weeks up to and including 43 weeks' gestation. Outcome statistics are presented in a variety of forms as discussed above.

Both tables show that prolonged pregnancy is associated with an increased risk of perinatal death. However, there is no consistency between studies as to the timing of that increased risk from fetal death before labour, to antepartum death to early neonatal death or even infant mortality. The studies summarized in Table 22.1 suggest that an increased risk of neonatal death is the main source of the increased perinatal risk. However, Table 22.2 shows that when pregnancies ending at 42 weeks are compared with those delivered at 41 weeks, every adverse outcome is increased with the exception of the 'estimated probability of intrapartum and neonatal death' from the Smith study [19]. When pregnancies ending at 41 weeks are compared with those ending at 40 weeks, this outcome is again unchanged, as is the neonatal mortality rate in multiparae in the Ingemarsson and Kallen [24] series and the infant mortality rate in the Hilder [10] series. All other outcomes deteriorate from 40 weeks to 41 weeks and again from 41 weeks to 42 weeks.

Effect of parity and birthweight

The series presented by Ingemarsson and Kallen [24] shows that the increasing risks of adverse outcome associated with advancing gestation age are more marked in nulliparae than in multiparae (Table 22.2). In an analysis of 181,524 singleton pregnancies with reliable dates delivered at 40 weeks or later in Sweden between 1 January 1987 and 31 December 1992, birthweight of 2 standard deviations or more below the mean for gestational age was associated with a significantly increased odds ratios for both fetal (odds ratios ranging from 7.1 to 10.0) and neonatal death (odds ratios from 3.4 to 9.4) [24]. The Norwegian cohort reported by Campbell *et al.* [25] also showed that small-for-gestational age babies were more vulnerable to the risks of prolonged pregnancy. In their series, babies weighing less than the 10th centile had a 5.68 (95% CI 4.37–7.38) relative risk of perinatal death at 42 weeks' gestation or later compared with babies between the 10th and 90th centile at the same gestational age. In this series, birthweight above the 90th centile was associated with the lowest relative risk of perinatal death (0.51; 95% CI 0.26–1.0).

Prolonged pregnancy and home birth

There is a lack of good quality epidemiological evidence on the outcome of post-term pregnancy when delivery occurs at home. Bastian *et al.* [26] used multiple methods of case identification and follow-up to assemble a population-based cohort of 7002 home births in Australia. Fifty perinatal deaths occurred, giving a perinatal mortality rate of 7.1 per 1000. Seven of 44 (15%) of perinatal deaths in women with a known gestational age occurred in women who were 42 weeks pregnant or more. A study conducted among Native Americans, examining an increase in perinatal mortality in home births attended by midwives compared with those attended by doctors identified post-dates pregnancies, breech deliveries and twins as the

source of the difference in mortality rates between the two groups [27].

Perinatal morbidity

Epidemiological studies identify birth after 41 weeks or after 42 weeks as a risk factor for a variety of adverse neonatal outcomes. Caughey *et al.* [28] conducted a retrospective, cohort study of all low-risk, term, cephalic, and singleton births that were delivered at the University of California, San Francisco, between 1976 and 2001. The incidence of adverse neonatal mortality outcomes at 40, 41 and 42 weeks' gestation was examined in a multivariate analysis and compared with the rates in pregnancies that were delivered at 39 weeks of gestation, after controlling for maternal demographics, length of labour, induction, mode of delivery, and birth weight (except macrosomia). Compared with the outcome at 39 weeks' gestation, the relative risk of meconium aspiration increased significantly from 2.18 at 40 weeks to 3.35 at 41 weeks and 4.09 (95% CI 2.07–8.08) at 42 weeks. A composite outcome of 'severe neonatal complications' including skull fracture and brachial plexus injuries, neonatal seizures, intracranial haemorrhage, neonatal sepsis, meconium aspiration syndrome, and respiratory distress syndrome, increased from a relative risk of 1.47 at 40 weeks to 2.04 at 41 weeks to 2.37 (95% CI 1.63–3.49) at 42 weeks.

A strong association between neonatal seizures and delivery at 41 weeks' gestation or more has been identified in previous case control studies. Minchom *et al.* [29] found that delivery after 41 weeks' gestation was associated with an odds ratio of 2.7 (95% CI 1.6–4.8). Curtis *et al.* [30] studied 89 babies with early neonatal seizures delivered after 42 weeks' gestation in Dublin. Twenty-seven were delivered after 42 weeks' gestation compared with 6 of 89 controls (odds ratio 4.73; 95% CI 2.22–10.05).

Cerebral palsy

Neonatal encephalopathy may be followed by the development of cerebral palsy, while other cases of cerebral palsy may occur following a clinically normal neonatal period. It is accepted that the presence of neonatal encephalopathy indicates that a neurological insult has taken place during labour or the early neonatal period, while its absence is thought to indicate an insult at some earlier time in pregnancy [31]. Gaffney *et al.* [32] examined the obstetric background of 141 children from the Oxford Cerebral Palsy Register. Forty-one children whose cerebral palsy was preceded by neonatal encephalopathy were compared with 100 who had not suffered from neonatal encephalopathy. The babies with neonatal encephalopathy were more likely to have been delivered at 42 weeks' gestation or more (odds ratio 3.5; 95% CI 1–12.1). Babies born at 42 weeks or more to nulliparous women were at particular risk of this sequence of events (odds ratio 11.0; 95% CI 1.2–102.5).

Other complications of labour

Dystocia, shoulder dystocia and obstetric trauma are all increased in post-term pregnancy [25]. Here, the risks increase with increasing fetal weight, but gestational age remains a risk factor independent of birthweight. In a case-matched study of 285 women with uncomplicated singleton post-term pregnancy and spontaneous onset of labour and 855 women with uncomplicated singleton term pregnancy, Luckas *et al.* [33] showed that Caesarean section was significantly more common in women with post-term pregnancy (relative risk = 1.90, 95% CI = 1.29–2.85). The increase was equally distributed between Caesarean sections performed for failure to progress in labour (RR = 0.74, 95% CI = 1.02–3.04) and fetal distress (RR = 2.00, 95% CI = 1.14–3.61). This finding is consistent with the hypothesis that some cases of prolonged pregnancy are associated with a defect in the physiology of labour, in addition to any increase in risk of fetal hypoxia. However, the possibility of bias in management arising out of the knowledge that a pregnancy is post-term cannot be excluded as a factor in the increase in Caesarean section rates.

Antenatal tests in prolonged pregnancies

The evidence of increased perinatal mortality and morbidity in prolonged pregnancy compared with delivery at 39 or 40 weeks' gestation inevitably leads to the conclusion that some cases of prolonged pregnancy should be prevented by earlier delivery. It would seem logical to use screening tests to identify pregnancies that are destined to have an adverse outcome and to intervene selectively in these pregnancies.

The ideal test of fetal well-being in prolonged pregnancy would allow identification of all fetuses at risk of adverse outcome, at a stage where delivery would result in a universally good outcome. Pregnancies testing 'negative' in this test would be safe *in utero* for an interval of a few days until either delivery or a repeat test occurred and would eventually deliver with a good outcome. At present, no method of monitoring post-term pregnancy is backed up by strong evidence of effectiveness. There is some observational evidence that some pregnancies at risk of adverse outcome can be identified, but less evidence that prediction of the adverse outcome confers prevention.

Ultrasound assessment of amniotic fluid

Ultrasound monitoring of amniotic fluid volume was first described in 1980 when a subjective classification of 'normal', 'reduced' or 'absent' amniotic fluid was described, based on the presence or absence of echo-free space between the fetal limbs and the fetal trunk or the uterine wall [34]. To test the value of the classification, 150 patients with pregnancies of 42 weeks or more duration underwent ultrasound examination in the 48 h prior to delivery. The patients classified as having 'reduced' or 'absent' amniotic fluid had a statistically significant excess incidence of meconium stained liquor, fetal acidosis, and birth asphyxia and meconium aspiration. Manning *et al.* [35] described a semiquantitative method based on the largest vertical pool of amniotic fluid and used a 1-cm pool depth as the cut-off for intervention in a population of babies with suspected growth retardation. This was subsequently modified to 2 cm to improve detection of the growth retarded infant [36]. Crowley *et al.* [37] found an increase in adverse outcomes in post-term pregnancies where the maximum pool depth was less than 3 cm. Fischer *et al.* [38] found that a maximum vertical pool of less than 2.7 cm was the best predictor of abnormal perinatal outcome.

Phelan [39] described the 'amniotic fluid index', which is the sum of the maximum pool depth in four quadrants. Fischer *et al.* [38] found that maximum pool depth performed better than amniotic index in predicting adverse outcomes in post-term pregnancies. Alfirevic [40] randomly allocated women with post-term pregnancy to monitoring using either maximum pool depth or amniotic fluid index (AFI). Both groups underwent computerized fetal heart rate monitoring every 3 days in addition to amniotic fluid measurements. The threshold for intervention was a maximum pool depth of less than 1.8 cm or an AFI of less than 7.3 cm. These figures had been identified as the 3rd centiles for the local population. The number of women found to have an abnormal AFI was significantly higher than the number found to have an abnormal maximum pool depth and more women underwent induction of labour in the AFI arm of the trial. There were no perinatal deaths and no statistically significant differences in perinatal outcome between the two groups.

Morris *et al.* [41] performed an observational study of 1584 pregnant women at or beyond 40 weeks' gestation in Oxford. Women underwent measurement of amniotic fluid, using both the single deepest pool and AFI. The results of these ultrasound measurements were concealed from caregivers. These authors agreed with Alfirevic *et al.* [40] that more women 'test positive' using AFI with single deepest pool. One hundred and twenty-five women (7.9%) had an AFI of less than 5 cm in contrast to 22 women (1.4%)

who had single deepest pool less than 2 cm. There were no perinatal deaths. There were seven cases of severe perinatal morbidity – an incidence of 0.44%. Two of these had an AFI of <5 cm and four had an AFI of less than 6 cm. None of the seven cases had a deepest pool measurement of less than 2 cm.

Locatelli *et al.* [42] conducted a similar study, but measured AFI twice weekly from 40 weeks until delivery. A composite adverse outcome of fetal death, 5 min Apgar <7, umbilical artery pH of <7, Caesarean section for fetal distress, occurred in 19.8% of those with an AFI of <5 compared with 10.7% of those with an AFI of >5 ($P = 0.001$).

These studies of amniotic fluid after 40 weeks suggest some association between reduction in volume and adverse outcome, but overall it performs with a poor sensitivity and specificity. There is no evidence to suggest that it can be relied on as a means of monitoring pregnancies after 41 weeks' gestation. In a meta-analysis of studies on the relationship of amniotic fluid with adverse fetal outcome, Chauhan *et al.* [43] concluded that there was some association between oligohydramnios and an increased risk of Caesarean section for non-reassuring fetal heart rate patterns and low Apgar scores; however, the data relating to neonatal acidosis were insufficient. The decline in confidence in ultrasound assessment of amniotic fluid volume is compounded by studies which show a poor correlation between ultrasound AFI and actual amniotic fluid volumes measured by dye dilution studies [44,45].

Biophysical profile

Observational studies indicate that low biophysical scores identify babies at higher risk of adverse outcome [46]. However, evidence of ability to predict adverse outcome must not be interpreted as proof of the ability to prevent these outcomes.

A systematic review of four trials, comparing biophysical profile scoring (BPS) with other forms of antepartum fetal monitoring, yields insufficient data to show that the biophysical profile is better than any other form of fetal monitoring [47]. Only one of these randomized controlled trials deals specifically with prolonged pregnancy [40]. This trial compares monitoring of prolonged pregnancy using a modified biophysical profile score (consisting of computerized cardiotocography, AFI and the rest of the components of the conventional biophysical profile) with simple monitoring using cardiotocography and measurement of amniotic fluid depth [40]. The more complex method of monitoring post-term pregnancy is more likely to yield an abnormal result, but does not improve pregnancy outcome as evidenced by umbilical cord pH.

An observational study of biophysical profile scoring in the management of prolonged pregnancy showed that the 32/293 women who had abnormal biophysical profiles had significantly higher rates of neonatal morbidity, Caesarean section for fetal distress and meconium aspiration than the women with reassuring biophysical profiles [48]. A further observational study of 131 prolonged pregnancies showed that a normal biophysical profile score was highly predictive of normal outcome, but an abnormal test had only a 14% predictive value of poor neonatal outcome [49].

Cardiotocography

Antenatal cardiotocography (CTG) has been widely used for more than 20 years to monitor moderate- to high-risk pregnancies. Observational studies have reported very low rates of perinatal loss in high-risk pregnancies monitored in this way [50,51]. Four randomized controlled trials comparing CTG with other methods of antepartum fetal monitoring were the subject of a Cochrane review [52]. Women with post-term pregnancy were included in these trials. On the basis of the information presented in this review, the antenatal CTG has no significant effect on perinatal outcome or on interventions such as elective delivery. Miyazaki and Miyazaki [53] reported a series of 125 women with post-term pregnancies where a reactive CTG was recorded within 1 week of delivery. Ten adverse outcomes were reported from this group – four antepartum deaths, one neonatal death, one case of neonatal encephalopathy and four cases of fetal distress on admission in early labour. The poor performance of antenatal CTG in this series and in the randomized trials may relate to errors in interpretation or excessive intervals between tests. Numerical analysis using computerized calculations of the baseline rate and variability may reduce the potential for human error [54]. Weiner *et al.* [55] compared the value of antenatal testing with computerized CTG, conventional CTG, Biophysical Profile Scores and Umbilical Artery Doppler. Three hundred and thirty-seven pregnant women who were delivered after 41 weeks' gestation and who had 610 antenatal tests were included in this study. Ten of 12 fetuses with reduced fetal heart rate variation on computerized CTG had a trial of labour. Nine of these 10 fetuses had fetal distress during labour. Seven of the 12 fetuses with reduced fetal heart rate variation were acidotic at delivery (umbilical artery pH < 7.2). Overall, there were 10 acidotic fetuses at delivery in the study group. Only two of them had an umbilical systolic/diastolic ratio >95th percentile, three had an amniotic fluid index ≤5, and five had fetal heart rate decelerations before labour. Fetuses who demonstrated an abnormal intrapartum fetal heart rate tracing or who were acidotic at delivery had a

Table 22.3 Randomized trials of routine versus selective induction at 41–42 weeks' gestation

Trial	Size	Gestation at trial entry	Method of induction	Method of fetal surveillance	Perinatal deaths
Augensen *et al.* [90]	409	290	Oxytocin and amniotomy	CTG	0
Bergsjo *et al.* [74]	188	284	Membrane sweep, oxytocin, amniotomy	Fetal movement, ultrasound, urinary oestriol	1 in induction arm 2 in selective arm
Cardozo *et al.* [75]	363	290	PGE2, oxytocin, amniotomy	Fetal movement, CTG	1 in selective arm 1 in induction arm
Chanrachakul & Herabutya [91]	249	290	Amniotomy and oxytocin	CTG, AFI	0
Dyson *et al.* [72]	302	287	PGE2, oxytocin, amniotomy	CTG, AFI	1 in selective arm
Hannah *et al.* [70]	3407	287	PGE2, oxytocin, amniotomy	Fetal movement, CTG, AFI	2 in selective arm
Heden *et al.* [92]	238	295	Amniotomy, oxytocin	CTG, AFI	0
Henry *et al.* [73]	112	290	Amniotomy and oxytocin	Amnioscopy	2 in selective arm
Herabutya *et al.* [93]	108	294	PGE2, oxytocin	CTG	1 in selective arm
James *et al.* [94]	74	287	Extra-amniotic saline if Bishop score <5; membrane sweep, amniotomy and oxytocin	Fetal movement, BPS	0
Katz *et al.* [71]	156	294	Amniotomy, oxytocin	Fetal movement, amnioscopy oxytocin challenge	1 in each arm
Martin *et al.* [95]	22	287	Laminaria, oxytocin	CTG, AFI	0
NICHD [96]	440	287	CTG, oxytocin, amniotomy	CTG, AFI	0
Roach & Rogers [97]	201	294	PGE2	CTG, AFI	0
Suikkari *et al.* [98]	119	290	Amniotomy, oxytocin	CTG, human placental lactogen, oestriol. AFI	0
Witter & Weitz [99]	200	287	Oxytocin, amniotomy	Oestriol, oxytocin challenge	0

significantly higher rate of reduced fetal heart rate variation or decelerations before labour. The authors conclude that computerized CTG may improve fetal surveillance in post-term pregnancy. The obvious criticism of this study is the 'circular argument' of using an antepartum CTG abnormality to predict an intrapartum CTG abnormality.

Fetal movement counting

This is yet another test used commonly in the supervision of post-term pregnancies (see Table 22.3) that is not backed up by firm evidence of efficacy. Two randomized trials have addressed the question of whether clinical actions taken on the basis of fetal movement improve fetal outcome [56,57]. The larger of these trials involved over 68,000 women [57]. These trials collectively provide evidence that routine formal fetal movement counting does not reduce the incidence of intrauterine fetal death in late pregnancy. Routine counting results in more frequent reports of diminished fetal activity, with a greater use of other techniques of fetal assessment, more frequent admission to hospital and an increased rate of elective delivery. It may be that fetal movement counting in post-term pregnancy will perform more effectively than it does in low-risk pregnancies. Women will be required to pay extra attention to

fetal movements for less than 1 week in the majority of cases and will usually be attending at intervals of 3 days for other tests.

Doppler velocimetry

Two studies of umbilical artery Doppler velocimetry [58,59] in prolonged pregnancy indicate that it is of no benefit. In a small observational study comparing the predictive values of CTG, AFI, biophysical profile scoring and the ratio of middle cerebral artery (MCA) Doppler to umbilical artery Doppler, Devine *et al.* [60] found that the MCA Doppler to umbilical artery Doppler ratio was the best predictor of 'adverse outcome' in this study, defined by meconium aspiration syndrome or Caesarean section for fetal distress or fetal acidosis.

Evidence-based management of prolonged pregnancy

Ultrasound to establish accurate gestational age

The first step towards managing prolonged pregnancy is to reduce the number of cases of prolonged pregnancy by providing ultrasound verification of gestational age for all pregnancies. A systematic review shows that routine second trimester ultrasound reduces the number of cases of prolonged pregnancy [8]. A recent randomized controlled trial of first versus second trimester ultrasound showed a lower rate of post-term pregnancy in pregnancies dated by first trimester ultrasound [61]. A secondary analysis of data from the FASTER Trial showed that first trimester ultrasound determination of gestational age by crown–rump length as opposed to LMP reduces the apparent incidence of pregnancies greater than 41 weeks from 22.1 to 8.2% [9].

Induction of labour for prolonged pregnancy

Obstetricians have responded in various ways to the apparently increased perinatal mortality and morbidity associated with prolonged pregnancy. Management options include induction at term to prevent pregnancies reaching 42 weeks, routine induction at 42 weeks or shortly before and selective induction at 42 weeks in cases identified by tests as being at risk of adverse outcome. Fortunately, the benefits and hazards of some of these strategies have been evaluated in randomized controlled trials. Randomized or quasi-random trials comparing elective induction at term versus expectant management, and elective induction after 41 weeks versus monitoring of post-term pregnancies were identified using the search strategy described by the Cochrane Pregnancy and Childbirth Group and formed the basis of a systematic review of management options in post-term pregnancy [62]. The main outcomes of interest are those already identified in the analysis of post-term pregnancy risks – perinatal mortality, neonatal encephalopathy, meconium stained amniotic fluid, Caesarean section. In addition, evidence was sought relating to the effect of the various management options on maternal satisfaction. Subsequently, Sanchez-Ramos *et al.* [63] published a systematic review of randomized trials comparing induction of labour with expectant management in pregnancies of 41 weeks gestation and more.

Induction at or before 40 weeks

Pre-emptive induction of labour, where women with uncomplicated pregnancies were routinely offered induction at or before 40 weeks, was practised in some obstetric units in some countries in the 1970s. Six randomized trials compare a policy of 'routine' induction at 39 weeks [64,65], or 40 weeks [66–69], with either 'expectant' management of an indefinite duration or expectant management until 42 weeks' gestation. These trials reveal no evidence of any major benefit or risk to 'routine' induction at 40 weeks. Two perinatal deaths of normally formed babies occurred

in the expectant arm of these trials and none in the induction arm. Obviously, this is not a significant difference. There was no effect on Caesarean section (odds ratio 0.60 95% CI 0.35–1.03), instrumental delivery or use of analgesia in labour. Not surprisingly, given the relationship between gestational age and meconium staining of the amniotic fluid in labour, induction around 40 weeks reduces the incidence of meconium staining in labour (odds ratio 0.50 (0.31–0.86). Unfortunately, the authors of these trials did not address the important question of women's views of induction of labour at this stage of pregnancy. The authors of these trials missed a golden opportunity in failing to measure women's satisfaction with their care. 'Routine' induction of labour at 40 weeks would no longer be considered a realistic option for the prevention of post-term pregnancy. The number of inductions at 40 weeks required to prevent an adverse outcome at 41 or 42 weeks would be excessive and intervention at this level would be unlikely to be welcomed by women, obstetricians or midwives.

Induction of labour at 41 weeks

Sixteen randomized trials comparing 'routine' induction of labour at a specified gestational age with a policy of selective induction of labour in response to an abnormal antepartum test are summarized in Table 22.3.

These trials form the basis of a systematic review by Sanchez-Ramos *et al.* [63]. Twelve of them had been previously included in the Cochrane Review by Crowley [62]. One trial is larger than all others and contributes considerable weight to both meta-analyses [70].

Both meta-analyses adopt an inclusive approach and include trials of variable size and quality. The gestational age at trial entry varies from 287 days to 294 days gestation. A variety of methods of antepartum fetal testing are used to supervise pregnancies in the expectant arm of the trials.

Perinatal mortality

Even the largest trial [70] has insufficient statistical power to detect a significant reduction in the perinatal mortality rate. To have an 80% chance of detecting a 50% reduction in a perinatal mortality rate of 3 per 1000, a sample size of 16,000 is required. Table 22.3 records the 13 perinatal deaths that occurred in the randomized trials, 3 among 3159 women allocated to induction and 10 among 3067 women allocated to selective induction. One normally formed baby, among those allocated to induction [71], died from asphyxia following emergency Caesarean section for meconium stained amniotic fluid and prolonged bradycardia 2 h following induction of labour. The other two deaths among those allocated to routine induction occurred in babies with lethal congenital anomalies. Three further deaths occurred in babies with anomalies among those allocated to selective induction. The other seven deaths occurred in normally formed babies. Two deaths in the Canadian Post-term Pregnancy Trial [70] occurred despite adherence to the monitoring protocol of daily movement counting and three times weekly CTG and ultrasound assessment of amniotic fluid volume. These babies were both small, weighing 2600 g and 3175 g. In the Dyson trial [72], a neonatal death from meconium aspiration occurred in a 43-week baby delivered for acute fetal bradycardia following spontaneous labour. Fetal heart rate monitoring and ultrasound assessment of amniotic fluid had been reassuring 48 h before the spontaneous onset of labour. One of the deaths in the Henry [73] trial was attributed to gestational diabetes. The second occurred due to meconium aspiration in a woman who refused induction following detection of meconium at amnioscopy. The deaths in the Bergsjo [74] and the Cardozo [75] trials were due to pneumonia and abruptio placentae, respectively.

The authors of the systematic reviews adopt a different approach to the inclusion of perinatal deaths in babies with fetal abnormalities. These are excluded in the Cochrane review [62] and included by Sanchez-Ramos [63]. Thus, the Cochrane systematic review shows that induction of labour is associated with an significant reduction in perinatal mortality in normally formed babies (odds ratio 0.23; 95% CI 0.06–0.90), while Sanchez-Ramos confirms the reduction in the risk of perinatal death (0.9 versus 0.33%) but with the 95% confidence intervals for the odds ratio of 0.41 crossing unity (95% CI of 0.14–1.28).

Other perinatal outcomes

Both systematic reviews report a significant reduction in the incidence of meconium stained amniotic fluid but this does not affect the rate of meconium aspiration (0.82; 95% CI 0.49–1.37) [62]. There is no effect on fetal heart rate abnormalities during labour. The odds ratio for neonatal jaundice 3.39 (95% CI 1.42–8.09), based on the small number of trials that reported this outcome, indicate that it is increased by induction. The systematic reviews do not show any beneficial or hazardous effects on Apgar scores, neonatal intensive care admission or neonatal encephalopathy.

Effect of induction of labour on risk of Caesarean section

Sanchez-Ramos *et al.* [63] report that induction of labour is associated with a reduction of the rate of Caesarean section (odds ratio 0.88; 95% CI 0.78–0.99). Crowley reported

a similar outcome, but interpreted it as evidence that a policy of 'routine' induction of labour *does not increase* the likelihood of Caesarean section. She believed that a postrandomization bias in the Hannah trial may have weighted the results towards a spurious reduction in risk of Caesarean section. Women in the expectant arm of the Hannah trial who required induction because of abnormal antenatal tests were denied vaginal prostaglandins whereas those allocated to 'routine' induction were treated with prostaglandin E2 (PGE2). This could potentially lead to an increase in dystocia or failed induction in those denied prostaglandins. However, this does not account for the 8.3% rate of Caesarean section for fetal distress in the selective induction arm of the Hannah trial compared to 5.7% in the routine induction arm. The effect of a policy of induction of labour on reducing the rate of Caesarean section for fetal distress is consistent across the trials reviewed. No significant heterogeneity was detected by Sanchez-Ramos *et al.* [63]. These authors also performed funnel plots, which were symmetric, indicating no evidence of publications bias.

Because the reduced rate of Caesarean section associated with induction of labour is contrary to a traditionally held view among obstetricians that induction of labour increases the likelihood of delivery by Caesarean section, a number of secondary analyses were carried out by Crowley [62]. These showed that induction of labour for post-term pregnancy does not increase the Caesarean section rate, irrespective of parity, cervical ripeness, method of induction or ambient Caesarean section rates.

Women's views of induction for post-term pregnancy

Regrettably, randomized trials give little information on women's views of induction versus conservative management. Only one trial assessed maternal satisfaction with induction of labour [75]. These authors showed that satisfaction was related to the eventual outcome of labour and delivery, rather than to the mode of onset of labour. Women's views are likely to be influenced by the local culture, by the attitude of their caregivers and by practical considerations such as the duration of paid maternity leave. Few obstetricians, midwives or childbirth educators are capable of giving women unbiased information about the risks of post-term pregnancy and the benefits and hazards of induction of labour. In a prospective questionnaire study of women's attitudes towards induction of labour for post-term pregnancy Roberts and Young [76] found that, despite a stated obstetric preference for conservative management, only 45% of women at 37 weeks' gestation were agreeable to conservative management if undelivered by 41 weeks. Of those undelivered by

41 weeks gestation 31% still desired conservative management. This significant decrease was unaffected by parity or certainty of gestational age. In a subsequent study, Roberts *et al.* [77] offered women a choice between induction and conservative management at 42 weeks. Forty-five per cent of women opted for conservative management.

Clinical guidelines for management of prolonged pregnancy

Following the publication of the Canadian Post-term Pregnancy Trial [70] and the Cochrane Review on Post-term Pregnancy Management [64] the Society of Obstetricians and Gynaecologists of Canada issued a clinical practice guideline [78] recommending that:

1 After 41 weeks' gestation, if the dates are certain, women should be offered elective delivery.

2 If the cervix is unfavourable, cervical ripening should be undertaken.

3 If expectant management is chosen, assessment of fetal health should be initiated.

The Royal College of Obstetricians and Gynaecologists (RCOG) issued a clinical guideline on induction of labour in 2001, which included recommendations on management of prolonged pregnancy [79]. These recommendations were:

• An ultrasound to confirm gestation should be offered prior to 20 weeks, as this reduces the need for induction for perceived post-term pregnancy.

• Women with uncomplicated pregnancies should be offered induction of labour beyond 41 weeks.

• From 42 weeks, women who decline induction of labour should be offered increased antenatal monitoring, consisting of a twice weekly CTG and ultrasound estimation of maximum amniotic pool depth.

The American College of Obstetricians and Gynecologists Practice Guidelines [80] are at considerable variance with those issued by RCOG and SOGC.

Level A recommendations

• Women with post-term pregnancies who have unfavourable cervices can either undergo labour induction or be managed expectantly.

• Prostaglandin can be used in post-term pregnancies to promote cervical ripening and induce labour.

• Delivery should be effected if there is evidence of fetal compromise or oligohydramnios.

Level C recommendations

• Despite a lack of evidence that monitoring improves perinatal outcome, it is reasonable to initiate antenatal surveillance of post-term pregnancies between 41 weeks and 42 weeks' of gestation because of evidence that perinatal morbidity and mortality increase as gestational age advances.

• Many practitioners use twice weekly testing with some evaluation of amniotic fluid volume beginning at 41 weeks' of gestation. A non-stress test and amniotic fluid volume (a modified biophysical profile (BPP)) should be adequate.

• Many authorities recommend prompt delivery in a post-term patient with a favourable cervix and no other complications.

The SOGC guidelines provoked an impassioned response [81]. The authors challenged the evidence of increased morbidity and mortality as pregnancy advances and the evidence from the randomized trials that induction of labour post-term does not increase Caesarean section rates and may reduce perinatal mortality rates. In particular, they were concerned that the recommendation from SOGC and RCOG that induction should be 'offered' at 41 weeks' gestation would be interpreted as a policy of mandatory induction at 41 weeks' gestation.

Practical management of prolonged pregnancy

The RCOG recommendations are an excellent guide to practice. Every effort should be made to ensure that dates are as accurate as possible. When the woman reaches 41 weeks she should meet with a consultant obstetrician. Women have a right to be informed of the small increase in risk associated with continuing the pregnancy after 41 weeks. Thornton and Lilford [82] showed that pregnant women are much more risk averse than are their caregivers. Following a vaginal examination, induction of labour should be offered on a date after 41 weeks that is acceptable to both the woman's wishes and the hospital resources. The vaginal examination could be accompanied by sweeping of the membranes, provided women are warned about the discomfort associated with this and are agreeable to proceed. Membrane sweeping reduces the need for 'formal' induction of labour [83]. The vaginal examination allows the obstetrician to inform the woman of the likely ease and success of induction of labour. For women who have previously delivered vaginally and for women with a favourable cervix, induction of labour is unlikely to be a difficult process. Women who wish to avoid induction of labour should be supported but should be made aware of the lack of reliability of antenatal tests and the lack of evidence that avoiding induction of labour reduces the risk of Caesarean section. As induction of labour with prostaglandins is associated with an increased risk of uterine scar dehiscence compared with a spontaneous onset of labour [84], women who have had a previous Caesarean section, especially those with no vaginal deliveries require carefully individualized management at 41 weeks' gestation.

References

1. World Health Organisation (2003) *International Classification of Disease. ICD-10. Chapter*, XV: 048.

2. Bierman J, Siegel E, French F & Simonian K (1965) Analysis of the outcome of all pregnancies in a community. *Am J Obstet Gynecol* **91**, 37–45.

3. Boyce A, Mayaux MJ & Schwartz D (1976) Classical and true gestational postmaturity. *Am J Obstet Gynecol* **125**, 911–3.

4. Butler NR & Bonham DG (1963) *Perinatal Mortality.* Edinburgh: Churchill Livingstone.

5. Chamberlain R, Chamberlain G, Howlett B & Masters K (1978) *British Births 1970*, Vol. 2. *Obstetric Care*. London: Heineman Medical.

6. Smith GC (2001) Use of time to event analysis to estimate the normal duration of human pregnancy. *Human Reprod* **16**, 1497–500.

7. Eik-Nes SH, Okland O, Aure JC & Ulstein M (1984) Ultrasound screening in pregnancy: a randomised controlled trial. *Lancet* **1**, 1347.

8. Neilson JP (1998) Ultrasound for fetal assessment in early pregnancy. *Cochrane Database Syst Rev* **4**, CD000182. DOI 10.1002/14651858CD000182.

9. Bukowski R, Saade G, Malone F, Hankins G & D'Alton M (2001) A decrease in postdate pregnancies is an additional benefit of first trimester screening for aneuploidy. *Am J Obstet Gynecol* **185**(Suppl) S148.

10. Hilder L, Costeole K & Thilaganathan B (1998) Prolonged pregnancy: evaluating gestation-specific risks of fetal and infant mortality. *Br J Obstet Gynaecol* **105**, 169–73.

11. Bakketieg LS & Bergsjo P (1989) Post-term pregnancy: magnitude of the problem. In: Chalmers I, Enkin M & Keirse MJNC (eds) *Effective Care in Pregnancy and Childbirth*, Vol. 1. Oxford: Oxford University Press, 165775.

12. Mogren I, Stenlund H & Hogberg U (1999) Recurrence of prolonged pregnancy. *Int J Epidemiol* **28**, 253–7.

13. Lockwood CJ, Moscarelli RD, Lynch L, Lapinski RH & Ghidini A (1994) Low concentrations of vaginal fetal fibronectin as a predictor of deliveries occurring after 41 weeks. *Am J Obstet Gynecol* **171**, 1–4.

14. Ramanathan GYuC, Osei E & Nicolaides KH (2003) Ultrasound examination at 37 weeks' gestation in the prediction of pregnancy outcome: the value of cervical assessment. *Ultrasound Obstet Gynecol* **22**, 598–603.

15. McLean M, Bisits A, Davies J, Woods R, Lowry P & Smith R (1995) A placental clock controlling the length of human pregnancy. *Nat Med* **1**, 460–3.

16. Buekens P, Delvoie P, Woolast E & Robyn C (1984) Epidemiology of pregnancies with unknown last menstrual period. *J Epidemiol Commun Health* **38**, 79–80.

17. Hall MH & Carr-Hill RA (1985) The significance of uncertain gestation for obstetric outcome. *Br J Obstet Gynaecol* **92**, 452–60.

18. Naeye RL (1978) Causes of perinatal mortality excess in prolonged gestations. *Am J Epidemiol* **108**, 429–33.

19. Smith GC (2001) Life-table analysis of the risk of perinatal death at term and post term in singleton pregnancies. *Am J Obstet Gynecol* **184**, 489–96.

20. Hilder L, Costeloe K & Thilaganathan B (2000) Prospective risk of stillbirth. Study's results are flawed by reliance on cumulative prospective risk. *Br Med J* **320**, 444–5.

21. Yudkin PL, Wood L & Redman CW (1987) Risk of unexplained stillbirth at different gestational ages. *Lancet* **8543**, 1192–4.

22. Cotzias CS, Paterson-Brown S & Fisk N (1999) Prospective risk of unexplained stillbirth in singleton pregnancies at term: population based analysis. *Br Med J* **319**, 287–8.

23. Yudkin P & Redman CW (2000) Impending fetal death must be identified and pre-empted. *Br Med J* **320**, 444.

24. Ingemarsson I & Kallen K (1997) Stillbirths and rate of neonatal deaths in 76,761 postterm pregnancies in Sweden, 1982–91: a register study. *Acta Obstetrica Gynecologica Scand 1997*, **76**, 658–62.

25. Campbell MK, Ostbye T & Irgens LM (1997) Post-term birth, risk factors and outcomes in a 10-year cohort of Norwegian births. *Obstet Gynecol* **89**, 543–8.

26. Bastian H, Keirse MJ & Lancaster PA (1998) Perinatal death associated with planned home birth in Australia: a population based study. *Br Med J* **317**, 384–8.

27. Mehl-Madrona L & Madrona MM (1997) Physician- and midwife-attended home births. Effects of breech, twin, and post-dates outcome data on mortality rates. *J Nurse Midwifery* **42**, 91–8.

28. Caughey AB, Washington AE & Laros RK (2005) Neonatal complications of term pregnancy: rates by gestational age increase in a continuous, not threshold, fashion. *Am J Obstet Gynecol* **192**, 185–90.

29. Minchom P, Niswander K, Chalmers I *et al.* (1987) Antecedents and outcome of very early neonatal seizures in infants born at or after term. *Br J Obstet Gynaecol* **94**, 431–9.

30. Curtis P, Matthews T, Clarke TA *et al.* (1988) The Dublin Collaborative Seizure Study. *Arch Dis Child* **63**, 1065–8.

31. MacLennan A (1999) A template for defining a causal relation between acute intrapartum events and cerebral palsy: international consensus statement. *Br Med J* **319**, 1054–9.

32. Gaffney G, Flavell V, Johnson A, Squier M & Sellers S (1994) Cerebral palsy and neonatal encephalopathy. *Arch Dis Child* **70**, F195–200.

33. Luckas M, Buckett W & Alfirevic Z (1998) Comparison of outcomes in uncomplicated term and post-term pregnancy following spontaneous labor. *J Perinat Med* **26**, 475–9.

34. Crowley P (1980) Non-quantitative estimation of amniotic fluid volume in suspected prolonged pregnancy. *J Perinatat Med* **8**, 249–51.

35. Manning FA, Hill LM & Platt LD (1981) Qualitative amniotic fluid volume determination by ultrasound: antepartum detection of intrauterine growth retardation. *Am J Obstet Gynaecol* **151**, 304–8.

36. Chamberlain PF, Manning FA, Morrison I, Harman CR & Lange IR (1984) Ultrasound evaluation of amniotic fluid. 1. The relationship of marginal and decreased amniotic fluid volumes to perinatal outcome. *Am J Obstet Gynecol* **150** 245–9.

37. Crowley P, O'Herlihy C & Boylan P (1980) The value of ultrasound measurement of amniotic fluid volume in the management of prolonged pregnancies. *Br J Obstet Gynaecol* **91**, 444–8.

38. Fischer RL, McDonnell M, Bianculli RN, Perry RL, Hediger ML & Scholl TO (1993) Amniotic fluid volume estimation in the postdate pregnancy: a comparison of techniques. *Obstet Gynecol* **81**, 698–704.

39. Phelan JP, Smith CV, Broussard P & Small M (1987) Amniotic fluid Volume assessment with the four quadrant technique at 36–42 weeks' gestation. *J Reprod Med* **32**, 540–2.

40. Alfirevic Z & Walkinshaw SA (1995) A randomised controlled trial of simple compared with complex antenatal fetal monitoring after 42 weeks of gestation. *Br J Obstet Gynecol* **102**, 638–43.

41. Morris JM, Thompson K, Smithey J *et al.* (2003) The usefulness of ultrasound assessment of amniotic fluid in predicting adverse outcome in prolonged pregnancy: a prospective blinded observational study. *Br J Obstet Gynaecol* **110**, 989–94.

42. Locatelli A, Zagarell A, Toso L, Assi F, Ghidini A & Biffi A (2004) Serial assessment of amniotic fluid index in uncomplicated term pregnancies: prognostic value of amniotic fluid reduction. *J Matern Fetal Neonat Medical* **15**, 233–6.

43. Chauhan SP, Sanderson M, Hendrix NW, Magann EF & Devoe LD (1999) Perinatal outcome and amniotic fluid index in the antepartum and intrapartum periods: a meta-analysis. *Am J Obstet Gynecol* **181**, 1473–8.

44. Chauhan SP, Magann EF, Morrison JC, Whitowrth NS, Hendrix NW & Devoe LD (1994) Ultrasonographic assessment of amniotic fluid does not reflect actual amniotic fluid Volume. *Obstet Gynecol* **84**, 856–60.

45. Magann EF, Chauhan SP, Barrilleaux PS, Whitworth NS & Martin JN (2000) Amniotic fluid index and single deepest pocket: weak indicators of abnormal amniotic Volumes. *Obstet Gynecol* **96**, 737–40.

46. Manning F, Morrison J, Lange IR, Harmann CR & Chamberlain PF (1985) Fetal assessment based on fetal biophysical profile. experience in 12,620 referred high-risk pregnancies. 1. Perinatal mortality by frequency and etiology. *Am J Obstet Gynecol* **151**, 343–50.

47. Alfirevic Z & Neilson JP (1996) Biophysical profile for fetal assessment in high risk pregnancies. *Cochrane Database Syst Rev* **1** CD000038. DOI 10.1002/14651858CD000038.

48. Johnson JM, Harman CR, Lange IR & Manning F (1986) Biophysical scoring in the management of the postterm pregnancy. An analysis of 307 patients. *Am J Obstet Gynecol* **154**, 269–73.

49. Hann L, McArdle C & Sachs B (1987) Sonographic biophysical profile in the postdate pregnancy. *J Ultrasound Med* **6**, 191–5.

50. Keegan KA & Paul RH (1980) Antepartum fetal heart rate testing. IV. The non-stress test as the primary approach. *Am J Obstet Gynaecol* **136**, 75–80.

51. Mendenhall HW, O'Leary J & Phillips KO (1980) The nonstress test: the value of a single acceleration in evaluating the fetus at risk. *Am J Obstet Gynecol* **136**, 87–91.

52. Pattison N & McCowan L (1999) Cardiotocography for antepartum fetal assessment. *Cochrane Database Syst Rev* **1**, CD001068. DOI 10.1002/14651858CD001068.

53. Miyazaki FS & Miyazaki BA (1981) False reactive nonstress tests in postterm pregnancies. *Am J Obstet Gynaecol* **140**, 269–76.

54. Dawes GS, Moullden M & Redman CWG (1991) System 8000: computerised antenatal FHR analysis. *J Perinat Med* **19**, 47–51.

55. Weiner Z, Farmakides G, Schulman H, Kellner L, Plancher S & Maulik D (1994) Computerized analysis of fetal heart rate variation in post-term pregnancy: prediction of intrapartum fetal distress and fetal acidosis. *Am J Obstet Gynecol* **171**, 1132–8.

56. Neldam S (1980) Fetal movement as an indication of fetal wellbeing. *Lancet* **8180**, 1222–4.

57. Grant A, Elbourne D, Valentin L & Alexander S (1989) Routine formal fetal movement counting and risk of antepartum late death in normally formed singletons. *Lancet* **8659**, 345–9.

58. Guidetti DA, Divon MY, Cavalieri RL, Langer O & Merkatz IR (1987) Fetal umbilical artery flow velocimetry in postdate pregnancies. *Am J Obstet Gynecol* **157**, 1521–3.

59. Stokes HJ, Roberts RV & Newnham JP (1991) Doppler flow velocity analysis in postdate pregnancies. *Aust NZ J Obstet Gynaecol* **31**, 27–30.

60. Devine PA, Bracero LA, Lysikiewicz A, Evans R, Womack S & Byrne DW (1994) Middle cerebral to umbilical artery Doppler ratio in post-date pregnancies. *Obstet Gynecol* **84**, 856–60.

61. Bennett KA, Crane JM, O'Shea P, Lacelle J, Hutchens D & Copel JA (2004) First trimester ultrasound screening is effective in reducing postterm labor induction rates: a randomized controlled trial. *Am J Obstet Gynecol* **190**, 1077–81.

62. Crowley P (2000) Interventions for preventing or improving the outcome of delivery at or beyond term. *Cochrane Database Syst Rev* **1**, CD000170. DOI 10.1002/14651858CD000170.

63. Sanchez-Ramos L, Olivier F, Delke I & Kaunitz AM (2003) Labor induction versus expectant management for postterm pregnancies: a systematic review with meta-analysis. *Obstet Gynecol* **101**, 1312–8.

64. Cole RA, Howie PW & MacNaughton MC (1975) Elective induction of labour. A randomised prospective trial. *Lancet* **1**, 767–70.

65. Martin DH, Thompson W, Pinkerton JHM & Watson JD (1978) Randomised controlled trial of selective planned delivery. *Br J Obstet Gynaecol* **85**, 109–13.

66. Breart G, Goujard J, Maillard F, Chavigny C, Rumeau-Rouquette C & Sureau C (1982) Comparison of two obstetrical policies with regard to artificial induction of labour at term. A randomised trial. *J Obstet Biol Reprod (Paris)* **11**, 107–12.

67. Egarter CH, Kofler E, Fitz R & Husselein PI (1989) Is induction of labour indicated in prolonged pregnancy? Results of a prospective randomised trial. *Gynecol Obstet Invest* **27**, 6–9.

68. Tylleskar J, Finnstrom O, Leijon I, Hedenskog S & Ryden G (1979) Spontaneous labor and elective induction – a

prospective randomized study. Effects on mother and fetus. *Acta Obstetrica Gynecologica Scand* **58**, 513–8.

69. Sande HA, Tuveng J & Fonstelien T (1983) A prospective randomized study of induction of labor. *Int J Gynecol Obstet* **21**, 333–6.

70. Hannah ME, Hannah WJ, Hellman J, Hannah WJ, Hewson S, Milner R & Willan A, Canadian Multicenter Post-Term Pregnancy Trial Group (1992) Induction of Labour as compared with serial antenatal monitoring in post-term pregnancy. A randomized controlled trial. *NEJM* **326**, 1587–92.

71. Katz Z, Yemini M, Lancet M, Mogilner BM, Ben-Hur H & Caspi B (1983) Non-aggressive management of post-date pregnancies. *Eur J Obstet Gynecol Reprod Biol* **15**, 71–9.

72. Dyson D, Miller PD & Armstrong MA (1987) Management of prolonged pregnancy: induction of labour versus antepartum testing. *Am J Obstet Gynecol* **156**, 928–34.

73. Henry GR (1969) A controlled trial of surgical induction of labour and amnioscopy in the management of prolonged pregnancy. *J Obstet Gynaecol Br Commonwealth* **76**, 795–8.

74. Bergsjo P, Gui-dan H, Su-qin Y, Zhi-zeng G & Bakketeig LS (1989) Comparison of induced vs non-induced labor in post-term pregnancy. *Acta Obstetrica Gynecologica Scand* **68**, 683–7.

75. Cardozo L, Fysh J & Pearce JM (1986) Prolonged pregnancy: the management debate. *Br Med J* **293**, 1059–63.

76. Roberts LJ & Young KR (1991) The management of prolonged pregnancy – an analysis of women's attitudes before and after term. *Br J Obstet Gynaecol* **98**, 1102–6.

77. Roberts L, Cook E, Beardsworth SA & Trew G (1994) Prolonged pregnancy: two years experience of offering women conservative management. *J Royal Army Med Corps* **140**, 32–6.

78. Society of Obstetricians and Gynaecologists of Canada (1997) Materno-fetal committee. Post-term pregnancy. *(Committee Opinion). SOGC Clinical Practice Guidelines*, no. 15.

79. Royal College of Obstetricians and Gynaecologists Evidence-based Clinical Guideline Number 7. RCOG 2001.

80. ACOG Practice Bulletin. Management of Postterm Pregnancy ACOG (2004) Practice Bulletin, 55. *Obstet Gynecol* **104**, 639–40.

81. Menticoglou S & Hall PF (2002) Routine induction of labour at 41 weeks gestation: nonsensus consensus. *Br J Obstet Gynaecol* **109**, 485–91.

82. Thornton J & Lilford R (1989) The caesarean section decision: patients' choices are not determined by immediate emotional reactions. *J Obstet Gynaecol* **9**, 283–8.

83. Boulvain M, Stan C & Irion O (2005) Membrane sweeping for induction of labour. *Cochrane Database Syst Rev* **1**, CD000451. DOI 10.1002/14651858CD000451.pub2.

84. Lydon-Rochelle M, Holt VL, Easterling TR & Martin DP (2001) Risk of uterine rupture during labor among women with a prior caesarean delivery. *N Engl J Med* **345**, 3–8.

85. Sue A, Quan AK, Hannah ME, Cohen MM, Foster GA & Liston RM (1999) Effect of labour induction on rates of stillbirth and caesarean section in post-term pregnancies. *CMAJ* **160**, 1145–9.

86. Fabre E, Gonzalez de Aguero R, de Agustin JL, Tajada M, Repolles S & Sanz A (1996) Perinatal mortality in term and post-term births. *J Perinat Med* **24**, 163–9.

87. Olesen AW, Basso O & Olsen J (2003) Risk of recurrence of prolonged pregnancy. *BMJ* **326**, 476.

88. Divon MY, Haglund B, Nisell H, Otterblad PO & Westgren M (1998) Fetal and neonatal mortality in the post-term pregnancy the impact of gestational age and fetal growth restriction. *Am J Obstet Gynecol* **178**, 726–31.

89. Caughey AB & Musci TJ (2004) Complications of term pregnancies beyond 37 weeks of gestation. *Obstet Gynecol* **103**, 57–62.

90. Augensen K, Bergsjo P, Eikeland T, Ashvik K & Carlsen J (1987) Randomized comparison of early versus late induction of labour in post-term pregnancy. *Br Med J* **294**, 1192–5.

91. Chanrachakul B & Herabutya Y (2002) Postterm with favourable cervix. Is induction necessary? *Eur J Obstet Gynecol Reprod Biol* **4367**, 1–4.

92. Heden L, Ingemarsson I, Ahlstrom H & Solum T (1991) Induction of labor vs conservative management in prolonged pregnancy: controlled study. *Int J Fetomaternal Med* **4**, 148–52.

93. Herabutya Y, Prasertsawat PO, Tongyai T & Isarangura Na Ayudthya N (1992) Prolonged pregnancy: the management dilemma. *Int J Gynecol Obstet* **37**, 253–8.

94. James C, George SS, Gaunekar N & Seshadri L (2001) Management of prolonged pregnancy: a randomized trial of induction of labour and antepartum foetal monitoring. *Nat Med J India* **14**, 270–3.

95. Martin JN, Sessums JK, Howard P, Martin RW & Morrison JC (1989) Alternative approaches to the management of gravidas with prolonged post-term postdate pregnancies. *J Miss State Med Assoc* **30**, 105–11.

96. National Institute of Child Health and Human Development Network of Maternal-Fetal Medicine Units (1994) A clinical trial of induction of labor versus expectant management in postterm pregnancy. *Am J Obstet Gynecol* **170**, 716–23.

97. Roach VJ & Rogers MS (1997) Pregnancy outcome beyond 41 weeks gestation. *Int J Gynaecol Obstet* **59**, 19–24.

98. Suikkari AM, Jalkanen M, Heiskala H & Koskela O (1983) Prolonged pregnancy: induction or observation. *Acta Obstet Gynecol Scand Suppl* **116**, 58.

99. Witter FR & Weitz CM (1987) A randomised trial of induction at 42 weeks of gestation vs expectant management for postdates pregnancies. *Am J Perinatol* **4**, 206–11.

Chapter 23: Induction and augmentation of labour

G. Justus Hofmeyr

Introduction

The culmination of normal pregnancy involves three stages: prelabour, cervical ripening and labour. These occur as a continuum rather than as isolated events [1]. Endogenous prostaglandins play a part in all these processes [2]. Interventions to artificially ripen the cervix, induce uterine contractions and augment labour once it is in progress also lack distinct boundaries. This chapter will briefly discuss reasons for these interventions and methods which may be used.

Labour induction and augmentation may be a source of conflict and distress. For most health workers they are seen as routine, technical procedures. For many women, they have emotive connotations, evoking a sense of personal inadequacy and eroded self-esteem. It is important for health workers to approach the question of labour induction with sensitivity, and to involve women in the decision-making process.

Labour induction is one of the most frequent medical procedures in pregnant women. It is a major intervention in the normal course of pregnancy, with the potential to set in motion a cascade of interventions, particularly Caesarean section. However, with modern methods of labour induction, this risk appears to have diminished.

When should labour be induced?

The decision to induce labour is a matter of rather complex clinical judgement. It usually constitutes a choice between three options: allowing the pregnancy to continue, inducing labour or performing elective Caesarean section. The decision takes into account a number of factors.

- Anticipated benefits to the mother, such as improving a medical condition which is caused or aggravated by pregnancy, including pre-eclampsia, placental abruption and certain respiratory, hepatic and cardiac disorders; relieving discomfort, such as from multiple pregnancy, polyhydramnios or spontaneous symphysiotomy; allowing essential treatment to be commenced, such as for cervical cancer; relieving emotional distress after intrauterine death; or alleviating anxiety about the baby's well-being.

- Estimated risks to the mother, such as increased pain and need for analgesia, uterine hyperstimulation, Caesarean section, infection, complications of the procedures, post-partum haemorrhage, uterine rupture (very rarely), anxiety if the induction is protracted or unsuccessful, and loss of self-esteem because of perceived failure to give birth normally.

- Anticipated benefits to the baby, such as improved growth and development when intrauterine growth is suboptimal, and reduced risk of intrauterine death from complications such as diabetes, prolonged pregnancy (beyond 41 weeks), amnionitis, prelabour ruptured membranes, rhesus immunization, fetal compromise and cholestasis of pregnancy.

- Estimated risks to the baby, such as prematurity and compromise from uterine hyperstimulation.

Several factors influence the decision.

- The condition of the mother.
- The condition of the baby.
- The gestational age of the baby, and level of certainty about the baby's age. When fetal lung maturity is uncertain, amniocentesis may be performed to assess markers for lung maturity such as the alcohol 'shake' test, lecithin/sphingomyelin ratio and phosphatidyl glycerol level.
- Previous Caesarean section.
- The preference of the mother.
- The likelihood that induction of labour will be efficient and vaginal delivery successful.

The last factor is in part dependent on the state of the uterine cervix, which is related to the imminence of spontaneous labour.

The 'ripeness' of the uterine cervix

The process of softening, shortening and partial dilation of the cervix usually takes place in the days or weeks prior to the onset of labour, but the timing of this process is variable. An unfavourable or 'unripe' cervix is one which has undergone minimal change and is more resistant to attempts at induction of labour. In the first trimester,

Table 23.1 Modified 'Bishop' cervical score

Score	0	1	2	3
Cervical dilation (cm)	0	1–2	3–4	5+
Cervical length (cm)	3	2	1	<1
Station of the presenting part or more	−3	−2	−1, 0	+1
Consistency	Firm	Moderate	Soft	
Position	Posterior	Midposition	Anterior	

50% of the dry weight of the cervix is tightly aligned collagen, 20% smooth muscle and the rest is ground substance composed of elastin and glycosaminoglycans (Chondroitin, dermatan sulphate and hyaluronidase) [3]. During pregnancy, hyaluronidase increases from 6 to 33%, whereas dermatan and chondroitin, which bind collagen more tightly, decrease. Collagenase and elastase enzymes increase, as do the vascularity and water content.

A standardized method of semiquantitative clinical scoring of the cervix was described by Bishop in 1964 [4], and has since been modified (see Table 23.1). A score of 6 or more predicts the likelihood of successful induction of labour. A score of 5 or less is regarded as being unfavourable for induction of labour, and use of artificial rupture of the amniotic sac and/or oxytocin infusion are unlikely to be successful. More recently, measurement of fibronectin in cervicovaginal secretions has been used to predict the imminence of labour, with variable success.

Royal College of Obstetricians and Gynaecologists guidelines

Guidelines developed by the Royal College of Obstetricians and Gynaecologists [5] recommend offering an ultrasound scan before 20 weeks to confirm the gestational age; membrane 'sweeping' after 40 weeks; routine labour induction after 41 weeks; if declined, fetal monitoring from 42 weeks with induction of labour recommended if the monitoring is abnormal. In the case of pregnancy complications, membrane sweeping or labour induction is offered at the appropriate gestation.

Methods of induction of labour with a favourable cervix [6]

The more favourable the cervix the greater the likelihood of efficient labour induction, irrespective of the method chosen. Artificial rupture of the membranes (amniotomy) using a toothed forceps or purpose-designed plastic hook, is a simple method of labour induction. Depending on the

urgency of the labour induction, oxytocin infusion may be started with the amniotomy or may be used only if progress after amniotomy is inadequate. Because of the considerable variability in sensitivity of the myometrium to oxytocin, oxytocin is administered as a variable dose infusion, titrated against uterine contractions. A typical dosage schedule would be 1 mU/min, doubling the rate of infusion every 20–30 min until adequate uterine contractions are achieved or a rate of 32 mU/min is reached. Once labour is established the infusion rate may be progressively reduced, as the myometrial sensitivity increases, to a rate of about 7 mU/min. Amniotomy should be avoided if the woman is not known to be free of infections such as HIV and hepatitis, in which case oxytocin infusion may be used with intact membranes.

Because amniotomy and/or oxytocin infusion tend to be ineffective when the cervix is unfavourable, it is customary to use amniotomy and/or oxytocin infusion for labour induction with favourable cervix and prostaglandins when the cervix is unfavourable. However, prostaglandins may equally be used when the cervix is favourable and in fact several trials (with rather small numbers) have shown various prostaglandins, including misoprostol, to be more efficient than oxytocin infusion for labour induction with favourable cervix and associated with greater satisfaction in the women.

Methods of induction of labour with an unfavourable cervix

The mainstay of induction of labour with an unfavourable cervix is the use of exogenous prostaglandins [7] or methods to stimulate the release of endogenous prostaglandins to 'ripen' the cervix and induce contractions.

Prostaglandins for labour induction

Labour induction with prostaglandin F2 alpha was introduced in the 1960s. Subsequently, formulations of prostaglandin E2 (PGE2, dinoprostone) were developed which largely replaced the use of F2 alpha. The most common route of administration is vaginal, and tablets, suppositories, gels and pessaries have been developed. A randomized comparison found similar effectiveness for a 10-mg PGE2 sustained release vaginal insert compared with 3 mg PGE2 vaginal tablets twice at a 6-h interval. In seven out of eight women with uterine hyperstimulation, removal of the vaginal insert was sufficient to normalize uterine activity. In the PGE2 tablet group eight out of nine with uterine hyperstimulation required medical treatment.

A wide variety of dosages and dosing intervals are in use. A limiting factor for the use of prostaglandin E2 preparations in many countries has been the cost.

The Royal College of Obstetricians and Gynaecologists recommend vaginal prostaglandins for the initiation of cervical ripening or labour induction for both unfavourable and favourable cervices [8]. PGE2 tablets (3 mg 6–8 hourly to a maximum dose of 6 mg) are recommended in preference to PGE2 gel (2 mg for nulliparous women with modified Bishop cervical score <4, 1 mg for all others, repeated 6 hourly to a maximum dose of 4 mg).

In the case of ruptured membranes, intravenous oxytocin is recommended as an alternative initiating agent, as detailed in p. The effectiveness of oxytocin is optimized with ruptured membranes. If oxytocin is used after PGE2, 6 h should elapse after the last vaginal dose of PGE2 to reduce the risk of uterine hyperstimulation.

Comparison of methods of induction of labour

Because vaginal PGE2 is widely recognized and accepted as a standard method of labour induction, alternative methods which are less well established will be compared with PGE2 as the 'gold standard'. Particular attention will be paid to misoprostol because of the controversy surrounding its use and the volume of recent research.

Comparisons of alternative methods are most reliably based on the results of randomized clinical trials. To manage the complexity of several hundred reported randomized trials comparing multiple combinations of 25 methods of labour induction, the Pregnancy and Childbirth Group of the Cochrane Collaboration, in collaboration with the Clinical Effectiveness Support Unit, Royal College of Obstetricians and Gynaecologists, developed a strategy to review well-defined clusters of comparisons in a series of systematic reviews using standardized outcomes and clinical subgroups [9]. For the purposes of this chapter, data comparing PGE2 administered vaginally (as the 'gold standard') with any other method have been extracted from these reviews (Table 23.2).

A problem fundamental to these comparisons is that one method may appear to be more effective than another simply because a large dosage has been used. What is most relevant is the relationship between effectiveness and the incidence of uterine hyperstimulation (with the attendant risks of fetal compromise and uterine rupture), for each method. In the last column of Table 23.2, the relative risk of failed delivery within 24 h is multiplied by the relative risk of uterine hyperstimulation with fetal heart rate changes. The result serves as a rough indication of efficiency (relationship between effectiveness and hyperstimulation) for each method, relative to PGE2 as the 'gold standard'. On the basis of this method, the efficiency of mechanical methods appears better, vaginal misoprostol worse and oral misoprostol and oxytocin with amniotomy similar to that

of PGE2. There were too few data on vaginal PGF2-alpha for comment.

Intracervical prostaglandins

PGE2 may be administered into the cervical canal, in smaller dosages than those used vaginally, with the objective of optimizing the local effect on the cervix. Administration is somewhat more cumbersome and no clear advantages over vaginal administration have emerged.

Intravenous oxytocin alone

Traditionally, the use of oxytocin has been accompanied by amniotomy. In countries with high HIV prevalence, amniotomy is avoided in women not known to be free of HIV infection. However, oxytocin without amniotomy is significantly less effective than vaginal PGE2 for labour induction in women with unfavourable cervices.

Amniotomy

Rupturing the amniotic membranes through the cervix has been documented as a method of labour induction for over 200 years. A rise in prostaglandin metabolites with a relationship to the induction–delivery interval following artificial rupture of membranes has been demonstrated. This method has the advantage that the use of exogenous uterine stimulants, with the risk of uterine hyperstimulation, is avoided, and the amniotic fluid may be observed. However, the procedure may be uncomfortable and it gives rise to the possibility of ascending infection. Prolonged rupture of the membranes may increase the risk of fetal infections including HIV, and the procedure itself might place the fetus at increased risk of HIV if the skin of the presenting part is scratched. With an unfavourable cervix, amniotomy is often not technically possible.

Intravenous oxytocin with amniotomy

The combination of intravenous oxytocin and amniotomy is commonly used in women with favourable cervices.

Misoprostol

Misoprostol, an orally active, stable prostaglandin E1 analogue, has entered clinical use in Obstetrics and Gynaecology on a wide scale without having been registered for such use [10].

The American College of Obstetricians and Gynecologists' Guidelines for induction of labour recommend that misoprostol 25 μg 3- to 6- hourly is effective for induction of labour (level A evidence), and 50 μg 6-hourly may be appropriate in some situations, though increased risk of complications has been reported (level B evidence).

Table 23.2 Various methods of labour induction compared with PGE2 administered vaginally as the 'gold standard', extracted from the respective systematic reviews in the Cochrane Library

Method compared with PGE2	Outcomes: relative risk (RR) (95% confidence interval) [n]					
	Vaginal delivery not achieved within 24 h	Uterine hyperstimulation with fetal heart rate changes	Caesarean section	Serious neonatal morbidity or perinatal death	Serious maternal morbidity or death	Efficacy (RR for vaginal delivery in 24 h × RR for uterine hyperstimulation)
Intravenous oxytocin	1.9 (1.4–2.4) [360]	0.35 (0.04–3.3) [767]	1.1 (0.95–1.3) [4649]	3.0 (0.3–29) [3084]	1.1 (0.15–7.6) [275]	0.7 (0.56–7.9)
Amniotomy		No events [260]	1.2 (0.38–3.8) [260]			
Intravenous oxytocin with amniotomy	0.9 (0.46–1.8) [42]	0.81 (0.45–1.5) [739]	1.06 (0.79–1.4) [1140]	1.00 (0.07–15) [612]	No events [378]	0.73 (0.21–2.7)
Vaginal misoprostol	0.80 (0.73–0.87) [2906]	2.0 (1.5–2.8) [3121]	0.97 (0.86–1.1) [3484]	6.0 (0.25–146) [360]		1.6 (1.1–2.4)
Vaginal PG F2-alpha	0.51 (0.05–5.4) [75]	1.0 (0.07–14) [106]	1.0 (0.47–2.2) [107]			0.51 (0.0035–76)
Oral misoprostol	1.2 (0.94–1.5) [691]	0.87 (0.49–1.6) [929]	0.90 (0.70–1.2) [959]	No events [267]	No events [962]	1.04 (0.46–2.4)
Mechanical methods	1.7 (1.2–2.5) [109]	0.14 (0.04–0.53) [484]	1.2 (0.94–1.6) [786]		No events [88]	0.24 (0.045–1.3)
Membrane sweeping			0.70 (0.44–1.1) [339]			
Extra-amniotic prostaglandins	1.26 (1.0–1.6) [261]	No events [261]	0.89 (0.42–1.9) [142]			
Oral prostaglandins			0.69 (0.33–1.5) [63]			
Oestrogens (with amniotomy)		5.0 (0.25–100) [60]	0.88(0.36–2.11) [60]			

Comparisons are expressed as relative risks (95% confidence intervals), [n]. A relative risk below 1 indicates that the outcome was less frequent with the method being compared with PGE2.

Effectiveness of misoprostol

In most of the dosage regimens used, misoprostol is at least as effective as conventional methods of labour induction. In doses above 25 μg 4–6-hourly vaginally, misoprostol is associated with fewer failures to deliver vaginally within 24 h than dinoprostone. The greater efficiency of misoprostol has been related to more rapid cervical ripening.

Oral versus vaginal route of administration of misoprostol

Oral compared with vaginal administration of misoprostol 400 μg has a shorter time to peak serum level (34 versus 80 min) and produces a higher peak, but has far briefer activity. This is reflected in more rapid and pronounced initial increase but less persistence in uterine tonus with the oral route. Because of the short duration of action with the oral route, we have studied oral misoprostol 2-hourly for labour induction, commencing with a dose of 20 μg, increased if necessary to 40 μg after 2–3 doses. To administer such small doses, we dissolved 200 μg misoprostol in 200 m water, and shook well before each administration. The solution was discarded after 12 h. In a multicentre randomized trial in 695 women, we found this method to be similar to vaginal dinoprostone 2 mg, repeated after 6 h, with respect to effectiveness, uterine hyperstimulation, Caesarean section rates and perinatal outcome. For consistency with commonly used dosages we have modified the dosage to 25 μg 2-hourly, increased, if necessary, in nulliparous women only to 50 μg 2-hourly.

Systematic review of randomized trials comparing oral with vaginal routes of administration has found the oral route to be associated with slower labours but fewer Caesarean sections.

Buccal or sublingual misoprostol

The sublingual route combines the shorter onset of the oral route and the longer duration and greater bioavailability of the vaginal route. The buccal route should be studied with caution as dosages may have to be reduced considerably to be safe.

Rectal misoprostol

In one small study, similar efficacy for labour induction was found when misoprostol was administered vaginally or rectally.

Dosage of vaginal misoprostol

Systematic review of trials comparing lower dosages (ranging from 25 μg 6-hourly to 50 μg 4-hourly) with higher dosages of vaginal misoprostol showed that the lower dosage regimens required more oxytocin use, had similar rates of delivery within 24 h and Caesarean section and were associated with significantly less uterine hyperstimulation. There is a strong case to be made for using a small dose (e.g. 25 μg) [11], at least initially.

Complications of misoprostol

Areas of concern regarding safety relate mainly to uterine hyperstimulation and possible effects of this on the mother and baby.

Uterine hyperstimulation

Systematic review has found vaginal misoprostol in the dosages used to be associated with more uterine hyperstimulation with non-reassuring fetal heart rate changes than is PGE2. As misoprostol was also more potent as a uterine stimulant in these trials, it is difficult to be sure whether the difference is pharmacological or purely dose related.

MECONIUM-STAINED LIQUOR

Meconium-stained liquor is significantly more common with labour induction with misoprostol than with either vaginal or intracervical PGE2. We have previously postulated that certain myometrial stimulants may cross the placenta to stimulate fetal bowel smooth muscle and cause meconium passage. However, misoprostol and dinoprostone have similar stimulatory effects on rat ileum relative to the myometrial effect [12]. An alternative explanation for the increased meconium passed during misoprostol induction of labour is that the resistance of misoprostol to placental 15-hydroxyprostaglandin dehydrogenase enables more misoprostol to enter the fetal circulation than does PGE2.

PRECIPITATE DELIVERY

Precipitate delivery (labour < 2 h) has been described as a complication of misoprostol. Most reviews and trials have not documented the occurrence of precipitate delivery. In fact 'mean time to delivery' is frequently given as a primary endpoint. Precipitate deliveries may contribute to apparently favourable mean induction to delivery times, without being identified as an unfavourable outcome. The importance of precipitate delivery is that it may be a marker for excessive uterine response to misoprostol and risk of uterine rupture.

RUPTURE OF THE UNSCARRED UTERUS

There have been numerous reports of rupture of an unscarred uterus following misoprostol labour induction, including a maternal death within 7 h of labour induction with one dose of misoprostol 50 μg vaginally in a healthy woman with uneffaced cervix. Without a reliable basis of comparison, it is unclear whether the risk of uterine rupture following misoprostol induction is greater or less than with other methods of labour induction.

WOMEN WITH PREVIOUS CAESAREAN SECTION

Several cases of rupture of uterine scars following misoprostol induction have been reported. A recent retrospective study found significantly more cases of uterine rupture or dehiscence following cervical ripening with misoprostol than when oxytocin or prostaglandin E2 were used. Misoprostol should not be used in women with uterine scars.

CAESAREAN SECTION

The relationship between misoprostol use and Caesarean section is a complex one. The trend in randomized trials has been an increase in Caesarean sections for fetal heart rate abnormality and a reduction for poor progress of labour, giving a reduction overall.

PERINATAL OUTCOME

Despite increases in uterine hyperstimulation, most reviews and trials have shown no significant difference in perinatal outcome following misoprostol labour induction versus other methods.

POST-PARTUM HAEMORRHAGE

Increased post-partum haemorrhage was noted in a retrospective study of misoprostol induction compared with the general obstetric population (58/1037 versus

394/11255) and in a randomized trial following labour induction with vaginal misoprostol 50 μg versus 25 μg 4-hourly (9.8 versus 2.2%).

Conclusion

Misoprostol is a highly effective agent for labour induction. Complications remain a matter of concern, particularly uterine hyperstimulation, precipitate labour, meconium-stained liquor, uterine rupture and post-partum haemorrhage. The available data suggest that risks can be minimized with the use of small dosages and that the starting dose should not exceed 25 μg vaginally or orally. Limited evidence favours the oral over the vaginal route. There is a need for large-scale randomized trials comparing low-dose misoprostol regimens with conventional methods to determine with more certainty the relative rates of rare adverse outcomes.

Mechanical methods of labour induction, including extra-amniotic Foley catheter

Mechanical methods of dilating the cervix are among the oldest known methods of labour induction. The presumed mechanism of action is physical stretching of the cervix and release of endogenous prostaglandins as a result of stimulation of the cervix and lower uterine segment. Placement of an extra-amniotic balloon catheter such as a Foley catheter or the 'Atad' double balloon catheter have been associated with somewhat slower effect than PGE2, less uterine hyperstimulation with fetal heart rate changes and fewer Caesarean sections. Compared with misoprostol 50 μg 4-hourly there were no differences in cervical ripening or labour induction success, fewer uterine contraction abnormalities and less meconium-stained liquor.

Extra-amniotic saline infusion

The stimulatory effect of the extra-amniotic balloon catheter may be enhanced by infusion of normal saline into the extra-amniotic space at 50 ml/h. In a randomized study, extra-amniotic saline infused through a Foley catheter compared with vaginal misoprostol, 25 μg 4-hourly was associated with shorter time to delivery, less frequent abnormal fetal heart rate tracings and less frequent tachysystole. There were no differences in the routes of delivery or neonatal outcomes. Oxytocin was used when necessary in both groups.

The limited data from randomized trials suggest that extra-amniotic saline infusion is an effective method of labour induction and may be safer than methods using exogenous uterine stimulants.

Membrane sweeping

Separating the membranes from the lower uterine segment by a circular motion of a finger inserted through the cervix is a common procedure used to curtail pregnancy. It is associated with an increase in circulating prostaglandins and reduced formal labour inductions, but is uncomfortable and not possible when the cervix is closed or very posterior.

Castor oil, bath, and/or enema

Castor oil, bath and enema were a time-honoured method of inducing labour. Only one randomized trial has evaluated castor oil with inconclusive results. We have shown an association between castor oil, a cathartic, and meconium passage possibly by a direct effect on the fetal bowel.

Other methods

For the following methods of labour induction, there is insufficient evidence either of effectiveness or of benefits over the methods outlined above: extra-amniotic prostaglandins, intravenous prostaglandins, oral prostaglandins, mifepristone, oestrogens, corticosteroids, relaxin, hyaluronidase, acupuncture, breast stimulation, sexual intercourse, and homoeopathic methods.

Induction of labour with previous Caesarean section

In a retrospective study the rates of rupture of a scarred uterus were: 2.5% for labours induced with prostaglandins; 0.77% for other methods of labour induction and 0.52% for spontaneous labour [13]. The Committee on Obstetric Practice of the American College of Obstetricians and Gynecologists have concluded that the risk of uterine rupture during attempts at vaginal birth after Caesarean section is substantially increased with the use of various prostaglandin agents for the induction of labour, and their use for this purpose is discouraged [14]. On the basis of the evidence above relating to uterine hyperstimulation, extra-amniotic saline infusion (or amniotomy alone when the cervix is favourable) may be the safest options for labour induction following Caesarean section. However, there is no direct evidence to substantiate this assumption.

Preterm labour induction

When labour is induced before term, the cervix is often unfavourable. A recent case-control study found shorter labours and fewer cases of severe post-partum haemorrhage in preterm than term or post-term pregnancies induced with PGE2 gel.

Augmentation of labour

Spontaneous labour is divided into a latent phase of variable duration and an active phase during which rapid dilation of the cervix takes place. The active phase on average commences when the cervix is 3 cm dilated and fully effaced.

Augmentation of the latent phase of labour

The latent phase of labour may be difficult to diagnose prospectively as late pregnancy painful contractions with all the appearances of true labour at times fail to progress to active labour. The decision to augment the latent phase of labour, therefore, is more similar to that for labour induction than for augmentation of the active phase of labour. The same attempts to balance potential benefits and risks should be applied, also taking into account the distress caused by ongoing uncertainty as to whether labour is or is not commencing. The latent phase of labour is usually augmented by amniotomy followed by oxytocin infusion either simultaneously or if the response to amniotomy alone is inadequate. For women not known to be free of HIV infection, oxytocin alone or prostaglandins may be used as for labour induction. Extra-amniotic saline infusion may be used if the cervix is narrow enough to retain the Foley catheter bulb.

Augmentation of the active phase of labour

The active phase of labour may be augmented routinely, as in the 'active management of labour' introduced by O'Driscoll and co-workers in the 1960s [15] or selectively when labour progress is considered to be inadequate and the cause thought to be inadequate uterine efficiency. The active management of labour involved stringent criteria for the diagnosis of labour, amniotomy, oxytocin infusion and a commitment to the labouring woman of one-to-one presence of a member of the health-care team, and an expedited delivery. Subsequent research has sought to isolate the individual effects of these interventions.

Routine amniotomy is associated with reduced labour duration (on average 1–2 h), use of oxytocin and low 5-min Apgar scores and a trend to increased Caesarean section.

The Cochrane systematic review of continuous support for women during labour and birth found a reduction in use of analgesia, operative delivery and dissatisfaction with the experience of childbirth, and a non-significant reduction in labour duration. Continuous support is recommended for all women during labour.

The essential factor in the use of augmentation to treat poor progress in labour is the diagnosis of ineffective uterine activity. A common problem is to distinguish between prolonged latent phase of labour and poor progress in the active phase. This may be reduced by stringency in the diagnosis of the active phase. Progress in the active phase of labour is best monitored with a graphical representation of cervical dilation and descent of the presenting part against time (the partograph). Various modifications of the partograph have come into use. Typically, labour progress is considered inadequate when cervical dilation is delayed by 2 or 4 h beyond the expected rate (1 cm/h). If there is no evidence of fetopelvic disproportion uterine activity is assumed to be inadequate and the labour augmented. In the event of uncertainty intrauterine pressure may be monitored to assess uterine activity objectively. Contractions occurring every 3 min, lasting 45 s, and reaching intrauterine pressures of 60–80 mmHg are considered optimal. External assessment of uterine contractions by palpation or with indirect tocography is useful for monitoring the duration and frequency of contractions, but not the intensity.

Labour augmentation for women with previous Caesarean section is controversial. For breech presentation, poor progress in the active phase of labour is regarded as a possible indicator of fetopelvic disproportion and Caesarean section recommended rather than labour augmentation.

When labour augmentation is decided upon, the usual method used is amniotomy (once HIV infection has been excluded) with or without oxytocin infusion as outlined in p. for labour induction.

Conclusion

The most important consideration with respect to labour induction is not how, but whether labour induction should be undertaken. Careful consideration must be given to potential benefits and risks to mother and baby, both physical and emotional, as well as to the state of the uterine cervix. When the cervix is unfavourable, oxytocin infusion and/or artificial rupture of the membranes are less likely to be effective in inducing labour. PGE2 administered vaginally in various formulations is the usual method of labour induction. Misoprostol is a less expensive method. At dosages around 25 µg 4-hourly vaginally, both effectiveness and side effects appear similar to PGE2. Oral misoprostol may have advantages over the vaginal route of administration.

Mechanical methods of labour induction stimulate the cervix and lower uterine segment to release endogenous prostaglandins. Infusion of saline through an extra-amniotic Foley catheter appears to be an effective method of labour induction with low rate of uterine hyperstimulation.

Several other methods of labour induction have not been adequately assessed by randomized trials to be able to be advocated for general use.

References

1. Calder AA (1999) Induction and augmentation of labour. In: Edmonds DK (ed) *Dewhurst's Obstetrics and Gynaecology*. Oxford: Blackwell Science.
2. Olson DM (2003) The role of prostaglandins in the initiation of parturition. *Best Prac Res Clin Obstetrics Gynaecol* **17**, 717–30.
3. Rayburn WF (2002) Preinduction cervical ripening: basis and methods of current practice. *Obstet Gynecol Surv* **57**, 683–91.
4. Bishop EH (1964) Pelvic scoring for elective induction. *Obstet Gynecol* **24**, 266–8.
5. Royal College of Obstetricians and Gynaecologists (RCOG) (2003) *Induction of Labour*. Evidence-based Clinical Guideline (no. 9). London: RCOG Press.
6. Crane JMG & Young DC (2003) Induction of labour with a favourable cervix and/or prelabour rupture of membranes. *Best Prac Res Clin Obstet Gynaecol* **17**, 795–809.
7. MacKenzie IZ & Burns E (1997) Randomised trial of one versus two doses of prostaglandin E2 for induction of labour: 1. Clinical outcome. *Br J Obstet Gynaecol* **104**, 1062–7.
8. Clinical Effectiveness Support Unit Royal College of Obstetricians and Gynaecologists (2001) Induction of labour. Evidence-*Based* Clinical Guidelines (No. 9). London: RCOG Press.
9. Hofmeyr GJ & Gulmezoglu AM (2002) Vaginal misoprostol for cervical ripening and induction of labour (Cochrane Review). *The Cochrane Library*. **1**, CD000941.
10. Goldberg AB, Greenberg MB & Darney PD (2001) Misoprostol and pregnancy. *N Engl J Med* 2001, 2002; **344**, 38–47.
11. Wing DA (2002) A benefit-risk assessment of misoprostol for cervical ripening and labour induction. *Drug Safety* **25**, 665–76.
12. Matonhodze BB, Katsoulis LC & Hofmeyr GJ (2002) Labor induction and meconium: *in vitro* effects of oxytocin, dinoprostone and misoprostol on rat ileum relative to myometrium. *J Perinatal Med* **30**, 405–10.
13. Lydon-Rochelle M, Holt VL, Easterling TR & Martin DP (2001) Risk of uterine rupture during labor among women with a prior cesarean delivery. *N Engl J Med* **345**, 3–8.
14. Committee opinion (2002) Induction of labor for vaginal birth after cesarean delivery. *Obstet Gynecol* **99**, 679–80.
15. O'Driscoll K, Foley M & MacDonald D (1984) Active management of labour as an alternative to cesarean section for dystocia. *Am J Obstet Gynecol* **63**, 485–90.
16. Alfirevic Z (2000) Oral misoprostol for induction of labour (Cochrane Review). *The Cochrane Library*, **4**, CD001338.
17. Hofmeyr GJ, Alfirevic Z, Kelly T *et al.* (2001) Methods for cervical ripening and labour induction in late pregnancy: generic protocol (Protocol for a Cochrane Review). *The Cochrane Library* **4**, CD002074.

Chapter 24: Malpresentation, malposition, cephalopelvic disproportion and obstetric procedures

S. Arulkumaran

Malpresentation and malposition

Introduction and definitions

The lowest pole of the fetus that presents to the lower uterine segment and the cervix is *presentation*. About 95% of fetuses at term present by the *vertex* in labour and hence is called normal presentation. The vertex is a diamond-shaped area defined by the two parietal eminences, anterior fontanellel and posterior fontanellel. When the presentation is other than the vertex, that is, breech, brow, face or shoulder they are termed *malpresentations*.

The definitive aetiology for malpresentations is not known in the majority of cases. They may be associated with contracted pelvis, large baby, polyhydramnios, multiple pregnancy, low-lying placenta, preterm labour, anomalies of the fetus (neck tumours), uterus (congenital or acquired, e.g. lower segment fibroids) or pelvis.

Position is defined by the relationship of the denominator of the presenting part to fixed points of the maternal pelvis. The fixed points of the pelvis are the sacrum posteriorly, sacro-iliac joint postero-laterally, ileo-pectineal eminences antero-laterally and symphysis pubis anteriorly. The denominator is the most definable peripheral point in the presenting part, for example, occiput in vertex, mentum in face and sacrum in breech presentation. Malposition is more applicable to cases of normal presentation, that is, the vertex. The vertex presents itself in the occipito-anterior (OA) – (right, left or direct OA) position in about 90% of the cases in the late first stage of labour at term and is called normal position. In these cases the head is well flexed and presents the smallest anteroposterior (suboccipito-bregmatic) and lateral (biparietal) diameters (9.5 × 9.5 cm^2) and the parietal eminences are at the same level in the pelvis (synclitism). If the occiput lies in the posterior half of the pelvis, then it is considered a malposition. They usually present with a slightly extended head with a larger anteroposterior diameter (occipito-frontal) of 11.5 cm (Fig. 24.1). They may also present with anterior or posterior asynclitism (parietal eminence in the anterior half of the pelvis and lower – anterior asynclitism and

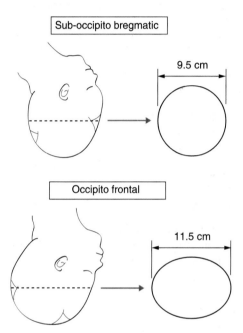

Fig. 24.1 Anteroposterior diameters of the vertex in the well-flexed head (suboccipito-bregmatic – usually OA positions) and slightly deflexed head (occipito-frontal – usually occipito-posterior or transverse positions). (Reproduced from the 1st edition of Dewhurst's textbook of Obstetrics and Gynaecology for Postgraduates.)

posterior – vice versa) when the saggital suture may be shifted more posteriorly or anteriorly (Fig. 24.2). Extension of the head with asynclitism presents a larger diameter and hence longer and difficult labours and more operative deliveries.

A vast majority of cases with malposition correct themselves to normal position due to flexion of the head at the atlanto-occipital joint and the occiput rotates forwards with additional uterine contractions. This is due to the thrust of the spinal column of the fetus on one side of the oval-shaped head which lies on the medially downwards sloping pelvic floor musculature of the levator ani. This natural mechanism of labour promotes spontaneous vaginal deliveries.

213

Asynolitism

The sagittal suture is lying behind
the symphysis pubis

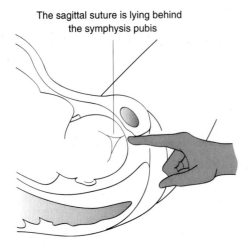

Fig. 24.2 Posterior asynclitism of the vertex – posterior parietal bone is prominent and the sagital suture is shifted much anterior in the pelvis.

Malpresentation (breech, face, brow, shoulder) in labour

Breech presentation

The incidence of breech varies according to the gestation and is 40% at 20 weeks, 6–8% at 34 weeks and 3–4% by term [1]. In most cases of breech there is no reason for the fetus to present by the breech. However, it is useful to look for factors that predispose to breech presentation and ultrasound is useful in this respect. Bicornuate uterus, uterine fibroid, low-lying placenta, multiple pregnancies, polyhydramnios and oligohydramnios are known causes. Rarely could breech presentation be due to congenital malformation such as spina bifida or hydrocephaly.

Identification of breech presentation

The breech commonly presents with flexion at the hip and extension at the knees (extended breech) followed by the breech presenting with flexion at the hips and knees (flexed or complete breech). At times one leg could be flexed and the other extended (incomplete breech). Rarely one or both feet may present (footling breech) and at times it may be knee presentation (Fig. 24.3). Because of the inappropriate fit of the presenting part of the breech to the pelvis, there is a greater chance of cord prolapse and it is higher with footling presentation when it may be as high as 10%. With careful palpation breech presentation is recognized in the antenatal period. Identification becomes easier with increasing gestation and if the mother is multiparous or has a thin abdomen. The fetus would be in the longitudinal lie with the head palpable as a spherical hard mass in the upper pole. The head is usually to one or the other side under the hypochondrium and is tender on deep palpation. The breech which is broader is felt above or within the pelvis. When the breech is extended there is difficulty in identifying the head. It is easier in earlier gestation as the head could be balloted. If the extended breech is in the pelvis it may be difficult to distinguish from a deeply engaged head. An ultrasound examination or vaginal examination will help to identify the head that is engaged. On auscultation with a stethoscope the fetal heart is located above the umbilicus but with a Doptone this may be deceptive as a transducer can pick up the fetal heart rate (FHR) below the umbilicus.

Antenatal management

Increased perinatal mortality and morbidity with breech presentation is well recognized. With routine prenatal

Flexed breech	Footing presentation	Extended (frank) breech
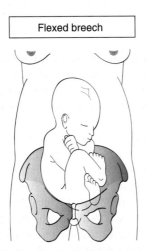	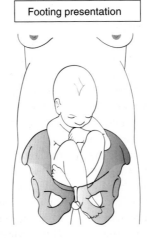	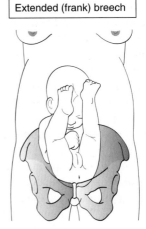

Fig. 24.3 Types of breech presentation.

screening congenital malformation has become a rarer cause leaving prematurity, birth asphyxia due to cord accidents and trauma as the main cause of morbidity. Although current literature recommends elective Caesarian section (CS) for term breeches [2] training in assisted vaginal delivery is needed as some mothers elect to have assisted vaginal births. The study did not address delivery of those who come in established labour with a breech presentation, preterm breeches or breech presentation in multiple pregnancies. There is evidence to suggest that breech presentation may signify an underlying pathology and the mode of delivery may not influence the final outcome [3]. However, the vast majority of cases do not have significant abnormality and delivery as a cephalic presentation or elective CS may reduce morbidity and mortality associated with assisted breech delivery. Hence external cephalic version, ECV, is offered after 36+ weeks as the chance of spontaneous version of breech to cephalic version after 37 weeks is estimated as 1 in 20 [1].

The couple needs adequate counselling of success rates and complications and the details of the procedure. ECV is contraindicated in those with placenta praevia, multiple pregnancies, history of antepartum haemorrhage, intrauterine growth restriction and in those with pre-eclampsia or hypertension. ECV is a relative contraindication for those with uterine scars.

ECV should only be performed in a setting where urgent CS is possible should there be evidence of fetal compromise during or soon after ECV. It is done in the delivery room after confirming by a scan that the fetus is still in breech presentation and after making a note of the side of the fetal back, type of breech presentation, fetal attitude, position of the placenta and the quantity of amniotic fluid. A cardiotocograph (CTG) done 20–30 min prior to ECV should indicate the fetus is not hypoxic. Multiparity, flexed breech presentation, adequate liquour volume and breech mobile above the brim favour the chance of success. Positioning the mother in the Trendelenberg position, intravenous hydration prior to the process with the hope of increasing amniotic fluid, use of vibro-acoustic stimulation and uterine relaxation with a short-acting tocolytic have been advocated to increase the success rates [4]. Forwards or backwards somersault is practised after disengaging the breech and shifting it to the opposite side to where the head is moved, followed by movement of the head to the lower pole. The average success rate is about 60% in multiparous women, less than 40% in primiparous women [5]. ECV has the potential risks of cord accidents, prelabour rupture of membranes, feto-maternal transfusion, placental separation and fetal compromise or death. If the mother was Rhesus negative, anti-D should be prescribed after the attempt of ECV and a Kleihauer-Betke test carried out to determine the adequacy of the dose.

The CTG after ECV for 30–40 min should show a reactive normal trace and no uterine irritability. There should be no bleeding, leaking of amniotic fluid per vagina or uterine tenderness prior to discharge. Those where ECV did not succeed need counselling regards the options of an elective CS or assisted vaginal breech delivery.

Intrapartum management

Careful selection of patients for assisted vaginal delivery is essential to achieve optimal outcome. Frank and complete breech with fetal weights <4000 g are favoured while those with footling should be advised regarding increased chance of cord prolapse. Pelvic adequacy should not be in doubt and clinical estimation appears adequate with no evidence to suggest that CT or X-ray pelvimetry increases the chance of success. Spontaneous onset of labour is preferred. Induction of labour with breech should be only in highly selected cases as CS may be a better option than induction.

Mothers are advised to attend the delivery unit when membranes rupture or with onset of painful contractions. Cord presentation or prolapse should be excluded on admission. The labour is conducted as for vertex presentation. Rate of cervical dilatation and descent of the breech and the FHR pattern are the key arbitrators to guide conduct of labour. If progress of labour was poor, adequacy of uterine contractions should be evaluated. Limited period of oxytocin augmentation could be of value and safe in selected cases. If the progress is poor in the first few hours of augmentation, it is better to opt for CS. The second stage needs full cooperation from the mother and assistance; hence epidural anaesthesia is recommended for pain relief and for management of the second stage.

In most cases of breech presentation there is a tendency for mothers to have early bearing down sensation and hence cervical dilatation should be checked and the mother encouraged to bear down only when the breech has reached the perineal phase of the second stage. It is important not to intervene early and to have the mother in lithotomy only after the anterior buttock and anus of the baby come into view over the mother's perineum with no retraction in between contractions. An episiotomy may not be essential in multipara with a distensible perineum but may be an advantage in a primigravida. This is done with the regional block or with pudendal block and local infiltration of the perineum.

Usually the fetus emerges in the sacro-lateral position. The mother should be encouraged to bear down with uterine contractions to deliver the fetus unassisted up to the level of the umbilicus. Assistance for the breech should be in the form of lateral manipulation with traction only for delivery of the head. In cases with extended knees (frank

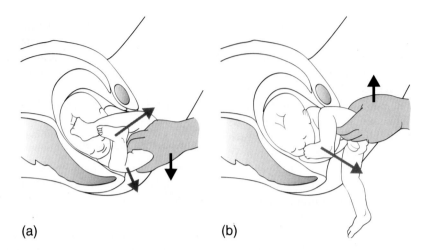

(a)   (b)

Fig. 24.4 Delivery of the extended legs by slight abduction of the thigh and flexion at the knees.

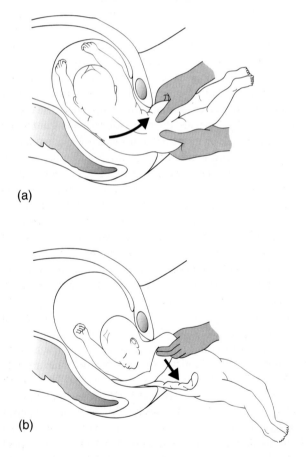

(a)

(b)

Fig. 24.5 Delivery of the arm by rotation of the body so that the posterior shoulder, which was below the sacral promontory, becomes anterior and below the pubic symphysis.

breech) the legs are delivered by slight abduction at the hip followed by flexion of the knees (Fig. 24.4). The body of the fetus is ideally kept with the dorsum facing upwards.

When the scapulae become visible, if the arms are flexed the forearms are delivered by sweeping it in front of the fetal chest. If the arms are extended adduction and flexion of the shoulder followed by extension at the elbow helps to bring down the forearm and hand. In case this was not possible, 'Lovset manoeuvre' is resorted to where the posterior shoulder, which is below the level of the sacral promontory, is brought anterior below the symphysis pubis by rotating the fetus clockwise by holding the baby with the thumbs on the sacrum and index fingers on the anterior superior iliac spines (Fig. 24.5). After delivery of the shoulder which has come anterior the fetus is turned in the anticlockwise direction to enable descent of the opposite shoulder. After delivery of the shoulder the dorsum of the fetus should face anterior and on vaginal examination the chin should be facing the sacrum.

The descent of the head in the pelvis is assisted by the weight of the fetus which is gently supported till the nape of the neck is seen under the symphysis pubis. This signals that the head is low in the pelvis and could be delivered by one of three methods (1) Swinging the trunk towards the maternal abdomen till the mouth and the nose of the fetus become visible; (2) Mauriceau–Smellie Veit manoeuvre can be employed where two fingers are pressed over the maxilla to flex the head and delivery is accomplished by shoulder traction (Fig. 24.6); (3) A Piper or Neville Barnes Forceps can be applied from below while an assistant holds the baby just below the horizontal and traction applied. Following any of the three methods delivery of the fetal head is completed after suctioning the oro-pharynx followed by nasopharynx and by ironing the perineum beyond the forehead.

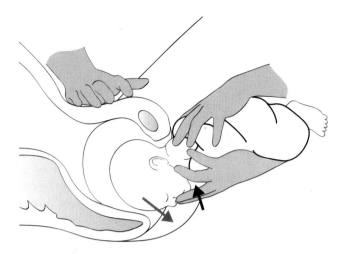

Fig. 24.6 Delivery of the head by jaw flexion and shoulder traction.

Conclusion

Current evidence supports elective CS for term breech presentation. There is not enough evidence to recommend the mode of delivery for preterm breeches. Morbidity and mortality may be more influenced by the gestation and estimated birthweight than the mode of delivery. Hence, it is important to have detailed counselling with the parents and consultation with the paediatricians in coming to an informed decision about the mode of delivery.

Some mothers may prefer assisted vaginal breech delivery and there are others who may be admitted in advanced labour. Their request and needs should be accommodated. The needed skills should be acquired by assisting others, practising assisted breech delivery at the time of CS and on mannequins. Having someone with experience would be more reassuring to the inexperienced accoucheur and to the couple.

Brow presentation

In brow presentation the head is half extended and presents to the pelvis with the largest anteroposterior diameter (mento-vertical – 13 cm). The lower most part of the head that is palpable on vaginal examination is the forehead but it is termed as brow because the orbital ridges and the bridge of the nose are the most definable part of the presentation. The incidence is rare and is about 1 in 1500–3000 deliveries.

The presentation may correct itself in labour by flexion and present as a vertex or undergo further extension and present as a face and may result in vaginal delivery. Persistence of brow presentation in labour at term is not compatible with vaginal delivery and necessitates a CS. In early labour, preparations should be undertaken for CS and time allowed to see whether flexion or extension

would take place. Failure to progress in the next few hours in labour with the persistence of brow presentation is an indication for CS and not for augmentation of labour with oxytocin. In extreme prematurity the fetus may descend as a brow and deliver as a brow or may convert to a face or vertex after it reaches the pelvic floor. Although vaginal delivery is possible in preterm fetuses there is a possibility of spinal cord damage and a CS is preferred. Complications in labour include cord prolapse with membrane rupture and rare incidence of uterine rupture in neglected cases. In cases of intrauterine fetal death and in those with lethal malformation in the extreme preterm period, where injury to the fetus is not a concern, labour may be allowed if there is good progress in anticipation of vaginal delivery. At term, destructive operations and vaginal delivery may be possible for cases of fetal death or lethal anomaly but CS is still preferred in the developed world for fear of genital tract trauma in the hands of those who are not familiar with these techniques.

Face presentation

Face presentation occurs in approximately 1:500 to 1000 deliveries. The general causes for malpresentations apply for face presentation. There is a small chance of congenital abnormality such as anencephaly or thyroid goitre and this need to be excluded by an ultrasound examination. In the majority it is due to extension of the head in a normal fetus. The possibility of face presentation can be suspected on abdominal examination if the prominence of the head is palpable more prominently at a higher level on the opposite side of the fetal spine. In a thin woman a deep groove may be palpable between the occiput and the back. Face presentation is confirmed on vaginal examination when the nose, eyes and the hard gum margins are palpated.

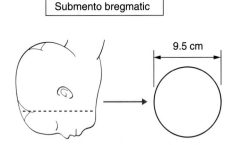

Fig. 24.7 The anteroposterior submento-bregmatic diameter of face presentation. (Reproduced from the 1st edition of Dewhurst's textbook of Obstetrics and Gynaecology for Postgraduates.)

Difficulties may be encountered in recognizing the presentation when the membranes are intact especially if the presenting part is high or in the presence of oedema due to few hours of labour.

The mechanism of labour has some similarity to that of the vertex. The transverse submento-bregmatic diameter enters the pelvis. In the vast majority it rotates forwards to be in the mento-anterior position with the chin behind the symphysis pubis. The presenting lateral (biparietal – 9.5 cm) and anteroposterior (submento-bregmatic – 9.5 cm) diameters are conducive for vaginal delivery (Fig. 24.7). Descent is possible posteriorly in the pelvis when the position is mento-anterior because of large space in the lateral sacral area.

The head is born with the chin emerging under the pubic arch followed by the forehead over the perineum. If the face rotates to a mento-posterior position, although the diameters are the same as mento-anterior, the lateral dimensions of the frontal bones are large and do not permit descent behind the narrow retropubic arch and hence a CS is advisable.

Even with favourable mento-lateral or anterior position if there is failure to progress the safer option for the fetus is CS in the first stage. In late second stage of labour with the face at the outlet in mento-anterior or lateral position outlet forceps delivery can be carried out by skilled personal if spontaneous delivery is not forthcoming.

Shoulder presentation

In multiparous women with singleton pregnancies shoulder presentation is more common without any cause due to the laxity of the uterus. However, there are known associations and they are preterm, congenital fetal or uterine malformation, fibroids, placenta praevia and polyhydramnios. The incidence at term is about 1:400. Transverse lie with shoulder presentation in the antenatal period corrects itself to longitudinal lie with the onset of labour due to increased muscular tone of the uterus. Should rupture of membranes take place with the fetus in the transverse lie, cord prolapse, shoulder presentation and arm prolapse are likely possibilities with progressive cervical dilatation.

In early labour with the membranes intact, one could wait in anticipation of spontaneous or assisted correction to longitudinal lie while making all the preparation for CS. If the membranes rupture and the fetus is still in the transverse lie, CS should be performed to avoid injury to the fetus or the uterus. In cases where the diagnosis is made late the fetus may be impacted in the transverse lie and safe delivery may be only possible by a CS with a midline vertical incision. It may be possible to deliver the fetus through a lower segment transverse incision with acute uterine relaxation using a short acting drug (e.g. 0.25 mg terbutaline in 5 cc saline given IV over 5 min) [6]. Following this treatment if the uterus does not contract despite oxytocics, a small dose of beta blocker such as Propranolol 1 mg IV may be needed to contract the uterus and to avoid post-partum haemorrhage [7]. Labour and spontaneous vaginal delivery is possible in extreme preterm and macerated fetuses.

Cephalopelvic disproportion

The diagnosis of cephalopelvic disproportion is usually retrospective after a well-conducted trial of labour. In the first stage of labour, failure of cervical dilatation despite good contractions, increasing caput and moulding, CTG changes suggestive of head compression and appearance of fresh meconium may suggest the possibility of disproportion. Traditionally one views the failure to progress due to problems with the passage, passenger and power. If the cervix does not dilate satisfactorily (<0.3 cm/h) with 6–8 h of oxytocin augmentation, one should exclude the issues related to power and search for issues related to the passage or passenger. Obvious problems with the passenger such as hydrocephalus, large baby or brow presentation should have been picked up prior to augmentation. Similarly congenitally small pelvis or deformed pelvis due to accident should be known earlier. The shape of the pelvis influences the labour outcome and rarely may it be due to an android or platypelloid pelvis (Fig. 24.8). More common is the relative disproportion caused by different degrees of deflexion or asynclitism of the head presenting a larger diameter. Adequate contractions for 6–8 h may help in flexion, correction of asynclitism and moulding resulting in a smaller diameter of the head. In addition it helps to maximize the pelvic 'give' by more separation of the symphysis pubis. These dynamic changes may result in progress of labour and delivery.

In the second stage of labour, failure of descent of the head with increasing caput and moulding in the presence of good contractions may indicate disproportion. If

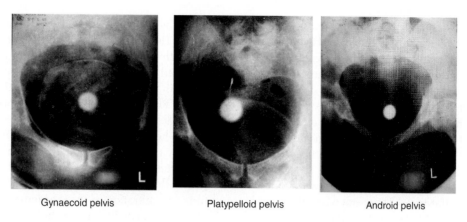

Gynaecoid pelvis   Platypelloid pelvis   Android pelvis

Fig. 24.8 Different pelvic shapes in xxx that influences outcome of labour. (Reproduced from the 1st edition of Dewhurst's textbook of Obstetrics and Gynaecology for Postgraduates.)

there is no progress with spontaneous contractions which are assessed to be inadequate, oxytocin augmentation may be tried for a period of 1 h. If the head is reasonably low that an instrumental delivery is possible then the woman may be encouraged to bear down. Failure of descent indicates disproportion. If this is due to malposition or asynclitism and the station is below spines it may be possible to deliver by forceps or ventouse. Failure to progress due to cephalopelvic disproportion in the first stage and in the second stage when the station is high, delivery is accomplished by CS.

Instrumental vaginal deliveries

The incidence of instrumental vaginal deliveries (IVD) varies from 6 to 12% and depends on the institution and the population. Commonest indications are delay in the second stage of labour, poor maternal effort and fetal distress including cord prolapse in the second stage of labour. Maternal indications include severe cardiac, respiratory or hypertensive disease or intracranial pathology where bearing down effort may be detrimental for her health.

Prolonged second stage may be due to inadequate uterine contractions, poor expulsive efforts by the mother, minor disproportion or malposition. The incidence of IVD is slightly more with the use of epidural analgesia and this may be due to inadequate uterine activity secondary to abolition of Ferguson's reflex due to the absence of reflex release of oxytocin due to stretching of the upper vagina [8]. Inadequate uterine activity in these women may be improved by oxytocin infusion to reduce IVD [9].

Certain prerequisites need to be fulfilled prior to performing an instrumental vaginal delivery. The condition of the mother and the fetus and the clinical situation should be considered carefully. The medical personal should introduce themselves to the woman and her partner and explain the reason for IVD. Assessment should be with a chaperone. The findings and the plan of action and the procedure that is to follow should be explained. Verbal or written consent should be taken based on the protocol after explaining the indication, advantages and disadvantages which should be recorded. It is a distressing time for the mother and her partner and sensitive explanation and counselling is needed.

General examination should include condition of the mother, pain relief and hydration. Analgesia in the form of pudendal block and local perineal infiltration (20 ml of 1% plain lignocaine) may be adequate for low forceps or ventouse deliveries. For midcavity instrumental deliveries an epidural and for a trial of instrumental delivery, spinal anaesthesia may be more suitable. Fetal condition should be evaluated based on clinical information and the degree of normality or otherwise of the auscultation or cardiotocographic findings. In cases of cord prolapse, antepartum bleeding or prolonged deceleration there is some urgency to deliver and actions should proceed with a brisk speed.

Abdominal examination is important to assess the size of the fetus, the fifth of head palpable and the adequacy of uterine contractions. Oxytocin infusion should be considered if uterine contractions are inadequate (less than four in ten minutes each lasting >40 s) in the absence of signs of fetal compromise. Bladder should not be palpable suggesting that it is empty. If not, it should be emptied by catheterization. If the fetus is felt to be large (depends on the size of the mother but should be considered large if the estimate suggests it to be >4.5 kg) extra caution need to be taken to avoid prolonged period of traction and to be prepared for possible shoulder dystocia.

Vaginal examination should confirm the cervix to be fully dilated with absent membranes. The colour and quantity of amniotic fluid should be noted. The presentation should be vertex. Excess caput (soft tissue swelling) or moulding may suggest the possibility of some disproportion. Overlapping of skull bones and inability to reduce it with gentle pressure is considered as moulding +++; ++ indicates overlapping of the bones that can be reduced by gentle digital pressure and + indicates meeting of the bones without any overlap. The position (e.g. left occipito-anterior (LOA) or occipito-transverse (LOT)) and station which is the leading bony part of the skull in relation to ischial spines should be identified. Ideally the station should be below spines with descent of the head with contraction and bearing down effort.

In three dimensional terms, the female pelvis accommodates the fetal head at term. Therefore when the head is 0/5'th palpable above the pelvic brim the leading part of the head should be below the ischial spines. In an obese mother and in those with occipito-posterior positions, palpation of the fifths above the brim may be difficult and may be deceptive. If (1/5)th or (0/5)th of the head was palpable above the brim but on vaginal examination the head was above spines then the small amount of head palpated may have been the fetal chin and the vertex may be in occipito-posterior position. IVD should not be attempted when the head is more than (1/5)th palpable and/or when the station is above spines.

The station and position will determine whether to proceed with IVD and the type of instrument to be used. The position is determined by palpating for the suture lines, posterior fontanelle and occiput. The inverted Y shaped suture lines or overlapping of parietal bones over the occipital bone help to identify the posterior fontanelle. The posterior fontanelle is small and the caput and moulding may make identification difficult. Anterior fontanelle is easily identified as a soft diamond-shaped depression recognized at the junction of the two parietal bones with the two frontal bones. If anterior fontanelle is felt easily around the centre of the pelvis it indicates the possibility of a deflexed head. In a well-flexed head the anterior fontanelle is likely to face the side wall of the pelvis. It is useful to confirm the position by palpating and flicking the fetal ear. The finger has to be moved from the direction of the occiput for the ear to flick. Palpation of the ear also indicates that the largest diameter of the head (i.e. the biparietal eminences) has descended below the midcavity. The sagittal suture should cut the pelvis into halves. If the sagittal suture is far posterior or anterior there is asynclitism and it suggests the reason for the delay and should warn the possible difficulties with IVD. The degree of descent and rotation of the head with contraction and bearing down effort should give some idea about the possibility of successful IVD.

IVD can be performed with the mother in the dorsal position and the legs flexed and abducted or in the left lateral position, but it is much easier when the mother is placed in lithotomy with the buttocks just beyond the edge of the bed. The adequacy of pain relief should be checked. The procedure should be done under antiseptic and aseptic conditions. The vulva and perineum should be cleansed and the bladder catheterized if necessary.

The pain relief needed may be judged by the station of the head. Regional anaesthesia in the form of epidural or spinal anaesthesia is preferred for *mid cavity IVD*, that is, when the head is engaged but the station is above +2 cm but below the ischial spines [10]. If the vertex is beyond +2 cm but not reached the pelvic floor it would be termed *low cavity IVD* and regional or pudendal block anaesthesia with local infiltration of the perineum may be adequate. *Outlet IVD* is carried out when the head is on the perineum with the scalp visible without any separation of the labia. In this situation the vertex would have reached the pelvic floor and would be in the direct, right or left occipito-anterior position needing no rotation or slight rotation of less than 45°. Pudendal block anaesthesia and local infiltration of perineum is generally adequate although some may prefer regional anaesthesia.

It is preferable to deliver by CS if the head is above ischial spines. When vertex is below the spines, IVD is possible and different types of forceps and vacuum could be used depending on the position and station of the vertex. In order to make comparison of outcome, there are suggestions to use the terminology of the specific station and the position (i.e. right occipito-transverse (ROT) at +2 or left occipito-posterior (LOP) at +3) at the time of instrumentation, instead of the broad categories of mid, low and outlet IVD [10].

Choice of instruments – forceps/ventouse

Different forceps and vacuum devices are used for IVD. The choice of forceps or vacuum instrument should depend on the operators experience, station and position of the vertex. Hence the assessment of the station and the position of the vertex are of great importance. For occipito-anterior positions in the mid- or low cavity or low direct occipito-posterior positions (to deliver as face to pubis) the Neville Barnes with or without axis traction handle or the Simpson's forceps can be used. Wrigley's forceps is ideal for outlet deliveries. If the position is occipito-lateral or posterior a Keilland's forceps is needed to achieve rotation without inflicting trauma to the fetus or the maternal passages. Vacuum devices such as silk, silastic or metal cup with the suction tubing arising from the dorsum of the cup, that is, anterior cup can be used for an occipito-anterior position. A posterior metal cup or rigid plastic cup with the suction tubing coming to the lateral side of the cup is needed for an occipito-posterior or lateral position so that the cup can be manipulated between the head and

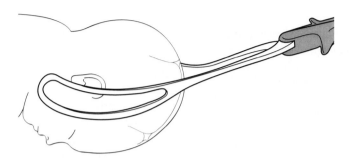

Fig. 24.9 Biparietal-bimalar application offers uniform grip on the two sides. The sagittal suture bisects the shank which is over the flexion point – about 3 cm anterior to the occiput. Not more than a finger can be inserted between the heel of the blade and the head.

the vaginal wall to reach the flexion point that is 3 cm in front of the occiput on the sagittal suture.

Forceps delivery

Most forceps have a pair of fenestrated blades with a cephalic and pelvic curve between the heel and toes (at the distal end) of the blades. The heel continues as a shank which ends in the handle. The handles of the two blades sit together so that they could be held by one hand and are kept in place by a lock on the shank. The cephalic curve is constructed to grasp the fetal head – with the toes of the blades over the maxilla or malar eminences while the length of the blade grasps the sides of the head from the malar area along the side of the head in front of the ear and the parietal bones in front of the occiput. This bimalar-biparietal application exerts uniform pressure on the head. In this position the shank is over the flexion point and thus allowing the correct direction of pull. If the posterior fontanelle is further backwards the blades can be slightly disengaged, lifted upwards and locked so that the downward pull will cause the flexion. The pelvic curve fits the pelvis and is minimal in those forceps used for rotation as in cases with malposition, for example, Kielland's forceps.

Prior to application of forceps the blades should be assembled to check whether they fit together as a pair. The handle which lies on the left hand is the left blade and in cases of direct or LOA positions, it is inserted first negotiating the pelvic and cephalic curve with a curved movement of the blade between the fetal head and the operator's hand kept along the left vaginal wall. The right blade is held by the right hand and is applied between the left hand that protects the vagina and the head by negotiating the cephalic and pelvic curve. If the blades were applied correctly, the handles should lie horizontally and lock easily. The three ESSENTIAL points of, sagittal suture in the midline (i.e. no asynclitism), occiput 3 to 4 cm above the shank (i.e. traction will be along the flexion point) and not more

than one finger space between the head and the heel of the blade (i.e. optimal application with uniform pressure on the head from beyond the malar to the parietal area) should be checked prior to traction (Fig. 24.9). Traction is in the direction of the pelvic curve and is synchronized with contractions and maternal bearing-down efforts. An episiotomy is usually needed when the head is crowning at the vulva. The direction of traction is upwards as the head is born by extension.

KEILLAND'S FORCEPS

Before Keilland's forceps are used, it is essential to identify abdominally the side of the baby's back and the occiput on vaginal examination. The forceps are applied with the 'knobs' facing towards the baby's occiput. The anterior or posterior blade may be applied first directly depending on the preference of the obstetrician. The anterior blade can be positioned by direct, reverse or classical and wandering method. In the wandering method the anterior blade is placed over the face and then moved to lie on the side of the fetal head. The posterior blade can be applied directly. The blades are locked and asynclitism corrected by sliding the shanks on each other till the sliding locks come to the same level. If there is no asynclitism the sagittal suture of the fetus will lie equidistant from the two blades of the forceps. If the blades cannot be locked easily the application of the forceps should be checked and reapplied.

An abnormal position (e.g. occipito-transverse) is corrected by rotating the handles of the forceps blades towards the baby's back and then directing the fetal occiput to the anterior position to emerge underneath the symphysis pubis. When the application is correct with the shank 2–3 cm below the occiput the head is flexed with the traction. An excessive twisting force should not be used. Rotational forceps and vacuum deliveries for malposition are best done by an experienced person or under supervision.

COMPLICATIONS OF FORCEPS

Forceps have been used with less frequency due to a greater incidence of maternal vaginal and perineal lacerations including 3rd and 4th degree tears compared with vacuum deliveries. Transient facial and scalp abrasions are not uncommon but clears in a few days. Paralysis of the VII nerve is rare and it usually resolves within days or weeks. Cephalhaematomas and fracture of the skull are rare and depressed fracture may need elevation by surgery.

Ventouse delivery

Ventouse or vacuum delivery is an alternative for forceps delivery for similar indications in the second stage of labour. The conditions that need to be satisfied for any instrumental delivery need to be checked prior to application. The cups come in different sizes and are usually 4, 5 or 6 cm in diameter. The cup is applied over the flexion point which is 3–4 cm in front of the occiput on the midline indicated by sagittal suture [11]. It is halfway between the two parietal eminences and hence promotes flexion to permit the minimal diameters for the vertex to descend through the pelvis. Application over the flexion point is a flexing median application (Fig. 24.10a). At this site the anterior margin of the cup is 3–4 cm behind the posterior margin of the anterior fontanelle along the sagittal suture. If the position is close to the occiput but not on the midline it is called flexing paramedian application (Fig. 24.10b). If it is in the midline but closer to the anterior fontanelle it is deflexing median (Fig. 24.10c) and if it is off the midline it is deflexing paramedian application (Fig. 24.10d). Deflexing applications expose larger diameters especially if they are paramedian applications.

It is important for the accoucheur to identify the position of the head and to know whether the head is asynclitic so that the cup can be applied correctly over the flexion point. A specially designed cup is needed for occipito-lateral or posterior positions. The tubing should emerge from the lateral aspect of the cup (posterior metal cup) or through a groove in the cup (e.g. Posterior rigid plastic cup – Omni cup) allowing the cup to be inserted and moved between the vaginal wall and the head to reach the flexion point [12]. Soft silk, plastic or anterior metal cup where the tubing comes from the centre of the cup is suitable for application when the head is in the occipito-anterior position as the flexion point is within reach when the labia are parted and the cup is advanced on to the head. These cups are not suitable for occipito-posterior or lateral positions as the lateral vaginal wall would not permit the central stem or suction tubing on the dorsum of the cup for the cup to be shifted to the occiput. Once the cup is placed firmly on the fetal scalp vacuum is created by a hand-held pump or a mechanical pump up to 0.2 bars or 150 mmHg or 0.2 kg/cm^2 negative pressure. The positioning in relation to the sagittal suture and the posterior fontanelle should be checked and inclusion of the vaginal or cervical tissue excluded. The vacuum is increased to 0.7–0.8 bars or 500–600 mmHg or 08. kg/cm^2 prior to commencement of traction with uterine contractions and bearing down effort. There is no need to create the vacuum in steps of 0.2 bar every few minutes or for the release of the vacuum in between traction efforts. The traction needs to be applied in a direction to cause flexion of the head and for it to descend along the axis of the pelvis. Descent of the head with flexion promotes auto-rotation of the head to a favourable occipito-anterior position from the occipito-lateral or posterior position.

Ventouse deliveries in proportion to forceps deliveries have increased over the last decade due to evidence suggesting less perineal trauma including third degree tears [13]. The soft tissue sucked into the cup remains as an elevated circular 'bump' called 'chignon'. This soft tissue swelling settles in the next 2–3 days. Neonatal injuries are scalp abrasions, retinal haemorrhages, haematoma confined to one of the skull bones, neonatal jaundice and rarely subgaleal haemorrhage which could cause severe morbidity and mortality [14]. There is also an increased incidence of neonatal jaundice. Follow-up studies of those who had low outlet instrumental deliveries have shown normal physical and neurological outcome [15].

It is not used in very preterm (<34 weeks) babies and those fetuses with possible haemorrhagic tendencies for fear of causing subgaleal haemorrhage and morbidity or mortality. Application of the ventouse prior to full

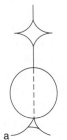
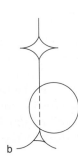
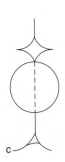
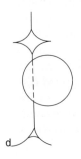

a   b   c   d

Fig. 24.10 Possible placement of the vacuum cup – most favourable to unfavourable (a) to (d); (a) flexing median; (b) flexing paramedian; (c) deflexing median; (d) deflexing paramedian.

dilatation but after 7–8 cm dilated in multiparous women has been practiced by experienced personal but should be treated with caution. In those with cardiac, respiratory or neurological disease where maternal expulsive efforts may cause compromise, forceps may be better than vacuum delivery.

Trial of instrumental delivery

At times it is difficult to assess whether instrumental delivery could be carried out safely or to opt for a CS. If fetal distress is present, CS may be a better option, as further delay may compromise the baby. Trial of instrumental delivery should be done in the theatre under good epidural or spinal anaesthesia and with the theatre team, anaesthetist and paediatrician present. The intent is to abandon IVD should there be any difficulty and to proceed to immediate CS. This should have been explicitly explained to the mother and her partner and appropriate consent obtained prior to the procedure, which should be undertaken by a senior person.

Caesarean section

Delivery of the baby by an abdominal and uterine incision known as Caesarean section (CS) is increasingly used for safe delivery for fetal or maternal reasons either electively or as an emergency. A small proportion is contributed by maternal request for non-medical reasons [16] or by monetary incentives [17]. Advent of blood transfusion with minimal incidence of cross reactions, improved anaesthesia, aseptic and antiseptic techniques and the invention of antibiotics have made it a safe procedure. Depending on the population and the facilities available the incidence varies between 10 and 25% in most developed countries.

INDICATIONS FOR CS

Based on the timing of CS at the time of decision making, the indications are grouped under one of four categories [18].

Category 1 or emergency CS – There is an immediate threat to the mother or the fetus. Ideally the CS should be done within the next 30 min. Some examples are; abruption, cord prolapse, scar rupture, scalp blood pH < 7.20 and prolonged FHR deceleration < 80 beats/min.

Category 2 or urgent CS – There is maternal or fetal compromise but was not immediately life threatening. Here the delivery should be completed within 60–75 min and cases with FHR abnormalities are those of concern.

Category 3 or scheduled CS – The mother needed early delivery but there was no maternal or fetal compromise. There may be concern that continuation of pregnancy is likely to affect the mother or fetus in hours or days to come. This group has a wide range of indications. It may be a case of failure to progress where the CS is planned within the next hour or two or it may be a case of growth-restricted fetus in the preterm period with absent end diastolic flow but a normal CTG or a case with pre-eclampsia where the liver or renal function tests are gradually deteriorating where the CS is planned for within hours to days. The timing of the CS would vary but some plan should be in place to deliver before further deterioration occurs.

Category 4 or elective CS – The delivery is timed to suit the mother and staff. These are cases where there is an indication for CS but there is no urgency and examples include placenta praevia with no active bleeding; malpresentations, (e.g. brow, breech); history of previous hysterotomy or vertical incision CS; past history of repair of vesico-vaginal or recto-vaginal fistulae or stress incontinence; HIV infection.

Placenta accreta is more common with anterior placenta praevia in women with a scar. This may result in massive haemorrhage and rarely the need for a hysterectomy and hence consent and preparations should be appropriate. Placement of intra-arterial catheters for embolization of uterine arteries at the time of CS should be considered where facilities exist.

Elective CS is generally done around 39 weeks as the incidence of tachypnoea of the newborn is much less after this gestation. However, the medical or obstetric condition determines the gestation at which the elective CS is planned – the main principle being to carry out the CS as late as possible in gestation without compromising the maternal or fetal health.

TYPES OF CAESAREAN SECTION

The CS is described based on the type of incision on the uterus.

Lower uterine segment incision

Lower segment CS involves a horizontal incision on the lower segment after reflecting the visceral peritoneum. This is the commonest CS procedure. The abdomen is opened by a low midline, paramedian and more commonly by a Pfannenstiel (suprapubic horizontal) incision and the peritoneal cavity opened. The bladder is reflected from the lower segment and a transverse incision is made on the lower uterine segment care being taken not to injure the fetus. The presenting part is delivered through the lower segment. A forceps can be used to assist delivery in a cephalic presentation.

Traditionally the lower uterine segment muscle is closed in two layers followed by closure of the visceral peritoneum. The merits of single versus two layer closure of the muscle and closure versus non-closure of the visceral peritoneum is currently being investigated by the 'Caesarian section surgical techniques (CAESAR)' randomized controlled study. Lower segment CS (LSCS) is the commonest procedure because it is easier to incise the lower segment, deliver the fetus from the point of incision and to approximate the layers because of the thin muscle layers compared with the upper segment. In addition the peritoneal layer can be closed and was thought to provide an advantage against infection. The blood loss and infection rate is much less with LSCS compared with an upper segment CS.

The uterine cavity should be cleaned not to leave any retained tissue. It should be made sure that the cervical os is open to allow drainage of blood. Closure of the uterine wound is followed by peritoneal toilet when any blood or liquor in the abdomen and pelvis is removed using suction or gauze swabs on a sponge holder. The opportunity is taken at this stage to inspect the ovaries and tubes. Prophylactic antibiotics and low molecular weight heparin against thromboembolism shall be routinely administered intra-operatively by the anaesthetists. If the mother is Rhesus negative and the baby is Rhesus positive, a dose of anti-D should be given and a Kleihauer-Betke test performed to determine the adequacy of the dose of Anti-D. Care of the mother should be similar to that after any major abdominal surgery.

Midline vertical incision

The midline vertical incision could be in the lower or upper segment of the uterus. Commonly it starts in the lower segment as a small buttonhole incision till the uterine cavity is reached and is extended upwards. Because of the difficulty in making the incision, increased blood loss, inadequate approximation at closure, increased post-operative morbidity and inability to offer a trial of vaginal delivery in the next pregnancy due to possible higher incidence of scar rupture, the midline incision is reserved for specific indications.

A midline approach is used when the lower segment approach is difficult because of fibroids or anterior placenta praevia with large vessels in the lower segment. Other indications are preterm breech with poorly formed lower segment, impacted transverse lie with ruptured membranes or transverse lie with a congenital anomaly of the uterus. An extreme example is a perimortem CS.

In special circumstances a lower or upper segment (or spanning both segments) vertical or an inverted T incision is made.

COMPLICATIONS ASSOCIATED WITH CS

Morbidity and mortality associated with the procedure cannot be totally avoided. The common complications are haemorrhage, anaesthesia-related complication and infection. Prophylactic antibiotics are administered to reduce the incidence of infection. Occasionally there is injury to bowel, bladder, ureters or the fetus. Thromboembolism is rare but could be fatal and hence pre-, intra- and post-operative precautions should be taken to avoid it. Intra operatively pneumatic inflatable boots are used for the legs and prophylactic dose of heparin is administered. Post-operatively the use of heparin, graded elastic stockings, mobilization and chest and leg physiotherapy are advocated to reduce the incidence of deep venous thrombosis (DVT).

Late complications of wound infection and secondary haemorrhage are not that uncommon. Vesico- or ureterovaginal fistulae due to visceral injury are extremely rare.

Anaesthetic complications are extremely rare due to the availability of experienced anaesthetists and most CS being performed under regional anaesthesia. Women may rarely complain of light general anaesthesia causing awareness which goes unnoticed by the anaesthetists as the women are paralysed. Other problems include vomiting on induction and post-operative lung atelectasis following general anaesthesia. Aspiration of gastric contents leads to Mendelson's syndrome which is a dreaded complication of general anaesthesia that can result in maternal mortality. To reduce such an event gastric contents are neutralized with 20 ml of 0.3 Sodium citrate and gastric emptying promoted with Metoclopramide 10 mg IV. For elective CS, Ranitidine 150 mg, an H_2 agonist is administered 2 h before surgery. In those who had a meal recently or who had opiates pre-operative emptying of the stomach is advocated to minimize risk of post-operative aspiration.

Caesarean hysterectomy is needed for uncontrollable post-partum haemorrhage, placenta accreta or uterine rupture and for cervical malignant disease as part of planned treatment. Maternal mortality is extremely low and is usually related to the reason for which a CS is done or due to anaesthetic or haemorrhagic complications and is estimated to be less than 0.33 per 1000.

Episiotomy and perineal lacerations

Perineal lacerations may occur with normal or instrumental vaginal delivery. Vulval and anterior vaginal tears do occur with vaginal delivery but posterior vaginal tear associated with perineal injury is more common and occurs with the delivery of the head and at times with the shoulders. Perineal tears are classified based on the involvement of the perineum.

First degree tear involves the skin only while the second degree involves the perineal muscle. Injury to anal sphincter is classified as third degree tear and is subdivided based on the degree of involvement. If less than half the thickness of the external anal sphincter is involved it is categorized as 3a and it becomes 3b if it is a full thickness involvement and 3c when the internal sphincter gets involved. When the tear damages the sphincter and involves the anal epithelium it is called fourth degree tear.

EPISIOTOMY

Episiotomy is an intentional surgical incision of the perineum after informed consent with the aim of increasing the soft tissue outlet dimensions to help with childbirth. It is not advocated for every delivery and the rate of episiotomy depends on the philosophy and judgement of the caregiver.

Episiotomy is advocated when anterior tears with bleeding or multiple perineal tears appear. When there is fetal distress it is carried out to expedite delivery. It facilitates instrumental vaginal deliveries although the need for an episiotomy is less with ventouse deliveries and a distensible perineum. If the delivery process is delayed and it is thought to be due to a rigid perineum an episiotomy may facilitate delivery. Whenever there are vaginal manipulations needed such as in some assisted breech deliveries and in cases of shoulder dystocia an episiotomy may be useful. Those women who had a previous pelvic floor or perineal surgery may also benefit by an episiotomy.

In the USA, a midline episiotomy starting from the fourchette for a few centimetres towards the anus is popular while a mediolateral episiotomy starting from the fourchette going laterally to 45° is carried out in the UK. A sharp scissors is used to make a single incision about 3–6 cm depending on the size of the perineum. The depth involves the superficial perineal muscles like a second degree tear. If episiotomy is performed with normal vaginal delivery then local perineal infiltration may be adequate. In cases of instrumental vaginal delivery the woman may have epidural or spinal anaesthesia. Whatever anaesthesia is used it is important to check whether she could feel the pain prior to the incision and if needed additional local infiltration should be used.

Although midline episiotomies are associated with minimal bleeding, easier to repair, has less pain post repair and heals well compared with the mediolateral episiotomy it is associated with more 3rd and 4th degree tears because of the straight easy extension into the anus.

Appreciable blood loss is not uncommon with episiotomy and is avoided by performing the episiotomy when the head crowns. Early incision increases blood loss and immediate repair after delivery will help to minimize blood loss.

PERINEAL REPAIR

The adequacy of pain relief should be rechecked prior to starting the repair which is made easy with good light and optimal exposure. The exposure and difficulty with seeing the edges of the vaginal skin due to bleeding from above can be overcome by placing a tampon or vaginal swab with a tail that comes outside the introitus. Care should be exercised to remove this tampon or swab after completion of the repair. The vagina is very vascular and the descending branches attached to the vaginal skin might retract and hence the apex of the tear or episiotomy should be secured by a suture above the apex to stop any bleeding. The suture is then threaded down at half to 1 cm intervals taking each vaginal wall in turn with a continuous locking suture using a synthetic suture material like 'vicryl rapide'. This helps in haemostasis and prevents vaginal shortening. The distance between sutures in the medial side may be longer compared with the lateral vaginal wall to bring about good approximation so that at the fourchette the hymenal membrane and the junction of the pink vaginal skin to pigmented outer skin margin at the introitus meet as it was before the tear or the episiotomy.

The perineal muscles can be approximated by continuous or interrupted sutures. The perineal skin is approximated by subcuticular suture as it is associated with less pain and heals well. Continuous, loose non-locking sutures to approximate perineal muscles and subcuticular structure has been found to be a suitable method with less pain and no need for removal of sutures [19]. A vaginal examination should confirm good approximation of the cut edges and good haemostasis. A rectal examination is not always necessary but helps to exclude accidental suture involvement of the rectum.

Before cleaning and placing a pad against the vagina an instrument, needle and swabs count should be carried out. Detailed documentation should include estimated blood loss and post repair care should include sufficient instructions for pain relief including appropriate analgesics.

Although rare, episiotomy and perineal tears may be complicated by bleeding, pain and haematoma formation necessitating additional medical or surgical intervention within hours of repair. Late complications include infection, breaking down of the repair, pain, scarring, dyspareunia and rarely fistula formation. Endometriosis of the scar is exceptional but should be entertained if a woman complains of cyclical pain at the site of the episiotomy.

THIRD AND FOURTH DEGREE TEARS

Careful examination will reveal the extent of damage as to whether it is 3 a, b, c or 4th degree tear. Once recognized as 3rd or 4th degree the repair has to be done in the operating theatre with good lighting, experienced assistance, appropriate instruments and under anaesthesia to relax the sphincter muscle as dissection and mobilization of the muscle is necessary. Anal epithelial tears are repaired with 3/0 vicryl rapid sutures and the knots are placed on the side of the lumen. 3/0 PDS suture with a round bodied needle is used for repair of the muscle. End to end or overlapping method can be used as shown in Fig. 24.11a,b [20].

Post-operative care is important and is managed with laxative, stool softener and antibiotic. The symptoms may persist and the repair may not be always successful with a risk of incontinence of faeces and flatus. Where facilities permit patients should have follow-up to evaluate their symptoms and if necessary to do suitable investigations such as endo-anal ultrasonograpy or anal manometry studies. If symptoms persist repair by an experienced colorectal surgeon may need to be considered.

References

1. Westgren M, Edvall H, Nordstrom L, Svalenius E & Ranstam J (1985) Spontaneous cephalic version of breech presentation in the last trimester. *Br J Obstet Gynaecol* **92**, 19–22.
2. Hofmeyer GJ & Hannah ME (2001) Planned Caesarean section for term breech delivery. *Cochrane Database Syst Rev* **1**, CD000166. Review. Update in: *Cochrane Database Syst Rev* (2003) **3**, CD000166.
3. Ingemarsson I, Arulkumaran S & Westgren M (1989) Breech delivery – management and long term outcome. In Tejani N (ed.) USA: CRC Press Inc, 143–59.
4. Annapoorna V, Arulkumaran S, Anandakumar C, Chua S Montan S & Ratnam SS (1997) External cephalic version at term with tocolysis and vibroacoustic stimulation. *Int J Obstet Gynecol* **59**, 13–8.
5. Hofmeyer G & Kulier R (2003) External cephalic version for breech presentation at term (Cochrane Review). *The Cochrane Library*, Issue **1**. Oxford:Update Software.
6. Chandraharan E & Arulkumaran S (2005) Tocolytics. *Curr Opin Obstet Gynaecol* **17**, 151–6.
7. Anderson K, Ingemansen I, Penson CG (1975) Effects of terbutaline on human uterine activity at term. *Acta Obstet Gynecol Scand* **54**, 165–72.
8. Ferguson JKW (1941) A study of the motility of the intact uterus at term. *Surg Gynecol and Obstet* **73**, 359–66.
9. Saunders N, Spiby H, Gilbert Z (1989) Oxytocin infusion during second stage of labour in primiparous women using epidurmal analgesia. A randomised controlled trial. *BMJ* **299**, 423–26.
10. ACOG Practice Bulletin (2000) Operative Vaginal Delivery. Clinical management guidelines for the obstetrician—Gynecologist, number 17, June 20.
11. Aldo Vacca (1992) Clinical principles in 'Handbook of Vacuum extraction in obstetric practice' Ed. Aldo Vacca, Edward Arnold Publishers, London 1992, 22–27.
12. Hayman R, Gilby J & Arulkumaran S (2002) Clinical evaluation of a 'handpump' vacuum delivery device. *Obstet Gynecol* **100**, 1190–5.
13. Johanson RB & Menon BKV (2002) Soft versus rigid vacuum extractor cups for assisted vaginal delivery (Cochrane review). *The Cochrane Library* Issue 4, Oxford: Update Software.
14. Uchil D & Arulkumaran S (2003) Neonatal subgaleal hemorrhage and its relationship to delivery by vacuum extraction. *Obstet Gynecol Surv* **58**(10), 687–93.
15. Murphy D, Lebling R, Veruty L, Swingler R & Patel R (2001) Early maternal and neonatal morbidity associated with operative delivery in second stage of labour: a cohort study. *Lancet* **358**, 1203–7.
16. Penna L & Arulkumaran S (2003) Cesarean section for non-medical reasons. *Int J Gynaecol Obstet* **82**(3), 399–409.
17. Finger C (2003) Caesarean section rates skyrocket in Brazil. *Lancet* **362**, (9384), 628.
18. RCOG Clinical effectiveness support unit (2001) *The National Sentinel Caesarean Section Audit Report. Classification of Urgency of Caesarean Section.* London: RCOG Press, 49–53.
19. Kettle C, Hills RK, Jones P, Darby L, Gray R & Johanson R (2002) Continuous versus interrupted perineal repair with standard or rapidly absorbed sutures after spontaneous vaginal birth: a randomized controlled trial. *Lancet* **359**, 2217–23.
20. Thakar R & Sultan AH (2005) The management and prevention of Obstetric perineal trauma. In: Arulkumaran S, Penna LK, & Bhasker Rao K (eds) *The Management of Labour* Chennai: Orient Longmans, 252–68.

Further reading

Baskett T & Arul Kumaran S (2002) Operative delivery and intrapartum surgery. *Best Prac Res Clin Obstet Gynaeco* **16** (1).

Ralpha W Hale (2001) *Dennen's Forceps Deliveries*, 4th edn. Washington: The American College of Obstetricians and Gynaecologists – Women's Health Care Physicians.

Society of Obstetricians and Gynecologists of Canada (2004) Clinical Practice Guidelines No 148 – Guidelines for operative vaginal birth. (www.sogc.org)

Baskett T & Arulkumaran S (2004) *Intrapartum Care for the MRCOG and Beyond.* RCOG Publication:

Chapter 25: Hypertensive disorders

Andrew Shennan

Introduction

Hypertension in pregnancy is a significant management problem for every obstetrician. In a minority of cases it is associated with proteinuria, and this usually indicates a multisystem disease, also known as pre-eclampsia. It is this syndrome that is associated with increased morbidity and mortality to both mother and baby. However, hypertension alone may be the first signs of pre-eclampsia and therefore cannot be presumed innocent. In addition it is increasingly recognized that chronic hypertension has associated perinatal problems.

Incidence, classification and definition

Pregnant women with hypertension can be broadly divided into one of three categories: chronic hypertension, non-proteinuric hypertension (sometimes known as pregnancy-induced hypertension) or pre-eclampsia. To distinguish between these is clinically useful as management and likely prognosis are disparate. In the United Kingdom fewer than ten women will die each year from pre-eclampsia [1] but this remains a relatively common cause of death in pregnany in the developed world. Only about one in two thousand women will have an eclamptic convulsion but the associated maternal mortality is 2% [2]. Eclampsia itself is not usually life threatening, but is associated with severe disease, and women will usually die from an unrelated complication of pre-eclampsia. Of all maternal deaths, fewer then half are associated with eclampsia. It has been estimated by the World Health Organization (WHO) that worldwide approximately 60,000 women will die each year from pre-eclampsia.

Hypertension in pregnancy is common occurring in approximately one in five women after 20 weeks' gestation. However, only a small minority of these have serious disease associated with morbidity. Concern about adverse effects results in intensive surveillance of a large number of women; as a result almost a quarter of antenatal admissions are a result of monitoring and managing women with hypertension. Obstetric day units help reduce the need for inpatient management. As the cause and onset of the disease is unpredictable, frequent assessment of women with pregnancy-induced hypertension remains the mainstay of safe clinical practice.

As delivery is the only cure for pre-eclampsia, it is the commonest cause of iatrogenic prematurity accounting for 15% of all premature births and approximately one in five very low birthweight infants (<1500 g) [3]. Size at birth is related to future health [4] and therefore pre-eclampsia may result in future adult disease for the baby. This includes an increased risk of hypertension and diabetes when they become adults. Maternal disease and fetal involvement do not always correlate, for example, in those women who have Eclampsia; at term they often have normal weight [2]. There is, however, a clear relationship between persistently raised blood pressure and morbidity and mortality; still-birth rates are higher at *any* gestation when the maternal diastolic pressure is equal to or greater than 95 mmHg [5].

In an average UK population the incidence of pre-eclampsia occurs in less than 1 in 20 women. In a primigravida population in Ireland the incidence was as low as 2% [6]. It is generally recognized that non-proteinuric hypertension occurs in at least three times as many people. Some studies from the United States have demonstrated the prevalence of pre-eclampsia to be nearer 10%, possibly related to the high-risk status population studied.

The key signs of pre-eclampsia are hypertension and proteinuria and these are used to define the disease. These are responses to end-organ damage and they are not always the most important nor fundamental aspects of the syndrome, but are used as they are easy to measure. For pragmatic reasons the threshold of abnormality of blood pressure and proteinuria is not high in order to avoid missing 'at risk' cases. The International Society for the Study of Hypertension in Pregnancy (ISSHP) uses the term gestational hypertension when women have previously been normotensive (Table 25.1). This definition is based on the original recommendations of Davey and MacGillvray [7].

Table 25.1 A summary of the ISSHP classification

A. Gestational hypertension and/or proteinuria developing during pregnancy, labour or the puerperium in a previously normotensive non-proteinuric woman
    1. Gestational hypertension (without proteinuria)
    2. Gestational proteinuria (without hypertension)
    3. Gestational proteinuric hypertension (pre-eclampsia)
B. Chronic hypertension (before the 20th week of pregnancy) and chronic renal disease (proteinuria before the 20th week of pregnancy)
    1. Chronic hypertension (without proteinuria)
    2. Chronic renal disease (proteinuria with or without hypertension)
    3. Chronic hypertension with superimposed pre-eclampsia (new onset proteinuria)
C. Unclassified hypertension and/or proteinuria
D. Eclampsia

Definitions:
Hypertension in pregnancy:
A. Diastolic BP $\geq$ 110 mmHg on any one occasion OR
B. Diastolic BP $\geq$ 90 mmHg on 2 or more consecutive occasions $\geq$4 h apart
Proteinuria in pregnancy:
A. One 24 h collection with total protein excretion $\geq$300 mg per 24 h OR
B. Two 'clean-catch – midstream' or catheter specimens of urine collected $\geq$4 h apart with $\geq$2 + on reagent strip

Table 25.2 Risk factors for pre-eclampsia at antenatal booking

	Relative risk	Confidence intervals
Antiphospholipid syndrome	9.72	4.34–21.75
Previous history of pre-eclampsia	7.19	5.83–8.83
Pre-existing diabetes	3.56	2.54–4.99
Multiple pregnancy	2.93	2.04–4.21
Nulliparity	2.91	1.28–6.61
Family history	2.90	1.70–4.93
Raised BMI		
(a) before pregnancy	2.47	1.66–3.67
(b) at booking	1.55	1.28–1.88
Age over 40	1.96	1.34–2.87
Raised diastolic blood pressure (>80 mmHg)	1.38	1.01–1.87

Pathophysiology

Pre-eclampsia has been known as 'The Disease of Theories', as the exact course of events that lead to the clinical syndrome have not been elucidated. However, there is an increasing understanding of these events. It is known that pre-eclampsia is fundamentally related to poor trophoblast invasion in the myometrium and this results in maternal spiral arteries being hampered in their normal physiological vasodilatation [8]. The maternal syndrome of pre-eclampsia must be related to additional factors as inadequate trophoblast invasion is also seen in pregnancies complicated by fetal growth restriction without maternal disease. It is clear that impaired intervillous blood flow results in inadequate perfusion and ischaemia in the second half of pregnancy. This probably results in the production of reactive oxygen species. Once the normal endogenous antioxidants are overwhelmed, a condition of oxidative stress exists. This is probably fundamental to the clinical syndrome of pre-eclampsia. Either through oxidative stress or other vasoactive substances being released from the placenta, activation of the vascular endothelium occurs [9]. The vascular endothelium is known to supply all organ systems and this explains the widespread aspects of the syndrome. Markers of endothelial damage are frequently raised. In addition there is abnormality in lipid profiles, such that triglycerides and free fatty acids are roughly doubled. There is an increase in lipid peroxidation both systemically and in the placenta suggesting that oxidative stress is fundamentally involved in the endothelial cell damage.

Management

Identifying those at risk: clinical risk factors

Although most women who get pre-eclampsia do not have risk factors, a significant proportion (>1 in 3) will. Taking a careful history will allow risk assessment. The National Institute of Clinical Excellence (NICE) antenatal guidelines suggests this is an important part of clinical management and recommends that at first contact a woman's level of risk for pre-eclampsia should be evaluated so that a plan for her subsequent schedule of antenatal appointments can be formulated. These guidelines have indicated the following as risk factors for developing pre-eclampsia; nulliparity, age 40 or older, a family history of pre-eclampsia (e.g. pre-eclampsia in a mother or sister), a prior history of pre-eclampsia, a body mass index (BMI) at or above 35 at first contact, a multiple pregnancy or pre-existing vascular disease (e.g., hypertension or Diabetes) [10]. A recent systematic review has quantified some of these risks at the booking visit [11] (Table 25.2).

As family history in a first degree relative is strongly related to pre-eclampsia, this illustrates the significant genetic influence. Exposure to the paternal antigen via either the fetus or the partner does have an influence suggesting an immunological element to the disease process. Pre-eclampsia is more common in first pregnancies and even miscarriages or termination of pregnancy will provide some reduction in risk [12]. Non-barrier methods of contraception and increased duration of sexual cohabitation have been reported to reduce risk [13,14]. Both teenage mothers and pregnancies conceived by donor insemination increase the risk [15]. If pregnant by a partner who has previously fathered an affected pregnancy the woman has nearly double the risk of pre-eclampsia [16]. These clinical observations are probably related to exposure to paternal antigens. Underlying medical diseases particularly those involving the cardiovascular system increase the risk of pre-eclampsia suggesting that maternal susceptibility is an important factor in response to the placental aetiology [17,18]. This includes glucose intolerance either in a form of gestational or established diabetes. Obesity is an independent risk factor for pre-eclampsia. Placental size may be important, as molar pregnancies are a rare cause of pre-eclampsia occurring prior to 20 weeks gestation. Pregnancies complicated by hydrops fetalis (mirror syndrome) or trisomy chromosomal component also have an increased risk. Previous pre-eclampsia is a strong risk factor, particularly if early onset; approximately one out of five women who have required delivery before 37 weeks will have a recurrence.

Identifying those at risk: investigations

Tests to predict pre-eclampsia can be broadly divided into biophysical and biochemical. The most promising biophysical test is that of uterine artery Doppler. This is a relatively quick and inexpensive test that can be performed at a similar time to the anomaly scan. It has the advantage of identifying poor placental perfusion, which is fundamental to the disease process. There is a relatively high resistant circulation with a notch apparent in the uterine artery Doppler (Fig. 25.1).

As change to a normal low-resistant circulation can be delayed the later the test is performed the better its predictive value. Approximately one in five women who have an abnormal Doppler at 20 weeks' gestation will develop pre-eclampsia [19]. At 24 weeks' gestation the prediction value is greater. Identifying women at risk will allow increase in surveillance and use of prophylactic therapies can be considered. If adequate preventative measures become available then these screening test will become increasingly important. However, the value of using such biophysical tests, in terms of improving outcome, has as yet not been established, and NICE do not recommend their use in low-risk women [10]. Doppler measurements are used more commonly in high-risk women, although the likelihood ratios are lower, and positive tests in both high- and low-risk women give similar absolute risks or positive predictive values, approximately 20%.

Other biophysical tests, such as the measure of blood pressure do have a predictive value when measured in early pregnancy [11]. Even within a normal blood pressure range the level of blood pressure is related to risk. However, this is seriously confounded by the poor technique in measuring blood pressure. Attempts have been made to improve this by using automated blood pressure measurement but at the moment these remain largely ineffective as they use an oscillometric technique to measure blood pressure which is inaccurate in pre-eclampsia [20]. Other biophysical test such as isometrics exercise testing and the "roll over test" have very poor predictive value and have to become established in clinical practice. The angiotensin II sensitivity tests involve assessing blood pressure response to infusing the vasoconstrictor angiotensin II but this was also not clinically practical both due to poor prediction and being a time consuming and costly investigation [21].

Numerous haematological and biochemical markers have been used to both predict and evaluate pre-eclampsia. The simple measurements of haemoglobin and haematocrit have a weak association with the development of pre-eclampsia as does plasma volume. In women who have chronic hypertension the measure of uric acid and platelets can help in determining those who get superimposed pre-eclampsia; again they lack sensitivity and specificity. Second trimester human chorionic gonadotropin and maternal serum alpha feto protein is

Abnormal (high resistance and notch)

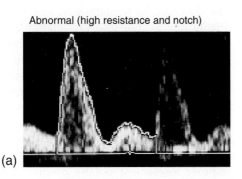

(a)

Normal (low resistance)

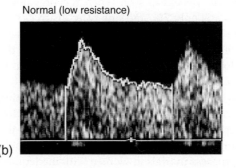

(b)

Fig. 25.1 A comparison of normal and abnormal fetal velocity waveforms.

associated with a twofold increase of pre-eclampsia. This is probably related to the disease process at the utero-placental interface. The predictor value again is not large enough to be clinically practicable. Endothelial activation does occur in pre-eclampsia and there are many markers that are increased that are related to endothelial damage. Some will increase prior to clinical manifestations of the disease but almost invariably there is overlap in women who are subsequently normal and those who have serious disease, again limiting the clinical usefulness. Investigation such as urinary excretion of calcium, microalbuminuria and prostacyclin metabolites have all been investigated. Combinations of markers may improve predictive values and future work is likely to consider combining endothelial and placental markers to develop algorithms that can be introduced in a practical way. However, until prophylactic measures that are clinically useful are introduced these tests will remain largely investigatory. Table shows markers that have been investigated in early pregnancy and how they change in relation to subsequent pre-eclampsia [22].

Prophylactic therapies

The key to modern management of pre-eclampsia is close surveillance and timely delivery prior to serious consequences. In an ideal world preventing the manifestation of the disease would be far more preferable. Aspirin, calcium, and antioxidants have all been investigated, with some evidence of success. Fish oils, magnesium and even rhubarb [23] have shown less promise.

Low-dose aspirin reverses the imbalance between the vasoconstrictor thromboxane A_2 and the vasodilator prostacyclin, which is known to occur in pre-eclampsia. There are 42 randomized controlled trials published in the Cochrane collaboration demonstrating a 15% relative risk reduction in pre-eclampsia when either aspirin or other antiplatelet agents are given. There is a similar reduction (14%) in the risk of death to the baby as well as an 8% reduction in the risk of preterm delivery [24]. It is generally accepted that aspirin should be considered in high-risk women. Benefit is seen when the prevalence of pre-eclampsia is only 7%, and one baby death can be prevented for every 250 treated [25]. The evidence demonstrates it is safe. There are ongoing investigations as to the appropriate dose and timing as well as the population to be targeted.

There are 10 trials in nearly 7000 women demonstrating the beneficial role of calcium as pre-eclamptic prophylaxis and overall there is a significant reduction in the incidence of pre-eclampsia [26]. However, this is largely related to the success in trials in women with inadequate calcium intake, and the benefit to the baby is not as clear as

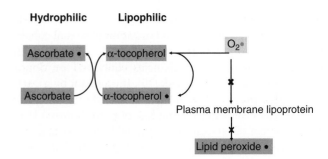

Fig. 25.2 Synergy between vitamin C and E: postulated mechanism for preventing oxidative stress damage.

aspirin. The WHO has recently completed a trial (results awaited) to see whether supplementation in developed countries is worthwhile. The investigations into the use of fish oils containing N3 fatty acid known to inhibit platelet thromboxane A2 have not shown a significant reduction in pre-eclampsia. As oxidative stress is known to be fundamental to the disease process one trial demonstrated that vitamin C and E supplementation in the second trimester of pregnancy may be beneficial, demonstrating more then a 50% reduction when high-risk women were treated [27]. This involved 1000 mg vitamin C and 400 IU vitamin E, which are known to act synergistically (Fig. 25.2); however, further studies which are currently ongoing need to confirm this.

COMBINING PREDICTION AND PREVENTION

A test does not have to be perfect to be a useful clinical tool. As pre-eclampsia has a relatively low prevalence, numbers needed to treat to prevent one case can be dramatically reduced when combining a relatively modest test in terms of predictive powers (e.g. 20%) with treatment. Figure 25.3 demonstrates the relationship between predication and relative risk reduction, in terms of the numbers needed to treat [28].

Assessment of the mother

The threshold of hypertension and proteinuria are relatively low to diagnose pre-eclampsia so the first key aspect of management involves confirming the diagnosis to ensure that iatrogenic morbidity does not ensue. Hypertension that occurs in early pregnancy, that is, before 28 weeks' gestation results in pre-eclampsia developing in approximately 50% of women. In contrast women who present at term with hypertension are unlikely to develop pre-eclampsia (approximately a 10% risk). Care in assessing both blood pressure and proteinuria can improve assessment as false positive and negative tests are commonplace.

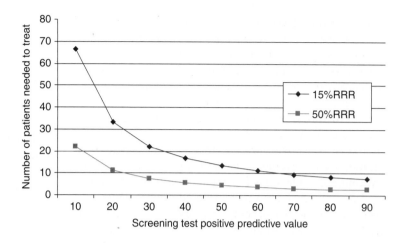

Fig. 25.3 Positive predictive value and relative risk reduction (RRR) on numbers needed to treat.

Digit preference (the practice of rounding the final digit of blood pressure to zero) occurs in the vast majority of antenatal measurements and simply taking care to avoid this will limit inaccurate diagnoses. Using a standard bladder in a sphygmomanometer cuff will systematically undercuff 25% of an average antenatal population. Having large cuffs available and using them will prevent the overdiagnosis of hypertension [29]. Keeping the rate of deflation to 2–3 mmHg will prevent overdiagnosing diastolic hypertension, as will using Korotkoff 5, which is now universally recommended for diagnosing diastolic hypertension. Korotkoff 4 (the muffling of the sound) is less reproducible, and randomized controlled trials confirmed that it is safe to abandon it, except in those rare situations when the blood pressure approaches zero [30,31]. Dipstick proteinuria is not only prone to false positive results but also an equal prevalence of false negatives. Twenty-four hour collections of urine are necessary to confirm the diagnosis. New automated devices can be used to assess proteinuria. They significantly improve predictive values [32]. Protein/creatinine ratios can be used for immediate assessment as they are similar to the accuracy of 24-h collections.

It is possible to have severe disease and normal blood pressure or proteinuria. In a survey in women with eclampsia, only just over half had a recent measurement indicating both significant proteinuria and hypertension [2]. The syndrome of pre-eclampsia is multisystemic, and other organ involvement must be carefully considered, including the placenta. Other signs of the disease have not been included in the definition for pragmatic reasons, but they are often equally important. A careful history should also include whether women have symptoms such as visual disturbance, headaches and epigastric pain. Sometimes nausea or even vomiting can be a presenting feature. However, at least 50% of women even with severe disease will be asymptomatic [2]. When managing women, particularly remote from term, involvement of all organ systems must be carefully investigated.

Platelets are consumed due to the endothelial activation. A falling count, particularly to less than $100 \times 10^9/l$ may indicate a need to consider delivery. Counts above 50 are likely to support haemostasis. An increasing haematocrit or haemoglobin indicates hypovolaemia, which is characteristic of severe disease. If labour is anticipated then clotting abnormalities should be checked as pre-eclampsia can cause disseminated intravascular coagulation. This is important if regional anaesthesia is used, which is preferable to general anaesthesia. Renal tubular function can be assessed by measuring uric acid, which is a marker of disease severity, although normal levels can occur in severe disease. Acute fatty liver can result in spuriously high levels of uric acid (along with high white cell count, and low glucose). Urea and creatinine are associated with late renal involvement and generally not useful as indicators of disease severity. Liver transaminases should be measured to indicate hepatocellular damage. Normal ranges of transaminases are approximately 20% lower than non-pregnant [33]. Subcapsular involvement of the liver can occur, resulting in epigastric pain with normal transaminase measurements. HELLP (Haemolysis, Elevated Liver Enzymes, Low Platelets) syndrome occurs when liver involvement is associated with haemolysis and low platelets. This is a severe variant of pre-eclampsia. When protein excretion exceeds 3 g in 24 h, the circulating albumin is likely to fall (nephrotic syndrome) and this increases the risk of pulmonary oedema. Lactate dehydrogenase levels will increase in the presence of haemolysis.

Antenatal corticosteroids should be given to enhance fetal lung maturity, and are not contraindicated in pre-eclampsia. Steroid therapy is also known to help recovery from HELLP syndrome and has been used in the post-partum period. Antenatal corticosteroids may actually improve biochemical markers in women with pre-eclampsia. The treatment of blood pressure should be reserved principally for severe hypertension, that is, blood pressures over 170/110 mmHg. However, this does require urgent therapy. Treatment of moderate hypertension may be detrimental to fetal growth [34], and moderate blood pressure should not be aggressively treated. Once fetal lung maturity is likely to be adequate, delivery should be considered, that is, after 32 weeks' gestation. Multiorgan involvement or fetal compromise would be indications for delivery. Close inpatient supervision is otherwise required and can be considered prior to 32 weeks' gestation or when the benefit of conservative management is judged to outweigh delivery. Conservative management will reduce neonatal morbidity, without substantially increasing maternal problems. Recent evidence suggests that under 30 weeks neonatal morbidity is high, and conservative management is desirable [35]. However, at least one third of women still need to be delivered for fetal reasons under 34 weeks.

The inability to control hypertension, deteriorating liver or renal function, progressive fall in platelet or albumin, or neurological complications would be indications for maternal delivery at any gestation.

Fetal assessment

Early onset pre-eclampsia is particularly involved with placental insufficiency, and more than half of babies born before 34 weeks will be growth restricted [35]. This also explains why abruption is more common, occurring in about 1 in 20 of these early onset cases. Fetal well-being should always be carefully considered in all cases of pre-eclampsia, and includes a symphyseal fundal height assessment, as well as a general enquiry as to fetal movements. At early gestations an ultrasound scan must be performed to assess fetal growth, and should include determination of the amniotic fluid index and umbilical artery Doppler waveforms. A non-reactive CTG with decelerations or a fetal condition that is deteriorating warrants delivery, as it is unlikely to improve with time and may worsen with antihypertensive therapy.

Intrapartum care of pre-eclampsia

Many units have now developed a severe pre-eclampsia protocol. Cases which require protocol determined management are often defined as those with severe hypertension (greater than 170/110 mmHg) or hypertension with an additional complication such as headache, visual disturbance, epigastric pain, clonus (more than three beats) or a platelet count less than 100 or AST more than 50 IU units per litre.

Table 25.3 Maternal mortality 1985–2002: immediate hypertensive deaths

Intracerebral haemorrage	24 (37%)
Pulmonary (ARDS/oedema)	43 (35%)
Other	35 (28%)
Total	123

The confidential enquiry into maternal deaths demonstrates that the two main reasons why women die are cerebral haemorrhage or adult/acute respiratory distress syndrome [1]. Table 25.3 demonstrates all data from these causes since 1985, when data was made available from the whole of the United Kingdom. The two most important factors that contribute to these deaths are therefore severe hypertension and fluid intake. The control of blood pressure and fluid balance is therefore critical. In contrast to pulmonary causes of death, in recent years, deaths related to intracerebral haemorrhage have not been reduced, suggesting control of blood pressure remains suboptimal through poor monitoring and treatment (Fig. 25.4).

Blood pressure control

Blood pressure should be measured frequently (at least every 15 min). Automated sphygmomanometers can be used to facilitate this, or alternatively intra-arterial readings can be assessed via a peripheral arterial pressure transducer. As non-invasive measurements are obtained principally by oscillometric blood pressure devices, which underestimate blood pressure in pre-eclampsia [20,36], significant changes in blood pressure should be confirmed using mercury sphygmomanometry. Some devices are now accurate, and only those specifically assessed for accuracy in pre-eclampsia should be purchased in the future [37]. On an individual patient basis the accuracy of any device used should be established against an observer using standard sphygmomanometry, preferably with a mercury sphygmomanometer. Mean arterial pressures (MAP) are generally used to guide management in protocols. Antihypertensive therapy should be instigated when the MAP is ≥125 mmHg, or urgently if >140 mmHg as above this cerebral autoregulation of pressure is not reliable. Either hydrallazine or labetalol can be used as a first line treatment, although labetalol is favoured [38]. As these are important emergency measures in preventing stroke, clinicians involved in the management of severe pre-eclampsia should be familiar with treatment regimes. Some protocols advocate infusing a colloid to protect the uteroplacental circulation if the baby is undelivered. This should be done with caution, and careful consideration to the impact of the overall fluid management, and preferably under central venous pressure (CVP) surveillance.

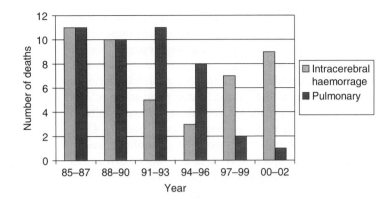

Fig. 25.4 Maternal mortality 1985–2002: immediate hypertensive deaths.

Control of fluid balance

Strict monitoring of input and output is essential in the sick pre-eclamptic patient. A combination of the reduced intravascular volume, leaking capillaries and low albumin make women prone to pulmonary oedema. Renal failure is a rare complication of pre-eclampsia but should be considered when there has been inadequate transfusion or profound hypotension following post-partum bleeding, as there is reduced intravascular volume. Oliguria is relatively common, and strict monitoring should be considered rather than aggressive blind fluid replacement. Administration of intravenous fluid in the oliguric patient must be done with caution. Most protocols will limit fluid intake to approximately 1 ml/kg/h. CVP monitoring and Foley catheter insertion should be used whenever possible. Repetitive fluid challenges should be avoided in the absence of invasive monitoring. Should the CVP be high (>8 mmHg) with persistent oliguria then a dopamine infusion can be considered (1 μ/kg/min.) Haemodialysis or haemofiltration may be necessary if the creatinine or potassium rises. Close communication with a renal physician should be sought. Administration of diuretics will only temporarily improve urine output, and confounds the reduced circulating volume. Frusimide should therefore be reserved for treating pulmonary oedema. Pulmonary artery catheterization should be considered in difficult cases.

Anticonvulsant management

An eclamptic fit is usually self-limiting; however, anticonvulsive therapy should be given to abort it when possible. Magnesium sulphate can be used to control such a fit (up to 8 mg given by slow intravenous infusion). Diazepam 10 mg can also be used but its anticonvulsant properties are short-lived as compared to its sedative properties. In those women who have prolonged fitting a brain scan is required to rule out an intracerebral bleed. Following an eclamptic fit magnesium sulphate is the prophylaxis of choice [39]. Magnesium sulphate has been demonstrated to reduce cerebral ischaemia by acting as membrane stabilizer and vasodilator and is superior to both diazepam and phenytoin in preventing further fits. It is also associated with a significant reduction in the need for maternal ventilation and intensive care admissions. Magnesium sulphate is given in a 2 g intravenous loading dose in an infusion of 1 g/h. Some protocols suggest 2 g/h but efficacy has been demonstrated at 1 g/h. It is renally excreted so therefore in cases of oliguria or rising urea care must be taken regarding toxicity and this is detected by absence of patellar reflexes. Respiratory arrest and muscle paralysis along with cardiac arrest can occur and an antidote is 10 ml of 10% calcium gluconate. Even with severe pre-eclampsia, eclamptic fits are rare and occur in less than 2%. The Magpie trial evaluated giving magnesium sulphate versus placebo in women with pre-eclampsia and there was a significant reduction in fits in those women receiving treatment; magnesium sulphate will roughly halve the incidence of eclampsia [40]. The evidence also suggests that there are less maternal deaths but trials have not been large enough to show that this is significantly so. The threshold for giving magnesium sulphate to a pre-eclamptic woman is uncertain but generally as the risk increases the benefit favours therapy.

Anaesthetic management

Endotracheal intubation can cause severe hypertension and general anaesthetic should be avoided [41]. Regional blockade is therefore the anaesthesia of choice; prior to insertion a coagulopathy should be excluded. Platelet level of more than 80×10^9 are likely to ensure haemostasis and most obstetric anaesthetists would be happy to perform this procedure under such circumstances. In women who have a Caesarean section a low threshold for invasive CVP monitoring is necessary. Careful management of fluid particularly following post-partum haemorrhage is essential. Following delivery one in three eclamptic fits will occur in the post-partum period most of these within 48 h [2]. Although eclampsia has been reported beyond this time it is not usually associated with serious morbidity and generally anticonvulsant prophylaxis can be stopped within a 48-h period. Blood pressure should be monitored carefully for at least 4 days following delivery as the highest reading can occur at this time [42]. Quite frequently it is necessary to give women antihypertensive therapy at home and follow-up is recommend at 6 weeks. Methyldopa has generally unwanted side effects and most common antihypertensive therapies can be used.

Post-natal management

At the post-natal follow-up both blood pressure and urine should be checked for underlying renal and cardiovascular abnormalities. It is now clear that women who had pre-eclampsia have a doubling of subsequent ischaemic heart disease probably related to underlying vascular pathology. This risk is greater the more growth restricted and premature her baby is. At the post-natal visit future pregnancies should be discussed as well as the need for screening for hypertension in later life.

References

1. Department of Health (2001) *Why Mothers Die*, 1197–1999. Report on Confidential Enquiries into Maternal Deaths in the United Kingdom. London: ROCG Press.
2. Douglas KA & Redman CWG Eclampsia in the United Kingdom. *Br Med J* **309**, 1395–400.
3. Project 27/28 (2003) *An Enquiry into Quality of Care and Its Effect on the Survival of Babies Born at 27–28 weeks*. London: London Stationery Office.
4. Barker DJP, Bull AR & Osmond C (1990) Fetal and placental size and risk of hypertension in adult life. *BMJ* **301**, 259–61.
5. Freidman EA & Neff RK (1996) Pregnancy outcome is related to hypertension, odema and proteinuria. In: Churchill D & Beevers DG (eds) *Hypertension in Pregnancy* London: BMJ Books.
6. Higgins JR, Walshe JJ, Halligan A, O'Brien E, Conroy R & Darling MR (1997) Can 24-hour ambulatory blood pressure measurement predict the development of hypertension in primigravidae? *Br J Obstet Gynaecol* **104**, 356–62.
7. Davey DA & MacGillivray I (1988) The classification and definition of the hypertensive disorders of pregnancy. *Am J Obstet Gynecol* **158**, 892–8.
8. Brosens IA (1977) Morphological changes in the utero-placental bed in pregnancy hypertension. *Clin Obstet Gynaecol* **77**, 573–93.
9. Roberts JM, Taylor RN, Musci TJ, Rodgers GM, Hubel CA & McLaughlin MK (1989) Pre-eclampsia: an endothelial cell disorder. *Am J Obstet Gynecol* **161**, 1200–4.
10. National Institute for Clinical Excellence (2003) *NICE Guideline CG6 Antenatal Care – Routine Care for the Healthy Pregnant Woman*. London: NICE.
11. Duckitt K & Harrington D (2005) Risk factors for pre-eclampsia at antenatal booking: systematic review of controlled studies. *Br Med J* **330**, 565.
12. Strickland DM, Guzick DS, Cox K, Gant NF & Rosenfeld CR (1986) The relationship between abortion in the first pregnancy and development of pregnancy-induced hypertension in the subsequent pregnancy. *Am J Obstet Gynecol* **154**, 146–8.
13. Klonoff-Cohen HS, Savitz DA, Cefalo RC & McCann MF (1989) An epidemiologic study of contraception and pre-eclampsia. *J Am Med Assoc* **262**, 3141–7.
14. Robillard PY, Hulsey TC, Perianin J, Janky E, Miri EH & Papiernik E (1994) Association of pregnancy-induced hypertension with duration of sexual cohabitation before conception. *Lancet* **344**, 973–5.
15. Need JA, Bell B, Meffin E & Jones WR (1983) Pre-eclampsia in pregnancies from donor insemination. *J Reprod Immunol* **5**, 329–38.
16. Lie RT, Rasmussen S, Brunborg H, Gjessing HK, Lie-Nielsen E & Irgens LM (1998) Fetal and maternal contributions to risk of pre-eclampsia: population based study. *BMJ* **316**, 1343–7.
17. Rey E & Couturier A (1994) The prognosis of pregnancy in women with chronic hypertension. *Am J Obstet Gynecol* **171**, 410–6.
18. McCowan LM, Buist RG, North RA & Gamble G (1996) Perinatal morbidity in chronic hypertension. *Br J Obstet Gynaecol* **103**, 123–9.
19. Mires GJ, Williams FL, Leslie J & Howie PW (1998) Assessment of uterine arterial notching as a screening test for adverse pregnancy outcome. *Am J Obstet Gynecol* **179**, 1317–23.
20. Penny JA, Shennan AH, Halligan AW Taylor DJ, de Swiet M & Anthony J (1997) Blood pressure measurement in severe pre-eclampsia. *Lancet* **349**, 1518.
21. Kyle PM, Buckley D, Kissane J, de Swiet M & Redman CW (1995) The angiotensin sensitivity test and low-dose aspirin are ineffective methods to predict and prevent hypertensive disorders in nulliparous pregnancy. *Am J Obstet Gynecol* **173**, 865–72.
22. Robyn North. Can we predict pre-eclampsia? In: *Pre-eclampsia*. London: RCOG Press, 257–75.
23. Zhang ZJ, Cheng WW & Yang YM (1994) [Low-dose of processed rhubarb in preventing pregnancy induced hypertension]. Zhonghua Fu Chan Ke Za Zhi **29**, 463–4.
24. Duley L, Henderson-Smart D, Knight M & King J (2001) Antiplatelet drugs for prevention of pre-eclampsia and its consequences: systematic review. *Br Med J* **322**, 329–33.
25. Duley L, Henderson-Smart DJ, Knight M & King JF (2003) Antiplatelet agents for preventing pre-eclampsia and its complications. *Cochrane Database Syst Rev* **4**, CD004659. DOI: 10.1002/14651858.CD004659.
26. Atallah AN, Hofmeyr GJ & Duley L (2002) Calcium supplementation during pregnancy for preventing hypertensive disorders and related problems. *Cochrane Database Syst Rev* **1**, CD001059. DOI 10.1002/14651858.CD001059. Cochrane calcium.
27. Chappell LC, Seed PT, Briley AL *et al.* (1999) Prevention of pre-eclampsia by antioxidants: A randomized trial of

vitamins C and E in women at increased risk of pre-eclampsia. *Lancet* **354**, 810–6.

28. Shennan AH (2003) Recent developments in antenatal care. *Br Med J* **327**, 604–8.

29. Shennan AH & Waugh J (2003) The measurement of blood pressure and proteinuria in pregnancy. In: *Pre-eclampsia*. London: RCOG press, 305–24.

30. Shennan A, Gupta M, Halligan A, Taylor DJ & de Swiet M (1996) Lack of reproducibility in pregnancy of Korotkoff phase IV as measured by mercury sphygmomanometry. *Lancet* **347**, 139–42.

31. Brown MA, Buddle ML, Farrell T, Davis G & Jones M (1998) Randomised trial of management of hypertensive pregnancies by Korotkoff phase IV or phase V. *Lancet* **352**, 777–81.

32. Waugh J, Bell SC, Kilby M, Seed P, Blackwell C & Shennan AH, Halligan AWF (2005) Optimal bedside urinalysis for the detection of proteinuria in hypertensive pregnancy – a study of diagnostic accuracy? *Br J Obstet Gynaecol* **112**(4), 412–7.

33. Girling JC, Dow E & Smith JH (1997) Liver function tests in pre-eclampsia: importance of comparison with a reference range derived for normal pregnancy. *Br J Obstet Gynaecol* **104**(2), 246–50.

34. Von Dadelszen P, Ornstein MP, Bull SB, Logan AG, Koren G & Magee LA (2000) Fall in mean arterial pressure and fetal growth restriction in pregnancy hypertension: a meta-analysis. *Lancet* **355**, 87–92.

35. Shear RM, Rinfret D & Leduc L (2005) Should we offer expectant management in cases of severe preterm preeclampsia with fetal growth restriction? *Am J Obstet Gynecol* **192**(4), 1119–25

36. Natarajan P, Shennan A, Penny J, Halligan A & de Swiet M (1999) A comparison of an oscillometric and auscultatory automated blood pressure monitor in pre-eclampsia. *Am J Obstet Gynaecol* **181**, 1203–10.

37. Golara M, Benedict A, Jones C, Randhawa M, Poston L & Shennan AH (2002) Inflationary oscillometry provides accurate measurement of blood pressure in pre-eclampsia. *Br J Obstet Gynaecol* **109**, 1143–7.

38. Magee LA, Cham C, Waterman EJ, Ohlsson A & von Dadelszen P (2003) Hydralazine for treatment of severe hypertension in pregnancy: meta-analysis. *Br Med J* **327**(7421), 955–60.

39. Which anticonvulsant for women with eclampsia? Evidence from the Collaborative Eclampsia Trial. *Lancet* 1995; **345**(8963), 1455–63.

40. The Magpie Trial Collaboration G (2002) Do women with pre-eclampsia, and their babies, benefit from magnesium sulphate? The Magpie Trial: a randomised placebo-controlled trial. *Lancet* **359**(9321), 1877–90.

41. Allen RW, James MF, Uys PC *et al.* (1991) Attenuation of the pressor response to trachael intubation in hypertensive proteinuric pregnant patients by lignocaine, alfentanil and magnesium sulphate. *Br J Anaesth* **66**, 216–23.

42. Atterbury JL, Groome LJ, Hoff C (1998) Yarnell JA. Clinical presentation of women readmitted with postpartum severe preeclampsia or eclampsia. *J Obstet Gynecol Neonatal Nurs* **27**(2), 134–41.

Chapter 26: Heart disease in pregnancy

Catherine Nelson-Piercy

Introduction

Although pregnancies complicated by heart disease are rare in the UK, Europe and the developed world, cardiac disease is now the leading cause of maternal death in the UK (CEMACH) [1]. There were 44 indirect deaths attributed to cardiac disease in 2000–2002, giving a death rate of 2.2 per 100,000 maternities. The maternal mortality rate from cardiac disease has continued to rise since the early 1980s. The major causes of cardiac deaths over the last 10 years are cardiomyopathy (predominantly peripartum), myocardial infarction (predominantly coronary artery dissection), dissection of the thoracic aorta and pulmonary hypertension. In the UK, rheumatic heart disease is now extremely rare in women of childbearing age and mostly confined to immigrants. There have been no maternal deaths reported from rheumatic heart disease since 1994.

Women with congenital heart disease, having undergone corrective or palliative surgery in childhood survive into adulthood, are encountered more frequently. These women may have complicated pregnancies. Women with metal prosthetic valves face difficult decisions regarding anticoagulation in pregnancy.

Because of significant physiological changes in pregnancy, symptoms such as palpitations and signs such as an ejection systolic murmur are very common and innocent findings. Not all women with significant heart disease are able to meet these increased physiological demands. The care of the pregnant and parturient woman with heart disease requires a multidisciplinary approach, involving obstetricians, cardiologists and anaesthetists, preferably in a dedicated antenatal cardiac clinic. This allows formulation of an agreed and documented management plan encompassing management of both planned and emergency delivery.

The most common and important cardiac conditions encountered in pregnancy are discussed below.

Physiological adaptations to pregnancy, labour and delivery

Blood volume starts to rise by the 5th week after conception secondary to oestrogen- and prostaglandin-induced relaxation of smooth muscle that increases the capacitance of the venous bed. Plasma volume increases and red cell mass rises, but to a lesser degree, thus explaining the physiological anaemia of pregnancy. Relaxation of smooth muscle on the arterial side results in a profound fall in systemic vascular resistance and together with the increase in blood volume, determines the early increase in cardiac output. Blood pressure falls slightly but by term has usually returned to the prepregnancy value. The increased cardiac output is achieved by an increase in stroke volume and a lesser increase in resting heart rate of 10–20 beats/min. By the end of the second trimester the blood volume and stroke volume have risen by between 30 and 50%. This increase correlates with the size and weight of the products of conception and is therefore considerably greater in multiple pregnancies as is the risk of heart failure in heart disease [2].

Although there is no increase in pulmonary capillary wedge pressure (PCWP), serum colloid osmotic pressure is reduced. The colloid oncotic pressure–pulmonary capillary wedge pressure gradient is reduced by 28%, making pregnant women particularly susceptible to pulmonary oedema. Pulmonary oedema will be precipitated if there is either an increase in cardiac pre-load (such as infusion of fluids), or increased pulmonary capillary permeability (such as in pre-eclampsia), or both.

In late pregnancy in the supine position, pressure of the gravid uterus on the inferior vena cava (IVC) causes a reduction in venous return to the heart and a consequent fall in stroke volume and cardiac output. Turning from the lateral to the supine position may result in a 25% reduction in cardiac output. Pregnant women should therefore be nursed in the left or right lateral position wherever possible. If the mother has to be kept on her back, the pelvis should be rotated so that the uterus drops forward and cardiac output as well as uteroplacental blood flow is optimized. Reduced cardiac output is associated with reduction in uterine blood flow and therefore in placental perfusion; this can compromise the fetus.

Labour is associated with further increases in cardiac output (15% in the first stage and 50% in the second stage). Uterine contractions lead to auto transfusion of 300–500 ml of blood back into the circulation and the sympathetic response to pain and anxiety further elevate heart rate and blood pressure. Cardiac output is increased more during contractions but also between contractions. The rise in stroke volume with each contraction is attenuated by good pain relief and further reduced by epidural analgesia and the supine position. Epidural analgesia or anaesthesia cause arterial vasodilatation and a fall in blood pressure [3]. General anaesthesia is associated with a rise in blood pressure and heart rate during induction but cardiovascular stability thereafter. Prostaglandins given to induce labour have little effect on haemodynamics but ergometrine causes vasoconstriction and syntocinon can cause vasodilation and fluid retention.

In the third stage up to a litre of blood may be returned to the circulation due to the relief of inferior vena cava obstruction and contraction of the uterus. The intrathoracic and cardiac blood volume rise, cardiac output increases by 60–80% followed by a rapid decline to pre-labour values within about 1 hour of delivery. Transfer of fluid from the extravascular space increases venous return and stroke volume further. Those women with cardiovascular compromise are therefore most at risk of pulmonary oedema during the second stage of labour and the immediate post-partum period. All the changes revert quite rapidly during the first week and more slowly over the following 6 weeks, but even at a year; significant changes still persist and are enhanced by a subsequent pregnancy [4].

Normal findings on examination of the cardiovascular system in pregnancy

These may include a loud first heart sound with exaggerated splitting of the second heart sound and a physiological third heart sound at the apex. A systolic ejection murmur at the left sternal edge is heard in nearly all women and may be remarkably loud and be audible all over the precordium. It varies with posture and if unaccompanied by any other abnormality it reflects the increased stroke output. Venous hums and mammary souffles may be heard. Because of the peripheral vasodilatation the pulse may be bounding and in addition ectopic beats are very common in pregnancy.

Cardiac investigations in pregnancy

The electrocardiographic (ECG) axis shifts superiorly in late pregnancy due to a more horizontal position of the heart. Small Q-waves and T-wave inversion in the right precordial leads are not uncommon. Atrial and ventricular ectopics are both common.

The amount of radiation received by the fetus during a maternal chest X-ray (CXR) is negligible and CXRs should never be withheld if clinically indicated in pregnancy. Transthoracic echocardiogram is the investigation of choice to exclude, confirm or monitor structural heart disease in pregnancy. Transoesophageal echocardiograms (TOE) are also safe with the usual precautions to avoid aspiration. Magnetic resonance imaging (MRI) and chest computerized tomography (CT) are safe in pregnancy. Routine investigation with electrophysiological studies and angiography are normally postponed until after pregnancy but angiography should not be withheld in, for example, acute coronary syndromes.

General considerations in pregnant women with heart disease

The outcome and safety of pregnancy are related to the
• presence and severity of pulmonary hypertension
• presence of cyanosis
• haemodynamic significance of the lesion
• functional class as determined by the level of activity that leads to dyspnoea [New York Heart Association, NYHA] [5].
Most women with pre-existing cardiac disease tolerate pregnancy well if they are asymptomatic or only mildly symptomatic (New York Heart Association class II or less) before the pregnancy, but important exceptions are pulmonary hypertension, Marfan's syndrome with a dilated aortic root and some women with mitral or aortic stenosis.

Cardiac events such as stroke, arrhythmia, pulmonary oedema and death complicating pregnancies in women with structural heart disease, are predicted by [6]
• a prior cardiac event or arrhythmia
• NYHA classification > II
• cyanosis
• left ventricular ejection fraction <40%
• left heart obstruction (mitral valve area <2 cm^2, aortic valve area <1.5 cm^2, aortic valve gradient (mean – non-pregnant) >30 mmHg).
These features therefore also act as reasons to refer to specialist centres for counselling and management of the pregnancy.

Women with cyanosis (oxygen saturation <80–85%) have an increased risk of intrauterine growth restriction, fetal loss, and thromboembolism secondary to the reactive polycythaemia. Their chance of a live birth in one study was less than 20% [7].

Women with the above risk factors for adverse cardiac or obstetric events should be managed and counselled by a multidisciplinary team including cardiologists with expertise in pregnancy, obstetricians with expertise in cardiac disease, fetal medicine specialists and paediatricians. There should be early involvement of obstetric anaesthetists and a carefully documented plan for delivery.

Specific cardiac conditions

Congenital heart disease

Asymptomatic acyanotic women with simple defects usually tolerate pregnancy easily. Many defects will have been treated surgically or by the interventional paediatric cardiologist but others are first discovered during pregnancy. Women with congenital heart disease are at increased risk of having a baby with congenital heart disease, and should therefore be offered genetic counselling if possible before pregnancy [8] and detailed scanning for fetal cardiac anomalies with fetal echocardiography by 18–20 weeks' gestation.

Acyanotic congenital heart disease

ATRIAL SEPTAL DEFECT

After bicuspid aortic valve (which is much commoner in males), secundum ASD (atrial septal defect) is the commonest congenital cardiac defect in adults. Paradoxical embolism is rare and arrhythmias do not usually develop until middle age. Mitral regurgitation caused by mitral leaflet prolapse develops in up to 15% of uncorrected ASDs. Pulmonary hypertension is rare.

No problems are anticipated during pregnancy but acute blood loss is poorly tolerated. It can cause massive increase in left-to-right shunting and a precipitous fall in left ventricular output, blood pressure, coronary blood flow and even cardiac arrest.

VENTRICULAR SEPTAL DEFECT AND PATENT ARTERIAL DUCT

Like regurgitant valve disease, these defects, which increase the volume load of the left ventricle, are well tolerated in pregnancy unless the defects are large and complicated by pulmonary vascular disease.

PULMONARY STENOSIS

Pulmonary stenosis does not usually give rise to symptoms during pregnancy. But, when severe and causing right ventricular failure, balloon pulmonary valvotomy has been successfully carried out during pregnancy. The procedure is best carried out during the second trimester with maximal uterine shielding.

AORTIC STENOSIS

Left ventricular outflow tract obstruction at any level can cause problems during pregnancy. Prepregnancy assessment is the ideal. Significant obstruction results if the aortic valve area is <1 cm^2 or if the non-pregnant mean gradient across the valve is >50 mmHg. Indications that pregnancy will be high risk include failure to achieve a normal rise in blood pressure without the development of ST- or T-wave changes during exercise, impaired left ventricular function and symptoms.

The ECG will normally show left ventricular hypertrophy and the Doppler transaortic valve velocity will rise during pregnancy if the stroke volume increases in a normal fashion. If the left ventricular systolic function is impaired the left ventricle may not be capable of generating a high gradient across the valve so that a low gradient may be falsely reassuring.

Any patient who develops angina, dyspnoea or resting tachycardia should be admitted to hospital for rest. Administration of a β-adrenergic blocking drug will increase diastolic coronary flow time and left ventricular filling with resultant improvement in angina and left ventricular function. If despite these measures angina, pulmonary congestion and left ventricular failure persist or progress, balloon aortic valvotomy needs to be considered [9]. These valves are intrinsically not ideal and severe aortic regurgitation may be created but, if successful, the procedure may buy time and allow completion of the pregnancy. The procedure can also be carried out for relief of discrete subaortic stenosis but with some risk of causing mitral regurgitation.

COARCTATION OF THE AORTA

Most cases encountered will already have been surgically corrected, although residual narrowing is not uncommon. Aortic coarctation may first be diagnosed during pregnancy and should always be excluded when raised blood pressure is recorded at booking.

Although the blood pressure can be lowered adequate control cannot be maintained during exercise which brings the risk of cerebral haemorrhage or aortic dissection. The woman should therefore be advised to rest and avoid exertion. The risk of dissection is increased in patients with pre-existing aortic abnormality associated with coarctation, Marfan syndrome or other inherited disorders of connective tissue.

Hypertension should be aggressively treated and to minimize the risk of rupture and dissection beta-blockers are the ideal agents. Left ventricular failure is unlikely in the absence of an associated stenotic bicuspid aortic valve or endocardial fibro-elastosis with impaired left ventricular function. Normal delivery is usually possible, although severe coarctation would indicate a shortened second stage.

MARFAN SYNDROME

Eighty percent of Marfan patients have some cardiac involvement most commonly mitral valve prolapse and regurgitation. Pregnancy increases the risk of aortic rupture or dissection usually in the third trimester or early post-partum. Progressive aortic root dilation and an aortic root dimension >4 cm are associated with increased risk (10%). Women with aortic roots >4.6 cm should be advised to delay pregnancy until after aortic root repair or root replacement with resuspension of the aortic valve [10].

Conversely, in women with minimal cardiac involvement and an aortic root <4 cm pregnancy outcome is usually good [11], although those with a family history of aortic dissection or sudden death are also at increased risk since in some families aortic root dissection occurs in the absence of preliminary aortic dilatation.

Management should include counselling regarding the dominant inheritance of the condition, monthly echocardiograms to assess the aortic root in those with cardiac involvement and beta-blockers for those with hypertension or aortic root dilation. Vaginal delivery for those with stable aortic root measurements is possible but elective Caesarean section with regional anaesthesia if there is an enlarged or dilating aortic root is recommended [11].

Cyanotic congenital heart disease

Cyanotic congenital heart disease in the adult is usually associated either with pulmonary hypertension as in the Eisenmenger syndrome, or with pulmonary stenosis as in the tetralogy of Fallot. Patients with single ventricle, transposition of the great arteries and complex pulmonary atresias with systemic blood supply to the lungs may all survive to adult life with or without previous palliative surgery.

TETRALOGY OF FALLOT

The association of severe right ventricular outflow tract obstruction with a large subaortic ventricular septal defect and overriding aorta causes right ventricular hypertrophy and right-to-left shunting with cyanosis. Pregnancy is tolerated well but fetal growth is poor with a high rate of miscarriage, prematurity and small-for-dates babies. The haematocrit tends to rise during pregnancy in cyanosed women because systemic vasodilatation leads to an increase in right-to-left shunting. Women with a resting arterial saturation of 85% or more, a haemoglobin below 18 g and a haematocrit below 55% have a reasonable chance of a successful outcome. The arterial saturation falls markedly on effort so rest is prescribed to optimize fetal growth but subcutaneous low molecular weight heparin (LMWH) should be given to prevent venous thrombosis and paradoxical embolism.

Women who have had a previous surgical correction of the tetralogy do well in pregnancy [12].

POST-OPERATIVE CONGENITAL HEART DISEASE

Survivors of neonatal palliative surgery for complex congenital heart disease need individual assessment. Echocardiography by a paediatric or adult congenital cardiologist enables a detailed assessment to be made.

Following the Fontan operation for tricuspid atresia or transposition with pulmonary stenosis, the right ventricle is bypassed and the left ventricle provides the pump for both the systemic and pulmonary circulations. Increases in venous pressure can lead to hepatic congestion and gross oedema but pregnancy can be successful.

EISENMENGER SYNDROME AND PULMONARY HYPERTENSION

Pulmonary vascular disease whether secondary to a reversed large left-to-right shunt such as a ventriculo-septal defect (VSD), (Eisenmenger's syndrome) or to lung or connective tissue disease (e.g. scleroderma) or due to primary pulmonary hypertension is extremely dangerous in pregnancy and women known to have significant pulmonary vascular disease should be advised from an early age to avoid pregnancy and be given appropriate contraceptive advice. Maternal mortality is 40% [13].

The danger relates to fixed pulmonary vascular resistance that cannot fall in response to pregnancy, and a consequent inability to increase pulmonary blood flow with refractory hypoxaemia. Pulmonary hypertension is defined as a non-pregnant elevation of mean (not systolic) pulmonary artery pressure equal to or greater than 25 mmHg at rest or 30 mmHg on exercise in the absence of a left-to-right shunt. Pulmonary artery systolic (not mean) pressure is usually estimated by using Doppler ultrasound to measure the regurgitant jet velocity across the tricuspid valve. This should be considered a screening test. There is no agreed relation between the mean pulmonary pressure and the estimated systolic pulmonary pressure. If the systolic pulmonary pressure estimated by Doppler is thought to indicate pulmonary hypertension, a specialist cardiac opinion is recommended. If there is pulmonary hypertension in the presence of a left-to-right shunt the diagnosis of pulmonary vascular disease is particularly difficult and further investigation including cardiac catheterization to calculate pulmonary vascular resistance is likely to be necessary. Pulmonary hypertension as defined by Doppler studies may also occur in mitral stenosis and with large left-to-right shunts that have not reversed. Women with pulmonary hypertension who still have predominant left-to-right shunts are at lesser risk and may do well during pregnancy, but although such women may not have pulmonary vascular disease and a fixed pulmonary vascular resistance (PVR) (or this may not have been established prior to pregnancy), they have the potential to develop it and require very careful monitoring.

In the event of unplanned pregnancy a therapeutic termination should be offered [13]. Elective termination carries a 7% risk of mortality, hence the importance of avoiding pregnancy if possible. If such advice is declined, multidisciplinary care, elective admission for bed rest, 60% oxygen and thromboprophylaxis with LMWH are recommended [14]. Fetal growth should be carefully monitored.

Most fatalities occur during delivery or the first week post-partum. There is no evidence that monitoring the pulmonary artery pressure pre- or intrapartum improves outcome, and indeed insertion of a pulmonary artery catheter increases the risk of thrombosis, which may be fatal in such women [15]. Vasodilators given to reduce the pulmonary artery pressure will (with the exception of inhaled nitric oxide and prostacyclin), inevitably result in a concomitant lowering of the systemic pressure exacerbating hypoxaemia.

There is no evidence that abdominal or vaginal delivery, or regional versus general anaesthesia improve outcome in pregnant women with pulmonary hypertension. Great care must be taken to avoid systemic vasodilatation. The patient should be returned to the intensive care unit (ITU) after delivery. Oximetry, subcutaneous heparin and passive physiotherapy should be continued and mobilization should proceed only slowly. Nebulized prostacycline can be used to try to prevent pulmonary vasoconstriction. When sudden deterioration occurs (usually in the post-partum period) resuscitation is rarely successful and no additional cause is found at autopsy although there may be concomitant thromboembolism, hypovolaemia or pre-eclampsia. Death is usually preceded by vagal slowing, a fall in blood pressure and oxygen saturation followed by ventricular fibrillation.

Acquired valve disease

MITRAL VALVE PROLAPSE

Floppy mitral valve may be sporadic or inherited as a dominant condition in some families with variants of Marfan syndrome. Pregnancy is well tolerated and antibiotic prophylaxis is only required if there is mitral regurgitation.

Rheumatic heart disease

MITRAL STENOSIS

Worldwide, mitral stenosis remains the most common potentially lethal pre-existing heart condition in pregnancy. There are many pitfalls because an asymptomatic patient may deteriorate in pregnancy, mitral stenosis

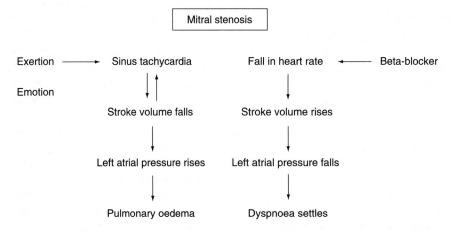

Fig. 26.1 Mitral stenosis.

may have increased in severity since a previous uncomplicated pregnancy, stenosis can reoccur or worsen after valvuloplasty or valvotomy and mitral stenosis that may previously not have been recognized may be missed during routine antenatal examination because the murmur is diastolic and submammary.

Women may deteriorate secondary to tachycardia (related to pain, anxiety, exercise or intercurrent infection), arrhythmias or the increased cardiac output of pregnancy. Sinus tachycardia at rest should prompt concern. Tachycardia is the reflex response to failure to increase stroke volume and it reduces the time for left atrial emptying so that the stroke volume falls, the reflex sinus tachycardia accelerates and the left atrial pressure climbs. This creates a vicious circle of increasing heart rate and left atrial pressure and can precipitate pulmonary oedema. The anxiety caused by the dyspnoea increases the tachycardia and exacerbates the problem (Fig. 26.1). Pulmonary oedema may also be precipitated by increased volume (such as occurs during the third stage of labour or following injudicious intravenous fluid therapy) [16]. The risks are increased with severe mitral stenosis (mitral valve area <1 cm^2), moderate or severe symptoms prior to pregnancy, and in those diagnosed late in pregnancy [16].

The ECG in mitral stenosis shows left atrial P waves and right axis deviation. The CXR shows a small heart but with prominence of the left atrial appendage and left atrium and pulmonary congestion or oedema. The diagnosis is confirmed with transthoracic echocardiography.

Women with severe mitral stenosis should be advised to delay pregnancy until after balloon, open or closed mitral valvotomy, or if the valve is not amenable to valvotomy, until after mitral valve replacement. Beta-blockers decrease heart rate, increase diastolic filling time and decrease the risk of pulmonary oedema [17] and should be given in pregnancy to secure and maintain a heart rate of under 90 beats/min. Diuretics should be commenced or continued if indicated.

In the event of pulmonary oedema, the patient should be sat up, oxygen should be given and the heart rate slowed by relief of anxiety with diamorphine, and 20 mg of intravenous frusemide administered. Digoxin should only be used if atrial fibrillation occurs as it does not slow the heart in sinus rhythm (because increased sympathetic drive easily overcomes its mild vagotonic effect).

If medical therapy fails or for those with severe mitral stenosis, balloon mitral valvotomy may be safely and successfully used in pregnancy if the valve is suitable [16] although this will require transfer to a hospital with major cardiac facilities. Percutaneous balloon valvotomy carries a risk of major complications of about 1%, whereas for surgical valvotomy the figures are: closed valvotomy – fetal mortality 5–15%, maternal 3% and open valvotomy – fetal

mortality 15–33%, maternal 5%. If an open operation on the mitral valve is going to be required, this should be deferred until after delivery [18].

Women with mitral stenosis should avoid the supine and lithotomy positions as much as possible for labour and delivery. Fluid overload must be avoided, and even in the presence of oliguria, without significant blood loss, the temptation to give intravenous colloid must be resisted. Cautious epidural analgesia or anaesthesia are suitable for the patient with mitral stenosis as is vaginal delivery but limitation of maternal effort with an instrumental delivery may be indicated.

REGURGITANT VALVE DISEASE

Patients with regurgitant valve disease either mitral or aortic tolerate pregnancy much better than patients with valvular stenosis. The systemic vasodilatation in pregnancy reduces regurgitant flow as does tachycardia in patients with aortic regurgitation. When the valve disease is of rheumatic origin the advent of sudden atrial fibrillation may precipitate pulmonary oedema.

Mechanical heart valves

Most women with prosthetic heart valves have sufficient cardiovascular reserve to accomplish pregnancy safely. The optimal strategy for anticoagulation in women with metal heart valve replacements in pregnancy is controversial since the interests of the mother and the fetus are in conflict. These women require life-long anticoagulation and this must be continued in pregnancy because of the increased risk of thrombosis.

If the international normalized ratio (INR) is meticulously controlled maternal risks from warfarin are hardly, if at all, increased. However, warfarin is associated with warfarin embryopathy (chondrodysplasia punctata) if given during the period of organogenesis (6 and 12 weeks gestation) [19], and fetal intracerebral haemorrhage at any time.

Overdosage results from a greater anticoagulant effect on the fetus than on the mother because the immature fetal liver produces only low levels of vitamin K-dependent clotting factors and maternal procoagulants do not cross the placenta due to their large molecular size. Warfarin also increases the risks of miscarriage and stillbirth [20].

The fetal risk from warfarin is dose dependent. Fortunately, most women require less than 5 mg daily. Women requiring more than this are at increased risk of teratogenesis, miscarriage and stillbirth [21].

Heparin and low molecular weight heparin do not cross the placenta and therefore are an attractive option. But even in full anticoagulant doses, they are associated with an increased risk of valve thrombosis and embolic events [19–22]. Heparins can also cause retroplacental haemorrhage so the risk of fetal loss is not eliminated. Further disadvantages of unfractionated heparin include a need for parenteral administration, powerful but short duration of action, narrow therapeutic index, a steep dose–response curve, increasing dose requirement during pregnancy and lack of agreed optimal test or target for safe and effective activity. Overshooting with incremental dosage brings a risk of bleeding. High doses of unfractionated heparin long term may also cause osteoporosis. LMWHs have a better safety profile in pregnancy but the manufacturers say they are specifically not recommended as anticoagulants in patients with prosthetic heart valves.

There are three basic options for anticoagulation management

1 Continue warfarin throughout pregnancy, stopping only for delivery. This is the safest option for the mother [19,20].
2 Replace the warfarin with high-dose unfractionated or low molecular weight heparin from 6 to 12 weeks' gestation to avoid warfarin embryopathy.
3 Use high dose unfractionated or low molecular weight heparin throughout pregnancy.

Which option is chosen will depend on several factors

1 *The type of mechanical valve.* The risk of thrombosis is less with the newer bi-leaflet valves (e.g. carbomedics) than with the first-generation ball and cage (e.g. Starr-Edwards), or second-generation single tilting disc (e.g. Bjork Shiley) valves.
2 *The position of the valve replacement.* Valves in the aortic rather than the mitral position are associated with a lower risk of thrombosis [23].
3 *The number of mechanical valves.* Two valves give a higher risk of thrombosis.
4 *The dose of warfarin* required to maintain a therapeutic INR.
5 *Any previous history of embolic events.*

If warfarin is used in pregnancy serial fetal scans are indicated to detect severe embryopathy with stippled epiphyses and intracerebral haemorrhage. Warfarin should be discontinued and substituted for LMWH for 10 days prior to delivery to allow clearance of warfarin from the fetal circulation. For delivery itself LMWH therapy is interrupted.

Conversion from LMWH back to warfarin should be delayed for at least 3–5 days post-partum to minimize the risk of obstetric haemorrhage.

In the event of bleeding or the need for urgent delivery in a fully anticoagulated patient, warfarin may be reversed with fresh frozen plasma (FFP) and vitamin K, and heparin with protamine sulphate. Vitamin K should be avoided if possible since it renders the woman extremely difficult to anticoagulate with warfarin after delivery.

Thrombolytic treatment can be used for prosthetic valve thrombosis during pregnancy, and although it may cause embolism or bleeding or placental separation, the risks are lower than those of cardiothoracic surgery.

Women with metal valve replacements all require antibiotic endocarditis prophylaxis for delivery regardless of the mode of delivery [24,25].

Coronary artery disease

When myocardial infarction occurs in pregnancy it usually develops without preceding angina because the underlying cause is more likely to be due to non-atherosclerotic conditions. Spontaneous coronary artery dissection and coronary artery thrombosis are the commonest causes [1,26] and sudden severe chest pain the usual manifestation. Most occur during late pregnancy or peripartum and affect the anterior wall of the heart.

Maternal death rate is 20%. Myocardial infarction has been attributed to the administration of oxytocic agents. Coronary thrombosis may be associated with drug abuse from crack cocaine. Embolic occlusion should always be considered and an embolic source such as mitral stenosis or infective endocarditis sought.

The risk factors for ischaemic heart disease in pregnancy are the same as for the non-pregnant. The risk is increased in multigravid women and in those who smoke and women with diabetes, obesity, hypertension and hypercholesterolaemia.

Management of acute myocardial infarction is as for the non-pregnant woman.

Coronary angiography should be undertaken without hesitation in order to define the pathology and determine management. Intravenous and intracoronary thrombolysis and percutaneous transluminal coronary angioplasty and stenting have all been successfully performed in pregnancy. Both aspirin and beta-blockers are safe in pregnancy. There are less data for clopidogrel and glycoprotein IIb/IIIa inhibitors although there are case reports of their successful use. Statins should be discontinued for the duration of pregnancy as they are associated with an increased risk of malformations [27].

Hypertrophic cardiomyopathy

Hypertrophic cardiomyopathy (HCM) is an autosomal dominant disease characterized by hypertrophy of the undilated left ventricle in the absence of an abnormal haemodynamic load and with underlying myocyte and myofibrillar disarray. Family studies, now sometimes aided by genetic identification of a responsible mutant gene, have indicated the broad spectrum of phenotypic abnormality that exists not only between individuals at different ages but within families. Patient series previously described from specialist centres represented a highly skewed population of high-risk patients referred because of disabling symptoms or a malignant family history. In the years before echocardiography only gross examples of the disorder could be identified but these patients formed the basis of many of the published natural history studies.

HCM is not infrequently first diagnosed in pregnancy when a systolic murmur leads to an ECG and echocardiographic study. Most patients are asymptomatic and do well. HCM used to be regarded as a rare disease with a high risk of sudden death but is now recognized to be relatively common, being found in 1 in 500 young adults in a recent study and in most patients the disorder is benign.

Patients with HCM respond well to pregnancy by a useful increase in their normally reduced left ventricular cavity size and stroke volume. The danger relates to left ventricular outflow tract obstruction that may be precipitated by hypotension or hypovolaemia. Symptoms of shortness of breath, chest pain, dizziness or syncope indicate the need for a β-blocking drug [28]. Ventricular arrhythmias commoner in older patients are uncommon in the young. Sudden death has only very rarely been reported during pregnancy. It is most important in all patients to avoid vasodilatation during labour and delivery and regional anaesthesia/analgesia. Any hypovolaemia will have the same effect and should be rapidly and adequately corrected. It is most unusual to find hypertrophy in the infants of mothers with HCM.

Peripartum cardiomyopathy

This pregnancy-specific condition is defined as the development of cardiac failure between the last month of pregnancy and 5 months post-partum, in the absence of an identifiable cause or recognizable heart disease prior to the last month of pregnancy, and left ventricular systolic dysfunction demonstrated by the following echocardiographic criteria [29].
- Left ventricular ejection fraction <45%
- Fractional shortening <30%
- LVEDP (left ventriculae end diastolic dimension) >2.7 cm/m^2

Echocardiography shows dilatation which usually involves all four chambers but is dominated by left ventricular hypokinesia which may be global or most marked in a particular territory.

The condition is rare but the true incidence is unknown as mild cases undoubtedly go unrecognized. Recognized risk factors include multiple pregnancy, hypertension (be

it pre-existing or related to pregnancy or pre-eclampsia), multiparity, increased age, and Afro-Caribbean race.

Peripartum cardiomyopathy does not differ clinically from dilated cardiomyopathy except in its temporal relationship to pregnancy. The severity varies from catastrophic to subclinical when it may be discovered only fortuitously through echocardiography. Diagnosis should be suspected in the peripartum patient with breathlessness, tachycardia or signs of heart failure. Fluid overload is often a major feature and may be precipitated by the use of syntocinon or by fluids given to maintain cardiac output during spinal anaesthesia for delivery. The CXR shows an enlarged heart with pulmonary congestion or oedema and often bilateral pleural effusions. Systemic embolism from mural thrombus may herald the onset of ventricular arrhythmias or precede the development of clinical heart failure and pulmonary embolism may further complicate the clinical picture.

The differential diagnosis includes pre-existing dilated cardiomyopathy, pulmonary thromboembolism, amniotic fluid embolism, myocardial infarction and β_2 agonist associated pulmonary oedema in patients who have been given such an agent to postpone premature delivery. Echocardiography immediately implicates the left ventricle and excludes pulmonary embolism as the cause.

Management is as for other causes of heart failure with oxygen, diuretics, vasodilators, and angiotensin converting enzyme (ACE) inhibitors if post-partum. Thromboprophylaxis is imperative. The cautious addition of a β-adrenergic blocking drug may be helpful if tachycardia persists, particularly if the cardiac output is well preserved. The most gravely ill patients will need intubation, ventilation and monitoring with use of inotropes and sometimes temporary support from an intra-aortic balloon pump or ventricular assist device. Heart transplantation may be the only chance of survival in severe cases.

About 50% of women make a spontaneous and full recovery. Most case fatalities occur close to presentation and cardiomyopathy is the cause of almost a quarter of maternal cardiac deaths [1]. Recent data show a 5-year survival of 94% [30]. Patients should remain on an ACE inhibitor for as long as left ventricular function remains abnormal. Prognosis and recurrence depend on the normalization of left ventricular size within 6 months of delivery [31]. Those women with severe myocardial dysfunction, defined as LV end diastolic dimension ≥6 cm and fractional shortening ≤21% are unlikely to regain normal cardiac function on follow-up [32]. Those whose LV function and size do not return to normal within 6 months and prior to a subsequent pregnancy are at significant risk of worsening heart failure (50%) and death (25%) or recurrent peripartum cardiomyopathy in the next pregnancy. They should therefore be advised against pregnancy [31].

Arrhythmias

Atrial and ventricular premature complexes (VPC) are common in pregnancy. Many pregnant women are symptomatic from forceful heart beats that occur following a compensatory pause after a VPC. Most women with symptomatic episodes of dizziness, syncope, and palpitations do not have arrhythmias [33].

A sinus tachycardia requires investigation for possible underlying pathology such as blood loss, infection, heart failure, thyrotoxicosis or pulmonary embolus. The commonest arrhythmia encountered in pregnancy is supraventricular tachycardia (SVT). First onset of SVT (both accessory pathway-mediated and AV nodal re-entrant) is rare in pregnancy but 22% of 63 women with SVT had exacerbation of symptoms in pregnancy [34]. 50% of SVTs do not respond to vagal manoeuvres.

Propranolol, verapamil and adenosine have Federal Drugs Agency (FDA) approval for acute termination of SVT. Adenosine has advantages over verapamil including probable lack of placental transfer and may be safely used in pregnancy for SVTs that do not respond to vagal stimulation [35,36]. Flecanide is safe and is used in the treatment of fetal tachycardias. Propafenone and amiodarone should be avoided [37], the latter because of interference with fetal thyroid function [38]. Temporary and permanent pacing, cardioversion, and implantable defibrillators are also safe in pregnancy [35].

Cardiac arrest

This should be managed according to the same protocols as used in the non-pregnant. Pregnant women (especially those in advanced pregnancy) should be 'wedged' to relieve any obstruction to venous return from pressure of the gravid uterus on the IVC. This can be most rapidly achieved by turning the patient into the left lateral position. If cardio-pulmonary resuscitation (CPR) is required then the pelvis can be tilted while keeping the torso flat to allow external chest compressions. Emergency Caesarean section may be required to aid maternal resuscitation.

Endocarditis prophylaxis

Infective endocarditis is rare in pregnancy but threatens the life of both mother and child. Fatal cases of endocarditis in pregnancy have occurred antenatally, rather than as a consequence of infection acquired at the time of delivery [1]. Treatment is essentially the same as outside pregnancy

Table 26.1 Stratification of cardiac conditions according to risk of bacterial endocarditis

High-risk	Prosthetic valves (metal, bioprosthetic and homografts)
Endocarditis prophylaxis recommended	Previous bacterial endocarditis, Complex cyanotic congenital heart disease (Fallot's, Transposition of great arteries) Surgical systemic/pulmonary shunt
Moderate-risk	Other congenital cardiac malformations, Acquired valvular disease
Endocarditis prophylaxis recommended	Hypertrophic cardiomyopathy Mitral valve prolapse with mitral regurgitation
Negligible-risk	Isolated secundum atrial septal defects, Surgically repaired ASD, VSD, PDA
Endocarditis prophylaxis not recommended	Mitral valve prolapse without regurgitation, Physiological heart murmurs, Cardiac pacemakers

Adapted from [25].

with emergency valve replacement if indicated. As always, the baby should be delivered if viable before the maternal operation.

Antibiotic prophylaxis is mandatory for those with prosthetic valves and for those with a previous episode of endocarditis [25]. Many cardiologists recommend that women with structural heart defects (e.g. VSD) also receive prophylaxis. Recommendations of the American Heart Association stratify cardiac conditions into high-, moderate- and negligible (not requiring antibiotic prophylaxis) risk [25] (Table 26.1).

The current UK recommendations (24) are amoxycillin 2 g i.v. plus gentamicin 120 mg i.v. at the onset of labour or ruptured membranes or prior to Caesarean section, followed by amoxycillin 500 mg orally (or i.m/i.v. depending on patient's condition) 6 h later.

For women who are allergic to penicillin, vancomycin 1 g i.v. or teicoplanin 400 mg i.v. may be used instead of amoxycillin [25].

References

1. de Swiet M & Nelson-Piercy C (2004) Cardiac disease. In: *Confidential Enquiries into Maternal and Child Health. Why Mothers Die, 2000–2002.* 6th Report of Confidential Enquiries into Maternal Deaths in UK. London: RCOG press.
2. Robson SC, Hunter S, Boys RJ & Dunlop W (1989) Serial study of factors influencing changes in cardiac output during human pregnancy. *Am J Physiol* **256**, H1060–65.
3. Robson SK, Hunter S, Boys R, Dunlop W & Bryson M (1986) Changes in cardiac output during epidural anaesthesia for caesarian section. *Anaesthesia* **44**, 465–79.
4. Clapp JF III & Capeless E (1997) Cardiovascular function before, during and after the first and subsequent pregnancies. *Am J Cardiol* **80**, 1469–73.

5. McCaffrey FM & Sherman FS (1995) Pregnancy and congenital heart disease: The Magee Women's Hospital. *J Mates Fet Med* **4**, 152–9.

6. Siu SC, Sermer M, Colman *et al.* (2001) Prospective multicenter study of pregnancy outcomes in women with heart disease. *Circulation* **104**, 515–21.

7. Presbitero P, Somerville J, Stone S *et al.* (1994) Pregnancy in cyanotic congenital heart disease. Outcome of mother and fetus. *Circulation* **89**, 2673–6.

8. Burn J, Brennan P, Little J *et al.* (1998) Recurrence risks in offspring of adults with major heart defects: results from first cohort of British Collaboration study. *Lancet* **351**, 311–16.

9. Presbitero P, Prever SB & Brusca A (1996) Interventional cardiology in pregnancy. *Eur Heart J* **17**, 182–8.

10. Lipscomb KJ, Clayton Smith J, Clarke B, Donnai P & Harris R (1997) Outcome of pregnancy in women with Marfan's syndrome. *Br J Obstet Gynaecol* **104**, 201–6.

11. Rossiter JP, Repke JT, Morales AJ *et al.* (1995) A prospective longitudinal evaluation of pregnancy in the Marfan syndrome. *Am J Obstet Gynecol* **173**, 1599–6.

12. Singh H, Bolton PJ & Oakley CM (1983) Outcome of pregnancy after surgical correction of tetralogy of Fallot. *Br Med J* **285**, 168.

13. Yentis SM, Steer PJ & Plaat F (1998) Eisenmenger's syndrome in pregnancy: maternal and fetal mortality in the 1990s. *Br J Obstet Gynaecol* **105**, 921–2.

14. Avila WS, Grinberg M, Snitcowsky R *et al.* (1995) Maternal and fetal outcome in pregnant women with Eisenmenger's syndrome. *Eur Heart J* **16**, 460–4.

15. Rosenthal & Nelson-Piercy C (2000) Value of inhaled nitric oxide in Eisenmenger syndrome during pregnancy (letter). *Am J Obstet Gynecol* **183**, 781–2.

16. Desai DK, Adanlawo M, Naidoo DP, Moodley J & Kleinschmidt I (2000) Mitral stenosis in pregnancy: a four-year experience at King Edward VIII Hospital. *Br J Obstet Gynaecol* **107**, 953–8.

17. al Kasab SM, Sabag T, al Zaibag M *et al.* (1990) Beta-adrenergic receptor blockade in the management of pregnant women with mitral stenosis. *Am J Obstet Gynecol* **163**, 37–40.

18. Oakley CM (1996) Valvular disease in pregnancy. *Curr Opin Cardiol* **11**, 155–9.

19. Chan WS, Anand S & Ginsberg JS (2000) Anticoagulation of pregnant women with mechanical heart valves. *Arch Intern Med* **160**, 191–6.

20. Sadler L, McCowan L, White H, Stewart A, Bracken M & North R (2000) Pregnancy outcomes and cardiac complications in women with mechanical, bioprosthetic and homograft valves. *Br J Obstet Gynaecol* **107**, 245–3.

21. Cotrufo M, De Feo M, De Santo L, Romano G, Della Corte A & Renzulli A (2002) Risk of warfarin during pregnancy with mechanical valve prostheses. *Obstet Gynecol* **99**, 35–40.

22. Meschengieser SS, Fondevilla CG, Santarelli MT & Lazzari MA (1999) Anticoagulation in pregnant women with mechanical heart valve prostheses. *Heart* **82**, 23–6.

23. Elkayam U (1999) Pregnancy through a prosthetic heart valve. *J Am Coll Cardiol* **33**, 1642–45.

24. Endocarditis Working Party of the British Society for Antimicrobial Chemotherapy (1982) The antibiotic prophylaxis of infective endocarditis. *Lancet* **2**, 1323–26.

25. Dajani AS, Taubert KA, Wilson W *et al.* (1997) Prevention of bacterial endocarditis. Recommendations by the American Heart Association. *J Am Med Assoc* **277**, 1794–801.

26. Roth A & Elkayam U (1996) Acute myocardial infarction associated with pregnancy. *Ann Int Med* **125**, 751–7.

27. Edison RJ & Muenke M (2004) Central nervous system and limb anomalies in case reports of first-trimester statin exposure. *N Engl J Med* **350**(15), 1579–82.

28. Oakley GD, McGarry K, Limb DG & Oakley CM (1979) Management of pregnancy in patients with hypertrophic cardiomyopathy. *Br Med J* **1**, 1749–50.

29. Pearson GD, Veille JC, Rahimtoola S *et al.* (2000) Peripartum cardiomyopathy. National Heart, Lung and Blood Institute and Office of Rare Diseases (NIH). Workshop Recommendations and Review. *J Am Med Assoc* **283**, 1183–88.

30. Felker GM, Thompson RE, Hare JM *et al.* (2000) Underlying causes and long-term survival in patients with initially unexplained cardiomyopathy. *N Engl J Med* **342**, 1077–84.

31. Elkayam U, Tummala PP, Rao K *et al.* (2001) Maternal and fetal outcomes of subsequent pregnancies in women with peripartum cardiomyopathy. *N Engl J Med* **344**, 1567–71.

32. Witlin AG, Mabie WC & Sibai BM (1997) Peripartum cardiomyopathy: a longitudinal echocardiographic study. *Am J Obstet Gynecol* **177**, 1129–32.

33. Shotan A, Ostrezega E, Mehra A, Johnson JV & Elkayam U (1997) Incidence of arrhythmias in normal pregnancy and relation to palpitations, dizziness and syncope. *Am J Cardiol* **79**, 1061–4.

34. Lee SH, Chen SA, Wu TJ *et al.* (1995) Effects of pregnancy on first onset and symptoms of paroxysmal supraventricular tachycardia. *Am J Cardiol* **76**, 675–8.

35. Page RL (1995) Treatment of arrhythmias during pregnancy. *Am Heart J* **130**, 871–6.

36. Mason BA, Ricci-Goodman J & Koos BJ (1992) Adenosine in the treatment of maternal paroxysmal supraventricular tachycardia. *Obstet Gynecol* **80**, 478–80.

37. James PR (2001) Cardiovascular disease. In: Nelson-Piercy C (ed) Prescribing in pregnancy. *Bailliere's Best Pract Res Clin Obstet Gynaecol* **15**, 903–11.

38. Magee LA, Downar E, Sermer M *et al.* (1995) Pregnancy outcome after gestational exposure to amiodarone. *Am J Obstet Gynecol* **172**, 1307–11.

Chapter 27: Diabetes and endocrine disease in pregnancy

Anne Dornhorst and Catherine Williamson

Introduction

Diabetes occurs in 2–5% of all UK pregnancies and its prevalence is rising. Forty years ago the majority of women with diabetes attending an antenatal clinic had type 1 diabetes and were young, non-obese and of low parity. Today the majority of women have type 2 diabetes, or gestational diabetes (GDM), and are older, more obese and of higher parity. These women also include a small proportion of individuals diagnosed as having the rarer monogenetic or mitochondrial forms of diabetes, who previously would have been misclassified as having type 1 or 2 diabetes.

The prevalence of type 2 diabetes among women of child-bearing years is predicted to increase due to current trends in obesity and physical inactivity. Type 2 diabetes must not be considered a less serious condition than type 1 diabetes as clinical experience over the last decade has consistently shown that the perinatal mortality and morbidity is higher among pregnancies associated with type 2 diabetes than type 1 diabetes [1].

The type of diabetes a woman has influences the obstetric management from pre-conceptual counselling through to post-natal care. As a generalization it is the degree of maternal hyperglycaemia that dictates fetal outcome, while it is the type of diabetes that influences maternal outcome. The main characteristics of the different types of diabetes encountered in obstetric practice are shown in Table 27.1.

The general principles for the management of diabetic pregnancies are discussed below. Specific issues relating to the screening and management of women with GDM are briefly discussed. The neonatal complications of a diabetic pregnancy and the long-term impact these pregnancies have on the future health of the child are also briefly considered.

General principles for the management of diabetic pregnancies

When maternal diabetes precedes the pregnancy it is associated with an increased risk of miscarriage, congenital abnormalities, accelerated fetal growth, late stillbirth, birth trauma, neonatal hypoglycaemia and long-term health problems for the child. Gestational diabetes is associated with those complications attributable to maternal hyperglycaemia arising in the latter half of pregnancy. The principal tenet for the management of all diabetic pregnancies, from the time of conception through to the time of delivery, is to strive for maternal euglycaemia. The need for good glycaemic control is based on evidence implicating hyperglycaemia with maternal and fetal complications, see Table 27.2. Although other maternal metabolic disturbances do occur that may be detrimental to pregnancy, such as changes in lipid metabolism, it is hyperglycaemia, not dyslipidaemia, that is particularly harmful to embryogenesis and it is glucose, not fat, that is the fetal fuel substrate responsible for fetal hyperinsulinaemia and accelerated fetal growth.

To achieve the level of glycaemic control required to minimize complications associated with diabetic pregnancies, hospitals require a multidisciplinary diabetic obstetric team working to local agreed guidelines that are based on national and international agreed best practice. The structured approach to the management of diabetic pregnancies is discussed below, see Table 27.3.

Prior to pregnancy

PRECONCEPTION COUNSELLING

When women with diabetes attend a pre-conception clinic, pregnancy outcomes are improved. These clinics provide an opportunity for glycaemic control to be intensively managed, high-dose folic acid supplements prescribed and information given on when to stop potentially harmful drugs, such as Angiotensin-converting enzyme (ACE) inhibitors and angiotensin receptor blockers. Women can also be assessed for diabetic complications, and aspirin or heparin considered for those at risk of pre-eclampsia or thrombophilia.

The importance for the best achievable glycaemic control prior to pregnancy is stressed by studies showing that

Table 27.1 The types of diabetes encountered in obstetric practice

Type 1 diabetes	Absolute insulin deficiency due to an autoimmune destruction of the pancreatic β-cell. Presents typically under the age of 20 years old, only 10% have a first degree relative affected. Not associated with obesity. Accounts for approximately 5% of all diabetes outside pregnancy.
Type 2 diabetes	Relative insulin deficiency due to increased insulin resistance. Presents typically over the age of 20, and >50% have a first degree relative affected. Associated with obesity. Accounts for approximately 90% of all diabetes outside pregnancy.
Monogenetic diabetes	MODY (Maturity Onset of Diabetes of the Young). Results from a single gene mutation causing defects in pancreatic β-cell insulin secretion. Present from birth and typically diagnosed under the age of 20, autosomal dominant with nearly 100% having a first degree relative affected. Not associated with obesity. Accounts for approximately 2% of all diabetes outside pregnancy.
Mitochondrial diabetes	Arises from a mutation in mitochondrial DNA leading to a defect in insulin secretion. Associated with a number of other medical problems including neural sensory deafness, a tendency for stroke and lactic acidosis. Diabetes develops at approximately 35 years of age and is maternally inherited. Not associated with obesity. Accounts for approximately 1% of all diabetes outside pregnancy.
Secondary diabetes	Diabetes due to other medical conditions, i.e. pancreatitis, cystic fibrosis, glucocorticoids and other drugs. Accounts for approximately 2% of all diabetes outside pregnancy.

Table 27.2 The role of maternal hyperglycaemia on maternal and fetal complications

	Influence of hyperglycaemia
1st trimester	
Implantation	Inhibits trophectoderm differentiation
Embryogenesis	Increases oxidative stress affecting expression of critical genes essential for embryogenesis
Organogenesis	Activates the diacylglycerol-protein kinase C cascade increasing congenital defects
Miscarriage	Increases premature programmed cell death of key progenitor cells of the blastocyst
2nd trimester	
Endocrine pancreas	Stimulates fetal β-cells
Fetal growth	Stimulates fetal hyperinsulinaemia that results in growth acceleration seen on ultrasound by 26 weeks
3rd trimester	
Fetal growth	A major fetal substrate and determinate for accelerated fetal growth
Adipose disposition	Stimulates hyperinsulinaemia that promotes fat disposition including intra-abdominal fat
Lung maturation	Stimulates hyperinsulinaemia that delays lung maturation by inhibiting surfactant proteins
Stillbirth	Is associated with defects in placental maturation that increase the risk of fetal hypoxia
Delivery	
Birth trauma	By causing accelerated fetal growth there is an increased risk of shoulder dystocia predisposing to birth trauma and asphyxia
Neonate	
Hypoglycaemia	Stimulates fetal hyperinsulinaemia that predisposes to neonatal hypoglycaemia
Hypocalcaemia	Alters the placental expression of calbindin mRNA that affects calcium status at birth
Polycythaemia	Stimulates fetal hyperinsulinaemia that enhances antepartum haemapoiesis as does fetal hypoxia
Cardiomyopathy	Stimulates fetal hyperinsulinaemia that predisposes to hypertrophic cardiomyopathy
Adolescence/adulthood	
Obesity	Intrauterine exposure predisposes to the metabolic syndrome, independent of any genetic susceptibility
Type 2 diabetes	Intrauterine exposure predisposes to type 2 diabetes, independent of any genetic susceptibility

when the HbA1c value, the measure of overall glycaemic control, are within the normal range the risk of congenital abnormalities approaches that of the non-diabetic population. To achieve this level of control requires women with type 1 diabetes, and many of those with type 2 diabetes, to have 4–5 insulin injections a day or an insulin pump. A long-acting basal insulin is usually given at night with a short-acting bolus insulin taken with each meal. For women with type 2 diabetes previously on oral hypoglycaemic agents switching to insulin remains standard practice; however, certain oral hypoglycaemic agents are now being prescribed to women with gestational diabetic pregnancies [2] and pregnant women with polycystic ovarian syndrome. While many women with type 2 diabetes require multiple daily injections of insulin others may achieve good glycaemic control using

Table 27.3 A structured approach to the management of diabetic pregnancies

Prior to pregnancy
  Preconception counselling
1st trimester
  Referral to a combined multidisciplinary diabetic obstetric
    antenatal clinic
  Dating scan
  Screening for diabetic complications
  Screening for non-diabetic co-morbidities
  Assessment and optimization of glycaemia
  Advice on hypoglycaemia prevention
2nd trimester
  Optimization of glycaemic control
  Screening for congenital abnormalities
  Surveillance for medical obstetric complications
  Assessment of fetal growth
3rd trimester
  Optimization of glycaemic control
  Assessment of fetal growth
  Timing and mode of delivery
Delivery
  Protocols for insulin during labour and delivery
Post-partum
  Adjustment of insulin dosage
  Breast feeding
  Discussing contraception

a twice-daily mixture of a short- and long-acting insulin, or alternatively a short-acting insulin three times a day with meals.

1st trimester

REFERRAL TO A COMBINED MULTIDISCIPLINARY DIABETIC OBSTETRIC ANTENATAL CLINIC

Pregnancy outcomes are improved when women with diabetes attend a multidisciplinary diabetic obstetric antenatal clinic. This team should comprise of an obstetrician, diabetologist, specialized midwife, diabetic nurse and dietician who are jointly involved with the care of all pregnant diabetic women attending the hospital. Immediate access to this combined clinic is essential as fetal organogenesis occurs within 12 weeks from conception and the need to normalize maternal glycaemia at this time is therefore critical. Each woman needs to be seen or phoned by the diabetic nurse on a weekly basis throughout the first trimester, even if they need to be seen less frequently by other members of the team.

DATING ULTRASOUND SCAN

As the majority of diabetic women have an elective delivery before term it is essential that the correct gestational age of the pregnancy is known. Ideally a dating scan should be performed within the first 10 weeks following conception as this allows both the viability of the pregnancy to be confirmed and an accurate gestational age obtained. Relying on ultrasound scanning later in a diabetic pregnancy is less accurate as either fetal growth restriction or growth promotion may be present.

SCREENING FOR DIABETIC COMPLICATIONS

Diabetic micro- and macrovascular complications increase with duration of diabetes. Many pregnant women with type 1 diabetes will have been diabetic for over 20 years and are likely to have, or have had, diabetic retinopathy. Women with type 2 diabetes are more prone to diabetic maculopathy that is less duration dependent than the background and proliferative retinopathy seen in type 1 diabetes. When glycaemic control rapidly improves, as may occur during the pre-conception period, retinopathy can worsen. A dilated retinal examination each trimester should be performed with referral to an ophthalmologist if retinopathy is present.

Diabetic renal disease is more common in women with type 1 than type 2 diabetes, and its frequency increases with increasing duration of diabetes. Microalbuminuria and proteinuria are indicators of diabetic renal involvement and if present, and not attributable to a urinary tract infection, a urinary creatinine ratio or 24 h urine collection should be performed to quantify the degree of proteinuria. A glomerular filtration rate (GFR) should be calculated on women with a raised plasma creatinine. The presence of proteinuria and or a reduced GFR is a significant risk factor for nephrotic syndrome, hypertension, pre-eclampsia, placental insufficiency, preterm delivery and neonatal morbidity and mortality.

Diabetic neuropathy also increases with duration of diabetes and is therefore more common in women with type 1 diabetes. Autonomic neuropathy is particularly problematic in pregnancy as it blunts the adrenergic and metabolic response to hypoglycaemia potentially leading to life-threatening episodes of hypoglycaemia. These are more likely to occur during the first half of pregnancy before maternal insulin resistance increases and helps minimize this risk.

Autonomic neuropathy also causes gastroparesis that increases the risk in early pregnancy of nausea and vomiting and may contribute to poor glycaemic control due to the erratic food absorption of meals.

Diabetes is associated with premature cardiovascular disease. By the age of 40 women with type 1 diabetes who have been diabetic for more than 20 years are likely to have coronary artery calcification and a degree of coronary artery disease (CAD), independently of any other risk factors. Older women with type 2 diabetes are also at increased risk of CAD. A previous history of CAD or its diagnosis in pregnancy is associated with significant maternal morbidity, see Chapter 26.

SCREENING FOR NON-DIABETIC CO-MORBIDITIES

Women with type 1 diabetes are more susceptible to other autoimmune diseases. The prevalence of autoimmune thyroid disease is sufficiently high to warrant all type 1 women, not known to have thyroid disease, to be screened for it early in pregnancy. The other autoimmune diseases associated with type 1 diabetes should only be screened for if clinically indicated.

Women with type 2 diabetes are likely to have the other components of the metabolic syndrome including obesity, hypertension, dyslipidaemia and insulin resistance. Obesity, independently of diabetes, is a risk factor for late stillbirth, birth trauma and maternal complications post-partum [3]. The hypertriglyceridaemia associated with the metabolic syndrome provides the fetus with glycerol and fatty acids that can be utilized by the fetus as a fuel substrate increasing the risk of accelerated fetal growth. Type 2 diabetic women who are obese should receive appropriate dietary management that should include advice to minimize excessive weight gain.

ASSESSMENT AND OPTIMIZATION OF GLYCAEMIA

The first HbA1c measurement taken in pregnancy provides a crude assessment of the risk of major congenital malformations, with the risk increasing with increasing HbA1c values. Keeping fasting glucose levels during the critical period of organogenesis below 5.8 mmol/l and postprandial glucose levels below 9.1 mmol/l has been shown to decrease the fetal malformations rate in a large Danish cohort of women with pregestational diabetes. The background risk overall of congenital malformations among diabetic pregnancies remains between 2 and 3 times that of non-diabetic pregnancies [4].

Normal physiological changes in pregnancy facilitate the maternal–fetal transfer of glucose, especially postprandially. When diabetes is present excess maternal glucose is preferentially transferred across the placenta rather than taken up in maternal muscle or fat. Circulating fetal glucose from the 12th week can stimulate fetal insulin secretion that functions as an intrauterine growth factor. To optimize maternal glycaemic control and minimize excess maternal glucose transfer requires the maintenance of fasting maternal plasma glucose levels below 6 mmol/l and 1 h postprandial levels below 8 mmol/l. This tight degree of glycaemic control usually requires a highly flexible insulin regime, best suited by giving multiple injections of short- and long-insulin injections throughout the day or an insulin pump. The newer quicker analogue insulins are well suited for targeting postprandial glycaemia. However their long-term safety in pregnancy is still being evaluated as is the use of the long-acting insulin analogues.

The adjustment of the insulin dose is based on frequent daily blood glucose monitoring that should include a fasting value, a 1-h postmeal value and a bedtime reading. The skill in adjusting the insulin dose around individual patients with varying lifestyles, durations or diabetes and diabetic complications is considerable. There is no one formula that is applicable for all type 1 or type 2 women, and the precise insulin regime and dose needed has to be formulated on an individual basis between the women, who are often extremely adept in doing this, and the diabetic team.

It is important to remind women with type 1 diabetes never to stop their insulin if not eating because of nausea, vomiting or for any other reason. Ketoacidosis develops more quickly in pregnancy and at lower blood glucose levels due to enhanced maternal lipolysis. All women with type 1 diabetes should know how and when to test for urinary ketones and to come to the hospital if they are unwell with persistent ketoneurea. In type 2 diabetes there is usually sufficient insulin to prevent ketoacidosis. However in pregnancy, due to the profound insulin resistance and enhanced maternal lipolysis, this can occur especially in the presence of vomiting. Diabetic ketoacidosis is associated with a high fetal loss.

ADVICE ON HYPOGLYCAEMIA PREVENTION

Maternal hypoglycaemia is frequent during early pregnancy in women taking insulin. Hypoglycaemia is not by itself harmful to the fetus but can be life threatening for the woman. During the last 15 years over half of all UK maternal deaths reported in the Confidential Enquiry into Maternal Deaths, among type 1 diabetic women have been attributed to hypoglycaemia. Risk factors for severe hypoglycaemia are type 1 diabetes of long duration, poor hypoglycaemic awareness, autonomic neuropathy, gastroparesis, renal impairment and sleeping alone. All women must be aware of the risk of hypoglycaemia as they intensify their insulin management. Individual advice on the timing of meals and snacks to minimize hypoglycaemia needs to be given and family members should be instructed on how and when to administer glucagon. Women should carry identification cards specifying that they are taking insulin and what to do if they become hypoglycaemic. Specific advice on driving should include the need to perform a blood test before getting into a car and not to drive if experiencing hypoglycaemic episodes without warning signs. Outside pregnancy the use of the very short analogue insulins is associated with fewer severe hypoglycaemic episodes, especially at night, and similar advantages have been reported in pregnancy.

2nd trimester

OPTIMIZATION OF GLYCAEMIC CONTROL

By the start of the second trimester in non-diabetic pregnancies there is a fall in fasting glucose and a rise in postprandial glucose values. By the middle of the second trimester maternal insulin resistance starts to increase due to high concentrations of circulating maternal fatty acids and placental hormones. By term, in non-diabetic women, insulin secretion has to increase 2–3 fold to control blood glucose levels postprandially.

Women with diabetes who start pregnancy well-controlled may not need to increase their overall insulin dosage until after 20 weeks' gestation, prior to this they may actually need to reduce their insulin due to nausea and decreased food intake. After this time insulin requirements begin to rise usually doubling or trebling by term. The diabetic nurses should ensure that the women have the knowledge and confidence to increase their insulin in response to their glucose monitoring readings. As the basal night time insulin is increased it may be necessary to give half this dose in the morning to avoid nocturnal hypoglycaemia.

Women with type 2 diabetes are usually insulin resistant prior to pregnancy. For those women taking oral hypoglycaemic agents during the first trimester by the second trimester when insulin resistance increases further these drugs are usually unable to secrete sufficient insulin to achieve adequate glycaemic control. By the end of pregnancy daily insulin doses in women with type 2 diabetes may exceed 300 units a day. Outside pregnancy Metformin is frequently prescribed to individuals with type 2 diabetes as it has a beneficial effect on insulin resistance and reduces the total insulin dose required. Although Metformin is not licensed for pregnancy, experience of its use in treating both pregnant women with polycystic ovaries, type 2 diabetes and GDM is increasing [5]. Today some centres are prescribing Metformin in addition to insulin in the management of obese type 2 diabetic women.

SCREENING FOR CONGENITAL ABNORMALITIES

A detailed anomaly ultrasound scan should be offered to all diabetic women between 18 and 20 weeks' gestation to look for major congenital abnormalities. This scan should specifically examine those structures most commonly affected in diabetic pregnancies, namely the spine, skull, kidneys and heart.

Fetal echocardiography between 20 and 24 weeks' gestation should be offered to view the four chambers of the heart together with the ventricular outflow tracts.

SCREENING FOR CHROMOSOMAL ANOMALIES

Chromosomal abnormalities such as Down's syndrome are not increased in women with diabetes. Calculating the risk of a fetus with Down's syndrome based on the standard formula of gestational age, the mother's age, and levels of unconjugated oestriol (uE3), alpha fetoprotein (AFP) and human chorionic gonadotropin (hCG) is less accurate, as both plasma levels of AFP and uE3 are lower in diabetic pregnancies. This also explains why the use of AFP to screen for neural-tube defects is also inaccurate.

Surveillance for medical obstetric complications

Women with diabetes have an increased risk of hypertension in pregnancy, including pre-eclampsia. In addition to serial clinic blood pressure measurements and urine analysis for protein, uterine artery Doppler wave-form analysis at 24 weeks may be helpful in identifying those women most at risk.

ASSESSMENT OF FETAL GROWTH

Ultrasound scans for assessment for fetal growth usually starts at the end of the second trimester and is repeated thereafter every 4 weeks, or more frequently if needed. Baseline measurement of fetal abdominal circumference at 26 weeks expressed as a percentile can be compared with later scans to provide evidence for growth acceleration or restriction. Measurement of liquor volume should also be serially recorded, as polyhydramnios is more common in diabetic pregnancies.

3rd trimester

OPTIMIZATION OF GLYCAEMIC CONTROL

During the third trimester maternal insulin resistance continues to increase along with insulin requirements. Achieving good glycaemic control tends to become easier as the insulin resistance protects women from severe hypoglycaemic episodes.

When glucocorticoid steroids are required for lung maturation insulin requirements over the next 72 h may need to double. It is important if two 12 mg Beclomethasone injections are required at 24-h intervals that the insulin dose is either proactively increased or the women admitted and an intravenous insulin sliding scale administered over the 72 h which can be given in addition to her normal insulin dose.

ASSESSMENT OF FETAL GROWTH

Evidence on serial ultrasounds of a rising abdominal circumference percentile in relation to the head circumference or bi-parietal diameter is indicative of accelerated fetal growth. This pattern of fetal growth is seen in association with poor maternal control and fetal hyperinsulinaemia. It is the fetal insulin that promotes excessive fat deposition within the abdomen and also stimulates enlargement of the liver and heart. While the term 'macrosomia' is widely used clinically and in the literature to describe infants of diabetic mothers, the precise definition of macrosomia remains poorly defined, with definitions varying from an absolute birthweight of >4 kg, 4.5 kg or >5 kg to a percentile birthweight of >90%, 95% or 97.5%. As birthweight is dependent on gestational age, sex, ethnic origin, parental height and maternal weight, any definition based on absolute weight is best avoided. With diabetes it is the pattern of fetal growth rather than the absolute or percentile birthweight that is important. The influence of maternal obesity alone accounts for many of the infants of type 2 diabetic mothers having high birthweights.

Serial ultrasounds can also help identify those women who have an infant with fetal growth restriction or asymmetrical growth restriction (poor increase in AC centile growth compared with the head circumference). Such growth patterns are indicative of utero-placental insufficiency and are frequently seen in Type 1 diabetic women with renal impairment, vascular disease or hypertension. If detected, serial biophysical tests on the fetus and regular maternal assessment of fetal movements should be commenced because delivery may be necessary if they are abnormal.

TIMING AND MODE OF DELIVERY

All pregnant women with diabetes should be made aware early in pregnancy that it is potentially harmful to the baby for the pregnancy to go beyond term. While women should be encouraged to be actively involved in their delivery plans they need to understand that the decision about the exact timing and mode of delivery is best deferred to around 36 weeks' gestation when a more informed discussion can take place based on maternal and fetal well-being.

The risk of late unexpected stillbirth among women with diabetes is approximately fourfold higher than for the non-diabetic population [6] and it is for this reason that most authorities advocate delivery between 38 and 39 weeks. Induction at 38 weeks' gestation in a nulliparous type 1 woman is often slow or unsuccessful. Caesarian section following failed induction is therefore high among type 1 diabetic women and this contributes to the overall high Caesarean rate, often >50% for many units. By contrast women with type 2 diabetes are more likely to be multiparous and therefore induction of labour before term is more likely to be successful.

The risk of birth trauma increases with increasing birthweight. The risk of shoulder dystocia is approximately 3% when the birthweight is between 4 and 4.5 kg, and 10–14% for a birthweight >4.5 kg. However, a Caesarean section policy based purely on estimated birthweight by ultrasound (4000 or 4500 g) would result in an unacceptable high rate. Planning delivery of a large baby of a diabetic mother detected on ultrasound needs to include maternal past obstetric history, her own size and personal preference.

Delivery

PROTOCOLS FOR INSULIN DURING LABOUR AND DELIVERY

As most women with diabetes will be given a day for delivery, be it for induction or Caesarean section, there need to be clear written guidelines for both the women and the labour ward on how insulin requirements are managed during labour. While there is not an absolute right or wrong way to give insulin during this period it is usual hospital policy to start an intravenous insulin sliding scale with a 5% glucose insulin infusion during active labour and during an operative delivery, and that is continued after delivery until the mother starts taking meals. During this time hourly blood glucose monitoring should be done. Once delivered the insulin dose must be halved, see below.

As most pregnant women prior to delivery are taking a night time long-acting basal insulin and quick-acting bolus insulin with their evening meal, women being admitted for a planned induction should be encouraged to take their normal insulin doses the night before. Once admitted they should continue with their short-acting bolus insulin to cover meals only switching to an intravenous insulin sliding scale once in labour or a decision has been taken to perform a Caesarean section.

Ideally elective Caesarean sections should be planned for early morning, with the women instructed to take their normal bolus insulin with their evening meal and two thirds of their usual basal insulin the night before admission. Once on the ward an intravenous insulin sliding scale can be started, with the dose adjusted downwards straight after delivery, p. 252.

Post-partum

Insulin requirements drop to prepregnancy values immediately following delivery of the placenta. For women with type 1 diabetes they can recommence their prepregnancy insulin regime as soon as they are eating and drinking normally. This dose of insulin should be clearly written in the notes as part of the delivery plan. For women who have type 2 diabetes previously on oral agents, these too can be restated immediately following pregnancy.

Insulin is not excreted into breast milk and is considered completely safe for use during breastfeeding. Insulin requirement often fall in mothers with type 1 diabetes who breastfeed due to the small increase in metabolic rate that occurs with lactation. The use of Metformin by breastfeeding mothers is also considered safe, as very little of the drug is excreted in breast milk. The sulphonylurea oral agents are highly protein bound and as this binding is nonionic are unlikely to be displaced by other drugs and to pass into breast milk. Theoretically the oral agents that are secretagogues could cause neonatal hypoglycaemia, and for this reason, metformin is favoured over the sulphonylurea drugs when an oral hypoglycaemic drug is needed while breastfeeding. The post-partum period is also a time when contraception advice should be offered.

SCREENING FOR AND THE MANAGEMENT OF GESTATIONAL DIABETES

Gestational diabetes is glucose intolerance first recognized in pregnancy. This definition includes women with previously undiagnosed diabetes at one end of the spectrum and those with mild disturbances of glucose intolerance resulting from the metabolic changes in late pregnancy at the other end. There is no controversy that women with undiagnosed diabetes should be as vigorously managed in pregnancy as those women known to have diabetes prior to pregnancy. As the background prevalence of undiagnosed type 2 diabetes increases the need to screen for diabetes early in pregnancy will also increase. A much smaller proportion of women of this age will be in the preclinical stages of type 1 diabetes and they too may present with GDM.

Internationally, there remains no agreement on how and who to screen for GDM. While different criteria exist across Europe and the USA for its diagnosis, there has been a general trend to move towards the World Health Organization (WHO) criteria based on a 75-g oral glucose tolerance test (OGTT), see Table 27.4. The decision to screen for GDM universally or to only target those women with recognized risk factors, see Table 27.5, has also not been resolved.

There is considerable debate on the benefits to pregnancy outcome on identifying and treating all women with lesser degrees of glucose intolerance, such as those that fulfil the WHO criteria for impaired glucose tolerance (IGT). An overall reduction in perinatal complications among women actively treated for GDM has recently been

Table 27.4 World Health Organization (WHO) criteria for glucose tolerance based on a 75 g oral glucose tolerance test (OGTT)

	Fasting plasma glucose	2 fasting h glucose
Normal glucose tolerance	<7.0 mmol/l	<7.8 mmol/l
Impaired glucose tolerance	<7.0 mmol/l	>7.8 <11.1 mmol/l
Diabetes*	>7.0 mmol/l	>11.1 mmol/l

*Definition requires either the fasting or 2 h value to be met.

Table 27.5 Risk factors for gestational diabetes

Body mass index >30 kg/m^2
Gestational diabetes in a previous pregnancy
Age: >25 years old
Family history of diabetes
Ethnicity – belonging to a non-white ethnic group
Previous delivery of a large baby
Previous stillbirth

demonstrated in an Australian randomized clinical trial involving 1000 women with GDM [7]. These women were diagnosed using the WHO criteria for IGT between 24 and 34 weeks' gestation and were then randomized to receive active intervention with diet, glucose monitoring and insulin, if required, or to no active intervention. This study also showed that the intervention group had a 10% higher rate of induction of labour than those receiving routine care; the Caesarean section rate, however, was similar.

The exact threshold of maternal glycaemia, if there is one, within the WHO range of IGT that warrants active treatment has still to be defined and another large multinational study involving 25,000 unselected pregnancies known as the HAPO (Hyperglycaemic Adverse Pregnancy Outcome) Study will hopefully provide information on this.

The glycaemic targets set for GDM in pregnancy should be similar to those for all diabetic women, namely fasting blood glucose below 6 mmol/l and postprandial glucose of <8 mmol/l. While some women with GDM can be controlled with diet and modest exercise alone, many require insulin to reach these targets. The exact role for the use of oral hypoglycaemic agents is controversial. Although the newer sulphonylurea agents appear safe when given after 15 weeks' gestation [2] their use with or without metformin is still felt by many to be less effective and flexible than prescribing insulin. Certainly in those parts of the world in which access to insulin is problematic, oral hypoglycaemic agents provide an alternative therapeutic option.

Women identified as having GDM, who do not have previously undiagnosed diabetes, usually revert to having normal glucose tolerance post-partum. However, over the subsequent 20 years the majority will develop type 2 diabetes. Lifestyle intervention that minimizes weight gain and encourages physical activity has been shown to halve the progression rate to diabetes over the subsequent 4–5 years. It is therefore important that women who have GDM receive basic lifestyle advice post-partum and are informed on the need to be screened annually for diabetes.

NEONATAL AND LONGER TERM CONSEQUENCES OF A DIABETIC PREGNANCY

The neonate of the diabetic mother in addition to the increased risk of congenital abnormalities is at increased risk of a number of transient metabolic disturbances as outlined in Table 27.2 [8]. The commonest of these is hypoglycaemia that is a consequence of persistent fetal hyperinsulinaemia occurring after birth when the maternal transfer of glucose has ceased. All of these metabolic conditions are transient and all can be attributed to the over exposure to maternal glucose and other fuel nutrients.

Recent studies on children of both type 1 and type 2 diabetic mothers have shown that there is an increased risk of childhood obesity and metabolic disturbances in adolescence including an increased risk of glucose intolerance [9]. This risk increases among children of poorly controlled diabetic mothers. As young adults, children of diabetic mothers have an increased risk of type 2 diabetes. The emergence of diabetes in these children is at an earlier age than that of their mother. Together these follow-up studies are highly suggestive that maternal diabetes can influence aspects of fetal metabolic programming, and stresses the importance of achieving exemplary glycaemic control in all diabetic pregnancies.

Endocrine disease

Thyroid disease is the commonest endocrine disorder in pregnant women and this will therefore be considered in more detail than other endocrinopathies. However, pituitary, adrenal and parathyroid disease may have serious consequences for the mother and fetus and these will also be discussed.

Thyroid disease

THYROID FUNCTION IN NORMAL PREGNANCY

The thyroid hormones thyroxine (T4) and tri-iodothyronine (T3) are synthesized within the thyroid follicles.

Table 27.6 Normal ranges for thyroid function tests in pregnancy

Gestation	FT4 (pmol/l)	FT3 (pmol/l)	TSH (mU/l)
Non-pregnant	11–23	4–9	0–4
1st trimester	11–22	4–8	0–1.6
2nd trimester	11–19	4–7	0.1–1.18
3rd trimester	7–15	3–5	0.7–7.3

[22–24].

Thyroid-stimulating hormone (TSH) stimulates synthesis and release of T3 and T4, in addition to uptake of iodide which is essential for thyroid hormone synthesis. Although T4 is synthesized in greater quantities, it is converted into the more potent T3 by deiodination in peripheral tissues.

During normal pregnancy the circulating levels of thyroid binding globulin increase, and as a consequence total T3 and T4 levels also increase. Therefore the free hormone levels should be measured in pregnant women. TSH levels should be interpreted with caution in the first trimester as hCG has a weak stimulatory effect on the TSH receptor. Table 27.6 summarizes the normal ranges for TSH, free T4 and free T3 in pregnancy.

The fetus cannot synthesize thyroxine and tri-iodothyronine until the 10th week of gestation, and it is therefore dependent upon transplacental transfer of the maternal hormone. There is increased maternal synthesis of thyroid hormones in the first trimester as a result of transplacental passage and the high levels of thyroid binding globulin, and this in turn results in an increased maternal requirement for iodide. In areas of relative iodide deficiency this may result in the development of maternal hypothyroxinaemia and goitre.

HYPOTHYROIDISM

Hypothyroidism affects approximately 1% of pregnant women. Providing thyroxine replacement therapy is adequate, hypothyroidism is not associated with an adverse pregnancy outcome for the mother or fetus. Older studies demonstrated an association between poorly controlled hypothyroidism and a variety of adverse outcomes, including congenital abnormalities, hypertension, premature delivery, fetal growth restriction and post-partum haemorrhage. These complications have not been reported in more recent studies, although inadequate treatment was associated with an increased risk of gestational hypertension in a study of 68 women with overt hypothyroidism or subclinical hypothyroidism [10]. Furthermore, a study that compared 404 women with subclinical hypothyroidism (i.e. raised TSH with normal FT4) with 16,894 controls demonstrated an association with placental abruption and premature delivery [11]. Overt hypothyroidism causes subfertility, and the presence of thyroid autoantibodies, even if the mother is euthyroid, is associated with an increased risk of miscarriage that was quantified as having an odds ratio of 2.3 (95%CI, 1.8–2.95) in a recent meta-analysis [12].

Severe hypothyroidism affects the subsequent intelligence of the offspring of affected mothers. A study that measured TSH levels in retrospectively collected midterm serum screening samples identified a subgroup of women with raised TSH and demonstrated that their children had neurodevelopmental delay at the age of 7–9 [13]. Other studies have also suggested that inadequately treated hypothyroidism may affect the subsequent intelligence of the offspring, and one recent study suggested that correction of hypothyroxinaemia in later pregnancy may prevent abnormal infant development [14].

Women with hypothyroidism should be given thyroxine replacement at a dose that ensures their thyroid function tests are normal with a FT4 at the upper end of the normal range appropriate for each trimester of pregnancy (Table 27.6). The exception is for women who have had a thyroidectomy for thyroid cancer as it is necessary to suppress TSH secretion, and in whom the thyroxine dose should be increased if required. Thyroxine absorption is decreased by certain drugs including iron and calcium supplements, thyroxine is best taken on an empty stomach and 4 h apart from any iron or other supplements.

HYPERTHYROIDISM

Hyperthyroidism affects 1 in 500 pregnant women, 90% of whom have Graves' disease. Graves' disease is caused by TSH receptor stimulating antibodies. Women with well-treated disease rarely have maternal complications of pregnancy. However, the disease may remit during the latter trimesters such that treatment may need to be reduced or stopped. In the post-partum period the disease may flare and require treatment with the same or higher doses of antithyroid medication. Poorly controlled hyperthyroidism is associated with several pregnancy complications, including maternal thyrotoxic crisis, miscarriage, gestational hypertension, pre-eclampsia and intrauterine growth restriction [15,16]. The risk of these complications is reduced if the disease is adequately controlled before delivery.

The principal drugs used to treat hyperthyroidism (propylthiouracil and carbimazole) inhibit thyroid hormone synthesis. The early reports of an association between carbimazole treatment and aplasia cutis in the fetus have not been confirmed by subsequent studies, and there is no other evidence that either drug is associated with congenital abnormalities. However, a greater proportion of carbimazole enters breast milk, and therefore propylthiouracil is usually the drug of choice if a woman is diagnosed as having hyperthyroidism for the first time during pregnancy. Both drugs may rarely cause neutropenia and agranulocytosis. Therefore patients should be aware that symptoms of infection, particularly sore throat, may be associated with bone marrow suppression and they must have a neutrophil count checked immediately should they occur. Once drug treatment has been commenced thyroid function tests should be carried out and checked regularly.

Propylthiouracil and carbimazole both cross the placenta. However, fetal hypothyroidism is rarely seen. TSH receptor stimulating antibodies also cross the placenta and may influence the fetal and neonatal thyroid status. The potential consequences of transplacental passage of thyroid stimulating antibodies (and the relevance of concurrent administration of antithyroid medication) are summarized in Fig. 27.1.

Women requiring antithyroid medication should not be discouraged from breastfeeding. However, if they are taking more than 15 mg carbimazole or 150 mg propylthiouracil daily the infant should be reviewed and they should be encouraged to feed before taking the medication and to take divided doses.

Thyrotoxic crisis, also called 'thyroid storm', is a medical emergency that can present with exaggerated features of hyperthyroidism in addition to hyperpyrexia, congestive cardiac failure, dysrhythmias and an altered mental state. It may be precipitated by infection, abrupt cessation of treatment, surgery, labour or delivery and must be treated immediately as it can be life threatening. Treatment involves administration of intravenous fluids, hydrocortisone, propranolol, oral iodine and carbimazole or propylthiouracil.

POST-PARTUM THYROIDITIS

Post-partum thyroiditis is associated with the presence of thyroid antiperoxidase antibodies. The quoted incidence varies between 2 and 16%. It is characterized by an initial hyperthyroid phase that classically occurs 1–3 months post-partum, followed by a hypothyroid phase, which usually resolves by 12 months after delivery. The hypothyroidism may require treatment with thyroxine, but treatment should be stopped after 1 year as many cases resolve. However, the likelihood of developing subsequent hypothyroidism in women who have had post-partum thyroiditis is quoted at 5% per year, so affected women should have their thyroid function checked regularly.

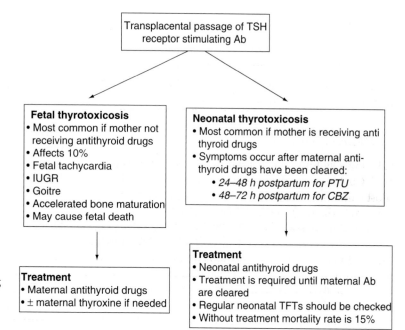

Fig. 27.1 Fetal and neonatal effects of transplacental passage of TSH receptor stimulating antibodies. Abbreviations: IUGR, intrauterine growth restriction; CBZ, carbimazole; PTU, propylthiouracil; TFT, thyroid function test.

Pituitary disease

The anterior pituitary secretes prolactin, growth hormone (GH), adrenocorticotrophic hormone (ACTH), follicle-stimulating hormone (FSH), luteinizing hormone (LH) and thyroid-stimulating hormone (TSH).

PITUITARY TUMOURS

Prolactinomas

In normal pregnancy the pituitary gland increases in size by 50–70% as a consequence of normal lactotroph hyperplasia, and therefore a tumour that did not cause pressure effects in the non-pregnant state may do so during pregnancy. The most frequently seen pituitary tumours in pregnant women are prolactinomas, although ACTH- or GH-secreting tumours or non-functioning (i.e. non-hormone secreting) tumours may also be seen. Common symptoms that occur as a consequence of enlargement of a pituitary tumour are headache and visual disturbance, in particular bitemporal field loss. Rarely a woman may develop pituitary apoplexy or diabetes insipidus.

Prolactinomas are subdivided according to their size. Tumours that measure <10 mm in diameter are defined as microprolactinomas and constitute the majority. In non-pregnant patients, 5% of tumours are defined as macroprolactinomas (>10 mm). Most women with microprolactinomas can be reassured that they rarely enlarge in pregnancy. It is not necessary to continue treatment with dopamine agonists once a woman with a microprolactinoma has conceived. Surveillance should include a clinical assessment each trimester that comprises assessment of the visual fields to confrontation and enquiry for symptoms suggestive of pituitary enlargement. Serum prolactin levels should not be checked as they increase by as much as 10-fold by the 25th week of gestation. Several studies have reported the frequency of symptomatic enlargement of microprolactinomas in pregnancy and when these data are combined, only 1.4% of 363 cases have symptoms of tumour enlargement [17]. In contrast, 26.2% of 84 women with macroprolactinomas had symptomatic tumour enlargement, and in 19 cases this resulted in treatment with a dopamine agonist or surgery. Sixty-seven women with macroprolactinomas had been treated with surgery or irradiation before pregnancy, and only two of these cases had symptomatic tumour enlargement [17].

Women with macroprolactinomas should continue to take dopamine agonists throughout pregnancy and the visual fields should be checked with formal perimetry on a regular basis, that is, at least once each trimester and more commonly if there are any concerns. Bromocriptine was the first dopamine agonist to be used, but its use is associated with relatively common side-effects, including nausea, vomiting and postural hypotension. Therefore cabergoline and quinagolide are now more commonly used as they are better tolerated, and cabergoline has the additional advantage of a longer half-life, allowing it to be given once or twice weekly. The data that are available indicate that bromocriptine and cabergoline are not associated with an increased risk of congenital abnormalities or other adverse pregnancy outcomes. However, there are insufficient data about the outcomes of pregnancies in which the mother was treated with quinagolide.

Women taking dopamine agonists are usually unable to lactate. However, breastfeeding is not contraindicated in women with microprolactinomas as it does not cause an increase in the size of these pituitary tumours.

ACTH-secreting tumours

Cushing's syndrome is caused by excess circulating cortisol. Cushing's syndrome in non-pregnant individuals is most commonly caused by ACTH-secreting tumours (i.e. Cushing's disease), while adrenal tumours are the commonest cause in pregnant women, and 21% of the adrenal tumours are malignant [18]. The predominance of adrenal tumours may be explained by reduced fertility in women with pituitary tumours. Cushing's syndrome caused by both pituitary and adrenal tumours will be considered in this section as many of the features overlap.

Plasma levels of cortisol, ACTH and cortisol-binding globulin are raised in pregnancy, as is the urinary free cortisol. Therefore it is important to refer to normal ranges for pregnancy when investigating the hypothalamo-pituitary axis in a pregnant woman. A review of case reports of maternal Cushing's syndrome reported premature delivery in 12 of 23 cases, one spontaneous abortion and two stillbirths [18]. A review of the management of Cushing's syndrome secondary to adrenal tumours demonstrated that the fetal and neonatal outcome is better if the tumour is removed during pregnancy rather than at completion of pregnancy [19].

Untreated Cushing's syndrome in pregnancy is associated with increased rates of maternal and fetal morbidity and mortality, and in particular the incidence of diabetes mellitus and hypertension is high. Treatment of Cushing's syndrome is primarily surgical. There have been reports of successful use of the medical agents metyrapone, ketoconazole and aminogluthemide all of which inhibit biosynthesis of cortisol, and of cyproheptadine which suppresses corticotrophin-releasing hormone. However, experience is limited due to the rarity of Cushing's syndrome in pregnancy.

Other pituitary tumours

GH-secreting tumours cause acromegaly which is associated with impaired fertility, and therefore pregnancy occurs rarely. Even in treated women there have been very few reports of pregnancy. Women with acromegaly usually have macroadenomas, and therefore the normal stimulation of adjacent lactotrophs may result in symptoms consistent with tumour expansion in pregnancy. It is therefore important to monitor the visual fields using formal perimetry as for women with pituitary macroadenomas. Women have an increased risk of impaired glucose tolerance, diabetes mellitus and hypertensive disease. Treatment options include dopamine agonists to reduce the size of adjacent lactotrophs, somatostatin analogues or surgery. The somatostatin analogue octreotide has been used in a small number of cases without adverse effects.

The most effective treatment for non-functioning pituitary tumours is surgery (possibly followed by radiotherapy).

DIABETES INSIPIDUS

Diabetes insipidus is caused by a deficiency of the posterior pituitary hormone vasopressin. A subgroup of affected women require an increased dose of desmopressin as a consequence of placental synthesis of vasopressinase. This may also explain why some cases present *de novo* in pregnancy. Desmopressin is more effective than vasopressin as it is more resistant to vasopressinase.

LYMPHOCYTIC HYPOPHYSITIS

Lymphocytic hypophysitis is an inflammatory disease of the pituitary that occurs more commonly in women and is associated with pregnancy. Approximately 60% of cases present with hypopituitarism and 20% present with diabetes insipidus [20]. It is important to distinguish lymphocytic hypophysitis from a pituitary adenoma as surgery may exacerbate hypopituitarism associated with the former. Lymphocytic hypophysitis may resolve spontaneously and approximately 50% of cases respond to corticosteroids, although the condition commonly recurs following cessation of treatment.

SHEEHAN'S SYNDROME

The term Sheehan's syndrome describes hypopituitarism that presents in the late post-partum period, and which is caused by haemorrhage and hypotension at the time of delivery. The hypotension results in avascular necrosis which affects the anterior pituitary more commonly than the posterior pituitary. Women most frequently present with a failure of lactation and subsequent amenorrhoea, but they may have any feature of hypopituitarism including the more subtle features of hypoadrenalism and hypothyroidism.

Adrenal disease

ADRENAL TUMOURS

Adrenal tumours are rare in pregnancy. The commoner tumours secrete corticosteroids, catecholamines or aldosterone, causing Cushing's syndrome, phaeochromocytoma or Conn's syndrome, respectively. Nonfunctioning tumours may rarely occur. Cushing's syndrome is more commonly caused by adrenal tumours in pregnant women as discussed above.

Phaeochromocytoma is rare but important to diagnose because the maternal and fetal mortality has been quoted as 50% if it is not treated adequately. The diagnosis should be suspected in women with hypertension that occurs in association with sweating, anxiety, headache or palpitations. The clinical features may be paroxysmal and some women have impaired glucose tolerance or diabetes. The diagnosis is made with 24-h urinary catecholamines which should be repeated several times if an initial test is normal. Other investigations that may be used are plasma catecholamines or a pentolinium suppression test, and there should be a low threshold for performing magnetic resonance imaging. Treatment should be with an alpha-blocker, for example, phenoxybenzamine, in the first instance followed by a beta-blocker, for example, propranolol. Definitive treatment is surgical removal, the timing of which is dictated by the gestational age at diagnosis, the response to medical treatment and the accessibility of the tumour.

CONN'S SYNDROME

Primary hyperaldosteronism, also called Conn's syndrome, is characterized by hypertension in association with low serum potassium, raised plasma aldosterone and suppressed renin activity. The pregnancy-specific reference ranges for these hormones should be used. Conn's syndrome usually improves in pregnancy. However, when symptomatic the hypertension may be treated with conventional antihypertensives. Spironolactone should not be used as this may cause feminization of the male fetus. Surgery is also a treatment option.

HYPOADRENALISM

Hypoadrenalism may result from haemorrhagic destruction, for example, as a consequence of severe obstetric haemorrhage or from autoimmune destruction (Addison's disease). It may present in an insidious manner with symptoms of fatigue, hypotension, nausea, vomiting, and ultimately with sepsis or circulatory collapse. Serum biochemistry may reveal hyponatraemia and a serum cortisol should be checked (ideally with a cortisol-binding globulin and in liaison with an endocrinologist). If a diagnosis of Addison's disease is made, it should be remembered that this commonly coexists with other autoimmune diseases, and there should be a low threshold for screening for conditions such as pernicious anaemia, thyroid disease or type

I diabetes. Glucocorticoid replacement is mandatory if the hypoadrenalism is suspected although this can usually be delayed until after the serum cortisol has been checked. The glucocorticoid dose should be increased to cover the stress of labour or intercurrent infections and the woman should carry a steroid card and medicalert bracelet.

CONGENITAL ADRENAL HYPERPLASIA

The term congenital adrenal hyperplasia describes several inborn errors of metabolism that affect glucocorticoid and mineralocorticoid synthesis, the commonest of which is 21-hydroxylase deficiency. They are associated with reduced fertility, particularly if associated with mineralocorticoid deficiency. Affected women who manage to conceive have increased risks of hypertension and pre-eclampsia. The steroid requirement rarely increases during pregnancy. However, the dose of glucocorticoids should be increased to cover labour. Women should receive genetic counselling prior to conception to discuss the merits of mutation screening in the partner (for 21-hydroxylase deficiency the carrier rate is 1 in 50) and the risk of having an affected fetus.

PARATHYROID DISEASE

Hyperparathyroidism is associated with a raised parathyroid hormone and may be primary, secondary or tertiary. Primary hyperparathyroidism is most commonly caused by a parathyroid adenoma, and is associated with hypercalcaemia and hypercalciuria. Secondary hyperparathyroidism is a normal physiological consequence of chronic hypocalcaemia, for example, in association with vitamin D deficiency or chronic renal failure. Tertiary hyperparathyroidism occurs when a clone of cells starts to function autonomously following long-standing secondary hyperparathyroidism. Primary hyperparathyroidism is commoner in women and 25% of cases occur in the childbearing years. Most pregnant women with the disease are asymptomatic, although they may have symptoms of hypercalcaemia including nephrolithiasis, pancreatitis or altered mental state. The condition does, however, have a high perinatal complication rate, with fetal death reported as 27–31% of conservatively managed pregnancies and neonatal tetany occurring in 50% of neonates of untreated mothers [21]. The perinatal complication rate is reduced considerably if the condition is treated and for most cases the appropriate therapy is surgical removal of the tumour, ideally in the first trimester.

Vitamin D deficiency

Vitamin D deficiency may be nutritional or secondary to a metabolic disease. Nutritional deficiency of vitamin D is particularly common in women of Asian and Somali origin in the UK, and it can present with osteomalacia and pathological fractures in pregnancy. Maternal vitamin D deficiency is associated with neonatal morbidity and impaired growth within the first year, and therefore vitamin D supplementation is recommended in at-risk groups. The WHO recommends 400 IU (10 μg) of vitamin D daily during pregnancy and lactation. Outside pregnancy, individuals with osteomalacia may be treated with intramuscular (IM) injections of vitamin D, but at present there are no data to indicate whether this form of vitamin D administration is associated with any risk in pregnancy. The authors suspect that IM treatment may be appropriate for women with resistant, symptomatic osteomalacia but do not recommend it as a routine treatment in pregnant women.

References

1. Clausen TD, Mathiesen E, Ekbom P, Hellmuth E, Mandrup-Poulsen T & Damm P. (2005) Poor pregnancy outcome in women with type 2 diabetes. *Diabetes Care* **28**: 323–8.
2. Langer O, Conway DL, Berkus MD, Xenakis EM-J, Gonzales O (2000) A comparison of glyburide and insulin in women with gestational diabetes mellitus. *N Engl J Med* **343**, 1134–8.
3. Kristensen J, Vestergaard M, Wisborg K, Kesmodel U & Secher NJ (2005) Pre-pregnancy weight and the risk of stillbirth and neonatal death. *Br J Obstet Gynaecol* **112**, 403–8.
4. Wender-Ozegowska E, Wroblewska K, Zawiejska A, Pietryga M, Szczapa J & Biczysko R (2005) Threshold values of maternal blood glucose in early diabetic pregnancy-prediction of fetal malformations. *Acta Obstet Gynecol Scand* **84**, 17–25.
5. McCarthy EA, Walker SP, McLachlan K, Boyle J & Permezel M (2004) Metformin in obstetric and gynecologic practice: a review. *Obstet Gynecol Surv* **59**, 118–27.
6. Lauenborg J, Mathiesen E, Ovesen P et al. (2003) Audit on stillbirths in women with pregestational type 1 diabetes. *Diabetes Care* **26**, 1385–9.
7. Crowther CA, Hiller JE, Moss JR, McPhee AJ, Jeffries WS, Robinson JS, Australian Carbohydrate Intolerance Study in Pregnant Women (ACHOIS) Trial Group (2005) Effect of treatment of gestational diabetes mellitus on pregnancy outcomes. *N Engl J Med* **352**, 2477–86 .
8. Nold JL & Georgieff MK (2004) Infants of diabetic mothers. *Pediat Clin North Am* **51**, 619–37.
9. Weiss PA, Scholz HS, Haas J, Tamussino KF, Seissler J, Borkenstein MH (2000) Long-term follow-up of infants of mothers with type 1 diabetes. evidence for hereditary and nonhereditary transmission of diabetes and precursors. *Diabetes Care* **23**, 905–11.
10. Leung AS, Millar LK, Koonings PP, Montoro M & Mestman JH (1993) Perinatal outcome in hypothyroid pregnancies. *Obstet Gynecol* **81**, 349–53.
11. Casey BM, Dashe JS, Wells CE et al. (2005) Subclinical hypothyroidism and pregnancy outcomes. *Obstet Gynecol* **105**(2), 239–45.
12. Prummel MF & Wiersinga WM (2004) Thyroid autoimmunity and miscarriage. *Eur J Endocrinol* **150**(6), 751–5.
13. Haddow JE, Palomaki GE, Allan WC et al. (1999) Maternal thyroid deficiency during pregnancy and subsequent neuropsychological development of the child. *N Engl J Med* **341**(8), 549–55.
14. Pop VJ, Brouwers EP, Vader HL, Vulsma T, van Baar AL & de Vijlder JJ (2003) Maternal hypothyroxinaemia during early pregnancy and subsequent child development: a 3-year follow-up study. *Clin Endocrinol (Oxf)* **59**(3), 282–8.
15. Millar LK, Wing DA, Leung AS, Koonings PP, Montoro MN & Mestman JH (1994) Low birth weight and preeclampsia in pregnancies complicated by hyperthyroidism. *Obstet Gynecol* **84**(6), 946–9.
16. Mestman JH (2004) Hyperthyroidism in pregnancy. *Best Pract Res Clin Endocrinol Metab* **18**(2), 267–88.
17. Molitch ME (2003) Pituitary tumours and pregnancy. *Growth Horm IGF Res* **13**(Suppl A), S38–44.
18. Pickard J, Jochen AL, Sadur CN & Hofeldt FD (1990) Management of Cushing's syndrome secondary to adrenal adenoma during pregnancy. *Obstet Gynecol Surv* **45**(2), 87–93.
19. Pricolo VE, Monchik JM, Prinz RA, DeJong S, Chadwick DA & Lamberton RP (1990) Management of Cushing's syndrome secondary to adrenal adenoma during pregnancy. *Surgery* **108**(6), 1072–7.
20. Thodu E, Asa SL, Kontogeorgos G, Kovacs K, Horvath E & Ezzat S (1995) Clinical Case Seminar: Lymphocytic hypophysitis: Clinicopathological findings. *J Clin Endocrinol Metab* **80**, 2302–11.
21. Schnatz PF & Curry FL (2002) Primary hyperparathyroidism in pregnancy: evidence-based management. *Obstet Gynecol Surv* **57**, 365–76.
22. Parker JH (1985) Amerlex free tri-iodothyronine and free thyroxine levels in normal pregnancy. *Br J Obstet Gynaecol* **92**, 1234–8.
23. Chan BY & Swaminathan R (1988) Serum thyrotrophin hormone concentration measured by sensitive assays in normal pregnancy. *Br J Obstet Gynaecol* **95**, 1332–6.
24. Kotarba DD, Garner P & Perkins SL (1995) Changes in serum free thyroxine, free tri-iodothyronine and thyroid stimulating hormone reference intervals in normal term pregnancy. *J Obstet Gynecol* **15**, 5–8.

Further reading

ACOG Committee on Practice Bulletins. ACOG Practice Bulletin (2005) Clinical Management Guidelines for Obstetrician-Gynecologists. Number 60, Pregestational diabetes mellitus. *Obstet & Gynecol* **105**, 675–85.

Butte NF (2000) Carbohydrate and lipid metabolism in pregnancy: normal compared with gestational diabetes mellitus. *Am J Clin Nutr* **71**(5 Suppl) 1256S-61S.

Galerneau F & Inzucchi SE (2004) Diabetes mellitus in pregnancy. *Obstet Gynecol Clin North Am.* **31**, 907–33, xi–xii.

Buchanan TA & Xiang AH (2005) Gestational diabetes mellitus. *J Clin Invest.* **115**, 485–91.

Lakasing L & Williamson C (2005) Obstetric complications due to autoantibodies. *Baillieres Best Pract Res Clin Endocrinol Metab* **19**, 149–75.

de Swiet M (2002) *Medical disorders in Obstetric Practice* Oxford: Blackwell Publishing Company.

Hague WM (2001) Drugs in pregnancy. Endocrine disease (including diabetes). *Best Pract Res Clin Obstet Gynaecol* **15**(6), 937–52.

Chapter 28: Renal disease

John Davison

To provide care for women with underlying renal disease contemplating pregnancy or those already pregnant, the obstetrician must have up-to-date knowledge about pregnancy physiology, antenatal care and technology for fetal surveillance as well as neonatology. Also it is essential to appreciate the need for teamwork in a centre with all the necessary facilities for dealing with 'high risk' patients and to strike a balance between 'what the patient wants to know' and 'what the clinician needs to know'. This chapter focuses on chronic renal disease, women on dialysis and kidney allograft recipients, aiming to provide the busy clinician with 'at a glance information' for counselling and the 'clinical watchpoints' necessary for timely decision-making.

What the patient wants to know

Ideally, it should be couples who should be encouraged to discuss all of the implications. The advice will vary according to the pathology and the clinical setting. Nevertheless, the questions are straightforward:

Should I get pregnant?
Will my pregnancy be complicated?
Will I have a live and healthy baby?
Will I have problems after my pregnancy?

The answers should be equally straightforward and must be based on fact, not on anecdote. Even if some of the answers are not favourable, many women will choose to go ahead for a pregnancy or with the pregnancy, in an effort to re-establish a normal life in the face of chronic illness. In some cases this may bring them into conflict with their medical advisers and indeed, some women do not seek advice until already pregnant. This may lead to ethical dilemmas regarding clinicians' duties of care towards women who ignore advice. Attempts are being made to differentiate 'healthy' and 'pathological' levels of assumed risk and to understand the psychology of women who pursue parenthood despite substantial risk to their own health and that of their unborn child.

What the clinician needs to know about normal pregnancy

Glomerular filtration rate (GFR), measured as 24-h creatinine clearance (C_{cr}), increases by 6–8 weeks' gestation. Serum creatinine (S_{cr}) and urea (S_{urea}), which average 70 μ mol/l and 5 mmol/l, respectively, in non-pregnant women, decrease to mean values of 50 μmol/l and 3 mmol/l during pregnancy. At term a 15–20% GFR decrement occurs, which affects S_{cr} minimally.

An S_{cr} of 80 μmol/l and urea of 6 mmol/l, which are acceptable when non-pregnant, are suspect in pregnancy. Caution is needed, however, when assessing kidney function by S_{cr} alone, especially if some decline in GFR has already accrued because creatinine is both filtered and secreted, with the creatinine clearance:inulin clearance (C_{cr} : C_{inulin}) ratio usually 1.1–1.2. With the progression of renal dysfunction a greater proportion of urinary creatinine is via secretion with the clearance ratio attaining 1.4–1.6 when $S_{cr} \geq 125$ μmol/l. Thus, GFR could be considerably overestimated.

Prediction equations, such as the Cockcroft-Gault (CG) Formula, which use S_{cr} in relation to sex, age and weight to calculate GFR are best avoided in pregnancy because of changing body weight. A relatively new formula, the Modification of Renal Disease 2 (MDRD2) equation excludes weight but it has not yet been validated in pregnancy. Ideally, therefore, evaluation of renal function in pregnancy should be based on C_{cr} and not S_{cr}. Furthermore, S_{cr} levels may increase up to 17 μmol/l shortly after ingestion of cooked meat (because cooking converts preformed creatine to creatinine), which has to be taken into account when timing blood sampling during a 24-h C_{cr} test.

In normal pregnancy 24-h urinary total protein excretion (TPE) increases and up to 300 mg (some would say 500 mg) can be regarded as normal. So-called significant proteinuria with TPE>300 mg/24 h may correlate with 30 mg/dl in a 'spot urine' but given the problems with dipstick testing, many still prefer a 24-h or some timed quantitative determination. Use of 'spot urine' protein/creatinine ratios ≥30 mg/μmol is, however, an alternative.

What the clinician needs to know about chronic renal disease

Consensus now is that provided non-pregnant renal function is only mildly compromised, proteinuria not in the nephrotic range (3 g/24 h) and hypertension absent or minimal, then obstetric outcome is usually successful with little or no adverse effect on long-term renal prognosis.

Renal dysfunction and the prospects for pregnancy and afterwards

A woman may lose up to 50% of her renal function and still maintain an S_{cr} less than 130 μmol/l because of hyperfiltration by the remaining nephrons but if renal function is more severely compromised then small further decreases in GFR will cause S_{cr} to increase markedly.

In women with renal disease the pathology may be both biochemically and clinically silent. Most individuals remain symptom-free until their GFR declines to less than 25% of normal, and many serum constituents are frequently normal until a late stage of disease. Degrees of functional impairment that do not cause symptoms or appear to disrupt homoeostasis in non-pregnant individuals can, however, jeopardize pregnancy. Normal pregnancy is rare when renal function declines such that the non-pregnant S_{cr} and S_{urea} exceed 275 μmol/l and 10 μmol/l, respectively.

The basic question for a woman with renal disease must be: *is pregnancy advisable*? If it is, then the sooner she starts to have her family the better, since in many cases renal function will decline with time. Women with suspected or known renal disease, not always counselled prior to pregnancy, may present already pregnant, as a *'fait accompli'*; then the question must be: *'does pregnancy continue?'*

Obstetric and long-term renal prognoses differ in women with different degrees of renal insufficiency, and the prospects for pregnancy are best considered by categories of functional renal status prior to pregnancy.

Women with normal or only mildly decreased prepregnancy renal function (S_{cr} < 125 μmol/l) usually have a successful obstetric outcome, and pregnancy does not appear to adversely affect the course of their disease. There are exceptions with most strongly advising against pregnancy in women with scleroderma and periarteritis nodosa. A few express reservations when the underlying renal disorder is lupus nephropathy, membranoproliferative glomerulonephritis, and perhaps IgA and reflux nephropathies.

Most women will augment GFR, but not as much as in normal pregnant women. Increased proteinuria is common, occurring in 50% of pregnancies (although this is unusual in women with chronic pyelonephritis), and exceeds the nephrotic range (3 g in 24 h) in 50% of women. Perinatal outcome can be jeopardized by uncontrolled hypertension and for some when nephrotic range proteinuria is already present in early pregnancy.

Outlooks are more guarded when renal function is moderately impaired (S_{cr} 125 – –250 μmol/l) before pregnancy and are very drastically curtailed with severe renal dysfunction (S_{cr} > 250 μmol/l). Indeed, it is now apparent that once S_{cr} > 125 μmol/l the next significant 'cut-offs' from the clinical viewpoint are S_{cr} > 180 μmol/l and >220 μmol/l (see Table 28.1). These women do, however, become pregnant and their awareness of progress in antenatal care and neonatal provision can encourage them to anticipate good outcomes.

The literature has slowly increased in the last 10–15 years and the messages are clear: hypertension is common by term (50%) as is significant proteinuria (40%), as well as deterioration in renal function (at times rapid and substantial) and although the infant survival rates are good (80–90%), rates of premature delivery (60%) and fetal growth restriction (40%) underscore the very high potential for obstetric complications in these women. Not previously realized so clearly were the facts that 30–50% of women with moderate insufficiency experience functional loss more rapidly than would be expected from the natural course of their renal disease, plus poorly controlled hypertension might be a harbinger of poor outcome. As alluded to, once S_{cr}>250 μmol/l there are big risks of unsuccessful obstetric outcome and accelerated loss of renal function and even terminating the pregnancy may not reverse the decline.

Dialysis has been advocated prophylactically during pregnancy to increase the chances of successful outcome but 'buying time' for fetal maturation in this way is independent of the inexorable declines in renal function ultimately to endstage failure. As extreme prematurity and disturbing, life-threatening maternal problems are commonplace such additional health risks are difficult to justify. Perhaps the aim should be to preserve what little renal function remains and to achieve renal rehabilitation via dialysis and transplantation, after which the question of pregnancy can be considered if appropriate. Some women, however, will be prepared to take a chance and even seek assisted conception in the face of their infertility. As mentioned earlier, this pursuit of pregnancy and the issues surrounding the clinician's obligation to accede to (or refute) care that poses a risk to the woman's health is generating much discussion.

Of utmost importance to all the current controversies is that the literature that forms the basis of our views is primarily *retrospective* with most patients described having only mild dysfunction and women with severe disease

Table 28.1 Chronic renal disease: functional status, prospects for pregnancy and afterwards

S_{cr} (μmol/l)	Complicated pregnancy(%)	Successful obstetric outcome(%)	Loss of renal function(%)		Renal failure within 1 year post-partum(%)
			In pregnancy	Persists post-partum	
<125	25	98	2	–	–
>125	50	90	40	20	2
>180	90	75	65	40	25
>220	100	60	75	60	40

S_{cr} non-pregnant serum creatinine. Estimates based on literature review (1990–2005) from 217 women in 269 pregnancies that attained at least 24 weeks' gestation.

being limited in number. Confirmation of guidelines, therefore, requires further adequate prospective trials.

Antenatal strategy and decision making

Patients should be seen at 2-week intervals until 32 weeks' gestation, after which assessment should be weekly. Routine serial antenatal observations should be supplemented with

1 assessment of renal function by 24-h creatinine clearance and protein excretion (see Chapter 25);
2 careful blood pressure monitoring for early detection of hypertension and assessment of its severity;
3 early detection of pre-eclampsia;
4 biophysical/ultrasound surveillance of fetal size, development, and well-being;
5 early detection of covert bacteriuria or confirmation of urinary tract infection (UTI).

The crux of management is the balance between maternal prognosis and fetal prognosis – the effect of pregnancy on a particular disease and the effect of that disease on pregnancy. The 'clinical watchpoints' specifically associated with particular renal diseases are summarized in Table 28.2. The following guidelines apply to all clinical situations.

RENAL FUNCTION

If renal function deteriorates significantly at any stage of pregnancy, then reversible causes, such as UTI, subtle dehydration, or electrolyte imbalance (occasionally precipitated by inadvertent diuretic therapy) should be sought. Near term, as in normal pregnancy, a decrease in function of 15–20%, which affects S_{cr} minimally, is permissible. Failure to detect a reversible cause of a significant decrement is grounds to end the pregnancy by elective delivery. When proteinuria occurs and persists, but blood pressure is normal and renal function preserved, pregnancy can be allowed to continue under closer scrutiny.

BLOOD PRESSURE

Blood pressure should be measured in the sitting position with a cuff which is large enough for a particular patient's arm. Phases I and V of the Korotkoff sounds are used. Hypertension is not a disease but one end of a continuous distribution of all individuals' blood pressures. The conventional dividing line for obstetric hypertension is 140/90.

Most of the specific risks of hypertension in pregnancy appear to be related to superimposed pre-eclampsia (see Chapter 25). There is confusion about the true incidence of superimposed pre-eclampsia in women with pre-existing renal disease. This is because the diagnosis cannot be made with certainty on clinical grounds alone; hypertension and proteinuria may be manifestations of the underlying renal disease. Treatment of mild hypertension (diastolic blood pressure less than 95 mmHg in the second trimester or less than 100 mmHg in the third) is not necessary during normal pregnancy, but many would treat women with underlying renal disease more aggressively, believing that this preserves kidney function. Most patients can be taught to take their own blood pressure, but there are still debates about the accuracy of automated devices and the role of ambulatory blood pressure measurements.

FETAL SURVEILLANCE AND TIMING OF DELIVERY

Serial assessment of fetal well-being is essential since renal disease can be associated with fetal growth restriction and, when complications do arise, the judicious moment for intervention can be assessed by fetal status. Current technology should minimize the incidence of intrauterine fetal death as well as neonatal morbidity and mortality. Regardless of gestational age, most babies weighing >1500 g survive better in a special care nursery than in a hostile intrauterine environment. Planned preterm delivery may be necessary if there are signs of impending intrauterine fetal death, if renal function deteriorates substantially, if uncontrollable hypertension supervenes, or if eclampsia

Table 28.2 Chronic renal disease and pregnancy

Renal disease	'Clinical watchpoints'
Chronic glomerulonephritis and focal glomerular sclerosis (FGS)	Can be high blood pressure late in pregnancy but usually no adverse effect if renal function is preserved and hypertension absent prepregnancy. Some disagree, believing coagulation changes in pregnancy exacerbate disease, especially immunoglobulin A (IgA) nephropathy, membranoproliferative glomerulonephritis, and FGS
IgA nephropathy	Some cite risks of sudden escalating or uncontrolled hypertension and renal deterioration. Most note good outcome when renal function is preserved
Chronic pyelonephritis (infectious tubulointerstitial disease)	Bacteriuria in pregnancy and may lead to exacerbation
Reflux nephropathy	Some have emphasized risks of sudden escalating hypertension and worsening of renal function. Consensus now is that results are satisfactory when prepregnancy function is only mildly affected and hypertension is absent. Vigilance for urinary tract infections is necessary
Urolithiasis	Ureteral dilatation and stasis do not seem to affect natural history, but infections can be more frequent. Stents have been successfully placed and sonographically controlled ureterostomy has been performed during gestation
Polycystic kidney disease	Functional impairment and hypertension are usually minimal in childbearing years
Diabetic nephropathy	No adverse effect on the renal lesion. Increased frequency of infections, oedema or pre-eclampsia. Advanced nephropathy can be a problem
Human immunodeficiency virus with associated nephropathy (HIVAN)	Renal component can be nephrotic syndrome or severe impairment. Scanty literature but given ravages of this epidemic then HIVAN should be considered when immuno-compromised proteinuria occurs suddenly, especially in immuno-compromised patients.
Systemic lupus erythematosus	Prognosis is most favourable if disease is in remission 6 months before conception. Some increase steroid dosage immediately postpartum
Periarteritis nodosa	Fetal prognosis is poor. Maternal death can occur. Therapeutic abortion should be considered
Scleroderma	If onset during pregnancy, there can be rapid overall deterioration. Reactivation of quiescent scleroderma can occur during pregnancy and post-partum
Previous urologic surgery	Depending on original reason for surgery, there may be other malformations of the urogenital tract. Urinary tract infection is common during pregnancy and renal function may undergo reversible decrease. No significant obstructive problem, but Caesarean section might be necessary for abnormal presentation or to avoid disruption of the continence mechanism if artificial sphincters or neourethras are present
After nephrectomy, solitary and pelvic kidneys	Pregnancy is well tolerated. Might be associated with other malformations of the urogenital tract. Dystocia rarely occurs with a pelvic kidney

occurs. Clinicians are still searching for antenatal tests that identify the fetus at risk of intrauterine hypoxia and death. Ideally, such a test should not only be reliable but performed easily and repeatedly.

ROLE OF RENAL BIOPSY IN PREGNANCY

Experience with renal biopsy in pregnancy is sparse, mainly because clinical circumstances rarely justify the risks. Biopsy is therefore usually deferred until after delivery. Reports of excessive bleeding and other complications in pregnant women have led some to consider pregnancy as a relative contraindication to renal biopsy. When renal biopsy is undertaken immediately after delivery in women with well-controlled blood pressure and normal coagulation indices, the morbidity is certainly similar to that reported in non-pregnant patients.

The few generally agreed indications for antepartum biopsy are as follows:

1 Sudden deterioration of renal function before 30 weeks' gestation with no obvious cause. Certain forms of rapidly progressive glomerulonephritis may respond to aggressive treatment with steroid 'pulses', chemotherapy, and/or perhaps plasma exchange, when diagnosed early.
2 Symptomatic nephrotic syndrome before 30 weeks' gestation. While some might consider a therapeutic trial of steroids in such cases, it is best to determine whether the lesion is likely to respond to steroids, because pregnancy is itself a hypercoagulable state prone to deterioration by such treatment. On the other hand, proteinuria alone, in a non-eclamptic pregnant woman with well-preserved renal function and without gross oedema and/or hypoalbuminaemia, suggests the need for close monitoring and deferring biopsy until the puerperium.
3 Presentation with active urinary sediment, proteinuria, and borderline renal function in a woman not evaluated in the past. This is a very controversial area and it could be

argued that diagnosis of a collagen disorder such as sclero-derma or periarteritis would be grounds for terminating the pregnancy, or that classifying the type of lesion in a woman with lupus could determine the type and intensity of therapy.

SPECIFIC RENAL DISEASES AND PREGNANCY

Table 28.2 lists specific diseases associated with pregnancy, the information having been derived from publications over the past 10–15 years. To recap, the crucial balance between obstetric outcome and long-term renal progno-sis depends on prepregnancy renal functional status, the absence or presence of hypertension (and its manage-ment) and the renal lesion itself, as well as better fetal surveillance, more timely delivery and ever improving neonatal care.

LONG-TERM EFFECTS OF PREGNANCY IN WOMEN WITH RENAL DISEASE

Pregnancy does not cause deterioration or otherwise affect rate of progression of disease beyond what might be expected in the non-pregnant state, provided prepreg-nancy kidney dysfunction was minimal or very well controlled and hypertension is absent during pregnancy. An important factor in long-term prognosis could be the sclerotic effect that prolonged gestational renal vasodila-tion might have in the residual (intact) glomeruli of the kidneys of these women. The situation may be worse in a single diseased kidney, where more sclerosis has usually occurred within the fewer (intact) glomeruli. Although the evidence in healthy women and those with mild renal disease argues against hyperfiltration-induced damage in pregnancy, there is little doubt that in some women with moderate dysfunction there can be unpredicted, accel-erated, and irreversible renal decline in pregnancy or immediately afterwards (see Table 28.1).

What the clinician needs to know about dialysis patients

Dialysis and the prospects for pregnancy and afterwards

Despite reduced libido and relative infertility, women on dialysis can conceive and must therefore use contracep-tion if they wish to avoid pregnancy. Although conception is not common (an incidence of 1 in 200 patients has been quoted), its true frequency is unknown because most pregnancies in dialysis patients probably end in early spontaneous abortion. The high therapeutic abortion rate in this group of patients, (although decreased from 40% in

the 1990s to under 20% today), still suggests that those who become pregnant do so inadvertently, probably because they are unaware that pregnancy is possible.

Many authorities do not advise conception or contin-uation of pregnancy if present when the woman has severe renal insufficiency. Clinicians are reluctant to pub-lish unsuccessful cases or those that end in disaster, but the literature has expanded in recent years. Pregnancy poses big risks for the mother who is prone to volume overload, major exacerbations of her hypertension or superimposed pre-eclampsia, with only a 40–50% chance of a successful obstetric outcome.

Antenatal strategy and decision making

Women on dialysis, if they become pregnant, may present for care in advanced pregnancy because it was not sus-pected by either the patient or her doctors. Irregular menstruation is common in dialysis patients and missed periods are usually ignored. Urine pregnancy tests are unreliable (even if there is any urine available). Ultrasound evaluation is needed to confirm and date pregnancy.

DIALYSIS POLICY

Some patients have gestational GFR increments despite renal function being insufficient to sustain life without dialysis. The planning of dialysis strategy has several aims:

1 Maintain plasma $S_{urea} < 20$ mmol/l (some would argue <15 mmol/l), as intrauterine fetal death is more likely if values are much in excess of 20 mmol/l. (Success has occa-sionally been achieved despite levels of around 28 mmol/l for many weeks.) Invariably weekly dialysis is ≥ 20 h per week with higher K, lower Ca and lower HCO_3 dialysate. Heparin can be used for anticoagulation.

2 Avoid hypotension during dialysis, which could be damaging to the fetus. In late pregnancy the enlarging uterus and the supine posture may aggravate this situation by decreasing venous return.

3 Ensure 'tight' control of blood pressure throughout pregnancy.

4 Avoid rapid fluctuations in intravascular volume, by limiting interdialysis weight gain to about 1 kg until late pregnancy.

5 Scrutinize carefully for preterm labour, as dialysis and uterine contractions are associated.

6 Watch serum calcium closely to avoid hypercalcaemia.

7 Pregnant women with endstage disease usually require a 50% increase in hours and frequency of dialysis, a policy which renders dietary management and control of weight gain much easier.

ANAEMIA

Dialysis patients are usually anaemic, invariably aggravated further in pregnancy. Unnecessary blood sampling should be avoided in the face of anaemia and lack of venepuncture sites. The protocol for tests usually performed in one's own unit should be followed strictly, with no more blood removed per venepuncture than is absolutely necessary. Blood transfusion may be needed, especially before delivery. Caution is necessary as transfusion can exacerbate hypertension and impair the ability to control circulatory overload, even with extra dialysis. Fluctuations in blood volume can be minimized if packed red cells are transfused during dialysis. Treatment of anaemia with rHuEpo has been used in pregnancy without ill effect, when requirements can be higher. The theoretical risks of hypertension and thrombotic complications have not been encountered, nor have adverse neonatal effects.

HYPERTENSION

Normotension prepregnancy is reassuring. Some patients have abnormal lipid profiles and possibly accelerated atherogenesis, so theoretically may not have the cardiovascular capacity required to tolerate pregnancy. Patients with diabetic nephropathy who become pregnant are those in whom cardiovascular problems are the most worrisome. As a generalization, blood pressure tends to be labile and hypertension is common, although control may be possible by careful dialysis.

NUTRITION

Despite more frequent dialysis, an uncontrolled dietary intake should be discouraged. A daily oral intake of 70 g protein, 1500 mg calcium, 50 mmol potassium, and 80 mmol sodium is advised, with supplements of dialysable vitamins and iron and folic acid supplements. Vitamin D supplements can be difficult to judge in patients who have had parathyroidectomy. All this poses risks for fetal nutrition as well as the impact of a uraemic environment.

FETAL SURVEILLANCE AND TIMING OF DELIVERY

The same applies as with chronic renal disease. Preterm labour is generally the rule and it may commence during dialysis. Caesarean section should be necessary only for obstetric reasons although it has been argued that elective Caesarean section in all cases would minimize potential problems during labour.

Peritoneal dialysis

Young women can be managed with this approach and successful pregnancies have now been reported. Although anticoagulation and some of the fluid balance and volume problems of haemodialysis are avoided, these women, nevertheless, face the same problems of hypertension, anaemia, placental abruption, term labour, and sudden intrauterine death. Outcome is not dependent on mode of dialysis (haemodialysis versus peritoneal) but there may be more infertility in women receiving continuous ambulatory peritoneal dialysis (PD). It should be remembered that peritonitis can be a severe complication of chronic ambulatory PD, accounting for the majority of therapy failures. This superimposed on pregnancy can present a confusing diagnostic picture and management dilemmas.

What the clinician needs to know about kidney allograft recipients

Transplantation and the prospects for pregnancy and afterwards

Renal, endocrine, and sexual functions return rapidly after transplantation and assisted conception techniques are also available. About 1 in 50 women of childbearing age with a functioning transplant become pregnant during their remaining childbearing era. Of the conceptions, about 25% do not go beyond the initial trimester because of spontaneous or therapeutic abortion, but of those pregnancies in well women that do, 97% end successfully. In early pregnancy there may be increased risk of ectopic pregnancy because of pelvic adhesions following surgery, PD, IUCD's and pelvic inflammatory disease consequent to immunosuppression. Diagnosis of ectopic pregnancy may be delayed as irregular bleeding and pain may be wrongly attributed to deteriorating renal function and the presence of the pelvic allograft.

Allografting has even been performed with surgeons unaware that the recipient was in early pregnancy. Obstetric success in such cases does not negate the importance of contraception counselling for all renal failure patients and the exclusion of pregnancy prior to the surgery.

A woman should be counselled from the time the various treatments for renal failure and the potential for optimal rehabilitation are discussed. Couples who want a child should be encouraged to discuss all of the implications, including the harsh realities of maternal survival prospects. Individual centres have their own guidelines (Tables 28.3 and 28.4). In most, a wait of 18 months to 2 years post-transplant is advised. By then, the patient will have recovered from the surgery and any sequelae, graft function will have stabilized, and immunosuppression will be at maintenance levels. Also, if function is well

Table 28.3 Kidney allograft recipients: functional status, prospects for pregnancy and afterwards

| S_{cr} (μmol/l) | Complicated pregnancy(%) | Successful obstetric outcome(%) | Loss of renal function(%) | | Graft loss within 2 year post-partum(%) |
			In pregnancy	Persists post-partum	
<125	30	97	15	<5	<5
>125	60	90	15	5	10
>160	90	80	30	20	60
>200	100	70	60	40	90

S_{cr} non-pregnant serum creatinine. Estimates based on literature review (1988–2004) from 613 women in 849 pregnancies that attained at least 24 weeks' gestation.

Table 28.4 Guidelines for prepregnancy counselling of renal transplant recipients

Good general health for about 2 years after transplantation
Stature compatible with good obstetric outcome
No or minimal proteinuria
No hypertension*
No evidence of graft rejection
No pelvicalyceal distension on recent ultrasonography or intra venous urogram (IVU)
Stable graft function: $S_{cr} \leq 180$ μmol/l, preferably ≤ 125 μmol/l
Drug therapy at maintenance levels: prednisolone $\leq$15 mg/day, azathioprine $\leq$2 mg/kg/day, cyclosporin $\leq$5 mg/kg/day and tacrolimus $\leq$0.1–0.2 mg/kg/day. The experience with the 'newer' immunosuppression is minimal

*Due to high incidence of hypertension in patients on calcineurin inhibitors 'well-controlled hypertension' may be more appropriate.

Table 28.5 Kidney allografts and pregnancy: 'Clinical watchpoints' (ABC . . .)

Accurate dating/early diagnosis
Bacterial and viral infections
Co-morbid medical condition
Delivery decision
Effects of medication
Fetal surveillance
Graft function and rejection
Hypertension/nephropathy
Immunosuppression
Joint management at tertiary centre

maintained at 2 years, there is a high probability of allograft survival at 5 years. As with chronic renal disease it is preferable if prepregnancy S_{cr} < 125 μmol/l as above that level there can be more complications and problems. Interestingly, the two significant higher 'cut-offs' are S_{cr} 160 and 180 μmol/l, which are at a lower level than the equivalent 'cut-offs' in chronic renal disease at 180 and 220 μmol/l.

Antenatal strategy and decision making

Management requires serial assessment of renal function, early diagnosis and treatment of rejection, blood pressure control, early diagnosis or prevention of anaemia, treatment of any infection, and meticulous assessment of fetal well-being (Table 28.5). As well as regular renal assessments, liver function tests, plasma protein, and calcium and phosphate should be checked at 6-weekly intervals. Cytomegalovirus and herpes hominis virus status should be checked during each trimester and HIV should be determined at the first attendance. Haematinics are needed if the various haematological indices show deficiency.

ALLOGRAFT FUNCTION

The sustained increase in GFR characteristic of early normal pregnancy is evident in renal transplant recipients. Immediate graft function after transplantation and the better the prepregnancy GFR, the greater the increment in pregnancy. Transient 20–25% reductions in GFR can occur during the third trimester and do not usually represent a deteriorating situation with permanent impairment. Significant renal functional impairment can, however, develop in some patients during pregnancy, and this may persist following delivery, invariably being related to prepregnancy S_{cr} (see Table 28.3). As a gradual decline in function is common in non-pregnant patients anyway, it is difficult to delineate the specific role of pregnancy. Most agree that pregnancy does not compromise long-term graft progression unless there was already graft dysfunction prepregnancy.

Proteinuria occurs near term in 40% of patients but disappears post-partum and, in the absence of hypertension, is not significant except if it exceeds 1 g/24 h which by some is considered to be a marker of suboptimal obstetric outcome and/or later deterioration.

Whether or not calcineurin inhibitors are more nephrotoxic in the pregnant compared to the non-pregnant patient is not known. Certainly the literature indicates that with the advent of these immunosuppressors prepregnancy S_{cr} levels are higher overall than in the azathioprine/steroids era.

TRANSPLANT REJECTION

Serious rejection episodes occur in 5% of pregnant women. While this incidence is no greater than that seen in non-pregnant individuals during a similar period, it is unexpected because it has been assumed that the privileged immunological status of pregnancy might benefit the allograft. Rejection often occurs in the puerperium and may be due to a return to a normal immune state (despite immunosuppression) or possibly a rebound effect from the altered gestational immunoresponsiveness.

Chronic rejection with a progressive subclinical course may be a problem in all recipients. Whether pregnancy influences the course of subclinical rejection is unknown: no factors consistently predict which patients will develop rejection during pregnancy. There may also be a non-immune contribution to chronic graft failure due to the damaging effect of hyperfiltration through remnant nephrons, perhaps even exacerbated during pregnancy. Important 'clinical watchpoints' are that rejection is difficult to diagnose, if any of the clinical hallmarks are present – fever, oliguria, deteriorating renal function, renal enlargement, and tenderness – then the diagnosis should be considered. Ultrasound assessment may be helpful but without renal biopsy, rejection cannot be distinguished from acute pyelonephritis, recurrent glomerulopathy, possibly severe pre-eclampsia, and even cyclosporin nephrotoxicity and therefore renal biopsy is indicated before embarking upon antirejection therapy.

IMMUNOSUPPRESSIVE THERAPY

Immunosuppressive therapy is usually maintained at prepregnancy levels. There are many encouraging Registry and single centre reports of (non-complicated) pregnancies in patients taking cyclosporine and tacrolimus (FK506 or Prograf). Numerous adverse effects are attributed to calcineurin inhibitors in non-pregnant transplant recipients, including renal toxicity, hepatic dysfunction, chronic hypertension, tremor, convulsions, diabetogenic effects, hemolytic uremic syndrome, and neoplasia. In pregnancy, some of the maternal adaptations that normally occur may theoretically be blunted or abolished by cyclosporine, especially plasma volume expansion and renal hemodynamic augmentation. There is good evidence to suggest that patients have more hypertension and smaller babies.

Finally, newer agents such as mycophenolate (MMF/CellCept), antithymocytic globulin, ATG (Atgam) and orthodione , OKTS are being prescribed more frequently for transplant recipients, but there is very little information about these agents in pregnancy. Some of these newer agents were originally considered to have a 'rescue role' only in kidney and kidney–pancreas transplants but nowadays they can be used as primary immunosuppressive agents.

HYPERTENSION AND PRE-ECLAMPSIA

Hypertension, particularly before 28 weeks' gestation, is associated with adverse perinatal outcome. This may be due to covert cardiovascular changes that accompany or are aggravated by chronic hypertension. The appearance of hypertension in the third trimester, its relationship to deteriorating renal function, and the possibility of chronic underlying pathology and pre-eclampsia is a diagnostic problem. Pre-eclampsia is actually diagnosed clinically in about 30% of pregnancies.

INFECTIONS

Throughout pregnancy patients should be monitored carefully for bacterial and viral infection. Prophylactic antibiotics must be given before any surgical procedure, however trivial.

DIABETES MELLITUS

As the results of renal transplantation have improved in those women whose renal failure was caused by juvenile onset diabetes mellitus, pregnancies are now being reported in these women. Pregnancy complications occur with at least twice the frequency seen in the non-diabetic patient, and this may be due to the presence of generalized cardiovascular pathology, which is part of the 'metabolic risk factor syndrome'. Successful pregnancies have been reported after combined pancreas–kidney allografts.

FETAL SURVEILLANCE AND TIMING OF DELIVERY

The points discussed under chronic renal disease are equally applicable to renal transplant recipients (page...). Preterm delivery is common (45–60%) because of intervention for obstetric reasons and the common occurrence of preterm labour or preterm rupture of membranes. Preterm labour is commonly associated with poor renal function, but in some it has been postulated that long-term immunosuppression may 'weaken' connective tissues and contribute to the increased incidence of preterm rupture of the membranes.

Vaginal delivery should be the aim; usually there are no obstructive problems normechanical injury to the transplant. Unless there are specific obstetric problems then

Table 28.6 Neonatal problems in the newborn of kidney allograft recipients

Preterm delivery or small for gestational age
Respiratory distress syndrome
Adrenocortical insufficiency
Septicaemia
Cytomegalovirus infection
Hepatitis B surface antigen carrier state
Depressed haematopoiesis
Lymphoid and thymic hypoplasia
Reduced lymphocyte passive haemagglutination assay
  reactivity
Reduced T lymphocyte levels
Reduced immunoglobulin levels
Chromosome aberrations in leukocytes
Congenital abnormalities
Immunologic problems

spontaneous onset of labour can be awaited. During labour careful monitoring of fluid balance, cardiovascular status, and temperature is mandatory. Aseptic technique is essential for every procedure. Surgical induction of labour (by amniotomy) and episiotomy warrant antibiotic cover. Pain relief can be conducted as for healthy women. Augmentation of steroids should not be overlooked. Caesarean section should be undertaken for obstetric reasons only.

Post-delivery management issues (Table 28.6)

PAEDIATRIC MANAGEMENT

Over 50% of live borns have no neonatal problems. Preterm delivery is common (45–60%), small for gestational age babies are delivered in at least 20–30% of pregnancies, and occasionally the two problems coexist. Lower birthweights are seen in infants born to recipients of less than 2 years post-transplant. The use of calcineurin inhibitors can be associated with birthweight depression.

BREASTFEEDING

There are substantial benefits to breastfeeding. It could be argued that because the baby has been exposed to immunosuppressives and their metabolites in pregnancy, breastfeeding should not be allowed. Little is known, however, about the quantities of these drugs and their metabolites in breast milk and whether the levels are biologically trivial or substantial. For cyclosporin, levels in breast milk are usually greater than those in a simultaneously taken blood sample. Until the many uncertainties are resolved, breastfeeding probably should not be encouraged.

LONG-TERM ASSESSMENT

There are theoretical worries about in utero exposure to immunosuppresives with eventual development of malignant tumours in affected offspring, autoimmune complications and abnormalities in the reproductive performance in the next generation. Thus evaluation of the immune system and paediatric follow-up are needed. To date, information about general progress in early childhood has been good.

Maternal follow-up after pregnancy

The ultimate measure of transplant success is the long-term survival of the patient and the graft. As it is only 35 years since this procedure became widely employed in the management of endstage renal failure, few long-term data from sufficiently large series exist from which to draw conclusions. Furthermore, the long-term results for renal transplants relate to a period when many aspects of management would be unacceptable by present-day standards. Average survival figures of large numbers of patients worldwide indicate that about 90% of recipients of kidneys from related living donors are alive 5 years after transplantation. With cadaver kidneys, the figure is approximately 60%. If renal function was normal 2 years after transplant, survival increased to about 80%. This is why women are counselled to wait about 2 years before considering a pregnancy even though a view is now emerging that 1 year would be sufficient.

A major concern is that the mother may not survive or remain well enough to rear the child she bears. Pregnancy occasionally and sometimes unpredictably causes irreversible declines in renal function (Table 28.3). However, the consensus is that pregnancy has no effect on graft function or survival. Also, repeated pregnancies do not adversely affect graft function or fetal development, provided that prepregnancy renal function is well preserved and hypertension minimal and well controlled (Table 28.4).

CONTRACEPTION

It is unwise to offer the option of sterilization at the time of transplantation. Oral contraception can cause or aggravate hypertension, thromboembolism and subtle changes to the immune system. This does not necessarily contraindicate its use but careful surveillance is essential. IUCDs may aggravate menstrual problems, which in turn may obscure symptoms and signs of early pregnancy abnormalities, such as threatened miscarriage or ectopic pregnancy. The increased risk of chronic pelvic infection in immunosupressed patients with IUCDs is a substantial problem.

Indeed, as the insertion or replacement of a coil can be associated with bacteraemia of vaginal origin, antibiotic cover is essential at this time. Finally, the efficacy of the intrauterine device is reduced in women taking immunosuppressive and anti-inflammatory agents but many still request this method.

GYNAECOLOGICAL PROBLEMS

There is a danger that symptoms secondary to genuine pelvic pathology may be erroneously attributed to the transplant, due to its location near the pelvis. Transplant recipients receiving immunosuppressive therapy have a malignancy rate estimated to be 100 times greater than normal and the female genital tract is no exception. This association is probably related to factors such as loss of immune surveillance, chronic immunosuppression allowing tumour proliferation and prolonged antigenic stimulation of the reticuloendothelial system. Regular gynaecological assessment is therefore essential and any gynaecological management should be on conventional lines, with the outcome unlikely to be influenced by stopping or reducing immunosuppression.

Further reading

Armenti VT, Moritz MJ, Cardonick EH & Davison JM (2002) Immunosuppression in pregnancy: choices for infant and maternal health. *Drugs* **62**, 2361–75.

Armenti VT, Radomski JS, Moritz MJ, Gaughan WJ, McGrory CH & Coscia LA (2003) Report from the National Transplantation Pregnancy Registry (NTPR): outcomes of pregnancy after transplantation. *Clin Transplant* 131–41.

Bar J, Ben-Haroush A, Mor E *et al.* (2004) Pregnancy after renal transplantation – effect on 15 year graft survival. *Hypertens Pregnancy* **23**(Suppl 1), 126.

Cardonick E, Moritz M & Armenti VT (2004) Pregnancy in patients with organ transplantation. *Obstet Gynecol Surv* **59**, 214–22.

Castillio AA, Lew SQ & Smith AM (1999) Women's issues in female patients receiving peritoneal dialysis. *Adv Ren Replace Ther* **6**, 327–32.

Crowe AV, Rustom R, Gradden C *et al.* (1999) Pregnancy does not adversely affect renal transplant function. *Q J Med* **92**, 631–6.

Davison JM (2001) Renal disorders in pregnancy. *Curr Opin Obstet Gynaecol* **13**, 109–14.

Davison JM & Bailey DJ (2003) Pregnancy following renal transplantation. *J Obstet Gynaecol Res* **29**, 227–33.

Davison JM & Homuth V, Jeyabalan A *et al.* (2004) New aspects in the pathophysiology of preeclampsia. *J Am Soc Nephrol* **15**, 2440–8.

Hou S & Firanek C (1998) Management of the pregnant dialysis patient. *Adv Ren Replace Ther* **5**, 24–9.

Hou S (2003) Pregnancy in renal transplant recipients. *Adv Ren Replace Ther* **10**, 40–7.

Jungers P & Chauveau D (1997) Pregnancy in renal disease. *Kidney Int* **52**, 871–80.

Kuller JA, D'Andrea N & McMahon MJ (2001) Renal biopsy and pregnancy. *Am J Obstet Gynecol* **184**, 1093–6.

LeRay C, Coulomb A, Elefant E, Frydman R & Audibert F (2004) Mycophenolate mofetil in pregnancy after renal transplantation: a case of major fetal malformations. *Obstet Gynecol* **103**, 1091–4.

Lindheimer MD, Davison JM & Katz AI (2001) The kidney and hypertension in pregnancy: twenty exciting years. *Semin Nephrol* **21**, 173–80.

Mckay DB & Josephson MA (2005) Reproduction and transplantation: report on AST consenous conference on reproductive issues and transplantation. *AM J Transplant* **5**, 1592–99.

Mckay DB & Josephson MA (2006) Pregnancy in recipients of solid organs-effects on mother and child. *N Eng J Med* **354**, 1281–93.

Moroni G & Ponticelli C (2003) The risk of pregnancy in patients with lupus nephritis. *J Nephrol* **16**, 161–7.

Okundaye IB, Abrinko P & Hou SH (1998) Registry of pregnancy in dialysis patients. *Am J Kidney Dis* **31**, 766–74.

Parmar MS (2002) Chronic renal disease. *Br Med J* **325**, 85–9.

Rashid M & Rashid HM (2003) Chronic renal insufficiency in pregnancy. *Saudi Med J* **204**, 709–14.

Ross LF (2006) Ethical considerations related to pregnancy in transplant recipients. *N Eng J Med* **354**, 1313–16.

Sibai BM (2002) Chronic hypertension in pregnancy. *Obstet Gynecol* **100**, 369–377.

Sibanda N, Briggs D, Davison, JM, Johnson RJ & Rudge CT (2004) Outcomes of pregnancy after renal transplantation: a report of the UK Transplant Pregnancy Registry. *Hypertens Pregnancy* **23**(Suppl 1), 136.

Sivaraman P (2004) Management of pregnancy in transplant recipients. *Transplant Proc* **36**, 1999–2000.

Stratta P, Canavese C, Giacchino F, Mesiano P, Quaglia M & Rossetti M (2003) Pregnancy in kidney transplantation: satisfactory outcomes and harsh realities. *J Nephrol* **16**, 792–806.

Thompson BC, Kingdom, EJ, Tuck SM, Fernando ON & Swerry P (2003) Pregnancy in renal transplant recipients: the Royal Free experience. *Q J Med* **96**, 837–44.

Chapter 29: Haematological problems in pregnancy

P. Clark, A.J. Thomson and I.A. Greer

Anaemia

A normochromic, normocytic anaemia may occur from the 7–8th week of gestation, due to the physiological increase in plasma volume that is relatively greater than the increase in red cell mass. However, the haemoglobin (Hb) should not fall to <11 g/dl in the first, or <10 g/dl in the second and third trimesters [1,2]. More marked anaemia may be due to iron, folate, or more rarely, vitamin B_{12} deficiency or haemoglobinopathy.

Haematinic requirements

Pregnancy requires an iron intake of around 2.5 mg/day throughout, with perhaps 3.0–7.5 mg/day required in the third trimester. An average Western diet supplies around 250 μg/day of folate; however, requirements increase to around 400 μg/day during pregnancy [3], with deficiency most commonly due to lack of folate-rich vegetables such as broccoli and peas, which is often linked to social deprivation. Folate deficiency is more common in multiple pregnancy, frequent childbirth, and adolescent mothers. The body stores around 3 mg of B_{12}, with a daily dietary requirement of 3μ g/day. The only B_{12} source is animal foodstuffs; thus, vegetarians and vegans are most at risk of dietary deficiency.

The effects of deficiency

The signs and symptoms of early deficiencies are non-specific, including tiredness and features of any underlying cause (Table 29.1). Aside from anaemia, folate and B_{12} deficiency are linked to neural tube defects [4,5]. The effect of iron deficiency (before anaemia) on maternal and fetal well-being is not fully understood, but mild deficiency is linked to increased delivery bleeding, poor fetal iron stores and an increased placenta:fetus weight ratio [6]. Severe maternal iron deficiency is associated with premature delivery and low birthweight [1], although this may relate to the underlying cause. Most subjects with folate deficiency are identified incidentally due to a raised red cell Mean Cell Volume (MCV), but folate deficiency

Table 29.1 Causes of iron, folate and B_{12} deficiency

Iron	Diet	Vegetarian/Vegan
	Blood loss	Menorrhagia
		Peptic ulceration
		Inflammatory bowel disease
		Haemorrhoids
		Varices
		Aspirin
		Anticoagulants
		von Willebrands disease
	Malabsorption	Coeliac
		Gastrectomy
Folate	Dietary	Alcoholism
		Poverty
		Adolescence
	Malabsorption	Gluten-induced enteropathy (Coeliac)
	Increased use	Chronic haemolysis
		Congenital red cell disorders
		Haemoglobinopathy
		Myeloproliferative disorders
	Loss	Dialysis
	Miscellaneous	Anticonvulsants
B_{12}	Dietary	Vegans
	Malabsorption	Pernicious anaemia
		Partial gastric resection
		Ileal resection
		Intestinal stagnant loop
		Crohn's disease
		Tapeworms
		Tropical sprue
	Miscellaneous	Folate deficiency

anaemia often coexists with iron deficiency and more often presents at the end of pregnancy or in the early puerperium. B_{12} deficiency can also result in a demyelinating neuropathy, although mild maternal B_{12} deficiency appears compatible with normal pregnancy [7].

Diagnosis of deficiency

As the MCV may increase with normal gestation, the reduction in MCV usually seen in iron deficiency is not reliable in pregnancy. Serum iron, Total Iron Binding

Table 29.2 Differential diagnosis of a raised MCV

B_{12} deficiency	Pregnancy
Folate Deficiency	Liver disease
Alcohol	Myelodysplasia
Hypothyroidism	Haemolysis

Capacity (TIBC), ferritin, serum transferrin receptor levels and red cell-derived protoporphyrin can be used to diagnose iron deficiency. However, normal pregnancy leads to a progressive fall in serum iron, ferritin and an increase in TIBC, free protoporphyrin and transferrin receptor levels [8]. Thus, a number of parameters may be required to diagnose mild deficiency, although a markedly reduced serum ferritin (<12 ug/l) remains diagnostic. Megaloblastic anaemia from B_{12} or folate deficiency is suggested by an MCV >100 fl, with right-shifted neutrophils on the blood film (Table 29.2). Serum folate is sensitive to deficiency, but may be reduced with very recent dietary folate lack and also reduces in pregnancy [9]. Red cell folate levels are less affected by recent diet, but may rise in otherwise normal pregnancy [10,11]. If necessary, megaloblastic erythropoiesis can be demonstrated by bone marrow examination. Serum B_{12} levels may fall by 30–50% during normal pregnancy, but this is probably not a true tissue deficiency [7]. Specific tests to diagnose intrinsic factor deficiency (from pernicious anaemia) involve radioisotope exposure and are contraindicated in pregnancy, but plasma intrinsic factor antibodies, if present, can point to a diagnosis of pernicious anaemia.

Prophylaxis

The Hb concentration is often used to screen for haematinic deficiency, with an assessment at presentation and again in the early third trimester. Whether routine iron supplementation is warranted is not resolved, as it is not clear whether the fetus benefits [1]. If required, supplementation can be achieved with 30–60 mg of iron/day, which produces few side effects. Side effects are mainly seen with replacement (200 mg/day) therapy. Furthermore, supplementation of more than 200 mg/day will not produce a supra-normal haemoglobin (Hb) or haematocrit (HCT). To prevent neural tube defects, folic acid supplementation (at 400μ g/day) is routinely given in the first trimester. It should also be taken for 3 months prior to conception in those planning pregnancy and a higher dose is needed if there is a previous child with a neural tube defect or a chronic red cell disorder. Such supplementation is also of value with regard to prophylaxis of anaemia in women with potential dietary deficiency. Folate should be continued through pregnancy in women on antiepileptic drugs that antagonize folate metabolism or in those with likely dietary deficiency.

Treatment

The treatment of established iron deficiency is with 200 mg/day of elemental iron. This may lead to gastrointestinal upset, which can be dose or product related and is usually ameliorated by either dose reduction (100 mg/day), or a change in the preparation. Iron absorption is maximized when combined with ascorbic acid such as taking the iron supplements with fresh orange juice or a vitamin C preparation. Therapy failure occurs in malabsorption and when loss exceeds intake, but is most commonly due to poor compliance. There are also liquid oral iron preparations and parenteral therapy. Parenteral therapy is useful in malabsorption and failed compliance, but otherwise does not produce a faster response than oral iron and side effects are common. Proven folate deficiency anaemia should be treated with folic acid (5 mg/day). In all such cases of anaemia, B_{12} deficiency must also be excluded, as folate may improve the anaemia of B_{12} deficiency, but exacerbate any associated neurological deterioration [12]. In B_{12} deficiency, a single dose of 1000 μg of intramuscular B_{12} should lead to a reticulocyte response within 3–7 days. Weekly injections should be employed until anaemia resolves and lifelong replacement is often required.

The thalassaemias

The thalassaemias are a heterogeneous group of genetic disorders of haemoglobin synthesis, named after the haemoglobin that is deficient. The mutation may result in a reduced rate of production of the affected gene or result in no chain synthesis at all (reviewed in [13]). The majority of thalassaemias are inherited in a Mendelian recessive manner. Given the diversity of genetic defects and the possibility of genetic combinations, thalassaemias, irrespective of their molecular basis, are often classified by their clinical effects into thalassaemia minor, thalassaemia intermedia and thalassaemia major. In general, thalassaemia carriers are often symptomless and fall into the minor category. Intermediate levels are more severely affected and may often have anaemia, although this does not require regular transfusion. In its major form, thalassaemia presents with a lifelong transfusion dependency.

Alpha thalassaemia

Women with one or two out of four alpha gene deletions are usually symptom free and have a normal pregnancy outcome. With Hb H Disease, where three of the four alpha-globin genes are absent, there are variable clinical features ranging from mild asymptomatic anaemia to severe transfusion-dependent anaemia, with jaundice, hepatosplenomegaly, growth restriction and bone abnormalities. Mild to moderate haemolysis is the predominant feature. This is worsened by pregnancy; so prophylactic folic acid (5 mg/day) is needed. Gallstones are not infrequent. Infections, drugs and fever may also worsen the anaemia. A fetus affected by Hb Barts with no alpha chain production (both parents carrying two alpha deletions on the same chromosome) will develop hydrops, polyhydramnios, and placentomegaly [14]. There is a high risk of pre-eclampsia in the mother. The fetus is also at risk of congenital abnormalities. Carriage of alpha thalassaemia is associated with an MCV of less than 80 fl (often less than 70 fl), a mean corpuscular haemoglobin (MCH) of less than 27 pg, with, very often, no evidence of anaemia and normal mean corpuscular haemoglobin concentration (MCHC). If iron deficiency is excluded, then carriage of thalassaemia should be suspected and the diagnosis confirmed with polymerase chain reaction (PCR) and globin gene analysis.

Beta thalassaemia

This condition is due to a defect in beta chain synthesis caused by heterogeneous point mutations within the beta-globin gene, with nearly 180 different mutations associated with its phenotype. It interferes with red cell maturation and increases red cell destruction within the marrow and spleen. Major forms have lifelong chronic dyserythropoietic anaemia with splenomegaly and skeletal deformity. With inadequate transfusion profound anaemia, marked skeletal deformity of the long bones and skull, recurrent infections and death occurs. With adequate transfusion anaemia is controlled but transfusion-related iron overload will result in endocrine abnormalities, pancreatic, hepatic and cardiac failure. This results in failure of pubertal growth, delayed sexual development and hypogonadotrophic hypogonadism affecting fertility. Thus only a small number of successful pregnancies are reported [15–17]. With significant left ventricular dysfunction or arrhythmias pregnancy may be best avoided. Serum ferritin reflects hepatic iron stores, but does not relate well to cardiac deposition, although MRI can now quantify cardiac iron deposition. When pregnancy does occur Caesarean section is common for cephalo-pelvic disproportion due to the small stature of the mother and the fact that the unaffected fetus has normal growth. Spinal abnormalities should be considered with neuraxial anaesthesia. With beta-thalassaemia intermedia there is a reasonable pregnancy success rate with well-controlled disease. Transfusion requirements

increase with increasing gestation with the aim to maintain Hb over 10 g/dl and thereby correct anaemia, suppress hyperactive erythropoiesis and inhibit iron absorption. Most often, chelating agents are discontinued on diagnosis of pregnancy, and restarted after delivery, but folic acid supplements are required throughout pregnancy.

Beta-thalassaemia minor is usually symptom free, but anaemia is common in pregnancy [18]. Carriers have normal / low Hb, low MCV and MCH but normal MCHC. More severe anaemias may be encountered in those with dietary deficiencies. Folic acid supplementation should be prescribed (and oral iron, if ferritin low) throughout pregnancy. There is also possibly an increased risk of neural tube defects.

Screening for thalassaemia

Population screening for haemoglobin disorders has been practised for over 20 years. Carriers are reliably detected by screening red cell indices, traditionally the MCV <83 fl, but an MCH <27 pg is more reliable. Electrophoresis is then used to make the diagnosis (increased HbF and HbA$_2$(3.5–7% in beta heterozygotes). If the haemoglobin A$_2$ percentage is within the normal range, and the MCH is less than 25 pg, the woman should be investigated for alpha thalassaemia trait [13]. Prenatal diagnosis (chorionic villous sample (CVS), amniocentesis, fetal blood sample (FBS)) is possible by a mutation specific polymerase chain reaction (n.b. pre-implantation diagnosis is also possible) and the diagnostic accuracy is high in specialist centres.

Sickle cell disease

Sickle cell disease varies in presentation from a lifelong crippling haemolytic disorder (characterized by crises caused by infection, aplasia, infarction and haemolysis), to a diagnosis only made on a routine blood film examination. This variation may be due to the co-inheritance of persistence of fetal haemoglobin. With repeated crises bone deformity, osteomyelitis, renal failure, myocardial infarction, leg ulceration, gallstones and cardiac failure may develop. With repeated transfusions there is an increased risk of blood borne infections and iron overload. The outcome of pregnancy in mothers with sickling disorders is heavily dependent upon the adequacy of maternal health care [19]. In the USA, a maternal mortality rate of 0.25–0.5% has been reported, with 99% of pregnancies, which were viable after 28 weeks, resulting in a live birth. Around half of the pregnancies are complicated by at least one painful crisis and hospital admission is often required. There is likely to be an increased risk of pre-eclampsia and of a small-for-date baby, possibly through placental infarction [20]. In developing countries the outcome of pregnancy with a major sickling disorder may be substantially worse with high maternal and perinatal mortality.

Sickle cell trait results in no change to the haematological indices. It is diagnosed by a positive sickle test and the demonstration of both an HbA and HbS band on gel electrophoresis.

Sickle cell disease is diagnosed by the presence of anaemia, the presence of sickled red cells on the blood film, blood film appearances of hyposplenism, a positive sickle test and the pattern of HbS and HbF, with no HbA, on haemoglobin electrophoresis. The presence of a microcytosis may suggest the co-inheritance of thalassaemia, or the presence of iron deficiency. Higher haemoglobin (11–13 g/dl) may indicate the presence of haemoglobin C or co-inheritance of another haemoglobin variant.

In all subjects with a major sickling disorder treatment includes the prevention of infection. This is achieved with prophylactic penicillin and the use of pneumococcal, meningococcal and Haemophilus influenzae vaccinations with antimalarial prophylaxis if appropriate. The management of a painful crisis involves adequate pain control, treatment of any infection, maintenance of oxygenation, hydration and thromboprophylaxis [21]. Regular blood transfusion is not usually required. If, however, haemoglobin is falling (indicating an increase in haemolysis) and, especially, if there is evidence of a falling reticulocyte count (indicating an impending aplastic phase), then transfusion should be given. When transfusion is required and the haemoglobin is already less then 5 g/dl, it may be that a top-up transfusion to 12–14 g/dl will result in sufficient dilution of the sickle cells to the desired target level of <30% of the circulating red cells. When transfusion is required at a higher haemoglobin level (8–10 g/dl), then a partial exchange transfusion should be carried out (removing 500 ml by phlebotomy while transfusing two red cell units). The mainstay of management of a pregnancy in women with a severe sickling disorder, is folic acid supplementation (throughout pregnancy), regular haemoglobin estimations, regular monitoring of fetal growth and consideration of the need for transfusion. Randomized studies have shown no benefit in prophylactic blood transfusions in pregnancy, although there may be a reduction in the frequency of vaso-occlusive events when prophylactic transfusion has been used [22]. Transfusion should be considered when there is an acute anaemia (Hb<5 g/dl), pre-eclampsia, septicaemia, acute renal failure, acute chest syndrome, recent cerebral ischaemia of arterial origin, and when preparing for surgery. Multiple pregnancy will require assessment for transfusion on a more regular basis.

Haemolytic disease of the newborn

The Rh antigens on red cells result from the action of two genes (RhD and RhC/RhE), leading to two haplotypes (combining c or C, D or no D, e or E). Of these, RhD is the most important in obstetrics. Around 15% of Caucasians are RhD negative. If an RhD negative mother carries an RhD positive child, the transplacental passage of blood and immunoglobulin may result in the development of maternal anti-RhD antibody that passes to the fetus. Indeed, there is a one in six chance of maternal anti-RhD formation in the absence of prophylaxis. Whether the mother develops such antibodies depends upon the amount of feto-maternal haemorrhage (FMH) and any feto-maternal ABO mismatch (as natural maternal anti-A or anti-B may clear fetal cells before immunization occurs). Haemolytic disease of the newborn (HDN) most often occurs in the second pregnancy, but occasionally significant haemolysis occurs in the first (reviewed in [23]).

Antenatal diagnosis and monitoring

All women should have their blood group determined at pregnancy presentation and again at 28–32 weeks gestation, with a further estimation between 34 and 36 weeks also recommended [24]. In an RhD negative women, if a potential sensitizing event occurs (Table 29.3), whether she has circulating anti-RhD should be determined and (if more than 20 weeks gestation or at delivery) an FMH estimation carried out. At delivery, the ABO/RhD type of the baby should be determined from a cord sample. If the baby is RhD positive any anti-RhD on the fetal cells should be detected by a direct antiglobulin test.

Anti-RhD detected early in pregnancy is more likely to result in HDN than if detected for the first time later on.

Table 29.3 RhD sensitizing events

Antepartum haemorrhage	
Abdominal trauma	
Ectopic pregnancy	
Fetal external version	
Delivery	
Invasive investigations	Amniocentesis
	Chorionic villous sampling
	Fetal blood sampling
	Embryo reduction
	Shunt insertion
Fetal loss	Intrauterine death
	Stillbirth
	Miscarriage with evacuation
	Complete or incomplete miscarriage >12/40
	Therapeutic termination

When any antibody associated with HDN is detected it should be quantified. For RhD, this should be by automated methods and reported in international units, rather than by manual titration [24]. In general, the absolute value is not as important as a rising titre. In addition, it is now possible to determine if the fetus is RhD positive (as well as its *Kell* and *c* status) from fetal DNA obtained from the maternal circulation [25,26]. Although this technique is in its infancy, a very high sensitivity has been reported. Although most non-invasive methods are not sufficiently sensitive, weekly velocimetry of the fetal middle cerebral artery may be predictive of moderate or severe anaemia [27] and has begun to replace serial amniocentesis to predict when fetal blood sampling is required.

Fetal presentation with HDN

Fetal presentation varies from mild anaemia to severe anaemia with jaundice, oedema, cardiac failure, effusions and pulmonary haemorrhage, neurological deficits and kernicterus, which may result in stillbirth, neonatal death, or complete resolution.

Intrauterine management

If fetal maturity permits, delivery of the fetus is indicated when there is evidence of a high level of bilirubin in the amniotic fluid. When fetal immaturity does not make delivery feasible, fetal transfusion (which has reduced the perinatal mortality from 95 to 50%) should be carried out and such transfusion is indicated when the HCT is <25% (at 18–26 weeks gestation) or <30% after 34 weeks. The blood used should be cross-matched against maternal serum, with a haematocrit of 75–90% and be both sero-negative for cytomegalovirus, and gamma-irradiated. The aim is to increase the HCT to ~45% and further transfusions may be required every 1 to 3 weeks. In some circumstances repeated maternal plasma exchange or high-dose Intravenous Human Normal Immunoglobulin (IVIgG) have been used, until fetal transfusion is possible.

Prevention of HDN

Sensitization can be prevented by suppression of the maternal immune response to the RhD antigen, by the timely administration of a passive antibody [28–30]. Intramuscular anti-RhD should be administered to all RhD negative women within 72 h of delivery and, if not, within 9–10 days [30]. The dose required should be determined by the level of FMH. Given intramuscularly, 125 IU of anti-RhD is sufficient to protect against 1 ml of RhD positive red cells and in the UK, 250 IU is routinely given for any

potential sensitizing event before 20 weeks and 500 IU for any event after 20 weeks. If a further sensitizing event occurs >7 days after a prophylactic anti-RhD dose, a further dose should be given. Routine post-delivery anti-RhD immunoprophylaxis has markedly reduced fetal deaths; however, cases of HDN (from other blood groups, unrecognized sensitization in a previous pregnancy, red cell or platelet transfusion and inadequate treatment, or unrecognized potential sensitization) still occur. Indeed, unrecognized events are now the most important cause of maternal sensitization in many developed countries. These may be amenable to routine administration of anti-RhD to all RhD negative women with no detectable anti-RhD antibodies in the third trimester [31].

Non-RhD antibodies

At least 40 red cell antigens have been associated with HDN, including Rh*c*, Rh*C*, Rh*E*, Kell, Duffy, MNS, Lutheran, Kidd and *U*. After anti-RhD, antibodies against *c*, Kell (K_1) or *E* are the most frequently encountered antibodies requiring treatment. The K_1 antigen is found in 9% of Caucasians (who are virtually all heterozygous) and 8–18% of pregnancies with detectable maternal anti-K_1 result in a K_1 positive fetus, with hydrops in ~30% of such cases. Management of such antibodies requires a combination of ultrasound, paternal genotyping, fetal blood sampling and intrauterine transfusion [32].

Thrombocytopaenia

Towards the end of pregnancy <5% of women have a platelet count $<150 \times 10^9/l$. This gestational thrombocytopaenia carries no significance, but requires exclusion of other disorders (Table 29.4). If the platelet count is $<100 \times 10^9/l$, further investigations are required (Table 29.5).

Immune thrombocytopaenic purpura

ITP results in thrombocytopaenia from autoantibody-mediated destruction of platelets. Such antibodies occur idiopathically and also in association with other disorders (Table 29.6). ITP most commonly presents as asymptomatic maternal thrombocytopaenia, but transplacental passage of antibodies can result in fetal thrombocytopaenia in 9–15% and intracerebral haemorrhage in 1.5% of babies with affected mothers. The diagnosis of ITP in pregnancy is by exclusion of other disorders [33].

TREATMENT

Spontaneous bleeding is unlikely with platelets $>20 \times 10^9/l$ and monitoring of the patient and platelet count

Table 29.4 Thrombocytopaenia in pregnancy

Spurious (i.e. clumping or poor sampling)
Gestational
Immune thrombocytopaenic purpura (ITP)
Heparin-induced thrombocytopaenia (HIT)
Post-transfusion purpura (PTP)
Acute fatty Liver of pregnancy
Pre-eclampsia (PET)/ HELLP syndrome
Thrombotic thrombocytopaenic purpura (TTP)/ Haemolytic
  uraemic syndrome (HUS)
Disseminated intravascular coagulation (DIC)
Drug induced thrombocytopenia
Systemic lupus erythematosis (SLE)/antiphospholipid
  syndrome
Viral (HIV/EBV/CMV)
Congenital thrombocythemias/thrombocytopaenia
Hypersplenism
Type IIb von Willebrands disease
Marrow dysfunction/haematinic deficiency

Table 29.5 Investigation of thrombocytopaenia

Blood film to exclude platelet clumps, MAHA or other
  haematological disorders
Coagulation screen (to include fibrinogen and D-dimer levels)
Renal and liver function tests
Antiphospholipid antibodies
Anti-DNA antibodies to exclude SLE (antinuclear antibody is
  sufficient as a screening test)

Table 29.6 Causes of ITP

Idiopathic
Helicobacter pylori
SLE
Lymphoma/chronic lymphocytic leukaemia
HIV
Drugs

Table 29.7 Causes of TTP/HUS

TTP	Congenital
	Pregnancy
	Drugs (e.g. clopidogrel, ticlopidine, tacrolimus)
	Combined contraceptive pill
	Bone marrow transplant
	SLE
	Malignancy
	HIV
	E. coli-0157
HUS	Pregnancy
	Infection (cytotoxin producing *E. coli* or Shigella)
	Drugs (e.g. cyclosporine, quinine, chemotherapy)

if essential, is best carried out between 13 and 20 weeks' gestation.

ITP: THE MANAGEMENT OF DELIVERY

The baby's platelet count cannot be reliably predicted from any maternal features. Furthermore, fetal sampling is hazardous or prone to spuriously low results. Thus, procedures in labour and at delivery that pose an additional bleeding risk should be avoided (fetal scalp electrode, fetal blood sampling, ventouse and rotational forceps). There is no evidence, however, that Caesarean section is safer for the thrombocytopaenic fetus than an uncomplicated vaginal delivery, as the nadir in platelets is most often 24–48 h after delivery. A cord blood platelet count should be determined in all babies and close monitoring is required over the next 2–5 days.

Thrombotic thrombocytopaenic purpura/haemolytic uraemic syndrome

Thrombotic thrombocytopaenic purpura (TTP) and Haemolytic Uraemic Syndrome (HUS) are characterized by thrombocytopaenia, microangiopathic haemolytic anaemia (MAHA) and multiorgan failure. TTP is more often associated with neurological abnormalities and non-renal organ ischaemia, while patients with HUS have predominantly renal manifestations and usually occurs post-partum. HUS can also be associated with haemolysis, elevated liver, enzymes, low platelets (HELLP) syndrome. However, there is a significant crossover and it is often difficult to distinguish between the two [34–36]. TTP occurs most often as an idiopathic single episode, although there is a congenital form that may recur. Like HUS, it may also occur secondary to other influences (Table 29.7).

Von Willebrand factor is, on release from the endothelium, cleaved by the metalloprotease, ADAMTS-13, resulting in the correct balance of vWF multimers. TTP/HUS is characterized by a failure of this cleavage. In TTP,

are often all that is required, with the aim often attaining an adequate platelet count for delivery. A spontaneous vaginal delivery or Caesarean Section can take place when platelets are $>50 \times 10^9$/l. If the woman wishes or requires epidural or spinal anaesthesia then a platelet count of $>80 \times 10^9$/l is recommended [33].

When required, treatment with either oral corticosteroids or IVIgG produces 50–70% response rates. The IVIgG response usually lasts 2–3 weeks and repeated dosing may be required. Secondary treatments include high-dose methylprednisolone or azathioprine, or a combination of these therapies with IVIgG. Other treatments (vinca alkaloids and cyclophosphamide) are not suitable in pregnancy and splenectomy is also best avoided, but this can be due to a congenital deficiency of ADAMTS-13, but is more commonly due to an acquired autoantibody. The resultant excess of circulating ultra-large multimers leads to platelet aggregation and consumption, leading to microvascular thrombosis. However, in HUS, and in many cases of TTP, ADAMTS-13 is normal and, indeed, a reduction in ADAMTS-13 is not specific to TTP/HUS. Consequently, the exact mechanism is not fully understood. However, the physiological coagulation changes in pregnancy may predispose to the condition.

DIAGNOSIS

HUS typically presents post-partum with thrombocytopaenia, haemolysis, and renal failure. While TTP is a classic pentad of fever, haemolysis, thrombocytopaenia, CNS signs and renal dysfunction, all five are only present in around 50% of cases. TTP, particularly recurrent TTP, usually presents before 24 weeks of pregnancy. Routine blood clotting tests are often normal in the early stages of TTP/HUS, but as the disease progresses there may be coagulation activation and DIC.

TREATMENT

With the exception of endotoxin-related HUS (where supportive care is the main requirement) and congenital TTP, it is unlikely that a clear distinction between the two syndromes will be possible in the majority of pregnancy-related cases. As a consequence, both are often considered as a single syndrome when considering therapy, particularly as there may be benefit in plasma exchange (PEX) in non-toxin-related HUS [37].

The mainstay of treatment is PEX, which should be instituted within 24 h of presentation and although the optimal regime and fluid replacement is not certain, fresh frozen plasma (FFP – virally inactivated if possible) is the common standard, although cryosupernatant may be preferred. When exchange is not immediately available, FFP alone may be beneficial and, indeed, may be sufficient in congenital disease. Intravenous methylprednisolone and aspirin (when platelets >50 × 10⁹/l) are often added to PEX therapy. However, platelet transfusions should be avoided in TTP. If the patient deteriorates, or does not respond, higher volume, or frequency of exchanges, or different replacement fluid is recommended.

Venous thromboembolism

Venous thromboembolism (VTE), the leading direct cause of maternal death occurs throughout pregnancy with an estimated antenatal and post natal incidence of 6–12 and 3–7 per 10,000 maternities, respectively, with a higher rate post-partum. The incidence of fatal pulmonary embolism in pregnancy has fallen from the 1950s in the UK, largely through a reduction in the number of women dying after vaginal deliveries. There has been less impact on deaths in the antenatal and intrapartum period and after Caesarean section [38]. Gestational deep venous thrombosis (DVT) usually occurs in the ileo-femoral veins (70 versus 9% in the non-pregnant) and is therefore more likely to result in pulmonary embolism (PE). Furthermore, it is also more likely to occur in the left leg (85 versus 55% in the non-pregnant), perhaps related to compression of the left iliac vein by the right iliac artery.

Pathogenesis and risk factors

PHYSIOLOGICAL CHANGES IN PREGNANCY

VTE is up to 10 times more common in pregnancy than in comparable non-pregnant subjects, which may relate to the physiological changes in maternal circulation and coagulation which occur in normal pregnancy as a preparation for delivery (Fig. 29.1). A number of clotting factors increase, accompanied by a reduction in fibrinolysis and the anticoagulant, protein S [39]. Furthermore, a substantial reduction in venous blood flow (more marked in the left common femoral vein than the right) occurs by the end of the first trimester, reaching a nadir at 34–36 weeks, returning to normal 6 weeks post-natally. The third factor underlying most venous thrombosis is vascular damage and trauma to the pelvic veins may occur during normal vaginal delivery and particularly so during abdominal or instrumental delivery [40].

RISK FACTORS FOR VTE IN PREGNANCY

A number of risk factors for pregnancy VTE are known (Table 29.8) such as age over 35 years (1.216 versus 0.615 per 1000 maternities) and Caesarean (particularly emergency) Section [41]. Around 50% of pregnancy VTE have an identifiable underlying heritable thrombophilia (Tables 29.8 and 29.9). In addition, acquired persistent

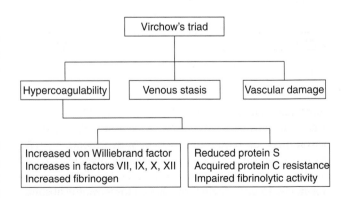

Fig. 29.1 The pathogenesis of pregnancy-associated VTE.

Table 29.8 Risk factors for venous thromboembolism in pregnancy

Age >35 years
Immobility
Obesity
Operative delivery
Pre-eclampsia
Parity >4
Surgical procedure in pregnancy or puerperium,
  e.g. post-partum sterilization
Previous DVT
Thrombophilia

Congenital	Antithromboin deficiency	
	Protein C deficiency	
	Protein S deficiency	
	Factor V Leiden	
	Prothrombin gene variant	
Acquired	Lupus anticoagulant	
	Anticardiolipin antibodies	

Excessive blood loss
Paraplegia
Sickle cell disease
Inflammatory disorders and infection, e.g. inflammatory bowel
  disease and urinary tract infection
Dehydration

Table 29.9 Prevalence rates of congenital thrombophilia in Western populations

Thrombophilia	Prevalence (per 1000 population)
Antithrombin deficiency	2.5–5.5
Protein C deficiency	2.0–3.3
Factor V Leiden (heterozygosity)	20–70
Prothrombin 20210A (heterozygosity)	20

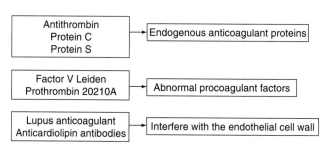

Fig. 29.2 Thrombophilia and risk of VTE.

antiphospholipid antibodies also increase pregnancy VTE risk (Fig. 29.2). From case-control and cohort studies the thrombotic risk is ~1:450 in FVL heterozygotes, ~1:200 in Prothrombin G20210A heterozygotes and ~1:113 with protein C deficiency. Hence, the absolute VTE risk is low for most common thrombophilias. However, the absolute risk is much higher with antithrombin deficiency (with a

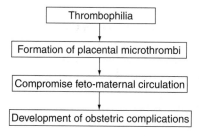

Fig. 29.3 Proposed mechanism of thrombophilia-related placental dysfunction.

VTE risk of 1:2.8 for type 1 and 1:42 for type 2 deficiency), FVL homozygotes (9–16:100) and combined defects (e.g. FVL/Porothrombin G20210A compound heterozygotes) have a pregnancy VTE risk of 4.6:100) [42].

THROMBOPHILIA AND OTHER COMPLICATIONS OF PREGNANCY

Maternal heritable thrombophilias are also associated with recurrent miscarriage, which is also a feature of antiphospholipid syndrome, where adverse pregnancy outcomes may be the result of poor placental perfusion due to localized thrombosis or increased thrombin generation. Antiphospholipid antibodies may also interfere with trophoblast invasion and, *in vitro*, heparin has been shown to ameliorate this effect. Low-dose aspirin and heparin is used for women with recurrent miscarriage and antiphospholipid syndrome [43]. The recently described associations between hereditable thrombophilias and miscarriage suggest that there may be a role for thromboprophylaxis in such cases. Thrombophilia may also result in placental dysfunction in later pregnancy, manifesting as growth restriction, pre-eclampsia, placental abruption and intrauterine fetal death, perhaps related to reduced placental perfusion, fibrin deposition and thrombus formation in uterine vessels and intervillous spaces (Fig. 29.3) [44]. In view of this, guidelines recommend thrombophilia screening for those with a history of recurrent pregnancy loss, second trimester miscarriage, intrauterine death, or severe/recurrent pre-eclampsia [42]. There is, as yet, however, no conclusive data that antithrombotic therapy will be beneficial, although some observational studies have indicated a benefit of Low Molecular Weight Heparin (LMWH) [45].

Thromboprophylaxis during pregnancy and the puerperium

VTE risk assessment should occur throughout pregnancy (and particularly pre- and post-delivery) since many risk factors (Table 29.8) may only become apparent as pregnancy advances and following delivery. Current guidelines recommend that if a previous VTE was associated with a temporary risk factor that is no longer present, and the event was not pregnancy or 'pill' related and there are no other risk factors, then antenatal thromboprophylaxis should not be routinely recommended [46]. However, thromboprophylaxis with LMWH should be employed in the puerperium. Antenatally, graduated elastic compression stockings or low-dose aspirin can also be used. In contrast, women with recurrent VTE, or a previous VTE and a family history of VTE (in a first-degree relative), or additional risk factors including thrombophilia, or where the previous event was idiopathic or pregnancy or 'pill' related should be offered antenatal LMWH thromboprophylaxis. A once-daily regime of LMWH (e.g. 40 mg enoxaparin, 5000 IU dalteparin) is appropriate, starting from their first presentation in pregnancy throughout the antenatal period and for at least 6 weeks post-partum. There is a lack of evidence to guide asymptomatic inherited or acquired thrombophilia management in pregnancy. These women may qualify for antenatal or post-natal thromboprophylaxis, depending on the specific thrombophilia and the presence of other risk factors. Women with previous VTE who are receiving long-term anticoagulant therapy should change to LMWH by 6 weeks' gestation to avoid teratogenesis. These women should be considered at very high risk of VTE and should receive 'treatment' doses of LMWH (e.g. enoxaparin 0.5–1 mg/kg/12 hourly or dalteparin 50–100 IU/kg/12 hourly-based on early pregnancy weight) throughout pregnancy.

Acute VTE in pregnancy – diagnosis and treatment

DIAGNOSIS

Features suggestive of DVT are common in normal pregnancy (Table 29.10), reflecting the physiological changes of pregnancy. Indeed less than 10% of women presenting

Table 29.10 The symptoms and signs of VTE

DVT	Leg pain or discomfort (especially the left leg)
	Swelling
	Tenderness
	Increased temperature and oedema
	Lower abdominal pain
	Elevated white cell count
PE	Dyspnoea
	Collapse
	Chest pain
	Haemoptysis
	Faintness
	Raised JVP
	Focal signs in the chest
	Associated symptoms and signs of DVT

with suspected DVT in pregnancy have the diagnosis confirmed and <6% with suspected PE are treated after completion of diagnostic imaging [47]. However, as mortality from untreated PE is high and clinical diagnosis of VTE unreliable, diagnostic imaging should be performed when VTE is suspected and anticoagulant treatment should be commenced (unless strongly contraindicated) until objective testing is concluded [48].

DVT

Real time/Duplex ultrasound is used to diagnose DVT. A negative ultrasound result with a low level of clinical suspicion should result in the discontinuation of anticoagulation. With a negative ultrasound, but a high level of clinical suspicion, anticoagulation should be continued and the ultrasound repeated in one week, or X-ray venography considered. If repeat testing is negative, anticoagulant treatment should be discontinued.

PE

If PE is suspected, ideally both ventilation/perfusion (V/Q) lung scanning and bilateral duplex ultrasound leg examinations should be performed (Table 29.11). When V/Q interpretation is difficult, then alternative imaging is warranted. This includes helical computerized tomography (CT) or pulmonary angiography, or magnetic resonance imaging. Helical CT delivers an average fetal radiation dose less than that with V/Q scanning (which is negligible in the context of the risk of PE) [49]. However, it is associated with radiation exposure to the woman's

Table 29.11 Investigation of DVT and PE in pregnancy

Test results	Management
V/Q scan reports a 'medium' or 'high' probability of PE	Anticoagulant treatment should be continued
'Low' probability of PE on V/Q scan but positive ultrasound for DVT	Anticoagulant treatment should be continued
V/Q scan reports a low risk of PE and there are negative leg ultrasound examinations	Anticoagulant treatment can be discontinued
V/Q scan reports a low risk of PE and there are negative leg ultrasound examinations, yet there is a high level of clinical suspicion	Anticoagulant treatment should continue with repeat testing in one week (V/Q scan and leg ultrasound examination)
If the clinical probability of PE is high, even if the V/Q scan shows 'low' probability and leg ultrasound examination is negative	Alternative imaging techniques should be considered (see text)

Table 29.12 Estimates of fetal radiation dose during diagnostic tests for VTE

Chest X-ray	<0.001 rad	
Limited venography	<0.05 rad	
V/Q scan (depends on isotopes used)	0.58 rad	
Low-dose perfusion scanning (omitting ventilation scanning)	<0.012 rad	
CT pulmonary angiography*	1st trimester	<0.002 rad
	2nd trimester	<0.008 rad
	3rd trimester	<0.013 rad

After Ginsberg *et al.* [51] except (*) from Winer-Muram et al., [49].

Table 29.13 The features of warfarin embryopathy

Mid-facial, particularly nasal, hypoplasia
Stippled chondral calcification
Short proximal limbs
Short phalanges
Scoliosis

thorax of over 2.0 rad, with 1 rad increasing her lifetime risk of breast cancer by 14% [50]. The radiation dose to the fetus with a CXR (chest X-ray) is small (Table 29.12), and this can safely be performed, principally to exclude other disorders [51]. The ECG is, however, of limited value and the interpretation of blood gases requires consideration of normal pregnancy physiology. D-dimer estimation has high negative predictive value as a screening test for VTE in the non-pregnant. However, elevated levels are seen during normal pregnancy [52]. Furthermore, even with a high sensitivity D-dimer assay around 4% of VTE will be missed. Thus, D-dimer results will not negate the need for an objective diagnostic test.

TREATMENT OF VTE IN PREGNANCY

Studies in non-pregnant patients show that LMWH is at least as safe and effective as unfractionated heparin (UFH) in both the initial treatment and subsequent prevention of recurrent VTE, but LMWH is preferable during pregnancy in view of the ease of administration, better bioavailability and safety (lower risk of heparin-induced osteoporosis and thrombocytopaenia) [48]. Thus LMWH is usually the treatment of choice in pregnancy. In the non-pregnant acute VTE, LMWH is administered once daily using a weight-adjusted dose, but as a decreased half-life occurs in pregnancy, twice-daily regimens are preferred (e.g. enoxaparin 1 mg/kg bid). Treatment with LMWHs can be monitored by measuring peak anti-Xa activity (3 h post-injection) with a therapeutic range of approximately 0.5–1.2 U/ml. However, for most patients such monitoring is considered unnecessary, as reliable results are found using a dose based on weight alone [53]. At extremes of body weight there may be a place for such monitoring. Treatment should be continued for at least 6 months and until at least 6 weeks post-partum. If the woman is still pregnant after 6 months treatment then there is

a case for reducing the dose to intermediate or prophylactic level, but this requires an individual assessment and consideration of continuing risk factors [54]. If UFH is used this can be by either intravenous infusion, followed by 6 months subcutaneous therapeutic LMWH, or adjusted-dose subcutaneous UFH, or adjusted-dose subcutaneous UFH or therapeutic LMWH for both initial and long-term treatment. There is a case for IV UFH in massive life-threatening PE with haemodynamic compromise (where thrombolytic therapy should also be considered). With UFH a mid-interval activated partial thromboplastin time (APTT) of 1.5–2.5 times control should be achieved. However, APTT testing is often poorly performed and an apparent heparin resistance in late pregnancy can lead to unnecessarily high doses. If a woman is treated exclusively with LMWH and has not previously been exposed to UFH there is no need to monitor the platelet count; otherwise this should be monitored after initiating treatment and at regular intervals [55]. Warfarin, which should be avoided antenatally, can be used post-partum.

RISKS OF ANTICOAGULANT THERAPY IN PREGNANCY

Both UFH and LMWH do not cross the placenta and are not associated with teratogenicity or fetal bleeding. In contrast, warfarin crosses the placenta and, if taken between 6 and 12 weeks of gestation, causes an embryopathy in approximately 6.4% of women, (Table 29.13), which can be avoided by heparin substitution [47]. The risk of embryopathy may be higher with >5 mg warfarin/day. Warfarin is also associated with fetal and neonatal haemorrhage. With fetal liver immaturity, maternal therapeutic warfarin (INR 2–3) is likely to result in excessive anticoagulation in the fetus. Warfarin during the second and third trimesters may also result in neurodevelopmental problems.

The maternal complications of anticoagulant therapy include haemorrhage, osteoporosis, thrombocytopaenia and allergy. With UFH, the rate of major bleeding in pregnant patients is 2% which is similar to heparin and warfarin when used for the treatment of DVT in the non-pregnant. One of the potential advantages of LMWH over UFH is an enhanced anti-Xa (antithrombotic):anti-IIa (anticoagulant) ratio, resulting in a theoretically reduced bleeding risk. UFH causes a dose-dependent loss of cancellous bone and, if administered for more than one month, symptomatic vertebral fractures occur in 2–3%, with significant density reduction evident in >30% with long-term therapy. LMWHs carry a much lower risk of symptomatic osteoporosis than UFH [56]. Around 3% of non-pregnant patients receiving UFH develop an idiosyncratic immune, IgG-mediated heparin-induced thrombocytopaenia (HIT), which is frequently complicated by extension of pre-existing VTE or new arterial thrombosis. The HIT risk is substantially lower with LMWH and considered negligible if LMWH is used exclusively (see p. 279). This condition should be suspected if platelets fall to $<100 \times 10^9/l$ (or to less than 50% of baseline), 5–15 days after commencing heparin (or sooner with recent heparin exposure). If ongoing anticoagulation is needed in such patients then the heparinoid, danaparoid sodium, is recommended. Routine platelet count monitoring is not required in obstetric patients who have received only LMWH, but if UFH (or LMWH after UFH) is used, platelets should be monitored every 2–3 days from day 4 to day 14, or until heparin is stopped [56]. Allergy to both UFH and LMWH usually take the form of itchy, erythematous lesions at the injection sites. Changing preparation or switching from a LMWH to UFH may help, although cross-reactivity can occur.

Labour and delivery

Heparin treatment should be discontinued 24 h prior to elective induction of labour or delivery by Caesarean section. If spontaneous labour occurs, the woman should not inject any further heparin until she has been assessed. If there is a high risk of haemorrhage, intravenous UFH should be employed (as prompt reversal occurs on discontinuation or with protamine). Similarly, if the woman has a very high risk of recurrent VTE (e.g. a VTE diagnosed near term) then therapeutic intravenous UFH can be initiated and discontinued 4 to 6 h prior to the expected time of delivery. The risk of epidural or spinal haematoma during neuraxial instrumentation in pregnant patients receiving LMWH has not been clearly quantified, but precautions are indicated (Table 29.14). Post-partum anticoagulants

(either heparin or warfarin) should be given for at least 6 weeks or until at least 6 months of anticoagulant therapy has been completed. Heparin and warfarin can both be used safely during breastfeeding.

Table 29.14 Heparin and neuraxial instrumentation

Wait 12 h after prophylactic dose LMWH before epidural instrumentation

Wait 24 h after the last therapeutic dose (e.g. 1 mg/kg 12 h enoxaparin) before epidural instrumentation

Wait 10–12 h from most recent LMWH injection before cannula removal

No LMWH for at least 4 h after epidural catheter removal

References

1. Haram, K, Nilsen S & Ulvik R (2001) Iron supplementation in pregnancy-evidence and controversies. *Acta Obstet Scand* **80**, 683–8.
2. Milman, N, Byg K-E & Agger A (2000) Hemoglobin and erythrocyte indices during normal pregnancy and postpartum in 206 women with and without iron supplementation. *Acta Obstet Scand* **79**, 89–98.
3. Ali S & Economides D (2000) Folic acid supplementation. *Curr Opin Obstet Gynecol* **12**, 507–12.
4. Hibbard E & Smithells R (1965) Folic acid metabolism and human embryopathy. *Lancet* **1**, 1254–6.
5. Ray J & Blom H (2003) Vitamin B12 insufficiency and the risk of fetal neural tube defects. *Q J Med* **96**, 289–95.
6. Hindmarsh P *et al.* (2000) Effect of early maternal iron stores on placental weight and structure. *Lancet* **356**, 719–23.
7. Pardo J *et al.* (2000) Evaluation of low serum vitamin B12 in the non-anaemic pregnant patient. *Hum Reprod* **15**, 224–6.
8. Van der Broek N *et al.* (1998) Iron status in pregnant women: which measurements are valid. *Br J Haematol* **103**, 817–24.
9. Ellison J *et al.* (2004) Effect of supplementation with folic acid throughout pregnancy on plasma homocysteine concentration. *Thromb Res* **114**, 25–7.
10. Andersson A *et al.* (1992) Decreased serum homocysteine in pregnancy. *Eur J Clin Chem Clin Biochem* **30**, 377–9.
11. Qvist I *et al.* (1986) Iron, zinc and folate status during pregnancy and two months after delivery. *Acta Obstetrica et Gynecologica Scandinavica* **65**, 15–22.
12. Commentary (1995) Does folic acid harm people with vitamin B12 deficiency. *Q J Med* **88**, 357–64.
13. Old J (2003) Screening and genetic diagnosis of haemoglobin disorders. *Blood Rev* **17**, 43–53.
14. Chui D & Waye J (1998) Hydrops fetalis caused by α-thalassaemia: an emerging health care problem. *Blood* **91**, 2213–22.
15. Aessopos A *et al.* (1999) Pregnancy in patients with well-treated beta-thalassaemia: outcome for mothers and newborn infants. *Am J Obstet Gynecol* **180**, 360–5.
16. Mordel N *et al.* (1989) Successful full-term pregnancy in homozygous β-thalassaemia major: case report and review of the literature. *Obstet Gynecol* **73**, 837–9.
17. Jensen C, Tuck S & Wonke B (1995) Fertility in β-thalassaemia major: a report of 16 pregnancies, preconceptual evaluation and a review of the literature. *Br J Obstet Gynaecol* **102**, 625–9.
18. Sheiner E *et al.* (2004) Beta-thalassaemia minor during pregnancy. *Obstet Gynecol* **103**, 1273–7.
19. Rahimy M *et al.* (2000) Effect of active prenatal management on pregnancy outcome in sickle-cell disease in an African setting. *Blood* **96**, 1685–9.
20. Koshy M (1995) Sickle cell disease and pregnancy. *Blood Rev* **9**, 157–64.

21. BCSH (2003) Guidelines for the management of the acute painful crisis in sickle cell disease. *Br J Haematol* **120**, 744–52.

22. Mahmood K (2004) Prophylactic versus selective blood transfusion for sickle cell anaemia during pregnancy (Cochrane Review). *The Cochrane Library*. Chichester, UK: John Wiley & Sons, Ltd.

23. Urbaniak S & Greiss M (2000) RhD haemolytic disease of the fetus and the newborn. *Blood Rev* **14**, 44–61.

24. BCSH (1996) Guidelines for blood grouping and red cell antibody testing during pregnancy. *Transfus Med* **6**, 71–74.

25. Finning K *et al.* (2002) Prediction of fetal D status from maternal plasma: introduction of a new noninvasive fetal RHD genotyping service. *Transfusion* **42**, 1079–85.

26. Lo Y *et al.* (1994) Prenatal determination of fetal rhesus D status by DNA amplification of peripheral blood of rhesus-negative mothers. *Ann N Y Acad Sci* **731**, 229–36.

27. Mari G *et al.* (2000) Noninvasive diagnosis by Doppler ultrasonography of fetal anemia due to maternal red-cell alloimmunization. Collaborative group for doppler assessment of the blood velocity in anemic fetuses. *New Engl J Med* **342**, 9–14.

28. National Institute for Clinical Excellence (2002) *Guidelines. Pregnancy-routine anti-D prophylaxis for rhesus negative women*. London: Nice.

29. Royal College of Obstetrics and Gynaecology (2002) *Green Top*. Guidelines Anti-D immunoglobulin for Rh prophylaxis. London: RCOG.

30. Bowman J (2003) Thirty-five years of Rh prophylaxis. *Transfusion* **43**, 1661–6.

31. MacKenzie I *et al.* (1999) Routine antenatal Rhesus D immunoglobulin prophylaxis: the results of a prospective 10 year study. *Br J Obstet Gynaecol* **106**, 492–7.

32. Daniels G *et al.* (2002) The clinical significance of blood group antibodies. *Transfus Med* **12**, 287–95.

33. BCSH (2003) Guidelines for the investigation and management of idiopathic thrombocytopaenic purpura in adults, children and in pregnancy. *Br J Haematol* **120**, 574–96.

34. George J (2003) The association of pregnancy with thrombotic thrombocytopenic purpura-hemolytic uremic syndrome. *Curr Opin Haematol* **10**, 339–344.

35. Esplin M & Branch DW (1999) Diagnosis and management of thrombotic microangiopathies during pregnancy. *Clin Obstet Gynecol* **42**, 360–7.

36. Veyradier A & Meyer D (2005) Thrombotic thrombocytopenic purpura and its diagnosis. *J Thromb Haemost* **3**, 2420–7.

37. BCSH (2003) Guidelines on the diagnosis and management of the thrombotic microangiopathic haemolytic anaemias. *Br J Haematol* **120**, 556–73.

38. Confidential Enquiry into Maternal and Child Health (2004) Stillbirth, neonatal and post neonatal mortality 2000–2002 England, *Wales and Northern Ireland*. London: CEMACH.

39. Clark P *et al.* (1998) Activated protein C sensitivity, protein C, protein S and coagulation in normal pregnancy. *Thromb Haemost* **79**, 1166–70.

40. Greer I & Thomson A (2001) Management of venous thromboembolism in pregnancy. *Best Pract Res Clin Obstet Gynaecol* **15**, 583–603.

41. McColl M, Ramsay J & Tait R (1997) Risk factors for pregnancy-associated venous thromboembolism. *Thromb Haemost* **78**, 1183–8.

42. Bates S *et al.* (2004) Use of antithrombotic agents during pregnancy: the Seventh ACCP Conference on Antithrombotic and thrombolytic therapy. *Chest* **163**, 627S–44S.

43. Rai R *et al.* (1997) Randomised controlled trial of aspirin and aspirin plus heparin in pregnant women with recurrent miscarriage associated with phospholipid antibodies (or antiphospholipid antibodies). *Br Med J* **314**, 253–7.

44. Kujovich J (2004) Thrombophilia and pregnancy complications. *Am J Obstet Gynecol* **191**, 412–24.

45. Younis J *et al.* (2000) The effect of thromboprophylaxis on pregnancy outcome in patients with recurrent pregnancy loss associated with factor V Leiden mutation. *Br J Obstet Gynaecol* **107**, 415–9.

46. Nelson-Piercy C (2004) Thromboprophylaxis during pregnancy labour and after vaginal delivery. *RCOG Guideline* no. 37. London: RCOG Press.

47. Chan W, Anand S & Ginsberg J (2000) Anticoagulation of pregnant women with mechanical heart valves: a systematic review of the literature. *Arch Int Med* **160**, 191–6.

48. Thomson A & Greer I (2001) Thromboembolic disease in pregnancy and the puerperium: acute management. *RCOG Guideline* no. 28. London: RCOG Press.

49. Winer-Muram H *et al.* (2002) Pulmonary embolism in pregnant patients: fetal radiation dose with helical CT. *Radiology* **224**, 487–92.

50. Remy-Jardin M & Remy J (1999) Spiral CT angiography of the pulmonary circulation. *Radiology* **212**, 615–36.

51. Ginsberg J *et al.* (1989) Risks to the fetus of anticoagulant therapy during pregnancy. *Thromb Haemost* **61**, 197–203.

52. Francalanci I *et al.* (1997) D-dimer plasma levels during normal pregnancy measured by specific ELISA. *Int J Clin Lab Res* **27**, 65–7.

53. Rodie V *et al.* (2002) Low molecular weight heparin for the treatment of venous thromboembolism in pregnancy – case series. *Br J Obstet Gynaecol* **109**, 1020–4.

54. Greer I & Hunt B (2004) Low molecular weight heparin in pregnancy: current issues. *Br J Haematol* **128**, 593–601.

55. Warkentin T & Greinacher A (2004) Heparin-induced thrombocytopenia: recognition, treatment, and prevention: the Seventh ACCP Conference on Antithrombotic and Thrombolytic Therapy. *Chest* **126**(Suppl 3), 311S–37S.

56. Greer I & Nelson-Piercy C (2005) Low-molecular weight heparins for thromboprophylaxis and treatment of venous thromboembolism in pregnancy: a systematic review of safety and efficacy. *Blood* **106**, 401–7.

Chapter 30: Miscellaneous medical disorders

Andrew McCarthy

Most medical conditions in this age group do not result in serious morbidity, though many have the potential to do so, that is, epilepsy, asthma and migraine. It is important that women receive good advice pre-pregnancy about the potential impact of their medical condition and enter pregnancy with appropriate confidence about routine medication or specific management plans to alter treatment in the first trimester. This necessitates that they have ready access to specialist help once they become pregnant. Some compromise in effectiveness of medical treatment for long-term conditions is potentially involved and it is clearly appropriate that these issues will have been addressed prior to pregnancy, that is, anticoagulation in high-risk patients or renal protection with angiotensin converting enzyme (ACE) inhibitors.

There are a variety of medical disorders which may impact on a mother's health during pregnancy and the puerperium. These may be classified as those that are incidental to the pregnancy and where no exacerbation is expected as a result of pregnancy and those that are clearly prone to exacerbation due to pregnancy. The latter are of greatest concern to obstetricians, but incidental problems leading to serious morbidity also require careful coordinated care and care pathways are often less robust for these conditions.

General considerations

Mean age of childbearing has increased steadily in recent years. This has the effect of increasing the chance of a pregnancy being complicated by coincidental medical conditions and increases the risk that such conditions can impact on women's health. In the United Kingdom [1] the latest figure collected over the triennium 2000–2002 reveals 3% of deliveries are to women 40 years of age and over. In some units 6% of women are 40 years and older. This reflects a major shift, increasing risk of morbidity from medical disorders, and may be a contributory factor in the increasing indirect deaths in the triennial maternal mortality enquiry.

Management of women with medical disorders is often best coordinated within clinics with both obstetric and medical opinions and midwifery input available. When problems arise such clinics make outpatient management much more convenient for the patient and facilitate good communication between the relevant medical teams. They also serve as a focal point with which the woman may make contact in early pregnancy when treatment changes may need to take place without delay or in later pregnancy if there are problems. The latest triennial enquiry emphasizes the importance of integrated care plans for women with medical disorders, good communication between specialties, and early and senior review and ensuring that women with complications are managed in centres with all relevant expertise.

Respiratory disorders

Women with respiratory disorders require careful assessment when they present for antenatal care. For those with a risk of respiratory compromise during pregnancy or delivery, investigation with pulmonary functions tests may be necessary or exclusion of associated pulmonary vascular disease by echocardiography. An anaesthetic opinion prior to the third trimester is valuable, including for those with possible respiratory compromise due to musculoskeletal problems.

Breathlessness can be one of the most difficult symptoms to interpret in pregnancy. Some increase in breathlessness arises during the course of a normal pregnancy, and yet the same complaint can be a manifestation of thromboembolism, cardiac disease or deterioration of background respiratory disease. Patients should have a careful clinical assessment by history and examination. Oxygen saturation, arterial blood gasses and chest X-rays may all help in differentiating physiological breathlessness from serious disease. Experienced medical opinion should be sought if there is concern about underlying pathology.

Management of acute respiratory compromise may require delivery. While the physiological adaptation to pregnancy is not critically dependent on any respiratory change, in the presence of pathology the negative impact of pregnancy including splinting of the diaphragm may mean that delivery is an important part of the treatment plan to ensure recovery. This may mandate Caesarean delivery in difficult circumstances and in such circumstances experienced obstetric, medical and anaesthetic input is required. Such patients may require general anaesthesia and intensive care post-delivery.

Asthma

Asthma is the most common respiratory disorder affecting 3% of women of childbearing age. Pregnancy has a variable effect on asthma but for the vast majority of women there is no impact whatsoever. The most common reason that their asthma symptoms deteriorate is patients reducing their treatment because of a belief that the medication may be harmful. All commonly used medications to control asthma are safe in pregnancy. All patients must be reassured that any flairs of their asthma must not be ignored and that treatment with medication such as steroids is safe both for themselves and for their fetus. With regard to the effect of asthma on fetal outcome, there is no evidence that there is any significant impact on fetal growth or outcome. Any patient whose asthma seems to be deteriorating, particularly in the third trimester, should be seen by an obstetric physician for review. It is obviously desirable that control of their asthma should be at its optimum prior to the onset of labour. Patients presenting in labour should be managed with an agreed protocol [2]. However, it is unusual for labour to be complicated by attacks of asthma and this is probably due to the increased secretion of cortisol during the process. However, attacks of asthma during labour can be managed by conventional treatment, such as inhaled beta-sympathomimetics. Patients who have been on maintenance glucocorticoids, for example, Prednisolone doses in excess of the equivalent of 5 mg Prednisolone daily, require hydrocortisone cover during labour. If an operative delivery is required, epidural anaesthesia is preferable to general anaesthesia but if a general anaesthetic is required, the anaesthetic care is the same as if the patient was not pregnant. Patients with severe asthma should be delivered in centres where appropriate backup facilities and medical expertise is available. Acute asthma is still a cause of maternal death and as such must be taken extremely seriously.

Pneumonia

Pneumonia can be a life-threatening illness in a woman of childbearing age. Acute pneumonia should be managed by experienced physicians and imaging should not be withheld if it is important to patient care. Most antibiotics are safe for the pregnant mother and it is important to treat infection vigorously rather than exercise restraint due to inappropriate fear of medication. The management objectives include prevention of respiratory compromise where there is a need for delivery as this will then be very high risk. It is also important to prevent the underlying infection developing into septicaemia with associated haemodynamic instability. Anaesthetic input is required from an early stage where delivery may need to be considered. Patients who have pneumonia have an increased risk of preterm labour, which presumably relates to the pyrexia and prostaglandin release.

Varicella pneumonia is a particular cause for concern for the pregnant woman requiring intravenous acyclovir. It can occur in association with encephalitis and hepatitis. Up to 10% of women affected by varicella will develop pneumonia and will require admission for intravenous treatment. There does not appear to be adverse sequelae for the fetus from acyclovir and case fatality rates have reduced to 1% or less with acyclovir treatment.

Tuberculosis

Pulmonary tuberculosis can present for the first time in pregnancy and the obstetrician must have a high index of suspicion when presented with symptoms of cough, malaise or weight loss in high-risk groups. Most treatment options appear to be safe including ethambutol, rifampicin, isoniazid with pyridoxine and also pyrazinamide. Streptomycin carries risks of VIII nerve damage and should be avoided. There is no conclusive evidence that the outcome of pregnancy is adversely affected by tuberculosis providing treatment is commenced in the first half of pregnancy. After birth, the neonate should be treated with prophylactic isoniazid for 3 months and thereafter BCG vaccination should be given, although its efficacy remains questionable.

Cystic fibrosis

Cystic fibrosis is not a common problem in pregnancy. However, an increasing number of women with cystic fibrosis are now surviving to an age where pregnancy is an option. Pre-conception counselling is essential and pulmonary function tests, echocardiography to exclude pulmonary hypertension and arterial blood gases are all essential in guiding the decision as to whether or not pregnancy is advisable. Chest infections during pregnancy require prompt and expert treatment and any associated problems such as diabetes require strict attention. The patient should be seen by an anaesthetist during pregnancy to assess pain relief and anaesthesia in labour and this is preferably by epidural anaesthetic. Most women with cystic fibrosis will have a good outcome to their pregnancy [3].

Respiratory failure post-partum

Respiratory failure can arise for the first time in the post-partum period. The differential diagnosis includes adult respiratory distress syndrome (ARDS), pulmonary oedema secondary to pre-eclampsia or nephrotic syndrome, amniotic fluid embolism, pulmonary embolism, infection and collapse and side effects of tocolysis. Often a single diagnosis is not reached and care is supportive. Care must be taken to exclude undiagnosed cardiac disease or peri-partum cardiomyopathy and protect the patient from thromboembolic complications. ARDS is still a recognized cause of maternal death.

Neurological conditions

Serious manifestations of neurological disease are fortunately rare in pregnancy, though cerebral haemorrhage remains a significant cause of maternal death. Epilepsy and migraine are common causes of morbidity.

Epilepsy

Women of childbearing age who suffer from epilepsy and are on maintenance therapy must have their treatment reviewed and monotherapy is recommended if at all possible. Antiepileptic drugs can cause teratogenicity and folic acid 5 mg daily is generally prescribed in view of the relative folate deficiency of many mothers on antiepileptic therapy. It is important that control of seizures is achieved to minimize maternal morbidity (fits can be fatal) and patients must be monitored during pregnancy to ensure that dose adjustments are made as appropriate. Sodium valproate is the major cause for concern in the second and third trimesters in the light of data suggesting increased educational needs in children exposed *in utero* [4,5]. All patients should receive anomaly ultrasound assessment to exclude specific abnormalities associated with their medication. These are specifically orofacial clefts, neural tube defects and craniofacial dysmorphism. Vitamin K is recommended to be given from 36 weeks onwards to prevent neonatal bleeding disorders. Epileptic seizures may occur during labour and as such may confuse the diagnostic situation that includes eclampsia. Epileptic seizures should be treated in these circumstances as they would be normally and may be reduced with the use of epidural anaesthesia. Post-partum drug doses may need to be adjusted if doses have been increased during pregnancy. Specific advice

must be given to epileptic women about childcare, for example, not bathing the baby on their own, and patient organizations offer information leaflets for patients, which are invaluable.

Migraine

Headaches are a common problem in pregnancy and migraine sufferers may find their symptoms worsen during the first trimester. Many patients may be using ergot alkaloids to treat migraine prior to the onset of pregnancy and they must be advised not to use these during pregnancy. Migraines may improve considerably in the second and third trimesters [6] but in patients in whom continuing problems exist, the strategies that are employed for prophylaxis are low-dose aspirin, paracetamol and codeine as pain relief and propranolol if attacks continue to be troublesome despite these measures. If focal migraine occurs as a new symptom in pregnancy an experienced opinion to exclude serious underlying causes must be sought.

Cerebrovascular disease

Cerebral haemorrhage is a major cause of maternal morbidity and mortality [1,7]. It can occur as a result of uncontrolled hypertension or due to vascular malformations. Patients presenting with neurological symptoms in association with pregnancy should be investigated in the same way as they would be in the non-pregnant state. Ischaemic strokes arise in pregnancy, but it is controversial as to whether this is associated with an increased incidence reflecting the coagulation changes of pregnancy. Investigation of any underlying thrombophilic state can be important and further thromboprophylaxis instigated.

In the maternal mortality triennial report published in 2004 [1], 17 out of 21 cases of intracranial haemorrhage were due to subarachnoid haemorrhage but none of the cases occurred during labour. In 7 of the 17 cases, an aneurysm was identified.

Cerebral vein thrombosis (CVT)

Cerebral vein thrombosis is rare in pregnancy [7], and it tends to present with a very severe headache and is most commonly found post-partum in association with dehydration. Magnetic resonance imaging (MRI) is mandatory although computer tomography (CT) scanning is the best method to detect acute intracerebral bleeding. The treatment is still somewhat controversial but increasingly anticoagulation is being used in spite of the history of haemorrhage.

Rheumatology

Antiphospholipid syndrome and systemic lupus erythematosus

Systemic lupus erythematosus (SLE) has an adverse effect on pregnancy outcome but it is significant that better outcomes are achieved in those who conceive when their condition is quiescent and worse for those with unstable disease or flares. Much of the impaired outcome can be explained as a result of secondary antiphospholipid syndrome (APS), with increased risks of intrauterine growth retardation, placental abruption and pre-eclampsia. Careful monitoring of immunosuppressive treatment is required and associated infection and flares must be treated promptly.

APS [8] is an acquired condition characterized by an increased tendency to thrombosis, recurrent miscarriage, impaired pregnancy outcome and thrombocytopaenia. Laboratory tests to confirm the diagnosis include anticardiolipin antibody levels and lupus anticoagulant. These tests must be positive on two consecutive occasions at least 6 weeks apart. This is because transient positivity can be found in association with viral illness. Treatment in pregnancy involves anti-platelet therapy with low-dose aspirin, and heparin. Autoantibodies to Ro and La which can complicate such pregnancies can be associated with congenital heart block and neonatal lupus syndrome.

Rheumatoid arthritis

In the presence of mild rheumatoid arthritis, a temporary improvement in the symptoms can arise during pregnancy, and this is presumed to be due to the steroidal properties of placental hormones. More women with moderate or severe disease are now willing to contemplate pregnancy. This is as a result, at least to some extent, of the increasing success of disease modifying drugs such as methotrexate, leflunomide and tumour necrosis factor (TNF) antagonists, but these must be withdrawn prior to or early in pregnancy. Pregnancy can prove more challenging in such cases and will require careful supervision with a rheumatologist or obstetric physician, and the involvement of an anaesthetist prior to delivery. For those on long-term steroid therapy, increased surveillance for gestational diabetes is necessary. Some consideration needs to be given to the extent of handicap which can arise from moderate or severe rheumatoid. This can seriously impair the ability of a mother to properly care for her newborn child. Early referral to an occupational therapist can ensure that the family is best prepared for any problems that may arise.

Scleroderma

Scleroderma and mixed connective tissue disease can also complicate pregnancy. Scleroderma/systemic sclerosis is a high-risk condition in pregnancy and will often be managed in very specialized units. Caution is required in assessing the cardiopulmonary status of such women when pregnancy is being planned. Hypertension and renal involvement are also common and require careful management. Mixed connective tissue disorders can also present problems, akin to those with lupus or other arthritic diseases.

Liver disorders

Liver disorders frequently complicate pregnancy, but fortunately rarely result in long-term morbidity. Cholestasis of pregnancy is the most common liver condition affecting pregnancy and it classically presents with an itch and consequent lack of sleep in the third trimester. From an obstetric viewpoint it is important to note that it is associated with an increased risk of intrauterine death, classically from 37 weeks' gestation, an increased risk of meconium passage and increased risk of preterm labour [9,10]. The mechanism of intrauterine death is uncertain but is likely to be related to a toxic effect on the fetus. Laboratory investigations include liver function tests and assay of serum bile acids. It is currently uncertain whether the bile acids themselves may be directly responsible for fetal demise. Treatment strategies include timely delivery, cool aqueous menthol cream to relieve itch, ursodeoxycholic acid and vitamin K. Ursodeoxycholic acid is currently the mainstay of treatment and is prescribed at doses commencing at 500 mg twice daily and may be increased to a maximum of 2 g daily. This condition has a high likelihood of recurrence (approximately 80%). Some women who present with this condition will have underlying liver disease and this is most likely to be noted with early onset disease or failure of liver function to return to normal after delivery.

Acute fatty liver of pregnancy (AFLP) is a serious but rare liver condition arising in pregnancy which can be very non-specific at time of presentation. It is associated with nausea, vomiting, abdominal pain and jaundice. Diagnosis is normally confirmed by a moderately elevated aspartate amino transferase (AST), and no direct evidence of pre-eclampsia. The diagnosis may be supported by imaging suggestive of fatty change. Manifestations of liver failure include coagulopathy, haemodynamic instability and hypoglycaemia. Hypoglycaemia is a common feature, especially in labour, and may be profound and requires immediate correction. Serial assessment of blood clotting is also important. Delivery must be achieved prior to the development of coagulation failure, where necessary at the expense of fetal maturity. It is often not possible to clearly distinguish AFLP from haemolysis, elevated liver enzymes, low platelets (HELLP) syndrome or pre-eclampsia.

Liver dysfunction in pregnancy can also be caused by incidental viral or autoimmune hepatitis. Where it is unexplained, serology for acute hepatitis must be sent and medical help requested. It is often difficult to determine whether liver dysfunction is due to a pregnancy related complication or incidental liver disease, and consideration must be given to delivery when there is uncertainty. Liver failure is rare in or after pregnancy. The more common causes include paracetamol overdose, viral hepatitis, HELLP syndrome and acute fatty liver of pregnancy. Correct diagnosis is important as early referral to a liver unit with a view to transplantation may be appropriate. Delivery will not affect the natural course of a viral hepatitis, but is likely to be beneficial with the latter two diagnoses. The issue of referral to specialist liver units most commonly arises after delivery if liver function continues to deteriorate. Such decisions should be made in consultation with a specialist unit.

Hyperemesis

Hyperemesis gravidarum is defined as vomiting in early pregnancy sufficient to warrant hospital admission. Vomiting is clearly very common in early pregnancy, but some women suffer disproportionately from it. This can occasionally result in serious sequelae including severe dehydration and increased risk of thromboembolism. Pregnancy outcome is generally unaffected, though there may be an increased incidence of intrauterine growth restriction (IUGR) where sustained vomiting results in maternal weight loss. Treatment options include small light snacks, intravenous rehydration and sometimes antiemetic treatment. Promethazine and metoclopramide are commonly used for this indication. There is uncertainty regarding the effectiveness of anitemetics [11], and they are generally best avoided unless hydration is compromised. It is important that B vitamins are replenished as Wernicke's encephalopathy can occur. Corticosteroids may have a role in exceptional cases. Ondansetron may also have a role in exceptional cases, but clear evidence of safety in the first trimester is still awaited. Total parenteral nutrition may be required, but this is very rare. It is difficult to predict recurrence risks in a subsequent pregnancy, but some women undoubtedly experience severe nausea and vomiting with every pregnancy.

It is very important that hyperemesis is regarded as a diagnosis of exclusion. Serious underlying causes for ongoing vomiting must be sought such as CNS pathology,

gastrointestinal disease or surgical problems. Peptic ulceration is rare in pregnancy but can arise. It is sometimes appropriate to consider endoscopy for women with persistent vomiting or a trial of treatment. Gastro-oesophageal reflux is a much more common problem. The diagnosis is not usually in doubt and the condition can be treated with antacids, sometimes metoclopromide, H2 antagonists and proton pump inhibitors.

Acute abdominal complications

Problems such as appendicitis, pancreatitis and cholecystitis can arise in pregnancy. They must be managed aggressively to minimize any risk of associated peritonitis which can result in premature labour and associated sepsis. Diagnosis of such complications can be difficult and requires an experienced opinion. It is generally recommended that early recourse to surgery for an acute appendicitis is the best option to prevent the development of peritonitis with possible serious sequelae, including preterm delivery.

Inflammatory bowel disease can also complicate pregnancy. Pregnancy outcome is in general satisfactory, though there may be some increased risk of preterm birth and IUGR, particularly if there is active disease. It is in general treated in the same way in pregnancy as in the non-pregnant state, with steroids and sulphasalazine the mainstays of treatment.

Supplementation of haematinics and vitamin D may be required. Possible sequelae such as perineal and perianal disease and intra-abdominal adhesions need to be considered when discussing mode of delivery.

Dermatoses of pregnancy

There are a number of specific dermatological conditions which arise in pregnancy only. The most common is termed polymorphic eruption of pregnancy affecting approximately 0.5% of pregnancies. This maculo-papular rash presents on the abdomen and thighs with umbilical sparing. It causes irritation and can be treated with steroid cream if localized, or systemic steroids. Skin biopsy is sometimes necessary in pregnancy, typically when there is a relatively early presentation and significant maternal symptoms. Polymorphic eruption tends to arise in the late third trimester and not to recur in subsequent pregnancies.

Pemphigoid gestationis in contrast is much rarer (1/60,000 incidence) and commences around the umbilicus. It commences as pruritic papules and plaques which develop into vesicles and bullae after a few weeks. It is thought to be immunological in origin and is associated with other autoimmune disorders. Severe cases should be treated with systemic steroids. This rash can be slow to resolve after delivery and has a high risk of recurrence in subsequent pregnancies, often at earlier gestations. This condition appears to be associated with some fetal risk and IUGR, and therefore fetal surveillance must be instituted.

Prurigo of pregnancy is another papular eruption affecting extensor surfaces and the abdomen. It may be associated with atopy and can be treated with antihistamines and topical steroids. There are other dermatoses which can arise specifically in pregnancy. Dermatological opinion and biopsy tend to be reserved for those that are particularly disabling, or have failed to respond to topical steroids.

Human immunodeficiency virus (HIV)

Routine antenatal testing for HIV is now the norm in most developed countries. This appears to be most effective if an opt-out approach is taken. Infection with HIV poses specific problems in pregnancy, and antiretroviral treatment must be supervised by experienced physicians. Infected women will be offered such treatment with the aims of reducing vertical transmission and minimizing disease progression [12]. Choice of antiretroviral treatment will depend on clinical status, viral load and CD4 counts. There is no evidence of reproducible congenital abnormality with different antiretroviral agents, but clearly some caution is required with newer agents and treatment regimes until long-term follow-up data become available. Risks of perinatal transmission are reduced by Caesarean delivery, appropriate intrapartum antiretroviral treatment, avoidance of breastfeeding and treatment for the neonate. These strategies have reduced mother to child transmission to 2%.

Psychiatric disorders in the antenatal period

It is increasingly clear that psychiatric problems can lead to maternal mortality and very significant morbidity [1]. Reference to the latest maternal mortality report confirms the major contribution psychiatric disease makes. Antenatal assessment must include an assessment of risk of psychiatric morbidity. This will involve review of any previous episodes of psychiatric care or social vulnerability. Patients at risk of such problems are often poor attendees for antenatal care and are disproportionately represented in refugee or ethnic minority subgroups. Language and culture are too often barriers to appropriate care. It is clear that health-care workers need to be aware of these factors, that systems need to be in place to ensure that such patients can access appropriate antenatal care and that plans are made to ensure provision of support in the puerperium.

Most psychotropic medication is relatively safe in pregnancy, with few overt congenital abnormalities described in association. The exceptions include lithium, which appears to be associated with an increased incidence of Ebstein's anomaly. This is a serious consideration for those patients with bipolar disorders, where a balanced judgement must be made reflecting psychiatric stability versus a 5% risk of a potentially surgically correctable anomaly. For many women suffering from anxiety disorders and mild depression, psychotherapy and counselling may be a better option than medication. Tricyclic antidepressants such as imipramine or amytryptaline appear to be safe in pregnancy, but there are arguments for reducing the dose or stopping treatment completely prior to delivery in view of the potential for anti-cholinergic side effects in the neonate. Benzodiazepines may carry some teratogenic risk and are best avoided. It is reasonable for many women on antidepressant medication at conception to have a trial off treatment provided this is supported by their psychiatrist.

Manic depressive illness and schizophrenia both carry substantial risks of relapse following delivery and care in the initial post-partum phase, including reintroduction of medication, must be planned in advance. Antipsychotic medication in pregnancy may carry some risk to the fetus, but this will often be outweighed by the need for stability. It is important that decisions on long-term therapy during pregnancy are made in consultation with a psychiatrist.

Substance abuse is another factor which can lead disadvantaged and vulnerable mothers to defaulting from care. It is important to detect substance abuse as there are specific programmes of care depending on the agent of abuse.

Conclusion

This chapter has involved discussion of many medical disorders which may affect pregnancy. It is easy to emphasize the importance of these issues by referring to the chapter on indirect deaths in the triennial enquiry into maternal death (Tables 30.1 and 30.2). This does not do justice, however, to the contribution that an interested obstetrician

Table 30.1 Rate of indirect maternal death/100,000 maternities

1985–87	3.7
1988–90	3.9
1991–93	4.3
1994–96	6.1
1997–99	6.4
2000–02	7.8

Table 30.2 Causes of indirect maternal death 2000–02

Diseases of CNS	**40**
Subarachnoid haemorrhage	17
Intracranial haemorrhage	3
Cerebral thrombosis	4
Epilepsy	13
Other	3
Infectious disease	**14**
HIV	4
Other	10
Diseases of respiratory system	**10**
Asthma	5
Other	5
Endocrine disease	**7**
Diabetes	3
Other	4
Gastrointestinal disease	**7**
Blood disease	**2**
Circulatory disease	**3**
Renal disease	**3**
Unknown	**4**
Total	**90**

or physician can make in managing these conditions. Managing these conditions well can lead to a woman having far greater confidence during her pregnancy, avoidance of unnecessary morbidity and avoidance of stillbirth associated with medical conditions such as obstetric cholestasis. Good quality antenatal care can also facilitate reduced difficulty in the puerperium, and avoidance of long-term morbidity when it is difficult for women to attend medical appointments and routine patterns of referral often break down.

References

1. Why Mothers Die 2000 – 2002. Report on confidential enquiries into maternal deaths in the United Kingdom. London: RCOG Press, 2004.
2. British Thoracic Society, Scottish Intercollegiate Guidelines Network (2003) British guideline on the management of asthma. *Thorax* **58**(Suppl 1), i1–94.
3. Boyd J, Mehta A & Murphy D (2004) Fertility and pregnancy outcomes in men and women with cystic fibrosis in the United Kingdom. *Hum Reprod* **19**(10), 2238–43.
4. Adab N, Kini U, Vinten J *et al.* (2004) The longer term outcome of children born to mothers with epilepsy. *J Neurol Neurosurg Psychiatry* **75**(11), 1575–83.
5. Kaplan P (2004) Reproductive health effects and teratogenicity of antiepileptic drugs. *Neurology* **63**(10 Suppl 4), S13–23.
6. Von Wald T & Walling A (2002) Headache during pregnancy. *Obstet Gynecol Surv* **57**(3), 179–85.
7. Jeng J, Tang S & Yip P (2004) Stroke in women of reproductive age: comparison between stroke related and unrelated to pregnancy. *J Neurol Sci* **221**(1–2), 25–9.
8. Wilson W, Gharavi A, Koike T *et al.* (1999) International consensus statement on preliminary classification criteria for definite antiphospholipid syndrome: report of an international workshop. *Arthritis Rheum* **42**(7), 1309–11.
9. Kenyon A, Piercy C, Girling J, Williamson C, Tribe R & Shennan A (2002) Obstetric cholestasis, outcome with active management: a series of 70 cases. *Br J Obstet Gynaecol* **109**(3), 282–8.
10. Williamson C, Hems L, Goulis D *et al.* (2004) Clinical outcome in a series of cases of obstetric cholestasis identified via a patient support group. *Br J Obstet Gynaecol* **111**(7), 676–81.
11. Jewell D & Young G (2003) Interventions for nausea and vomiting in early pregnancy. *Cochrane Database Syst Rev* **4**, CD000145.
12. Semprini A & Fiore S (2004) HIV and pregnancy: is the outlook for mother and baby transformed? *Curr Opin Obstet Gynecol* **16**(6), 471–5.

Further reading

(2002) In: Michael de Swiet (ed.) *Medical Disorders in Obstetric Practice*, 4th edn, Blackwell Publishing.

Chapter 31: Obstetric statistics

Jim G. Thornton

Introduction

Doctors do two main things; they diagnose and they treat patients. To do both they need to count what they are doing. We begin with the counting.

Counting

Everyone needs to count what they are doing. This tells them what is going on, and lets them allocate resources wisely and detect warning trends. To do this effectively we need unambiguous definitions. This is not always easy. The UK, like all other countries, has its own legal definitions which sometimes differ from those in other countries and also alter from time to time. The World Health Organization (WHO) tries to coordinate international statistics by producing agreed definitions in its International Classification of Diseases (ICD) publications which are updated at approximately 10 yearly intervals. Here are a few of the more important definitions used in obstetric epidemiology. This chapter uses the same definitions as the UK Office of National Statistics (ONS) and consider some of the difficulties that they cause statisticians.

Live birth

In the UK this is defined simply as 'a child born alive'. WHO says the same thing in more words – 'the complete expulsion or extraction from its mother of a product of conception, which after such separation, breathes or shows any other evidence of life, such as the beating of the heart, pulsation of the umbilical cord, or definite movement of voluntary muscles, whether or not the umbilical cord has been cut or the placenta is attached; each product of such a birth is considered live born. Twins both born alive count as two live births but a child who dies from asphyxia caused by shoulder dystocia after delivery of the head but before delivery of the body is not a live birth'.

There is no lower gestational age limit to the UK definition so a child of any gestational age which shows signs of life should be registered. This can occasionally lead to anomalies when for example a fetus of say 12 weeks is noticed to have a heart beat for some minutes after it has miscarried; although strictly a live birth, which should be registered as such and counted in the birth statistics, this offends against common sense.

The WHO does not interfere in national birth registrations but recommends that births only be included in national statistics if they weigh at least 500 g or have a gestational age of at least 22 weeks, so the problem does not arise. There were 639,721 live births registered in England and Wales in 2004.

Stillbirth

The UK definition is wordy; 'a child which has issued forth from its mother after the 24th week of pregnancy and which did not at any time after being completely expelled from its mother breathe or show any other sign of life.' WHO uses the synonym 'fetal death' and defines this as 'death prior to the complete expulsion of extraction from its mother of a product of conception, irrespective of the duration of pregnancy; the death is indicated by the fact that after such separation the fetus does not breathe or show any other evidence of life, such as beating of the heart, pulsation of the umbilical cord, or definite movement of voluntary muscles'. Again such fetal deaths should only be included in national statistics if the weight was at least 500 g or the gestation at least 22 weeks.

The UK policy of including all fetuses delivered after a certain time point also leads to anomalies. A fetus that dies at 20 weeks but is delivered at 26 weeks should be registered as a stillbirth. But what about a twin pregnancy at 8 weeks in which one fetus dies at 12 weeks and at term a minute nodule of presumed fetus papyraceous is identified by microscopic examination of the placenta? Strictly this also should be registered as a stillbirth, but fortunately common sense usually prevails.

Birth

Once we have agreed what a live birth and a stillbirth are, birth is easy. It is defined as 'a live birth or a stillbirth'. Note that pregnancies are not recorded systematically in the UK, or most other countries, unless they end in live birth, stillbirth or legal abortion. Spontaneous miscarriages are rarely recorded at all, for the obvious reason that many happen at home some of which may not be recognized for what they are even by the mother.

Maternal deaths

WHO defines a maternal death as 'the death of a woman while pregnant or within 42 days of termination of pregnancy, irrespective of the duration and the site of the pregnancy, from any cause related to or aggravated by the pregnancy or its management, but not from accidental or incidental causes'. Since some deaths caused by pregnancy can occur much later than 42 days WHO defines *late maternal death* as those related to or aggravated by the pregnancy between 42 days and 1 year after delivery. For some purposes it may be useful to count all deaths among women who are pregnant or recently delivered, so there is also a category of *pregnancy related deaths* which includes all deaths from whatever cause during pregnancy or within 42 days of termination of pregnancy.

Finally maternal deaths are subdivided into *direct deaths* arising from the pregnancy itself or its complications or treatment, and indirect deaths from pre-existing disease or disease unrelated to the pregnancy.

We express maternal deaths as the ratio of deaths to 100,000 live births, rather than as a rate per 100,000 pregnancies. The latter might seem more logical since many maternal deaths occur in the absence of a live birth, but is not possible because pregnancies are not registered. The maternal mortality ratio in the UK, and most similar developed countries is around 10 per 100,000 live births, while in much of Africa and the developing world it lies between 500 and 1000 per 100,000. No other health statistic differs so much between developed and developing countries.

In the UK more detailed causes of deaths are collected in the long established triennial Confidential Enquiries into Maternal Deaths (CEMD) and the more recent Confidential Enquiries into Stillbirths and Deaths in Infancy (CESDI). The value of these sorts of studies is repeatedly shown. For example, it has recently been discovered that many previously unrecognized pregnancy-related deaths were probably suicides, making this the leading cause of maternal death in the UK [1].

The reliability of statistics on some other areas of medical activity is relatively poor and periodic national censuses are required. For example, national statistics on Caesarean delivery are not routinely collected in the UK but the National Sentinel Caesarean Section Audit filled in many gaps.

Diagnosing

The single skill which most clearly differentiates doctors from members of other clinical specialties is their expertise in diagnosis. Only when we have made a diagnosis can we apply effective treatment – if there is any.

When we first meet a patient we are rarely, if ever, certain of the diagnosis and we have to carry out tests. A 'test' in this context is any item of information that can help us. It includes items from the history, and observations from the clinical examination, as well as such things as laboratory blood tests and X-ray examinations.

Unfortunately tests are rarely perfect: some people with a positive result will not have the disease, and conversely some with a negative result will have it. This is why interpretation may be difficult.

Before we can describe how good a test is, we need to decide what outcome we wish it to predict. We call this the 'reference standard'. Tests are applied to populations, and for obstetricians the population is often pregnant women so for them reference standards might include perinatal death or Down's syndrome or less important endpoints, such as low birthweight or low Apgar scores. If our test is only validated against such less important endpoints, we must always remember that these are not what we are really interested in.

Consider first a test that is either positive or negative and a reference standard that is present or absent. Let us imagine 100 pregnant women undergoing a test of fetal condition. The test is designed to predict whether the baby will live or die. If we apply the test to all 100 women and wait to see what happens, we might get a result like this:

This is the information that a scientist will have after completing research on a test. It is often called a 2×2 table. We can use such a table both to see how well the test performs, and to see what the risk of bad outcome is, for an individual with a particular result.

Test performance

By counting vertically in Fig. 31.1 we can see what proportion of the babies who did die (reference standard positive) were detected by the test (Fig. 31.2a). This is the sensitivity or true positive rate (TPR). For this hypothetical test it is 90%. We can also see how many of the babies that lived were correctly predicted by the test (Fig. 31.2b). This is the specificity or true negative rate (TNR). For our hypothetical test it is 80%.

	Reference standard +ve Baby dies	Reference standard −ve Baby lives		
Test +ve	18	16	34	
Test −ve	2	64	66	
	20	80	100	

Fig. 31.1 "Two by two" table of test results.

	Reference standard +ve Baby dies	Reference Standard −ve Baby lives		
Test +ve	18	16	34	
Test −ve	2	64	66	
	20	80	100	
	TPR 18/20 = 90%			

(a)

	Reference standard +ve Baby dies	Reference Standard −ve Baby lives		
Test +ve	18	16	34	
Test −ve	2	64	66	
	20	80	100	
		TNR 64/80 = 80%		

(b)

Fig. 31.2 (a) Sensitivity = True Positive Rate. (b) Specificity = True Negative Rate.

These test characteristics do not vary with the prevalence of the disease and are thus a stable measure of test performance. However they do vary with the cut-off value at which we call a test 'positive' or 'negative'. We will look at both these effects below, but first let us look at the results in another way, to predict an individual patient's risk.

Predicting an individual patient's risk

Sensitivity (TPR) and specificity (TNR) describe to the scientist how well the test works, but they are not of much use to the doctor who knows the test result (positive or negative) and wants to know how likely it is that the patient has the disease – or, in our example, that the baby will die. To estimate this we read Fig. 31.1 horizontally rather than vertically.

	Reference standard +ve	Reference standard −ve		
Test +ve	18	16	34	PVP 18/34 =53%
Test −ve	2	64	66	
	20	80	100	

(a)

	Reference standard +ve	Reference standard −ve		
Test +ve	18	16	34	
Test −ve	2	64	66	PVN 64/66 = 97%
	20	80	100	

(b)

Fig. 31.3 (a) Predictive value positive. (b) Predictive value negative.

First let us look at all the women with a positive result (Fig. 31.3a). Eighteen of the 34 babies actually died, so the predictive value of a positive result is 18 out of 34 or 53%. Note that the predictive value positive is NOT the same as the sensitivity (TPR), which we have already noted was 90%. (Although changing word order sometimes alters meaning in English, *predictive value positive* is exactly the same as *positive predictive value*.)

Of those who had a negative test (Fig. 31.3b), 64 out of 66 babies eventually survived. The predictive value of a negative result is thus 64 out of 66 or 97%. Again this is NOT the same as the specificity (TNR). We will see later that the predictive value of a test varies with the prevalence of the disease in the population.

The effect of varying the test cut-off point

So far we have been discussing 'dichotomous' tests, that is, tests that are simply either positive or negative. Most tests, however, give a range of results from strongly positive to strongly negative or, let us imagine for our test, a result between 0 and 100. Figure 31.4a shows the distribution of results for patients with and without disease, that is, 'Reference standard' positive and negative. If we take a cut-off value of 40, and call higher values 'positive', and lower 'negative' we get the same test characteristics as before.

Imagine what would happen if we varied the cut-off. The performance rates would change (Fig. 31.4b). We could, for example, move the cut-off value right up to 75 so that all the results were negative. The false negative and true negative rates would then both be 100%. If we moved the cut-off down to a value of 5 so that all the results were called positive the true and false positives would both be 100% (Fig. 31.4c).

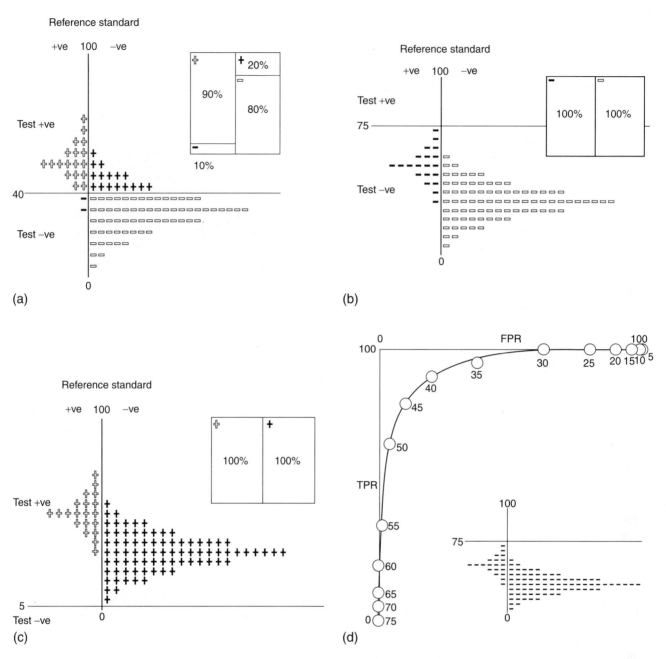

Fig. 31.4 (a) The original cut off value of 4.0. (b) Varying the cut-off value: High – No false positives but sensitivity zero. (c) Varying the cut-off value: Low – No false negatives but specificity zero. (d) Receiver Operator Characteristic (ROC) curve.

To see what is happening we can plot how the true and false positive rates vary with the cut-off level (Fig. 31.4d). We call the result a receiver operator characteristic or ROC curve. Figure 31.5a–d shows the 2 × 2 tables for a perfect and a useless test and their corresponding ROC curves.

The name Receiver Operator Characteristic arose during the Battle of Britain in 1940 when the German air force regularly flew bombing raids over London and Southern England. The British had just developed an early version of RADAR which was only a moderately good test for discriminating between reference standard positive – a flight of bombers, and reference standard negative – a flock of seagulls. The operators soon learned that by setting their dials to be very sensitive they never missed any incoming bombers but often called out their own pilots unnecessarily to defend against seagulls. If they set the dials to be more specific there were fewer false alarms but occasionally they would fail to detect the bombers in time. They called the discriminatory ability of each RADAR

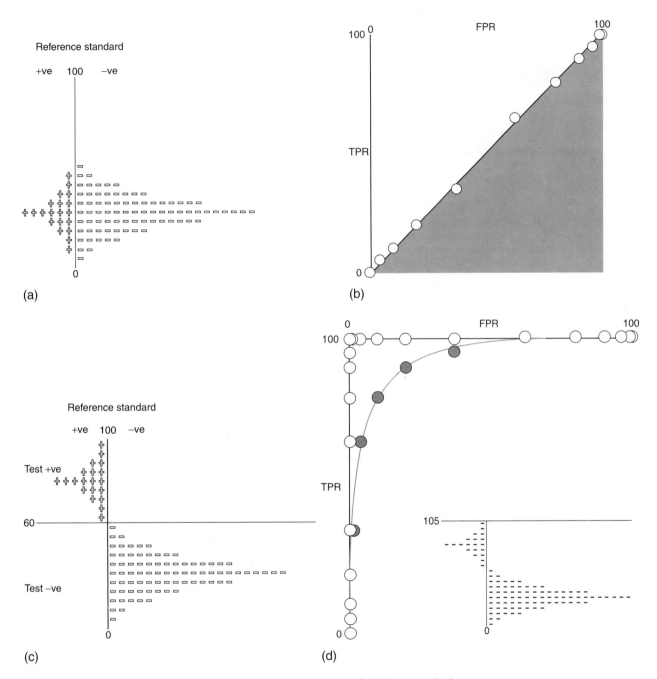

Fig. 31.5 (a) Useless test. (b) ROC curve – Useless test. (c) Perfect test. (d) ROC curve – Perfect test.

machine its 'receiver operator characteristic' (ROC) and the name stuck.

THE EFFECT OF DIFFERENT DISEASE PREVALENCE ON THE INTERPRETATION OF TEST RESULTS

The predictive value of a test result varies with the disease prevalence. As clinicians often say, 'Common things are common'.

Bayes theorem and likelihood ratios

Calculating the predictive value of a test result directly from the 2 × 2 table as we did earlier, is only possible if the patient in front of you comes from a population with the same disease prevalence as that of the patients on whom the test was originally developed. This is rarely the case. Tests are frequently developed on high-risk patients in teaching hospitals, and then applied to patients in a low-risk practice. Occasionally the reverse may happen,

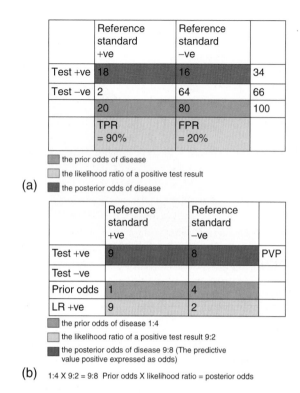

Fig. 31.6 (a) Bayes' theorem. (b) Bayes' theorem (ratios simplified).

if we apply a test to someone we already know to be at particularly high risk.

Doctors need a way of calculating the predictive value of a test from the information that they are likely to have available, namely the prevalence of the disease in their population and the test characteristics.

It can be done! We will change all our rates to odds for the following section since this makes the mathematics easier. A risk of 1 in 4 is the same as odds of 1:3. A risk of 90% is the same as odds of 90:10 or 9:1.

Let us return now to our original 2 × 2 table redrawn to show the crucial information (Fig. 31.6a,b). These two figures are identical except that in Fig. 31.6b the ratios have been simplified (divided by their lowest common denominator). The top row gives us the information we need – the predictive value positive. With a positive test the odds of having the disease are 18:16 or 9:8 (or slightly better than evens). The disease prevalence gives us the odds before the test result, that is 20:80 or 1:4. We call these the prior odds. What we need from the test is a single measure, the diagnostic value, which changed the prior odds of 1:4 to posterior odds of 9:8.

The answer is the ratio between the true positive rates (90%) and the false positive rate (20%). This is called the likelihood ratio of a positive result (LR +ve) because it is the ratio between the likelihood of having a positive result

if the disease is present, against the likelihood of having a positive result if the disease is absent. The LR +ve for this test is thus 9:2. The relationship between these three figures is:

Prior odds × likelihood ratio = posterior odds.

$$1:4 \qquad 9:2 \qquad 9:8$$

This is one of the most famous theorems in statistics, named the Bayes Theorem after its author, the Reverend Thomas Bayes. It comes in a number of different versions but this one, the odds-likelihood ratio form, is the most useful for doctors.

A dichotomous test (one that is either positive or negative) will have two likelihood ratios, one for a positive result and one for a negative result. If the test has a range of results the LR will vary also with the cut-off point chosen. It is possible to plot ROC curves as likelihood ratios.

If the doctor knows the LR for the test result and the prior odds, calculation of the individual patient's risk is easy. Here is an example.

Bayes and pregnancy tests; the Bayesian's wife

My wife felt pregnant but had a negative pregnancy test. Her doctor told her that 10% of pregnant women had a negative result on first testing but she was still disappointed. I calculated the probabilities as follows. I asked her how sure she had been that she was pregnant before the test and she said 95% certain. This gave prior odds of pregnancy of 19:1 which I rounded to 20:1. I assumed that the false positive rate was virtually nil so I got a LR for a negative test of 1:10 (likelihood of a negative result given pregnancy = 10%: likelihood of negative result given no pregnancy = 100%). This gave posterior odds that she was in fact pregnant of 20:1 × 1:10 = 2:1 and I converted this for her benefit into a probability of two in three. This estimate cheered her up and a couple of weeks later the pregnancy was confirmed. Adapted from [2].

Treating

Effective treatments

Some treatments such as insulin for diabetes, salpingectomy for ruptured tubal pregnancy, or *in vitro* fertilization for bilateral tubal blockage work so much better than the alternatives, that no one doubted early reports of their effectiveness. Few treatments, however, are so clear cut. More commonly, disease definitions are hazy, the prognosis is variable no matter what is done, and treatment is only partially effective. How is the practising doctor to choose?

The best way to measure the effectiveness of a treatment is to compare a group of patients given the treatment (the intervention or treatment group), with another group not given it (the control group). If there is already an established treatment for the disease, the control group will usually be given this treatment and the experimental group the new treatment. If the two groups are otherwise similar, and the treated patients have better outcomes, we conclude that the treatment was effective.

Difficulties arise if the two groups were not really comparable, or the play of chance misled us.

Bias

We call a systematic difference between the groups bias. It cannot be eliminated simply by increasing the sample size. There are many potential sources of bias.

If a new treatment is compared with treatments used in the past, the comparison will be subject to bias if other aspects of patient care are improving. Comparisons between patients treated by different doctors or in different hospitals are often biased. The doctor evaluating the treatment is often an expert whose patients will do better than those treated by other doctors. Conversely an expert may be referred the more difficult cases, biasing the results against the new treatment. Yet again, an expert with special diagnostic skills may make the diagnosis in milder cases, thus biasing results in favour of the new treatment.

Even if the same doctor administers the treatment, a non-randomized comparison of treatments may mislead. For example, comparisons of women who underwent amniotomy early in labour with those who did not will be bedevilled by subtle differences between the groups resulting from the reasons they underwent the amniotomy.

In theory, if we know what factors influence the outcome of treatment, the cases and controls can be matched for these factors to make the two groups similar. For example cases of cancer can be matched for the stage of the disease. A staging procedure, however, may not cover all the variation in say, spread of cancer. Two cancers may both be at the same stage but one may be a lot faster growing than the other. If the larger ones within each stage were more likely to be in the control group, the trial would be biased against the treatment. In practice we rarely know about all the possible factors that might affect outcome. An unknown factor can still bias results if it was unequally distributed between groups.

Bias must have affected many non-randomized studies of the effect of hormone replacement therapy in the 1980s and 1990s. Even after adjustment for known risk factors, such studies had suggested that hormone replacement therapy reduced heart attack and strokes. However, at least nine randomized controlled trials have now shown that it increases both [3]. The earlier results must have been due to bias in unknown risk factors.

The only way to ensure that two groups of patients are matched for unknown risk factors is to select them at random. This means using the toss of a coin, random number tables, or other forms of computer-generated random numbers, to select who gets the new treatment.

Allocation to treatment or placebo groups alternately, by day of the week, or last digit of hospital number is unsatisfactory since the doctors know the group allocation when they enter the trial, giving them scope for entry bias. For example, a trial comparing oxytocin infusion with prostaglandin pessary, as treatment for pregnant women whose membranes ruptured before labour began, used allocation by the final digit of the hospital number and got a biased result. The reason was that some staff believed, rightly or wrongly, that prostaglandin was the better treatment if the cervix was unripe. Women with a soft open cervix were entered in the trial without problems, but those with an unripe cervix were entered only if the digit was even (allocation to prostaglandin). If the final digit was odd the staff knew the allocation would be to oxytocin and some therefore did not enter the patient into the trial at all. Instead they gave prostaglandin anyway outside the trial. Thus, women in the trial allocated to oxytocin had riper cervices. Not surprisingly prostaglandin appeared to give worse results.

Bias can also occur if patients are more likely to be excluded from the trial in one group than the other. For example, we might wish to compare two policies for dealing with the membranes in labour; leave them intact or rupture them. Women are allocated at random in early labour – half to have the membranes ruptured, and half left intact. Some women allocated to the membrane rupture group are likely to make slow progress and eventually get the membranes ruptured anyway. If we remove them from analysis we will bias results against the membrane rupture policy, because we will be removing women with difficult labours from the 'leave intact' group. The situation will be even worse if some women in the 'membrane rupture' group labour so quickly that there is no time to artificially rupture the membranes. If we exclude them from the 'membrane rupture' group we will again be biasing results against rupture, by excluding the most favourable cases from that group.

We avoid the problem by analysing the trial by 'intention to treat'. This means comparing the two groups as chance allocated them. It may seem strange to include the results for some women who had the membranes left intact in the 'membrane rupture' group and some women who had them ruptured in the 'leave intact' group, but there is no other way to avoid bias. Of course we must ensure that compliance is high, if we really want to find out if a drug or procedure can work.

Biased assessment of outcome

Even if the two groups of patients in a trial are exactly comparable, bias may creep in if the investigators recording the outcomes know what treatment was received. For example, it is widely believed that amniotomy causes neonatal infection. If the doctors caring for the babies know that the membranes were ruptured early in labour they might do more tests for infection, and make the belief a self-fulfilling prophecy. If the doctors are not told which group the patient is in, they are said to be blinded, and their assessment of outcome can not be influenced.

If the patient believes that the treatment she has received works, that may also result in a self-fulfilling prophecy, the placebo effect. Trials of many treatments for premenstrual tension have shown high cure rates among patients given inactive medicine. Usually the active treatment has been no better, and investigators have concluded that the treatment was ineffective. If no placebo had been used, the treatment might have been wrongly given the credit for the improvement. Patients are also said to be 'blinded' when they do not know which treatment they are receiving. A trial is said to be 'double blind' when neither the patient nor the investigator knows which treatment is being given.

Blinding is not always necessary. If the end point is unambiguous – like death, or Caesarean section – blinding at the stage of outcome assessment is unnecessary, although it may still be necessary during the treatment period. If blinding is not possible, but the outcome is susceptible to observer bias, it may be possible to eliminate it by having independent observers make the assessment.

Statistical problems – avoiding being misled by the play of chance

Random variation differs from bias in that increasing the sample size will reduce it. There are two ways that the play of chance can mislead.

1 We may think there is a difference, when all we saw was chance variation. This is called a type 1, or alpha, error.

2 We may fail to realize that there is a real difference. This is called a type 2, or beta, error.

A number of statistical tests have been used to avoid making these errors.

TYPE 1 ERROR

The results of an experiment usually take the form of a series of observations on a treatment and control group. These may be continuous measures such as birthweights or dichotomous variables such as death rates. We will concentrate on dichotomous outcomes.

If the mortality rates are identical between treatment and control groups we won't be misled into a false belief that the treatment was effective. The difficulty arises when there is a difference and we want to know whether it occurred by chance or was caused by the treatment. Most statistical tests tell us how likely it was to occur by chance. This is the familiar P-value. By convention we call $P < 0.05$ 'statistically significant'. This means that there was a less than 5% chance that the difference we observed would occur by chance if the treatments were equally effective.

Although hallowed by tradition, this method of presenting results simply tells us that we have not made a type 1 error. If P is greater than 0.05 we do not know whether there really is no important difference, or whether our trial was too small. Nor does the P value tell us the likely size of any difference. A very small and clinically unimportant difference may be statistically highly significant if a large study has been performed.

TYPE 2 ERROR

Here we are concerned with the probability that a trial has failed to show a real effect, that is, a false negative result. The size of effect that it would matter to miss is a clinically meaningful effect – one that would cause doctors to change treatment. The probability of a negative result depends on the size of this minimum treatment effect we wish to detect. A particular trial can exclude a large effect more reliably than a small effect. We can measure the probability of failing to detect a particular size of effect. We call this the type 2 or beta error. The inverse of the type 2 error, the probability that the trial will indeed detect this size effect if it is really there is called the power of the trial.

ODDS RATIOS AND THEIR CONFIDENCE INTERVALS

A good way to look at treatment effects is to consider the risks or 'odds' of the bad outcome after treatment versus control therapy. The effect of the treatment is given in the form of a relative risk (RR) or an odds ratio (OR).

An OR of 1 indicates that the treatment does not alter the adverse outcome. An OR below 1 indicates that the chances of adverse outcome are reduced by treatment. An OR above 1 indicates that treatment increases these odds. An OR of 0.5 indicates a halving of the odds and an OR of 2 a doubling.

The 95% confidence intervals (CI) can be calculated. An OR of 0.5 with 95% CI '0.25–1', indicates that we have found a halving in the odds of the outcome and can be 95% confident that the true effect lies between an OR of 0.25 and 1.

Review: Prophylactic corticosteroids for preterm birth
Comparison: 01 Corticosteroids versus placebo or no treatment
Outcome: 02 Neonatal death

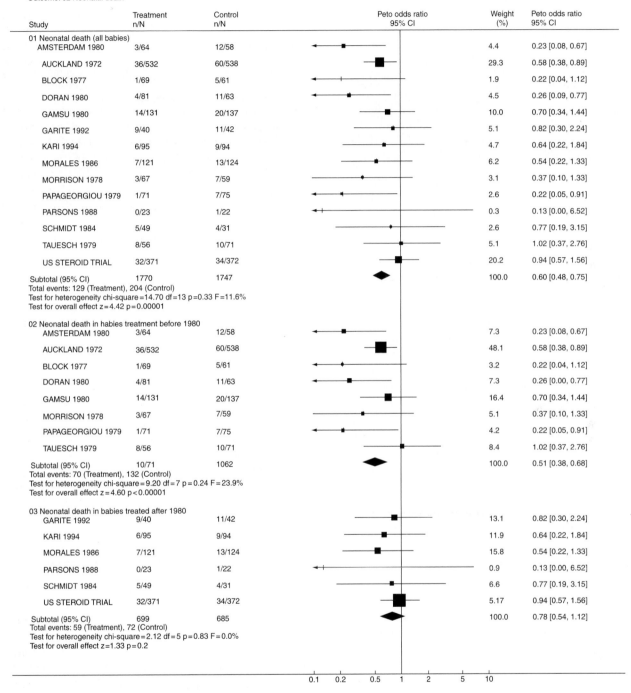

Fig. 31.7 Systematic review of randomized trials of the effect of corticosteroids for preterm on neonatal death.

This corresponds to a *P*-value of 0.05 since the confidence interval just includes 1. If the 95% CI fail to reach 1, the *P*-value is less than 0.05, that is. it is significant. If the 95% CI includes 1 the *P*-value is greater than 0.05, that is, the result is not statistically significant.

META-ANALYSIS

Type 2 errors are minimized by very large trials. Unfortunately these are difficult and expensive to perform. One solution is to combine the results of small and medium sized trials. The results can be conveniently presented as ORs for each trial separately and then beneath them the typical OR and CI for all the trials combined, the meta-analysis.

Figure 31.7, a version of one of the most famous meta-analysis graphs in obstetrics, is reproduced from the Cochrane collaboration review of the effect of corticosteroids to prevent neonatal death from respiratory distress syndrome after preterm labour. This type of graphical representation of the results of all the randomized trials of a particular intervention in a disease is now one of the most popular ways to summarize and present the best evidence of effectiveness.

References

1. Oates M (2003) Suicide: the leading cause of maternal death. *Br J Psychiatry* **183**, 279–81.
2. Gabriel Sánchez R, Carmona L, Roque M, Sánchez Gómez LM & Bonfill X (2005) Hormone replacement therapy for preventing cardiovascular disease in post-menopausal women. *Cochrane Database Syst Rev* 2, CD002229. DOI. 10.1002/14651858.CD002229.pub2.
3. Khan KS & Chien PF (2001) Evaluation of a clinical test. I. Assessment of reliability. *Br J Obstet Gynaecol* **108** 562–7.
4. Chien PF & Khan KS (2001) Evaluation of a clinical test. II. Assessment of validity. *Br J Obstet Gynaecol* **108** 568–72.

Further reading

Birth counts by Macfarlane and Mugford is one of the best guides and most convenient data sources for obstetric epidemiology. A pair of articles in *Br J Obstet Gynaecol* [3,4] are a good starting point for evaluating studies of test accuracy, although conventional statistical text books will be better guides to using tests in clinical practice. The Cochrane collaboration and its various guides and databases should be the first port of call for anyone wishing to find out about the effectiveness of a particular treatment.

Crowley P (1996) Prophylactic corticosteroids for preterm birth. *Cochrane Database Syst Rev* **1**, CD000065. DOI. 10.1002/14651858.

Department of Health (1998) *Why Mothers Die.* Report on Confidential Enquiries into Maternal Deaths in the United Kingdom, pp. 1994–6. London: Her Majesty's Stationery Office

Macfarlane A & Mugford M (2000) Birth Counts. *Statistics in Pregnancy and Childbirth*, 2nd edn. Vols 1 and 2.

National Institute for Clinical Excellence (2001) *Why Mothers die 1997–99. The Confidential Enquiries Into Maternal Deaths in the United Kingdom (CEMD).* London: RCOG Press.

Chapter 32: Contraception

Anna Glasier

Introduction

Contraceptive prevalence in the UK in the early twenty-first century is high. Only 2% of sexually active, potentially fertile women not wishing to conceive, reported not using a method of contraception in 2003/04 (Table 32.1) [1]. The average age of first intercourse in the UK for both men and women is 16 years, and the average age of first childbirth is 27. Since the mean age of menopause is 51 and the total fertility rate in the UK is 1.7, most women will need to use contraception for more than 30 years. Contraceptive choice varies with age, ethnicity, marital status, fertility intentions and education. In the UK in 2004 the oral contraceptive pill was the most popular method (25% of women use it) while the next most popular method was the male condom (23%) (Table 32.1). Long-acting reversible (LARC) methods of contraception (injectables, implants, intrauterine devices and systems) are used by less than 10% of women. The National Institute for Clinical Excellence (NICE) has recently produced guidance on LARC including an analysis of cost-effectiveness.

Despite high contraceptive prevalence, unintended pregnancy is common. In England and Wales the abortion rate in 2003 was 17.5 per 1000 women of reproductive age and 31.4 per 1000 for women aged 20–24. Not all unintended pregnancies end in abortion. As many as 30% of pregnancies which end in childbirth are unplanned when they are conceived. Most couples in the UK use contraceptive methods associated with relatively high failure rates when used typically. Among women using a reversible method, just under half are using oral contraception with typical-use failure rates of 8% (Table 32.2). Well over half are using a barrier method, periodic abstinence (natural family planning) or withdrawal, with typical-use failure rates of between 15% (male condom) and 32% (cap). Most data suggest that true method failure accounts for fewer than 10% of unintended pregnancies, the rest arising either because no method was used at the time of conception (30–50%) or because the method was used inconsistently or incorrectly.

Table 32.1 Current use of contraception by women aged 16–49 in Great Britain

Current use of contraception	%
Pill*	25**
Progestogen-only	5**
Combined pill	17**
Male condom	23**
Withdrawal	3**
IUD	4**
Injection/implant	3**
NFP	1**
Cap/diaphragm	1**
Foams/gels	1**
Hormonal IUS	1**
Female condom	0**
Emergency contraception	1**
Total at least one method	52**
Sterilized	11**
Partner sterilized	12**
Total at least one method	75**

From Dawe and Rainford [1].
* Includes women who did not know the type of pill used.
** Percentages sum to more than 100 as respondents could give more than one answer.

Currently available reversible methods of contraception fall into two broad categories, hormonal and non-hormonal. Certain issues are common to all methods.

Efficacy and effectiveness

The effectiveness of a method of contraception is expressed by the failure rates associated with its use. The rates in Table 32.2 are based on US studies and estimate the percentage of couples experiencing an unintended pregnancy during the first year of use of each method [2]. The effectiveness of a contraceptive depends on how it works and how easy it is to use. If a method prevents

Table 32.2 Effectiveness of contraceptive methods: percentage of women experiencing an unintended pregnancy during the first year of use and percentage continuing use at the end of the first year (USA)

Method	% Pregnant	
	Typical use	Perfect use
No method	85	85
Spermicides	29	18
Withdrawal	27	4
Periodic abstinence	25	
Calendar	9	
Ovulation method	3	
Sympto-thermal	2	
Cap, parous women	32	26
nulliparous women	16	9
Diaphragm	16	6
Condom, female	21	5
male	15	2
Combined pill and minipill	8	0.3
Combined hormonal patch (Evra)	8	0.3
Combined hormonal ring (NuvaRing)	8	0.3
DMPA (Depo-Provera)	3	0.3
IUD, copper T	0.8	0.6
LNG-IUS (Mirena)	0.1	0.1
Implant	0.05	0.05
Female sterilization	0.5	0.5
Male sterilization	0.15	0.10

From Trussell [2].

ovulation in every cycle in every woman it should have an efficacy of 100%, since if there is no egg there can be no conception. Only if a mistake is made, or if the method is used inconsistently, will a pregnancy occur. The contraceptive implant Implanon®, and combined oral contraceptive pill both inhibit ovulation. Pregnancy rates for perfect use of the pill are around 1 in 1000; failures are due to incomplete inhibition of ovulation among women who metabolize the pill rapidly. However, if pills are missed ovulation can occur and typical-use failure rates are 8 per 100. In contrast Implanon® makes no demands on compliance, use can only ever be perfect, and perfect-use and typical-use failure rates are virtually the same. For implants and intrauterine devices (IUDs) typical-use failures occur because the provider has failed (the IUD perforated the uterus or the woman was already pregnant when the implant was inserted, for example).

Pregnancy rates are still often described by the Pearl Index, the number of unintended pregnancies divided by the number of women years of exposure to the risk of pregnancy while using the method. Most rates are derived from clinical trials. There are some problems with this. The longer a cohort of couples using a method of contraception is followed, the lower the pregnancy rate is likely to be since the cohort increasingly comprises of couples unlikely to fall pregnant (because they are highly motivated to avoid pregnancy, good at using the method or subfertile). Furthermore, failure rates in clinical trials are often underestimated because all of the months of use of the method are taken into account when calculating failure rates, regardless of whether or not intercourse has occurred during that cycle. Additionally people who participate in trials do not represent the general public and compliance is atypically good. For long-acting methods of contraception such as IUDs and implants, pregnancy rates with time (cumulative pregnancy rates) are reported.

Compliance/adherence/concordance

Many couples use contraception inconsistently and/or incorrectly. Some methods are easier to use than others. The IUD/IUS (intrauterine system) and implants are inserted and removed by a health professional and are entirely independent of compliance for efficacy. Depo-Provera® lasts 12 weeks but correct use demands the motivation and organizational skills required to attend a clinic for repeat doses. Compliance with the oral contraception is not easy. In one study, 47% of women reported missing one or more pills and 22% two or more pills per cycle [3]. In a study using electronic diaries to record compliance, 63% of women missed one or more pills in the first cycle, and 74% in the second cycle of use [4]. Typical-use failure rates are even higher with condoms, diaphragms, withdrawal and natural family planning which rely on correct use with every act of intercourse.

Discontinuation

In an international review of discontinuation rates, after one year of use of hormonal contraception, rates varied from 19% (for Norplant) to 62% (the combined pill). Good data specific to the UK are lacking. Discontinuation rates are higher for methods which do not require removal by a health professional as is clear from Table 32.3, which shows the percentage of couples in the USA still using each method at the end of 1 year [2]. In a US study 50% of women discontinued the pill during the first three months of use [5]. Reasons for discontinuation are often associated with perceived risks and real or perceived side effects. The commonest reason for discontinuation is for bleeding dysfunction. In a Swedish study of 656 women followed for 10 years, between 28 and 35% of women (depending on age) stopped taking the pill because of fear of harmful side effects. Thirteen to seventeen percent of women stopped because of menstrual dysfunction,

Table 32.3 Percentage of US women continuing using each method at the end of the first year

Method	% of women continuing use at 1 year
No method	
Spermicides	42
Withdrawal	43
Periodic abstinence	51
Cap	
Parous women	46
Nulliparous women	57
Diaphragm	57
Condom	
Female	49
Male	53
Combined pill and minipill	68
Evra patch	68
NuvaRing	68
Depo-Provera	56
Lunelle	56
IUD	
Copper T	78
Mirena (LNG-IUS)	81
Implant	84
Female sterilization	100
Male sterilization	100

From Trussell [2].

15–20% because of weight gain and 14–21% because of reported mood change [6].

Contraindications

Most contraceptive users are young and medically fit and can use any available method safely. A few medical conditions, however, are associated with theoretical increased health risks with certain contraceptives, either because the method adversely affects the condition or because the condition, or its treatment, affects the contraceptive. The combined pill, for example, may increase the risk of a woman with diabetes developing cardiovascular complications; some anticonvulsants interfere with the efficacy of the combined pill. Since most trials of new contraceptive methods deliberately exclude subjects with serious medical conditions, there is little direct evidence on which to base sound prescribing advice. In an attempt to produce a set of international norms for providing contraception to women and men with a range of medical conditions which may contraindicate one or more contraceptive methods, the World Health Organization (WHO) developed a system addressing medical eligibility criteria (MEC) for contraceptive use [7]. Using evidence-based systematic reviews, conditions are classified into one of four categories. Category 1 includes conditions for which

there is no restriction for the use of the method while category 4 includes conditions representing an unacceptable health risk if the contraceptive method is used (absolutely contraindicated). Classification of a condition as category 2 indicates that the method may generally be used but that more careful follow-up is required. Category 3 conditions are those for which the risks of the combined oral contraceptive (COC) generally outweigh the benefits (relatively contraindicated). Provision of a method to a woman with a category 3 condition requires careful clinical judgement since use of that method is not recommended unless there is no acceptable alternative. The document is available on the web www.who.int/reproductive-health/publications/mec/index.htm and a system is in place to incorporate new data into the guideline as they become available.

Health benefits of contraception

Most couples use contraception for over 30 years. Additional health benefits beyond pregnancy prevention offer significant advantages and influence acceptability. In a nationwide sample of 943 US women, satisfaction with oral contraception was increased among women aware of the non-contraceptive benefits of the pill [8]. The commonest benefit of hormonal methods is an improvement in menstrual bleeding patterns including amenorrhoea (which many women in the UK appreciate). Barrier methods, particularly condoms, protect against sexually transmitted infections, including cervical cancer. When contraceptives are being used for their beneficial side effects or in the management of a medical problem such as menorrhagia, the risk–benefit ratio changes.

Hormonal contraception

Hormonal methods of contraception can be divided into combined and progestogen-only methods.

Combined hormonal contraception

THE METHODS

Combined hormonal contraception can be administered orally (the combined oral contraceptive pill, COCP), transdermally (the contraceptive patch), systemically (combined injectables) and via the vaginal route (the combined contraceptive vaginal ring, CCVR). In 2005 only the pill and the patch are marketed in the UK.

All methods contain both oestrogen – in the case of all but one brand of pills, the patch and the ring, ethinylestradiol (EE) – and a progestogen (synthetic progesterone). Although there are much less data available on the other delivery systems the mode of action, side effects and risks are similar.

Oral

The dose of oestrogen in the combined oral contraceptive pill varies from 50 to 15 μg. Only one 50 μg pill is marketed in the UK and it contains mestranol. Most women now use the so-called low-dose pills containing 30–35 μg. Low-dose pills are potentially safer since the cardiovascular risks of the pill are mainly due to oestrogen. Although the lowest-dose pill currently available (15 μg ethinylestradiol) has the same efficacy as 30 μg pills, cycle control is less effective and breakthrough bleeding more common. The progestogens used in currently available pills fall broadly into three groups, first and second generation progestins (e.g. norethindrone and levonorgestrel respectively) and the third generation series including gestodene, desogestrel and norgestimate. The newest COCP in the UK (Yasmin®) contains a progestogen with both anti-androgenic and anti-mineralocorticoid activity (drospirenone). Dianette® is a drug containing EE in combination with the anti-androgen cyproterone acetate which is licensed for the treatment of severe acne and hirsutism. It is contraceptive and has over the years often been regarded as just another combined pill. It is useful for women with symptoms of hyperandrogenism who require contraception but should not be used routinely for other women as it is associated with an increased risk of venous thrombosis.

The pill is taken for 21 days followed by a 7-day break when withdrawal bleeding usually occurs. Everyday (ED) preparations, in which a placebo tablet is taken during the pill free interval (PFI), may improve compliance but are more expensive and not widely used in the UK. Combined pills are available as monophasic preparations in which every pill in the packet contains the same dose of steroids and biphasic and triphasic preparations in which the dose of both steroids changes once or twice during the cycle. Phasic pills were introduced to reduce the total dose of progestogens and in the belief that a regimen which mimicked the normal cycle would produce better cycle control. There is no evidence for this and they are more expensive. Increasing number of women run packets of pills together for three months (tricycling) or more because they like the associated amenorrhoea. This is particularly useful for women who experience symptoms associated with the withdrawal bleed such as dysmenorrhoea or menstrual migraine and for women on enzyme-inducing drugs (such as some anticonvulsants) which theoretically reduce pill efficacy. In the US an 84-day preparation of pills (Seasonale®) is now marketed.

Transdermal

Only one contraceptive patch is currently available, 20 cm^2 in size, it delivers 20 μg EE and 150 μg/day norelgestromin (17-deacetyl norgestimate) daily. Each patch lasts seven days, three patches are used consecutively with a placebo patch or patch-free interval in week four when withdrawal bleeding occurs. Contraceptive protection lasts for up to ten days, allowing for errors in changing the patch. In a randomized trial comparing the patch with a COCP, effectiveness was not significantly different – the overall Pearl Index for the patch was 1.24/100 women years and for the COC was 2.18 [9]. In a large non-randomized trial four of the six pregnancies that occurred were in women weighing over 90 kg, suggesting that efficacy may be reduced among heavier women. After the first few cycles of use bleeding patterns and side effects are similar to those associated with the combined pill. Self-reported 'perfect use' was significantly better with the patch (88%) than with the pill (78%) in the randomized trial although whether this is so with use outside a clinical trial remains to be seen.

Vaginal

A combined contraceptive vaginal ring (Nuvaring®, Organon) releasing 15 μg EE and 120 μg etonorgestrel/day is now licensed in much of Europe. The ring is made of soft ethylene-vinyl-acetate (EVA) copolymer, has an outer diameter of 54 mm and a cross-sectional diameter of 4 mm. Designed to last for 3 weeks, a 7-day ring-free interval is associated with bleeding patterns which appear superior to those associated with the OC (Oral Contraceptive). In a comparison with a combined pill containing 30 μg EE and levonorgestrel 150 μg, the incidence of irregular bleeding in the Nuvaring® was significantly less (<5% versus 38.8% in each cycle). In all other respects, including efficacy, the ring is no different from the pill; however, there may be advantages in terms of demands on compliance.

Injectable

A once per month injectable contraceptive containing 25 mg medroxyprogesterone acetate and 5 mg oestradiol cypionate (Lunelle® Pharmacia) is available in some parts of the world including the USA. Injections are administered intramuscularly every 28 days. Bleeding patterns and efficacy are comparable with the COC. Bleeding episodes can be anticipated 18–22 days after injection and are induced by a decline in oestrogen concentrations to 50 pg/ml or less. Approximately 70% of women experience one bleeding episode per month, with only 4% experiencing amenorrhoea over three treatment cycles.

MODE OF ACTION

The principle mode of action of combined hormonal contraception (CHC) is the inhibition of ovulation. Oestrogen inhibits pituitary FSH (Follicle-Stimulating Hormone), suppressing the development of ovarian follicles, while progestogen inhibits the development of the LH (Luteinizing Hormone) surge. Pills, patches and rings are all administered for 21 days followed by a 7-day hormone-free interval (HFI). In some women the 7-day interval is long enough to allow follicle growth and 25% of pill users have ultrasound evidence of follicles 10 mm in diameter on the last day of the interval. If the interval is extended beyond 7 days, these follicles will continue to develop and, despite restarting contraception, ovulation may occur. For women who appear to have conceived as a result of a genuine method failure but who wish to continue using CHC, the HFI can be shortened to 4 days to ensure suppression of follicular development.

Additional contraceptive properties include changes in cervical mucus characteristics interfering with sperm transport, a possible alteration in tubal motility, endometrial atrophy and impaired uterine receptivity.

EFFICACY

See Table 32.2

CONTRAINDICATIONS

The absolute contraindications (MEC category 4 conditions) and relative (MEC category 3 conditions) to the combined pill and patch are listed in Tables 32.5 and 32.4, respectively.

RISKS AND SIDE EFFECTS

Minor side effects

Combined hormonal contraception affects almost every system in the body. Contraceptive steroids are metabolized by the liver and affect the metabolism of carbohydrates, lipids, plasma proteins, amino acids, vitamins and clotting factors.

Many of the reported side effects, particularly headache, weight gain and loss of libido, are common among women not using hormonal contraception. Those likely to be directly related to the contraceptive steroids include fluid retention, nausea and vomiting, chloasma, mastalgia and breast enlargement. All but chloasma (which gets worse with time) improve within 3 to 6 months. A different dose of oestrogen or type of progestogen or a different delivery system may help if time alone does not solve

Table 32.4 WHO Medical Eligibility Criteria category 3 conditions (relative contraindications) for use of the combined oral contraceptive pill

Multiple risk factors for arterial disease
Hypertension: systolic blood pressure 140–159 or diastolic pressure 90–99 mmHg, or adequately treated to below 140/90 mmHg
Some known hyperlipidemias
Diabetes mellitus with vascular disease
Smoking, <15 cigarettes/day, and age ≥35
Obesity
Migraine, without aura, and ≥35
Breast cancer >5 years ago without recurrence
Breastfeeding until 6 months post-partum
Post-partum and not breastfeeding, until 21 days after childbirth
Current or medically treated gallbladder disease
History of cholestasis related to combined oral contraceptives
Mild cirrhosis
Taking rifampicin (rifampin) or certain anticonvulsants

From WHO [7].

Table 32.5 WHO Medical Eligibility Criteria category 4 conditions (absolute contraindications) for use of the combined oral contraceptive pill

Breastfeeding <6 weeks post-partum
Smoking ≥15 cigarettes/day and age ≥35
Multiple risk factors for cardiovascular disease
Hypertension: systolic ≥160 or diastolic ≥100 mmHg
Hypertension with vascular disease
Current or history of deep-vein thrombosis/pulmonary embolism
Major surgery with prolonged immobilization
Known thrombogenic mutations
Current or history of ischaemic heart disease
Current or history of stroke
Complicated valvular heart disease
Migraine with aura
Migraine without aura and age ≥35 (continuation)
Current breast cancer
Diabetes for ≥20 years or with severe vascular disease or with severe nephropathy, retinopathy or neuropathy
Active viral hepatitis
Severe cirrhosis
Benign or malignant liver tumours

From WHO [7].

the problem. For women with persistent nausea on the pill, the patch is indicated. Side effects (real or perceived) often lead to discontinuation; 73% of British women of all ages quote weight gain as being a disadvantage of the pill.

Serious side effects

Cardiovascular disease. The combined pill is extremely safe. In a 25 year follow-up of 46,000 women in the UK the overall risk of death from any condition was the same for COC users and non-users [10]. Among current and recent [within 10 years] users, the COC was associated with an increased risk of death from only two conditions, cervical cancer (RR 2.5) and cerebrovascular disease (RR 1.9).

CHC increases the tendency to thrombosis in both the venous and arterial circulation. The adverse effect on clotting is related to the dose of oestrogen and, for pills, lower doses are theoretically associated with a reduced risk.

There is a three to fivefold increase in the risk of venous thromboembolism (VTE) associated with COCP use which is apparently independent of the dose of oestrogen, certainly if it is <50 μg. The risk is unaffected by age, smoking or duration of pill use, but is higher in obese women (BMI >25 kg/m^2) and in women with a history of pregnancy-induced hypertension (PIH). Four studies published in 1995 and 1996 demonstrated a differential risk of VTE depending on the type of progestogen in the pill. Combined pills containing either gestodene or desogestrel were shown to have a roughly twofold increased risk of VTE when compared with first or second generation combined pills. Although often attributed to confounding or bias, there is some biological plausibility for this differential risk. Regarded as second choice in the UK, these pills should be prescribed only for women intolerant of other types of combined pill and prepared to accept the increased risk of VTE. Whichever progestogen is used, the absolute risk of VTE is small (15/100,000 women years for pill users compared with 5/100,000 for non-users), and much less than that associated with pregnancy (60/100,000 women years). The risk is greatest during the first year of use of the COCP – perhaps due to the unmasking of inherited thrombophilias such as Factor V Leiden mutation. Screening for known thrombophilias is not cost effective and, although asking about a family history of VTE is routine when prescribing the pill, this too fails to detect most women at risk of VTE.

Although non-oral routes of administration avoid the first pass through the liver thereby theoretically having less effect on clotting factors, in the absence of contrary evidence, the patch, ring and combined injectable methods carry the same warning as the COCP.

Arterial disease is much less common but more serious. It is related to age, and the risk is strongly influenced by smoking. Pooled data from four large phase II clinical trials suggest that the COCP has a negligible effect on blood pressure [11]. The relationship between COCP use and myocardial infarction (MI) is controversial. While there is widespread agreement that there is an increased risk of MI among women who smoke or have hypertension,

some studies have demonstrated an increased risk among normotensive non-smokers while others have not [12,13]. In a recent meta-analysis of 23 studies, the adjusted odds ratio (OR) of MI was 2.48 (95% CI; 1.91–3.22) for current COCP users compared to never users [14]. The risk among past users was not significantly increased. The risk of MI was significant for users of second, but not third, generation pills. There was also a dose response relationship with EE, with pills containing 20 μg EE associated with no increase in risk. The risk of MI was significantly increased by smoking (OR 9.3, 95% CI 3.89–22.23) compared with non-smokers (many other studies have shown this) and for women with a history of hypertension (OR 9.9, 95% CI 1.83–53.53) and hypercholesterolemia (OR 2.08, 95% CI 1.5–2.9). The absolute risk of MI in women of reproductive age, even those with known risk factors, is however extremely small.

Use of the COC increases the risk of ischaemic stroke twofold; however, the risk of haemorrhagic stroke is unchanged. Smoking and hypertension increase the risk of stroke by three to ten times. However, stroke is also rare in women of reproductive age.

The COC is also contraindicated in migraine with aura. In a recent meta-analysis of 17 good-quality observational studies migraine was associated with a relative risk of stroke of 2.16 (95% CI: 1.89–2.48) and users of oral contraceptives had an eightfold increase in the risk of stroke when compared with non-users [15]. Many people incorrectly describe their headaches as migraine and it is important therefore to take a detailed history before refusing to prescribe the COC for someone with a history of 'migraine'.

Malignant disease

Breast cancer: Published data on CHC and breast cancer are difficult to interpret because pill formulations, patterns of reproduction (particularly age at first pregnancy and family size), diet and average weight have changed with time. A meta-analysis of 54 studies involving over 53,000 women with breast cancer and 100,000 control subjects concluded that use of the COCP was associated with a small increase in the risk of breast cancer. The increased risk persists for 10 years after stopping the pill [16]. The relative risk for current users was 1. 24; for 1–4 years after stopping, 1.16; and for 5–9 years after stopping, 1.07. After 10 years the relative risk was the same as that of non-users. Although the relative risk was higher for women who started the pill at a young age, there was little added effect from the duration of use, dose or type of hormone. Ever-users were significantly less likely (RR 0. 88) to have metastatic disease even if they had stopped the pill more than 10 years earlier. A more recent case control study involving 8000 women including women over 35, suggested no increased risk of breast cancer (RR 1.0 95% CI 0.8–1.3); however, the upper limit of the confidence interval is in keeping with the much larger meta-analysis. In the RCGP study no increase in the risk of death from breast cancer was detected [10]. It has been suggested that starting to use the pill may accelerate the appearance of breast cancer in susceptible women. Alternatively women using the pill might have their tumours diagnosed earlier although it is difficult to explain why a tendency to earlier diagnosis would persist for years after stopping. A biological effect of combined hormonal contraception remains a possibility.

Cervical cancer: Data on the risk of cervical cancer among pill users are also difficult to interpret since barrier methods confer some protection and any association identified in epidemiological studies may be simply the result of inadequate adjustment for sexual behaviour. In a recent meta-analysis of 10 case control studies, women with persistent infection with human papilloma virus (HPV) using hormonal contraception (mainly combined) for more than 5 years had an increased relative risk of cervical cancer of 2.8. Hormonal contraceptive use for longer than 10 years increased the relative risk to 4.0. Thus, despite concerns that sexual behaviour among women using different methods of contraception may be confounding, evidence is mounting for a real association between the use of CHC and cervical cancer. However, pill users are a captive population for cervical screening.

Recent evidence has suggested an increased risk of adenocarcinoma among long-term users but this is a rare tumour.

Liver cancer: Benign hepatic adenoma is a rare consequence of COC use.

Ovarian, endometrial and colon cancer: There is substantial evidence that COCP use protects against ovarian and endometrial cancer. There is a 50% reduction in the risk of epithelial ovarian cancer after 5 years use of the COC. The protective effect lasts for at least 10 years after pill use stops. The effect may be related to the reduction in the total number of ovulations, and therefore rupture of the ovarian capsule, experienced in a lifetime. COCP use also reduces the risk of endometrial cancer. The effect is strongly related to the duration of use (20% reduction in risk after 1 year, 50% after 4 years) and is sustained for perhaps as long as 15 years after stopping the pill. There is also some evidence to suggest that CHC may confer protection against colon cancer.

PRACTICAL PRESCRIBING

WHO has recently updated their evidence-based guideline on how to use contraceptives – The Selected Practice Recommendations for Contraceptive use [17]. Adapted slightly by the FFPRHC [18] for UK practice, this document gives advice on practical aspects of use of all methods of contraception.

The FFPRHC recommends a 30 μg EE containing pill in combination with a second generation progestogen as the pill of choice for new users on the grounds that such pills are the safest and cheapest (all pill types appear to be equally effective) [19].

Women should be carefully instructed as to how to use the pill or patch and what to do when mistakes are made. Many women choose or are advised to have a break from using hormonal contraception for a few months. While most cardiovascular risks decline when the method is stopped, they recur as soon as it is restarted and unplanned pregnancies commonly occur during such breaks. Most women who stop the pill regain normal fertility within 3 months. Secondary amenorrhoea is almost always the result of abnormalities present before the method was started (such as polycystic ovarian syndrome) but regular withdrawal bleeds mask these conditions. There is no evidence for any adverse effect on the fetus as a result of past or current pill use.

Key points

- CHC is available in a range of delivery systems.
- The main action of CHC is to suppress ovulation.
- The length of the hormone-fnt free interval is crucial to efficacy.
- The COC reduces the risk of ovarian and endometrial cancer by 50%.
- CHC is contraindicated in women with arterial and venous disease.
- Third generation progestogens may increase the risk of venous thromboembolism.
- Current users of the COC have an increased risk of breast cancer (RR 1.24).
- The perfect-use failure rate for the COC is 0.1/HWY, the typical-use failure rate is 8 per 100.

PROGESTOGEN-ONLY CONTRACEPTION

Progestogen-only contraception (POC) avoids the side effects of oestrogen. It is available in a wide variety of delivery systems including oral, injectables, implants and intrauterine systems (IUS). Implants and the IUS last for 3 and 5 years respectively. POC is much less commonly used than combined hormonal contraception and there are fewer data, particularly on the risks associated with long-term use.

THE METHODS

Oral

A number of types of progeotogen only pills (POP) (often called mini-pills) are available in the UK. The older formulations of POP contain a very low dose of second generation progestogen which inconsistently inhibits ovulation. The newest POP (Cerazette®) contains the third generation progestogen desogestrel at a dose sufficient to inhibit ovulation in almost every cycle [20].

Injectable

Long-acting injections of norethisterone-enanthate (NET-En) and depot medroxyprogesterone acetate (DMPA, Depo-Provera®)are both highly effective. Depo-Provera® is given by deep intramuscular injection, 150 mg every 12 weeks. NET-En is administered every 8 weeks (at least initially). It is not licensed for long-term use in the UK and has to be warmed before it can be drawn up into the syringe. A new micronized preparation of DMPA is likely to become available in 2007. Since it is a lower dose (104 mg DMPA), it is administered subcutaneously and can be self-administered.

Subdermal

The first contraceptive implant to become available was Norplant® but this has not been marketed in the UK for over 5 years. Implanon® is a single rod, containing 68 mg 3-keto-desogestrel (a metabolite of desogestrel) providing contraception for 3 years. The initial release rate of 60–70 μg/day falls gradually to around 25–30 μg/day at the end of 3 years. Implanon® is preloaded into a sterile disposable inserter and is inserted subdermally on the inner aspect of the non-dominant arm above the elbow. It is inserted and removed using local anaesthetic.

Intrauterine

The IUS (Mirena®) has a T-shaped plastic frame with a reservoir on the vertical stem containing 52 mg levonorgestrel (LNG) releasing 20 μg LNG/day for at least 5 years [21]. The IUS is inserted and removed using the same procedures as for copper IUD insertion (see Intrauterspine device, p.310) although the stem of the IUS is bigger and difficulties with insertion may be experienced particularly in women with a small uterus (such as following prolonged use of DMPA). Mirena® is licensed for the management of menorrhagia and is increasingly being used to deliver the progestogen component of hormone replacement therapy.

MECHANISM OF ACTION

All methods of POC have a number of mechanisms of action. Depo-Provera® Implanon® and Cerazette® inhibit ovulation. Lower-dose methods (older pill formulations and Norplant®) inhibit ovulation only inconsistently. All POC, regardless of the route of administration, affect cervical mucus reducing sperm penetrability and transport, and all (but particularly the LNG-IUS which has little effect on ovarian activity but causes marked endometrial atrophy) have an effect on the endometrium compromising implantation if ovulation and fertilization occur.

EFFICACY

Failure rates for the progestogen-only methods are shown in Table 32.2. The older POPs (containing low doses of second generation gestogens) have higher failure rates than the combined pill. The reduced efficacy is due partly to the fact that many women continue to ovulate, and partly because the POP has a shorter half-life in the circulation so that missing even just one pill may interfere with contraceptive efficacy. The desogestrel-containing POP is believed to have failure rates equivalent to those of the COCP as ovulation is consistently inhibited. The LNG-IUS lasts for 5 years but there are data demonstrating continued effectiveness for up to 7 years. Although not licensed beyond 5 years, extended use for up to 7 years may be discussed with older women who have amenorrhoea since the risks of perforation, expulsion and infection are all highest during the first few weeks after insertion (and re-insertion). Implanon® is effective (and licensed) for 3 years; there are no data on use beyond this time.

INDICATIONS AND CONTRAINDICATIONS

POC is commonly prescribed for women in whom estrogen is absolutely or relatively contraindicated, for example women with cardiovascular disease, migraine, diabetes or mild hypertension. In the UK, breastfeeding women are advised to use POC since estrogen impairs milk production. Contraindications (MEC conditions 3) which apply to all progestogen-only methods are shown in Table 32.6. In many countries regulatory authorities still insist on a long list of contraindications which apply to the combined pill.

SIDE EFFECTS

Minor side effects

Bleeding disturbances. The commonest side effect and cause for discontinuation of POC is an unacceptable bleeding pattern. This includes amenorrhoea if women have

Table 32.6 WHO Medical Eligibility Criteria category 3 conditions (relative contraindications) for use of progestogen-only methods

Breastfeeding at less than 6 weeks post-partum (all methods)
Current deep-vein thrombosis (DVT) pulmonary embolism (all methods)
Previous breast cancer with no evidence of disease for 5 years (all methods)
Active viral hepatitis (all methods)
Benign hepatic adenoma (all methods)
Severe decompensated cirrhosis (all methods)
Benign hepatic adenoma (all methods)
Malignant hepatoma (all methods)
Current or history of ischaemic heart disease or stroke (injections, starting or continuing; continuation of progestogen-only pills or implants)
Migraine with aura (continuation of all progestogen-only methods)
Unexplained vaginal bleeding (injections and implants)
Use of certain drugs: rifampicin (rifampin), griseofulvin, phenytoin, carbamazine, barbiturates, primidone (progestogen-only pills; implants)
Multiple risk factors for arterial cardiovascular disease (injections only)
Systolic blood pressure >160 or diastolic >100 mmHg (injections only)
Vascular disease (injections only)
Diabetes with nephropathy, other vascular disease or disease duration of >20 years (injections only)

not been forewarned that it may happen or find that they do not like it. Low-dose progestogen-only methods (pills and implants) are associated with a high incidence of irregular vaginal bleeding. This is due partly to their effect on ovarian function. In the normal cycle ovulation determines regular menstruation. Inconsistent ovulation and fluctuating endogenous oestrogen production from irregular follicle growth provide a recipe for irregular bleeding. However, there is also evidence to suggest that progestogen-only methods directly affect the vasculature of the endometrium increasing the chance of bleeding. Bleeding patterns differ according to the dose of progestogen and the route of administration.

Oral: Around 50% of women using the classical POPs continue to ovulate and therefore they menstruate regularly. Ten percent will experience complete suppression of follicular development and will have amenorrhoea. The rest will have inconsistent ovulation (often with a short luteal phase), or follicular development only and will bleed irregularly. Up to 20% of women using the desogestrel-containing POP will experience amenorrhoea while the rest are likely to have irregular bleeding since ovulation is inhibited.

Injectable: The high dose of progestogen in Depo-Provera® inhibits ovulation and by the end of 1 year of use, 70% of women have either infrequent scanty vaginal bleeding or amenorrhoea. Heavy prolonged bleeding may be a problem in around 2% of women. The cause is unknown and often leads to discontinuation of the method.

Subdermal: Menstrual disturbance is the norm; up to 20% of users experience amenorrhoea and almost all the rest will have irregular, unpredictable bleeding. Heavy bleeding is uncommon and measured blood loss is much less than that experienced during a normal menstrual cycle. Many women do not like the unpredictability of the bleeding; even very light bleeding is unacceptable if it lasts for days on end. Patterns do not become more regular with time as the dose of progestogen remains sufficient to inhibit ovulation for the full 3 years (unlike Norplant®).

Intrauterine: While women using the LNG-IUS continue to develop ovarian follicles and ovulate, most have amenorrhoea or only very light occasional bleeding because the presence of high concentrations of LNG in the uterine cavity induces endometrial atrophy. However, it takes time for atrophy to occur and most women experience frequent and often persistent spotting for 3 to 6 months after IUS insertion. LNG-IUS users can be reassured that bleeding patterns will improve with time.

Long-term use of both implants and the IUS (for which upfront costs are high) is essential for cost-effectiveness, and careful counselling about menstrual irregularities is vital to avoid premature discontinuation.

Irregular bleeding in association with both Depo-Provera® and Implanon® can be temporarily alleviated by the administration of oestrogens (simply by adding the combined pill) but this is only suitable as a short-term solution. Aspirin and vitamin E have both been shown to be ineffective for this purpose.

Persistent follicles/follicular cysts. The effect of the low-dose POCs on ovarian activity also results in a relatively high incidence of functional ovarian cysts or, more accurately, persistent follicles. It has been estimated that one in five women using the POP will have a 'cyst' demonstrable by ultrasound, and they are common among IUS users. Usually asymptomatic, persistent follicles can cause abdominal pain or dyspareunia. Most will disappear with menstruation and so treatment should be conservative.

Other 'hormonal' side effects. These include headache, nausea, bloating, breast tenderness and weight and mood change – all common in women not using hormonal contraception. They often settle with time but if not may be alleviated by changing to a different progestogen. Depo-Provera®, however, is associated with weight gain and women may gain as much as 16 kg after 2 years of use. Oily skin and acne can be a problem particularly with the more androgenic progestogens – LNG and NET. Some studies have suggested an increased risk of ectopic pregnancy. This has not been confirmed although methods of contraception which do not prevent ovulation are more likely to be associated with ectopic pregnancies than those which prevent ovulation.

Delay in the resumption of fertility.   Fertility returns rapidly after stopping low-dose POC. It may take up to 1 year, however, for normal fertility to return following cessation of Depo-Provera®. Women often complain of 'feeling premenstrual' despite continuing amenorrhoea. They can be assured that there is no permanent impairment of fertility but this delay makes Depo-Provera® an inappropriate method for women wishing short-term contraception.

Sexually transmitted infection.   A number of studies undertaken in the late 1980s and early 1990s suggested that the use of hormonal contraception may be associated with an increased risk of chlamydia and gonorrhoea. Hormonal contraceptive use is common and so are sexually transmitted infections (STI). Most of the studies have been cross-sectional in design, have used insensitive tests for chlamydia infection and most have failed to control for potential confounding factors such as sexual behaviour. A study involving over 800 women in the USA [22] suggested that the use of Depo-Provera® but not of oral contraception was significantly associated with an increased risk of chlamydia and gonorrhoea after adjusting for other risk factors (HR for Depo-Provera 3.6; 1.6–8.5: HR for the OC 1.5; 0.6–3.5). It has been suggested that since Depo-Provera® causes hypo-oestrogenism, thinning of the vaginal epithelium may increase the risk of infection. Further studies need to be done to determine whether the link between and STIs is causal or merely related to sexual behaviour.

Serious side effects

Because progestogen-only methods are much less widely used than the combined pill, data on long-term risks are sparse. Long-term (5 years) follow-up of over 16,000 women using Norplant reported no significant excess of any health problems including cardiovascular disease and neoplasia.

Cardiovascular disease.   There is no evidence for an increase in the risk of stroke, myocardial infarction or VTE in association with POC. Any association between VTE and progestogen used for the treatment of gynaecological conditions such as anovulatory dysfunctional uterine bleeding may be due to prescriber bias since the COC – often the method of choice – is contraindicated in women with known risk factors for VTE.

Malignant disease.   Depo-Provera® confers a high degree of protection against endometrial carcinoma but although it should theoretically also protect against ovarian cancer there are as yet no data to support this. There are no data on risks of cervical cancer although it is thought that all hormonal contraception may play a promoting role. Recent concern that the progestogen component of HRT may contribute to the increased risk of breast cancer has raised concerns about POC. The large meta-analysis on breast cancer and hormonal contraception included a small percentage of POP (0.8%) and injectable (1.5%) users [16]. Use of the POP within the last 5 years was associated with a very small but statistically significant increase in relative risk of breast cancer (1.17%). The same increase among injectable-users was not, however, significant. For both methods the relative risk had returned to normal 5 years after stopping.

Bone mineral density.   Complete inhibition of ovulation by Depo-Provera® causes hypo-oestrogenism and amenorrhoea. Hypo-oestrogenism is associated with a reduction in bone mineral density (BMD). It has been recognized for some time that current use of Depo-Provera® is associated with a loss of BMD when compared with non-users. This may be more of an issue with very young women who have not yet achieved peak bone mass. Results of cross-sectional studies are limited and inconsistent; however, two prospective studies have reported statistically significant decreases in BMD over two years among Depo-Provera® users aged between 12 and 21 compared with users of non-hormonal contraception [23,24]. While current DMPA users in older age groups do seem to have a decreased BMD compared with non-users, limited evidence suggest that women who stop using DMPA before the menopause can regain lost bone mass. There is, however, some concern about women over 40, who may not recover normal BMD after stopping Depo-Provera® before they inevitably lose more bone when they reach the menopause. While the data on BMD across all age groups is consistent, only one study has examined fracture risk and this was among women of a mean age of 21. There was no significant association between use of Depo-Provera® and the risk of stress fractures after adjusting for baseline BMD. In the UK the Committe on Safety of Medicines (CSM) has very recently advised that
• In adolescents, Depo-Provera® may be used as first-line contraception but only after other methods have been

discussed with the patient and considered to be unsuitable or unacceptable.

- In women of all ages, careful re-evaluation of the risks and benefits of treatment should be carried out in those who wish to continue use for more than 2 years.
- In women with significant lifestyle and or medical risk factors for osteoporosis, other methods of contraception should be considered.

The CSM does not advise how women who wish to continue Depo-Provera® should be evaluated after 2 years of use. However, the Faculty of Family Planning and Reproductive Healthcare in the UK cautions against using BMD scans which are unlikely to help in the decision-making process.

There are no sound data which demonstrate an effect of low-dose progestogen-only methods on BMD. Whether women who experience amenorrhoea while using Implanon® or the POP are at any risk is unknown.

Key points

- POC is available in a wide range of delivery systems.
- The dose of progestogen determines the mode of action and side effects.
- Irregular vaginal bleeding is a common reason for discontinuation of low-dose POC which do not inhibit ovarian activity completely.
- Despite normal ovarian activity the LNG-IUS is associated with amenorrhoea because of endometrial atrophy.
- Depo-Provera® inhibits ovarian activity completely and most users have amenorrhoea.
- There are few data on long-term safety. Theoretically POC are safer than CHC.
- POC does not increase the risk of cardiovascular disease.
- Depo-Provera® is associated with decreased BMD.
- Depo-Provera® may be associated with an increased risk of some sexually transmitted infections.

Intrauterine device

Seven copper-containing intrauterine devices (IUD) are currently available in the UK. Six have a plastic frame with copper wire wound round the stem or copper sleeves on the end of the arms. The amount of copper varies from 250 to 375 mm². One IUD is frameless (GyneFix®) and consists of six copper beads on a nylon thread. A knot at the top end of the thread is inserted into the fundal myometrium, the top and bottom copper beads are crimped to hold the string of beads in place. In all devices a tail protrudes through the cervical canal into the upper part of the vagina allowing easy removal. IUDs containing at least 300 mm² of copper have the lowest failure rates. Devices containing 250 mm² are licensed for 3 years, the T-Safe Cu 380A

for 8 years and the remainder for 5 years. The FFPRHC advises that an IUD inserted at or after the age of 40 can be retained until contraception is no longer required (i.e. beyond the licensed duration) [25]. There are good data to demonstrate efficacy up to 10 years for some devices and since the risks of perforation, infection and expulsion are all highest around the time of IUD insertion it makes sense to discuss prolonged continuation with the user.

Efficacy

In a WHO sponsored study of an IUD containing 380 mm² copper, the failure rate was 1 per 100 women in the first year of use. Over 5 years of use, cumulative pregnancy rates for devices containing at least 300 mm² are around 2%.

Mechanism of action

IUDs stimulate a marked inflammatory reaction in the uterus. The concentration of macrophages and leucocytes, prostaglandins and various enzymes in both uterine and tubal fluid increase significantly. It is thought that these effects are toxic to both sperm and egg and interfere with sperm transport. If a healthy fertilized egg reaches the uterine cavity implantation is inhibited.

Contraindications

There are very few women for whom a copper IUD is contraindicated. A history of malignant trophoblastic disease, endometrial cancer or pelvic TB and current STI or PID (pelvic inflammatory disease) are the only WHOMEC category 4 conditions. Women at risk of STI and women with HIV or AIDS can use a copper IUD but should be carefully counselled about safe sex and additional condom use should be promoted. Unexplained vaginal bleeding should be investigated before IUD insertion and a distorted uterine cavity (due for example to fibroids) may make insertion impossible.

Side effects

MENSTRUAL DISTURBANCE

The effect of the IUD – particularly the effect on local prostaglandins – on the endometrium tends to cause increased menstrual bleeding and dysmenorrhoea. Bleeding can be both heavier and more prolonged particularly during the first 3 to 6 months of use. In clinical trials up to 15% of women will discontinue for these reasons. Removal rates for bleeding and pain are similar when the frameless Gynefix® is compared with a framed device containing 380 mm² copper.

DYSMENORRHOEA

The presence of an IUD in the uterus is associated with an increased incidence of dysmenorrhoea. There is no good evidence that dysmenorrhoea is less among women using the frameless device.

ECTOPIC PREGNANCY

A meta-analysis of case control studies demonstrated no increase in the risk of ectopic pregnancy among current users, but the risk was increased among past users (OR 1.4; 95% CI 1.23–1.59) [26]. The absolute risk of *any* pregnancy is very low among IUD users and the annual ectopic pregnancy rate is 0.02 per 100 women years compared with 0.3–0.5 for women not using contraception.

PELVIC INFECTION

The risk of pelvic infection associated with IUD use has been overestimated. A meta-analysis suggested that the risk had halved during the 1980s [27]. Infection is most likely to occur during the first 20 days following insertion. Thereafter the risk of developing infection is not significantly higher than that among women using no contraception (<1.5 per 1000 women years). The risk can be reduced by using aseptic techniques during insertion and by restricting the method to women who do not have multiple partners and whose partners do not have multiple partners. Marital status and parity are really irrelevant to the risk of PID. Screening for STI is recommended prior to insertion in areas where the prevalence of infection is high and among individual women with known risk behaviours (including women under 25). Pelvic actinomyscosis can rarely occur in association with IUD use. Actinomyscosis-like organisms (ALOs) are sometimes seen on smears but if the patient is symptom free the IUD can be left and the smear repeated 6–12 months later. If there are symptoms the IUD should be removed avoiding contamination from the vagina and, after cutting off the tails which will be contaminated, sent for culture.

Insertion and removal

An IUD can be inserted at any time in the cycle if it can be reasonably certain the woman is not pregnant. Otherwise insertion should be limited to the first 7 days of the cycle. Post-partum insertion should be delayed until 4 weeks after childbirth for all women including breast-feeding women. An IUD can be inserted immediately after spontaneous or therapeutic abortion although expulsion rates may be higher in second trimester abortions. Unless pregnancy is desired, removal should only be undertaken in the late luteal phase or in the first 7 days of the cycle. In menopausal women the IUD should be left in for one year after the last menstrual period. If the IUD threads are not visible or snap during removal it may be possible to remove the device with a specially designed hook or a pair of artery forceps.

PERFORATION

Perforation of the uterus may occur at the time of insertion although it is often unnoticed. In large clinical trials it occurs in 1.3 of every 1000 insertions. Routine follow-up 6 weeks after insertion allows perforations to be detected. Absent threads should be investigated by ultrasound. At this stage the IUD can often be retrieved laparoscopically; left for months, local adhesion formation often necessitates laparotomy. The length of the uterine cavity should be measured using a sound and a tenaculum should be used at insertion to reduce the risk of perforation.

EXPULSION

The risk of expulsion is around 1 in 20. It is most common in the first 3 months of use and usually occurs during menstruation. Many clinicians advise that IUD users should regularly check to feel the IUD strings to detect expulsion. In reality this is often not easy to do and probably results in more anxiety than it prevents unrecognized expulsion.

Key points

- The IUD is a very effective method of contraception, lasting for at least 5 years, which can be used by unmarried, nulliparous women.
- Devices containing less than 300 mm^2 copper have higher failure rates and should not be used routinely.
- If an IUD is inserted after age 40 it can be left in place until contraception is no longer required.
- The commonest side effect (and commonest reason for premature removal) is heavy bleeding.
- The risk of ectopic pregnancy is enormously reduced compared with women using no contraception.
- The risk of pelvic infection has been overemphasized and by 3 weeks after insertion is not increased. Women with risk factors for STI should be screened before insertion but the IUD is not contraindicated.

Emergency contraception

Emergency contraception (EC) is defined as any drug or device used after intercourse to prevent pregnancy. One marketed hormonal method (levonelle-2, LNG 1.5 mg taken as a single dose within 72 h of intercourse) is available in the UK. The Yuzpe regimen, a combination of 100 μg ethinyloestradiol and 0.5 mg LNG taken twice with the two doses separated by 12 h is no longer marketed, but the same hormones are available in some brands of COC if levonelle-2 is unavailable.

Mechanism of action

Levonorgestrel 1.5 mg (LNG-EC) inhibits or delays ovulation if it is taken in the early to mid-follicular phase of the cycle. The risk of pregnancy at this time is less than 20%. Within 48 h of ovulation, when the risk of pregnancy is around 30%, LNG-EC appears to be ineffective in inhibiting ovulation. If ovulation does occur abnormalities of the luteal phase are common but the effect of these on fertility is unclear. There is no evidence that LNG-ED interferes with implantation.

Efficacy

There has never been a placebo-controlled trial of EC effectiveness and accurate estimates of efficacy are difficult to make. Many women are unsure of the exact date of their last menstrual period and most do not ovulate on exactly the same day each cycle. The majority of women who use emergency contraception are of unproven fertility and many use it after an accident with a condom which may not in fact have resulted in the leakage of seminal fluid. The chance of conception following one act of intercourse has been calculated to be around 27% per cycle so that even without emergency contraception over 70% of women will not conceive. While it has been suggested that LNG-EC may prevent as many as 90% of pregnancies, particularly if it is used soon after intercourse, this figure is probably a huge overestimate. Beyond 72 h after intercourse, given the likely mechanism of action, LNG-EC is even less effective.

Side effects

LNG-EC is free from side effects. Subsequent menses normally occur at the expected time. Few data are available on the safety of LNG-EC but the World Health Organization advises that there are no contraindications to its use [7]. There is no evidence that the regime is teratogenic should it fail to prevent pregnancy.

The copper IUD (but not the LNG-IUS) is a highly effective emergency contraceptive with failure rates of less than 1%. In the UK it is used for up to 5 days after the estimated day of ovulation, which may be more than 5 days after intercourse. It is particularly appropriate for women who wish to continue the IUD as a long-term method of contraception. Most women requesting

emergency contraception are however young and nulliparous and it can sometimes be difficult to insert a device. Simultaneous antibiotic treatment for chlamydia infection is recommended for women at risk.

Use of emergency contraception

In 2003 6% of women of reproductive age had used emergency contraception at least once in the past year. Among women aged 16–17 that figure rose to 20%. A number of studies suggest that around 11% of women presenting for abortion in the UK used emergency contraception to try to prevent the pregnancy. More than seven studies, undertaken in a variety of countries and settings, and using a variety of methods of emergency contraception, have shown that advanced provision of EC (giving a supply to be kept until needed) increases use. It also encourages earlier use and, except in adolescents, does not lead to the abandonment of more reliable methods of contraception. Increased use of EC, however, has not as yet been shown to reduce abortion rates.

Key points

- LNG-EC can be given within 72 h of unprotected intercourse.
- LNG-EC inhibits ovulation if given early in the cycle but not if given in the peri-ovulatory phase. There is no evidence that it inhibits implantation.
- Efficacy of LNG-EC is uncertain and has probably been exaggerated.
- Advanced provision of EC encourages use.
- A copper IUD can be inserted up to 5 days after ovulation for post-coital use and is about 99% effective.

Sterilization

In Britain almost 50% of couples aged 35–44 are using either male or female sterilization as their method of contraception. Vasectomy is safer, cheaper and performed under local anaesthesia. The ability to check for efficacy (with semen analysis) is a clear advantage when male is compared with female sterilization. Male fertility, however, continues well beyond that of women and these differences should be discussed during counselling. For detailed evidence-based guidance on male and female sterilization see the RCOG (Royal College of Obsteticians and Gynaecologists) Clinical Guideline [28].

Female sterilization

Female sterilization usually involves blocking both Fallopian tubes via laparotomy, mini-laparotomy, or more commonly by laparoscopy. Bilateral salpingectomy or hysterectomy may be preferable when there is coexistent gynaecological pathology. Mini-laparotomy and laparoscopic sterilization are probably equally safe and effective although laparoscopy is quicker and associated with less minor morbidity. Mini-laparotomy is preferred when sterilization is performed immediately post-partum when the uterus is large, the pelvis very vascular, and the risks of laparoscopy increased. A variety of techniques exists for occluding the tube; for laparoscopic sterilization Filshie clips or rings should be the method of choice. The preferred method of tubal occlusion during laparotomy and mini-laparotomy is the Pomeroy technique where a loop of tube is tied and excised. Diathermy of the tubes is associated with an increased risk of ectopic pregnancy and is more difficult to reverse. Moreover there can be serious complications if adjoining structures (most commonly bowel) are burnt. Rings are associated with a higher risk of haemorrhage from, or avulsion of, the tube and because of ischaemia of the loop caught in the ring cause much more post-operative pain. The RCOG recommends topical application of local anaesthesia to the Fallopian tubes whenever mechanical occlusive devices are being applied (even when general anaesthesia is used) since this reduces post-operative pain. Clips destroy less length of tube than rings but the higher failure rate in the USA study may reflect the fact that clip placement is technically more difficult than the application of rings or diathermy. Filshie clips are easier to apply than the Hulka Clemens variety and allow occlusion of thicker tubes. Post-partum sterilization using mechanical occlusion rather than partial salpingectomy has a much higher failure rate.

A number of chemical agents have been tested for their ability to occlude the Fallopian tube when instilled into the tube either directly or transcervically via the uterus. A quinacrine pellet (252 mg) is inserted into the uterine cavity through a modified IUD inserter passed through the cervix. Two insertions, 1 month apart, are made during the follicular phase of the cycle. Inflammation and fibrosis cause occlusion of the intramural segment of the tube and a failure rate of 2.6% after 1 year of follow-up is reported. The method is cheap and can easily be performed by non-medical personnel. However, the safety of quinacrine sterilization has not yet been determined and morbidity appears to be higher than with surgical procedures. Although widely used in some parts of Asia, the technique has not been approved in any developed country.

A new method of female sterilization has become available in the US and some parts of Europe. It is being provided in some areas of the UK, but is still under evaluation. The device, ESSURE® is an expanding spring measuring 2 mm in diameter and 4 cm in length made of titanium, stainless steel and nickel containing dacron fibres. Using hysteroscopy under local anaesthesia or mild sedation in an outpatient setting, the device is inserted via the cavity of the uterus into the proximal section of the Fallopian tube. The device induces a local inflammatory response and, eventually, fibrosis of the intramural tubal lumen. A number of studies have evaluated the efficacy, safety and acceptability of this procedure as an alternative to laparoscopic tubal sterilization, which usually requires general anaesthesia and hospitalization. Bilateral device placement is achieved in between 85 and 95% of patients. As yet follow-up is limited, but one trial from Australia reported no pregnancies among 111 women followed-up for 2 years.

EFFICACY

A prospective study of over 10,000 women in the USA compared the cumulative pregnancy rate 10 years after sterilization with a variety of different methods [29]. The overall pregnancy rate after 10 years was 18.5/1000 procedures. In this survey 33% of the pregnancies which occurred (excluding luteal phase pregnancies) were ectopic and the failure rate was higher among women sterilized before the age of 28. The longest period of follow-up data available for the Filshie clip suggests a failure rate of 2–3/1000 procedures after 10 years. The RCOG recommends telling women that the lifetime risk of failure is 1 in 200.

THE TIMING OF FEMALE STERILIZATION

Should sterilization be undertaken in association with pregnancy, women should be made aware of the possibility of regret and of potential increased failure rates. The RCOG advised that consent for sterilization should be obtained at least 1 week prior to Cesarean section if the two procedures are to be combined. It is seldom possible to arrange sterilization for a particular time of the cycle and women should continue using their current method of contraception until surgery. It is not necessary to stop the combined pill before sterilization as the risk of thromboembolic complications is negligible. If an IUD is in situ it should be removed at the time of sterilization, unless the operation is being done at midcycle and intercourse has taken place within the previous few days in which case it can be removed after the next menstrual period. The date of the last menstrual period should be checked pre-operatively. The RCOG recommends a routine pregnancy test on the day of sterilization as this significantly reduces the rate of undetected luteal phase pregnancies. Dilatation and curettage (D&C) at the time of sterilization is not usually performed. If it is intended as a means to terminate a luteal phase pregnancy it might be illegal unless the terms of the Abortion Act are being met. It may also be ineffective since the blastocyst is tiny and may be missed.

IMMEDIATE COMPLICATIONS

1 The mortality from laparoscopic sterilization is less than 8 per 100,000 operations. The commonest cause of death is anaesthesia.
2 Damage to major blood vessels, bowel or other internal organs may occur during the procedure and is usually recognized at the time of operation.
3 Gas embolism.
4 Thromboembolic disease is rare, but more likely immediately post-partum.
5 Wound infection.
It has been suggested that the operative complication rate is higher when sterilization is done at the same time as therapeutic abortion; however, the rate is less than that of the two separate procedures added together, but there is an increase in the failure rate.

LONG-TERM COMPLICATIONS

1 Menstrual disorders – A number of studies have demonstrated an increased incidence of gynaecological consultation and of hysterectomy following sterilization despite no demonstrable change in menstrual blood loss. Changes in menstrual bleeding patterns are inevitable with advancing age and after stopping the combined pill. Women who have been sterilized may be more likely to seek or accept hysterectomy as they are no longer capable of childbearing.
2 Abdominal pain and dyspareunia may occur after sterilization and are said to be more common after cautery. Repeat laparoscopy usually fails to demonstrate any pathology and the symptoms may sometimes be a manifestation of regret.
3 Psychological and psychosexual problems are rare and when they do arise tend to do so in those who have had problems before sterilization. Many studies report a better mental state after sterilization.
4 Bowel obstruction from adhesions is a very rare complication.

Vasectomy

Division or occlusion of the vas deferens prevents the passage of sperm. Division alone is associated with a high failure rate; it should be accompanied by fascial interposition or diathermy. The vas can be ligated or occluded with clips or by diathermy; clips appear to be associated with a higher failure rate and are not recommended. Percutaneous injection of sclerosing agents or occlusive

substances such as silicone is used in China. It has been claimed that the silicone plug can be removed and the vasectomy successfully reversed. No one method seems to be more effective than any other but the 'no scalpel vasectomy,' which obviates the need for a skin incision, is associated with a reduced incidence of haemorrhage and infection. No scalpel vasectomy is recommended in the RCOG guidelines.

The success of the procedure is verified by the absence of sperm from two consecutive samples of ejaculate collected at least 4 weeks apart. Histological examination of the excised portion of the vas is not necessary unless there is doubt about their identity. The time taken for azoospermia development depends on the frequency of intercourse; it is estimated that some 20 ejaculations are required and in the UK seminal fluid is usually examined at 12 and 16 weeks. Contraception must be continued until confirmation of two negative results has been received.

EFFICACY

Even after azoospermia has been confirmed there is a failure rate of around 1 in 2000 procedures. In a small number of men non-motile sperm persist after vasectomy. No pregnancies have been reported when less than 10,000 non-motile sperm/ml are found in a fresh specimen produced at least 7 months after the vasectomy.

IMMEDIATE COMPLICATIONS

Scrotal bruising occurs in almost everyone, haematoma (1–2%) and wound infection (up to 5%) are common minor complications.

LATE COMPLICATIONS

1 The development of antisperm antibodies (thought to be in response to leakage of sperm) occurs in most men and appears to be harmless unless restoration of fertility is desired.
2 Small inflammatory granulomata can form at the cut ends of the vas – presumably also in response to leaked sperm. Sperm granulomas may be painful and persistent but can be effectively excised.
3 Chronic testicular pain of unknown cause can persist in a very small number of men for years after a vasectomy.
4 Concerns have been raised in the past linking vasectomy with an increased risk of atherosclerosis, testicular cancer and other, mainly autoimmune, diseases. Several large studies have failed to substantiate these concerns. However, an increased risk of prostate cancer has also been suggested. Only epidemiological evidence is available and

Table 32.7 Points to cover when counselling for male or female sterlization

The reason for the request – some women seek sterilization as a cure for menstrual dysfunction, sexual problems or abdominal pain
Age – people under 30 are more likely to regret the decision
Family size and the possibility of wanting children/more children – couple with no children more likely to experience regret
Previous and current contraception and any problems experienced. Some women request sterilization because they are unable to find any other acceptable method of contraception. It is particularly important to discuss long-acting methods which are equally effective but reversible
Which partner should be sterilized
The stability of the relationship and the possibility of its breakdown
The quality of the couples' sex life
The procedure
The failure rate
The risks and side effects
Reversibility
The practical arrangements, e.g. continued use of interim contraception

there seems to be no biological plausibility for such a link, but further research is required.

Counselling for sterilization

Most couples seeking sterilization have been thinking about the operation for some considerable time. As many as 10% of couples may regret being sterilized and 1% request reversal. Couples sterilized at a young age, immediately post-partum or after therapeutic abortion are more likely to experience regret. A change of partner is the commonest reason for requesting reversal. As more than one in three marriages end in divorce in the UK and many couples now do not bother to get married, the stability of the couples' relationship as well as other factors (listed in Table 32.7) should be explored during counselling.

Reversal of sterilization

Reversal of female sterilization involves laparotomy, does not always work (microsurgical techniques are associated with around 70% success), and carries a significant risk of ectopic pregnancy (up to 5%). Reversal of vasectomy is technically feasible in many cases with patency rates of almost 90% being reported in some series. Pregnancy rates are much less (up to 60%) perhaps as a result of the presence of antisperm antibodies. Ovulation should be confirmed and a normal semen analysis obtained before

reversal is undertaken. Reversal is unlikely to be available on the NHS in most parts of the UK.

Key points

- Male and female sterilization are common in the UK.
- Female sterilization has a failure rate of 1 in 200 and vasectomy 1 in 2000 after 10 years.
- Menstrual disorders are common after female sterilization but are related to cessation of other methods of contraception (which affect menstrual bleeding) and ageing and not to sterilization itself.
- It has been suggested that vasectomy may be associated with an increased risk of prostate and testicular cancer but neither has been proven.
- Counselling for sterilization is essential.
- Reversal of sterilization is not always successful.

Barrier methods

Barrier methods work by preventing the passage of sperm into the female genital tract.

Male and female condoms

The male condom remains one of the most popular methods of contraception in the UK, 27% of couples use it as their main method (Table 32.1). Use increased significantly after the mid-1980s because of concern over the spread of HIV and AIDS. The latex condom is cheap, widely available over the counter and with the exception of the occasional allergic reaction, is free from side effects. Polyurethane condoms have not yet proved as effective for contraception but offer an alternative for people with latex sensitivity. Condoms are effective in preventing STI, including HIV [30].

Spermicide alone is not recommended for prevention of pregnancy as it is only moderately effective. Nonoxynol 9 (N-9) is a spermicidal product sold as a gel, cream, foam, film or pessary for use with diaphragms or caps. Many male condoms are lubricated with N-9. In response to data suggesting that frequent use of N-9 might increase the risk of HIV transmission, the WHO recommends that women who have multiple daily acts of intercourse or who are at high risk of HIV infection should not use N-9 (WHO website). For women at low risk of HIV infection N-9 is probably not unsafe. Since there is no evidence that lubricating male condoms with N-9 improves efficacy, such condoms should no longer be promoted.

The female condom is a polyurethane sheath the open end of which is attached to a flexible polyurethane ring. A removable ring inside the condom acts as an introducer and helps keep the device inside the vagina. It comes in one size with a non-spermicidal lubricant. It is designed for single use and is expensive. Failure rates are similar to those of the male condom (Table 32.2). Designed primarily with the prevention of sexually transmitted infections in mind, the female condom has not become popular in the UK.

Diaphragm and cervical cap

The diaphragm (and cap) is much less popular than male condoms. Both must be fitted by a doctor or nurse and do not confer the same degree of protection against STI since the vaginal skin is not covered. Selecting the correct size of diaphragm is similar to selecting the right size of vaginal ring for the management of vaginal prolapse (a skill which appears to be a closely guarded secret). On vaginal examination with the middle finger in the posterior fornix, the point at which the symphysis pubis abuts the ulnar border of the index finger is noted. The distance between that point and the tip of the middle finger is a guide to the appropriate size of diaphragm. Latex allergy, recurrent vaginal infections such as bacterial vaginosis or candida and recurrent urinary tract infection (UTI) are the only side effects.

Caps fit snugly over the cervix. They are very seldom used. A new device developed in the USA has limited availability in the UK (from Family Planning Sales Ltd, £12.95 each). Femcap® is a silicone rubber device shaped like an American sailor's hat. The design was intended to make the cap easier to fit, and less likely to slip, than the traditional diaphragm. Since it is said to confer less pressure on the surrounding vaginal walls it was also supposed to reduce the risk of UTI. In a randomized multicentre study comparing it with a traditional diaphragm, the failure rate of Femcap® was almost double (1.96 times that for diaphragm users). Although Femcap® users did have a lower risk of UTI (odds ratio 0.6, 95% CI 0.4–1.0) they were much more likely to find the device difficult to insert and remove and much more likely to experience dislodgement.

Key points

- Barrier methods all have high failure rates when used typically.
- Condoms are obtainable over the counter so provision is not dependent on a health professional.
- Diaphragms and caps must be fitted by a health professional.
- Male condoms reduce the risk of sexually transmitted disease including HIV/AIDS.
- Spermicides should not be used alone and if used frequently and in large quantities may increase the risk of HIV transmission.

Fertility awareness methods/natural family planning

Few couples in the UK use so-called natural methods of family planning (NFP) although in some parts of the world these methods are common. All involve the avoidance of intercourse during the fertile period of the cycle (periodic abstinence). Methods differ in the way in which they recognize the fertile period. The simplest is the calendar or rhythm method in which the woman calculates the fertile period according to the length of her normal menstrual cycle. The first day of the fertile period is calculated as being the length of the woman's shortest cycle minus 20 days, and the last day of the fertile period is the longest cycle minus 11 days. If therefore cycle length varies from 25–31 days the potential fertile period and days when intercourse should be avoided are days 5–20.

Other approaches use symptoms which reflect fluctuating concentrations of circulating oestrogen and progesterone. The mucus or Billings method relies on identifying changes in the quantity and quality of cervical and vaginal mucus. As circulating oestrogens increase with follicle growth the mucus becomes clear and stretchy allowing the passage of sperm. With ovulation, and in the presence of progesterone, mucus becomes opaque, sticky and much less stretchy or disappears altogether. Intercourse must stop when fertile-type mucus is identified and can start again when infertile-type mucus is recognized. Progesterone secretion is also associated with a rise in basal body temperature (BBT) of about 0.5°C. The BBT method is thus able to identify the end of the fertile period. Other signs/symptoms such as ovulation pain, position of cervix and degree of dilatation of the cervical os can be used additionally to help define the fertile period.

Whatever method is used, many couples find it difficult always to abstain from intercourse during the fertile period. Failure rates are high (Table 32.2) and most of the failures are due to conscious rule breaking. Perfect use of the mucus method is associated with a failure rate of only 3.4%. In a study of the mucus method couples who had completed their families had lower failure rates than couples who were using NFP as a method of birth spacing.

There is no evidence that pregnancies conceived with ageing gametes (i.e. towards the end of the fertile period) are associated with a higher risk of congenital malformations.

Lactational amenorrhoea method

Breastfeeding delays the resumption of fertility after childbirth and the length of the delay is related to the frequency and duration of breastfeeding episodes and the timing of the introduction of food other than breast milk (e.g.

solids). Prolonged breastfeeding can postpone ovulation, and therefore the risk of pregnancy, for more than a year. A woman who is fully or nearly fully breastfeeding and who remains amenorrhoeic has less than a 2% chance of pregnancy during the first 6 months after childbirth. The lactational amenorrhoea method or LAM is an algorithm which enables a woman to determine whether or not her pattern of infant feeding combined with her pattern of menstruation, confers effective contraception.

Prospective studies of LAM have demonstrated failure rates of 0.5–0.6%. In developed countries where average durations of breastfeeding are short, and where few women practice full or nearly full breastfeeding beyond 4 months post-partum, LAM is unlikely to be a practical method of contraception. In developing countries, however, where women breastfeed for much longer, and where modern methods of contraception may be expensive and difficult to obtain, the potential to use LAM is much greater.

Key points

- Periodic abstinence using a variety of fertility awareness methods can prevent pregnancy but depends heavily on compliance.
- LAM is associated with a 2% pregnancy rate.

References

1. Dawe F & Rainford L (2004) Contraception and sexual health 2003 A report on research using the ONS Omnibus Survey produced by the Office for National Statistics on behalf of the Department of Health, London. Office for National Statistics. 2004
2. Trussell J (2004) The essentials of contraception: efficacy, safety, and personal considerations. In: Hatcher RA, Trussell J, Stewart F *et al.* (eds) *Contraceptive Technology*, 18th revised edn. New York, USA: Ardent Media, Inc.
3. Rosenberg MJ & Waugh MS (1999) Causes and consequences of oral contraceptive noncompliance. *Am J Obstet Gynecol* **180**, S276–9.
4. Potter L, Oakley D, de Leon-Wong E & Canamanr R (1996) Measuring compliance among oral contraceptive users. *Fam Plann Perspect* **28**, 154–8.
5. Rosenberg MJ & Waugh MS (1998) Causes and consequences of oral contraceptive noncompliance. *Am J Obstet Gynecol* **180**, S276–9.
6. Larsson G, Blohm F, Sundell G *et al.* (1997) A longitudinal study of birth control and pregnancy outcome among women in a Swedish population. *Contraception* **56**, 6–16.
7. WHO (2004) Improving Access to Quality Care in Family Planning. *Medical Eligibility Criteria for Contraceptive Use*, 3rd edn. Geneva: Reproductive Health and Research, World Health Organization. Also available on the web at www.who.int/reproductive-health/publications/index.htm
8. Rosenburg MJ, Waugh MS & Meehan TE (1995) Use and misuse of oral contraceptives: risk indicators for poor pill taking and discontinuation. *Contraception* **51**, 283–8.
9. Audet Mc, Morean M, Koltun WD *et al.* for the ORTHO/EVRA Study Group (2001) Evaluation of contraceptive efficacy and cycle control of a transdermal contraceptive patch vs an oral contraceptive. A randomized controlled trial. *JAMA* **285**, 2347–54.
10. Beral V, Hermon C, Kay C, Hannaford P, Darby S & Reeves G (1999) Mortality associated with oral contraceptive use: 25 year follow up of a cohort of 46, 000 women from Royal College of General Practitioners' oral contraception study. *Br Med J* **318**, 96–100.
11. Endrikat J, Gerlinger C, Cronin M *et al.* (2001) Blood pressure stability in a normotensive population during intake of monophasic oral contraceptive pills containing 20 μg ethinyl oestradiol and 75 μg desogestrel. *Eur J Contracep Reprod Health Care* **6**, 159–66.
12. Tanis BC, Van der Bosch MAAJ, Kemmeren JM, Cats VM *et al.* (2001) Oral contraceptives and the risk of myocardial infarction. *New Engl J Med* **345**, 1787–93.
13. Dunn N, Thorogood M, Faragher B, de Caestecker L *et al.* (1999) Oral contraceptives and myocardial infarction: results of the MICA case control study. *Br Med J* **318**, 1579–84.
14. Khader YS, Rice J, John L & Abueita O (2003) Oral contraceptive use and risk of myocardial infarction: a meat-analysis. *Contraception* **68**, 11–7.
15. Etminan M, Takkouche B, Isorna FC & Samii A (2005) Risk of ischaemic stroke in people with migraine: systematic review and meta-analysis of observational studies. *Br Med J* **330**, 63–5.
16. The Collaborative Group on Hormonal Factors in Breast Cancer (1996) Breast cancer and hormonal contraceptives: a collaborative re-analysis of individual data on 53, 297 women with breast cancer and 100, 239 women without breast cancer from 54 epidemiological studies. *Lancet* **347**, 1717–27.
17. WHO (2005) Improving Access to Quality Care in Family Planning. Selected Practice Recommendations. Geneva: Reproductive Health and Research, World Health Organization. Also available on the web at www.who.int/reproductive-health/publications/index.htm
18. Faculty of Family Planning and Reproductive Healthcare (2002). UK Selected Practice Recommendations for Contraceptive Use. www.ffprhc.org.uk
19. Faculty of Family Planning and Reproductive Healthcare Clinical Effectiveness Unit (2003) FFPRHC Guidance (October 2003). First Prescription of Combined Oral Contraception *JFFPRHC* **29**, 209–23.
20. Rice CF, Killick SR, Dieben T & Coelingh Bennink HC (1999) A comparison of the inhibition of ovulation achieved by desogestrel 75μg and levonorgestrel 30μg daily. *Hum Reprod* **14**, 982–5.
21. Faculty of Family Planning and Reproductive Healthcare Clinical Effectiveness Unit (2004) FFPRHC Guidance (April 2004). The levonorgestrel intrauterine system (LNG-IUS) in contraception and reproductive Health. *JFFPRHC* **30**, 99–109.

22. Morrison C (2004) Hormonal contraceptive use, cervical ectopy and the acquisition of cervical infections. *Sex Transm Dis* **31**, 561–7.

23. Cromer BA, Blair JM, Mahan JD, Zibners L & Naumovski Z (1996) A prospective comparison of bone density in adolescent girls receiving depot medroxyprogesterone acetate (Depo-Provera). *J Pediatr* **129**, 671–6.

24. Lara-Torre E, Edwards CP, Perlman S & Hertwick SP (2004) Bone mineral density in adolescent females using depomedroxyprogesterone acetate. *J Pediatr Adolesc Gynecol* **17**, 17–21.

25. Faculty of Family Planning and Reproductive Healthcare Clinical Effectiveness Unit (2004). FFPRHC Guidance (April 2004). The copper intrauterine device as long-term contraception and reproductive health. *JFPRHC* **30**, 29–41.

26. Sivin I (1991) Dose and age-dependent ectopic pregnancy risks with intrauterine contraception. *Obstet Gynecol* **78**, 291–8.

27. Farley TMM, Rosenberg MJ, Rowe PJ, Chen JH & Meirik O (1992) Intrauterine devices and pelvic inflammatory disease: an international perspective. *Lancet* 339, 785–8.

28. Royal College of Obstetricians and Gynaecologists (2004) Male and Female Sterilisation. Evidence based Clinical Guideline No 4. London UK: RCOG.

29. Peterson HB, Xia Z, Hughes JM, Wilcok LS, Ratliff Tylor L & Trussel J (1996) The risk of pregnancy after tubal sterilization: findings from the US Collaborative review of sterilization. *Am J Obstet Gynecol* **174**, 1161–70.

30. Weller S & Davis K (2004) Condom effectiveness in reducing heterosexual HIV transmission. *Cochrane Database Syst Rev* **4**, 2002; (1):CD003255.

31. Steiner MJ, Dominik R, Rountree W, Nanda K & Dorflinger L (2003) Contraceptive effectiveness of a polyurethane condom and a latex condom: a randomised controlled trial. *Obstet Gynecol* **101**, 539–47.

Chapter 33: Termination of pregnancy

Gillian Flett and Allan Templeton

Termination of pregnancy is one of the most commonly practised gynaecological procedures in Great Britain. Surgical abortion by vacuum aspiration or dilatation and curettage was the method of choice from the 1960s. However, the late 1980s and 1990s saw exciting new developments in medical methods for early abortion and an improvement of medical methods for midtrimester termination with the introduction of mifepristone, which has been one of the most significant developments in fertility control in recent years. The result has been an extension of patient choice and a diversification in the provision of abortion services. 186,000 terminations are performed annually in England and Wales [1] and around 11,500 in Scotland [2]. Around 1 in 3 British women will have had an abortion by the age of 45 [3]. In Britain, over 98% of abortions are undertaken on the grounds that the pregnancy threatens the mental or physical health of the woman or her children [1,2]. It is these abortions which form the focus for this chapter. A minority of abortions are undertaken because of fetal abnormality and the special legal, ethical and service issues relating to these merit separate consideration.

The availability of NHS abortion provision varies considerably and improving timely access to abortion services is a major sexual health priority.

The law and abortion

The legal criteria surrounding abortion are specific to the country of practice. The abortion legislation in Great Britain is based on the 1967 Abortion Act [4] as amended by the Human Fertilisation Embryology Act 1990 [5]. Before an abortion can proceed, a certificate must be signed by two medical practitioners authorizing the abortion and this certificate requires to be retained for a period of at least 3 years. A notification form, which is forwarded to the Chief Medical Officer (CMO) for the relevant country, must be signed by the doctor taking responsibility for the procedure, although with medical termination it is frequently members of the nursing team who administer the drugs which have been preprescribed by the doctor. Most abortions are undertaken on the statutory grounds C or D which state that the pregnancy has not exceeded its 24th week and where continuance of the pregnancy would involve risks greater than if the pregnancy were terminated or injury to the physical or mental health of the women or of the existing children of her family (Table 33.1). It should be noted that the Abortion Act does not apply in Northern Ireland. A judicial review clarify the legal basis for providing terminations in situations to save the life of the mother or to prevent grave permanent injury to her physical or mental health. An appeal hearing on a judicial review in 2004 directed consultation with professionals, relevant agencies and women to provide clarification about state of current practice and provision of abortion services. Findings from the consultation will inform development of guidance materials for professionals about the provision of termination services in Northern Ireland.

Table 33.1 Statutory grounds for termination of pregnancy

A	The continuance of the pregnancy would involve risk to the life of the pregnant woman, greater than if the pregnancy were terminated
B	The termination is necessary to prevent grave permanent injury to the physical or mental health of the pregnant woman
C	The pregnancy has not exceeded its 24th week and the continuance of the pregnancy would involve risk, greater than if the pregnancy were terminated, of injury to the physical or mental health of the pregnant woman
D	The pregnancy has not exceeded its 24th week and the continuance of the pregnancy would involve risk, greater than if the pregnancy were terminated, or injury to the physical or mental health of the existing child (ren) of the family of the pregnant woman
E	There is a substantial risk that if the child were born it would suffer from such physical or mental abnormalities as to be seriously handicapped
F	To save the life of the pregnant woman
G	To prevent grave permanent injury to the physical or mental health of the pregnant woman

Doctors looking after women requesting abortion care should apply principles of good practice as described in the General Medical Council (GMC) document – Duties of a Doctor [6]. There is a conscientious objection clause within the Abortion Act and the British Medical Association (BMA) have produced a useful overview on the legal and ethical position [7]. Where practitioners have a conscientious objection they should provide advice and organize the first steps for arranging an abortion, where the request meets the legal requirements, and this would usually include prompt referral to another doctor as appropriate. Doctors and nurses can refuse to take part in an abortion but cannot refuse to take part in any emergency treatment.

Before an abortion proceeds, a clinician will certainly wish to be certain that all legal statute is fulfilled but it is also important to be sure that a woman has considered all her options carefully and is sure of her decision and gives informed consent. In recent years, sexual and reproductive health services and abortion providers have become more aware of the specific needs of young women and a competent young person can give her own consent, although encouragement is given for the involvement of parents.

Counselling and pre-assessment for abortion

Gestation is a major determinant of options available for terminating a pregnancy and a decision is usually reached by the woman in consultation with her medical carers and pregnancy counsellors. The termination method chosen has to be acceptable to the woman as well as being safe and effective. Full guidelines on good practice for the care of women requesting induced abortion have been published by the Royal College of Obstetricians and Gynaecologists (RCOG) [8]. Choice is an integral part of abortion care and provision of information along with sensitive counselling is essential to help the woman to select an abortion method that is right for her and which will optimize the abortion experience. Increasingly, women are referred to dedicated abortion services offering care separately from other gynaecological patients but with the full support of a gynaecological service should that be required. There is strong evidence supporting a lower risk of complications for abortions undertaken at earlier gestations. Because of this, services need to be organized to offer arrangements which minimize unnecessary delay.

At the pre-assessment consultation, counselling and choice of procedure are likely to dominate, but it is also an opportunity to screen for any pre-existing medical conditions which might require cross specialty liaison and,

despite the sensitivities of abortion, it is unusual for a woman to withhold her permission for this to happen. For serious medical conditions the risks of abortion are going to be lower than the risks of a continued pregnancy. The pre-assessment also provides an opportunity to enquire about previous contraceptive methods and to plan for intended use of contraception in the future. It is usual to check the body mass index and blood pressure for all patients and physical examination can be limited to auscultation of chest and heart for patients opting for general anaesthetic surgical termination. Although an idea of gestational age would have been gained from the menstrual history, it is well recognized that menstrual recall may be inaccurate and bimanual examination is very limited for assessing gestation. The greater accuracy of either abdominal or vaginal ultrasound as relevant to the anticipated gestation means that ultrasound is, in many centres, routine practice. Viability and pregnancy location can also be confirmed. It is important that this scan is undertaken in a sensitive setting and manner and the patient is advised that it is not necessary for her to watch the ultrasound examination in progress. A full blood count is recommended to screen for anaemia and also acts as a baseline for comparison should there be significant blood loss associated with the termination. It is also a useful opportunity to confirm immunity to rubella and to offer subsequent immunization if not immune. All patients have blood sent for confirmation of ABO and rhesus status with antibody screening. All unsensitized rhesus negative women should be given anti-D prophylaxis. Some centres offer testing for human immunodeficiency virus (HIV), hepatitis B and hepatitis C at this time, but unless a policy for routine screening has been adopted and accepted, it is recommended to undertake additional counselling and, at the present time, such testing remains on a selective basis. Cervical screening is not essential to abortion care but again there is an opportunity to check that screening is up to date and, where it is not, opportunistic cervical screening can be offered, but it is important to ensure that the result can be communicated to the woman and appropriate action taken on any abnormal result.

Screening for genital tract infection is helpful to identify pathogens which increase the risk of post-abortion infection and pelvic inflammatory disease, as well as the long-term sequelae of tubal factor infertility and ectopic pregnancy. The most important infecting organisms are *C. trachomatis* and *N. gonorrhoea*. Bacterial vaginosis is also associated with increased infection risk. Control group data from trials of prophylactic antibiotics for abortion suggests that infection complications occur in up to 1 in 10 termination cases. A full infection screen, including for sexually transmitted infections (STI), allows the opportunity for patient follow-up and partner notification and treatment to avoid reinfection. Prophylactic antibiotics at the time of abortion are advocated by some and a meta-analysis by Sawaya *et al.* [9] showed a reduction in risk for subsequent infective morbidity of around 50%. However, that approach still leaves the women at-risk from reinfection from an unrecognized and untreated partner. A third, and possibly ideal strategy, with a 'belt and braces' approach would provide a prophylactic regimen effective against bacterial vaginosis and *Chlamydia* along with a full vaginal STI screen [10]. Prophylaxis and a 'screen and treat' policy have been compared in a randomized trial which concluded that universal prophylaxis is at least as effective as a policy of screen and treat in reducing the short-term infective complications of abortion and could be provided at lower direct cost [11].

The RCOG Guideline Development Group in the UK [8] recommended that all abortion services should adopt a strategy to reduce post-abortion infective problems and the very minimum recommendation is for antibiotic prophylaxis against *Chlamydia* and bacterial vaginosis. Metronidazole 1 gm rectally at the time of abortion with 1 gm oral Azithromycin post-procedure would be one suitable regimen. Azithromycin seems to be increasingly favoured over a 7-day course of doxycycline where patient compliance can be more problematic. However, the evidence for specific prophylactic antibiotic regimes remains limited.

Choosing the method of abortion

The determining factors in an individual woman's choice for medical or surgical abortion are complex. Some women see the advantages of the surgical methods to be that they are simple and quick and associated with a relatively low risk of complication or failure. Medical methods are often favoured because they appear more physiological, like a miscarriage and avoid the need for uterine instrumentation and also share the advantages of low rates of complication and failure. Some women feel that they lack control where a surgical procedure is undertaken, whereas others specifically wish to remain unaware and have the procedure undertaken by their clinician. In 1991, the antiprogestogen mifepristone was licensed for termination up to 9 weeks' gestation and since then an extensive literature has built up to support the safety, efficacy and acceptability of the medical regimen for early first trimester abortion [12–15]. 1995 saw an extension of licence to include pregnancies over 13 weeks' gestation. At present, the medical regimen is not licensed for use in women over 9 and up to 13 weeks' gestation and the majority of abortions at these gestations remain surgical. There is randomized trial evidence comparing medical and surgical termination at 10–13 weeks' gestation confirming that the medical regimen is an effective alternative to surgery with high acceptability [16] and increasing numbers of units now offer medical termination as an alternative choice at these gestations. While ideally abortion services should be able to offer a choice of recommended methods across all the gestation bands, the minimum recommended by the RCOG guideline is that a service should be able to offer abortion by one of the recommended methods in a particular gestation band (Fig. 33.1).

Clinical practice in three larger Scottish units indicates that more than half of eligible women opt for medical methods when given a choice at early gestations up to 9 weeks and Scottish abortion statistics reveal that over 50% of all terminations in Scotland are now performed medically [2]. Medical abortion has been more patchy in its introduction in England and Wales and there continues to be significant variation in its provision across Health Authorities. Interestingly, the introduction of medical termination has not affected the overall abortion rate. That women value choice of method appropriate to the gestation of their pregnancy has been confirmed from patient surveys [17,18].

The RCOG guidelines recommend that conventional suction termination should be avoided at very early gestations under 7 weeks because the procedure is three times more likely to fail to remove the gestation sac than where the termination is performed between 7 and 12 weeks [19]. Although medical termination has been advocated at these very early gestations under 7 weeks, there is renewed interest in manual vacuum aspiration (MVA) under local anaesthetic using strict protocols to identify tissue and track subsequent serum beta hCG levels. The selection of medical or surgical method for later abortions beyond 15 weeks depends on the availability of health-care personnel who are trained and willing to participate in late dilatation and evacuation (D + E). There are fewer abortions at these gestations and they tend to be undertaken within the specialist independent sector. It is the case that as gestational age increases the safety of second trimester surgical abortion depends highly on the operator's skill and experience. Clinics and clinicians usually set the limits for operative care based on these considerations. It should be noted that there has been no formal comparison in randomized trials between second trimester D + E and the modern methods of medical midtrimester termination. Hysterotomy with its high associated morbidity and mortality has disappeared from practice.

Day-case care is recognized as a cost-effective model of service provision and a typical abortion service will be able to manage 90% of its patients on a day-care basis. Pre-existing medical problems, social factors, geographical distance and the possibility of a planned day case subsequently requiring overnight stay because of surgical

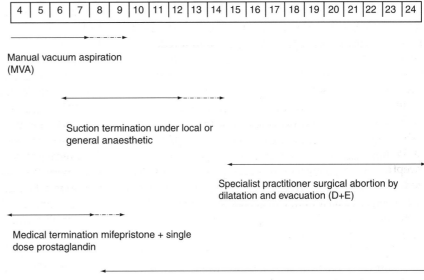

| 4 | 5 | 6 | 7 | 8 | 9 | 10 | 11 | 12 | 13 | 14 | 15 | 16 | 17 | 18 | 19 | 20 | 21 | 22 | 23 | 24 |

Manual vacuum aspiration
(MVA)

Suction termination under local or
general anaesthetic

Specialist practitioner surgical abortion by
dilatation and evacuation (D+E)

Medical termination mifepristone + single
dose prostaglandin

Medical termination mifepristone and repeated
doses of prostaglandin

Fig. 33.1 Methods of abortion suitable at different gestations.

or medical problems will, of course, influence the day-care rate. Those women undergoing a midtrimester procedure in particular should be advised of the possible need for an overnight stay.

Medical termination in the first trimester

The anti-progestogen mifepristone is used in combination with prostaglandin doses to achieve medical abortion. There are few contraindications to medical termination and they include: suspected ectopic pregnancy, chronic adrenal failure, long-term steroid use, haemorrhagic disorders, treatment with anticoagulants, known allergy to mifepristone or misoprostol, smokers over 35 with ECG abnormalities and breastfeeding women. Medical abortions require to be performed in hospitals or premises registered for abortion. The patient attends briefly to take the mifepristone dose and attends subsequently for day-patient admission, usually 36 to 48 h later. It is customary for legal reasons to supervise the swallowing of the mifepristone tablets, but side effects are trivial and the women can leave after 10 min. Women may bleed slightly in the 48 h following the mifepristone dose and, particularly at early gestations, a very small number may miscarry. The route of prostaglandin administration and regimens vary, but it is customary for the women to remain under supervision for 4–6 h after prostaglandin administration, during which time the majority will have expelled the pregnancy (Table 33.2). The nursing staff supervising the procedure confirm passage of the products. The amount of bleeding can be variable, but is often similar

to a heavy period and increases with the gestation. It is usual for women to have some lower abdominal cramp

Table 33.2 Medical methods

Up to 9 weeks (63 days) gestation
*Mifepristone 200 mg orally followed 1–3 days later by
  misoprostol 800 μg vaginally either by the woman or clinician

7–9 weeks (49–63 days) gestation
If abortion has not occurred 4 h after misoprostol
  administration, a second dose of 400 μg misoprostol may be
  administered vaginally or orally (depends upon bleeding or
  preference)

Other licensed regimen
Mifepristone 600 mg orally followed 36–48 h later by
  gemeprost 1 mg vaginally

9–13 weeks gestation
*Mifepristone 200 mg orally followed 36–48 h later by
  misoprostol 800 μg vaginally – a maximum of four further
  doses of misoprostol 400 μg may be administered at 3 h
  intervals, vaginally or orally depending on amount of
  bleeding

Midtrimester (abortion (13–24 weeks gestation)
*Mifepristone 200 mg orally, followed 36–48 h later by
  misoprostol 800 mg vaginally then misoprostol 400 μg orally,
  3 h intervals, to a maximum of four oral doses

Other licensed regimen
Mifepristone 600 mg orally, followed 36–48 h later by
  gemeprost. 1 mg vaginally every 3 h, to a maximum of five
  pessaries

---

*These regimens are unlicensed.

which will require administration of oral analgesia and a minority (less than 5%) might require opiate analgesia. The length of gestation influences the efficacy and complete abortion rate for the procedure, as well as complications, but this is more of an issue at 9–13 weeks' gestation. The risk of a continuing pregnancy, particularly in the 9–13 week gestation band remains a problem, and those units undertaking medical termination at these gestations are careful in counselling women regarding this. Where women pass only minimal or no products of conception, ultrasound should be carried out. An unrecognized ongoing pregnancy would be of particular concern because of the risk of fetal abnormality associated with misoprostol use.

Early medical abortion at gestations up to 9 weeks

Single agents have been abandoned in favour of combined regimens with mifepristone plus prostaglandin. The conventional prostaglandin analogue used for medical abortion is gemeprost, but a disadvantage is its cost and the fact that it is unstable at room temperature. The manufacturer's summary of product characteristics for mifepristone recommends a dose of 600 mg prior to prostaglandin administration for early medical abortion. A Cochrane review concluded that the dose could be lowered to 200 mg without significantly decreasing efficacy and a multicentre trial conducted by the World Health Organization (WHO) has further assessed the effect of reducing the dose of Mifepristone [20,21]. Although gemeprost is the conventional prostaglandin analogue used for abortion the alternative E₁ analogue misoprostol is also effective. Misoprostol is more effective if administered vaginally rather than orally [22–24]. A large review of 2000 women undergoing medical abortion up to 63 days' gestation using mifepristone 200 mg followed by a single dose of misoprostol 800 μg given vaginally achieved a complete abortion rate of 97.5% [25]. It was noticed, however, that efficacy significantly decreased at gestations greater than or equal to 49 days. A subsequent large-case series has shown that mifepristone in combination with two doses, rather than a single dose of misoprostol abolishes this gestation effect [26].

Medical abortion in the late first trimester (9–13 weeks)

Data are accumulating for the high uptake, acceptability and efficacy of medical termination at 9–13 weeks and, although still unlicensed at these gestations, it is likely to be offered as a choice for women undergoing abortion in many units. A randomized trial [27] comparing vacuum aspiration under general anaesthetic with medical abortion using a regimen of mifepristone 200 mg followed 36–48 h later by up to five doses of misoprostol showed that complete abortion rates for women not requiring a second procedure were 94.6% in the medical group and 97.9% in the surgical group, which was not a statistically significant difference. The same group has subsequently reported a consecutive series of 1076 women at 64–91 days of gestation managed using the same regimens. The complete abortion rate for the series was 95.8% with an ongoing pregnancy rate of 1.5% and a clear gestation effect was apparent [28].

Midtrimester medical abortion

Midtrimester medical abortion with mifepristone followed by prostaglandin has been shown to be safe and effective with shorter induction to abortion intervals than previous methods with prostaglandin alone or supplemented by oxytocin infusion. Again randomized trial evidence supports use of a 200 mg mifepristone dose [29]. The induction abortion interval tends to be longer with increasing gestation [30] and reported cumulative experience suggests that 97% of women abort successfully on the day of treatment within five doses of misoprostol. A second or third day of treatment may be required to complete the termination medically and patients should be forewarned of this possibility. Surgical evacuation of the uterus is not required routinely following midtrimester medical abortion and should only be undertaken where there is clinical evidence that the abortion is incomplete and this is likely to be required in only about 8% of cases [30].

Analgesia requirements

Abdominal pain is a common accompaniment to medical abortion. Analgesia requirements have been reported to be higher for women of younger age, higher gestation and longer-induction abortion interval, while women with a previous live birth(s) are less likely to use analgesia [31]. In a series of over 4000 women undergoing medical abortion up to 22 weeks' gestation, 72% used analgesia, the majority (97%) using oral analgesia and only 2.3% requiring intramuscular opiate [31]. The role of pre-emptive analgesia use needs to be evaluated, although the RCOG Guideline Group took the view that requirements for analgesia vary and there was no benefit for routine administration of a prophylactic analgesic. However, it is important that a range of oral and parenteral analgesics are available to meet women's needs.

Surgical termination

Surgical termination is performed in either a hospital setting or dedicated facility in a designated clinic. General anaesthetic is standard practice in the UK, although use of local anaesthetic, paracervical block, with or without sedation, is increasingly being offered. Vacuum aspiration is the standard procedure using a plastic cannula for aspiration with complete avoidance of using sharp instruments within the uterus, thereby minimizing the risk of uterine damage. Suction termination may be safer under local anaesthesia, but studies comparing the safety of local and general anaesthesia have been observational or only partially randomized.

Many clinicians avoid surgical termination under 7 weeks' gestation because of the risk of failure to remove the pregnancy. However, with the increased sensitivity of pregnancy tests, many women now present at very early gestations, shortly after a first period has been missed. For these women, it is not acceptable to defer the abortion until a suitable gestation for surgery and their preference might not necessarily be for medical termination or indeed, in certain circumstances, there could be contraindications to medical abortion. Suction terminations performed at less than 7 weeks' gestation are three times more likely to fail to remove the gestation sac than those performed between 7 and 12 weeks [19].

The 1990s saw renewed interested in MVA which had its origins back in the 1960s in relation to the practice of 'menstrual extraction'. MVA does take longer than electronic vacuum procedures, especially as the gestation increases towards 9 weeks. For MVA, uterine evacuation is accomplished using a 4, 5 or 6 mm flexible cannula attached to a 50 cc manual vacuum syringe. MVA had largely been abandoned after the legalization of abortion because of its failure rate, but modern protocols relying on human chorionic gonadodatrophin (hCG) assay, high-resolution ultrasound pre- and post-procedure and careful immediate tissue inspection are effective. Although the technique is well established in the USA, there is also renewed interested in introducing these early surgical abortion techniques in the UK. Creinin and Edwards report a continuing pregnancy rate of only 0.13% [32] but other series have reported 2.3% rates [33] and certainly, if conventional suction termination is the only method available within a service, the RCOG guideline group recommendation is to defer the procedure until the pregnancy has exceeded 7 weeks' gestation. It should be noted that there is no randomized trial evidence comparing MVA with medical termination at present.

Conventional suction termination is appropriate at 7–15 weeks' gestation although, possibly reflecting the skills and experience of practitioners, many units adopt medical abortion at gestations above 12–13 weeks.

Table 33.3 Cervical priming agents for surgical termination

*Misoprostol 400 μg $(2 \times 200\ \mu$g tablets) administered vaginally, either by the woman or clinician, 3 h prior to surgery
Gemeprost 1 mg vaginally, 3 h prior to surgery
Mifepristone 600 mg orally 36–48 h prior to surgery

*This regimen is unlicensed.

Cervical priming prior to surgical abortion reduces the complications of cervical injury, uterine perforation, haemorrhage and incomplete evacuation. Younger patient age is a risk factor for cervical damage and increasing gestation, particularly in multiparous women, is associated with uterine perforation. Mifepristone and the prostaglandin E_1 analogues, gemeprost and misoprostol are effective cervical priming agents (Table 33.3). In the UK, gemeprost is the licensed preparation, although there is evidence that misoprostol is an effective lower cost alternative. Mifepristone has also been shown to be an effective priming agent [34]. Mifepristone has higher efficacy than gemeprost and misoprostol when given 48 h ahead of surgery, but mifepristone has the disadvantage of requiring administration 36–48 h ahead of the abortion and there could be problems with preoperative bleeding. Misoprostol remains the most popular priming agent in the UK and the optimal time interval for administration is at least 3 h before surgery [35]. More recent work suggests that the sublingual route of administration is also effective for cervical priming, but is associated with an increased rate of gastrointestinal side effects.

Performing surgical abortion

Good technique is fundamental and aseptic technique should be observed with careful and gentle instrumentation to avoid injury to cervix or uterus. The operation itself is straightforward with low complication rates but skill and experience are important so that serious complications are quickly recognized and remedied. Precise techniques vary among operators. After confirming the position, size and shape of the uterus by bimanual examination, it is usual to apply a volsellum or tenaculum to the cervix and to dilate the cervix. The suction cannula should be positioned in the mid to upper fundus and when the operator is sure of correct placement, suction can be turned on. The cannula is gently rotated in a back and forth motion withdrawing only as far as the internal os until the flow of tissue and fluid has ceased and a gritty sensation is felt as the cannula moves against the wall of the contracted empty uterus. Sometimes sponge forceps may be required to remove products from the cervical canal. Sharp curettage should be avoided. Because of low rates of haemorrhage, oxytocics are not routinely administered.

The surgeon should ascertain that the major elements of the pregnancy are removed and are in keeping with the gestation of the pregnancy.

The risk of uterine perforation at the time of surgical abortion is of the order of 1–4 in 1000 from reports of large reviewed case series. The potential consequences resulting from visceral damage are so serious that if a perforation is suspected a laparoscopy should be undertaken as a minimum to confirm whether or not there is a perforation and certainly, where there is any possibility or suspicion of bowel injury, formal surgical laparotomy should be undertaken. The advantages of cervical priming in reducing the risk of cervical injury have been outlined. Precise rates are difficult to state because of the varying definitions of cervical injury and variable data collection. Overall, the rate of cervical injury is not thought to be greater than 1% for first trimester vacuum aspiration [8]. Cervical injury is more frequent and more serious with D + E in the second trimester. Failure to remove the pregnancy with ongoing pregnancy is a recognized association with surgical termination and the quoted failure rate is around 2.3 in 1,000 surgical abortions [19]. The rate is increased for multiparous women, for abortions undertaken at less than 7 weeks' gestation, where small cannula are used or in the presence of a uterine anomaly or where the procedure is undertaken by an inexperienced clinician.

Surgical abortion after the first trimester

Late D + E is practised extensively in the US and there are skilled practitioners in England, the Netherlands, France and parts of Australia. Otherwise, it is not widely performed and, for example, in Scotland, midtrimester terminations are almost exclusively undertaken using modern medical termination methods. D+E has not found favour among NHS gynaecologists in England, but is more widely used by the non-NHS providers. Conventional first trimester surgical evacuation can be used up to 15 weeks gestation, but thereafter specific techniques of cervical preparation and special instruments need to be used. More modern methods of aggressive cervical preparation, coupled with extensive clinical experience of the procedure, have improved safety. The use of real-time ultrasound scanning during the procedure can reduce the perforation rate. A retrospective cohort study compared complication rates of D+E and contemporary methods of medical abortion using misoprostol, but even excluding women in the medical group who had surgical evacuation of retained placental tissue, the complication rates were greater in the medical termination group as opposed to D + E (22% versus 4%) [36]. Historically, it was felt that D + E was a risk factor for subsequent adverse pregnancy outcome

with pregnancy loss and preterm delivery. A recent retrospective case analysis suggests that this is not the case [37]. The procedure can really only be safely undertaken by gynaecologists who have been trained specifically in the technique and have an adequate clinical throughput to maintain their skills.

Future directions

Studies from the USA have reported high efficacy and acceptability of medical abortion in home settings and home care is increasingly established in the USA. Evaluation in the context of a randomized trial has not occurred. A multicentre, questionnaire survey, sponsored by the Family Planning Association to assess women's views on the home administration of misoprostol for medical abortion indicated that there is acceptability and support for this approach [38]. Pilot work for home self-administration of misoprostol at early gestations up to 56 days has also confirmed feasibility and acceptability in a UK setting [39] and although further research is required, it is a development which could radically change the provision of abortion services and might have important cost implications.

Complications and problems

Legal abortion in developed countries is extremely safe. Sadly, illegal, unsafe abortion remains a major contributor to maternal mortality on a global basis. Complications do increase with older age, multiparity and increasing gestational age. Complications are usually categorized into those which occur immediately at the time of the procedure and those which arise subsequently. Most of the immediate complications have been discussed directly in relation to the medical and surgical procedures. The most common complication to occur following termination is for the patient to present with problematic bleeding or pain and it is important for retained products and infection to be excluded. Ultrasound is extremely useful in helping to resolve the situation. Trials of prophylactic antibiotics for abortion do suggest a reduction in infective complications. Major reviews have been undertaken regarding subsequent risk for breast cancer after termination and the conclusion goes against any causal relationship between induced abortion and subsequent increased risk for breast cancer [40,41].

Women often have concerns regarding their future reproductive health. Evidence continues to confirm that there is no proven association with subsequent ectopic pregnancy, placenta previa or infertility. Published literature regarding an association with preterm birth has been conflicting with the earlier studies suggesting no effect but more recent studies showing a positive link [42,43]. Many women report a sense of relief following abortion while others report complex emotional feelings in the 2–3 weeks immediately afterwards, although these subsequently settle. Most services offer follow-up support counselling as required. Some studies suggest higher rates of psychiatric illness or self-harm among women who have previously had an abortion, but interpretation needs to be careful as the situation may reflect a continuation of pre-existing conditions [42].

Post-abortion follow-up

First and foremost it is important to offer contraceptive advice prior to discharge and to provide starter supplies or initiate method immediately following termination. Women should also be given a written account of the symptoms which they could experience following abortion and which would require urgent medical consultation. A 24 h telephone helpline number should be available if women have concerns about pain, bleeding or high temperatures. Urgent emergency gynaecology assessment and admission needs to be available to back up abortion services. It is usual practice to offer a 2-week follow-up appointment with either the abortion service or the referring clinician. In practice many women seem to default on this appointment.

The discharge letter on the day of termination should contain sufficient information about the procedure to allow another practitioner to deal with any complications. Counselling support should be available for any woman who wishes following termination and for women who have a previous history of mental health problems. Women who experience particular difficulty after termination are often those who have been ambivalent prior to the procedure, who lack a supportive partner, who have a previous mental health problem or who have held strong opinions and considered abortion to be wrong.

Summary

Abortion is one of the most frequent but safest procedures in modern medicine. Complications and failure are not completely avoidable, but can be minimized by careful attention to detail at the pre-screening visit and with careful medical and surgical practice based on the available published evidence and guidelines. It is important that the gestation is accurately assessed. If prophylactic antibiotics are not used, infection screening including for STIs should be undertaken. For surgical procedures, sound aseptic techniques should be employed. The clinicians involved should be experienced and comfortable with the procedures which they perform. There should be a high index of suspicion for possible complications and the patient must have good access to clinical services for post-abortion advice and management of complications. Abortion is a necessary part of fertility control, but efforts aimed at improving accessibility and availability of emergency contraception and regular contraception should remain a sexual health priority.

References

1. Department of Health (2003) *Abortion Statistics, England and Wales: 2002.* Statistical Bulletin 2003/23. London: Department of Health. (http://www.publications.doh.gov.uk/public/sb0323.htm).
2. Scottish Health Statistics Abortions (2002) (http://www.isdscotland.org/isd/info3.jsp?pContentID=1919p_applic=CCC&p_service=Content.show&)
3. Birth Control Trust (1997) *Abortion Provision in Britain – How Services are Provided and How they could be improved.* London: Birth Control Trust.
4. Abortion Act 1967 (1967) London: HMSO.
5. Human Fertilisation and Embryology Act 1990 (1990) London: HMSO.
6. General Medical Council (1998) *Maintaining Good Medical Practice.* London: GMC.
7. British Medical Association (1997; revised 1999) *The Law and Ethics of Abortion: BMA Views.* London: BMA.
8. Royal College of Obstetricians and Gynaecologists (2004) *The Care of Women Requesting Induced Abortion 2000, revised 2004.* Evidence-based Guideline no 7. London: RCOG Press.
9. Sawaya GF, Grady D, Kerlikowske K & Grimes DA (1996) Antibiotics at the time of induced abortion: the case for universal prophylaxis on a meta-analysis. *Obstet Gynecol* **87**, 884–90.
10. Blackwell AL, Thomas PD, Wereham K & Emery SJ (1993) Health gains from screening for infection of the lower genital tract in women attending for termination of pregnancy. *Lancet* **342**, 206–10.
11. Penney GC, Thomson M, Norman J et al. (1998) A randomised comparison of strategies for reducing infective complications of induced abortion. *Br J Obstet Gynaecol* **105**, 599–604.
12. Spitz IM, Barden CW, Benton L & Robins A (1998) Early pregnancy termination with mifepristone and misoprostol in the United States. *N Engl J Med* **338**(18), 1241–7.
13. Bartley J, Tong S, Everington D & Baird DT (2000) Parity is major determinant of success rate in medical abortion: a retrospective analysis of 3161 consecutive cases of early medical abortion treated with reduced doses of mifepristone and vaginal gemeprost. *Contraception* **62**(6), 297–303.
14. Ashok PW, Templeton A, Wagaarachchi PT & Flett GM (2002) Factors affecting the outcome of early medical abortion: a review of 4132 consecutive cases. *Br J Obstet Gynaecol* **109**(11), 1281–9.

15. Slade P, Heke S, Fletcher J & Stewart P (1998) A comparison of medical and surgical termination of pregnancy: choice, emotional impact and satisfaction with care. *Br J Obstet Gynaecol* **105**(12), 1288–95.

16. Ashok PW, Kidd A, Flett GM, Fitzmaurice A, Graham W & Templeton A (2002) A randomised comparison of medical abortion and surgical vacuum aspiration at 10–13 weeks gestation. *Hum Reprod* **17**(1), 92–8.

17. Howie FL, Henshaw RC, Naagi SA *et al.* (1997) Medical abortion or vacuum aspiration? Two year follow up of a patient preference trial. *Br J Obstet Gynaecol* **104**, 829–33.

18. Penney GC, Templeton A & Glazier A (1994) Patients' views on abortion care in Scottish Hospitals. *Health Bulletin* **52**, 431–8.

19. Kaunitz AM, Rovira EZ, Grimes DA & Schuz KF (1985) Abortions that fail. *Obstet Gynaecol* **66**, 533–7.

20. Kulier R, Gulmezoglua AM, Hofmeyr GJ, Cheng LN & Campana A (2004) Medical methods for first trimester abortion. *Cochrane Database Syst Rev* **2**, CD002855.

21. World Health Organisation Task Force on Post-Ovulatory Methods for Fertility Regulation (2001) Lowering the doses of mifepristone and gemeprost for early abortion: a randomised controlled trial. *Br J Obstet Gynaecol* **108**, 738–42.

22. Grimes DA (1997) Medical abortion in early pregnancy: a review of the evidence. *Obstet Gynecol* **89**, 790–6.

23. el-Refaey H, Rajasekar D, Abdulla M, Calder L & Templeton A (1995) Induction of abortion with mifepristone (RU486) and oral or vaginal misoprostol. *N Engl J Med* **332**, 983–7.

24. el-Refaey H & Templeton A (1995) Induction of abortion in the second trimester by a combination of misoprostol and mifepristone: a randomised comparison between two misoprostol regimes. *Hum Reprod* **10**, 475–8.

25. Ashok PW, Penney GC, Flett GM & Templeton A (1998) An effective regimen for early medical abortion: a report of 2000 consecutive cases. *Hum Reprod* **13**, 2962–5.

26. Ashok PW, Templeton A, Wagaarachchi PT & Flett GMM (2002) Factors affecting the outcome of early medical abortion: a review of 4132 consecutive cases. *Br J Obstet Gynaecol* **109**, 1281–9.

27. Ashok PW, Kidd A, Flett GMM, Fitzmaurice A, Graham W & Templeton A (2002) A randomised comparison of medical abortion and surgical vacuum aspiration at 10–13 weeks of gestation. *Hum Reprod* **17**, 92–8.

28. Hamoda H, Ashok PW, Flett GM & Templeton A (2005) Uptake and efficacy of medical abortion over 9 and up to 13 weeks gestation: a review of 1076 consecutive cases. *Contraception* **71**, 327–32.

29. Webster D, Penney GC & Templeton A (1996) A comparison of 600 and 200 mg mifepristone prior to second trimester abortion with the prostaglandin misoprostol. *Br J Obstet Gynaecol* **103**, 706–9.

30. Ashok PW, Templeton A, Wagaarachchi PT & Flett GM (2004) Mid trimester medical termination of pregnancy: a review of 1002 consecutive cases. *Contraception* **69**(1), 51–8.

31. Hamoda H, Ashok PW, Flett GM & Templeton A (2004) Analgesia requirements and predictors of analgesia use for women undergoing medical abortion up to 22 weeks of gestation. *Br J Obstet Gynaecol* **111**, 996–1000.

32. Creinin MD & Edwards J (1997) Early abortion: surgical and medical options. *Curr Probl Obstet Gynecol Fertil* **20**, 6–32.

33. Paul ME, Mitchell CM, Rogers AJ, Fox MC & Lackie EG (2002) Early surgical abortion; efficacy and safety. *Am J Obstet Gynecol* **187**, 407–11.

34. Henshaw RC & Templeton AA (1991) Pre-operative cervical preparation before 1st trimester vacuum aspiration; a randomised controlled comparison between gemeprost and mifepristone (RU486). *Br J Obstet Gynaecol* **98**, 1025–30.

35. Fong YF, Singh Kuldip & Prasad RNV (1998) A comparative study using two dose regimens (200 μg and 400 μg) of vaginal misoprostol for preoperative cervical dilatation in first trimester nulliparae. *Br J Obstet Gynaecol* **105**, 413–7.

36. Autry AM, Hayes EC, Jacobson GF & Kirby RS (2002) A comparison of medical induction and dilatation in evacuation for second-trimester abortion. *Am J Obstet Gynecol* **187**, 393–7.

37. Kalish RB, Chasen ST, Rosenzweig LB, Rashbaum WK & Chervenak FA (2002) Impact of mid-trimester dilatation and evacuation on subsequent pregnancy outcome. *Am J Obstet Gynecol* **187**, 882–5.

38. Hamoda H, Critchley HOD, Paterson K, Guthrie K, Rodger M & Penney GC (2005) The acceptability of home medical abortion to women in UK settings. *Br J Obstet Gynaecol* **112**, 781–5.

39. Hamoda H, Ashok PW, Flett GMM & Templeton A (2005) Home self-administration of misoprostol for medical abortion up to 56 days gestation. *J Fam Plann Reprod Health Care* **31**, 189–92.

40. American College of Obstetrics and Gynecology Committee on Gynecology Practice (2003) ACOG Committee Opinion. Induced abortion and breast cancer risk. *Int J Gynaecol Obstet* **83**, 233–5.

41. Beral V, Bull D, Doll R, Peto R, Reeves G & Collaborative group on hormonal factors in Breast Cancer (2004) Breast cancer and abortion; collaborative reanalysis of data from 53 epidemiological studies, including 83,000 women with breast cancer from 16 countries. *Lancet* **363**, 1007–16.

42. Thorpe GM Jr, Hartmann KE & Shadigian E (2002) Long-term physical and psychological health consequences of induced abortion: review of the evidence. *Obstet Gynecol Surv* **58**, 67–79.

43. Henriet L & Kaminski M (2001) Impact of induced abortions on subsequent pregnancy outcome: the 1995 French national perinatal survey. *Br J Obstet Gynaecol* **108**, 1036–42.

Chapter 34: Normal and abnormal development of the genital tract

D. Keith Edmonds

Sexual differentiation and its control are vital to the continuation of our species and for the gynaecologist an understanding of the development of the genital organs is clearly important. Our understanding of this process has greatly increased in recent years and with it the understanding of normal and abnormal sexual development. Following fertilization the normal embryo contains 46 chromosomes, including 22 autosomes derived from each parent. The basis of mammalian development is that a 46XY embryo will develop as a male and a 46XX embryo will differentiate into a female. It is, however, the presence or absence of the Y chromosome which determines whether the undifferentiated gonad becomes a testis or an ovary.

There are several genes involved in the formation of the bipotential gonad and later the testis and the ovary. In the conversion of mesoderm to the bipotential gonad WT1 (Wilms' tumour suppressor gene) and NR5A1 (nuclear receptor 5 gene group A1) are the two most important. It has been proven that the testis determining factor is on chromosome Yp11.31 and this gene is termed the SRY (sex-determining region of the Y chromosome). This gene triggers testis formation from the indifferent gonad [1]. SRY is just one member of a family of genes which exist within a homeobox known as HMG. This group of genes have now become known as SOX genes and a number of other genes as well as SRY have now been shown to be associated with the differentiation of the gonad to a testis. Mutations of SRY cause pure gonadal dysgenesis or hermaphroditism. Male sex determination in the absence of a Y chromosome results in XX sex reversed individuals. There are two main types, SRY positive XX males and SRY negative XX males and the majority are SRY positive with the SRY gene being located on the X chromosome (Fig. 34.1).

Ovarian differentiation seems to be determined by the presence of two X chromosomes and the ovarian determinant is located on the short arm of the X chromosome and this was discovered as a result of the absence of the short arm results in an ovarian agenesis [2]. It is believed at the present time that DAX1 is the gene which determines that

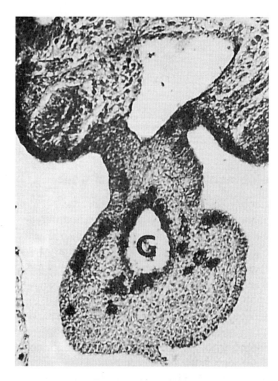

Fig. 34.1 Section of a 3.5 mm (28-day-old) human embryo stained with alkaline phosphatase. The picture shows the primitive gut, marked 'G', above which is the root of the mesentery. Above this again on either side is the intermediate mesoderm in which the genital organs develop. Germ cells are stained black and seen on either side of the primitive gut. Reproduced from [34] with permission.

the bipotential gonad will become an ovary. Other autosomal loci, as in the male, are certainly also involved in ovarian development. The development of the Müllerian and Wolffian structures must also be under genetic control and this is thought to be a polygenic multifactorial inheritance, although autosomal recessive genes may also be involved [3]. The influence of the differentiated gonad on the development of other genital organs is thus fundamental and the presence of a testis will lead to male genital organ development, but if the testes do not form

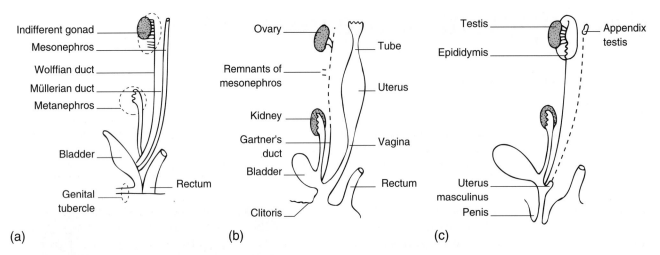

Fig. 34.2 Diagrammatic representation of genital tract development. (a) Indifferent stage; (b) female development; (c) male development.

the individual will develop female genital organs whether ovaries are present or not.

Development of the genital organs

Most embryological accounts agree on the principles of genital tract development, although some different views are held on the development of the vagina.

The genital organs and those of the urinary tract arise in the intermediate mesoderm on either side of the root of the mesentery beneath the epithelium of the coelom. The pronephros, a few transient excretory tubules in the cervical region, appears first but quickly degenerates. The duct, which begins in association with the pronephros, persists and extends caudally to open at the cloaca, connecting as it does so with some of the tubules of the mesonephros shortly to appear. The duct is called the mesonephric (Wolffian) duct. The mesonephros itself, the second primitive kidney, develops as a swelling bulging into the dorsal wall of the coelom of the thoracic and upper lumbar regions. The mesonephros in the male persists in part as the excretory portion of the male genital system; in the female only a few vestiges survive (Fig. 34.2). The genital ridge in which the gonad of each sex is to develop is visible as a swelling on the medial aspect of the mesonephros; the paramesonephric (Müllerian) duct from which much of the female genital tract will develop forms as an ingrowth of the coelomic epithelium on its lateral aspect; the ingrowth forms a groove and then a tube and sinks below the surface.

Uterus and fallopian tubes

The two paramesonephric ducts extend caudally until they reach the urogenital sinus at about 9 weeks' gestation.

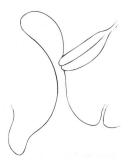

Fig. 34.3 Paired paramesonephric ducts protruding into the urogenital sinus as the Müllerian tubercle at 9 weeks of intrauterine life.

The blind ends project into the posterior wall of the sinus to become the Müllerian tubercle (Fig. 34.3). At the beginning of the third month the Müllerian and Wolffian ducts and mesonephric tubules are all present and capable of development. From this point onwards in the female there is degeneration of the Wolffian system and marked growth of the Müllerian system. In the male the opposite occurs as the result of production of Müllerian-inhibitory substance (MIS) produced by the fetal testis. The lower ends of the Müllerian ducts come together in the midline, fuse and develop into the uterus and the cervix. The cephalic ends of the duct remain separate to form the fallopian tubes. The thick muscular walls of the uterus and cervix develop from proliferation of mesenchyme around the fused portion of the ducts.

Vagina

At the point where the paramesonephric ducts protrude their solid tips into the dorsal wall of the urogenital sinus as the Müllerian tubercle there is marked growth of tissue from which the vagina will form, known as the vaginal plate. This plate grows in all dimensions greatly increasing the distance between the cervix and the urogenital sinus, and later the central cells of this plate break down to form the vaginal lumen. The complete canalization of the vagina does not usually occur until around the 20th to 24th week of pregnancy and failure of complete canalization may lead to a variety of septae, which cause outflow tract obstruction in later years. The debate which continues surrounds the portion of the vagina which is formed from the Müllerian ducts and that from the urogenital sinus by the growth of the sinovaginal bulb. Some believe that the upper four-fifths of the vagina is formed by the Müllerian duct and the lower fifth by the urogenital sinus, while others believe that the sinus upgrowth extends to the cervix displacing the Müllerian component completely the vagina thus derived wholly from the endoderm of the urogenital sinus. It seems certain that some of the vagina is derived from the urogenital sinus, but it is not certain whether the Müllerian component is involved or not.

External genitalia

The primitive cloaca becomes divided by a transverse septum into an anterior urogenital portion and a posterior rectal portion. The urogenital portion of the cloacal membrane breaks down shortly after division is complete and this urogenital sinus develops into three portions (Fig. 34.4). There is an external expanded phallic part, a deeper narrow pelvic part between it and the region of the Müllerian tubercle and a vesicourethral part connected superiorly to the allantois. Externally in this region the genital tubercle forms a conical projection around the anterior part of the cloacal membrane. Two pairs of swellings, a medial part (genital folds) and a lateral pair (genital swellings), are then formed by proliferation of mesoderm around the end of the urogenital sinus. Development up to this time (10 weeks, gestation) is the same in the male and the female. Differentiation then occurs. The bladder and urethra form from the vesicourethral portion of the urogenital sinus, and the vestibule from the pelvic and phallic portions. The genital tubercle enlarges only slightly and becomes the clitoris. The genital folds become the labia minora and the genital swellings enlarge to become the labia majora. In the male greater enlargement of the genital tubercle forms the penis and the genital folds fuse over a deep groove formed between them to become the penile part of the male urethra. The genital swellings enlarge, fuse and form the scrotum.

The final stage of development of the clitoris or penis and the formation of the anterior surface of the bladder and anterior abdominal wall up to the umbilicus is the result of the growth of mesoderm, extending ventrally around the body wall on each side to unite in the midline anteriorly.

Gonads

The primitive gonad appears in embryos at around 5 weeks' gestation. At this time coelomic epithelium develops on the medial aspect of the urogenital ridge and following proliferation leads to the establishment of the gonadal ridge. Epithelial cords then grow into the mesenchyme (primary sex cords) and the gonad now possesses an outer cortex and an inner medulla. In embryos with an XX complement, the cortex differentiates to become the ovary and the medulla regresses. The primordial germ cells develop by the 4th week in the endodermal cells of the yolk sac and during the 5th week they migrate along the dorsal mesentery of the hindgut to the gonadal ridges, eventually becoming incorporated into the mesenchyme and the primary sex cords by the end of the 6th gestational week.

The differentiation of the testis is evident at about 7 weeks by the disappearance of germ cells from the peripheral zone and gradual differentiation of remaining cells into fibroblasts, which form the tunica albuginea. The deeper parts of the sex cords give rise to the rete testis and the seminiferous and straight tubules. The first indication that the gonad will become an ovary is failure of these testicular changes to appear. The sex cords below the epithelium develop extensively with many primitive germ cells evident in this active cellular zone (Fig. 34.5). The epithelial cells in this layer are known as pregranulosa cells. The active growth phase then follows, involving the pregranulosa cells and germ cells, which are now very much reduced in size. This proliferation greatly enlarges the bulk of the gonad and the next stage (by 20 weeks onwards) shows the primitive germ cells, now known as oocytes, becoming surrounded by a ring of pregranulosa cells; stromal cells develop from the ovarian mesenchyme later, surround the pregranulosa cells and become known as granulosa cells and follicle formation is complete (Fig. 34.6). An interesting feature of the formation of follicles and the development of stroma is the disintegration of those oocytes which do not succeed in encircling themselves with a capsule of pregranulosa cells.

The number of oocytes is greatest during pregnancy and thereafter declines. Baker [4] found that the total population of germ cells rose from 600,000 at 2 months to a peak of 7 million at 5 months. At birth the number falls to 2 million, of which half are atretic. After 28 weeks or so of intrauterine life, follicular development can be seen at various stages and various sizes of follicles are also seen [5] Figs 34.7 and 34.8.

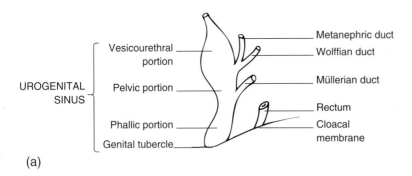

(a)

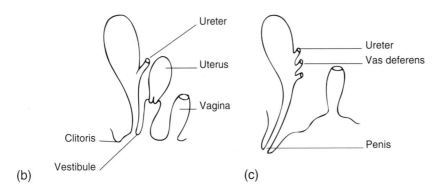

(b)   (c)

Fig. 34.4 Diagrammatic representation of lower genital tract development. (a) Indifferent stage; (b) female development; (c) male development.

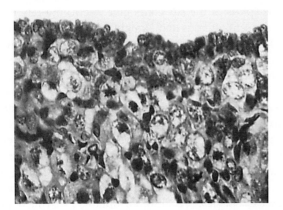

Fig. 34.5 Detail of immature ovary showing small epithelial cells (pregranulosa cells) and larger germ cells.

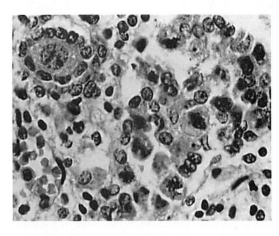

Fig. 34.6 A later ovary (31 weeks) showing a well-formed primary follicle (top left) and a germ cell (centre right) which is not yet completely surrounded by granulosa cells.

Genital tract malformations

Numerous malformations of the genital tract have been described, some of little clinical significance and others of considerable importance. Although many attempts have been made to explain malformation in terms of variation of the normal development, it is doubtful if there is any merit in this since malformations are by definition abnormal, and many curious malformations may be seen, for which variations of the normal development do not offer a convincing explanation.

Uterine anomalies

ABSENCE OF THE UTERUS

The uterus may be absent or of such rudimentary development as to be incapable of function of any kind. This condition is known as the Mayer-Rokitansky Kuster Hauser syndrome (MRKH). This type of anomaly is usually found when the vagina is absent also, the presenting symptom being one of primary amenorrhoea. These patients

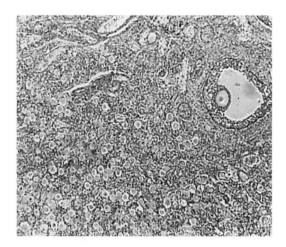

Fig. 34.7 Numerous primary follicles and one showing early development in the ovary of a child stillborn at 38 weeks.

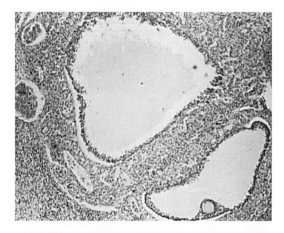

Fig. 34.8 Ovary from a child stillborn at 41 weeks showing a mature Graafian follicle, and a cystic follicle. Courtesy of the *Journal of Pathology and Bacteriology.*

have a 46XX chromosome complement and normal ovarian function. However, cases of absence of the uterus with development of the lower part of the vagina ending blindly and an absence or scanty appearance of pubic hair must raise the suspicion of androgen insensitivity. Unfortunately, no treatment is currently possible for such uterine abnormalities and in those cases where the diagnosis is androgen insensitivity removal of any testicular tissue must be undertaken to avert long-term risk of malignant change. However, whether the patient is XY or XX careful attention to psychological aspects of management is an extremely important facet of care.

FUSION ANOMALIES

Fusion anomalies of various kinds are not uncommon (Fig. 34.9) and may present clinically either in association with pregnancy or not. The lesser degrees of fusion defects are quite common, the cornual parts of the uterus remaining separate, giving the organ a heart-shaped appearance known as the bicornuate uterus. There is no evidence that such minor degrees of fusion defects give rise to clinical signs or symptoms. The presence of a septum extending over some or all of the uterine cavity, however, is likely to give rise to clinical features. Such a septate or subseptate uterus may be of normal external appearance or of bicornuate outline. Clinically, it may present with recurrent spontaneous abortion or malpresentation. A persistent transverse lie of the fetus in late pregnancy may suggest a uterine anomaly since the fetus tends to lie with its head in one cornu and the breech in the other.

In more extreme forms of failure of fusion the clinical features may be less, rather than more, marked. Two almost separate uterine cavities with one cervix are probably less likely to be associated with abnormalities than are the lesser degrees of fusion defect. Complete duplication of the uterus and cervix (uterus didelphys), if associated with a clinical problem, may prevent descent of the head in late pregnancy, or obstruct labour by the non-pregnant horn.

Rudimentary development of one horn may give rise to a very serious situation if a pregnancy is implanted there. Rupture of the horn with profound bleeding may occur as the pregnancy increases in size. The clinical picture will resemble that of a ruptured ectopic pregnancy with the difference that the amenorrhoea will probably be measured in months rather than weeks, and shock may be profound. A poorly developed or rudimentary horn may give rise to dysmenorrhoea and pelvic pain if there is any obstruction to communication between the horn and the main uterine cavity or the vagina. Surgical removal of this rudimentary horn is then indicated.

Vaginal anomalies

ABSENCE OF THE VAGINA

Absence of the vagina is generally associated with absence of the uterus or a rudimentary uterus. This is known as MRKH syndrome. Rarely the uterus may be present and the vagina, or a large part of it, absent. In the more common circumstances of absence of both vagina and uterus the patient will probably present between age 12 and 16 years with primary amenorrhoea. Secondary sexual characteristics will be present as the ovaries are normally developed and functional. This combination of normal secondary sexual development and primary amenorrhoea suggests an anatomical cause, such as an imperfect or absent vagina, for the failure to menstruate. Inspection of the vulva and abdominal examination will be required

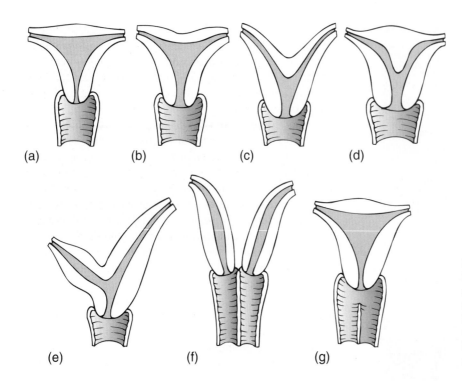

(a)   (b)   (c)   (d)

(e)   (f)   (g)

Fig. 34.9 Various fusion abnormalities of the uterus and vagina. (a) Normal appearance; (b) arcuate fundus with little effect on the shape of the cavity; (c) bicornuate uterus; (d) subseptate uterus with normal outline; (e) rudimentary horn; (f) uterus didelphys; (g) normal uterus with partial vaginal septum.

to exclude the presence of any retained blood in the upper part of the genital tract and will delineate the abnormality. Vulval development is normal, as may be seen in Fig. 34.10. The presumptive diagnosis of absent vagina can generally be made without difficulty at first examination. A very short vagina arising from androgen insensitivity may be mistaken for simple absence; so in every case of apparent vaginal absence a karyotype should be performed and if chromosome analysis confirms an XY sex chromosome complement the case should be managed appropriately.

All patients with abnormalities of the lower genital tract should have the renal tract investigated. Some 40% of patients with lower genital tract abnormalities will be found to have renal abnormalities, 15% of whom have an absent kidney. All patients should have a renal ultrasound performed to determine whether there is absence of a kidney and if more detailed analysis of the urinary tract is required this may be performed by intravenous urography. It is extremely rare for laparoscopy to be required to determine the abnormality and great care must be taken when performing a laparoscopy in case a pelvic kidney should exist because this may be injured with the trocar or laparoscope at the time of entry. Once the diagnosis is certain management may be divided into two sections, the first devoted to psychological counselling and the second aspect which involves the creation of a new vagina. Occasionally, patients present having already attempted intercourse and it may be that the sexual act is entirely enjoyable at the time of presentation, such that no further

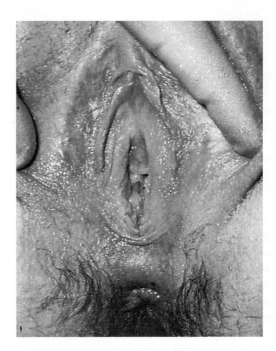

Fig. 34.10 Vulval appearances in a case of absence of the vagina.

therapy is required. It is very important to assess these couples or the patients themselves with great care so that appropriate therapy is applied at the correct time and it is not mandatory that all patients should have vaginas created. Circumstances determine whether or not this is a wise procedure.

COUNSELLING

The psychological problems that these patients manifest are generally devastating and profound. The reaction by both the patients and the parents varies considerably with the age of the girl, but they are generally frightened and confused and they express feelings of rejection and 'feeling like freaks'. They feel isolated and lonely and that nobody could possibly understand their feelings. They have concerns about sexual activity and fertility and also manifest great difficulty in maintaining heterosexual relationships. Most mothers of these children express great guilt and worry that they have been the perpetrator of this abnormality through some fault in pregnancy and great pressure may be put upon the gynaecologist to correct the problem in order to return the girl to normal. It is extremely dangerous and fraught with failure if an attempt at treatment is made before the patient is ready. In general these patients, if under the age of 17 years, do less well. Management requires an integrated health-care team and patients require continuing support and encouragement if they are to achieve the aims necessary. Support groups are invaluable and should be encouraged.

DIRECT THERAPY

The management of these cases is usually by non-surgical methods initially and then if necessary a surgical approach [6]. The technique of non-surgical treatment of the absent vagina was pioneered by Frank [7] and a review by Broadbent and Woolf [8] suggests a success rate of 90% with appropriate patient selection. The largest series reported in the world is of 242 patients with an 85% success [6]. The principle of the method is that the region which the vagina should occupy is a potential space filled with comparatively loose connective tissue which is capable of considerable indentation. The patient is instructed to use graduated glass dilators (Fig. 34.11) which are placed against the introitus and the blind vagina and gentle pressure is exerted in a posterior direction for approximately 10–20 min twice a day. Gradually the dilators will go further and further into the space and the dilators may be then increased in size and length until a 'neovagina' is created. In general, it takes between 8 and 10 weeks of repeated use of vaginal dilators to achieve a satisfactory result. The sexual satisfaction associated with this non-surgical procedure far exceeds that of the operative vaginoplasty [9].

In those patients who fail the non-surgical technique a vaginoplasty will need to be performed. A number of techniques have been used to create a vagina artificially, the most widely used being that of McIndoe and Read [10]. In this procedure a cavity is created between the bladder

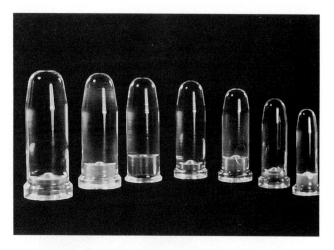

Fig. 34.11 Graduated glass dilators.

and bowel at the site where the natural vagina would have been, and this cavity is then lined by a split-thickness skin graft taken from the thigh and applied to the space on a plastic mould. The anatomical result can be very successful and remarkably good sexually. A review of 1311 reported cases gave a success rate of 92% [6]. However, there are a number of difficulties and disadvantages of this technique, not least the post-operative period, which is painful and sometimes protracted. The graft does not always take well and granulation may form over part of the cavity giving rise to discharge. Pressure necrosis between the mould and the urethra, bladder or rectum may lead to fistula formation, but the most important disadvantage is the tendency for the vagina to contract unless a dilator is worn or the vagina is used for intercourse regularly. It is therefore ideal to perform this procedure when sexual intercourse is desired soon afterwards because the procedure will fail if the patient does not maintain the vagina with the use of dilators. A further disadvantage of the use of split-thickness skin grafts is that the graft donor site remains as visible evidence of the vaginal problem and most women prefer not to have any external scarring.

In order to avoid the scar of the split-thickness skin graft, amnion has been used to line the neovagina and the results have been equally successful [11]. A recent review of our own series of well over 100 cases of amnion vaginoplasty have shown success rates of 85% satisfactory sexual activity following surgery [12].

The operation of vulvovaginoplasty pioneered by Williams [13] has some advantages as the procedure is simple, quick and relatively comfortable for the patient. The principle of the technique is the apposition of the labia majora in front of the neovagina to create a pouch into which the penis may be placed and sexual intercourse

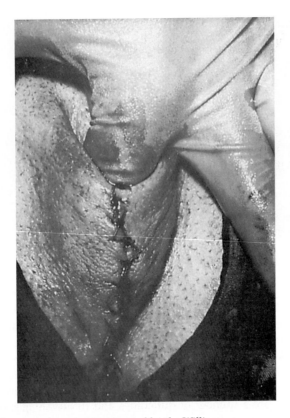

Fig. 34.12 A vagina constructed by the Williams vulvovaginoplasty method.

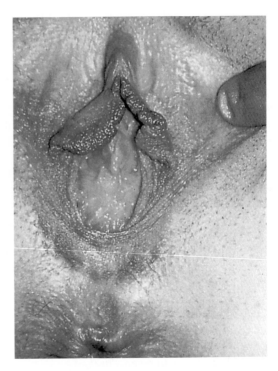

Fig. 34.13 An imperforate membrane occluding the vaginal introitus in a case of haematocolpos. Note the hymen clearly visible immediately distal to the membrane.

achieved (Fig. 34.12). The disadvantages of this technique are the unusual angle of the vagina, although this may lead to maximum clitoral stimulation at intercourse, and more importantly the destruction of the normal anatomy in a patient who previously had normal external genitalia. The psychological alteration in the external appearance of the vulva may be disturbing to some patients who find establishing relationships difficult in view of the abnormal anatomy.

A number of other techniques have been used to create a neovagina including the use of bowel and skin flaps. A procedure known as Vecchietti's operation has been popular in Europe for many years and this involves the use of a small olive which is placed in the dimple of the absent vagina. Laparoscopically wires can be brought out through the abdominal wall and then pressure exerted through a spring device, thereby creating a neovagina in a way that mimics the technique of Frank. It does, however, not rely on the woman herself using the dilators and after 7–9 days the olive is removed and the stretched vaginal skin is further dilated with glass dilators. Again, a recent review of the surgical techniques revealed success rates of approximately 90% [6].

HAEMATOCOLPOS

An imperforate membrane may exist at the lower end of the vagina, which is loosely referred to as the imperforate hymen, although the hymen can usually be distinguished separately (Fig. 34.13). These abnormalities of vertical fusion are seldom recognized clinically until puberty when retention of menstrual flow gives rise to the clinical features of haematocolpos, although rarely they may present in the newborn as a hydrocolpos. The features of haematocolpos are predominantly abdominal pain, primary amenorrhoea and occasionally interference with micturition. The patient is usually 14–15 years old, but may be older, and a clear history may be given of regular cyclical lower abdominal pain for several months previously. The patient may also present as an acute emergency if urinary obstruction develops. Examination reveals a lower abdominal swelling, and per rectum a large bulging mass in the vagina may be appreciated (Fig. 34.14). Vulval inspection may reveal the imperforate membrane which may or may not be bluish in colour depending upon its thickness. Diagnosis may be more difficult if the vagina is imperforate over some distance in its lower part or if there is obstruction in one-half of a septate vagina.

Treatment may be relatively simple or rather complex. If the membrane is thin, then a simple excision of the membrane and release of the retained blood resolve the

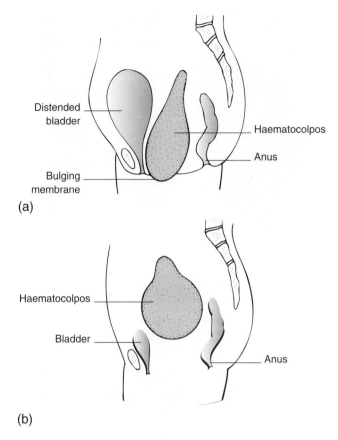

(a)

(b)

Fig. 34.14 (a) Diagrammatic view of haematocolpos. Note how the blood collecting in the vagina presses against the urethra and bladder base, ultimately causing retention of urine. (b) Haematocolpos associated with absence of the lower portion of the vagina. Note that the retained blood is now above the bladder base and retention of urine is unlikely.

problem. Redundant portions of the membrane may be removed but nothing more should be done at this time. Fluid will then drain naturally over some days. Examination a few weeks later is desirable to ensure that no pelvic mass remains which might also suggest haematosalpinx. In fact, haematosalpinx is most uncommon except in cases of very long standing and associated with retention of blood in the upper vagina. On these rare occasions, when a haematosalpinx is discovered, laparotomy is desirable, the distended tube being removed or preserved as seems best. Haematometra scarcely seems to be a realistic clinical entity, the thick uterine walls permitting comparatively little blood to collect therein. The subsequent menstrual history and fertility of patients who are successfully treated are probably not significantly different from that of unaffected women, although patients who develop endometriosis may have some fertility problems.

When the obstruction is more extensive than a thin membrane and a length of vagina is absent, diagnosis

and management are less straightforward and the ultimate interference with fertility is greater. Resection of the absent segment and reconstruction of the vagina may be done by either an end-to-end anastomosis of the vagina or a partial vaginoplasty.

The combination of absence of most of the lower vagina together with a functioning uterus presents a difficult problem. The upper part of the vagina will collect menstrual blood and a clinical picture similar in many ways to haematocolpos will be seen. Urinary obstruction is rare, however, since the retained blood lies above the level of the bladder base (Fig. 34.14). Diagnosis is more difficult and it may not be at all certain how much of the vagina is absent or how extensive the surgery would need to be to release the retained fluid and recreate the normal anatomy. Imaging may be by ultrasound or by the use of magnetic resonance imaging (MRI), and both these techniques may be successful in determining the exact anatomical relationships prior to surgery being performed. However, in the clinical situation the surgical approach is rarely entirely through the perineum and usually involves a laparotomy to establish finally how best the anatomy can be recreated.

Treatment is difficult and a dissection upwards is made as in the McIndoe-Read procedure. The blood is released, but its discharge for some time later may interfere with the application for a mould and skin graft. If possible, the upper and lower portions of the vagina should be brought together and stitched so that the new vagina with its own skin is created obviating the risk of contraction. However, the upper fragment tends to retract upwards resulting in a narrow area of constriction some way up the vagina, and this results in subsequent dyspareunia.

LONGITUDINAL VAGINAL SEPTUM

A vaginal septum extending throughout all or part of a vagina is not uncommon; such a septum lies in the sagittal plain in the midline, although if one side of the vagina has been used for coitus the septum may be displaced laterally to such an extent that it may not be obvious at the time of examination. The condition may be found in association with a completely double uterus and cervix or with a single uterus only. In obstetrics this septum may have some importance if vaginal delivery is to be attempted. In these circumstances the narrow hemivagina may be inadequate to allow passage of the fetus and serious tears may occur if the septum is still intact at this time. It is therefore prudent to arrange to remove the vaginal septum as a formal surgical procedure whenever one is discovered, either before or during pregnancy. The septum may occasionally be associated with dyspareunia when similar management is indicated.

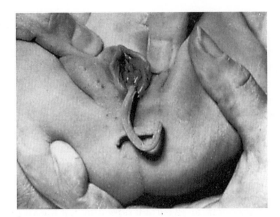

Fig. 34.15 Ectopic opening of the anus at the fourchette.

Occasionally, a double vagina may exist in which one side is not patent, and a haematometra and haematocolpos may occur in a single side. Under these circumstances the vaginal septum must be removed to allow drainage of the obstructed genital tract and the results are in general excellent.

Vulval anomalies

Rarely, anomalies in the development of bowel or bladder may give rise to considerable abnormality in the appearance of the vulva. The anus may open immediately adjacent to the vulva or just within it (Fig. 34.15). Bladder exstrophy will give rise to a bifid clitoris and anterior displacement of the vagina, in addition to bladder deformities themselves. Further discussion of these complex problems may be found in Edmonds [14].

Wolffian duct anomalies

Remnants of the lower part of the Wolffian duct may be evident as vaginal cysts, or remnants of the upper part as thin-walled cysts lying within the layers of the broad ligament (paraovarian cysts). It is doubtful if the vaginal cyst per se calls for surgical removal, although removal is usually undertaken. The cysts may cause dyspareunia and this is the most likely reason for their discovery and surgical removal. Cysts situated at the upper end of the vagina may be found to burrow deeply into the region of the broad ligament and the base of the bladder and should be approached surgically with considerable caution. A painful and probably paraovarian cyst will require surgical exploration and its precise nature will be unknown until the abdomen is opened. Such cysts normally come out easily from the broad ligament.

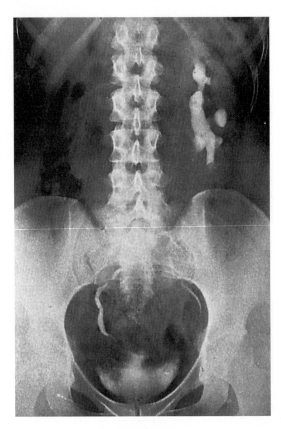

Fig. 34.16 An intravenous pyelogram in a patient with absence of the vagina, showing a single kidney and a gross abnormality of the course of the ureter.

Renal tract abnormalities

The association between congenital malformations of the genital tract and those of the renal tract is mentioned above. When a malformation of the genital organs of any significant degree presents some investigation to confirm or exclude a renal tract anomaly would be wise. An ultrasound scan can be arranged without any upset to the patient and will probably be sufficient in the first instance; however, if any doubt arises, an intravenous pyelogram may be performed. Lesions such as absence of a kidney, a double renal element on both or one side, a double ureter or a pelvic kidney (Fig. 34.16) may not call for immediate treatment but may do so later; moreover, it is as well to be aware of such abnormalities if the abdomen is to be opened for exploration or treatment of the genital tract lesion itself.

Ectopic ureter

One abnormality which apparently presents with gynaecological symptoms is the ectopic ureter (Fig. 34.17). A ureter opening abnormally is usually an additional one,

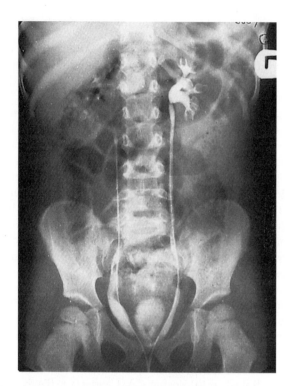

Fig. 34.17 An intravenous pyelogram in a child with an imperforate vagina. Both ureters open ectopically into the posterior urethra.

although sometimes a single one may be ectopic. The commonest site of the opening is the vestibule, followed closely by the urethra and then the vagina. Other sites are less common. The main symptom is uncontrollable wetness. The amount of moisture appearing at the vulva may, however, be small and is sometimes mistaken for a vaginal discharge. This confusion together with difficulties in confirming the diagnosis of an ectopic ureter, even when one is suspected, may lead to many patients being investigated for years before the condition is recognized. Diagnosis can sometimes be easy but is usually not so. The orifice at the vestibule may be clearly visible but more often careful search is necessary to locate it, if it can be seen at all. Cystoscopy and urethroscopy may be necessary to establish if normal ureteric openings exist in the bladder. Radiological study may be helpful by indicating a double element on one or both sides. Treatment will involve the help of a urological surgeon, and partial nephrectomy and ureterectomy or reimplantation of the ectopic ureter into the bladder may be undertaken.

Intersex disorders

There are three factors which determine an individual's sexual development. These are the effect of the sex chromosomes on the differentiation of the gonad, the proper functioning of the differentiated testis and the response of the end organ to this testicular function. The testes carry out their intrauterine function by producing two substances, testosterone and MIS.

Testosterone stimulates the development of the Wolffian duct, which differentiates into the internal male genitalia and also to the masculinization of the cloaca. MIS inhibits the development of the Müllerian structures which are always present and capable of development. MIS is a glycoprotein produced by the Sertoli cells [15] and its action seems to be mediated by the release of hyalunidase by the Müllerian duct cells, and local destruction occurs. There may also be inhibition of growth factor stimulation, presumably through specific cell membrane-associated receptors, as the regression is quite specific. MIS may have unilateral action so that each testis appears to produce the hormone, which results in regression of the Müllerian structures on its own side. The sensitivity of Müllerian structures to MIF is present only during the first 8 weeks of gestation.

The manner in which testosterone, produced by developing testes, is utilized to bring about masculinization of the cloaca is through conversion of testosterone to dihydrotestosterone through the action of the enzyme 5α-reductase. Wolffian structures, however, are capable of utilizing testosterone directly and are therefore independent of 5α-reductase activity. Thus, in those patients with 5α-reductase deficiency abnormal development of the external genitalia will occur and an intersex state results. For effective utilization of both testosterone and 5α-reductase it is necessary for the testosterone to be bound to the receptors on the cell membranes and ineffective binding of testosterone leads to abnormal sexual differentiation in disorders known as androgen insensitivity.

It is therefore evident that sexual development may be abnormal in the following circumstances:

1 There may be sex chromosome abnormalities interfering with testicular differentiation; the only common one is 46X/46XY mosaicism, giving rise to one of the forms of gonadal dysgenesis.

2 Testes may be incapable of producing testosterone, either because of complete failure of testicular differentiation (anatomical testicular failure) or a biosynthetic defect of testosterone production (enzymatic testicular failure).

3 The end organs may be incapable of utilizing testosterone because of 5α-reductase deficiency or because the androgen receptor is abnormal and therefore testosterone cannot bind to the cell wall (androgen insensitivity).

4 The production of Müllerian inhibitor may be deficient, leading to the growth of Müllerian structures in an otherwise normal male.

5 In a genetic female masculinization of the external genitalia may result in cases of excessive androgen production *in utero*, for example, congenital adrenal hyperplasia.

6 Rarely, in a genetic female, genes capable of producing the H-Y antigen may be found on an autosome, leading to the condition known as the 46XX male.

7 True hermaphroditism, i.e. the presence of testicular and ovarian tissue in the same individual, may be present and such patients are commonly genetically female with mosaicism, though genetic male variants also exist.

Clinical presentation

The child with ambiguous genitalia may present in a number of ways:

1 a masculinized female due to congenital adrenal hyperplasia (CAH) or androgen stimulation from another source;

2 an undermasculinized male for one of the reasons discussed above; or

3 a true hermaphrodite.

The masculinized female is usually caused by CAH; she may be unable to retain salt and water and die within a few weeks of birth from salt loss and dehydration if the diagnosis is not made. An important generalization concerns the age of presentation. If, as is usually the case, the patient presents at birth with sexual ambiguity it is important that full investigations be undertaken at once to choose the appropriate sex of rearing. The reasons for this are first, if the child has CAH she may die if not correctly treated, and second, whatever the diagnosis, the orientation of the child in the chosen sex of rearing will be better if she or he is placed in that gender role as soon as possible after birth and is allowed to grow up in it without further doubts about gender being expressed. Parents in these circumstances are extremely anxious to know the sex of their child and the prognosis for the future, but it is wise not to assign a gender role until all the information is available as an attempt at a later stage to change the sex of rearing may cause considerable psychological trauma. It is important to understand that it is extremely difficult to establish the correct diagnosis through superficial examination of the external genitalia. It is important that thorough investigation be carried out with the swiftest possible means to establish the correct diagnosis.

Presentation in the neonatal period

The first diagnosis to be confirmed or refuted is CAH. It must be admitted that, if a testis can be palpated with certainty, the likelihood of CAH is very small, but it should still be formerly excluded by the appropriate investigations.

CONGENITAL ADRENAL HYPERPLASIA

CAH is the most common cause of female intersex and is an autosomal recessive disorder resulting in enzyme deficiency related to the biosynthesis of cortisol and aldosterone. The commonest enzyme defect is 21-hydroxylase deficiency which results in a failure of conversion of 17α-hydroxyprogesterone to desoxycortisol and also failure of conversion of progesterone to desoxycorticosterone (Fig. 34.18). Two other enzyme deficiencies are recognized, although less common: 3β-hydroxysteroid hydrogenase deficiency and 11β-hydroxylase deficiency. In 21-hydroxylase deficiency, which accounts for 90% of cases of CAH, the deficiency results in an increase in progesterone and 17α-hydroxyprogesterone, which is therefore converted to androstenedione and subsequently to testosterone.

21-hydroxylase deficiency is an autosomal recessive disorder. Its relationship to human leucocyte antigen (HLA) type was established by Dupont *et al.* [16], and this has allowed mapping of the gene, which is located on the short arm of chromosome 6 [17]. It is located between HLA-B and HLA-DR, and subgroups of HLA-B have been closely linked to salt-losing CAH and HLA-BW51 with the simple virilizing form. Studies by Donohoue *et al.* [18] have shown that there are two hydroxylase genes (21-OHA and 21-OHB). Only 21-OHB is active and they both lie between the fourth components of complements C4A and C4B. A variety of mutations have been reported, including gene deletions of 21-OHB [19], gene conversions [18] and point mutations [20]. The incidence of 21-hydroxylase deficiency is between 1 in 5000 and 1 in 15,000.

Affected females are born with enlargement of the clitoris and excessive fusion of the genital folds, which obscure the vagina and urethra (Fig. 34.19), forming in the process an artificial urogenital sinus which has a single opening at some point on the perineum, usually near the base of the clitoris, although sometimes along its ventral surface and rarely at the tip. Thickening and rugosity of the labia majora are evident and they bear some resemblance to a scrotum. There is much variation of the thickness of the fused labial folds and in extreme cases they are very thick, with narrowing of the lower part of the vagina (Fig. 34.20). The uterus, fallopian tubes and vagina are always present and the vagina opens at some point in the urogenital sinus; in more severe cases it may be very difficult to identify this opening precisely. These clinical changes of masculinization are secondary to the elevated levels of androgens as a result of the enzyme defect.

In some infants a dangerous salt-losing syndrome may arise because of associated aldosterone deficiency and the child may die of wasting and vomiting within a few weeks of life if the diagnosis is not appreciated.

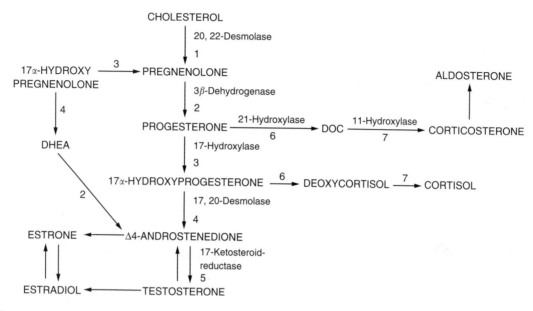

Fig. 34.18 Diagram of the enzyme steps necessary to convert cholesterol through its various intermediate stages to aldosterone, cortisol and testosterone. Note that 3β-dehydrogenase (labelled 2) is active at two places, as are 17-hydroxylase (labelled 3) 17,20-desmolase (labelled 4), 21-hydroxylase (labelled 6) and 11-hydroxylase (labelled 7).

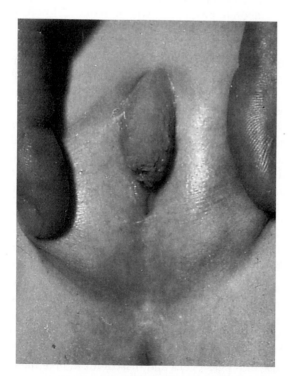

Fig. 34.19 The external genitalia of a child with CAH. Note the clitoral enlargement and the excessive fusion of labial folds which have resulted in only a single opening on the perineum.

When an infant is born with ambiguous genitalia, management also includes counselling the parents. It is helpful to reassure them that the child is healthy but there is a developmental anomaly of the genitalia. If the initial examination of the child fails to identify palpable gonads it is most likely that the child is female and the parents should be informed as such and the likelihood of CAH may be raised. The diagnosis must then be made with as much haste as possible to alleviate parental anxiety.

Investigation of a suspected case of CAH should include:

1 karyotyping, which may be performed on cord blood and results rapidly obtained;

2 measurement of 17α-hydroxyprogesterone in blood, which will be elevated in 21-hydroxylase deficiency;

3 examination of electrolytes to check the possibility of a salt-losing syndrome, and if the salt-losing state is present, sodium and chloride may be low and potassium raised; and

4 pelvic ultrasound to discover the presence of a uterus and vagina. This is not only reassuring to the parents, but highly indicative of the correct diagnosis.

The immediate management of such a child should always be undertaken by or in cooperation with the paediatrician. Cortisol or one of its related synthetic compounds must be given to suppress adrenocorticotrophic hormone secretion. If the child is a salt loser then salt loss must be very carefully controlled. For further management of the endocrine disorder the reader is referred to standard paediatric texts.

The surgical attention required for congenital adrenal hyperplasia patients has become extremely complex in recent years. In the past it has been standard practice to carry out two corrective procedures. First, the reduction

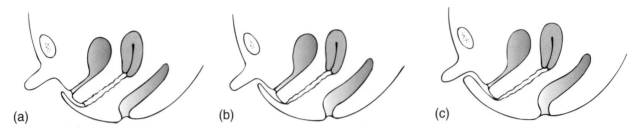

Fig. 34.20 Diagrammatic representation of clitoral enlargement and excessive fusion of labial folds to show (a) the different thickness of the folds, (b) the narrowing of the vagina in the most marked cases, and (c) variations in the point at which the urogenital sinus opens.

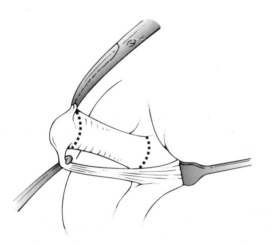

Fig. 34.21 Identification of the corpora cavernosa which are excised following preservation of the nerve and blood supply to the glans.

in the size of the clitoris if it is enlarged and, second, the division of the fused labial folds to expose the urethra and vagina beneath. Clitoral reduction which involves the removal of the shaft of the clitoris with preservation of the neurovascular bundle and the glands has been a standard procedure carried out by paediatric urologists for the last 30 years and has usually been carried out soon after birth or within the first few months of birth (Fig. 34.21). In collaboration with surgery to the labial folds, the fused labial folds may be divided and exposed (Fig. 34.22). However, these procedures have been carried out from a cosmetic point of view and also for the intention of deciding the gender of rearing and the physical reinforcement of that gender selection. A number of ethical issues have arisen in recent years challenging the practice of clitoral reduction. Minto *et al.* [21] reported that sexual function can be compromised following clitoral surgery suggesting all had sexual difficulty. While this study failed to address other reasons for sexual satisfaction other than the physical ability, it raises the question as to whether or not a surgical approach in early life is wise. Certainly, further

research is needed to ensure that the outcome for these individuals is optimized and individualized.

The division of the fused labial folds is simple if they are thin, when it may be performed at almost any age. However, in more complex cases, division at this early stage may give an indifferent result and the operation may need to be repeated later when the patient is beyond puberty, but surgery at this stage can be rather difficult. If the folds are very thick and especially if the vagina is narrowed more elaborate procedures will be required to open the introital ring and achieve a functional vaginal result.

Careful supervision by the paediatrician will be required throughout childhood such that normal menstrual and fertility patterns can be established. Grant *et al.* [22], in a review of menstrual and fertility patterns, indicated that menarche is often delayed by up to 2 years. The age of menarche is directly related to the hormonal control of the disease, although menstrual irregularity, including oligomenorrhoea and even amenorrhoea, may occur in spite of good control [23]. Fertility is reduced to some extent, although this seems to be a greater problem for salt losers [24].

OTHER CAUSES OF MASCULINIZATION IN GENETIC FEMALES

These cases of masculinized genetic females are now rare. There are cases of androgen-secreting tumours that have occurred in pregnancy, which have resulted in virilization of the fetus, especially luteomy [25], polycystic ovaries [26] and Krukenberg tumours [27]. The association between the use of progestogens and masculinization of the fetus is extremely rare.

It should be mentioned that the features of the genetic female masculinized from other androgen sources are not likely to be significantly different from those seen in CAH as far as the degree of masculinization is concerned (Fig. 34.23). There will, however, be no other metabolic defect and no salt-losing syndrome will be recognized but the management of such a case is to exclude CAH as the

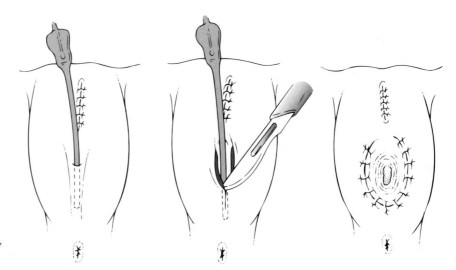

Fig. 34.22 Diagrammatic representation of division of fused labial folds. Courtesy of Dr R.R. Gordan and Bailliere Tindall.

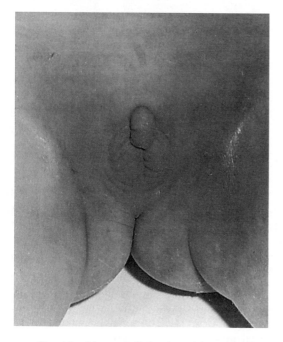

Fig. 34.23 Considerable masculinization of the external genitalia of a female child whose mother was treated with methyltestosterone in early pregnancy.

cause of the ambiguity and, having done this, the infant may be reared in her correct female role and surgical treatment carried out as for CAH. If no source of androgen can be identified, consideration must be given to the possibility of the child being a 46XX true hermaphrodite and if the degree of external masculinization is considerable it would be wise to consider gonadal biopsy. Rarely, no obvious androgenic source can be detected to explain the masculinization of the genitalia.

Male intersex and true hermaphrodites

If masculinization of a genetic female from CAH exogenous androgens has been excluded, which is done within the 1st week of life, distinction must be made between an undermasculinized male and a true hermaphrodite with ovarian and testicular tissue. The distinction can be made for certain only by laparotomy and gonadal biopsy. Laparoscopic biopsy is not adequate for establishing the nature of a gonad in an intersex child. The organ may be an ovotestis and, unless a representative biopsy is taken along the length of the gonad, it must be stressed that the biopsy of the gonad is not undertaken to determine what the sex of rearing should be. This decision is principally made on the suitability of external genitalia for sexual life in one or other gender role. It is necessary to know the nature of the gonad, however, so that if gonadal tissue is present which is inappropriate to the chosen gender role, as it always will be in a true hermaphrodite and in a male intersex being brought up as a female, gonadal tissue can be removed. Various conditions present under the general heading of male intersex and true hermaphroditism and these will now be considered.

XY FEMALES

Faults in androgen production

In this group of patients androgen production may fail from either anatomical or enzymatic testicular failure.

Anatomical testicular failure. Failure of normal testicular differentiation and development may be the result of a chromosome mosaicism affecting the sex chromosomes or possibly associated with an abnormal isochromosome [28], but usually the sex chromosomes appear to be normal and the condition is referred to as pure gonadal dysgenesis. Clinically such cases show variable features depending on how much testicular differentiation is present. Since differentiation is often poor, most patients have mild masculinization or none at all, and the uterus, tubes and vagina are generally present [29]. The presence of the uterus in this condition contrasts with the other forms of XY female described below.

Management of this group of patients is concerned with the reconstruction of the external genitalia in the manner described in previously and removal of the streak or rudimentary gonad in view of their raised potential for cancer. The degree of masculinization of such patients is often minimal and, if it is limited to a minor degree of clitoral enlargement with little or no fusion of the genital folds, surgery need not be undertaken. The risk of malignancy in the rudimentary testes is probably in the order of 30% and gonadal removal during childhood would be wise. Around the age of puberty replacement oestrogen–progestogen therapy must be started to produce secondary sexual development and menstruation.

Enzymatic testicular failure   Several metabolic steps are necessary for the complete formation of testosterone from cholesterol (Fig. 34.18). A number of biosynthetic defects have been reported at each stage of the process. As a result, clinical features are somewhat varied but since such enzyme defects are generally incomplete there is external genital ambiguity of varying degrees, the uterus, tubes and upper vagina being absent since the production of MIS by the testes is normal.

The decision on the sex of rearing will depend upon the degree of masculinization of the external genitalia but the female role is often the chosen one (Fig. 34.24). Surgical management is as already described. The identification of the precise enzyme defect can be difficult, but may be approached through human chorionic gonadotrophin stimulation of the gonads and measurement of various androgens to determine where the enzyme block occurs.

END-ORGAN INSENSITIVITY

In this group of conditions the end organ may be insensitive to androgen production because of 5α-reductase deficiency or from partial androgen insensitivity.

5α-Reductase deficiency

As described above, normal masculinization of the external genitalia requires the conversion of testosterone to dihydrotestosterone by 5α-reductase. Although the Wolffian structures respond directly to testosterone, in the presence of 5α-reductase deficiency a male infant will

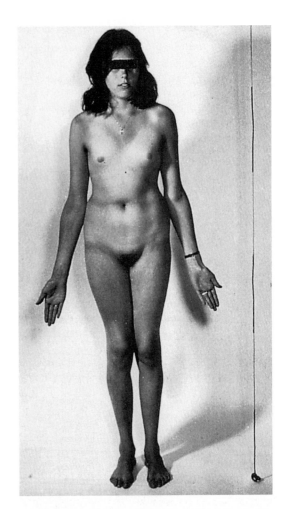

Fig. 34.24 A patient with enzymatic testicular failure believed to be due to 17-ketosteroid-reductase deficiency. Reproduced from [35] with permission.

have poor masculinization of external genitalia but the uterus, tubes and upper vagina will always be absent since MIS production will be normal. As a rule, the degree of genital masculinization is small or at worst moderate and most children are initially placed in the female role (Fig. 34.25). At puberty, however, the testes produce increased amounts of testosterone and there is greater virilization, perhaps to an extent that the patient may wish to change the gender role from female to male. Penis size tends to remain barely adequate, however, and the female gender role will often be a better one for such patients. 5α-Reductase deficiency is a familial disorder due to an autosomal recessive gene, so that the evidence of other similar affected members in the family often assists the diagnosis. If there is no such history, precise diagnosis may be attempted by human chorionic gonadotrophin stimulation of the gonad for 3 days with measurement of testosterone at the beginning and end of each test.

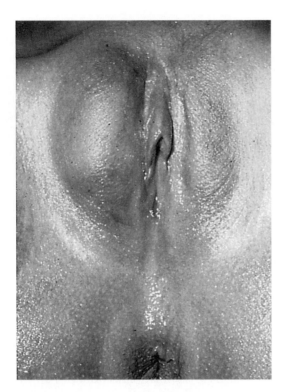

Fig. 34.25 The external genitalia of a 10-year-old 46XY child with 5α-reductase deficiency. Reproduced from [35] with permission.

Androgen insensitivity. This syndrome is seen only in the newborn if the enzyme defect giving rise to it is partial. Presentation in later life is described in p. 344 When patients in the partial form present at birth as of ambiguous sex, the principles of management are those outlined in p. 342 for 5α-reductase deficiency.

True hermaphrodites

True hermaphrodites are rare in Europe and the USA, but in some countries, notably South Africa, they appear to be much more common. They present with varying degrees of sexual ambiguity (Fig. 34.26) – maleness predominates in some patients, femaleness in others. In the majority the uterus and vagina are present. The karyotype in most true hermaphrodites is that of an apparently normal female (46XX); this occurred in 58% of the 172 cases reviewed by Van Niekerk [30] and Van Niekerk and Retief [31]. The next most frequent karyotype was 46XX/XY which appeared in 13%, followed by 46XY (11%) and 46XY/47XXY (6%) with other mosaics accounting for 10%.

Distribution of the gonads is interesting in that the commonest combination is for an ovotestis to be present on one side and an ovary on the other, with a testis on

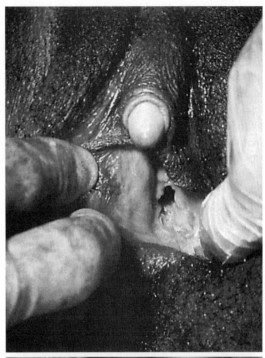
(a)

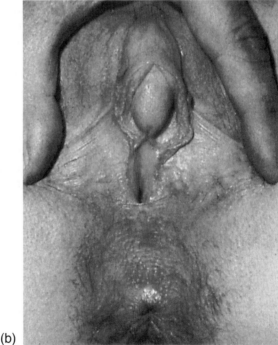
(b)

Fig. 34.26 External genitalia in two true hermaphrodites. (a) Behind a considerable degree of clitoral enlargement it is possible to identify the urethra (not shown in the figure) and the vagina, which is illustrated. (b) An equivalent amount of clitoral enlargement, but the excessive fusion of labial folds has led to only a single perineal opening and it is not possible to identify the urethra and vagina separately.

one side and an ovary on the other being almost as frequent. Ovotestis may be bilateral or combined with a testis. Diagnosis of true hermaphroditism can only be made by gonadal biopsy to demonstrate that ovarian and testicular tissue are both present. Sex of rearing is determined on the functional capability of the external genitalia, after which inappropriate organs are removed. In some cases it may be possible to identify the ovarian and testicular portions of an ovotestis for certain and to remove only that part which is unwanted. If this is not possible both must be removed. If the patient then requires to be brought up in the gender role for which there is no appropriate gonadal tissue replacement hormone therapy at puberty will be required.

Patients presenting after infancy

Doubt about an individual's sex may arise for the first time some years after birth, generally around puberty, when some heterosexual feature may become evident or a pre-existing minor feature becomes more profound. Sometimes an older patient is seen whose intersexual state had been recognized at birth but not investigated. The investigation of such patients follows the general pattern outlined above and is different in only minor respects. If, for example, a patient is seen with late-onset CAH about the time of puberty, the likelihood of a salt-losing syndrome is minimal and investigation of this aspect need not be intensive. Management is different in one particular and very important respect. The patient, of necessity, will have lived in one or other sex role for some time and may have become so well adjusted that no attempts should be made to change this gender role. This aspect of the matter is best illustrated by 46XY patients with androgen insensitivity discussed next. Such patients have no masculinization of external genitalia at all and in most instances are well-developed, phenotypic females. To suggest that they should change to the male role because they have male karyotypes and intra-abdominal testes would be the height of folly.

Androgen insensitivity

The intersexual condition most likely to be evident for the first time at or after puberty, but which may sometimes be encountered earlier in childhood, is the condition of androgen insensitivity. This was formerly known as testicular feminization. It will be evident from the discussion in p. 337 that there are several mechanisms by which a patient who has testes may be feminized, so this term is no longer appropriate. Since the basis of the condition is insensitivity to androgen, this term is a much more satisfactory one. The clinical picture of complete androgen insensitivity is remarkably uniform, although it now seems probable that two distinct mechanisms of insensitivity are present.

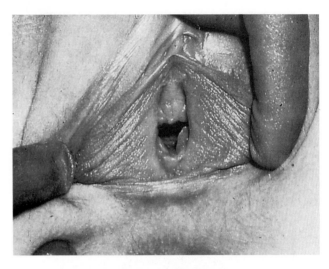

Fig. 34.27 The external genitalia of a patient with androgen insensitivity.

Most patients with androgen insensitivity present for the first time after puberty when, despite normal breast development, there is primary amenorrhoea. Further clinical examination will reveal absent or scanty pubic and axillary hair, a normal vulva (Fig. 34.27) but a short blind vagina with no cervix palpable. If a laparoscopy or laparotomy is performed, the uterus will be found to be absent and the testes are generally to be found within the abdomen in the inguinal canal or occasionally in the labia. Examination of the karyotype will disclose a normal 46XY male pattern.

Endocrine investigation reveals testosterone levels within the normal male range. Oestrogen levels are generally within the range where normal male and normal female values overlap. Luteinizing hormone values are generally elevated due, it is believed, to the insensitivity of the hypothalamus and the pituitary gland to testosterone. Follicle-stimulating hormone levels are more variable but are usually within the normal male range or slightly raised.

The aetiology of this condition may be due to complete absence of the gene for the androgen receptor or due to mutations or defects in the gene itself, leading to a receptor that cannot function. Thus the condition may be complete in those patients who have an absent androgen receptor whereby no interpretation of testosterone can occur at the cell membrane or in some cases, where the androgen receptor mutation is not complete, some receptivity may persist and, as a result of that, partial androgenization may occur. In these cases it is known as partial androgen insensitivity syndrome. Although most patients present some time after puberty because of primary amenorrhoea, the condition is occasionally seen in the child when a testis is found to occupy a hernial sac or when the presence of the

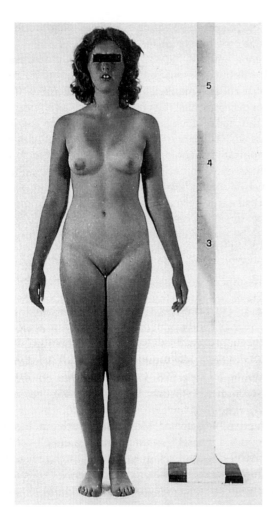

Fig. 34.28 The external appearance of a 46XY individual with androgen insensitivity. Note the excellent breast development and complete absence of pubic hair.

full blown syndrome in another sister leads to examination of a younger one and the male karyotype is revealed.

Management of the patient with androgen insensitivity depends upon the age at which the patient is seen. If seen after puberty when breast development is complete (Fig. 34.28), whether or not to remove the testes is considered. It seems likely that such patients have a raised potential for cancer, which is probably of the order of 5% during their lives [32]. Most would agree that this risk is sufficiently high to warrant gonadectomy and, therefore, this is advised. Discussion with the patient about the nature of her gonads will depend on the individual case. All patients should be informed of the nature of their condition when it is felt appropriate, but this depends on the maturity of the patient at the time of presentation. These women whose gonads are removed will question this procedure in the future. It is extremely important that

an appropriate explanation is given at the correct time. The clinician should take great care to ensure that the explanation given is correct and in appropriate language, so that the patient can understand the nature of her condition. It is important to emphasize that they are entirely female in spite of their chromosomal make up. Counselling of these women is often required and they should be referred to appropriate centres for management. None of these women should be left following gonadectomy without long-term follow-up and access to a specialist with an interest in this area.

Following gonadectomy, hormone replacement therapy with oestrogen should be given and this need not be cyclical since the uterus is absent. If the patient is seen for the first time in childhood and a diagnosis of complete androgen insensitivity is made, it can confidently be stated that feminization will occur at puberty and nothing need be done until that time. If, however, there are heterosexual features present it is very likely that masculinization will occur to some extent at puberty. This will have a profound psychological effect on the patient when she has been brought up in the female role. In these circumstances gonadectomy in childhood is wise, followed by induction of puberty with hormone replacement therapy at the appropriate time (Fig. 34.29). Surgery is seldom necessary in these women to elongate the vagina as it is usually functional, but should elongation be required graduated dilatation using Frank's procedure is the treatment of choice.

Other disorders encountered in the older patient

When the disorders discussed in pp. 337–334 as presenting at birth are seen in later life, certain differences in clinical features of management must be emphasized. The patient with CAH who has been reared as a female is unlikely to have sufficient masculinization of the external genitalia (Fig. 34.30) so reconstructive surgery is less commonly necessary. Secondary sexual development is apt to be poor or absent, but once the diagnosis has been made and the condition controlled by cortisol, spontaneous secondary sexual development should follow. If, however, a serious error has been made at birth because of an extreme degree of masculinization, the child being placed in the male role, management depends entirely upon the orientation of the patient to the male sex. If this is good and the phallus of a size judged suitable for intercourse, it may be wiser to allow the patient to continue in that gender role. It should be remembered, however, that if cortisol is used to inhibit the excess adrenocorticotrophic hormone activity, the apparent male will probably begin to menstruate so total hysterectomy and oophorectomy will be needed,

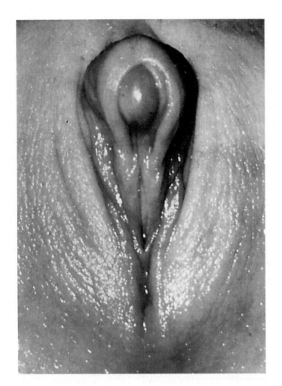

Fig. 34.29 External genitalia of a 7-year-old 46XY child with a degree of masculinization. Reproduced from [35] with permission.

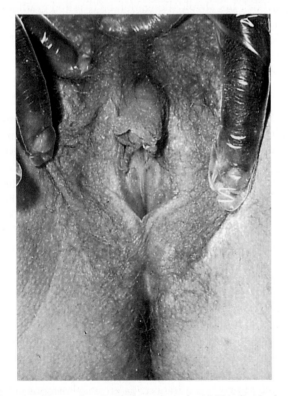

Fig. 34.30 External genital appearance of a 46XX individual with CAH seen for the first time at the age of 16 years.

testosterone should be administered and, if appropriate, a testicular prosthesis inserted.

Patients with 5α-reductase deficiency placed in the female role but otherwise untreated are likely to have male type puberty and may wish to change sex. An extremely difficult decision must then be made since, as already indicated, the phallic size is seldom sufficient for coitus. Many patients wish to change their gender role nonetheless, and this important psychological aspect of management must be fully assessed in deciding what to do for the best.

Menstruation and/or breast development may occur at puberty in a true hermaphrodite who has been thought to be male. In such a case, the adjustment to masculinity is likely to be good so mastectomy and hysterectomy with the removal of the ovary will be indicated.

Two other conditions require brief mention, although they are unlikely to be seen by the gynaecologist. Phenotypic males are rarely found to have a 46XX karyotype. Wachtel and Bard [33] refer to more than 80 cases reported in the literature. Those who have been appropriately examined have been shown to be H-Y antigen-positive and there is little clinical ambiguity in this group, the external genitalia being generally normal, although underdeveloped, and hypospadias has been mentioned several times.

Isolated deficiency of Müllerian inhibition has also been reported but such cases do not present clinically as examples of doubtful sex unless some unrelated surgical procedure reveals the surprising presence of Müllerian structures in an otherwise normal or near normal male.

References

1. Sinclair AH, Berta P, Palmer MS, Hawkins JR, Griffiths BL, Smith MJ, Foster JW, Frischauf AM, Lovell-Badge R, Goodfellow PN (1990) A gene from the human sex determining region encodes a protein with homology to DNA-binding motif. *Nature* **346**, 240–4.

Bennett MJ & Dewhurst CJ (1983) The use of ultrasound in the management of congenital malformations of the genital tract. *Pediatr Adolesc Gynecol* **1**, 25–8.

2. Simpson JL (1987) Genetic control of sex differentiation. *Semin Reprod Med* **5**, 209–20.

3. Elias S, Simpson JL, Carson SA *et al.* (1984) Genetic studies in incomplete Müllerian fusion. *Obstet Gynecol* **63**, 276–81.

4. Baker TG (1963) A quantitative and cytological study of germ cells in human ovaries. *Proc R Soc* **158**, 417–28.

5. Pryse-Davies J & Dewhurst CJ (1971) The development of the ovary and uterus in the fetus, newborn and infant. *J Pathol* **103**, 5–25.

6. Edmonds DK (2003) Congenital malformations of the genital tract and their management. *Best Pract Res Clin Obstet Gynaecol* **17**, 19–40.

7. Frank RT (1938) The formation of the artificial vagina without operation. *Am J Obstet Gynecol* **35**, 1053–6.

8. Broadbent RT & Woolf RM (1984) Non-operative construction of the vagina. *Plast Reconstr Surg* **73**, 117–22.

9. Nadarajah S, Quek J, Rose GL, Edmonds DK (2005) Sexual function in women treated with dilators for vaginal agenesis. *J Pediater Adolesc Gynecol* **18**, 39–42.

10. McIndoe AH & Bannister JB (1938) An operation for the cure of congenital absence of the vagina. *J Obstet Gynaecol Br Commonwlth* **45**, 490–5.

11. Morton KE & Dewhurst CJ (1986) Human amnion in the treatment of vaginal malformations. *Br J Obstet Gynaecol* **93**, 50–4.

12. Edmonds DK (2000) Congenital malformations of the genital tract. *Obstet Gynecol Clin N Am* **27**, 49–62.

13. Williams EA (1964) Congenital absence of the vagina. A simple operation for its relief. *J Obstet Gynaecol Br Commonwlth* **71**, 511–17.

14. Edmonds DK (2001) Sexual developmental anomalies and their reconstruction upper and lower tracts. In: Sanfilippo JS (ed.) *Pediatric and Adolescent Gynecology*, 2nd edn. Philadelphia: Saunders, 553–83.

15. Josso N, Picard JY & Tran D (1977) The anti-Müllerian hormone. *Recent Prog Horm Res* **33**, 117–60.

16. Dupont B, Obefield SE, Smithwik EM *et al.* (1977) Close genetic linkage between HLA and congenital adrenal hyperplasis. *Lancet* **ii**, 1309–12.

17. Bias WB, Urban MD, Migeon CJ *et al.* (1981) Intra HLA recommendations localising the 21-hydroxylase deficiency gene within the HLA complex. *Hum Immunol* **2**, 139–45.

18. Donohoue PA, Van Dop C, Jospe N & Migeon CJ (1986) Congenital adrenal hyperplasia – molecular mechanisms resulting in 21-hydroxylase deficiency. *Acta Endocrinol* **279**(Suppl), 315–20.

19. Werkmeister JW, New MI, Dupont B *et al.* (1986) Frequent deletions and duplications of the 21-hydroxylase genes. *Am J Hum Genet* **39**, 461–8.

20. Amor M, New MI & Wite PC (1987) A single base change in the OH21-B gene causing steroid 21-hydroxylase deficiency. *Endocrinology* **120** (suppl.), 272–4.

21. Minto CL, Laio KL, Conway GS & Creighton SM (2003) Sexual function in women with complete androgen insensitivity syndrome. *Fertil Steril* **80**, 157–64.

22. Grant D, Muram D & Dewhurst J (1983) Menstrual and fertility patterns in patients with congenital adrenal hyperplasia. *Pediatr Adolesc Gynecol* **1**, 97–103.

23. Klingensmith GJ, Jones HW & Blizzard RM (1977) Glucocorticoid treatment of girls with congenital adrenal hyperplasia: effect on height, sexual maturation and fertility. *J Pediatr* **90**, 996–1004.

24. Mulaikal RM, Migeon CJ & Rock JA (1987) Fertility rates in female patients with congenital adrenal hyperplasia due to 21-hydroxylase deficiency. *N Engl J Med* **316**, 178–81.

25. Hensleigh PA & Woodrugg DA (1978) Differential maternal fetal response to androgenising luteoma. *Obstet Gynecol Surv* **33**, 262–71.

26. Fayez JA, Bunch TR & Miller GL (1974) Virilisation in pregnancy associated with polycystic ovaries. *Obstet Gynecol* **44**, 511–21.

27. Forrest MG, Orgiazzi J, Tranchant D *et al.* (1978) Approach to the mechanism of androgen production in a case of Krukenberg tumour during pregnancy. *J Clin Endocrinol Metab* **47**, 428–34.

28. Simpson JL (1976) *Disorders of Sexual Differentiation.* New York: Academic Press, 199.

29. Edmonds DK (1989) Intersexuality. In: *Dewhurst's Practical Paediatric and Adolescent Gynaecology*. London: Butterworths, 17–20.

30. Van Niekerk W (1976) True hermaphroditism. *Am J Obstet Gynecol* **126**, 890–907.

31. Van Niekerk W & Retief A (1981) The gonads of human true hermaphrodites. *Hum Genet* **58**, 117–22.

32. Jones HW & Scott WW (1971) Male pseudohermaphroditism. In *Hermaphroditism, Genital Anomalies and Related Endocrine Disorders*, 2nd edn. Baltimore, MD: Williams & Wilkins, 261–75.

33. Wachtel SS & Bard J (1981) The 46XX male. In: Josso N (ed.) *The Intersex Child*. Basel: Karger, 116.

34. Jirasek JE & Leigh Simpson J (1976) *Disorders of Sexual Differentiation*. New York: Academic Press.

35. Dewhurst CJ (1980) *Practical Paediatric and Adolescent Gynaecology*. New York: Marcel Dekker.

Further reading

Gidwani G & Falconi T (1999) *Congenital Malformations of the Female Genital Tract. Diagnosis and Management*. Philadelphia: Lippincott, Williams and Wilkins.

Sanfilippo J (1999) *Pediatric and Adolescent Gynecology*. Philadelphia: W.B. Saunders.

Chapter 35: The menstrual cycle

William L. Ledger

Introduction

The human female is monotocous. The complex and highly regulated sequence of events that manifests as regular monthly menstruation exists to ensure that only one oocyte is ovulated in any one cycle and that implantation of an early embryo can arrest the process of endometrial shedding and ensure its survival. Monthly menstruation is an obvious marker that the various levels of interaction between hypothalamus, pituitary, ovary and uterus are functional. Interruption of this axis at any point leads to disordered menses. Gynaecologists will frequently have to investigate and treat such disorders. A clear understanding of the regulation of the normal cycle is therefore necessary to guide rational management when things go wrong.

Although termed the 'menstrual cycle', since menstruation is the obvious monthly event during reproductive life, the normal menstrual cycle is mostly a reflection of ovarian events. The selection and growth of the dominant follicle leads to increasing concentrations of oestrogens in the blood, stimulating endometrial growth. Later, following the luteinizing hormone (LH) surge, ovarian oestrogens and progesterone from the corpus luteum induce endometrial secretory changes and the decline in luteal steroid production in the absence of pregnancy leads to the onset of menstruation. Hence a description of clinical relevance of the menstrual cycle should focus on ovarian physiology, while not overlooking events in the hypothalamus and pituitary and at the level of the uterus.

The menstrual cycle is regulated at both endocrine and paracrine levels. Endocrinologically, there are classical feedback loops that modulate release of gonadotropin hormones from the pituitary with the ovarian steroids as the afferent arm. More recent studies have begun to elaborate a complex series of paracrine processes that operate within the tissues of the ovary and uterus to impose local regulation.

Step one: ensuring monovulation

Folliculogenesis and the 'Follicular Phase'

At birth, the human ovaries contain approximately 1,000,000 primordial follicles, arrested at prophase of the first meiotic division. This number already reflects considerable attrition from the maximum size of about 7,000,000 in the follicle 'pool' at 5 months of fetal life [1]. Further depletion of the follicle pool will continue throughout reproductive life, with regular escape of follicles from the primordial 'resting phase' by re-entry into meiosis. The process of 'escape' from the resting state is not dependent on extra-ovarian influences: follicle depletion occurs before and after menarche, during use of the oral contraceptive pill and during pregnancy and whether or not regular menstruation occurs. The majority of follicles will never develop beyond the pre-antral stage, travelling instead towards atresia. Of the original pool of 7,000,000 primordial follicles, only about 400 will ever acquire gonadotropin receptors and the possibility of ovulation. This dramatic attrition defines the female arm of natural selection, mirrored by the huge 'wastage' of spermatogenesis in the male in which millions of sperm are produced each day during fertile life with only a tiny proportion ever fertilizing an oocyte.

The early stages of follicle development in the human are independent of gonadotropins. Studies using transgenic animal species have begun to elucidate the contribution of locally acting intra-ovarian paracrine regulators of primordial follicle development including growth differentiation factor-9 (GDF-9), anti-Mullerian hormone (AMH) and the Bax family of regulators of apoptosis (Table 35.1).

Such studies are of more than theoretical interest: understanding the mechanisms regulating rate of entry into the pool of growing follicles should help to explain such common clinical problems as 'idiopathic' premature ovarian failure and early onset of menopause, as

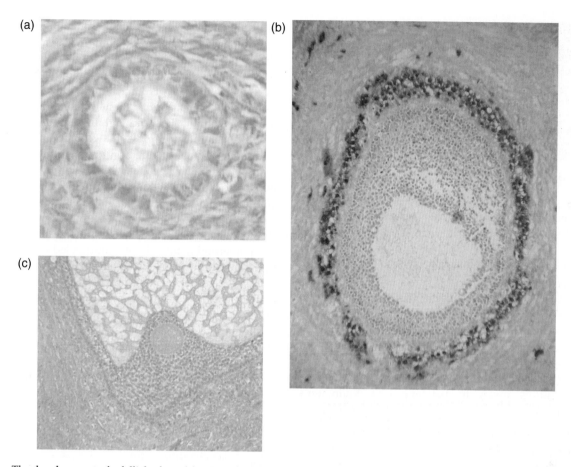

Fig. 35.1 The development of a follicle, from (a) primordial, (b) small antral and (c) pre-ovulatory stages. (a) The primordial follicle is surrounded by a single layer of undifferentiated epithelial cells and is insensitive to gonadotropins. (b) The early antral follicle has well-differentiated theca (immunostained brown) and granulosa cell layers surrounding the developing antral cavity with the oocyte. (c) The pre-ovular follicle with the oocyte surrounded by the cumulus oophorus with well-differentiated granulosa and theca cell layers.

Table 35.1 Specific gene 'knockouts' and their effects on ovarian function in the mouse

Transgenic/mutant mouse	Ovarian phenotype
c-kit deficiency, *Kit ligand* deficiency	Loss of germ cells (migration/proliferation failure)
Zfx, Atm, Dazla knockout	Loss of germ cells (proliferation failure)
WT-1 knockout	Failure of gonadal development
GDF-9 knockout	Folliculogenesis arrest (primary stage)
IGF-1 knockout	Folliculogenesis arrest (before antral follicle stage)
Fsh-β knockout	Folliculogenesis arrest (preantral stage)
ER-knockout	Failure to ovulate
Wnt-4 knockout	Reduced germ cell number masculinization

well as suggesting means of prolonging the reproductive lifespan.

Once a developing follicle reaches the pre-antral stage of development, further progression to the antral and pre-ovulatory stages appear to be absolutely dependant upon the presence of gonadotropins. The temporary elevation in circulating concentration of follicle stimulating hormone (FSH) seen in the early follicular phase of the ovarian cycle allows a limited number of pre-antral follicles to reach this stage of maturity, creating a 'cohort' of practically synchronously developing follicles. However, only one 'lead' follicle will acquire significant aromatase enzyme activity within its granulosa cells, leading to increased synthesis and secretion of oestradiol from androgenic precursor. The 'two-cell, two gonadotropin' hypothesis specifies the need for both LH, to stimulate production of precursor androgens, particularly androstenedione, by the theca cell layer, with FSH driving aromatization to oestradiol within

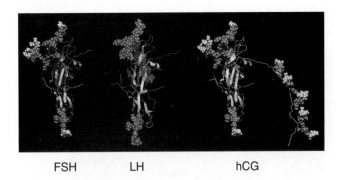

FSH   LH   hCG

Fig. 35.2 Molecular structure of FSH, LH and hCG.
(Reproduced by kind permission of Dr Bernadette Mannaerts,
Organon Ltd.)

the adjacent granulosa cell layer [3]. FSH, LH and hCG
(human chorionic gonadotropin) are structurally similar,
sharing an identical alpha subunit. Their specificity lies in
structural differences in the beta subunit (Fig. 35.2). Hence
assays for these molecules use antibodies directed against
beta-subunit epitopes.

The necessity for both LH and FSH at this stage of
the cycle is demonstrated when exogenous gonadtrophin
replacement is given to patients with Kallmann's
syndrome. These patients are unable to secrete gona-

dotropins into the circulation, but have normal ovarian
physiology. The results of a study of such a patient are
shown in Fig. 35.3. The patient had Kallmann's syndrome
with anosmia, primary amenorrhoea and hypogonadal
hypogonadism. Ovulation induction was undertaken
using two different preparations of gonadotropin. Treatment with both FSH and LH in the form of human
menopausal gonadotropins (HMG) induces both normal
follicle growth, monitored by transvaginal ultrasound
(bottom panel) and oestradiol secretion (top left panel),
leading to high luteal phase progesterone concentrations
after an artificial LH surge with hCG injection. This indicates that successful ovulation and luteinization occurred.
In contrast, treatment with FSH in the absence of LH,
using a recombinant FSH preparation led to identical follicle development on ultrasound but little elevation in
circulating oestradiol concentration in the phase of follicular growth and no increase in progesterone after hCG
injection.

The pituitary secretes the gonadotropin hormones LH
and FSH in response to pulses of gonadotropin releasing hormone (GnRH) from the hypothalamus, which
travel to the anterior pituitary via the hypothalamo-
hypophyseal portal tract. LH secretion appears to be

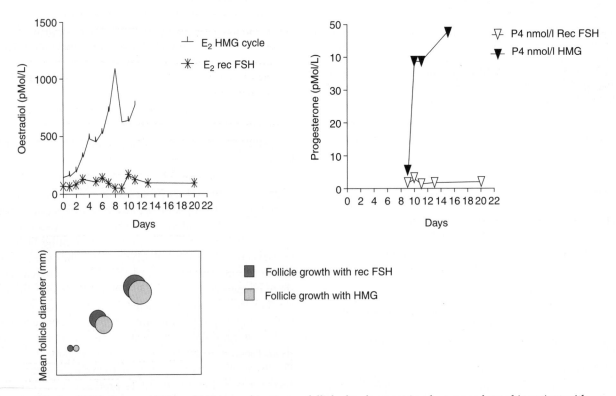

Fig. 35.3 Effects of FSH alone and FSH and LH in combination on follicle development in a hypogonadotrophic patient with
Kallmann's Syndrome. (Reproduced with kind permission from Dr Gillian Lockwood).

(a)

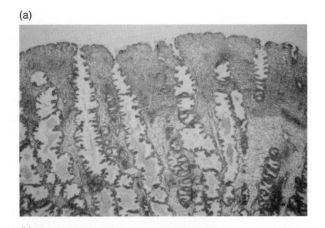

(b)

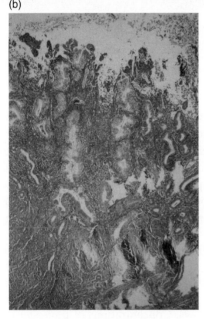

Fig. 35.4 Histological appearance of (a) late secretory and (b) menstrual endometrium (see p. 354). (Courtesy of Professor M Wells, University of Sheffield.)

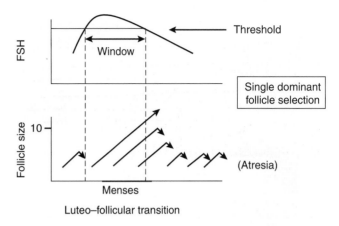

Fig. 35.5 The 'threshold concept' illustrating dependance of advanced follicle growth and maturation on a rise in circulating FSH concentration above an arbitrary threshold, with subsequent suppression of FSH preventing multiple follicle development. (Reproduced with kind permission from 'Archives of Medical Research', [5].)

closely regulated by GnRH pulsatility, while secretion of FSH is co-regulated by hypothalamic GnRH and other factors which act directly on the pituitary, possibly including the inhibins and activins. In the normal follicular phase, GnRH pulse frequency is approximately once per 90 min. GnRH pulses are less frequent in the luteal phase, occurring approximately once in 4 h.

Disorders that slow GnRH pulsatility, such as anorexia nervosa, result in failure of secretion of pituitary gonadotropins and a state of hypogonadal hypogonadism with undetectable serum LH and FSH and amenorrhoea.

Once the concentration of serum oestradiol begins to rise in the mid-follicular phase, there is a rapid suppression of pituitary FSH production by negative feedback. Recent studies have suggested that suppression of pituitary FSH secretion in the follicular phase might be co-mediated by rising serum concentrations of inhibin B, a glycoprotein secreted by the granulosa cells of the developing dominant follicle. It is perhaps not surprising that a dual mechanism to control follicular phase FSH secretion has evolved [4]. The resulting decrease in circulating concentration of FSH withdraws gonadotropin 'drive' from the remainder of the growing cohort of follicles. The result is progression to atresia for all but the dominant follicle, leading to mono-ovulation.

The mechanism by which this selection of a single dominant follicle occurs has been described by the 'threshold' concept, in which the rising concentration of FSH exceeds the threshold and thereby opens a 'window' allowing one follicle to continue growth and development. Suppression of FSH concentration then closes the window, preventing growth of multiple mature follicles (Fig. 35.5).

The threshold concept is useful in understanding the pitfalls of 'superovulation', in which daily injections of high doses of FSH are given as part of *in vitro* fertilization (IVF) treatment. The aim is to produce a cohort of eight or more mature follicles suitable for ultrasound guided oocyte retrieval. However, if the follicle pool is small (e.g. if the patient is nearing menopause), then the yield of mature follicles will be disappointing, while if the follicle pool is large (e.g. if the patient has polycystic ovary syndrome), then there is a danger of over-response with hyper-stimulation syndrome.

(a)
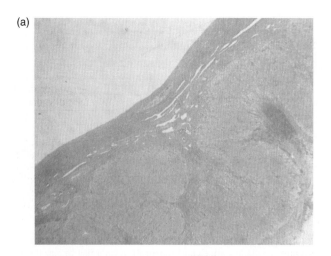

(b)
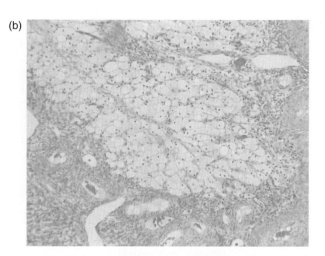

Fig. 35.6 The histological appearances of the corpus luteum, showing (a) an active corpus luteum and (b) regression of the corpus luteum with histiocyte infiltration. (Kindly provided by Professor M Wells, University of Sheffield.)

Step two: ensuring maintenance of very early pregnancy

The LH surge and ovulation

Final maturation of the oocyte only occurs after initiation of the LH surge. This ensures that the oocyte is mature and ready for fertilization when released from the follicle. The LH surge represents a coordinated discharge of LH from the gonadotroph cells of the anterior pituitary. This occurs in response to the rapid rise in oestradiol during the latter days of the follicular phase of the ovarian cycle. Pulses of GnRH from the hypothalamus increase in both magnitude and frequency, triggering the LH surge with a rapid outpouring of LH and, to a lesser extent, FSH from the anterior pituitary.

The LH surge is also preceded by a rise in serum concentration of progesterone. The contribution of this rise to the peri-ovulatory phase of the cycle is unclear, but prevention of the pre-ovular rise in serum progesterone concentration using the progesterone receptor antagonist mifepristone prevents efficient ovulation. Compounds with effects similar to mifepristone are being tested as possible contraceptive agents, possibly acting both by inhibiting ovulation and implantation.

The LH surge initiates final maturation of the oocyte with completion of meiosis and extrusion of the first polar body, which contains one of the two haploid sets of chromosomes from the oocyte. The LH surge also induces an inflammatory type reaction at the apex of the follicle adjacent to the outer surface of the ovarian cortex. A process of new blood vessel formation, with associated release of prostaglandins (PGs) and cytokines leads to rupture of the follicle wall and ovulation about 38 h after the initiation of the LH surge. A chemotactic effect of ovarian cytokines draws the fimbria of the Fallopian tube to within close proximity to the rupturing follicle. A thin mucus strand seems to join the mouth of the Fallopian tube to the ovular follicle, forming a bridge for transit of the oocyte into the tube.

The 'empty' follicle rapidly fills with blood and the theca and granulosa cell layers of the follicle wall luteinize, with formation of the corpus luteum (Fig. 35.6). A rapid synthesis of progesterone, along with oestradiol, follows. Concentrations of progesterone in serum rise to above 25 nmol/l, one of the highest concentrations seen for any hormone in the circulation. These concentrations rise still further if pregnancy follows.

Endometrial development during the menstrual cycle and early pregnancy

Progression through the follicular phase of the cycle is characterized by appearance of increasing amounts of oestradiol in the circulation. This acts on the basalis layer of endometrium, which persists from cycle to cycle in contrast to the monthly shedding of the more superficial layers of endometrium. The new, proliferative endometrium grows rapidly under the influence of oestradiol, in synchrony with the growth and maturation of the oocyte and its follicle. An organized architecture appears, with

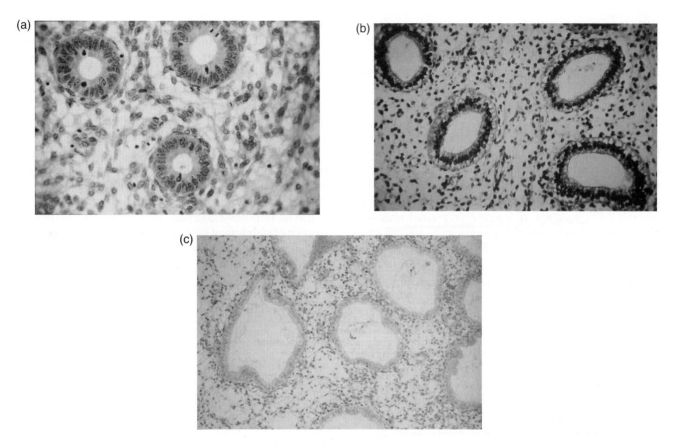

Fig. 35.7 The histological appearances of the endometrial cycle, showing proliferative, early secretory, mid-secretory phases equivalent to the images a, b and c. (Kindly provided by Professor M Wells, University of Sheffield.)

endometrial glands and stromal compartments, in preparation for the development of secretory endometrium permissive of implantation following the LH surge, luteinization of the ruptured follicle and formation of the corpus luteum, with secretion of large amounts of progesterone.

A key element in growth of healthy endometrium is formation of new blood vessels (endometrial angiogenesis), which seems to occur by elongation and expansion from pre-existing small vessels in the basalis. Endometrial angiogenesis can be divided into three stages, first during menstruation to reform the vascular bed, second, during the proliferative phase to develop endometrial vascular supply, and finally with spiral arteriole growth and coiling with the aim of providing an adequately vascularized site for implantation (Fig. 35.7) [6]. Therefore, in contrast to most vascular beds, which keep a persistent structure throughout life, the endometrial vascular network grows and regresses during each menstrual cycle. Numerous angiogenic and angiostatic factors have been identified in the human endometrium. Most

of these studies have focused on vascular endothelial growth factor (VEGF) and interleukins, which may be directly responsive to changing concentrations of ovarian steroids.

The development of a healthy secretory endometrium is essential for implantation and successful development of pregnancy. In the human, the oocyte is fertilized in the ampullary portion of the Fallopian tube and then travels to enter the uterus on day 3, at the morula stage of development. The blastocyst, with distinct trophectoderm and inner cell mass, forms on day 4. The blastocyst sheds the zona pellucida and then adheres to the endometrial epithelium, beginning the process of implantation. Implantation is the first step in the interaction between the cells of the blastocyst and endometrium, that is, between the mother and the fetus. Hence this interaction is critical to successful pregnancy, and a number of endometrial proteins have been identified as potential regulators of blastocyst development and implantation. These include endometrial integrins, glycosylated cell adhesion molecule 1 (GlyCAM-1) and osteopontin [7]. Continuous exposure of the endometrium to progesterone in early pregnancy downregulates progesterone receptors in the epithelium, a process which is associated with loss of the cell-surface mucin MUC1 and induction of secreted adhesion proteins. 'Rescue' of the corpus luteum by hCG secreted from the trophoblast of the developing pregnancy is essential for its continuance.

Interruption of progesterone synthesis and secretion by the corpus luteum, for example, using the progesterone receptor antagonist mifepristone, is used in clinical practice to induce termination of early pregnancy. In contrast, 'luteal phase support' in the form of hCG injection or injected or vaginal progestogens is used to support IVF pregnancies, since normal luteinization is interrupted by the GnRH agonist drugs used to prevent premature LH surges and unwanted ovulation.

Menstruation

Menstruation refers to the shedding of the superficial layers of the endometrium, with subsequent repair in preparation for regrowth from the basalis layer. Menstruation is initiated by a fall in circulating concentration of progesterone that follows luteal regression – failure of 'rescue' of the corpus luteum by an implanted early pregnancy. Luteal progesterone synthesis is dependent on LH from the pituitary gland. During luteolysis, progesterone secretion falls despite maintained serum concentrations of LH, since the corpus luteum becomes less sensitive to gonadotrophic support and becomes increasingly unable to maintain production of progesterone. In contrast, in a conception cycle, the increasing block to progesterone synthesis is overcome by the rapidly increasing concentrations of hCG which act on the corpus luteum through its LH receptors.

In the immediate pre-menstrual phase, progesterone withdrawal activates a complex series of intrauterine signals which include expression of chemotactic factors, which draw leucocytes into the uterus, expression of matrix metalloproteinase (MMP) enzymes, PGs and other compounds that act on the uterine vessels and smooth muscle. The 'invasion' of leucocytes and subsequent expression of inflammatory mediators has led to menstruation being likened to an inflammatory event [8,9]. The PGs of the E and F series are present in high concentrations in the endometrium and their synthesis is regulated by the ovarian steroids. Increased production of $PGF_{2\alpha}$ produces the myometrial contractions and vasoconstriction seen at menstruation, while E series PGs increase pain and

oedema, and are vasodilatory. PGE_2 also appears to induce synthesis of the cytokine IL-8 (interleukin-8), another key inflammatory and chemotactic mediator [10]. Pronounced vasoconstriction in turn leads to localized tissue hypoxia, further reinforcing release of inflammatory mediators. The end result of this cascade of events is constriction of the spiral arterioles with contraction of the uterine muscle, leading to expulsion of the shed tissue (Fig. 35.4).

These studies have clear relevance to clinical management of menorrhagia and other menstrual disorders. Inhibitors of PG synthesis are widely used in these conditions, with good scientific basis. However, PG synthesis is also an important component of ovulation, and use of powerful inhibitors of PG synthesis, such as non-steroidal anti-inflammatory agents, can lead to anovular cycles and involuntary infertility.

Conclusion

Although complex, the endocrine and paracrine events that regulate the normal ovarian and uterine cycles are well understood. This chapter illustrates several examples by which understanding of the basic physiology of the cycle has led to scientifically based therapeutics. Further exploration of these regulatory mechanisms will produce new approaches to diagnosis and treatment for gynaecologists and their patients.

References

1. Baker TC (1963) A quantitative and cytological study of germ cells in human ovaries. *Proc R Soc Biol* **158**, 417.
2. Block E (1951) Quantitative morphological investigations of the follicular system in women. *Acta Endocrinol* **8**, 33.
3. Baird DT (1987) A model for follicular selection and ovulation: lessons from superovulation. *J Steroid Biochem* **27**, 1.
4. Groome NP, Illingworth PJ, O'Brien M *et al.* (1996) Measurement of dimeric inhibin B throughout the human menstrual cycle. *J Clin Endocrinol Metab* **81**, 1401–5.
5. Macklon NS & Fauser BCJM (2001) Follicle-stimulating hormone and advanced follicle development in the human. *Arch Med Res* **32**, 595–600.
6. Rogers PAW & Gargett CE (1999) Endometrial angiogenesis. *Angiogenesis* **2**, 287–29.

7. Lessey BA (2002) Adhesion molecules and implantation. *J Reprod Immunol* **55**, 101–12.

8. Kelly RW (1994) Pregnancy maintenance and parturition: the role of prostaglandin in manipulating the immune and inflammatory response. *Endocr Rev* **15**, 684–706.

9. Kelly RW, King AE & Critchley HOD (2001) Cytokine control in human endometrium. *Reproduction* **121**, 3–19.

10. Sales KJ & Jabbour HN (2003) Cyclooxygenase enzymes and prostaglandins in pathology of the endometrium. *Reproduction* **126**, 559–67.

Chapter 36: The role of ultrasound in gynaecology

Joanne Topping

Introduction

The introduction of ultrasound into medicine and specifically into gynaecology has been an important development in the diagnosis and management of many common gynaecological disorders. Its use has revolutionized the management of problems in early pregnancy, decreased the need for more invasive procedures in postmenopausal and dysfunctional uterine bleeding and allowed significant advances in the management of infertility with ultrasound guided techniques in *in vitro* fertilization (IVF). Ultrasound examination of the pelvis is one of the most commonly used interventions in gynaecology at the present time.

The impact of 3D real-time imaging in gynaecology has yet to be fully investigated; this chapter will therefore concentrate on 2D real-time imaging.

Knowledge of the basic principles of ultrasound allows the operator to understand how the machine acquires an image and this leads to appropriate use of the controls to obtain the best possible image quality. It should also ensure the operator understands that high levels of ultrasound can produce biological damage such as cavitation and heating.

Ultrasound techniques

Ultrasound is so named because the sound waves are of such a high frequency (above 20 kHz) that they cannot be heard by the human ear. Higher frequency probes produce a narrower beam width; this allows better resolution but poorer penetration and, therefore, should be used for structures close to the probe. In gynaecology transabdominal (TA) probes tend to range from 3 to 5 MHz and transvaginal (TV) probes from 5 to 8.0 MHz.

The advantages and disadvantages of the TA versus TV route of ultrasound scanning are well known and summarized here (Table 36.1). Transvaginal ultrasound is the method of choice for the assessment of problems in early pregnancy and pelvic pain. Transabdominal scanning,

Table 36.1 Transabdominal versus transvaginal route of ultrasound scanning

Advantages	Disadvantages
Transabdominal ultrasound	
Wide field of view	Requires full bladder
Non-invasive	Low probe frequency
Suitable for large masses	therefore poorer resolution
Suitable for all ages	Bowel gas may obscure view
Chaperone not required	Images affected by maternal
	habitus
Transvaginal ultrasound	
High probe frequency giving	Internal examination
increased resolution of pelvic	Possible discomfort
structures	Not suitable for all patients
Diagnosis of early pregnancy	Chaperone required
viability approximately	
1 week before TA scan	
Empty bladder	
Not dependant on habitus	

however, is the only technique available for examining those women who are unable to tolerate a vaginal examination. It is also the technique of choice for assessing large pelvic masses. Thus, it is important that any practitioner performing ultrasound examinations is comfortable with both approaches.

Transvaginal method

The bladder needs to be empty (even a small amount of urine in the bladder can displace the pelvic organs), and women should be asked to empty their bladder before the examination begins. A small amount of gel is applied to the transducer tip and the tip and shaft of the probe covered with a non-spermicidal condom; apply a small amount of lubricant gel to allow easy insertion of the probe. When a transvaginal examination is being performed, palpation can be used to modify the position of pelvic structures to optimize the image quality.

Transabdominal method

To perform a pelvic ultrasound using the abdominal route requires the woman to have a full bladder, this pushes the uterus out of the pelvis; acts as an acoustic window and displaces bowel superiorly so preventing gas from the bowel scattering the ultrasound beam. When performing longitudinal scans with TA approach, the bladder is conventionally shown on the right of the image on the ultrasound monitor.

The position and relationship of the female pelvic organs varies considerably. The large size and central position of the uterus allows it to be used as a landmark for orientation. The uterine wall consists of three layers, the parametrium, myometrium and endometrium. The parametrium is highly echogenic and allows the uterus to be clearly outlined on ultrasound. The myometrium is the muscular layer of the uterus, which is normally homogenous and echodense. The echogenicity of other structures, for example, ovarian cysts are compared to that of the myometrium.

The role of ultrasound

Ultrasound is an extension of the clinical examination in gynaecology; it is unlikely that a woman with a normal pelvic examination and negative ultrasound has a significant gynaecological abnormality. Ultrasound should only be used when there is a clinical question to be answered. Incidental findings such as ovarian cysts are not uncommon in asymptomatic women and if ultrasound findings are taken in isolation they can be misleading.

Investigation of pelvic mass

Ultrasound is of paramount importance in evaluating a suspected pelvis mass. It is particularly useful when the mass is not well defined or when pelvic examination is limited by discomfort or patient habitus. The assessment of a pelvic mass is a good demonstration that neither the TA or TV route of examination should be used at the exclusion of the other; rather the two techniques are complimentary. The TA route allows for assessment of large tumours (beyond the range of the vaginal probe), evaluation of their relationship to other organs and assesses the presence of ascites. More detailed morphological assessment of a mass is better with transvaginal scan (TVS).

ENLARGED UTERUS

The commonest pathology seen on scanning the non-pregnant uterus is the presence of uterine fibroids. The vast majority lie within the myometrium, though some can be pedunculated or lie within the broad ligament.

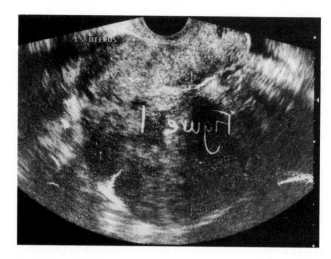

Fig. 36.1 Longitudinal section of a uterus, with a large posterior wall subserosal fibroid, with characteristic shadowing.

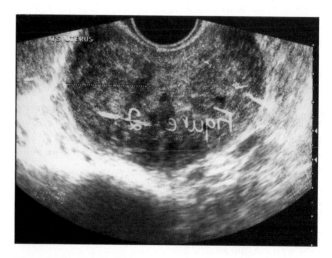

Fig. 36.2 Transverse section of a uterus showing bilateral intramural fibroids.

- Intramural – Within the myometrium without distorting the endometrial cavity or serosal surface.
- Submucous – Distort the endometrial cavity.
- Subserous – Distort the serosal surface.

Ultrasound helps define the number and size of fibroids and also their situation within the myometrium. In the majority of patients with fibroids there are multiple tumours. Ultrasound features of fibroids are that they are well circumscribed lesions that appear hypoechoic compared to the surrounding myometrium. They may contain foci of calcification with characteristic shadowing (Figs 36.1 and 36.2).

If a fibroid is pedunculated it is sometimes difficult to differentiate from a solid ovarian tumour. The demonstration of two normal ovaries or the use of Doppler to demonstrate that the blood supply originates from the uterus would identify the lesion as uterine in origin.

Ultrasound diagnosis of fibroids and their location helps to determine the relationship to presenting symptomatology, what treatment modalities are suitable and also for monitoring treatment in cases where gonadotrophin-releasing hormone (GnRH) analogues are used to shrink fibroids.

Leiomyosarcomas are the malignant counterpart of benign fibroids, and ultrasound *can not* reliably be used to determine sarcomatous change, although a change within the vascular pattern may be detected using Doppler.

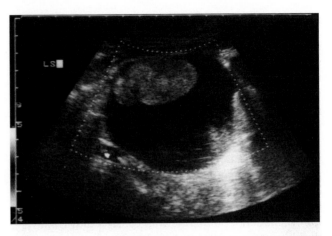

Fig. 36.3 A dermoid cyst showing characteristic appearance of hair and sebum as a "white ball".

OVARIAN CYSTS

The primary value of ultrasound in the management of ovarian cysts is to differentiate between a physiological cyst and a pathological cyst, and how likely it is that any pathological tumour is malignant. Several studies have concluded that ultrasound is the best imaging technique for the assessment of ovarian cysts. The following information should be gained from an ultrasound examination of an ovarian tumour.

• The side of the lesion unilateral or bilateral.
• The size – three dimensions if possible.
• Consistency – cystic or solid (size and regularity of solid components).
• Internal structures – unilocular, multilocular, complex. Nature of septa thin/thick.
• Internal wall – smooth, irregular presence of papillary projections, (solid projections into the cyst cavity from the cyst wall >3 mm in height).
• Echogenicity – in comparison to myometrium.

It is suggested that certain ultrasound features can be used to predict histological diagnosis [1]. Dermoid cysts are a good example and they are easily recognized on ultrasound owing to their fat and hair content. The most characteristic feature is the presence of a 'white ball' in the corner of the cyst (Fig. 36.3); this corresponds to hair and sebum. Hair that is free within the cyst shows as long echoic lines. There is often significant shadowing making it difficult to assess accurately the size of the cyst.

Endometriomas tend to be unilocular and have an echogenic ground glass appearance. Experienced gynaecological ultrasonographers can reliably differentiate benign from malignant cysts and are probably better at predicting malignancy than mathematical models [2]. Ultrasonic signs of malignancy include multilocular or multiple cysts, thick or irregular septa or cyst walls, papillary projections and the presence of solid components. [3]

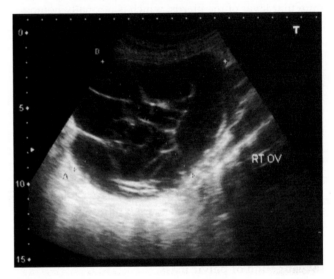

Fig. 36.4 A mucinous cystadenocarcinoma showing multiple locules.

The more complex a tumour, that is, the more septa and solid components it contains, the higher the risk of malignancy. Granberg *et al.* 1989 [4] found the frequency of malignancy in unilocular cysts to be 0.3% while in multilocular solid cysts it was 73% (Figs 36.4 and 36.5). Colour flow Doppler has been shown to be a useful adjunct in assessing the possibility of malignancy in ovarian tumours. The Doppler criteria for diagnosing malignancy are not clearly defined; however, malignant tumours will generally have lower blood flow impedance and higher blood flow velocity. This is due to the paucity of smooth muscle in the walls of blood vessels and the presence of arterio-venous shunting.

Sonographic findings can be used in conjunction with menopausal status/age and serum CA125 levels to give

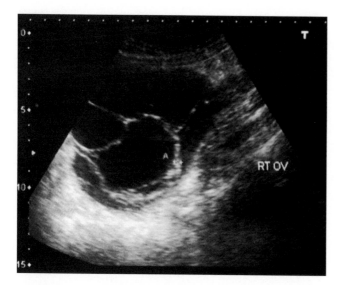

Fig. 36.5 The same cyst showing separate measuring 4.2 mm.

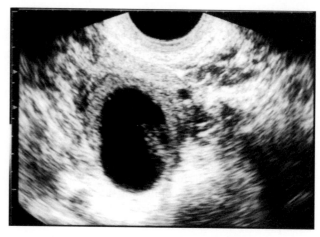

Fig. 36.7 Ovarian cysts showing the differing appearances of a haemorrhage. Figure 7 shows organised dot mimicking a solid component.

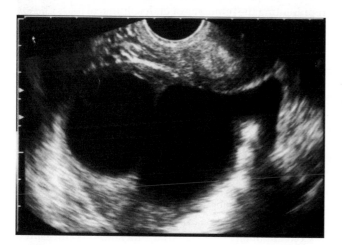

Fig. 36.6 A simple bilocular cyst, which is sonorlucent with normal surrounding ovarian tissue.

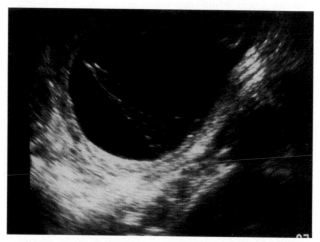

Fig. 36.8 Ovarian cysts showing the differing appearances of a haemorrhage. Figure 8 the typical "Spiders web" appearance.

score on the risk of malignancy index (RMI); this can be used as a triage for suspected ovarian cancers.

Pelvic pain

It is very important to take a good history of the nature and location of pelvic pain and determine by clinical examination what the likely differential diagnosis is prior to performing an ultrasound examination. There are many causes of pelvic pain and ultrasound findings taken in isolation may be misleading. For example, the majority of simple ovarian cysts are an incidental finding; however, ultrasound can help determine those patients in whom surgical intervention is required. The commonest pathologies in which ultrasound may be of use are cyst accidents, pelvic infection and endometriosis.

OVARIAN CYSTS

Ovarian cysts are relatively common in women during reproductive life. Ovarian cysts *per se* are not painful; however, a cyst accident be it haemorrhage, rupture or torsion may lead to pelvic pain.

Haemorrhage within a cyst can have a variety of ultrasound appearances, depending on the size and organization of the area of haemorrhage. Acute haemorrhage on ultrasound may be seen as particulate fluid; as the clot organizes there may be a hyperechoic area mimicking a solid component within the cyst and as the clot resolves it demonstrates a web of low-amplitude strands (Figs 36.6 and 36.7). A haemorrhagic corpus luteal cyst is a common cause of pain in women of reproductive age, but resolves spontaneously.

Torsion of the adenexae tends to be more common when there is a lesion within the adenexae – either an ovarian cyst or hydrosalpinx. However, it may occur with no associated pathology, and this is more common in adolescents.

The features of torsion on ultrasound scan can be nonspecific. The diagnosis relies on comparison of the torted ovary with the opposite side. The ovary appears congested and oedematous; multiple small cysts may be seen at the periphery of a markedly enlarged ovary. The most common torted cysts are dermoids and benign cyst adenomas. Doppler may be of use by confirming the absence of blood flow; however, this is not universal as torsion may be incomplete or intermittent. Free fluid will be present in about one-third of cases.

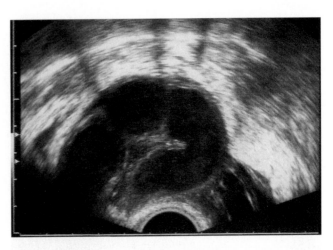

Fig. 36.9 A pyosalpinx with thickened walls.

ENDOMETRIOSIS

Endometriosis while sometimes asymptomatic it is often associated with chronic pelvic pain. Routine sonography is unlikely to detect peritoneal endometriotic deposits. Nodules in the pouch of Douglas may be visualized using a transrectal approach. It is possible to demonstrate endometriotic cysts (endometriomas) within the ovary which have a typical appearance. The cyst tends to be thick walled and the contents have a 'ground glass' appearance, the cyst being filled with homogenous hypoechoic low-level echoes. It is important to remember that endometriotic cysts are bilateral in 30–50% of cases.

PELVIC INFLAMMATORY DISEASE

Acute pelvic infection is a clinical diagnosis, with a history of pelvic pain, vaginal discharge, pyrexia adenexal tenderness and a raised white cell count. In early/mild disease the uterine appearance on ultrasound is rather non-specific with a decrease in endometrial reflectivity and the presence of fluid in the cavity. Typical features have been described if the adenexae are affected [4]. A normal fallopian tube is not usually visualized at ultrasound examination. A pyosalpinx has a very typical appearance of a thick-walled cystic 'sausage' shaped structure, with the appearance of incomplete septa, correlating with kinks or folds in the dilated tube. A lack of peristalsis allows differentiation from a loop of bowel (Fig. 36.9). Swollen mucosal folds protrude into the lumen giving the tube a cogwheel appearance when visualized in cross section. The appearance of a tube-ovarian abscess is very variable from a unilocular thick-walled cyst resembling an endometrioma to a multi-loculated solid mass; it is often impossible to visualize any normal ovarian tissue.

A hydrosalpinx is a feature of chronic disease; this is demonstrated as a dilated thin-walled tube containing anechoic fluid. One may see small hyperreflective nodules representing the remnants of endosalpingeal folds ('beads on a string').

Ultrasound assessment of abnormal uterine bleeding

POSTMENOPAUSAL BLEEDING

Transvaginal ultrasound offers an opportunity to individualize the management of postmenopausal bleeding, and decrease the need for invasive testing. There is good evidence that women who present with postmenopausal bleeding in whom a TV ultrasound has demonstrated an endometrial thickness of ≤4 mm have a very small risk of endometrial carcinoma [5].

Conventionally endometrial thickness is measured with a longitudinal section of the uterus measuring the endometrium at its thickest point. To ensure the view is a true longitudinal representation, the entire length of the cavity line should be visualized (Fig. 36.10). Measurement of thickness includes both layers of the endometrium as it can be difficult to identify the interface between the anterior and posterior layers. If there is any fluid within the uterine cavity the thickness of the fluid layer should be subtracted from the endometrial thickness. Those women with an endometrial thickness ≥5 mm should have endometrial sampling or hysteroscopy [6,7].

The appearance of the endometrium is important in assessing the possibility of malignancy (Table 36.2). Evidence of invasion into the myometrium is highly suggestive of malignancy (Figs 36.11 and 36.12).

The role of ultrasound in the assessment of women with abnormal pre- or peri-menopausal bleeding is not as clearly defined. The endometrial thickness alters with the different stages of the menstrual cycle. Endometrial polyps

Table 36.2 Ultrasound features of abnormal endometrium

Endometrial cancer	Endometrial hyperplasia
Endometrium thick and echogenid	Uniformly thick and echogenic
Endometrial/myometrial border irregular	Midline echo lost
Invasion of myometrium may be seen	Multiple cysts 1–2 mm diameter
Thickness >15 mm in postmenopausal woman highly suggestive of malignancy	Thickness >14 mm
Local areas of necrosis may be seen	

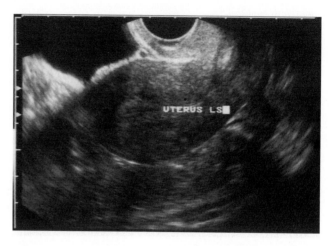

Fig. 36.10 A longitudinal section of the uterus showing normal endometrium.

or submucous fibroids are the only causes of abnormal bleeding that are likely to be demonstrated by ultrasound.

Abnormalities of the uterine cavity or the endometrium such as an endometrial polyp may be more clearly demonstrated using the technique of sonohysterography where fluid is injected into the uterine cavity to outline structures.

Early pregnancy

Ultrasound is an essential diagnostic tool in the assessment of early pregnancy complications. The gestational sac is the first sonographic evidence of a pregnancy. With TV sonography it is possible to visualize the gestation sac from 32 to 34 days following the last menstrual period. The sac at this stage measures 2–4 mm, is hypoechoic and surrounded by a hyperechoic rim. It is typically located in the upper part of the decidualized endometrium in an eccentric position (Fig. 36.10). The yolk sac becomes visible in the 5th week and by the end of the 5th week the embryo is seen. Initially the embryo appears as a bright linear echo adjacent to the yolk sac; growth rate at this stage is approximately 1 mm a day and by the time the embryo has reached a CRL of >6 mm it can be seen separately from the yolk sac (Fig. 36.13) and cardiac activity can be seen. If TA scanning is used each of the landmarks are seen approximately 1 week later. The use of ultrasound in the diagnosis of miscarriage is covered in the management of miscarriage.

Ectopic pregnancy

In conjunction with the use of serial beta human chorionic gonadotrophin (βHCG) estimation the use of transvaginal scanning facilitates a much earlier diagnosis of ectopic pregnancy, thus permitting the use of laparoscopic surgery or medical management. The absence of a gestation sac is a primary factor in diagnosing an ectopic. All units

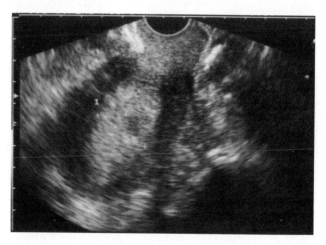

Fig. 36.11 Demonstrates the findings in abnormal endometrium. Figure 11 shows endometrial thickness of 27.2 mm.

need to define at what level of BHCG with the ultrasound machines they have available in their unit one can reliably identify an intrauterine gestation sac. The appearance of an ectopic mass is very variable; this is comprehensively covered in Chapter 14.

Infertility

Ultrasound has made significant improvement in the modern management of infertility. It has a role in the initial assessment of the infertile woman, in monitoring of treatment cycles and the performance of ultrasound guided procedures.

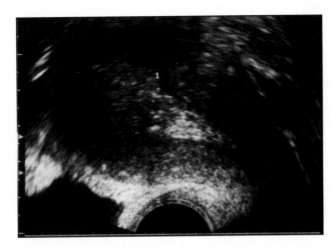

Fig. 36.12 Demonstrates the findings in abnormal endometrium. Figure 12 evidence of myometrial invasion.

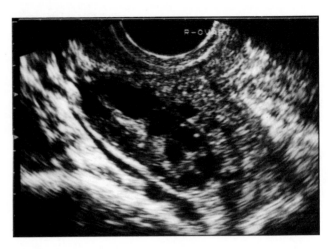

Fig. 36.14 A polycystic ovary with numerous small peripheral follicles and an echodensa stroma.

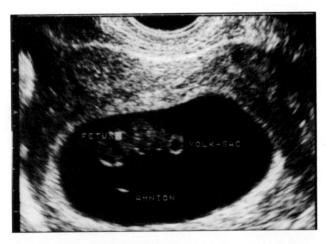

Fig. 36.13 Appearance of a normal early pregnancy of 8 weeks 1 day gestation.

INITIAL ASSESSMENT

A TV ultrasound allows assessment of the uterus for any obvious abnormalities or for the presence endometrial polyps or submucous fibroids. With a skilled operator hystero-contrast-sonography (HyCoSy) has comparable results to hysterosalpingography (HSG). It should be considered in those women at low risk of tubal disease as it has the advantage of being able to assess the ovaries at the same time while avoiding the use of radiation. In this procedure TV ultrasound is performed with the instillation of an echogenic contrast medium into the uterine cavity. One of the limitations of HyCoSy is the difficulty in storing information; images need to be recorded in real time.

Assessment of the ovaries is important especially in women with oligomenorrhoea as one may find polycystic ovaries which have a typical ultrasound appearance with the presence of 12 or more follicles measuring 2–9 mm in one or both ovaries and an ovarian volume greater than 10 ml. [8] (Fig. 36.12). An ultrasound appearance of polycystic ovaries does not equate to a diagnosis of polycystic ovarian syndrome. This diagnosis can only be made if the patient is symptomatic. At present ultrasound is not recommended as a tool for assessing ovulation (NICE 2004).

Ultrasound has a significant role in the monitoring of women undergoing infertility treatment especially those patients undergoing superovulation; there are details in the chapter on IVF.

Screening for ovarian malignancy

Throughout this text we have stated that ultrasound should only be used if a patient is symptomatic due to the high incidence of incidental findings in asymptomatic women. The one where this doesn't apply is screening for ovarian malignancy.

Malignant ovarian tumours are the most common cause of gynaecological cancer related deaths in the Western Europe; 4000 deaths occur every year in the UK from ovarian cancer. Transvaginal ultrasound is fundamental to any screening programme either as a single modality or in conjunction with serum tumour markers. An ovarian volume over 20 cm³ in pre-menopausal women and 10 cm³ in post-menopausal women is considered abnormal. The use of ultrasound screening for ovarian cancer is discussed in Chapter 55.

With continuing advances in technology, it is unlikely that the use of ultrasound as a diagnostic tool has reached its full potential. Further advances are eagerly awaited by most practitioners. However, one must always remember that ultrasound is an adjunct to and not a replacement for a good clinical history and examination. The normal appearance of pelvic organs alters throughout reproductive life under the influence of hormonal regulation. It can also be influenced by exogenous hormones such as hormone replacement theory (HRT) or the oral contraceptive pill. This information is therefore required for accurate interpretation of ultrasound images.

References

1. Jeremy K, Luise C, Bourne T (2001) The characterization of common ovarian cysts in premenopausal women. *Ultrasound Obstet Gynecol* **17**, 140–44.
2. Timmerman D, Schwarzler P, Collins WP Claerhout P Coenen M Amant F et al (1999) Subjective assessment of adenexal masses using ultrasonography: an analysis of intraobserver variability and experience. *Ultrasound Obstet Gynecol* **13**, 11–16.
3. Timmerman D (2004) The use of mathematical models to evaluate pelvic masses, can they beat an expert operator? *Best Pract Res Clin Obstet Gynecol* **18**, 91–104.
4. Timmerman D, Valentin L, Bourne TH et al (2000) Terms, definitions and measurements to describe the sonographic features of adenexal tumours: a consensus opinion from the International Ovarian Tumour Analysis (IOTA) group. *Ultrasound in Obstetrics and Gynecology* **16**, 500–505.
5. Granberg S, Wikland M, Jansson I (1989) macroscopic characterization of ovarian tumours and the relation to the histological diagnosis, criteria to be used in ultrasound evaluation. *Gynecol Oncol* **35**, 139–144.
6. Timor-Tritsch IE, Lerner JP, Monteagudo A et al (1998) Transvaginal sonographic markers of tubal inflammatory disease. *Ultrasound in Obstetrics and Gynaecology* **12**, 56–66.
7. Smith-Bindman R, Kerlikowske K, Feldstein VA, Subak L, Scheindler J, Segal M, Brand R, Grady D (1998) Endovaginal ultrasound to exclude endometrial cancer and other endometrial abnormalities. *JAMA* **280**, 1510–7.
8. Karlsson B, Milsom I, Granberg S (2003) Can ultrasound replace dilatation and curettage? A longitudinal evaluation of postmenopausal bleeding and transvaginal sonographic measurement of the endometrium as predictors of endometrial cancer. *Am J Obstet Gynecol* **188**(2), 401–8.
9. Consensus Statement Fertil Steril (2004) **81**, 19–25.

Further reading

European federation of Societies for Ultrasound in Medicine and Biology (EFSUMB). www.efsumb.org

Collaborative trial of Ovarian Cancer Screening. www.ukctocs.org.uk

Fertility assessment and treatment for people with fertility problems. www.nice.org.uk

Chapter 37: Gynaecological disorders of childhood and adolescence

D. Keith Edmonds

Gynaecological problems in the prepubertal child and at adolescence create great levels of anxiety in parents particularly, but fortunately very few of these disorders could be considered common. However, when they do present it is important that the clinician has an understanding so that appropriate advice may be given to the patient and management is frequently through simple means. The disorders fall into two groups, those related to prepuberty and those of adolescence.

Prepubertal child

Vulvovaginitis

This is the only gynaecological disorder of childhood which can be thought of as common. Its aetiology is based on opportunistic bacteria colonizing the lower vagina and inducing an inflammatory response. At birth the vulva and vagina are well oestrogenized due to the intrauterine exposure of the fetus to placental oestrogen. This oestrogenization causes thickening of the vaginal epithelium, which is entirely protective against any bacterial invasion. However, within 2–3 weeks of delivery the resultant hypo-oestrogenic state leads to changes in the vulval skin, which becomes thinner and the vagina epithelium also becomes much thinner. The vulval fat pad disappears and the vaginal entrance becomes unprotected. The vulval skin is thin, sensitive and easily traumatized by injury, irritation, infection or any allergic reaction that may ensue. The lack of labial protection and the close apposition of the anus mean that the vulva and lower vagina are constantly exposed to faecal bacterial contamination. The hypo-oestrogenic state in the vagina means that there are no lactobacilli and therefore the vagina has a resulting pH of 7 making it an ideal culture medium for low virulent organisms. The childhood problems of poor local hygiene compound the risk of low-grade non-specific infection. Children also have the habit of exploring their genitalia and in some cases masturbating. This chronic habit may lead to vulvovaginitis, which can prove extremely difficult to treat.

The possibility that vulvovaginitis may occur in childhood in those who have an impaired local host defence deficiency remains a possibility and the lack of an innate protective response from neutrophils.

The causes of vulvovaginitis in children are shown in Table 37.1 The vast majority of cases are due to non-specific bacterial contamination, although the other causes should be remembered. Candidal infection in children is extremely rare, although because it is a common cause of vulvovaginitis in the adult it is a common misdiagnosis in children. *Candida* in children is usually associated with diabetes mellitus or immunodeficiency and almost entirely related to these two medical disorders. The presence of viral infections, for example, herpes simplex or condyloma acuminata, should alert the clinician to the possibility of sexual abuse. Vulval skin disease is not uncommon in children, particularly atopic dermatitis in those children who also have eczema. Referral to a dermatologist is appropriate in these circumstances. Lichen sclerosis is also seen in children and may cause persistent vulval itching. The skin undergoes atrophy and fissuring and is very susceptible to secondary infection.

Table 37.1 Causes of vulvovaginitis in children

Bacterial
Non-specific – common
Specific – rare
Fungal – rare
Candida of vulva only
Viral — rare
Dermatitis
Atopic
Lichen sclerosis
Contact
Sexual abuse
Enuresis
Foreign body

Sexual abuse in children may present with vaginal discharge. Any child who has recurrent attacks of vaginal discharge should alert the clinician to this possibility. However, as non-specific bacterial infection is a common problem in children the clinician must proceed with considerable caution in raising the possibility of sexual abuse. Only those bacterial infections related to venereal disease, for example, gonorrhoea, may be cited as diagnostic of sexual abuse.

It is important that the clinician remembers that many girls suffer from urinary incontinence, particularly at night, and this creation of a moist vulva allows secondary irritation by bacteria leading to vulvovaginitis.

DIAGNOSTIC PROCEDURES

There are two aspects of the diagnosis in this condition in children. The first is inspection of the vulva and vagina. It is imperative that the clinician has good illumination, particularly if there is a history of the possibility of a foreign body being in the vagina. It is usually possible to examine the vagina through the hymen using an otoscope. This may well allow the diagnosis of a foreign body to be made.

The second aspect of diagnosis involves the taking of bacteriological specimens. This can be extremely difficult in a small child, as it is unlikely that the child will be cooperative. Any object which touches the vulva causes distress. The best way to take a bacteriological specimen is to use a pipette, which is much less irritating than a cotton wool swab. The pipette allows 1–2 ml of normal saline to be expelled into the lower part of the vagina, the tip of the pipette having been passed through the hymenal orifice. The fluid is then aspirated and sent for bacteriology. If a diagnosis of pin worms is to be excluded, then a piece of sticky tape over the anus early in the morning before the child gets out of bed will reveal the presence of eggs on microscopy. Results of bacteriological testing in children with vulvovaginitis are extremely difficult to interpret and while it is possible that specific organisms may be identified and appropriate antibiotic treatment be instigated, this is rarely the case.

The vast majority of children do not have a pathological organism. The primary treatment in this group is advice about perineal hygiene. All parents of children with chronic vaginal disease are extremely worried that this may cause long-term detrimental effects to their daughters, particularly in the fear of sexual dysfunction or subsequent infertility. There is no evidence that this is the case and therefore parents should be reassured that this is a local problem only. Management of these children is directed towards proper care of the perineum. The child must be taught to clean her vulva, particularly after defaecation from front to back, as this avoids the transfer of enterobacteria to the vulval area. After micturition the mother and child should be instructed to clean the vulva completely and not to leave the vulval skin wet as this damp, warm environment is an ideal culture surface for bacteria that cause vulvovaginitis. The mother must also be informed that vulval hygiene through daily washing should be performed, but that the soap should be gentle and not scented. Excessive washing of the vulva must be avoided as this leads to recurrent exfoliation and vulval dermatitis. During acute attacks of non-specific recurrent vulvovaginitis, children often complain of burning during micturition due to the passage of urine across the inflamed vulva. The use of barrier creams in these circumstances may be very useful.

Labial adhesions

Labial adhesions are usually an innocent finding and a trivial problem, but its importance is that it is frequently misdiagnosed as congenital absence of the vagina. The physical signs of labial adhesions are easily recognized. In the postdelivery hypo-oestrogenic state the labia minora stick together in the midline, usually from posterior forwards until only a small opening is left anteriorly through which urine is passed. Similar adhesions sometimes bind down the clitoris. It may be difficult to distinguish the opening at all. The vulva has the appearance of being flat, and there are no normal tissues beyond the clitoris evident. However, a translucent, dark, vertical line in the midline where the adhesions are thinnest can usually be seen, and these appearances are quite different from congenital absence of the vagina. There are usually no symptoms associated with this condition, although older children may complain that there is some spraying when they pass urine. The aetiology of the hypo-oestrogenic state means that they are never seen at birth, and instead occur during early childhood. As late childhood ensues and ovarian activity begins there is spontaneous resolution of the problem. In the majority of cases no treatment is required and the parents should be reassured that their daughters are entirely normal. In those children in whom there are some clinical problems local oestrogen cream can be applied for about 2 weeks. There is usually complete resolution of the labial adhesions. In some rare circumstances this will not resolve the problem, but at the end of the oestrogen therapy the midline is so thin that gentle separation of the labia may be undertaken using a probe, and this procedure causes no discomfort to the child. Application of a bland barrier cream at this stage will prevent further adhesion formation. Finally, in taking a history it is important to establish that there has not been any trauma to the vulva as very rarely labial adhesions may be the result of sexual abuse.

Puberty

Puberty is defined as the period of time during which secondary sexual characteristics develop, menstruation begins and the psychological outlook of the girl changes as she develops a more adult aspect to herself. The end result of puberty is the establishment of the fully physically mature adult woman capable of reproductive performance and fully psychologically developed as an adult. The physical changes of puberty are divided into five stages: breast growth, pubic hair growth, axillary hair growth, the growth spurt and menarche. Breast development, pubic hair and axillary hair development are classified by the Tanner system into five stages. Tanner stage 5 describes the mature breast, full pubic hair development and the establishment of axillary hair. The growth spurt in children occurs about 2 years earlier in girls than boys and in most girls in the UK occurs around the age of 11.5–12 years. Growth velocity at this stage reaches a peak of 8 cm/year, but the production of oestrogen from the ovary at this time eventually closes the epiphyses such that final height is achieved at around the age of 14.5 years.

Menarche in girls in the UK is around 12.6 years, but the onset of menstruation is influenced by a number of factors. There is no doubt that this is genetically controlled, and the release of gonadotrophin-releasing hormone (GnRH) by the neurones in the arcuate nucleus of the hypothalamus is controlled by central factors influencing DNA within the cells. It is hypothesized that neurotransmitters, endorphins, interleukins, leptin and other paracrine and autocrine factors modulate the onset of puberty and new data suggest that growth factors including transforming growth factor alpha and epidermal growth factor appear to play key roles in this regulatory process. The process is linked to an increase in percentage body fat and this percentage body fat is influenced by a number of external factors, for example, socio-economic status, allowing good nutrition or psychological problems to influence body weight, for example, anorexia nervosa [1]. However, there is little doubt that body fat is intimately involved in the coordination of the onset of GnRH release.

Early menstrual cycles are in the majority anovulatory, and cycle length may vary for some considerable years after menarche. It may take some 5–8 years before menstrual cycle normality is established. Therefore, it is again not uncommon that this primary dysmenorrhoea often post-dates menarche. As the anovulatory state is due to failure of luteinization of follicles and subsequent ovulation the lack of production of progesterone means

Table 37.2 Causes of precocious puberty

Idiopathic
Neurological
Cerebral tumours
Hydrocephalus
Postmeningitis
McCune-Albright syndrome
Ovarian tumours
Adrenal tumours
Gonadotrophin-secreting tumours
Exogenous oestrogen

that there is endometrial hyperplasia. In many girls their menstrual loss can be very heavy.

Precocious puberty

Precocious puberty is defined as the onset of secondary sexual characteristics prior to the age of 8 years. The aetiology of this is varied, as seen in Table 37.2.

In the vast majority of girls the cause is unknown. This idiopathic group constitutes 95% of all cases of precocious puberty. It is likely that this is solely due to initiation of the normal process of puberty at a premature age. As discussed in p., the onset is genetically predetermined. If this genetic determinant is inappropriately timed then the normal process of puberty will occur whenever the initiation occurs.

Some children with neurological disorders like cerebral tumours, hydrocephalus or postmeningitis or encephalitis may have an early puberty due to activation of the hypothalamus by the disease process. The mechanism by which this occurs remains obscure; although in the McCune-Albright syndrome, which is a disorder involving cystic bony change (polyostotic fibrous dysplasia), there is also associated endocrine dysfunction particularly of the hypothalamus and pituitary and in this condition precocious puberty is common. Various ovarian and adrenal tumours may be hormone secreting thus inducing secondary sexual characteristic changes, but these are not truly pubertal and are reversible on removal of the tumour. Cases of ingestion of exogenous oestrogen by children have also been reported, and this will indeed result in the onset of some menstrual loss in some children and again must not be considered as true precocious puberty.

TREATMENT

In those cases of idiopathic precocious puberty the clinician is faced with the problem of reversing the normal onset of puberty. There can be little doubt that the treatment of choice is the use of GnRH analogues, which are extremely effective at obliterating follicle-stimulating hormone (FSH) production by the pituitary. By doing this, the prepubertal state is re-established and the child can remain on this therapy until aged about 11.5–12 years when the therapy can be withdrawn and the normal onset of puberty will ensue. Any breast or pubic hair development that has occurred prior to the diagnosis will usually be reversible as the hypo-oestrogenic state prevents further growth and in most cases this results in some resolution of early change. However, if the secondary sexual characteristic changes have been much greater and development is beyond Tanner stage 3, little effect can be expected by this therapy on the physical changes. Similar success can be achieved with those children with neurological problems. Children who are found to have ovarian or adrenal tumours or gonadotrophin-secreting tumours should be treated surgically and their problems will resolve. It is important for the gynaecologist who is presented with these problems to remember that precocious puberty is socially undesirable and social management of the case is essential. Very rarely would a gynaecologist opt to treat a child with precocious puberty without the help of a paediatrician. In fact, cases of precocious puberty are now usually managed medically by paediatric endocrinologists.

Adolescence

The adolescent gynaecological patient usually presents with one of three disorders. First, there are those problems associated with the menstrual cycle and menstrual dysfunction, dysmenorrhoea and premenstrual syndrome are the main group of disorders. Second, the patient may present with primary amenorrhoea (see Chapter 38) and third, is the problem of teenage hirsutism.

Menstrual problems

As can be seen in the description of puberty, menstrual cycles are rarely established as normal ovulatory cycles from the beginning of puberty. It can take many years before the normal ovulatory menstrual cycle is established. This phenomenon is extremely important for the gynaecologist to understand, as the management of these cases is usually without active treatment but by support and understanding of the condition and the child.

Heavy menstruation

Faced with a mother and her daughter giving a story of heavy menstrual loss, it is important that the clinician takes an accurate history from the child if possible. This is often difficult if the mother is present throughout and it must be remembered that the perception of heavy menstruation is often not reflected in studies that have looked at actual menstrual loss. Normal menstrual loss should not exceed 80 ml during a period, although in 5% of individuals it is heavier than this and causes no trouble. The clinician is faced in these circumstances with attempting to assess whether or not the child truly has menstrual loss that is serious as a medical condition or menstrual loss that is irritating and distressing without being medically harmful. The best way to establish which of these is the case is to measure the haemoglobin. If the haemoglobin level is normal, that is, greater than 12 g/l, then an explanation should be given to the mother and child of the normal physiology of menstrual establishment that the manifestation of the menstrual loss is normal and that it may take some time for the cycle to be established. This condition requires no active treatment. However, it is imperative that the child is followed up at 6-monthly intervals until the pattern of menstruation is established as reassurance is the most important part of the management process of these girls.

In those girls with haemoglobin levels between 10 and 12 g/l it is apparent that they are losing more blood at menstruation than is desirable. Again, an explanation is required so that the mother and daughter understand the cause of the problem and the child should be administered iron therapy to correct what will be mild iron deficiency anaemia. In terms of management, menstrual loss needs to be reduced and this may be achieved by using either progestogens cyclically for 21 days in every 28-day cycle or to use the combined oral contraceptive pill. It would be unusual for either of these therapies to be unsuccessful in controlling the menstrual loss. If they are used, these therapies should be stopped on an annual basis so that assessment may be made as to whether or not the normal pattern of menstruation has been established through maturation of the hypothalamopituitary-ovarian access. Thereafter, the child requires no further medication. Again follow-up is essential if reassurance is to be given appropriately.

Finally, in the child with a haemoglobin count of less than 10 g/l, it is obvious that serious anaemia has resulted from menstrual loss. This again requires an explanation but more urgent attention from a medical point of view. Progestogens are very much less likely to be effective in this group and the oral contraceptive pill is by far the treatment of choice. It may be given continuously for a short period of time so that the anaemia can be corrected using oral iron and then the pill may be used in the normal way so that menstrual loss occurs monthly, if desired.

Any girl who continues to have menstrual loss which is reported to be uncontrolled by these management strategies should have an ultrasound scan performed to exclude a uterine pathology. These pathologies are extremely rare and the reader is referred to other texts for further information.

Primary dysmenorrhoea

Primary dysmenorrhoea is defined as pain which begins in association with menstrual bleeding. The management of dysmenorrhoea in the teenager is no different from that of the adult (see Chapter 34). Both the use of non-steroidal anti-inflammatories and the oral contraceptive pill is pertinent in teenagers, but again failure of these medications to control dysmenorrhoea should alert the clinician to the possibility of uterine anomaly and ultrasound imaging of the uterus should be performed to establish whether or not an anomaly exists.

Premenstrual syndrome

This is a difficult problem in adolescence as the psychological changes that are occurring during this time of a woman's life are often complex and stressful. It is established that premenstrual syndrome is a stress-related disorder. Therefore in teenage girls undergoing puberty the stresses and emotional turbulence that are associated with this, not surprisingly, may lead to premenstrual problems. These are very difficult to manage and are usually not medically treated but addressed through the help of psychologists if reassurance from the gynaecologist and an understanding of the process to the mother is not successful.

Hirsutism

Hair follicles cover the entire body and different types of hair are found in different sites. Androgens affect some areas of the human body and increase hair growth rate and also the thickness of terminal hairs. Androgens are also involved in sebum production and may cause this to be excessive. In some women excessive hair growth may occur on the arms, legs, abdomen, breasts and back such that it constitutes the problem of hirsutism. This may also be associated with acne, which may occur not only on the face but on the chest and back.

DIFFERENTIAL DIAGNOSIS

There are four major groups of disorders which may cause hirsutism in adolescence (Table 37.3). Those androgenic causes include congenital adrenal hyperplasia and its late

Table 37.3 Causes of hirsutism in adolescents

Androgenic causes
Congenital adrenal hyperplasia
● Classic
● Late onset
Androgen-secreting tumours
Polycystic ovarian syndrome
Idiopathic
XY gonadal dysgenesis

onset variant and also androgen-secreting tumours. The commonest group are women with polycystic ovarian syndrome and, while this is sometimes a difficult diagnosis to make in adolescents, it by far constitutes the greatest problem group. The diagnosis of XY gonadal dysgenesis is something that should be borne in mind when considering a child with hirsutism but a large percentage of patients have idiopathic hirsutism. It is important to remember that some girls will have a constitutional basis for their hirsutism and familial body hair patterns should be borne in mind when considering whether or not a young patient does in fact have hirsutism. Treatments for hirsutism are as in the adult and are covered in Chapter 47. In adolescence the mainstay of androgen excess treatment has been the oral contraceptive pill and without doubt this remains the main form of treatment. As the majority of these girls have some ovarian dysfunction, be that polycystic ovarian syndrome or an undefined problem, suppression of ovarian activity is very effective at circulating androgen. If this is insufficient to gain control of hair growth, then the use of cyproterone acetate or spironolactone may be considered.

In those patients who are not considered to have hirsutism due to a medical disorder, drug therapies may be ineffective and supportive measures may be necessary for cosmetic benefit. These include hair removal by shaving, waxing or electrolysis to those areas which are particularly cosmetically sensitive and also the use of bleaches to change hair colour thereby gaining cosmetic benefit.

Reference

1. Traggiai C & Stanhope R (2003) Disorders of pubertal development. *Best Pract Res Clin Obstet Gynaecol* **17**, 41–56.

Further reading

Balen A (2004) *Paediatric and Adolescent Gynaecology. A Multidisciplinary Approach.* Cambridge: Cambridge University Press.

Sanfilippo J (1999) *Pediatric and Adolescent Gynecology.* Philadelphia: W.B. Saunders.

Chapter 38: Primary amenorrhoea

D. Keith Edmonds

For the majority of pubertal girls menstruation is the final result of a series of events, which result in sexual maturity. Maturation of the hypothalamus through several years of late childhood begins a cascade of events which finally result in the establishment of the normal menstrual cycle and menstruation. Amenorrhoea will result when there is a failure of function in any of the organs involved in this cascade. Management of patients with primary amenorrhoea therefore demands a knowledge and understanding of the embryology of female development and the endocrinology of puberty, but also an ability to assess an adolescent girl in her entirety. Details of embryology and normal pubertal development can be found in Chapter 34.

Definition

There is considerable difficulty in defining the term primary amenorrhoea, other than the obvious statement that it is the failure to establish menstruation. The difficulty of definition relates to the time frame in which this definition is applied. To look at primary amenorrhoea as an isolated event is misleading as it is part of the whole development of puberty. Of the five changes that occur at puberty, menstruation is but one and may normally occur any time between ages 10 and 18 years. However, it occurs in conjunction with the development of other secondary sexual characteristics. It is therefore more useful to look upon secondary sexual development as the criteria for investigation and management in association with primary amenorrhoea. As a general rule, therefore, failure of the development of any secondary sexual characteristic by the age of 14 years should be investigated. In the presence of secondary sexual characteristics, menstruation ought to occur within 2 years of the establishment of this development. Failure to do so would warrant investigation. However, any child brought by its mother at any stage because of concern over the failure to establish either secondary sexual characteristics or menstruation should be investigated at that time. There are usually very good reasons why a mother will bring her daughter for investigation. This often relates to the fact that a sibling completed her pubertal development at an earlier age than the patient. While investigations may not lead to a diagnosis of abnormality, the proof of normality is also extremely important (Figs 38.1 and 38.2). It can be seen therefore that the term primary amenorrhoea is really not very meaningful in terms of definition, and a more useful term would be delayed puberty. This term encompasses the completion of the processes involved in reaching sexual maturity and allows a much more pragmatic approach to the management.

Normal puberty

Puberty is the time when one becomes functionally able to reproduce. This includes both physical and psychological development, but it is important to understand that there is a wide range of ages between which these changes take place. There are five changes that occur, known as the secondary sexual characteristics. In girls these are breast, pubic hair, axillary hair development, the growth spurt and the onset of menstruation; only subsequently does ovulation become established.

Breast growth is divided into five stages (Tanner classification; [1]) and it begins around 9 years of age, the full development taking around 5 years. It is unusual for no breast tissue to develop by 13 years of age. Pubic hair occurs almost in parallel with breast development and is also classified as five stages. Axillary hair only has three stages and this development tends to occur later at around the age of 13. The growth spurt occurs at between 10 and 14 years and most girls will reach their maximum height between these ages. The peak height velocity occurs around 12.1 years [2]. Finally menstruation occurs in 95% of girls in the UK by the age of 13 years, although delay in the remainder up to age 16 must be considered as normal [3]. There are many factors influencing the age of menarche (see Chapter 37). All of the physical

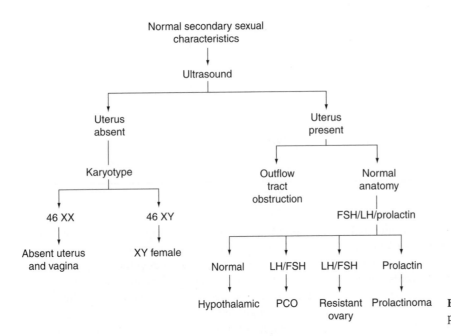

Fig. 38.1 Investigative pathway for a patient with normal sexual characteristics.

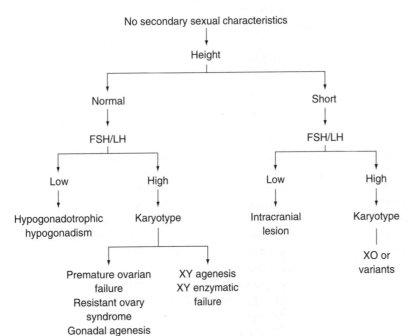

Fig. 38.2 Investigative pathway for a patient with no secondary sexual characteristics.

changes of puberty occur as a result of endocrine maturation. During childhood gonadotrophin levels are low, both in terms of pulse frequency and pulse amplitude but finally the establishment of a mature hypothalamus and gonadotrophin-releasing hormone (GnRH) release leads to a normal endocrine environment [4]. This results in ovarian stimulation and the production of oestradiol from the follicles which begin to develop at around the age of

8.5 years [5]. This rise in oestrogen leads to secondary sexual development of the breasts and the establishment of menstruation. The secretion of androgen (primarily dihydroepiandrosterone (DHEA) and dihydroepiandrosterone sulphate (DHEAS)) begins to rise at around the age of 6 (adrenarche) and continues to rise until the age of 12 years. These seem to be the prime instigators of pubic and axillary hair growth.

Aetiology of primary amenorrhoea

From a clinical aspect it is probably best to classify the aetiologies of primary amenorrhoea based on the presence or absence of secondary sexual characteristics. This will be used as the basis of a classification system (Table 38.1), and finally there is a group of patients in whom there is heterosexual development.

Table 38.1 Classification of primary amenorrhoea

Secondary sexual characteristics normal
Imperforate hymen
Transverse vaginal septum
Absent vagina and functioning uterus
Absent vagina and non-functioning uterus
XY female – androgen insensitivity
Resistant ovary syndrome
Constitutional delay

Secondary sexual characteristics absent
Normal stature
  Hypogonadotrophic hypogonadism
    Congenital
  Isolated gonodotrophin-releasing hormone deficiency
  Olfactogenital syndrome
    Acquired
  Weight loss/anorexia
  Excessive exercise
  Hyperprolactinaemia
Hypergonadotrophic hypogonadism
  Gonadal agenesis
  XX agenesis
  XX or XY agenesis
  Gonadal dysgenesis
  Turner mosaic
  Other X deletions or mosaics
  XY enzymatic failure
  Ovarian failure
  Galactosaemia
Short stature
  Hypogonadotrophic hypogonadism
    Congenital
  Hydrocephalus
    Acquired
  Trauma
  Empty sella syndrome
  Tumours
  Hypergonadotrophic hypogonadism
  Turner syndrome
  Other X deletions or mosaics

Heterosexual development
Congenital adrenal hyperplasia
Androgen-secreting tumour
5α-Reductase deficiency
Partial androgen receptor deficiency
True hermaphrodite
Absent Müllerian inhibitor

Secondary sexual characteristics normal

IMPERFORATE HYMEN

The imperforate hymen may present at two ages of development. It may present in early childhood when the infant presents with a bulging hymen behind which is a mucocele, the vagina expanded by vaginal secretions of mucus. This is easily released and does not subsequently cause any problems following hymenectomy. It may also present in later life when a pubertal girl complains of intermittent abdominal pain, which is usually cyclical. The pain is due to dysmenorrhoea associated with the accumulation of menstrual blood within the vagina. The vagina's very distensible features allow quite large quantities of blood to collect in some cases. This situation is known as haematocolpos. It is very unusual for much blood to accumulate within the uterus as the uterus is a muscular organ which is difficult to distend. When some blood does accumulate within the cavity it is known as a haematometra. As the mass enlarges there may be associated difficulty with micturition and defaecation. Examination will reveal on occasions an abdominal swelling and observation of the introitus will display a tense bulging bluish membrane which is the hymen.

TRANSVERSE VAGINAL SEPTUM

In circumstances where the vagina fails to cannulate the upper and lower parts of the vagina are separate. These girls present with cyclical abdominal pain due to the development of a haematocolpos, but the thickness of the transverse vaginal septum means that the clinical appearance is very different from that of an imperforate hymen. Again, an abdominal mass may be palpable but inspection of the vagina shows that it is blind ending and, although it may be bulging, it is pink not blue. The hymenal remnants are often seen separately. Transverse vaginal septum may occur at three levels, known as a lower, middle or upper third septum. If the space between the upper and lower vagina is considerable, no introital swelling may be visible and rectal examination may disclose a mass. The management is very different from imperforate hymen and very careful assessment must be made before embarking on any management strategy.

ABSENT VAGINA AND THE FUNCTIONING UTERUS

This is a rare phenomenon when embryologically the uterine body has developed normally, but there is failure of development of the cervix. This leads to failure of the development of the upper vagina. The presenting symptom is again cyclical abdominal pain, but there is no pelvic mass to be found because there is no vagina to be distended. Although a small haematometra may be present, retrograde menstruation occurs leading to the development of endometriosis and in some patients pelvic adhesions.

ABSENT VAGINA AND A NON-FUNCTIONING UTERUS

This is the second most common cause of primary amenorrhoea, second only to Turner syndrome. Secondary sexual characteristics are normal as would be expected as ovarian function is unaffected. Examination of the genital area discloses normal female external genitalia but a blind ending vaginal dimple which is usually not more than 1.5 cm in depth. This is known as the Meyer-Rokitansky-Kuster-Hauser syndrome (or the MRKH syndrome) and the uterine development is usually very rudimentary. Often small uterine remnants (anlage) are found on the lateral pelvic side walls. It is important to remember that 40% of these patients have renal anomalies, 15% of which are major, for example, an absent kidney, and there are also recognizable skeletal abnormalities in association with this syndrome [6].

XY FEMALE

There are a number of ways in which an individual may have an XY karyotype and a female phenotype. These are failure of testicular development, enzymatic failure of the testis to produce androgen, particularly testosterone, and androgenic receptor absence or failure of function. In androgen insensitivity there is a structural abnormality with the androgen receptor, due to abnormalities of the androgen receptor gene, which results in a non-functional receptor. This means that the masculinizing effect of testosterone during normal development is prevented and patients are therefore phenotypically female with normal breast development. This occurs because of peripheral conversion of androgen to oestrogen and subsequent stimulation of breast growth. Pubic hair is very scanty in these patients as there is no androgen response in target tissues. The vulva is normal and the vagina is usually short. The uterus and tubes are absent in this particular version of the XY female. The testes are usually found in the lower abdomen, but occasionally may be found in hernial sacs in childhood, which alerts the surgeon to the diagnosis [7]. Other versions of this syndrome are not associated with secondary sexual development (see below).

RESISTANT OVARY SYNDROME

This is an extremely rare condition as a cause of primary amenorrhoea, but it has been described. There are elevated levels of gonadotrophin in the presence of apparently normal ovarian tissue; patients do have some degree of secondary sexual characteristic development, but never produce adequate amounts of oestrogen to result in menstruation. It is believed that these women have an absence or malfunction of follicle-stimulating hormone (FSH) receptors in the ovarian follicles, and are unable to respond properly to FSH.

CONSTITUTIONAL DELAY

There are, however, a number of girls in whom normal secondary sexual characteristics exist. There is no anatomical anomaly and endocrine investigations are all normal. If serial sampling is carried out during a 24-h period these young women are found to have immature pulsatile release of GnRH. This is the sole reason for their constitutional delay. These young women will eventually menstruate spontaneously as the maturation process proceeds.

Secondary sexual characteristics absent (normal height)

ISOLATED GNRH DEFICIENCY (THE OLFACTOGENITAL SYNDROME, KALLMAN SYNDROME)

In this condition the hypothalamus lacks the ability to produce GnRH and therefore there is a hypogonadotrophic state. The pituitary gland is normal and stimulation with exogenous GnRH leads to normal release of gonadotrophins. This condition arises due to a maldevelopment of neurones in the arcuate nucleus of the hypothalamus. These neurones are derived embryologically from the olfactory bulb, and therefore some patients may also have failure of development of the ability to smell (anosmia). When this occurs it is known as Kallman syndrome. The genetic basis of Kallman syndrome is slowly being discovered and so far two possibilities exist which are either mutations of the X chromosome KAL1 gene (encoding anosmin) or the fibroblast growth factor receptor 1 gene (FGFR1), which both lead to agenesis of the olfactory and GnRH-secreting neurones [8]. There may well be other mutations and other genes involved which still need to be discovered.

WEIGHT LOSS/ANOREXIA

Weight loss is more commonly associated with secondary amenorrhoea than primary amenorrhoea, but unfortunately it is increasingly apparent that young girls may suffer from anorexia nervosa in the prepubertal state. This leads to failure of the activation of the gene which initiates GnRH release in the hypothalamus, and therefore a persistent hypogonadotrophic state exists. The growth spurt is not usually influenced by this, but secondary sexual characteristics are absent.

EXCESSIVE EXERCISE

Over recent years it has become increasingly recognized that excessive exercise in pubertal children leads to a decreased body fat content, without necessarily affecting body mass. Development of muscle contributes to overall weight, and therefore weight alone cannot be used as the parameter to discover whether or not there is an aetiology for their amenorrhoea through this mechanism. A number of examples of this exist including ballet dancers, athletes and gymnasts. These girls fail to menstruate and may actually develop frank anorexia nervosa.

HYPERPROLACTINAEMIA

This is an unusual cause of primary amenorrhoea and much more commonly seen as a cause of secondary amenorrhoea. There may be a recognizable prolactinoma in the pituitary, but often no apparent reason is seen. Imaging may reveal an anomaly.

GONADAL AGENESIS

In this situation there is complete failure of development of the gonad. These girls may be either 46XX or 46XY. The 46XX pure gonadal dysgenesis is an autosomal recessive disorder and other genes other than those located on the X chromosome are involved. The location of these genes remains unclear and in all these patients their genotype does not affect their phenotype, all of them being female. In 46XY or 45X/46XY, when the absence of testicular determining factor or its receptor are postulated as the cause of the failure of differentiation of the gonad, there is absence of testicular development. They, therefore, fail to produce any androgen or Müllerian inhibitor. Therefore Wolffian structures regress and Müllerian structures persist and menstruation will occur when oestrogen is administered. The external genitalia reflect normal female phenotype. Height is normal as the growth spurt occurs at the normal time. However, in those girls who are 46XY the failure of production of androgen or oestrogen means that their long bones do not undergo epiphyseal closure at the normal time and therefore final height may be excessive.

OVARIAN FAILURE

These unfortunate girls have ovarian failure as a result of either chemotherapy or radiotherapy for childhood malignancy.

GALACTOSAEMIA

This inborn error of galactose metabolism is due to the deficiency of galactose-1-phosphate uridyl transferase. The aetiology of the association between this and hypogonadotrophic hypogonadism is still to be clarified but these patients have galactose-1-phosphate uridyltransferase and this acute toxic syndrome causes ovarian cellular destruction which is thought to be due to the accumulation of galactose metabolites which may induce programmed cell death (apoptosis).

GONADAL DYSGENESIS

The gonad is described as dysgenetic if it is abnormal in its formation. This encompasses a spectrum of conditions which vary with the degree of differentiation. The commonest is Turner syndrome, which is a single X chromosome giving 45X as the karyotype. The missing chromosome may be either X or Y. There are other circumstances in which the gonadal dysgenesis may be associated with a mosaic. Here two cell lines exist within one individual, the most common being 45X/46XX. There are other structural chromosomal anomalies associated with gonadal dysgenesis known as deletions. If the deletion involves the part of the long arm of the X chromosome or the short arm then loss of this genetic material may affect gonadal development. In Turner's syndrome ovarian development is normal until 20 weeks' of gestation and at this stage oocytes are found in the ovaries. However, further maturation is impaired and a massive atresia occurs during the latter part of pregnancy. The ovaries in most individuals consist solely of stroma and are unable to produce oestrogen. There is a normal female phenotype and internal genital development is also normal. The loss of an X chromosome results in short stature as the genes for height are on the short arm of the X chromosome. In mosaicism the proportion of each cell line determines the manifestation of the condition. The higher the percentage of 45X cells the more likely are the features of Turner syndrome.

In XY individuals there may be a dysgenetic gonad associated with enzymatic failure. In this situation testosterone fails to be produced. This is usually associated with normal production of Müllerian inhibitor. Therefore internal development leads to Müllerian atrophy, but external development fails to masculinize due to the lack of testosterone. Wolffian structures also fail to develop. The external phenotype, therefore, is female with a short vagina.

Secondary sexual characteristics absent (short stature)

CONGENITAL INFECTION

The most common aetiology in this group is hydrocephalus, as a result of childhood or neonatal infection. It is believed that this aetiology damages the hypothalamus and renders the GnRH-secreting neurones functionless, thereby creating a hypogonadotrophic hypogonadic state.

TRAUMA

Trauma to the skull base may also damage the hypothalamus, and prevent GnRH secretion.

EMPTY SELLA SYNDROME

In this unusual condition the sella turcica is found to be empty and there is congenital absence of the pituitary gland or at least part of it leading to failure to produce gonadotrophins. Thus secondary sexual characteristics do not develop.

TUMOURS

A number of tumours have been described in the pituitary which may lead to destruction of the gland. The most common of which is craniopharyngioma. This is a tumour which usually arises in childhood and results in destruction of the pituitary gland. These children present already on maintenance therapy for other hormonal deficiencies and are hypogonadotrophic.

TURNER SYNDROME

In pure Turner syndrome the chromosome complement is 45X and here a syndrome of short stature and ovarian failure lead to the typical features of this syndrome. These children usually present in the teenage years, either because of failure of development of secondary sexual characteristics or more commonly referred from growth clinics for induction of secondary sexual characteristics. Attempts to improve height have proved difficult to achieve.

Heterosexual development

CONGENITAL ADRENAL HYPERPLASIA

This anomaly occurs as a result of an enzyme deficiency in the steroid pathway of the adrenal gland (see Chapter 34) and children with this condition require steroid replacement [9,10]. It is imperative that they have good control of their congenital adrenal hyperplasia at puberty if they are to go through the process of secondary sexual characteristic development at the appropriate time. However, many of these girls fail to comply with their steroid therapy and they are therefore uncontrolled. As a result of that, they fail to establish the normal process of puberty. It is therefore

quite common to find that puberty is delayed and steroid control needs to be addressed [11,12].

ANDROGEN-SECRETING TUMOURS

These extremely rare situations arise when the ovary contains an arrhenoblastoma. Here excessive production of androgen results in virilization and removal of the tumour resolves the problem.

5α-REDUCTASE DEFICIENCY

This form of XY female results from an enzyme deficiency, which prevents the conversion of testosterone to 5-hydroxytestosterone, which is a necessary biochemical step in the development of the external genitalia in the male. The cloaca can only respond to this testosterone derivative and not to testosterone itself. The external genitalia are therefore female, but the internal genitalia are normal male as Müllerian inhibitor secretion leads to Müllerian agenesis. These patients are therefore amenorrhoeic.

TRUE HERMAPHRODITE

In this condition the child has the presence of both testicular and ovarian tissue. This may occur either in isolation, such that there is an ovary and a testis in the same individual, or the gonad may contain both ovarian and testicular tissue. This leads to intersex problems at birth (see Chapter 34), and subsequently, if not resolved at birth, amenorrhoea due to androgen production at puberty, thereby preventing the development of the normal menstrual cycle.

ABSENT MÜLLERIAN INHIBITOR

There is a rare condition in which an XY individual may not produce Müllerian-inhibitory substance (MIS) which means that the internal genitalia are female with persistence of the Müllerian structures and also because testosterone is produced the Wolffian structures also persist. In this extremely rare syndrome there is dual internal organ persistence.

Evaluation and management

Having understood the classification of these syndromes, it becomes apparent that most of the conditions are rare and constitutional delay without doubt is the most common diagnosis. However, as the rest of the diagnoses have serious implications this diagnosis of constitutional delay should only be made when all other syndromes have been excluded. It is important to record a full history and examination including most importantly the development of secondary sexual characteristics and height. Secondary sexual characteristics should be classified according to the staging system of Tanner. Individuals can then be classified according to their secondary sexual characteristics.

Normal secondary sexual characteristics

The presence of normal secondary sexual characteristics should alert the clinician to the concept that outflow tract obstruction may be occurring. This is the most common cause of primary amenorrhoea in the presence of normal secondary sexual characteristics. It is thus appropriate to carry out investigations to make this diagnosis. It is inappropriate to perform any physical pelvic examination on these young adolescents and imaging techniques should be used. It is simple to arrange for a pelvic ultrasound to assess the pelvic anatomy, and only in rare circumstances where this cannot be delineated by ultrasound should it be necessary to use magnetic resonance imaging (MRI) or computed tomography (CT) scanning. If the uterus is absent the karyotype should be performed and if this is 46XX then the Rokitansky syndrome is the most likely diagnosis. If the chromosome complement is 46XY the patient is, by definition, an XY female. If the uterus is present on ultrasound then there may be an associated haematocolpos and haematometra and appropriate reconstructive surgery should be carried out. If the pelvic anatomy is normal then it is essential to assess gonadotrophin and prolactin levels as this would tend to indicate a hypothalamic cause for the amenorrhoea, so-called constitutional delay. In some conditions the luteinizing hormone (LH) to FSH ratio may be elevated, for example, polycystic ovaries, and if resistant ovary syndrome is the diagnosis these gonadotrophin levels will be elevated. Elevation of prolactin levels suggests a prolactinoma.

MANAGEMENT

Patients with an absent uterus require special psychological counselling and their care should be managed in a centre able to offer the complete range of psychological psychosexual and gynaecological expertise. These young girls will have major problems with future sexual activity and their infertility. They require very careful counselling. At the appropriate time a vagina may be created either non-surgically or surgically. In 85% of cases the use of vaginal dilators is successful (see Chapter 37).

In girls who are found to have an XY karyotype, careful counselling is necessary over the malignant potential of their gonads, this being reported at around 30%. It is therefore necessary for them to have their gonads removed and this must be performed at a time when counselling is complete. Sharing the information of the karyotype with the patient should be entertained at that time when the relationship between the clinician and the patient warrants it. Not all women wish this information when they are young, but if directly requested it should be shared with them. At some stage it is probably best that all patients be informed of their karyotype.

In outflow tract obstruction surgical management may occur at various levels. The simplest form is an imperforate hymen and in this condition a cruciate incision in the hymen allows drainage of the retained menstrual blood. Transverse vaginal septae are much more difficult to deal with and require specialist reconstruction to create a vagina which is subsequently functional (see Chapter 37) [13].

If investigations suggest constitutional delay and secondary sexual characteristic development is complete, there is no need to suggest any treatment other than annual review. These young women very much appreciate the opportunity to return for monitoring until such times as their menstruation commences. In some circumstances it may be useful to promote a menstruation using the oral contraceptive pill for one cycle to prove that menstruation can occur and this can be extremely reassuring. If the diagnosis of a resistant ovary syndrome is suspected, then diagnosis can really only be made by ovarian biopsy and subsequent histology confirming or illustrating the absence of oocytes. Finally, elevated prolactin levels should provoke the clinician to perform an imaging of the pituitary fossa, probably best done by CT scan or MRI to determine the presence or absence of a microadenoma and management subsequently with bromocriptine.

Absence of secondary sexual characteristics

In this particular situation, it is extremely important to make an assessment of the patient's height. If the patient is of normal height for age, measurement of gonadotrophin will reveal levels that are either low or high. Low levels of gonadotrophins confirm the diagnosis of hypogonadotrophin hypogonadism, and elevated levels should provoke the clinician to perform a karyotype. The 46XX patient will have premature ovarian failure, the resistant ovary syndrome or gonadal agenesis while the XY female will have 46XY gonadal agenesis or testicular enzymatic failure. If stature is short gonadotrophin levels will either be low, as associated with an intracranial lesion or high which, following a karyotype, will almost certainly indicate Turner syndrome or a Turner mosaic.

MANAGEMENT

In patients with hypogonadotrophic hypogonadism treatment should be towards managing any avoidable problem or in the isolated GnRH deficiency hormone replacement therapy will need to be instituted to induce secondary sexual characteristic development. These patients can be informed that they are infertile and that ovulation induction in the future can be invoked using various fertility regimes. Hormone replacement therapy is essential and regimes exist for the induction of secondary sexual characteristics over 3–5 years. Oestrogen should be used alone for about 2 years, and then 2–3 years of gradual introduction of progestogens thereby establishing normal breast growth over a time frame that is equivalent to normal. Any attempt to accelerate breast growth by using higher doses of oestrogen will result in abnormal breast growth and this should be avoided at all costs. Patients with an XY dysgenesis or enzymatic failure should have gonadectomies performed to avoid malignancy.

It must always be remembered that any chronic medical illness which prevents normal growth will result in delayed onset of puberty and these causes must be considered in any patient presenting in this way.

References

1. Tanner JM (1962) *Growth at Adolescence*. Oxford: Blackwell Scientific Publications.
2. Marshall WA & Tanner JM (1969) Variation in the pattern of pubertal changes in girls. *Arch Dis Child* **44**, 291.
3. Marshall WA (1974) Growth and secondary sexual characteristics and related abnormalities. *Clin Obstet Gynecol* **1**, 593.
4. Lee PA, Plotnick LP, Migeon CJ *et al.* (1978) Integrated concentrations of follicle stimulating hormone and puberty. *J Clin Endocrinol Metab* **46**, 488.
5. Stanhope R, Adams J, Jacobs HS & Brook CGD (1985) Ovarian ultrasound assessment in normal children and idiopathic precocious puberty. *Arch Dis Child* **60**, 116.
6. Edmonds DK (2003) Congenital malformations of the genital tract and their management. *Best Practice Res Clin Obstet Gynaecol* **17**, 19–40.
7. Dewhurst CJ & Spence JEH (1977) The XY female. *Br J Hosp Med* **17**, 498.
8. Karges B & de Roux N (2005) Molecular genetics of isolated hypogonadotropic hypogonadism and Kallmann syndrome. *Endocr Dev* **8**, 67–80.
9. White PC, Grossberger D & Onufer BJ (1985) Two genes encoding steroid 21-hydroxylase are located near the genes encoding the fourth component of complement in man. *Proc Natl Acad Sci* **82**, 1089.
10. Donohoue PA, Van Dop, Jospe N *et al.* (1986) Congenital adrenal hyperplasia: molecular mechanisms resulting in 21 hydroxylase deficiency. *Acta Endocrinol* Suppl **279**, 315.
11. Grant D, Muram D & Dewhurst CG (1983) Menstrual and fertility patterns in patients with congenital adrenal hyperplasia. *Pediatr Adolesc Gynecol* **1**, 97.
12. Edmonds DK (1989) *Dewhurst's Practice Paediatric and Adolescent Gynaecology*. London: Butterworths.
13. Edmonds DK (1993) Sexual developmental abnormalities and their reconstruction. In: Sanfillipo J (ed.) *Pediatric and Adolescent Gynaecology*. Philadelphia: Saunders.

Further reading

Timmreck LS & Reindollar RH (2003) Contemporary issues in primary amenorrhoea. *Obstet Gynecol Clin North Am* **30**, 287–302.

Fenichel P (2004) Delayed puberty. In: Sultan C (ed.) *Pediatric and Adolescent Gynecology. Evidence-based Clinical Practice*, Vol. 7. Basel: Karger, 106–28.

Chapter 39: Polycystic ovary syndrome and secondary amenorrhoea

Adam H. Balen

Introduction: defining polycystic ovary syndrome and secondary amenorrhoea

In this chapter we shall first describe in detail our current understanding of polycystic ovary syndrome (PCOS), which is a condition that presents with ovarian dysfunction and endocrine problems and is also associated with hyperinsulinaemia and metabolic disease. The polycystic ovary syndrome is a heterogeneous condition which is defined by the presence of two out of the following three criteria [1]: oligo- and/or anovulation [2], hyperandrogenism (clinical and/or biochemical) [3], polycystic ovaries, with the exclusion of other aetiologies. PCOS therefore encompasses symptoms of menstrual cycle disturbance and as such is the commonest cause of secondary amenorrhoea. The second part of the chapter will discuss the pathophysiology and management of other causes of secondary amenorrhoea.

Amenorrhoea is the absence of menstruation, which might be temporary or permanent. It may occur as a normal physiological condition such as before puberty, during pregnancy, lactation or the menopause, or as a feature of a systemic or gynaecological disorder. Primary amenorrhoea may be a result of congenital abnormalities in the development of ovaries, genital tract or external genitalia or a perturbation of the normal endocrinological events of puberty (and these are described in Chapter 37). Furthermore, most of the causes of secondary amenorrhoea can also cause primary amenorrhoea, if they occur before the menarche.

Examination and investigation of patients with PCOS and secondary amenorrhoea

A thorough history and a careful examination should always be carried out before investigations are instigated – looking particularly at stature and body form, signs of endocrine disease, secondary sexual development and the external genitalia. A history of secondary amenorrhoea may be misleading, as the 'periods' may have been the result of exogenous hormone administration in a patient who was being treated with hormone replacement therapy (HRT) for primary amenorrhoea. In most cases, however, a history of secondary amenorrhoea excludes congenital abnormalities. A family history of fertility problems, autoimmune disorders or premature menopause may also give clues to the aetiology.

EXCLUDE PREGNANCY

It is always important to exclude pregnancy in women of any age and whereas some may think that this statement superfluous, it is usual to see one or two patients a year who are pregnant despite denying the possibility.

EXAMINATION

Measurement of height and weight should be done in order to calculate a patient's body mass index (BMI). The normal range is 20–25 kg/m^2, and a value above or below this range may suggest a diagnosis of weight-related amenorrhoea (which is a term usually applied to underweight women).

Signs of hyperandrogenism (acne, hirsutism, balding (alopecia)) are suggestive of the PCOS, although biochemical screening helps to differentiate other causes of androgen excess. It is important to distinguish between hyperandrogenism and virilization, which is additionally associated with high circulating androgen levels and causes deepening of the voice, breast atrophy, increase in muscle bulk and cliteromegaly (see Virilization p. 378). A rapid onset of hirsutism suggests the presence of an androgen secreting tumour of the ovary or adrenal gland. Hirsutism can be graded and given a 'Ferriman-Gallwey Score', by assessing the amount of hair in different parts of the body (e.g. upper lip, chin, breasts, abdomen, arms and legs). It is useful to monitor the progress of hirsutism, or its response to treatment, by making serial records, either using a chart or by taking photographs of affected areas of the body.

A total testosterone is adequate for general screening (Table 39.1). It is unnecessary to measure other androgens

Table 39.1 Endocrine normal ranges

Follicle stimulating harmone (FSH)*	1–10 IU/l (early follicular)
Luteinizing hormone (LH)*	1–10 IU/l (early follicular)
Prolactin*	<400 mIU/l
Thyroid stimulating hormone*	0.5–5.0 IU/l
Thyroxine (T4)	50–150 nmol/l
Free T4	9–22 pmol/l
Tri-iodothyronine (T3)	1.5–3.5 nmol/l
Free T3	4.3–8.6 pmol/l
Thyroid binding globulin (TBG)	7–17 mg/l
Testosterone (T)*	0.5–3.5 nmol/l
Sex hormone binding globulin (SHBG)	16–120 nmol/l
Free androgen index ([T × 100] ÷ SHBG)	<5
Dihydrotestosterone	0.3–1 nmol/l
Androstenedione	2–10 nmol/l
Dehydroepiandrosterone sulphate	3–10 μmol/l
Cortisol: 8 a.m.	140–700 nmol/l
midnight	0–140 nmol/l
24 h urinary	<400 nmol/24h
Oestradiol	250–500 pmol/l
Oestrone	400–600 pmol/l
Progesterone (mid-luteal)	>25 nmol/l to indicate ovulation
17-hydroxyprogesterone	1–20 nmol/l

* Denotes those tests performed in routine screening of women with amenorrhoea.

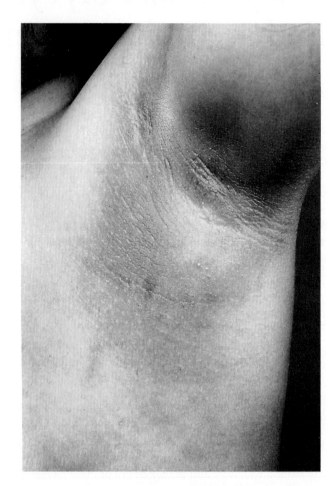

Fig. 39.1 Acanthosis nigricans, as seen typically in the skin folds (axilla, neck, elbow, vulva). Reproduced from *Infertility in Practice*, 2nd edn., Balen & Jacobs, Churchill Livingstone 2003, with permission.

unless total testosterone is >5 nmol/l. Insulin suppresses SHBG, resulting in a high free androgen index (FAI) in the presence of a normal total *T*. The measurement of SHBG is not required in routine practice and will not affect management.

One should be aware of the possibility of Cushing's syndrome in women with stigmata of the PCOS and obesity as it is a disease of insidious onset and dire consequences; additional clues are the presence of central obesity, moon face, plethoric complexion, buffalo hump, proximal myopathy, thin skin, bruising and abdominal striae (which alone are a common finding in obese individuals). Acanthosis nigricans is a sign of profound insulin resistance and is usually visible as hyperpigmented thickening of the skin folds of the axilla and neck; it is associated with PCOS and obesity (Fig. 39.1).

Virilization

A testosterone concentration greater than 5 nmol/l should be investigated to exclude androgen secreting tumours

of the ovary or adrenal gland, Cushing's syndrome and late-onset congenital adrenal hyperplasia (CAH). While CAH often presents at birth with ambiguous genitalia (see Chapter 34), partial 21-hydroxylase deficiency may present in later life, usually in the teenage years with signs and symptoms similar to PCOS. In such cases testosterone may be elevated and the diagnosis confirmed by an elevated serum concentration of 17-hydroxyprogesterone (17-OHP); an abnormal ACTH stimulation test may also be helpful (250 μg ACTH will cause an elevation of 17-OHP, usually between 65 and 470 nmol/l).

In cases of Cushing's syndrome a 24-h urinary free cortisol will be elevated (>700 nmol/24 h). The normal serum concentration of cortisol is 140–700 nmol/l at 8 a.m. and less than 140 nmol/l at midnight. A low-dose dexamethasone suppression test (0.5 mg 6-hourly for 48 h) will cause a suppression of serum cortisol by 48 h. A simpler screening test is an overnight suppression test, using a single midnight dose of dexamethasone 1 mg (2 mg if obese) and measuring the serum cortisol concentration at 08.00 h when it should be less than 140 nmol/l. If Cushing's syndrome is confirmed a high-dose dexamethasone suppression test (2 mg 6-hourly for 48 h) should suppress serum cortisol by 48 h if there is a pituitary ACTH-secreting adenoma (Cushing's disease); failure of suppression suggests an adrenal tumour or ectopic secretion of ACTH – further tests and detailed imaging will then be required.

The measurement of other serum androgen levels can be helpful. Dehydroepiandrosterone sulphate (DHEAS) is primarily a product of the adrenal androgen pathway (normal range <10 μmol/l). If the serum androgen concentrations are elevated the possibility of an ovarian or adrenal tumour should be excluded by ultrasound or CT scans.

Amenorrhoeic women might have hyperprolactinaemia and galactorrhoea. It is important, however, not to examine the breasts before taking blood as the serum prolactin concentration may be falsely elevated. If there is suspicion of a pituitary tumour, the patient's visual fields should be checked, as bitemporal hemianopia secondary to pressure on the optic chiasm requires urgent attention. General, vaginal, breast examinations and stress can all cause a temporary elevation in serum prolactin concentration.

Thyroid disease is common and the thyroid gland should be palpated and signs of hypothyroidism (dry thin hair, proximal myopathy, myotonia, slow-relaxing reflexes, mental slowness, bradycardia, etc.) or hyperthyroidism (goitre with bruit, tremor, weight loss, tachycardia, hyperreflexia, exopthalmos, conjunctival oedema, ophthalmoplegia, etc.) elicited.

A bimanual examination is inappropriate in a young woman who has never been sexually active, and examination of the external genitalia of an adolescent should be undertaken in the presence of the patient's mother. Furthermore, it may be more appropriate to defer this from the first consultation to assure the patient's confidence in future management. A transabdominal ultrasound examination of the pelvis is an excellent non-invasive method of obtaining valuable information in these patients and while an examination under anaesthetic is sometimes indicated for cases of intersex with primary amenorrhoea, it is rarely required in cases of secondary amenorrhoea.

Endocrine investigations (Table 39.1)

A baseline assessment of the endocrine status should include measurement of serum prolactin and gonadotropin concentrations and an assessment of thyroid function. Prolactin levels may be elevated in response to a number of conditions, including stress, a recent breast examination, or even having a venepuncture. The elevation,

however, is moderate and transient. A more permanent, but still moderate elevation (greater than 700 mIU/l) is associated with hypothyroidism and is also a common finding in women with PCOS, where prolactin levels up to 2500 mIU/l have been reported [1]. PCOS may also result in amenorrhoea, which can therefore create diagnostic difficulties, and hence appropriate management, for those women with hyperprolactinaemia and polycystic ovaries. Amenorrhoea in women with PCOS is secondary to acyclical ovarian activity and continuous oestrogen production. A positive response to a progestogen challenge test (e.g. medroxyprogesterone acetate 10 mg daily for 5 days), which induces a withdrawal bleed will distinguish patients with PCOS related hyperprolactinaemia from those with polycystic ovaries and unrelated hyperprolactinaemia, because the latter causes oestrogen deficiency and therefore failure to respond to the progestogen challenge.

A serum prolactin concentration of greater than 1500 mIU/l warrants further investigation. Computerized tomography (CT) or magnetic resonance imaging (MRI) of the pituitary fossa may be used to exclude a hypothalamic tumour, a non-functioning pituitary tumour compressing the hypothalamus or a prolactinoma. Serum prolactin concentrations greater than 5000 mIU/l are usually associated with a macroprolactinoma which by definition are greater than 1 cm in diameter.

The patient's oestrogen status may be assessed clinically by examination of the lower genital tract, or by means of a progestogen challenge. Serum measurements of oestradiol are unhelpful as they vary considerably, even in a patient with amenorrhoea. If the patient is well oestrogenized the endometrium will be shed on withdrawal of the progestogen.

Serum gonadotropin measurements help to distinguish between cases of hypothalamic or pituitary failure and gonadal failure. Elevated gonaotrophin concentrations indicate a failure of negative feedback as a result of primary ovarian failure. A serum follicle stimulating hormone (FSH) concentration of greater than 15 IU/L that is not associated with a preovulatory surge suggests impending ovarian failure. FSH levels of greater than 40 IU/L are suggestive of irreversible ovarian failure. The exact values vary according to individual assays, and so local reference levels should be checked [2]. It is important also to assess serum gonadotropin levels at baseline, that is during the first 3 days of a menstrual period. In patients with oligo/amenorrhoea it may be necessary to perform two or more random measurements, although combining assessment of endocrinology with an ultrasound scan on the same day aids the diagnosis.

An elevated luteinizing hormone (LH) concentration, when associated with a raised FSH concentration, is indicative of ovarian failure. However, if LH is elevated alone (and is not attributable to the preovulatory LH surge), this suggests PCOS. This may be confirmed by a pelvic ultrasound scan. Rarely an elevated LH in a phenotypic female may be due to androgen insensitivity syndrome (AIS), although this condition presents with primary amenorrhoea.

Failure at the level of the hypothalamus or pituitary is reflected by abnormally low levels of serum gonadotropin concentrations, and gives rise to hypogonadotrophic hypogonadism. Kallman's syndrome is the clinical finding of hyposmia and/or colour blindness associated with hypogonadotrophic hypogonadism – usually a cause of primary amenorrhoea. It is difficult to distinguish between hypothalamic and pituitary aetiology as both respond to stimulation with gonadotropin releasing hormone (GnRH). A skull X-ray should be performed and CT or MRI if indicated.

Karyotype and other tests

Women with premature ovarian failure (under the age of 40 years) may have a chromosomal abnormality (e.g. Turner's syndrome [45X, or 46XX/45X mosaic] or other sex chromosome mosaicisms) (Plate 39.1 *facing p. 562*). A number of genes have also been associated with familial POF, but are not assessed in routine clinical practice. An autoantibody screen should also be undertaken in women with a premature menopause, although it can be difficult to detect antiovarian antibodies many will have evidence of other autoantibodies (e.g. thyroid), which then indicates the need for further surveillance.

A history of a recent endometrial curettage or endometritis in a patient with normal genitalia and normal endocrinology, but with absent or only a small withdrawal bleed following a progestogen challenge, is suggestive of Asherman's syndrome. A hysterosalpingogram (HSG) may be helpful and a hysteroscopy will confirm the diagnosis (Fig. 39.2).

Measurement of bone mineral density (BMD) is indicated in amenorrhoeic women who are oestrogen deficient. Measurements of density are made in the lumbar spine and femoral neck. The vertebral bone is more sensitive to oestrogen deficiency and vertebral fractures tend to occur in a younger age group (50–60 years) than fractures at the femoral neck (70+ years). However, it should be noted that crush fractures can spuriously increase the measured BMD. An X-ray of the dorsolumbar spine is therefore often complimentary, particularly in patients who have lost height.

Amenorrhoea may also have long-term metabolic and physical consequences. In women with PCOS and prolonged amenorrhoea, there is a risk of endometrial hyperplasia and adenocarcinoma. If, on resumption of

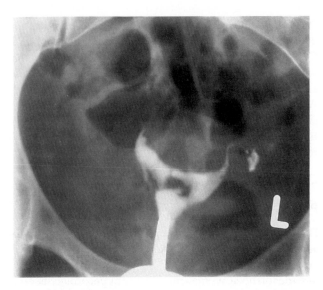

Fig. 39.2 Conventional X-ray HSG demonstrating Ashermann's syndrome, with intrauterine synechiae. There is no flow of contrast through the right tube, although thickening of the cornula end of the tube suggests the possibility of tubal spasm. There is flow to the end of the left fallopian tube, although no free spill into the peritoneal cavity. This raises the possibility of sacculated adhesions around the fimbrial end of the tube. Reproduced from *Infertility in Practice*, 2nd edn., Balen & Jacobs, Churchill Livingstone 2003, with permission.

menstruation there is a history of persistent intermenstrual bleeding or on ultrasound there is a postmenstrual endometrial thickness of greater than 10 mm then an endometrial biopsy is indicated.

Serum cholesterol measurements are important because of the association of an increased risk of heart disease in women with premature ovarian failure. Women with PCOS [3], although not oestrogen deficient, may have a subnormal HDL:total cholesterol ratio. This is a consequence of the hypersecretion of insulin that occurs in many women with PCOS, and may increase the lifetime risk of heart disease.

Glucose tolerance

Women who are obese, and also many slim women with PCOS, will have insulin resistance and elevated serum concentrations of insulin (usually <30 mU/l fasting). A 75 g oral glucose tolerance test (GTT) should be performed in women with PCOS and a BMI > 30 kg/m^2, with an assessment of the fasting and 2-hour glucose concentration (Table 39.2). It has been suggested that South Asian women should have an assessment of glucose tolerance if their BMI is greater than 25 kg/m^2 because of the greater risk of insulin resistance at a lower BMI than seen in the Caucasian population.

Table 39.2 Definitions of glucose tolerance after a 75 g glucose tolerance test (GTT)

	Diabetes mellitus	Impaired glucose tolerance (IGT)	Impaired fasting glycaemia
Fasting glucose (mmol/l)	≥7.0	<7.0	≥6.1 and <7.0
2 h glucose (mmol/l)	≥11.1	≥7.8 and ≤11.1	<7.8

Polycystic ovary syndrome

The polycystic ovary syndrome (PCOS) is a heterogeneous collection of signs and symptoms that gathered together form a spectrum of a disorder with a mild presentation in some, while in others a severe disturbance of reproductive, endocrine and metabolic function. The pathophysiology of the PCOS appears to be multifactorial and polygenic. The definition of the syndrome has been much debated. Key features include menstrual cycle disturbance, hyperandrogenism and obesity. There are many extra-ovarian aspects to the pathophysiology of PCOS, yet ovarian dysfunction is central. At a recent joint ESHRE/ASRM (European Society for Human Reproduction and Embryology/American Society for Reproductive Medicine) consensus meeting a refined definition of the PCOS was agreed: namely the presence of two out of the following three criteria:

1 Oligo- and/or anovulation;

2 Hyperandrogenism (clinical and/or biochemical);

3 Polycystic ovaries (The Rotterdam ESHRE/ASRM-sponsored PCOS consensus workshop group, 2004).

Other aetiologies of hyperandrogenism and menstrual cycle disturbance should be excluded by appropriate investigations, as described within this chapter. The morphology of the polycystic ovary, has been redefined as an ovary with 12 or more follicles measuring 2–9 mm in diameter and increased ovarian volume (>10 cm^3) [4] on transvaginal ultrasound.

There is considerable heterogeneity of symptoms and signs among women with PCOS and for an individual these may change over time [1] (Table 39.3). The PCOS is familial and various aspects of the syndrome may be differentially inherited. The PCOs can exist without clinical signs of the syndrome, which may then become expressed in certain circumstances. There are a number of factors that affect expression of PCOS, for example, a gain in weight is associated with a worsening of symptoms while weight loss may ameliorate the endocrine and metabolic profile and symptomatology [5].

Genetic studies have identified a link between PCOS and disordered insulin metabolism, and indicate that the syndrome may be the presentation of a complex genetic trait disorder. The features of obesity, hyperinsulinaemia, and hyperandrogenaemia which are commonly seen in PCOS are also known to be factors which confer an increased risk of cardiovascular disease and non-insulin dependent diabetes mellitus (NIDDM) [6]. There are studies which indicate that women with PCOS have an increased risk for these diseases which pose long-term risks for health, and this evidence has prompted debate as to the need for screening women for PCOS [7].

Various factors influence ovarian function and fertility is adversely affected by an individual being overweight or having elevated serum concentrations of LH. Strategies to induce ovulation include weight loss, oral antioestrogens (principally clomifene citrate), parenteral gonadotropin therapy and laparoscopic ovarian surgery. There have been no adequately powered randomized studies to determine which of these therapies provide the best overall chance of an ongoing pregnancy. Women with PCOS are at risk of ovarian hyperstimulation syndrome (OHSS) and so ovulation induction has to be carefully monitored with serial ultrasound scans. The realization of an association between hyperinsulinaemia and PCOS has resulted in the use of insulin lowering and sensitizing agents, such as metformin, which appear to ameliorate the biochemical profile and improve reproductive function.

Defining the polycystic ovary (Fig. 39.3)

Polycystic ovaries are commonly detected by ultrasound or other forms of pelvic imaging, with estimates of the prevalence in the general population being in the order of 20–33% [8,9]. Although the ultrasound criteria for the diagnosis of polycystic ovaries have not, until now, been universally agreed, the characteristic features are accepted as being an increase in the number of follicles and the amount of stroma as compared with normal ovaries, resulting in an increase in ovarian volume. The 'cysts' are not cysts in the sense that they do contain oocytes and indeed are follicles whose development has been arrested. The actual number of cysts may be of less relevance than the volume of ovarian stroma or of the ovary itself, which has been shown to closely correlate with serum testosterone concentrations [10].

At the recent ESHRE/ASRM consensus meeting a refined definition of the PCOS was agreed, encompassing a description of the morphology of the polycystic ovary. According to the available literature, the criteria fulfilling sufficient specificity and sensitivity to define the polycystic ovary (PCO) are the presence of 12 or more follicles measuring 2–9 mm in diameter and increased ovarian volume (>10 cm^3) [4]. If there is a follicle greater than 10 mm in diameter, the scan should be repeated at a time of ovarian

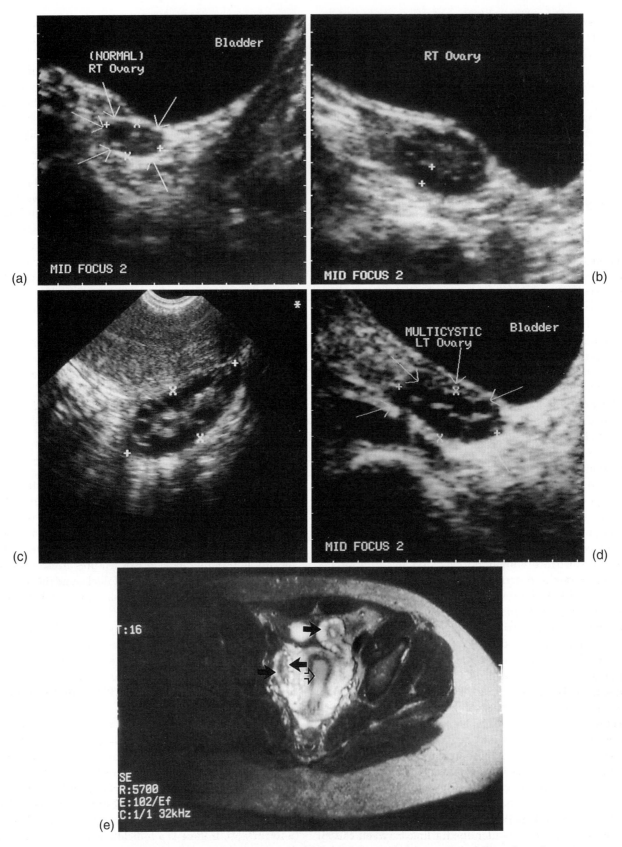

Fig. 39.3 (a) Transabdominal ultrasound scan of a normal ovary. (b) Transabdominal ultrasound scan of a polycystic ovary. (c) Transvaginal ultrasound scan of a polycystic ovary. (d) Transabdominal ultrasound scan of a multicystic ovary. (e) Magnetic resonance imaging (MRI) of a pelvis, demonstrating two polycystic ovaries (closed arrows) and a hyperplastic endometrium (open arrow). Reproduced from *Infertility in Practice*, 2nd edn., Balen & Jacobs, Churchill Livingstone 2003, with permission.

quiescence to calculate volume and area. The presence of a single polycystic ovary is sufficient to provide the diagnosis. The distribution of the follicles and the description of the stroma are not required in the diagnosis. Increased stromal echogenicity and stromal volume are specific to PCO, but it has been shown that the measurement of the ovarian volume (or area) is a good surrogate for the quantification of the stroma in clinical practice. A woman having PCO in the absence of an ovulation disorder or hyperandrogenism ('asymptomatic PCO') should not be considered as having PCOS, although she may develop symptoms over time, for example, if she gains weight.

Genetics of PCOS

The PCOS has long been noted to have a familial component [11]. Genetic analysis has been hampered by the lack of a universal definition for PCOS. Most of the criteria used for diagnosing PCOS are continuous traits, such as, degree of hirsutism, level of circulating androgens, extent of menstrual irregularity, and ovarian volume and morphology. To perform genetic analyses these continuous variables have to be transformed into nominal variables. Family studies have revealed that about 50% of first-degree relatives have PCOS suggesting a dominant mode of inheritance [12]. Commonly first-degree male relatives appear more likely to have premature baldness and metabolic syndrome. As hyperandrogenism is a key feature of PCOS it is logical to explore the critical steps in steroidogenesis and potential enzyme dysfunction. Some studies have found an abnormality with the cholesterol side chain cleavage gene (*CYP11a*), which is the rate limiting step in steroidogenesis.

It has been hypothesized that polymorphisms in the insulin receptor (*INSR*) gene that induce mild changes in insulin receptor function may contribute to the development of PCOS, as it is unlikely that a major mutation is present given the wide variability of insulin resistance in women with PCOS. The insulin gene variable number of tandem repeats (*VNTR*) minisatellite locus lies 5'-to the insulin gene on chromosome 11p15.5, and regulates the expression of the insulin gene. The class III allele of the insulin *VNTR* gene is associated with anovulatory PCOS.

Further discussion of this complex area is beyond the scope of this chapter and much research is being performed to provide a more detailed account of the various genetic abnormalities that may be involved in the pathogenesis of PCOS.

The pathophysiology of PCOS

Hypersecretion of androgens by the stromal theca cells of the polycystic ovary leads not only to the cardinal clinical manifestation of the syndrome, hyperandrogenism, but is also one of the mechanisms whereby follicular growth is inhibited with the resultant excess of immature follicles. Hypersecretion of luteinizing hormone (LH) by the pituitary – a result both of disordered ovarian-pituitary feedback and exaggerated pulses of GnRH from the hypothalamus – stimulates testosterone secretion by the ovary. Furthermore, insulin is a potent stimulus for androgen secretion by the ovary which, by way of a different receptor for insulin, does not exhibit insulin resistance. Insulin therefore amplifies the effect of LH, and additionally magnifies the degree of hyperandrogenism by suppressing liver production of the main carrier protein sex hormone binding globulin (SHBG), thus elevating the 'free androgen index'. It is a combination of genetic abnormalities combined with environmental factors, such as nutrition and body weight, which then affect expression of the syndrome.

Racial differences in expression of PCOS

The highest reported prevalence of PCO has been 52% among South Asian immigrants in Britain, of whom 49.1% had menstrual irregularity [13]. Rodin *et al.* [13] demonstrated that South Asian women with PCO, had a comparable degree of insulin resistance to controls with established type 2 diabetes mellitus. Insulin resistance and hyperinsulinaemia are common antecedents of type 2 diabetes, with a high prevalence in South Asians. Type 2 diabetes also has a familial basis, inherited as a complex genetic trait that interacts with environmental factors, chiefly nutrition, commencing from fetal life. South Asians with anovulatory PCOS have greater insulin resistance and more severe symptoms of the syndrome than anovulatory white Caucasians with PCOS [14]. Furthermore, women from South Asia, living in the UK appear to express symptoms at an earlier age than their Caucasian British counterparts.

Heterogeneity of PCOS

The findings of a large series of more than 1700 women with polycystic ovaries detected by ultrasound scan, are summarized in Table 39.4 [1]. All patients had at least one symptom of the PCOs. Thirty-eight percent of the women were overweight (BMI >25 kg/m^2). Obesity was significantly associated with an increased risk of hirsuitism, menstrual cycle disturbance and an elevated serum testosterone concentration. Obesity was also associated with an increased rate of infertility and menstrual cycle disturbance. Twenty-six percent of patients with primary infertility and 14% of patients with secondary infertility had a BMI of more than 30 kg/m^2.

Table 39.3 Signs and symptoms of polycystic ovary syndrome

Symptoms
Hyperandrogenism (acne, hirsutism, alopecia – *not* virilization)
Menstrual disturbance
Infertility
Obesity
Sometimes: asymptomatic, with polycystic ovaries on ultrasound scan

Serum endocrinology
↑ Fasting insulin (not routinely measured; insulin resistance or impaired glucose tolerance assessed by GTT)
↑ Androgens (testosterone and androstenedione)
↑ Luteinizing hormone (LH), usually normal follicle stimulating hormone (FSH)
↑ Sex hormone binding globulin (SHBG), results in elevated 'free androgen index'
↑ Oestradiol, oestrone (neither measured routinely as very wide range of values)
↑ Prolactin

Possible late sequelae
Diabetes mellitus
Dyslipidaemia
Hypertension, cardiovascular disease
Endometrial carcinoma
Breast cancer

Table 39.4 Characteristics of 1741 women with ultrasound-detected polycystic ovaries

Age (years)	31.5 (14–50)
Ovarian volume (cm^3)	11.7 (4.6–22.3)
Uterine area (cm^2)	27.5 (15.2–46.3)
Endometrium (mm)	7.5 (4.0–13.0)
BMI (kg/m^2) [19–25]*	25.4 (19.0–38.6)
FSH IU/l [1–10]*	4.5 (1.4–7.5)
LH IU/l [1–10]*	10.9 (2.0–27.0)
Testosterone nmol/l [0.5–2.5]*	2.6 (1.1–4.8)
Prolactin [<350 mU/l]*	342 (87–917)

Mean and 5–95 percentiles (*normal range).

Approximately 30% of the patients had a regular menstrual cycle, 50% had oligomenorrhoea and 20% amenorrhoea. A rising serum concentration of testosterone was associated with an increased risk of hirsuitism, infertility and cycle disturbance. The rates of infertility and menstrual cycle disturbance also increased with increasing serum LH concentrations greater than 10 IU/L. The serum LH concentration of those with primary infertility was significantly higher than that of women with secondary infertility and both were higher than the LH concentration of those with proven fertility. Ovarian morphology appears to be the most sensitive marker of the PCOS,

compared to the classical endocrine features of raised serum LH and testosterone, which were found in only 39.8 and 28.9% of patients, respectively, in this series [1].

Health consequences of polycystic ovary syndrome

Obesity and metabolic abnormalities are recognized risk factors for the development of ischaemic heart disease (IHD) in the general population, and these are also recognized features of PCOS. The question is whether women with PCOS are at an increased risk of IHD, and whether this will occur at an earlier age than women with normal ovaries. The basis for the idea that women with PCOS are at greater risk for cardiovascular disease is that these women are more insulin resistant than weight-matched controls and that the metabolic disturbances associated with insulin resistance are known to increase cardiovascular risk in other populations. Insulin resistance is defined as a diminution in the biological responses to a given level of insulin. In the presence of an adequate pancreatic reserve, normal circulating glucose levels are maintained at higher serum insulin concentrations. In the general population cardiovascular risk factors include insulin resistance, obesity, glucose intolerance, hypertension, and dyslipidaemia.

There have been a large number of studies demonstrating the presence of insulin resistance and corresponding hyperinsulinaemia in both obese and non-obese women with PCOS [6]. Obese women with PCOS have consistently been shown to be more insulin resistant than weight-matched controls. It appears that obesity and PCOS have an additive effect on the degree and severity of the insulin resistance and subsequent hyperinsulinaemia in this group of women. The insulin resistance causes compensatory hypersecretion of insulin, particularly in response to glucose, so euglycaemia is usually maintained at the expense of hyperinsulinaemia. Insulin resistance is restricted to the extra-splanchnic actions of insulin on glucose dispersal. The liver is not affected (hence the fall in SHBG and HDL), neither is the ovary (hence the menstrual problems and hypersecretion of androgens) nor the skin, hence the development of acanthosis nigricans. Women with PCOS who are oligomenorrhoeic are more likely to be insulin resistant than those with regular cycles – irrespective of their BMI, with intermenstrual interval correlating with the degree of insulin resistance [15].

Women with PCOS have a greater truncal abdominal fat distribution as demonstrated by a higher waist:hip ratio. The central distribution of fat is independent of BMI and associated with higher plasma insulin and triglyceride concentrations, and reduced HDL (high-density cholestrol) concentrations. From a practical point of view, if the measurement of waist circumference is greater than

88 cm, there will be excess visceral fat and an increased risk of metabolic problems.

Thus there is evidence that insulin resistance, central obesity and hyperandrogenaemia have an adverse effect on lipid metabolism, yet these are surrogate risk factors for cardiovascular disease. However, Pierpoint *et al.* [16] reported the mortality rate in 1028 women diagnosed as having PCOS between 1930 and 1979. All the women were older than 45 years and 770 women had been treated by wedge resection of the ovaries. Seven hundred and eighty-six women were traced; the mean age at diagnosis was 26.4 years and average duration of follow-up was 30 years. There were 59 deaths, of which 15 were from circulatory disease. Of these 15 deaths, 13 were from ischaemic heart disease. There were six deaths from diabetes as an underlying or contributory cause compared with the expected 1.7 deaths. The standard mortality rate both overall and for cardiovascular disease was not higher in the women with PCOS compared with the national mortality rates in women, although the observed proportion of women with diabetes as a contributory or underlying factor leading to death was significantly higher than expected (odds ratio 3.6, 95% CI 1.5–8.4). Thus despite surrogate markers for cardiovascular disease, in this study, no increased rate of death from CVS disease could be demonstrated.

PCOS in younger women

The majority of studies which have identified the risk factors of obesity and insulin resistance in women with PCOS have investigated adult populations, commonly including women who have presented to specialist endocrine or reproductive clinics. However, PCOS has been identified in much younger populations [9], in which women with increasing symptoms of PCOS, however, were found to be more insulin resistant. These data emphasize the need for long-term prospective studies of young women with PCOS to clarify the natural history, and to determine which women will be at risk of diabetes and cardiovascular disease later in life. A study of women with PCOS and a mean age of 39 years followed over a period of 6 years, found that 9% of those with normal glucose tolerance developed impaired glucose tolerance (IGT) and 8% developed NIDDM [17]. While 54% of women with IGT at the start of the study had NIDDM at follow-up. The risks of disease progression, not surprisingly, were greatest in those who were overweight.

ENDOMETRIAL CANCER

Endometrial adenocarcinoma is the second most common female genital malignancy but only 4% of cases occur in women less than 40 years of age. The risk of developing endometrial cancer has been shown to be adversely influenced by a number of factors including obesity, long-term use of unopposed oestrogens, nulliparity and infertility. Women with endometrial carcinoma have had fewer births compared with controls and it has also been demonstrated that infertility *per se* gives a relative risk of 2 [18]. Hypertension and Type 2 diabetes mellitus have long been linked to endometrial cancer, conditions that are now known also to be associated with PCOS. The true risk of endometrial carcinoma in women with clearly defined PCOS, however, is difficult to ascertain [19].

Endometrial hyperplasia may be a precursor to adenocarcinoma, although the rate of progression is difficult to predict. Although the degree of risk has not been clearly defined, it is generally accepted that for women with PCOS who experience amenorrhoea, or oligomenorrhoea, the induction of artificial withdrawal bleeds to prevent endometrial hyperplasia is prudent management (RCOG Guidelines). Indeed it is considered important that women with PCOS shed their endometrium at least every 3 months. For those with oligo-/amenorrhoea who do not wish to use cyclical hormone therapy we recommend an ultrasound scan to measure endometrial thickness and morphology every 6–12 months (depending upon menstrual history). An endometrial thickness greater than 10 mm in an amenorrhoeic woman warrants an artificially induced bleed, which should be followed by a repeat ultrasound scan and endometrial biopsy if the endometrium has not been shed. Another option is to consider a progestogen secreting intrauterine system, such as the Mirena IUS®.

BREAST CANCER

Obesity, hyperandrogenism, and infertility occur frequently in PCOS, and are features known to be associated with the development of breast cancer. However, studies examining the relationship between PCOS and breast carcinoma have not always identified a significantly increased risk. The study by Coulam *et al.* [20] calculated a relative risk of 1.5 (95% CI 0.75–2.55) for breast cancer in their group of women with chronic anovulation which was not statistically significant. After stratification by age, however, the relative risk was found to be 3.6 (95% CI 1.2–8.3) in the postmenopausal age group. Pierpoint *et al.* [16] assessed mortality from the national registry of deaths and standardized mortality rates (SMR) calculated for patients with PCOS compared with the normal population. The average follow-up period was 30 years. The SMR for all neoplasms was 0.91 (95% CI 0.60–1.32) and for breast cancer 1.48 (95% CI 0.79–2.54). In fact breast cancer was the leading cause of death in this cohort.

OVARIAN CANCER

In recent years there has been much debate about the risk of ovarian cancer in women with infertility, particularly in relation with the use of drugs to induce superovulation for assisted conception procedures. Inherently the risk of ovarian cancer appears to be increased in women who have multiple ovulations – that is those who are nulliparous (possibly because of infertility) with an early menarche and late menopause. Thus it may be that inducing multiple ovulations in women with infertility will increase their risk – a notion that is by no means proven. Women with PCOS who are oligo-/anovulatory might therefore be expected to be at low risk of developing ovarian cancer if it is lifetime number of ovulations rather than pregnancies that is critical. Ovulation induction to correct anovulatory infertility aims to induce unifollicular ovulation and so in theory should raise the risk of a woman with PCOS to that of a normal ovulating woman. The polycystic ovary, however, is notoriously sensitive to stimulation and it is only in recent years with the development of high-resolution transvaginal ultrasonography that the rate of unifollicular ovulation has attained acceptable levels. There are a few studies which have addressed the possibility of an association between polycystic ovaries and ovarian cancer. The results are conflicting, due to problems with the study designs. In the large UK study of Pierpoint *et al.* [16], the standardized mortality rate for ovarian cancer was 0.39 (95% CI 0.01–2.17).

Management of the polycystic ovary syndrome

OBESITY

The clinical management of a woman with PCOS should be focused on her individual problems. Obesity worsens both symptomatology and the endocrine profile and so obese women (BMI >30 kg/m^2) should therefore be encouraged to lose weight. Weight loss improves the endocrine profile, the likelihood of ovulation and a healthy pregnancy. Much has been written about diet and PCOS. The right diet for an individual is one that is practical, sustainable and compatible with her lifestyle. It is sensible to keep carbohydrate content down and to avoid fatty foods. It is often helpful to refer to a dietician. Anti-obesity drugs may help with weight loss. Metformin has not been shown to be valuable to aiding weight reduction.

MENSTRUAL IRREGULARITY

Amenorrhoeic women with PCOS are not oestrogen deficient and are not at risk of osteoporosis. Indeed they are oestrogen replete and at risk of endometrial hyperplasia (see p. 385). The easiest way to control the menstrual cycle is the use of a low-dose combined oral contraceptive preparation (COCP). This will result in an artificial cycle and regular shedding of the endometrium. An alternative is a progestogen (such as medroxyprogesterone acetate [Provera] or dydrogesterone [Duphaston]) for 12 days every 1–3 months to induce a withdrawal bleed. It is also important once again to encourage weight loss.

HYPERANDROGENISM AND HIRSUTISM

The bioavailability of testosterone is affected by the serum concentration of SHBG. High levels of insulin lower the production of SHBG and so increase the free fraction of androgen. Elevated serum androgen concentrations stimulate peripheral androgen receptors, resulting in an increase in 5alpha reductase activity directly increasing the conversion of testosterone to the more potent metabolite, dihydrotestosterone. Women with PCOS do not become virilized (i.e. do not develop deepening of the voice, increased muscle mass, breast atrophy or clitoromegaly).

Hirsutism is characterized by terminal hair growth in a male pattern of distribution, including chin, upper lip, chest, upper and lower back, upper and lower abdomen, upper arm, thigh and buttocks. A standardized scoring system, such as the modified Ferriman and Gallwey score may be used to evaluate the degree of hirsutism before and during treatments (Fig. 39.4). Many women attend having already tried cosmetic techniques and so it may be difficult to obtain a baseline assessment.

Drug therapies may take 6–9 months or longer before any improvement of hirsutism is perceived. Physical treatments including electrolysis, waxing and bleaching may be helpful while waiting for medical treatments to work. Electrolysis is time-consuming, painful and expensive and should be performed by an expert practitioner. Regrowth is not uncommon and there is no really permanent cosmetic treatment. Laser and photothermolysis techniques are more expensive but may have a longer duration of effect. Comparative studies, however, have not been performed. Repeated treatments are required for a near permanent effect because only hair follicles in the growing phase are obliterated at each treatment. Hair growth occurs in three cycles so 6–9 months of regular treatments are typical.

Medical regimens should stop further progression of hirsutism and decrease the rate of hair growth. Adequate contraception is important in women of reproductive age as transplacental passage of antiandrogens may disturb the genital development of a male fetus. First line therapy has traditionally been the preparation Dianette, which contains ethinyloestradiol (30 μg) in combination with cyproterone acetate (2 mg). Addition of higher doses of the synthetic progestogen cyproterone acetate (CPA, 50–

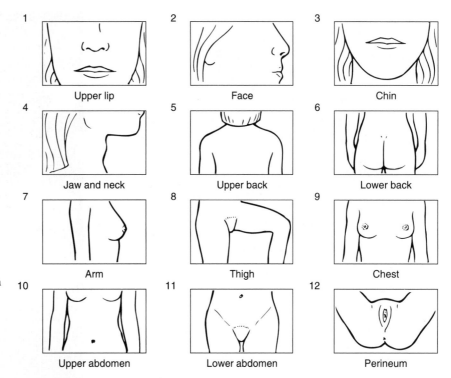

Fig. 39.4 The Ferriman-Gallwey Hirsutism Scoring System. The chart is used both to provide an initial score, with a scale of 0–3 at each of 12 points, depending on severity, and for the monitoring of progress with therapy. Reproduced from *Infertility in Practice*, 2nd edn., Balen & Jacobs, Churchill Livingstone 2003, with permission.

100 mg) do not appear to confer additional benefit [21], but are sometimes prescribed for the first 10 days of each 21-day cycle for women who are particularly resistant to treatment with Dianette alone. The effect on acne and seborrhoea is usually evident within a couple of months. Cyproterone acetate can rarely cause liver damage and liver function should be checked regularly (after 6 months and then annually). Once symptom control has been obtained it is advisable to switch to a combined oral contraceptive pill containing a lower dose of ethinyl oestradiol, because of concerns about increased risk of thromboembolism with Dianette.

Spironolactone is a weak diuretic with antiandrogenic properties and may be used in women in whom the COCP is contraindicated at a daily dose of 25–100 mg. Drosperinone is a derivative of spironolactone and contained in the new COCP, Yasmin®, which may also be beneficial for women with PCOS.

Other antiandrogens such as ketoconazole, finasteride and flutamide have been tried, but are not widely used in the UK for the treatment of hirsutism in women due to their adverse side effects. Furthermore they are no more effective than cyproterone acetate.

INFERTILITY

Improvement in lifestyle with a combination of exercise and diet to achieve weight reduction is important to improve the prospects of both spontaneous and drug-induced ovulation. In addition, overweight women with PCOS are at increased risk of obstetrical complications, including gestational diabetes mellitus and pre-eclampsia. Ovulation can be induced with the antioestrogen clomifene citrate (50–100 mg) taken from days 2–6 of a natural or artificially induced bleed. While clomifene is successful in inducing ovulation in over 80% of women, pregnancy only occurs in about 40%. Clomifene citrate should only be prescribed in a setting where ultrasound monitoring is available (and performed) to minimize the 10% risk of multiple pregnancy and to ensure that ovulation is taking place [22,23]. A daily dose of more than 100 mg rarely confers any benefit and can cause thickening of the cervical mucus, which can impede passage of sperm through the cervix. Once an ovulatory dose has been reached, the cumulative conception rate continues to increase for up to 10–12 cycles [22].

The therapeutic options for patients with anovulatory infertility who are resistant to antioestrogens are either parenteral gonadotropin therapy or laparoscopic ovarian diathermy. Because the polycystic ovary is very sensitive to stimulation by exogenous hormones, it is very important to start with very low doses of gonadotropins and follicular development must be carefully monitored by ultrasound scans. The advent of transvaginal ultrasonography has enabled the multiple pregnancy rate to be reduced to less than 5% because of its higher resolution

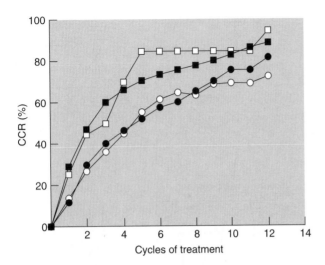

Fig. 39.5 Cumulative conception rates over successive cycles in normal women (triangle) and after ovulation induction in 103 women with anovulatory polycystic ovary syndrome (circle), 77 women with hypogonadotrophic hypogonadism (diamond) and 20 patients with weight-related amenorrhoea (square). While patients with weight-related amenorrhoea conceive readily after ovulation induction we now believe that their management should be weight gain before conception (see text). From Balen *et al.* [24].

and clearer view of the developing follicles. Cumulative conception and livebirth rates after 6 months may be 62% and 54%, respectively, and after 12 months 73% and 62%, respectively [24] (Fig. 39.5). Close monitoring should enable treatment to be suspended if more than two mature follicles develop, as the risk of multiple pregnancy increases (Fig. 39.6).

Women with the polycystic ovary syndrome are also at increased risk of developing the ovarian hyperstimulation syndrome (OHSS). This occurs if too many follicles (>10 mm) are stimulated and results in abdominal distension, discomfort, nausea, vomiting and sometimes difficulty breathing. The mechanism for OHSS is thought to be secondary to activation of the ovarian renin-angiotensin pathway and excessive secretion of vascular epidermal growth factor (VEGF). The ascites, pleural and pericardial effusions exacerbate this serious condition and the resultant haemoconcentration can lead to thromboembolism. The situation worsens if a pregnancy has resulted from the treatment as hCG from the placenta further stimulates the ovaries. Hospitalization is sometimes necessary for intravenous fluids and heparin to be given to prevent dehydration and thromboembolism. Although the OHSS is rare it is potentially fatal and should be avoidable with appropriate monitoring of gonadotropin therapy.

Ovarian diathermy is free of the risks of multiple pregnancy and ovarian hyperstimulation and does not require

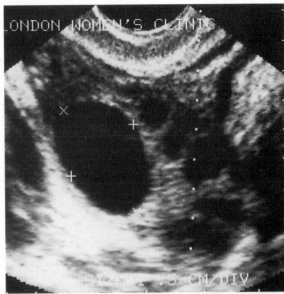

(a)

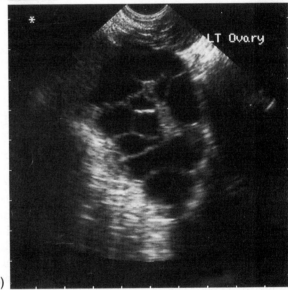

(b)

Fig. 39.6 (a) Transvaginal ultrasound scan of unifollicular development in a polycystic ovary and (b) an overstimulated polycystic ovary. Reproduced from *Infertility in Practice*, 2nd edn., Balen & Jacobs, Churchill Livingstone 2003, with permission.

intensive ultrasound monitoring (Plate 39.2, *facing p. 562*). Laparoscopic ovarian diathermy has taken the place of wedge resection of the ovaries (which resulted in extensive peri-ovarian and tubal adhesions), and carries a reduced risk of multiple pregnancy compared with gonadotropin therapy in the treatment of clomiphine-insensitive PCOS. A meta-analysis has shown that pregnancy rates are greater with 6 months gonadotropin therapy compared with 6 months after laparoscopic ovarian diathermy, although by 12 months the pregnancy rates are similar [25].

INSULIN-SENSITIZING AGENTS AND METFORMIN

A number of pharmacological agents have been used to amplify the physiological effect of weight loss, notably metformin. This biguanide inhibits the production of hepatic glucose and enhances the sensitivity of peripheral tissue to insulin, thereby decreasing insulin secretion. It has been shown that metformin ameliorates hyperandrogenism and abnormalities of gonadotropin secretion in women with PCOS and can restore menstrual cyclicity and fertility.

A Cochrane review has confirmed a beneficial effect of metformin in improving rates of ovulation when compared with placebo and also improving both rates of ovulation and pregnancy when used with clomifene citrate compared with clomifene citrate alone [26]. The data indicate that serum concentrations of insulin and androgens improve although, contrary to popular belief, body weight does not fall.

Metformin therapy may be commenced after appropriate screening and advice about diet, lifestyle and exercise for anovulatory women with PCOS who have failed to conceive. The usual dose is either 850 mg bd or 500 mg tds. Baseline investigations should include an oral GTT, full blood count (FBC), urea and electrolytes (U&E) and liver function tests (LFTs). Side effects are predominantly gastrointestinal (anorexia, nausea, flatulence and diarrhoea) and may be reduced by taking metformin just before food and gradually increasing the dose from 850 mg nocte to 850 mg bd after 1 week. Metformin therapy is not thought to cause lactic acidosis in non-diabetic women with PCOS and normal renal and liver function. Metformin should be discontinued for 3 days after iodine-containing contrast medium has been given. Metformin is usually discontinued in pregnancy although there is no evidence of teratogenicity and preliminary reports from retrospective studies of a reduced rate of gestational diabetes.

More studies are required to assess the potential benefits of metformin and other insulin-sensitizing agents on other symptoms of the PCOS. All studies to date are of short duration – at most 6 months and usually much shorter – and there are no data on long-term use and the potential to reduce progression of impaired glucose tolerance to type 2 diabetes or ameliorate other long-term sequelae.

Key points

- PCOS is the commonest endocrine disorder in women (prevalence 15–20%).
- PCOS runs in families and affects approximately 50% of first-degree relatives.
- PCOS is a heterogeneous condition. Diagnosis is made by two out of the following three criteria: (1) oligo- and/or anovulation, (2) hyperandrogenism (clinical and/or biochemical), (3) polycystic ovaries, with the exclusion of other aetiologies.
- Management is symptom orientated.
- If obese, weight loss improves symptoms and endocrinology and should be encouraged. A GTT should be performed if the BMI is >30 kg/m^2 (or >25 kg/m^2 if Asian). Dietary advice and exercise are essential components of a weight-reducing programme. Anti-obesity drugs or surgery may be indicated.
- Menstrual cycle control may be achieved by cyclical oral contraceptives or progestogens.
- Ovulation induction may be difficult and require progression through various treatments which should be monitored carefully to prevent multiple pregnancy.
- Hyperandrogenism is usually managed with Dianette, containing ethinyloestradiol in combination with cyproterone acetate. A new COCP, Yasmin may also be of benefit. Alternatives include spironolactone. Flutamide and finasteride are not routinely prescribed because of potential adverse effects. Reliable contraception is required.
- Insulin-sensitizing agents (e.g. metformin) are showing promise for ovulation induction but require further long-term evaluation and should only be prescribed by endocrinologists/reproductive endocrinologists. Weight loss is not guaranteed.

Secondary amenorrhoea

Cessation of menstruation for 6 consecutive months in a woman who has previously had regular periods, is the usual criteria for investigation. However, some authorities consider 3 or 4 months amenorrhoea to be pathological but here we enter the grey area between amenorrhoea and oligomenorrhoea. Women with secondary amenorrhoea must have a patent lower genital tract, an endometrium that is responsive to ovarian hormone stimulation and ovaries that have responded to pituitary gonadotropins.

Secondary amenorrhoea is best classified according to its aetiological site of origin and can be subdivided into disorders of the hypothalamic-pituitary-ovarian-uterine axis and generalized systemic disease. The principal causes of secondary amenorrhoea are outlined in Table 39.5. The frequency with which these conditions present can be seen in Table 39.6.

Management of secondary amenorrhoea

GENITAL TRACT ABNORMALITIES

Asherman's syndrome

Asherman's syndrome is a condition in which intrauterine adhesions prevent normal growth of the endometrium

Table 39.5 Classification of secondary amenorrhoea

Uterine causes	Asherman's syndrome
	Cervical stenosis
Ovarian causes	Polycystic ovary syndrome
	Premature ovarian failure (genetic, autoimmune, infective, radio/chemotherapy)
Hypothalamic causes *(hypogonadotrophic hypogonadism)*	Weight loss
	Exercise
	Chronic illness
	Psychological distress
	Idiopathic
Pituitary causes	Hyperprolactinaemia
	Hypopituitarism Sheehan's syndrome
Causes of hypothalamic/ pituitary damage *(hypogonadism)*	Tumours (craniopharyngiomas, gliomas, germinomas, dermoid cysts)
	Cranial irradiation
	Head injuries
	Sarcoidosis
	Tuberculosis
Systemic causes	Chronic debilitating illness
	Weight loss
	Endocrine disorders (thyroid disease, Cushing's syndrome etc.)

Table 39.6 The aetiology of secondary amenorrhoea in 570 patients attending an endocrine clinic (Balen *et al.* 1993).

Polycystic ovary syndrome	36.9%
Premature ovarian failure	23.6%
Hyperprolactinaemia	16.9%
Weight-related amenorrhoea	9.8%
Hypogonadotrophic hypogonadism	5.9%
Hypopituitarism	4.4%
Exercise-related amenorrhoea	2.5%

[27]. This may be the result of a too vigorous endometrial curettage affecting the basalis layer of the endometrium or adhesions may follow an episode of endometritis. It is thought that oestrogen deficiency increases the risk of adhesion formation in breastfeeding women who require a puerperial currettage for retained placental tissue. Typically amenorrhoea is not absolute, and it may be possible to induce a withdrawal bleed using a combined oestrogen/progestagen preparation. Intrauterine adhesions may be seen on a hysterosalpingogram (HSG) (Fig. 39.2). Alternatively, hysteroscopic inspection of the uterine cavity will confirm the diagnosis and enable treatment by adhesiolysis. The adhesions bridge the anterior and posterior walls of the uterine cavity and are usually avascular, although may contain vessels, muscle and even endometrium. Following surgery, a 3-month course of cyclical progesterone/oestrogen should be given. Some

clinicians insert a foley catheter into the uterine cavity for 7–10 days post-operatively [28], or an intrauterine contraceptive device for 2–3 months [29], to prevent recurrence of adhesions.

In a series of 292 infertile women who were thought to have intrauterine adhesions, as detected by HSG, 46% conceived without treatment but only 53% delivered a live infant and 13% had placenta accreta [30]. It has been suggested that the pregnancy rates after hysteroscopic treatment of intrauterine adhesions depends upon the degree of the initial problem [31] being 93% for mild and 57% for severe disease. The outcome of the pregnancy would appear to depend upon the post-treatment contour of the uterine cavity.

Cervical stenosis

Cervical stenosis is an occasional cause of secondary amenorrhoea. It was relatively common following a traditional cone biopsy for the treatment of cervical intraepithelial neoplasia. However, modern procedures such as laser or loop diathermy have less post-operative cervical complications [32]. Treatment for cervical stenosis consists of careful cervical dilatation.

OVARIAN CAUSES OF SECONDARY AMENORRHOEA

Polycystic ovary syndrome

See earlier sections.

Premature ovarian failure. Ovarian failure by definition, is the cessation of periods accompanied by raised gonadotropin level prior to the age of 40 years. It may occur at any age. The exact incidence of this condition is unknown as many cases go unrecognized, but estimates vary between 1 and 5% of the female population. Studies of amenorrhoeic women report the incidence of premature ovarian failure to be between 10 and 36%.

Chromosomal abnormalities are common in women with primary amenorrhoea. Hague *et al.* [33] found chromosomal abnormalities in 70% of patients with primary amenorrhoea and in 2–5% of women with secondary amenorrhoea due to premature ovarian failure. Ovarian failure occurring before puberty is usually due to a chromosomal abnormality, or a childhood malignancy that required chemotherapy or radiotherapy. Adolescents who loose ovarian function soon after menarche, are often found to have a Turner's mosaic (46XX/45X) or an X-chromosome trisomy (47, XXX) (also see Plate 39.1, *facing p. 562*). There are some genetic anomalies that run in families with premature ovarian failure (POF), although these are not assessed in routine clinical practice.

Overall, the most common cause of POF is autoimmune disease; with infection, previous surgery, chemo- and radiotherapy also contributing ovarian autoantibodies can be measured and have been found in up to 69% of cases of POF. However, the assay is expensive and not readily available in most units. It is therefore important to consider other autoimmune disorders, and screen for autoantibodies to the thyroid gland, gastric mucosa parietal cells and adrenal gland if there is any clinical indication.

Prior to the absolute cessation of periods of true premature ovarian failure, some women experience an intermittent return to menses, interspersed between variable periods of amenorrhoea. Gonadotropin levels usually remain moderately elevated during these spontaneous cycles, with plasma FSH levels of 15–20 iμ/l. This occult ovarian failure, or resistant ovary syndrome, is associated with the presence of primordial follicles on ovarian biopsy, and pregnancies are sometimes achieved, although the ovaries are usually resistant to exogenous gonadotropins as they are to endogenous hormones. It is probable that reports of pregnancy in women with POF represent cases of fluctuating ovarian function rather than successes of treatment [34].

It is, however, possible to achieve pregnancy by oocyte donation, as part of *in vitro* fertilization treatment. Experimental work in animals has succeeded in transplanting primordial follicles into irradiated ovaries, with subsequent ovulation and normal pregnancy [35]. The prospect of transplantation of cryopreserved ovarian tissue is coming close to fruition in humans and should soon offer the chance of fertility to women who have received radiotherapy or chemotherapy.

The diagnosis and consequences of premature ovarian failure require careful counselling of the patient. It may be particularly difficult for a young woman to accept the need to take oestrogen preparations that are clearly labelled as being intended for older postmenopausal women, while at the same time having to come to terms with the inability to conceive naturally. The short- and long-term consequences of ovarian failure and oestrogen deficiency are similar to those occurring in the fifth and sixth decade. However, the duration of the problem is much longer and therefore hormone replacement therapy is advisable to reduce the consequences of oestrogen deficiency in the long term.

Younger women with premature loss of ovarian function have an increased risk of osteoporosis. A series of 200 amenorrhoeic women between the ages of 16–40 demonstrated a mean reduction in bone mineral density of 15% as compared with a control group and after correction for body weight, smoking and exercise [36]. The degree of bone loss was correlated with the duration of the amenorrhoea and the severity of the oestrogen deficiency rather than the underlying diagnosis, and was worse in patients with primary amenorrhoea compared with those with secondary amenorrhoea. A return to normal oestrogen status may improve bone mass density, but bone mineral density is unlikely to improve more than 5–10% and it probably does not return to its normal value. However, it is not certain if the radiological improvement seen will actually reduce the risk of fracture, as remineralization is not equivalent to the restrengthening of bone. Early diagnosis and early correction of oestrogen status is therefore important.

Women with POF have an increased risk of cardiovascular disease. Oestrogens have been shown to have beneficial effects on cardiovascular status in women. They increase the levels of cardioprotective HDL but also total triglyceride levels, while decreasing total cholesterol and low-density lipoprotein (LDL) levels. The overall effect is of cardiovascular protection.

The HRT preparations prescribed for menopausal women are also preferred for young women. The reason for this is that even modern low dose combined oral contraceptive (COC) preparations contain at least twice the amount of oestrogen that is recommended for HRT, in order to achieve a contraceptive suppressive effect on the hypothalamic-pituitary axis. HRT also contains 'natural' oestrogens rather than the synthetic ethinyloestradiol that is found in most COCs.

Pituitary causes of secondary amenorrhoea

Hyperprolactinaemia is the commonest pituitary cause of amenorrhoea. There are many causes of a mildly elevated serum prolactin concentration, including stress, and a recent physical or breast examination. If the prolactin concentration is greater than 1000 mμ/l then the test should be repeated and if still elevated it is necessary to image the pituitary fossa (CT or MRI scan). Hyperprolactinaemia may result from a prolactin-secreting pituitary adenoma, or from a non-functioning 'disconnection' tumour in the region of the hypothalamus or pituitary, which disrupts the inhibitory influence of dopamine on prolactin secretion. Large non-functioning tumours are usually associated with serum prolactin concentrations of less than 3000 mμ/l, while prolactin-secreting macroadenomas usually result in concentrations of 8000 mμ/l or more. Other causes include hypothyroidism, polycystic ovary syndrome (up to 2500 mU/l) and several drugs (e.g. the dopaminergic antagonist phenothiazines, domperidone and metoclopramide).

In women with amenorrhoea associated with hyperprolactinaemia the main symptoms are usually those of oestrogen deficiency [37]. In contrast, when hyperprolactinaemia is associated with PCOS, the syndrome is characterized by adequate oestrogenization, polycystic ovaries on ultrasound scan and a withdrawal bleed in response to a progestogen challenge test. Galactorrhoea may be found in up to a third of hyperprolactinaemic patients, although its appearance is neither correlated with prolactin levels or with the presence of a tumour [38]. Approximately 5% of patients present with visual field defects [39].

A prolactin-secreting pituitary microadenoma is usually associated with a moderately elevated prolactin (1500–4000 mIU/L) and is unlikely to result in abnormalities on a lateral skull X-ray. On the other hand, a macroadenoma, associated with a prolactin greater than 5000–8000 mIU/L and by definition greater than 1 cm diameter, may cause typical radiological changes – that is, an asymmetrically enlarged pituitary fossa, with a double contour to its floor and erosion of the clinoid processes. The CT and the MRI scans now allow detailed examination of the extent of the tumour and, in particular, identification of suprasellar extension and compression of the opitic chiasm or invasion of the cavernous sinuses. Prolactin is an excellent tumour marker and so the higher the serum concentration the larger the size of the tumour expected on the MRI scan. In contrast a large tumour on the scan with only a moderately elevated serum prolactin concentration (2–3000 mIU/L) suggests a non-functioning tumour with 'disconnection' from the hypothalamus (Fig. 39.7).

The management of hyperprolactinaemia centres around the use of a dopamine agonist, of which bromocriptine is the most widely used. Of course, if the hyperprolactinaemia is drug induced stopping the relevant preparation should be commended. This may not, however, be appropriate if the cause is a psychotropic medication, for example, a phenothiazine being used to treat schizophrenia. In these cases it is reasonable to continue the drug and prescribe a low dose COC preparation to counteract the symptoms of oestrogen deficiency. Serum prolactin concentrations must then be carefully monitored to ensure that they do not rise further.

Most patients show a fall in prolactin levels within a few days of commencing bromocriptine therapy and a reduction of tumour volume within 6 weeks. Side effects can be troublesome (nausea, vomiting, headache, postural hypotension) and are minimized by commencing the therapy at night for the first 3 days of treatment and taking the tablets in the middle of a mouthful of food. Longer term side effects include Raynauds, constipation, and psychiatric changes – especially aggression, which can occur at the start of treatment.

Bromocriptine should be commenced at a dose of half a tablet at night (1.25 mg) and increased gradually, every 5 days to 2.5 mg at night and then 1.25 mg in the morning with 2.5 mg at night until the daily dose is 7.5 mg (in two or three divided doses). The maintenance dose should be

Table 39.7 Drug therapy for hyperprolactinaemia

Bromocriptine	2.5–20 mg daily, divided doses	Maintenance usually 5–7.5 mg/day
Cabergoline	0.25–1 mg twice weekly	Maintenance usually 1 mg/day

the lowest that works and is often lower than that needed initially to initiate a response.

Longer-acting preparations (e.g. twice weekly cabergoline) may be prescribed to those patients who develop unacceptable side effects. Cabergoline generally appears to be better tolerated and more efficacious than bromocriptine but is currently not recommended for women trying to conceive (Table 39.7).

Surgery, in the form of a *trans*sphenoidal adenectomy, is reserved for cases of drug resistance and failure to shrink a macroadenoma or if there are intolerable side effects of the drugs (the most common indication). Non-functioning tumours should be removed surgically and are usually detected by a combination of imaging and a serum prolactin concentration of less than 3000 mμ/l. When the prolactin level is between 3000 and 8000 mμ/l a trial of bromocriptine is warranted and if the prolactin level falls it can be assumed that the tumour is a prolactin-secreting macroadenoma. Operative treatment is also required if there is suprasellar extension of the tumour that has not regressed during treatment with bromocriptine and a pregnancy is desired. With the present day skills of neurosurgeons in transsphenoidal surgery, it is seldom necessary to resort to pituitary irradiation, which offers no advantages and long-term surveillance is required to detect consequent hypopituitarism (which is immediately apparent if it occurs after surgery).

Women with a microprolactinoma who wish to conceive can be reassured that they may stop bromocriptine when pregnancy is diagnosed and require no further monitoring, as the likelihood of significant tumour expansion is very small (less than 2%). On the other hand, if a patient with a macroprolactinoma is not treated with bromocriptine the tumour has a 25% risk of expanding during pregnancy. This risk is probably also present if the tumour has been treated but has not shrunk, as assessed by CT or MRI scan. The first line approach to treatment of macroprolactinomas is therefore with bromocriptine combined with barrier methods of contraception. In cases with suprasellar expansion, follow-up CT (or MRI) scan should be performed after 3 months of treatment to ensure tumour regression, before it is safe to embark upon pregnancy. Bromocriptine can be discontinued during pregnancy, although if symptoms suggestive of tumour re-expansion occur an MRI scan should be performed and if there is continuing suprasellar expansion it is necessary

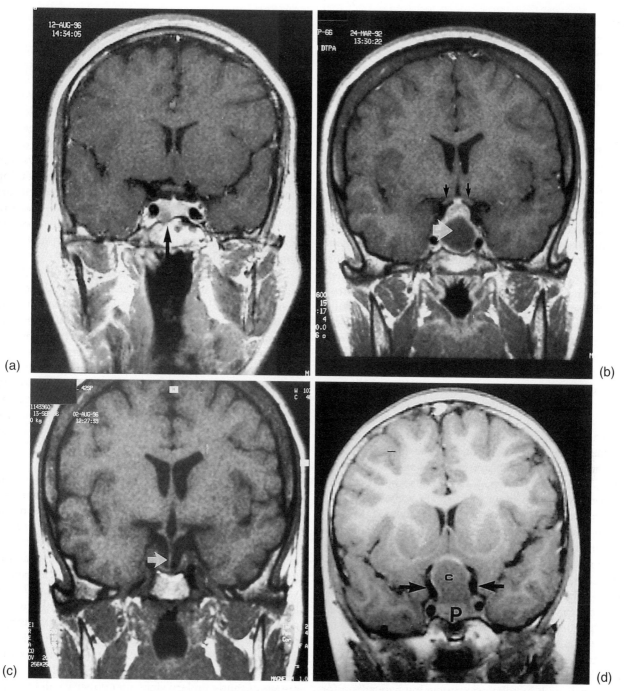

Fig. 39.7 (a) Pituitary microadenoma. Cranial magnetic resonance imaging (MRI). A coronal section T1-weighted spin echo sequence after i.v. gadolinium. The normal pituitary gland is hyperintense (bright) while the tumour is seen as a 4-mm area of non-enhancement (grey) in the right lobe of the pituitary, encroaching up to the right cavernous sinus. It is eroding the right side of the sella floor (arrow). Pituitary macroadenoma. MRI scans of a pituitary macroadenoma before and after bromocriptine therapy: (b) T1-weighted image post gadolinium enhancement demonstrating a macroadenoma with a large central cystic component (large arrow). There is suprasellar extension with compression of the optic chiasm (small arrows). (c) After therapy the tumour has almost completely resolved and there is tethering of the optic chiasm (arrow) to the floor of the sella. (d) Craniopharyngioma. Cranial MRI: Coronal T1-weighted section after gadolinium enhancement. The tumour signals intensity on the T1 image and only part of the periphery of the tumour enhances. The carotid arteries have a low signal intensity (black arrows) due to the rapid flow within them and are deviated laterally and superiorly by the mass (C), which arises out of the pituitary fossa (P). Reproduced from *Infertility in Practice*, 2nd edn., Balen & Jacobs, Churchill Livingstone 2003, with permission.

to recommence bromocriptine therapy. These patients also require expert assessment of their visual fields during pregnancy [39].

If the serum prolactin is found to be elevated and the patient has a regular menstrual cycle, no treatment is necessary unless the cycle is anovulatory and fertility is desired. Amenorrhoea is the 'bioassay' of prolactin excess and should be corrected for its sequelae, rather than for the serum level of prolactin.

Hypothalamic causes of secondary amenorrhoea

Hypothalamic causes of amenorrhoea may be either primary or secondary. Primary hypothalamic lesions include craniopharyngiomas, germinomas, gliomas and dermoid cysts. These hypothalamic lesions either disrupt the normal pathway of prolactin inhibitory factor (dopamine), thus causing hyperprolactinaemia or compress or destroy hypothalamic and pituitary tissue. Treatment is usually surgical, with additional radiotherapy if required. Hormone replacement therapy is required to mimic ovarian function, and if the pituitary gland is damaged either by the lesion or by the treatment, replacement thyroid and adrenal hormones are required.

Secondary hypogonadotrophic hypogonadism may result from systemic conditions including sarcoidosis, tuberculosis as well as following head injury or cranial irradiation. Sheehan's syndrome, the result of profound and prolonged hypotension on the sensitive pituitary gland, enlarged by pregnancy, may also be a cause of hypogonadotrophic hypogonadism in someone with a history of a major obstetric haemorrhage [40]. It is essential to assess the pituitary function fully in all these patients and then instigate the appropriate replacement therapy. Ovulation may be induced with pulsatile subcutaneous GnRH or human menopausal gonadotropins (hMG). The administration of pulsatile GnRH provides the most 'physiological' correction of infertility caused by hypogonadotrophic hypogonadism and will result in unifollicular ovulation, while hMG therapy requires close monitoring to prevent multiple pregnancy. Purified or recombinant FSH preparations are not suitable for women with hypogonadotrophic hypogonadism (or pituitary hypogonadism) as these patients have absent endogenous production of LH and so while follicular growth may occur, oestrogen biosynthesis is impaired [41]. Thus hMG, which contains FSH and LH activity, is necessary for these patients.

Systemic disorders causing secondary amenorrhoea

Chronic disease may result in menstrual disorders as a consequence of the general disease state, weight loss or by the effect of the disease process on the hypothalamic-pituitary axis. Furthermore, a chronic disease that leads to immobility such as chronic obstructive airways disease, may increase the risk of amenorrhoea associated osteoporosis.

Some diseases affect gonadal function directly. Women with chronic renal failure have a discordantly elevated LH [42], possibly as a consequence of impaired clearance [43]. Prolactin is also elevated in these women, due to failure of the normal inhibition by dopamine. Liver disease affects the level of circulating sex hormone binding globulin, and thus hormone levels, thereby disrupting the normal feedback mechanisms. Metabolism of various hormones including testosterone, are also liver dependent; both menstruation and fertility return after liver transplantation [44].

Endocrine disorders such as thyrotoxicosis and Cushing's syndrome are commonly associated with gonadal dysfunction [45]. Autoimmune endocrinopathies may be associated with premature ovarian failure, because of ovarian antibodies. Diabetes mellitus may result in functional hypothalamic-pituitary amenorrhoea [46].

Management of these patients should concentrate on the underlying systemic problem and on preventing complications of oestrogen deficiency. If fertility is required, it is desirable to achieve maximal health and where possible to discontinue teratogenic drugs.

Weight-related amenorrhoea

Weight can have profound effects on gonadotropin regulation and release. Weight and eating disorders are also common in women. A regular menstrual cycle will not occur if the BMI is less than 19 kg/m^2. Fat appears to be critical to a normally functioning hypothalamic-pituitary-gonadal axis. It is estimated that at least 22% of body weight should be fat to maintain ovulatory cycles [47]. This level enables the extra ovarian aromatization of androgens to oestrogens, and maintains appropriate feedback control of the hypothalamic-pituitary-ovarian axis [48]. Therefore, girls who are significantly underweight prior to puberty may have primary amenorrhoea, while those who are significantly underweight after puberty will have secondary amenorrhoea. The clinical presentation depends upon the severity of the nutritional insult and its age of onset. To cause amenorrhoea the loss must be 10–15% of the women's normal weight for height. Weight loss may be due to a number of causes including self-induced abstinence, starvation, illness and exercise.

Whatever the precipitating cause, the net result is impairment of gonadotropin secretion. In severe weight loss, oestrogen may be catabolized to the antioestrogen 2-hydroxy-oestrone, rather than to the usual oestradiol, which may further suppress gonadotropin secretion. This pathway is enhanced by cigarette smoking. Weight-related gonadotropin deficiency is more pronounced with LH than FSH [49]. This and the reduction in pulsatility of gonadotropin secretion may result in a 'multicystic' pattern in the ovary. This appearance is typical of normal puberty and is seen when there are several cysts (about 5–10 mm in diameter) together with a stroma of normal density.

Anorexia nervosa is at the extreme end of a spectrum of eating disorders and is invariably accompanied by menstrual disturbance, and indeed may account for between 15 and 35% of patients with amenorrhoea. Women with anorexia nervosa should be managed in collaboration with a psychiatrist, and it is essential to encourage weight gain as the main therapy.

An artificial cycle, may be induced with the COC. However, this may corroborate in the denial of weight loss being the underlying problem. Similarly, while it is possible to induce ovulation with GnRH, or exogenous gonadotropins, treatment of infertility in the significantly underweight patient is associated with a significant increase in intrauterine growth retardation and neonatal problems. Furthermore, since three quarters of the cell divisions that occur during pregnancy do so during the first trimester, it is essential that nutritional status is optimized before conception. Low birthweight is also now being related to an increased risk of cardiovascular disease, diabetes PCOS in adult life [50].

Weight-related amenorrhoea may also have profound long-term affects on bone mineral density. The age of onset of anorexia nervosa is important, as prolonged amenorrhoea before the normal age at which peak bone mass is obtained (~25 years) increases the likelihood of severe osteoporosis.

Worldwide, involuntary starvation is the commonest cause of reduced reproductive ability, resulting in delayed pubertal growth and menarche in adolescents [51] and infertility in adults. Acute malnutrition, as seen in famine conditions and during and after the Second World War has profound effects on fertility and fecundity [48]. Ovulatory function usually returns quickly on restoration of adequate nutrition. Chronic malnutrition, common in developing countries has less profound effects on fertility, but is associated with small and premature babies.

PSYCHOLOGICAL STRESS

Studies have failed to demonstrate a link between stressful life events and amenorrhoea of greater than 2 months. However, stress may lead to physical debility such as weight loss which may then cause menstrual disturbance.

Exercise-related amenorrhoea

Menstrual disturbance is common in athletes undergoing intensive training. Between 10 and 20% have oligomenorrhoea or amenorrhoea, compared with 5% in the general population [52]. Amenorrhoea is more common in athletes under 30 years and is particularly common in women involved in the endurance events (such as long distance running). Up to 50% of competitive runners training 80 miles per week may be amenorrhoeic [53].

The main aetiological factors are weight and percentage body fat content, but other factors have also been postulated. Physiological changes are consistent with those associated with starvation and chronic illness.

Ballet dancers provide an interesting subgroup of sportswomen, because their training begins at an early age. They have been found to have a significant delay in menarche (15.4 compared to 12.5 years) and a retardation in pubertal development which parallels the intensity of their training [54]. Menstrual irregularities are common and up to 44% have secondary amenorrhoea [55]. In a survey of 75 dancers 61% were found to have stress fractures and 24% had scoliosis; the risk of these pathological features was increased if menarche was delayed or if there were prolonged periods of amenorrhoea [55]. These findings may be explained by delayed pubertal maturation resulting in attainment of a greater than expected height and a predisposition to scoliosis, as oestrogen is required for epiphyseal closure.

Exercise-induced amenorrhoea has the potential to cause severe long-term morbidity, particularly with regard to osteoporosis. Studies on young ballet dancers have shown that the amount of exercise undertaken by these dancers does not compensate for these osteoporotic changes [55]. Oestrogen is also important in the formation of collagen and soft tissue injuries are also common in dancers [56]. Whereas moderate exercise has been found to reduce the incidence of postmenopausal osteoporosis, young athletes may be placing themselves at risk at an age when the attainment of peak bone mass is important for long-term skeletal strength. Appropriate advice should be given, particularly regarding diet, and the use of a cyclical oestrogen/progestogen preparation should be considered.

Iatrogenic causes of amenorrhoea

There are many iatrogenic causes of amenorrhoea, which may be either temporary or permanent. These include malignant conditions that require either radiation to the abdomen/pelvis or chemotherapy. Both these treatments may result in permanent gonadal damage; the amount of damage being directly related to the age of the patient, the cumulative dose and the patient's prior menstrual status.

Gynaecological procedures such as oophorectomy, hysterectomy and endometrial resection inevitably result in amenorrhoea. Hormone replacement should be prescribed for these patients where appropriate. Hormone therapy itself can be used to deliberately disrupt the menstrual cycle. However, iatrogenic causes of ovarian quiescence have the same consequences of oestrogen deficiency due to any other aetiology. Thus the use of GnRH analogues in the treatment of oestrogen-dependent conditions (e.g. precocious puberty, endometriosis, uterine fibroids) results in a significant decrease in bone mineral density in as little as 6 months. Although the demineralization is reversible with the cessation of therapy, especially for the treatment of benign conditions in young women who are in the process of achieving their peak bone mass, the concurrent use of an androgenic progestogen or oestrogen 'add-back' therapy may protect against bone loss.

Key points

- Secondary amenorrhoea is usually considered to be amenorrhoea of 6 or more months duration during reproductive years.
- Aetiology and treatment can be conveniently catagorized into hypothalamic, pituitary, ovarian, uterine causes or systemic illness, which in essence causes secondary hypothalamic amenorrhoea.
- Correct diagnosis is readily made if a logical protocol is applied.
- The polycystic ovary syndrome is the commonest cause and is the only major cause of amenorrhoea that is not associated with oestrogen deficiency.
- The amenorrhoea of polycystic ovary syndrome should be treated to either enhance fertility or prevent endometrial hyperplasia/adenocarcinoma.
- Oestrogen deficiency results in the long-term sequelae of osteoporosis and cardiovascular disease and so the cause of amenorrhoea should be corrected early and hormone replacement therapy administered if necessary.
- Fertility can be achieved either after ovulation induction or, in cases of premature ovarian failure with oocyte donation/*in vitro* fertilization.

References

1. Balen AH, Conway GS, Kaltsas G *et al.* (1995) Polycystic ovary syndrome: the spectrum of the disorder in 1741 patients. *Human Reprod* **10**, 2107–11.
2. Seth J, Hanning I, Jacobs HS & Jeffcoate SL (1989) Measuring serum gonadotropins: a cautionary note. *Lancet* **i**, 671.
3. Conway GS (1990) Insulin resistance and the polycystic ovary syndrome. *Contemp Rev Obstet Gynaecol* **2**, 34–9.
4. Balen AH, Laven JSE, Tan SL & Dewailly D (2003) Ultrasound assessment of the polycystic ovary. *Int Consensus Definitions Human Reprod Update* **9**, 505–14.
5. Clark AM, Ledger W, Galletly C *et al.* (1995) Weight loss results in significant improvement in pregnancy and ovulation rates in anovulatory obese women. *Human Reprod* **10**, 2705–12.
6. Rajkowha M, Glass MR, Rutherford AJ, Michelmore K & Balen AH (2000) Polycystic ovary syndrome: a risk factor for cardiovascular disease? *Br J Obstet Gynaecol* **107**, 11–8.
7. RCOG (2003) *Long-term Consequences of Polycystic Ovary Syndrome.* RCOG Guideline number 33.
8. Polson DW, Wadsworth J, Adams J & Franks S (1988) Polycystic ovaries: a common finding in normal women. *Lancet* **ii**, 870–2.
9. Michelmore KF, Balen AH, Dunger DB & Vessey MP (1999) Polycystic ovaries and associated clinical and biochemical features in young women. *Clin Endocrinol Oxf* **51**, 779–86.
10. Kyei-Mensah A, Tan SL, Zaidi J & Jacobs HS (1998) Relationship of ovarian stromal Volume to serum androgen concentrations in patients with polycystic ovary syndrome. *Human Reprod* **13**, 1437–41.
11. Legro RS & Strauss JF (2002) Molecular progress in infertility: polycystic ovary syndrome. *Fertil Steril* **78**, 569–76.
12. Legro RS (1999) Polycystic ovary syndrome, phenotype and genotype. *Endocrinol Metab Clin North Am* **28**(2), 379–96.
13. Rodin DA, Bano G, Bland JM, Taylor K & Nussey SS (1998) Polycystic ovaries and associated metabolic abnormalities in Indian subcontinent Asian women. *Clin Endocrinol* **49**(1), 91–9.
14. Wijeyaratne CN, Balen AH, Barth J & Belchetz PE (2002) Clinical manifestations and insulin resistance (IR) in polycystic ovary syndrome (PCOS) among South Asians and Caucasians: is there a difference? *Clin Endocrinol* **57**, 343–50.
15. Conway GS, Agrawal R, Betteridge DJ & Jacobs HS (1992) Risk factors for coronary artery disease in lean and obese women with the polycystic ovary syndrome. *Clin Endocrinol* **37**, 119–25.
16. Pierpoint T, McKeigue PM, Isaacs AJ, Wild SH & Jacobs HS (1998) Mortality of women with polycystic ovary syndrome at long-term follow-up. *J Clin Epidemiol* **51**, 581–6.
17. Norman RJ, Masters L. Milner CR, Wang JX & Davies MJ (1995) Relative risk of conversion from normoglycaemia to impaired glucose tolerance or non-insulin dependent diabetes mellitus in polycystic ovary syndrome. *Hum Reprod* **16**, 1995–98.
18. MacMahon B (1974) Risk factors for endometrial cancer. *Gynecol Oncol* **2**, 122–9.
19. Balen AH (2001) Polycystic ovary syndrome and cancer. *Human Reprod Update* **7**, 522–5.
20. Coulam CB, Annegers JF & Kranz JS (1983) Chronic anovulation syndrome and associated neoplasia. *Obstet Gynecol* **61**, 403–7.
21. Barth JH, Cherry CA, Wojnarowska F & Dawber RPR (1991) Cyproterone acetate for severe hirsutism: results of a

double-blind dose-ranging study. *Clin Endocrinol* **35**, 5–10.

22. Kousta E, White DM & Franks S (1997) Modern use of clomifene citrate in induction of ovulation. *Human Reprod Update* **3**, 359–65.

23. Balen AH (2003) Ovulation induction – optimizing results and minimizing risks. *Human Fertil* **6**, S42–51.

24. Balen AH, Braat DDM, West C, Patel A & Jacobs HS (1994) Cumulative conception and live birth rates after the treatment of anovulatory infertility. *Human Reprod* **9**, 1563–70.

25. Farquhar C, Vandekerckhove P & Lilford R (2002) Laparoscopic 'drilling' by diathermy or laser for ovulation induction in anovulatory polycystic ovary syndrome (Cochrane Review). *The Cochrane Library*. Issue 4. Oxford: Update Software.

26. Lord JM, Flight IHK & Norman RJ (2003) Metformin in polycystic ovary syndrome. systematic review and meta-analysis. *Br Med J* **327**, 951–5.

27. Asherman JG (1950) Traumatic intrauterine adhesions. *J Obstet Gynaecal Br Emp* **57**, 892–6.

28. Doody KM & Carr BR (1990) Amenorrhea. In: Chihal HJ & London SN (eds) *Menstrual Cycle Disorders*. Philadelphia: W.B. Saunders, *Obstet Gynecol Clin N Am* **17**, 361–87.

29. Jewelewicz R & van de Wiele RL (1980) Clinical course and outcome of pregnancy in 25 patients with pituitary microadenomas. *Am J Obstet Gynecol* **136**, 339–43.

30. Schenker JG & Margalioth EJ (1992) Intrauterine adhesions: an updated appraisal. *Fertil Steril* **37**, 593–610.

31. Valle RF & Sciarra JJ (1988) Intrauterine adhesons: hysteroscopic diagnosis, classification, treatment and reproductive outcome. *Am J Obstet Gynecol* **158**, 1459–70.

32. Baggish MS (1980) High power density carbon dioxide laser therapy for early cervical neoplasia. *Am J Obstet Gynaecol* **136**, 117–25.

33. Hague WM, Tan SL, Adams J & Jacobs HS (1987) Hypergonadotrophic amenorrhoea – etiology and outcome in 93 young women. *Int J Gynaecol Obstet* **25**, 121–5.

34. Check JH, Nowroozi K, Chase JS, Nazari A, Shapse D & Vaze M (1990) Ovulation induction and pregnancies in 100 consecutive women with hypergonadotrophic amenorrhoea. *Fertil Steril* **53**, 811–6.

35. Gosden RG (1990) Restitution of fertility in sterilized mice by transferring primordial ovarian follicles. *Human Reprod* **5**, 499–504.

36. Davies MC, Hall M & Davies HS (1990) Bone mineral density in young women with amenorrhoea. *Br Med J* **301**, 790–3.

37. Jacobs HS (1981) Management of prolactin-secreting pituitary tumours. In: J Studd, (eds) *Progress in Obstetrics and Gynaecology*, Vol. 1 Edinburgh: Churchill Livingstone, 263–76.

38. Jacobs HS, Franks S, Murray MAF, Hull MGR, Steele SJ & Nabarro JDN (1976) Clinical and endocrinological features of hyperprolactinaemic amenorrhoea. *Clin Endocrinol* **5**, 439–54.

39. Soule SG & Jacobs HS (1995) Prolactinomas: present day management. *Br J Obstet Gynaecol* **102**, 178–81.

40. Sheehan HL (1939) Simmond's disease due to post-partum necrosis of the anterior pituitary. *Q J Med* **8**, 277.

41. Shoham Z, Balen AH, Patel A & Jacobs HS (1991) Results of ovulation induction using human menopausal gonadotropin or purified follicle-stimulating hormone in hypogonadotropic hypogonadism patients. *Fertil Steril* **56**, 1048–53.

42. Steinkampf MP (1990) Systemic illness and menstrual dysfunction. In: HJ Chihal, SN London (eds) *Menstrual Cycle Disorders*. Philadelphia: W.B. Saunders. *Obstet Gynecol Clin N Am* **17**, 311–9.

43. de Kretser DM, Atkins RC & Paulsen CA (1973) Role of the kidney in the metabolism of luteinising hormone. *J Endocrinol* **58**, 425.

44. Cundy TF, O'Grady JG & Williams R (1990) Recovery of menstruation and pregnancy after liver transplantation. *Gut* **31**, 337–8.

45. Kaufman FR, Kogut MD, Donnell GN, Goebelsmann U, March C & Koch R (1981) Hypergonadotrophic hypogonadism in female patients with galactosemia. *N Engl J Med* **304**, 994–8.

46. Djursing H (1987) Hypothalamic-pituitary-gonadal function in insulin treated diabetic women with and without amenorrhoea. *Dan Med Bull* **34**, 139.

47. Frisch RE (1976) Fatness of girls from menarche to age 18 years, with a nomogram. *Hum Biol* **48**, 353–9.

48. Van der Spuy ZM (1985) Nutrition and reproduction. In: Jacobs, HS (ed.) *Reproductive Endocrinology, Clinics in Obstetrics and Gynaecology*, vol. 12. London: W.B. Saunders, 579–604.

49. Warren MP & Vande Wiele RL (1973) Clinical and metabolic features of anorexia nervosa. *Am J Obstet Gynecol* **117**, 435–49.

50. Barker DJP (1990) The fetal and infant origins of adult disease. *Br Med J* **301**, 111.

51. Kulin HE, Bwibo N, Mutie D & Santner SJ (1982) The effect of chronic childhood malnutrition on pubertal growth and development. *Am J Clin Nutr* **36**, 527–36.

52. Schwartz B, Cumming DC, Riordan E, Selye M, Yen SSC & Rebar RW (1981) Exercise-associated amenorrhoea: a distinct entity? *Am J Obstet Gynecol* **141**, 662–70.

53. Cumming DC & Rebar RW (1983) Exercise and reproductive function in women. *Am J Indust Med* **4**, 113–25.

54. Warren MP (1980) The effects of exercise on pubertal progression and reproductive function in girls. *J Clin Endocrinol Metab* **51**, 1150–7.

55. Warren MP, Brooks-Gunn J, Hamilton LH, Warren LF & Hamilton WG (1986) Scoliosis and fractures in young ballet dancers. *N Engl J Med* **314**, 1348–53.

56. Bowling A (1989) Injuries to dancers: prevalence, treatment and perception of causes. *Br Med J* **298**, 731–4.

57. Harrington DJ, Smith KK & Balen AHA (1996) Case of premature menopause in an ovulating 46XY female patient. *Contemp Rev Obstet Gynecol* **8**, 465–9.

Further reading

Adams J, Franks S, Polson DW *et al.* (1985) Multifollicular ovaries. clinical and endocrine features and response to pulsatile gonadotropin releasing hormone. *Lancet* ii, 1375–8.

Adams J, Polson DW & Franks S (1986) Prevalence of polycytic ovaries in women with anovulation and idiopathic hirsuitism. *Br Med J* **293**, 355–9.

Armar NA, McGarrigle HHG, Honour JW, Holownia P, Jacobs HS & Lachelin GCL (1990) Laparoscopic ovarian diathermy in the management of anovulatory infertility in women with polycystic ovaries. endocrine changes and clinical outcome. *Fertil Steril* **53**, 45–9.

Balen AH, Conway GS, Kaltsas G, Techatraisak K, Manning PJ, West C & Jacobs HS (1995) Polycystic ovary syndrome: the spectrum of the disorder in 1741 patients. *Hum Reprod* **10**, 2705–12.

Balen AH & Jacobs HS (1994) A prospective study comparing unilateral and bilateral laparoscopic ovarian diathermy in women with the polycystic ovary syndrome. *Fertil Steril* **62**, 921–5.

Balen AH, Shoham Z & Jacobs HS (1993) Amenorrhoea – causes and consequences. In: Asch RH & Studd JJW (eds) *Annual Progress in Reproductive Medicine*. Carnforth, Lancashire: Parthenon Press, 205–34.

Balen AH (2000) Surgical management of PCOS: pros and cons. *Obstet Gynaecol* **2**, 17–20.

Balen AH, Tan SL & Jacobs HS (1993) Hypersecretion of luteinising hormone – a significant cause of infertility and miscarriage. *Br J Obstet Gynaecol* **100**, 1082–9.

Bridges NA, Cooke A, Healy MJR, Hindmarsh PC & Brook CGD (1993) Standards for ovarian Volume in childhood and puberty. *Fertil Steril* **60**, 456–60.

Brinsden PR, Wada I, Tan SL, Balen AH & Jacobs HS (1995) Diagnosis, prevention and management of the ovarian hyperstimulation syndrome. *Br J Obstet Gynaecol* **102**, 767–72.

Cameron IT, O'Shea FC, Rolland JM, Hughes EG, de Kretser DM & Healy DL (1988) Occult ovarian failure: a syndrome of infertility, regular menses and elevated follicle-stimulating hormone concentrations. *J Clin Endocrinol Metab* **67**, 1190–4.

Carey AH, Chan KL, Short D, White D, Williamson R & Franks S (1993) Evidence for a single gene defect causing polycystic ovaries and male pattern baldness. *Clin Endocrinol* **38**, 653–8.

Clayton RN, Ogden V, Hodgekinson J *et al.* (1992) How common are polycystic ovaries in normal women and what is their significance for the fertility of the population? *Clin Endocrinol* **37**, 127–34.

Farquhar CM, Birdsall M, Manning P & Mitchell JM (1994) Transabdominal versus transvaginal ultrasound in the diagnosis of polycystic ovaries on ultrasound scanning in a population of randomly selected women. *Ultrasound Obstet Gynaecol* **4**, 54–9.

Fox R, Corrigan E, Thomas PA & Hull MGR (1991) The diagnosis of polycystic ovaries in women with oligo-amenorrhoea: predictive power of endocrine tests. *Clin Endocrinol* **34**, 127–31.

Gadir AA, Mowafi RS, Alnaeser, Alrashid AH, Aloneziom & Shaw RW (1990) Ovarian electrocautery versus hMG and pure FSH therapy in the treatment of patients with PCOS. *Clin Endocrinol* **33**, 585–92.

Hall JG, Sybert VP & Williamson RA (1982) Turner's syndrome. *West J Med* **137**, 32.

Hull MGR, Knuth UA, Murray MAF & Jacobs HS (1979) The practical value of the progestogen challenge test, serum oestradiol estimation or clinical examination in assessment of the oestrogen state and response to clomifene in amenorrhoea. *Br J Obstet Gynaecol* **86**, 799–805.

Jacobs HS, Hull MGR, Murray MAF & Franks S (1975) Therapy-orientated diagnosis of secondary amenorrhoea. *Hormone Res* **6**, 268–87.

Jonard S, Robert Y, Cortet-Rudelli C, Decanter C & Dewailly D (2003) Ultrasound examination of polycystic ovaries: is it worth counting the follicles? *Hum Reprod* **18**, 598–603.

Kiddy DS, Hamilton-Fairly D, Seppala M *et al.* (1989) Diet induced changes in sex hormone binding globulin and free testosterone in women with normal or polycystic ovaries: correlation with serum insulin-like growth factor 1. *Clin Endocrinol* **31**, 757–63.

Lunenfeld B & Insler V (1974) Classification of amenorrhoea states and their treatment by ovulation induction. *Clin Endocrinol* **3**, 223–37.

Lutjen P, Trounson A, Leeton J, Findlay J, Wood C & Renou P (1984) The establishment and maintenance of pregnancy using *in vitro* fertilization and embryo donation in a patient with primary ovarian failure. *Nature* **307**, 174–5.

RCOG (2004) *Guidelines on the Initial Investigation and Management of Infertility*. London: RCOG Press, NICE, London.

Rossaminth WG, Keckstein J, Spatzier K & Lauritzen C (1991) The impact of ovarian laser surgery on the gonadotropin secretion in women with PCOD. *Clin Endocrinol* **34**, 223–30.

Rossing MA, Daling JR, Weiss NS, Moore DE & Self SG (1994) Ovarian tumours in a cohort of infertile women. *N Engl J Med* **331**, 771–6.

Sampaolo P, Livien C, Montanari L, Paganelli A, Salesi A & Lorini R (1994) Precocious signs of polycystic ovaries in obese girls. *Ultrasound Obstet Gynaecol* **4**, 1–6.

Fauser B, Tarlatzis B, Chang J *et al.* (The Rotterdam ESHRE/ASRM-sponsored PCOS consensus workshop group) (2004) Revised 2003 consensus on diagnostic criteria and long-term health risks related to polycystic ovary syndrome (PCOS). *Human Reprod* **19**, 41–7.

Turner HH (1938) A syndrome of infantilism, congenital webbed neck, and cubitus valgus. *Endocrinol* **23**, 566.

Van der Spuy ZM, Steer PJ, McCusker M, Steele SJ & Jacobs HS (1998) Outcome of pregnancy in underweight women after spontaneous and induced ovulation. *Br Med J* **296**, 962–5.

Chapter 40: Menstrual problems: menorrhagia and primary dysmenorrhagia

Margaret C.P. Rees

Introduction

Menorrhagia and dysmenorrhoea form a significant part of gynaecological work. This is not surprising since women will each experience about 400 menstruations between the menarche and the menopause. Menorrhagia is the main presenting complaint in women referred to gynaecologists and accounts for most hysterectomies and nearly all endometrial ablative procedures.

Menorrhagia (heavy blood loss)

Menorrhagia comes from the Greek 'men' meaning month and 'rhegynai' to rush out. It is a complaint of heavy cyclical menstrual blood loss over several consecutive cycles without any intermenstrual or post-coital bleeding [1]. In objective terms it is a blood loss greater than 80 ml per period [2]. While various pathologies have been implicated in menorrhagia, in 50% of cases of objective menorrhagia no pathology is found at hysterectomy (Table 40.1). Although 'unexplained' menorrhagia is a very appropriate term the label dysfunctional uterine bleeding which implies endocrine abnormalities is often given. However, most cases of menorrhagia are associated with regular ovulatory cycles and anovular cycles tend mainly to occur soon after the menarche or in the perimenopause.

Presentation and assessment

Patients with menorrhagia commonly complain of increased menstrual loss requiring more sanitary protection or the passage of clots and flooding. Assessment is detailed in Table 40.2. Of note women find it very difficult to assess accurately the amount of blood loss. Thus, in clinical practice only 40% of women complaining of menorrhagia have measured losses greater than 80 ml [3]. The alkaline haematin method is considered to be the 'gold standard' for measuring menstrual blood loss [2]. Here sanitary devices are soaked in 5% sodium hydroxide to convert the blood to alkaline haematin whose optical density is then measured. Since it is not routinely available various pictorial scoring systems have been proposed but reliability is conflicting [3–5]. Furthermore

Table 40.1 Causes of menorrhagia

Uterine
Fibroids
Endometrial polyps
Endometriosis
Pelvic inflammatory disease

Systemic
Coagulation disorders
Von Willebrand's disease
Idiopathic thrombocytopaenia purpura
Factor V, VII, X and XI deficiency
Hypothyroidism

Iatrogenic
Progestogen only contraceptives
Intrauterine contraceptive devices
Anticoagulants

Table 40.2 Initial assessment

History
How long have periods been heavy
Is there flooding or passage of clots
How long do periods last and how often do they occur
Has there been any change
Is there any intermenstrual bleeding or post-coital bleeding
Is there pelvic pain or dyspareunia
What contraception is being used
Are cervical smears up to date (according to local screening
  programmes)

Assessment
Undertake pelvic examination and cervical smear (according to
  local screening programmes)
Haematology and biochemistry
Imaging
Endometrial sampling
Hysteroscopy

recent technological changes in the manufacture of sanitary towels mean that these pictorial methods need to be revalidated. Measurement of total menstrual fluid by means of a weighing technique has been described as sufficiently accurate for clinical purposes, but needs further evaluation [5].

Investigations

HAEMATOLOGY AND BIOCHEMISTRY

A full blood count should be performed in all women complaining of menorrhagia, since it is a common cause for anaemia [1]. Ferritin is not recommended routinely. Testing for bleeding disorders should only be undertaken if clinically indicated, for example, menorrhagia since the menarche and a history of bleeding after dental extractions and childbirth [4,6]. Thyroid function tests should only be undertaken if clinically indicated. No other endocrine investigations are warranted.

IMAGING

Transvaginal sonography (TVS) is usually the first investigation. TVS measures endometrial thickness and diagnoses polyps and leiomyomata with a sensitivity of 80% and specificity of 69% [7]. It is well established that endometrial thickness measured by TVS is indicative of pathology in postmenopausal women. However, the exact cut-off values for endometrial thickness measurement in premenopausal women to predict endometrial neoplasia are subject to continuing debate. The British 'RCOG Guideline Development Group' analysed a number of studies and concluded that 10–12 mm was a reasonable cut-off when using TVS, preferably undertaken in the follicular phase, as a method prior to more invasive procedures of endometrial assessment [5,8]. TVS can be enhanced using sonohysterography or colour flow Doppler but availability may be limited [9,10].

ENDOMETRIAL SAMPLING

The purpose of endometrial sampling in menorrhagia is to exclude or diagnose endometrial cancer or hyperplasia. Endometrial sampling is recommended in women aged more than 40 years and those with increased risk of endometrial malignancy. Significant risk factors for development of an endometrial carcinoma are obesity, diabetes mellitus, hypertension, chronic anovulation, nulliparity with a history of infertility, a family history of endometrial and colonic cancer and tamoxifen therapy [5]. In younger women endometrial sampling can also be indicated if abnormal bleeding does not resolve with medical treatment. In polycystic ovary syndrome in which endometrial

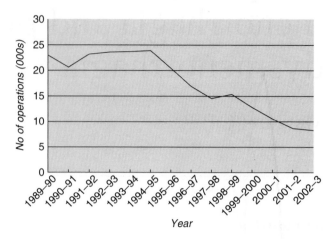

Fig. 40.1 Numbers of hysterectomies for menorrhagia between 1989/90 and 2002/3 in NHS Trusts in England. (Reid and Mukri [12]). Reproduced with permission from the BMJ Publishing Group.

hyperplasia is a common finding, endometrial assessment may be necessary if abnormal bleeding is a presenting symptom, or suspicious sonographic endometrial features are observed [5,8].

The most common methods of endometrial sampling are:
- Aspiration curettage (Pipelle, Vabra)
- Dilatation and curettage (D&C)
- Hysteroscopy

'One-stop' outpatient services based on initial TVS may reduce the need for further procedures such as hysteroscopy [11].

Management

Management has changed over the past two decades with the introduction in the mid-1980s of therapeutic endoscopic endometrial destructive procedures and in 1995 of the levonorgestrel-releasing intrauterine device in the UK. The number of hysterectomies for menorrhagia have been estimated to have fallen by 36% between 1989 and 2002/3 [6,12] (Fig. 40.1). Also an inverse social gradient in hysterectomy has been observed with surgery being inversely related to social class and education, especially at younger ages [7,13].

Drug therapy

The aims of therapy are to reduce blood loss, reduce the risk of anaemia and improve quality of life. Medical therapy is indicated when there is no obvious pelvic abnormality and the woman wishes to retain her fertility. Since menstrual loss, in the absence of pathology, does not change markedly treatment is long term. Thus the drug

Table 40.3 Non-hormonal
treatments for menorrhagia

Non-steroidal anti-inflammatory drugs
Mefenamic acid
Meclofenamic acid
Naproxen
Ibuprofen
Flurbiprofen
Diclofenac

Antifibrinolytics
Tranexamic acid
Epsilon-amino caproic acid

Etamsylate

Table 40.4 Hormonal treatments
for menorrhagia

Progestogens
Norethisterone
Medroxyprogesterone acetate
Dydrogesterone

Intrauterine progestogens
Levonorgestrel IUS (Mirena)
Progesterone IUS (Progestasert)

Combined oestrogen/ progestogens
Oral contraceptives
Hormone replacement therapy

Other
Danazol
Gestrinone
GnRH analogues

regimen chosen must be effective, have few or mild side effects and must be acceptable to the patient. It is important to assess drug therapies in terms of reduction of measured menstrual blood loss because of the poor correlation between objective and subjective assessment of menstrual blood loss (see Presentation and Assessment, p. 399).

Medical therapies can be divided into two main classes: non-hormonal and hormonal. The former includes non-steroidal anti-inflammatory drugs and antifibrinolytics, and the latter progestogens, oral contraceptives, hormone replacement therapy, danazol, gestrinone and GnRH analogues (Tables 40.3 and 40.4). Non-hormonal treatment is taken during menstruation itself and should be a first line in primary care using either mefenamic acid or tranexamic acid; both can be used together, but there are no good studies of the effect of the combination. Referral should be considered if neither inhibitors of prostaglandin synthesis or antifibrinolytic agents are effective after 3 months' therapy [1].

NON-HORMONAL

Non-steroidal anti-inflammatory drugs

The cyclooxygenase (COX) pathway with its two enzymes cyclooxygenase-1 (COX-1) and cyclooxygenase-2 (COX-2) represents one of the major routes for oxidative metabolism of arachidonic acid to prostaglandins. The demonstrated involvement of prostaglandins in the genesis of menorrhagia points to cyclooxygenase inhibitors as a potentially effective treatment. Cyclooxygenase inhibitors, commonly referred to as non-steroidal anti-inflammatory drugs (NSAIDs), can be chemically classified into two main groups – COX-1 inhibitors: salicytes (aspirin), indolacetic acid analogues (indometacin), aryl proprionic acid derivates (naproxen, ibuprofen), fenamates (mefenamic acid, flufenamic acid, meclofenamic acid) and COX-2 inhibitors: coxibs (celecoxib). Various NSAIDs have been evaluated in a number of randomized trials and have to date been limited to COX-1 inhibitors. In a Cochrane review, five of seven randomized trials showed that mean menstrual blood loss was less with NSAIDs than with placebo, and two showed no difference [8,14]. Furthermore, there was no evidence that one NSAID (naproxen or mefenamic acid) was superior to the other. The fenamates (e.g. mefenamic acid) are the most extensively studied NSAIDs. They have the unique property to inhibit prostaglandin synthesis as well as to bind to prostaglandin receptors, which, are significantly increased in the uteri from women with menorrhagia [15]. Reductions in menstrual blood flow range from 22 to 46% with this therapy. With regards to long-term therapy, a follow-up of 12 to 15 months after commencing treatment showed continuing efficacy of the NSAID mefenamic acid [16]. Reduction of menstrual blood loss has also been evaluated for other NSAIDs such as naproxen, ibuprofen, sodium diclofenac and flurbiprofen. The percentage of blood loss reduction varied from 25 to 47% depending on the agent and dosage used [15]. Furthermore, they are also effective in women with a copper or non-hormonal intrauterine contraceptive device. An additional beneficial effect is that these drugs will also alleviate symptoms from dysmenorrhoea.

Optimal doses and schedules are difficult to define. Most studies, however, analysed regimens starting on the first day of menstruation and continuing for 5 days or until cessation of menstruation. Common side effects of NSAIDs are gastrointestinal irritation and inhibition of platelet aggregation. Specific inhibitors of COX-2 might also be effective in the treatment of menorrhagia, but there is great uncertainty about the safety of this class of drugs [17].

Antifibrinolytics

Plasminogen activator inhibitors have therefore been promoted as a treatment for menorrhagia because of increased endometrial fibrinolytic activity in women with menorrhagia.

Tranexamic acid is a synthetic lysine derivate that exerts its antifibrinolytic effect by reversibly blocking lysine binding sites on plasminogen and thus preventing fibrin degradation [18]. Tranexamic acid 2 to 4.5 g/day for 4 to 7 days reduces menstrual blood flow by 34 to 59% over two to three cycles. The effect is superior to placebo, mefenamic acid, flurbiprofen, ethamsylate and oral luteal phase norethisterone at clinically relevant dosages [9,19]. Antifibrinolytics are also effective in women with copper or non-hormonal intrauterine devices [18,19]. Tranexamic acid is usually well tolerated. Side effects are mainly limited to mild gastrointestinal complaints. A Cochrane review found no significant increase in reported events with antifibrinolytic therapy in comparison to placebo or other treatments [9,19]. Earlier theoretical concerns about thromboembolism caused by antifibrinolytic action of tranexamic acid have been refuted by long-term studies.

Ethamsylate

Ethamsylate is thought to act by reducing capillary fragility, though the precise mechanisms are uncertain. Studies with objective MBL measurement using the currently recommended doses show that it is ineffective [1,5,8].

HORMONAL TREATMENTS

Progestogens

The use of progestogens is based on the erroneous concept that women with menorrhagia principally have anovulatory cycles and that a progestogen supplement is required. Progestogens are a common prescription for women complaining of menorrhagia. Oral, intrauterine and intramuscular depot injections are employed. The last are used mainly for contraception and there is little information regarding menorrhagia.

Oral administration. Traditionally administration was in the luteal phase. However, studies with measured menstrual loss with luteal administration for 7 days of norethisterone 5 mg twice daily show either a decrease or even an increase in flow [10,20]. However, norethisterone 5 mg three times daily from day 5–26 is effective [21]. Side effects include weight gain, headache and bloatedness.

Intrauterine administration. Intrauterine administration especially of levonorgestrel (LNG) is very effective. There are currently two progestogen-impregnated devices: the Mirena® intra uterine system (IUS) (Schering, Germany), which delivers 20 μg of LNG over 24 h for about 5 years and the Progestasert® (Alza Pharmaceuticals, USA) which releases about 65 μg of progesterone over 24 h for about 16 months. Other newer so-called frameless devices are currently being evaluated.

The Mirena IUS (LNG-IUS) reduces menstrual blood loss by up to 96 and 20% of women using the LNG-IUS are reported to be amenorrheic after 1 year [11,22]. Over a 3-year period 65% of women with an LNG-IUS continue to report improved menstrual bleeding. Apart from lowering menstrual blood loss the LNG-IUS may alleviate symptoms of dysmenorrhoea and reduce the incidence of pelvic inflammatory disease. The LNG-IUS also provides very effective contraception. Results are comparable with endometrial resection [12,23] and it can be employed as an alternative to hysterectomy [24].

The main adverse effects associated with LNG-IUS are frequently occurring variable bleeding and spotting, particularly within the first few months of use. LNG-IUS is also sometimes associated with the development of ovarian cysts, but these are usually symptomless and show a high rate of spontaneous resolution. When compared with other medications and hysterectomy, the LNG-IUS is much cheaper per menstrual cycle unless it is removed before 5 years. The LNG-IUS showed similar efficacy and patient satisfaction at much lower costs ($1530 for IUS versus $4222 for hysterectomy) [24]. It also preserves fertility while providing contraception and provides the progestogen for systemic hormone replacement therapy in perimenopausal women.

The Progestasert was the first hormonally impregnated device but prospective randomized studies in menorrhagia are lacking. The main disadvantage of this device is its association with an increased risk of ectopic pregnancy.

Oestrogen/progestogen

From clinical experience oral contraceptine pills (OCPs) are generally considered to be effective in the management of dysfunctional menstrual bleeding. However, there are few available data to support this observation [13,25]. Data regarding hormone replacement therapy are scant.

Androgens

Danazol. Danazol is an isoxazol derivative of 17α-ethinyl-testosterone which acts on the hypothalamic pituitary axis as well as on the endometrium to produce atrophy. Danazol reduces menstrual blood loss by up to 80% from baseline. Higher doses of Danazol (≥200 mg/day) seem to be more successful than low-dosage therapy [26]. Its clinical use is limited by androgenic side effects which are experienced by up to three quarters of patients.

Gestrinone. Gestrinone is a 19-testosterone derivative which has anti-progestogenic, anti-oestrogenic and androgenic activity. In a placebo-controlled study it reduced menstrual blood loss in 79% patients with objective menorrhagia [27]. However, it also has androgenic side effects.

Gonadotropin-releasing hormone agonists

Gonadotropin-releasing hormone (GnRH) agonists, administered continuously or in depot form, downregulate expression of GnRH receptors, which blocks gonadotropin secretion from the anterior pituitary. This leads to ovarian suppression. GnRH have been mainly used in fibroid-associated bleeding [28]. Concerns about the long-term effects of ovarian suppression such as osteoporosis generally limit use beyond 6 months even when add-back therapy and oestrogen/progestogen hormone replacement therapy is used in conjunction.

Anti-progestational agents

Mifepristone (RU-486) is a synthetic 19-norsteroid with anti-progestogen activity that is known to inhibit ovulation and to disrupt endometrial integrity. Systematic review shows that it induces amenorrhoea and reduces leiomyoma size [29]. However, a notable adverse effect was development of endometrial hyperplasia.

Surgery

Surgery may be necessary to deal with pelvic abnormalities such as polyps, fibroids, chronic pelvic inflammatory disease or endometriotic masses. Operations should be as conservative as possible in women who wish to retain their fertility. Surgery includes removal of endometrial polyps, endometrial destruction, myomectomy and ultimately hysterectomy. Submucous fibroids or endometrial polyps should be removed hysteroscopically.

HYSTERECTOMY

The three choices are abdominal (TAH), vaginal (VH) or laparoscopically (LAVH) assisted with the first being the most common [14,30]. The last has the potential for short hospital stay (1 day or less) but currently is infrequently used in the UK [14,30]. Hysterectomy should only be offered to women whose family is complete. Complications of hysterectomy are often underestimated. The VALUE study in England and Wales is a recent assessment of complications [14,30]. Unfortunately only 45% of cases were reported. Overall operative complications occurred in 3.5% with 9% getting a post-operative complication. The death rate at 6 weeks after surgery was 0.38 per 1000. Visceral damage occurred in 0.76% after TAH, 0.61% after VH and 1.13% after LAVH. Significant bleeding was found in 2.3% of TAH cases, 1.9% after VH and 4.2% after LAVH. Following LAVH 1.5% of women returned to theatre compared to 0.7% after TAH or VH.

In a study from the USA fever rate after TAH was 30% and 15% needed a blood transfusion [31]. Pyrexia occurred in 15% after VH. Bowel injury occurred in 3/1000 women following abdominal hysterectomy and 6/1000 after vaginal hysterectomy. The urinary tract was damaged in 3/1000 after abdominal hysterectomy but 14/1000 with the vaginal route. Mortality was 1/1000.

Long-term sequelae

Hysterectomy may or may not be accompanied by oophorectomy and may be total or subtotal. Even if the ovaries are conserved there are concerns that the menopause may occur early. Other concerns include mental well-being, psychosexual dysfunction and urinary tract and bowel symptoms.

Bilateral oophorectomy or surgical menopause results in an immediate menopause which may be intensely symptomatic. Hysterectomy without oophorectomy can induce ovarian failure either in the immediate postoperative period, where in some cases it may be temporary, or at a later stage where it may occur sooner than the time of natural menopause, that is, 51. Early ovarian failure increases the risk of developing cardiovascular disease and osteoporosis. The diagnosis of ovarian failure is more difficult in the absence of menstrual function. A case could be made for annual follicle stimulating hormone (FSH) estimation in women who have had a hysterectomy before the age of 40.

There is currently a vogue for subtotal hysterectomy, with the understanding that sexual function is better preserved than with total hysterectomy. The downside is that cervical smears have to be continued. Also there may be some endometrium in the cervical stump and this has been reported in 7% of women [15,32]. This UK randomized trial found that neither subtotal nor total abdominal hysterectomy adversely affected urinary, bowel or sexual function at 12 months [15,32]. A Dutch study found that sexual pleasure improves after vaginal hysterectomy, subtotal abdominal hysterectomy, and total abdominal hysterectomy. The prevalence of one or more bothersome sexual problems 6 months after vaginal hysterectomy, subtotal abdominal hysterectomy, and total abdominal hysterectomy was 43% (38/89), 41% (31/76), and 39% (57/145), respectively [16,33].

In the late 1970s it was believed from retrospective studies that hysterectomy increased psychiatric morbidity but was refuted by subsequent prospective studies. This has been confirmed in a study of total versus subtotal hysterectomy [34]. All women showed an improvement in psychological symptoms following both operations and no difference was found between the two procedures.

ENDOMETRIAL ABLATION

There are two classes of methods with second generation not requiring hysteroscopic skills (Table 40.5). The advantage of these methods is that hospital stay is much shorter being 1 day rather than 5–6 for VH or TAH. Like hysterectomy, these treatments should only be offered to women who desire no further children. There are several factors which affect clinical outcome. Women older than 45 years are more likely to become amenorrhoeic. Adenomyosis has been associated with a higher failure rate of first-generation techniques. The reported incidence of intra-operative complications is relatively low being about 1%. The most common complications are haemorrhage, perforation, need for emergency surgery and absorption of distending medium (radiofrequency-induced thermal ablation, microwaves and thermal balloons do not use a distending medium). The MISTLETOE study (Minimally Invasive Surgical Technique-Laser, Endothermal or Endoresection) showed that uterine perforation and haemorrhage were more common with TCRE, and fluid overload occurred more frequently with laser ablation. While some of the variability in the rates of complications can be explained by inherent differences between the treatment modalities, there were also considerable differences in training and supervision, as 52% of doctors using the

resectoscope started out unsupervised in contrast to only 7% using laser. Most complications were encountered in the first 100 cases undertaken by an individual surgeon [17,35].

A concern is need for repeat surgery such as hysterectomy. Reported rates vary being of the order of 21% at 6.5 years [36]. Systematic review has found few significant differences between the outcomes of first- and second-generation techniques including bleeding, satisfaction and quality-of-life measures and repeat surgery rates. Second-generation techniques had significantly shorter operating and theatre times and there appear to be fewer serious perioperative adverse effects [18,37].

While the likelihood of pregnancy after endometrial ablation is low, the frequency has been reported to be 0.7%, with a variety of complications and adverse outcomes for the fetus. Women who undergo this procedure should therefore be advised to use effective contraception.

Decision aids

Increasing patient participation in treatment decision is important in view of the wide choices available. Decision aids come in a variety of formats including leaflets, audiotapes, decision boards, computer programs, videos, websites, and structured interviews. These were examined in a randomized controlled trial with 2 years of follow-up of 894 women [19,38]. Women were randomized to the control group, information alone group (booklet and video), or information plus interview group (interview). Hysterectomy rates were lower for women in the interview group (38%) (adjusted odds ratio [OR], than in the control group (48%) and women who received the information alone (48%). The interview group had lower mean costs ($1566) than the control group ($2751) (mean difference, $1184; 95% CI, $684–$2110) and the information group $2026 (mean difference, $461; 95% CI, $236–$696). Thus, providing women with information alone did not affect treatment choices; however, the addition of an interview to clarify values and elicit preferences had a significant effect on women's management and resulted in reduced costs.

Dysmenorrhoea

Derived from the Greek meaning difficult monthly flow, the word dysmenorrhoea has come to mean painful menstruation. Dysmenorrhoea can be classified as either primary or secondary. In the former type there is no pelvic pathology while the latter implies underlying pathology which leads to painful menstruation. This chapter will deal with primary dysmenorrhoea since secondary dysmenorrhoea is dealt with in chapters on disease states.

Table 40.5 Methods of endometrial ablation

First generation
Trans Cervical Resection of the Endometrium (TCRE)
Endometrial Laser Resection (ELA)
Roller Ball Endometrial Ablation (REA)

Second generation
Thermal Balloons (Thermachoice, Cavatherm)
Microwave Endometrial Ablation (MEA)
Circulating Hot Saline (Hydro therm Ablator)
Cryotherapy

Primary dysmenorrhoea

The prevalence of dysmenorrhoea is high. A Swedish study found that 72% of 19-year-old women reported dysmenorrhoea, nearly 40% regularly used medication for the pain and 8% stayed absent from work or school at every period [39]. According to an American study, 60% of menstruating young women suffered from dysmenorrhoea and 14% regularly missed school [40].

Primary dysmenorrhoea is associated with uterine hypercontractility characterized by excessive amplitude and frequency of contractions and a high 'resting' tone between contractions. During contractions endometrial blood flow is reduced and there seems to be a good correlation between minimal blood flow and maximal colicky pain, favouring the concept that ischaemia due to hypercontractility causes primary dysmenorrhoea. Prostaglandin and leukotriene levels are elevated in menstrual fluid and uterine tissue of women with dysmenorrhoea as are systemic levels of vasopressin.

Presentation and assessment

In general primary dysmenorrhoea appears 6–12 months after the menarche when ovulatory cycles begin to become established. The early cycles after the menarche are usually anovular and tend to be painless. The pain usually consists of lower abdominal cramps and backache and there may be associated gastrointestinal disturbances such as diarrhoea and vomiting. Symptoms occur predominantly during the first 2 days of menstruation.

The diagnosis of primary dysmenorrhoea is one of exclusion (Table 40.6). If symptoms are typical of primary dysmenorrhoea, a therapeutic trial may be embarked on before considering any examination and investigation especially in adolescents. If clinical evaluation raises suspicion of secondary dysmenorrhoea transvaginal sonography (TVS) or magnetic resonance imaging (MRI) or laparoscopy should be considered. Similarly, if symptoms of primary dysmenorrhoea are not alleviated with either

Table 40.6 Assessment

How long have periods been painful
Has there been any change
When does the pain occur
Is there pelvic pain at other times or dyspareunia
Is there flooding or passage of clots
How long do periods last and how often do they occur
Is there any intermenstrual bleeding or post-coital bleeding
Is there a history of infertility or pelvic inflammatory disease
What contraception is being used
Are cervical smears up to date (according to local screening
 programmes)

NSAIDs or the combined oral contraceptive pill or the combination of the two, secondary causes of dysmenorrhoea need to be considered. Secondary dysmenorrhoea should also be suspected if symptoms initially typical of primary dysmenorrhoea worsen in duration (starting premenstrually) and intensity.

Management

Women will usually seek medical advice when self-help measures such as heat and over the counter NSAIDs have failed [41]. The mainstays of treatment are NSAIDs and the combined oral contraceptive pill, the latter especially when fertility control is required.

NON-STEROIDAL ANTI-INFLAMMATORY DRUGS

Meta-analysis shows that COX-1 inhibitors such as mefenamic acid, naproxen, ibuprofen and aspirin are all effective [20,21,42,43]. Ibuprofen is the preferred analgesic because of its favourable efficacy and safety profiles [20,42,44]. Commencing treatment before the onset of menstruation appears to have no demonstrable advantage over starting treatment when bleeding starts. This observation is compatible with the short plasma half-life of NSAIDs. The advantage of starting treatment at the onset of menstruation is that it prevents the patient treating herself when she is unknowingly pregnant which would only become apparent when a period is missed.

It is interesting to note that traditional healers have used plants with significant COX-inhibitory activity to treat menstrual pain [45].

THE COMBINED ORAL CONTRACEPTIVE PILL

Although commonly used, clinical trial evidence supporting the efficacy of combined oral contraceptives in primary dysmenorrhoea is limited. They are thought to act by inhibiting ovulation and decreasing endometrial production of prostaglandins and leukotrienes by inducing endometrial atrophy and therefore reducing the amount of endometrial tissue available to produce these mediators [23,46,47]. However, most of the clinical trials were undertaken with contraceptives with higher doses of hormones than those currently used [23,46].

OTHER HORMONAL METHODS

Although primarily designed for parous women, the LNG-IUS may be an effective treatment for nulliparous women who have a contraindication to either NSAIDs or the combined oral contraceptive. In women aged 25–47 years, the frequency of menstrual pain decreased from

60 to 29% after 36 months use of the device [48]. Other alternatives include depot progestogens used for contraception. Clinically they are effective since they render most women amenorrhoeic, but clinical trial data are scant. Of some of the new progestogen only contraceptive pills (e.g. 75 mcg desogestrel) effectively inhibit ovulation and thus probably relieve symptoms of dysmenorrhoea.

OTHER METHODS

A number of other pharmaceutical agents exist that alleviate the symptoms of dysmenorrhoea. An orally active vasopressin receptor antagonist has been shown to be effective [49].

Beta-adrenergic agonists and calcium channel blockers can reduce uterine contractility and thus are potentially effective but clinical trials have not been undertaken [50,51]. Transdermal glyceryl trinitrate has also been evaluated [52]. A placebo-controlled trial found both placebo and vitamin E are effective in relieving symptoms due to primary dysmenorrhoea, but the effects of vitamin E are more marked [53]. A randomized control study found supplementation with omega-3 polyunsaturated fatty acids beneficial in the management of dysmenorrhoea in adolescents [54]. The mode of action is presumed to involve altered prostaglandin biosynthesis.

References

1. Royal College of Obstetricians and Gynaecologists (1998) *The Initial Management of Menorrhagia*. Evidence-based guidelines 1. London: RCOG Press.
2. Hallberg L, Hogdahl AM, Nilsson L & Rybo G (1996) Menstrual blood loss–a population study. Variation at different ages and attempts to define normality. *Acta Obstet Gynecol Scand* **45**, 320–51.
3. Fraser IS, McCarron G & Markham R (1984) A preliminary study of factors influencing perception of menstrual blood loss volume. *Am J Obstet Gynecol* **149**, 788–93.
4. Reid PC, Coker A & Coltart R (2000) Assessment of menstrual blood loss using a pictorial chart: a validation study. *BJOG* **107**, 320–2.
5. Mansfield PK, Voda A & Allison G (2004) Validating a pencil-and-paper measure of perimenopausal menstrual blood loss. *Womens Health Issues.* **14**, 242–7.
6. Philipp CS, Faiz A, Dowling N et al. (2005) Age and the prevalence of bleeding disorders in women with menorrhagia. *Obstet Gynecol* **105**, 61–6.
7. Vercellini P, Cortesi I, Oldani S, Moschetta M, De Giorgi O & Crosignani PG (1997) The role of transvaginal ultrasonography and outpatient diagnostic hysteroscopy in the evaluation of patients with menorrhagia. Hum Reprod **12**, 1768–71.
8. Royal College of Obstetricians and Gynaecologists (1999) The Management of Menorrhagia in Secondary Care. Evidence-based guidelines 5. London: RCOG Press.
9. Dijkhuizen FP, De Vries LD, Mol BW et al. (2000) Comparison of transvaginal ultrasonography and saline infusion sonography for the detection of intracavitary abnormalities in premenopausal women. *Ultrasound Obstet Gynecol* **15**, 372–6.
10. Levine D (1999) Pelvic doppler. *Semin Ultrasound CT MR* **20**, 239–49.
11. Jones K & Bourne T (2001) The feasibility of a 'one stop' ultrasound-based clinic for the diagnosis and management of abnormal uterine bleeding. *Ultrasound Obstet Gynecol* **17**, 517–21.
12. Reid PC & Mukri F (2005) Trends in number of hysterectomies performed in England for menorrhagia: examination of health episode statistics, 1989 to 2002–3. *Br Med J* **330**, 938–9.
13. Marshall SF, Hardy RJ & Kuh D (2000) Socioeconomic variation in hysterectomy up to age 52: national, population based, prospective cohort study. *Br Med J* **320**, 1579.
14. Lethaby A, Augood C & Duckitt K (2002) Nonsteroidal anti-inflammatory drugs for heavy menstrual bleeding. *Cochrane Database Syst Rev* **1**, CD000400.
15. Adelantado JM, Rees MCP, Lopez-Bernal A & Turnbull AC (1988) Increased uterine prostaglandin E receptors in menorrhagic women. *Br J Obstet Gynaecol* **95**, 162–5.
16. Fraser IS, McCarron G, Markham R, Robinson M & Smyth E (1983) Long-term treatment of menorrhagia with mefenamic acid. *Obstet Gynecol* **61**, 109–12.
17. Psaty BM & Furberg CD (2005) COX-2 Inhibitors – lessons in drug safety. *N Engl J Med* **352**, 113–5.
18. Wellington K & Wagstaff AJ (2003) Tranexamic acid: a review of its use in the management of menorrhagia. *Drugs* **63**, 1417–33.
19. Lethaby A, Farquhar C & Cooke I (2000) Antifibrinolytics for heavy menstrual bleeding. *Cochrane Database Syst Rev* **4**, CD000249.
20. Lethaby A, Irvine G & Cameron I (2000) Cyclical progestogens for heavy menstrual bleeding. *Cochrane Database Syst Rev* **2**, CD001016.
21. Irvine GA, Campbell-Brown MB, Lumsden MA, Heikkila A & Walker JJ, Cameron IT (1998) Randomised comparative trial of the levonorgestrel intrauterine system and norethisterone for treatment of idiopathic menorrhagia. *Br J Obstet Gynaecol* **105**, 592–8.
22. Lethaby AE, Cooke I & Rees M (2000) Progesterone/progestogen releasing intrauterine systems versus either placebo or any other medication for heavy menstrual bleeding. *Cochrane Database Syst Rev* **2**, CD002126.
23. Rauramo I, Elo I & Istre O (2004) Long-term treatment of menorrhagia with levonorgestrel intrauterine system versus endometrial resection. *Obstet Gynecol* **104**, 1314–21.
24. Hurskainen R, Teperi J, Rissanen P et al. (2001) Quality of life and cost-effectiveness of levonorgestrel-releasing intrauterine system versus hysterectomy for treatment of menorrhagia: a randomised trial. *Lancet* **357**, 273–7.
25. Iyer V, Farquhar C & Jepson R (2000) Oral contraceptive pills for heavy menstrual bleeding. *Cochrane Database Syst Rev* **2**, CD000154.
26. Beaumont H, Augood C, Duckitt K & Lethaby A (2002) Danazol for heavy menstrual bleeding. *Cochrane Database Syst Rev* **1**, CD001017.

27. Turnbull AC & Rees MC (1990) Gestrinone in the treatment of menorrhagia. *Br J Obstet Gynaecol* **97**, 713–5.

28. Moghissi KS (2000) A clinician's guide to the use of gonadotropin-releasing hormone analogues in women. Medscape Womens Health **5**, 5.

29. Steinauer J, Pritts EA, Jackson R & Jacoby AF (2004) Systematic review of mifepristone for the treatment of uterine leiomyomata. *Obstet Gynecol* **103**, 1331–6.

30. Maresh MJA, Metcalfe MA, McPherson K *et al.* (2002) The VALUE national hysterectomy study: description of the patients and their surgery. *Br J Obstet Gynaecol* **109**, 302–12.

31. Krebs HB (1986) Intestinal injury in gynecologic surgery: a ten year experience. *Am J Obstet Gynecol* **155**, 509–14.

32. Thakar R, Ayers S, Clarkson P, Stanton S & Manyonda I (2002) Outcomes after total versus subtotal abdominal hysterectomy. *N Engl J Med* **347**, 1318–25.

33. Roovers JP, van der Bom JG, van der Vaart CH & Heintz AP (2003) Hysterectomy and sexual wellbeing: prospective observational study of vaginal hysterectomy, subtotal abdominal hysterectomy, and total abdominal hysterectomy. *Br Med J* **327**, 774–8.

34. Thakar R, Ayers S, Georgakapolou A, Clarkson P, Stanton S & Manyonda I (2004) Hysterectomy improves quality of life and decreases psychiatric symptoms: a prospective and randomised comparison of total versus subtotal hysterectomy. *BJOG* **111**, 1115–20.

35. Overton C, Hargreaves J & Maresh M (1997) A national survey of the complications of endometrial destruction for menstrual disorders: the MISTLETOE study. Minimally invasive surgical techniques – laser, endoThermal or endoresection. *Br J Obstet Gynaecol* **104**, 1351–9.

36. Phillips G, Chien PF & Garry R (1998) Risk of hysterectomy after 1000 consecutive endometrial laser ablations. *Br J Obstet Gynaecol* **105**, 897–903.

37. Garside R, Stein K, Wyatt K, Round A & Price A (2004) The effectiveness and cost-effectiveness of microwave and thermal balloon endometrial ablation for heavy menstrual bleeding: a systematic review and economic modelling. *Health Technol Assess* **8**, 1–155.

38. Kennedy AD, Sculpher MJ, Coulter A *et al.* (2002) Effects of decision aids for menorrhagia on treatment choices, health outcomes, and costs: a randomized controlled trial. *JAMA* **288**, 2701–8.

39. Andersch B & Milsom I (1982) An epidemiologic study of young women with dysmenorrhea. *Am J Obstet Gynecol* **144**, 655–60.

40. Klein JR & Litt IF (1981) Epidemiology of adolescent dysmenorrhea. *Pediatrics* **68**, 661–4.

41. Campbell MA & McGrath PJ (1999) Non-pharmacologic strategies used by adolescents for the management of menstrual discomfort. *Clin J Pain* **15**, 313–20.

42. Zhang WY & Li Wan Po A (1998) Efficacy of minor analgesics in primary dysmenorrhoea: a systematic review. *Br J Obstet Gynaecol* **105**, 780–9.

43. Marjoribanks J, Proctor ML & Farquhar C (2003) Nonsteroidal anti-inflammatory drugs for primary dysmenorrhoea. *Cochrane Database Syst Rev* **4**, CD001751.

44. Daniels SE, Talwalker S, Torri S *et al.* (2002) Valdecoxib, a cyclooxygenase-2-specific inhibitor, is effective in treating primary dysmenorrhea. *Obstet Gynecol* **100**, 350–8.

45. Lindsey K, Jager AK, Raidoo DM *et al.* (1999) Screening of plants used by Southern African traditional healers in the treatment of dysmenorrhoea for prostaglandin-synthesis inhibitors and uterine relaxing activity. *J Ethnopharmacol* **64**, 9–14.

46. Proctor ML, Roberts H & Farquhar CM (2001) Combined oral contraceptive pill (OCP) as treatment for primary dysmenorrhoea. *Cochrane Database Syst Rev* **4**, CD002120.

47. Fraser IS & Kovacs GT (2003) The efficacy of non-contraceptive uses for hormonal contraceptives. *Med J Aust* **178**, 621–3.

48. Baldaszti E, Wimmer-Puchinger B & Loschke K (2003) Acceptability of the long-term contraceptive levonorgestrel-releasing intrauterine system (Mirena): a 3-year follow-up study. *Contraception* **67**, 87–91.

49. Brouard R, Bossmar T, Fournie-Lloret D *et al.* (2000) Effect of SR49059, an orally active V1a vasopressin receptor antagonist, in the prevention of dysmenorrhoea. *Br J Obstet Gynaecol* **107**, 614–9.

50. Bulletti C, de Ziegler D, de Moustier B *et al.* (2001) Uterine contractility: vaginal administration of the beta-adrenergic agonist, terbutaline. Evidence of direct vagina-to-uterus transport. *Ann N Y Acad Sci* **943**, 163–71.

51. Bakheet DM, El Tahir KE, Al-Sayed MI *et al.* (1999) Studies on the spasmolytic and uterine relaxant actions of *n*-ethyl and *n*-benzyl-1,2-diphenyl ethanolamines: elucidation of the mechanisms of action. *Pharmacol Res* **39**, 463–70.

52. Moya RA, Moisa CF, Morales F *et al.* (2000) Transdermal glyceryl trinitrate in the management of primary dysmenorrhea. *Int J Gynecol Obstet* **69**, 113–8.

53. Ziaei S, Faghihzadeh S, Sohrabvand F *et al.* (2001) A randomised placebo-controlled trial to determine the effect of vitamin E in treatment of primary dysmenorrhoea. *Br J Obstet Gynaecol* **108**, 1181–3.

54. Harel Z, Biro FM, Kottenhahn RK *et al.* (1996) Supplementation with omega-3 polyunsaturated fatty acids in the management of dysmenorrhea in adolescents. *Am J Obstet Gynecol* **174**, 1335–8.

Further reading

Duckitt K & McCully K (2003) Menorrhagia. *Clin Evid* 2151–69.

Garry R (2005) The future of hysterectomy. *Br J Obstet Gynaecol.* **112** 133–9.

Oehler MK & Rees MC (2003) Menorrhagia: an update. *Acta Obstet Gynecol Scand* **82**, 405–22.

Proctor M & Farquhar C (2003) Dysmenorrhoea. *Clin Evid* 1994–2013.

Vilos GA (2004) Hysteroscopic and nonhysteroscopic endometrial ablation. *Obstet Gynecol Clin North Am* **31**, 687–704, xi.

Chapter 41: Premenstrual syndrome

P.M.S. O'Brien

Introduction

Premenstrual *symptoms* occur in most women. There may have been evolutionary benefit for this in that intercourse would have occurred more frequently at the time of ovulation and less likely to once ovulation had passed when the female becomes less receptive to the male. As with all biological parameters there are extremes and so some women have minimal or no symptoms (5–10%). A similar number have such extreme symptoms that there is a major impact on their life, that of their family, their interpersonal relationships and normal day to day functioning. This extreme is premenstrual syndrome.

Definition

The terminology of premenstrual disorders is complex. Premenstrual tension was the original medical term but has now become the usual lay term; premenstrual syndrome (PMS) is the medical term most often used in the United Kingdom. Premenstrual dysphoric disorder (PMDD) is the extreme predominantly psychological end of the PMS spectrum estimated to occur in 3–9% of women [1] (Table 41.1). It is the term used increasingly by psychiatrists in the United States. Strictly speaking these are research and not clinical diagnostic criteria; it should be noted that much recent research into aetiology and treatment has been undertaken on women who fulfil the criteria for PMDD. Women designated as having PMDD also fulfil criteria for PMS but not necessarily vice versa. The term PMDD may become more established in Europe.

The term premenstrual syndrome (PMS) is defined in the *Tenth Revision of the International Classification of Disease (ICD-10)* [2]. A woman is considered to have premenstrual syndrome if she complains of recurrent psychological or somatic symptoms (or both), occurring specifically during the luteal phase of the menstrual cycle and which resolve in the follicular phase at least by the end of menstruation.

Table 41.1 DSM-IV research diagnostic criteria for PMDD (1994)

A. In most menstrual cycles, five (or more) of the following symptoms are present, with at least one of the symptoms being either (1), (2), (3), or (4)

  1 Markedly depressed mood, feelings of hopelessness, or self-deprecating thoughts

  2 Marked anxiety, tension, feeling of being 'keyed up' or 'on edge'

  3 Marked affective lability (e.g. feeling suddenly sad or tearful or increased sensitivity to rejection)

  4 Persistent and marked anger or irritability or increased interpersonal conflicts

  5 Subjective sense of difficulty in concentrating

  6 Decreased interest in usual activities (e.g., work, school, friends, hobbies)

  7 Lethargy, easy fatigability, or marked lack of energy

  8 Marked change in appetite, overeating, or specific food cravings

  9 Hypersomnia or insomnia

  10 A sense of being overwhelmed or out of control

  11 Other physical symptoms, such as breast tenderness or swelling, headaches, joint or muscle pain, a sensation of 'bloating', weight gain

B. Interference with work, school, or social relationships

C. Symptoms of PMDD must be present for most of the time during the last week of the luteal phase (premenses) and absent during the week after menses

D. The disturbance cannot merely be an exacerbation of the symptoms of another disorder

E. Confirmation by prospective daily ratings for two consecutive menstrual cycles

Symptoms

A wide range of symptoms has been described but it is their timing and severity that are most important, more so than the specific character [3].

Depression, irritability, anxiety, tension, aggression, inability to cope and feeling out of control are typical psychological symptoms. Bloatedness, mastalgia and headache are classical physical symptoms.

Calendar of premenstrual experiences (COPE)

Day of cycle	1	2	3	4	5	6	7	8	9	10	11	12	13	14	15	16	17	18	19	20	21	22	23	24	25	26	27	28	29	30	31	32	33	34
Day of month																																		
Irritability	3	3	3	1	1	1	0	0	0	0	0	0	0	0	0	0	0	0	1	1	3	3	3	2	3	3	2	3	2	3	2	1	1	1
Mood swings	3	3	3	1	1	1	0	0	0	0	0	0	0	0	0	0	0	0	1	1	3	3	3	2	3	3	2	3	2	3	2	1	1	1
Depression	0	0	0	1	1	0	0	0	0	0	0	0	0	0	0	0	0	0	0	0	0	0	0	0	0	0	0	0	0	0	0	0	0	0
Hostility	3	3	3	1	1	1	0	0	0	0	0	0	0	0	0	0	0	0	1	1	3	3	3	2	3	3	2	3	2	3	2	1	1	1
Sadness	3	3	3	1	1	1	0	0	0	0	0	0	0	0	0	0	0	1	1	1	3	3	3	2	3	3	2	3	2	3	2	1	1	1
Negative thoughts	3	3	3	1	1	1	0	0	0	0	0	0	0	0	0	0	0	0	1	1	3	3	3	2	3	3	2	3	2	3	2	1	1	1
Bloating	3	3	3	1	1	1	0	0	0	0	0	0	0	0	0	0	0	0	1	1	3	3	3	2	3	3	2	3	2	3	2	1	1	1
Breast pain	3	3	3	1	1	1	0	0	0	0	0	0	0	0	0	0	0	0	1	1	3	3	3	2	3	3	2	3	2	3	2	1	1	1
Appetite changes	3	3	3	1	1	1	0	0	0	0	0	0	0	0	0	0	0	0	1	1	3	3	3	2	3	3	2	3	2	3	2	1	1	1
Carbohydrate cravings	3	3	3	1	1	1	0	0	0	0	0	0	0	0	0	0	0	0	1	1	3	3	3	2	3	3	2	3	2	3	2	1	1	1
Hot flashes	0	0	0	1	1	0	0	0	0	0	0	0	0	0	0	1	0	0	0	1	0	0	0	0	1	0	0	0	0	0	0	0	0	1
Insomnia	3	3	3	1	1	1	0	0	0	0	0	0	0	0	0	0	0	0	1	1	3	3	3	2	3	3	2	3	2	3	2	1	1	1
Headache	0	0	0	1	1	0	0	0	0	0	0	0	0	0	0	0	0	0	0	0	0	0	0	0	0	0	0	0	0	0	0	0	0	0
Fatigue	3	3	3	1	1	1	0	0	0	0	0	0	1	1	1	1	1	1	1	1	3	3	3	2	3	3	2	3	2	3	2	1	1	1
Confusion	0	0	0	1	1	0	0	0	0	0	0	0	0	0	0	0	0	0	0	0	0	0	0	0	0	0	0	0	0	0	0	0	0	0
Poor concentration	0	0	0	1	1	1	0	0	0	0	0	0	0	0	0	0	0	0	1	0	0	0	2	0	3	0	0	0	0	0	2	1	1	1
Social withdrawal	0	0	0	1	1	0	0	0	0	0	0	0	0	0	0	0	0	0	0	0	0	0	0	0	0	0	0	0	0	0	0	0	0	0
Hyperphagia	0	0	0	1	1	0	0	0	0	0	0	0	0	0	0	0	0	0	0	0	0	0	0	0	0	0	0	0	0	0	0	0	0	0
Arguing	3	3	3	1	1	1	0	0	0	0	0	0	0	0	0	0	0	0	1	1	3	3	3	2	3	3	2	3	2	3	2	1	1	1
Decreased interest	0	0	0	1	1	0	0	0	0	0	0	0	0	0	0	0	0	0	0	0	0	0	0	0	0	0	0	0	0	0	0	0	0	0

Day 1 is the first day of cycle. (i.e. first day of menses)
Use one chart for each menstrual cycle
Luteal phase and thus, ovulation occurs 14 days before menses

Severity code: 0 = none
1 = mild
2 = moderate
3 = severe

Fig. 41.1 A chart prospectively completed by a patient suffering with PMS. Note the cyclicity of symptoms, occurring mainly premenstrually and the absence of symptoms in the follicular phase.

Because most normal women have some degree of symptomatology in the days leading up to the period it is considered that it is the severity of symptoms, namely that they significantly disrupt normal functioning, that distinguishes those women with PMS from those with no more than physiological premenstrual symptoms.

Diagnosis

There are no objective tests (physical, biochemical or endocrine) to assist in making the diagnosis. Prospectively completed specific symptom charts are required (Fig. 41.1). This is partly because the retrospective reporting of symptoms is inaccurate and because significant numbers of women who present with PMS have another underlying problem such as the perimenopause, thyroid disorder, migraine, chronic fatigue syndrome, irritable bowel syndrome, seizures, anaemia, endometriosis, drug or alcohol abuse, menstrual disorders as well as psychiatric disorders such as depression, bipolar illness, panic disorder, personality disorder and anxiety disorder.

The confirmation of luteal phase timing with the relief of symptoms by the end of menstruation is diagnostic providing the symptoms are of such severity to impact on the patient's normal functioning. It is also important to exclude patients who have a premenstrual exacerbation (PME) of an underlying psychological disorder among several others.

Validated assessment instruments include the calendar of premenstrual experiences (COPE) (Fig. 41.1) and the daily rating of severity of problems (DRSP) form.

PMS is characterized by a consistent pattern of absent symptoms during the follicular phase of the cycle.

GnRH agonists in diagnosis

The use of the so-called GnRH analogue test may be of benefit in clarifying the diagnosis. Although there are several studies to demonstrate that this group of drugs successfully eradicates PMS symptoms it has never been proven scientifically as a true test. It is used extensively by gynaecologists (off license and with due discussion with the patient) for the purposes of removing the ovarian cycle to determine which of a patient's symptoms are clearly related to the endocrine cycle and which (i.e. those which persist) are not. This is also a valuable way of demonstrating whether symptoms or medical problems such as premenstrual migraine, asthma and epilepsy are truly related to the hormone cycle. If a woman was undergoing a hysterectomy for a gynaecological indication, such information may help the patient make the decision to conserve or retain her ovaries. If any PMS or other premenstrual symptom is eradicated by GnRH, it is likely (though not guaranteed) that she would also benefit from removal of ovaries if the hysterectomy is being undertaken. This information would be valuable in the final pre-operative counselling.

Aetiology

Premenstrual syndrome is not due to a single factor. Genetic, environmental, and psychological are important factors in mood disorders as well as hormonal influence.

The principal cause of PMS is uncertain; it is strongly considered that the cyclical endogenous progesterone produced in the luteal phase of the cycle is responsible for symptoms in women who are unusually sensitive to normal progesterone levels [4]. Indeed, no differences have been demonstrated in progesterone levels between women with and without PMS [5]. It has been hypothesized that the mechanism of this increased sensitivity is related to an abnormal neuroendocrine factor and most evidence points to a dysregulation of serotonin metabolism [4].

Throughout reproductive life progesterone production seems to have an influence on women's physical/psychological health. Progesterone and its metabolites such as allopregnanolone are produced by the ovary and the adrenals, and also *de novo* in the brain. These hormones themselves are neurosteroids that readily cross the blood–brain barrier. Progesterone has a sedative effect when administered.

Women have no PMS before puberty, during pregnancy or after the menopause – these are times where ovarian hormone cycling has not begun or has ceased.

Suppression of the ovarian endocrine cycle with danazol, following administration of analogues of GnRH or by bilateral oophorectomy results in the suppression of PMS symptoms. Therefore, the hypothesis that ovarian steroids have a role in the pathophysiology of the syndrome is intuitively obvious.

Conversely, the use of progestagens in sequential hormone replacement therapy (HRT) provokes cyclicity in the negative mood and physical symptoms similar to those seen in PMS.

Research, none of which is recent, into PMS has generated data which could support theories of progesterone deficiency, oestrogen/progesterone imbalance or progesterone excess. However, the consensus is that serum ovarian steroid concentrations are normal in these women and interactions of fluctuating levels of ovarian steroids or their metabolites with neurotransmitter systems or receptor imbalances in the brain are directly relevant to the pathogenesis of PMS [6]. This is believed to render women more sensitive to physiological levels of progesterone.

Neurotransmitters

Oestrogen has clear effects on several neurotransmitters, including serotonin, acetylcholine, noradrenaline and dopamine. It cumulatively acts as an agonist on serotonergic function by increasing the number of serotonin receptors, serotonin (5-HT) postsynaptic responsiveness and neurotransmitter transport and uptake. It also increases serotonin synthesis and boosts the levels of the metabolite 5-hydroxy indole acetic acid (5-HIAA). It is well known that the serotonergic system plays a substantial role in regulating mood, sleep, sexual activity, appetite and cognitive ability. Serotonin is a major component in the development of depression. Our knowledge of the role of serotonin in depression has been extended into PMS research [4] and several studies demonstrated altered 5-HT metabolism in these patients. Blood levels and platelet uptake of 5-HT have been found to be low in PMDD patients, and acute depletion of tryptophan, the precursor of serotonin, aggravates symptoms of PMS and PMDD. This hypothesis is supported indirectly by the observation that serotonin-receptor concentrations vary with changes in oestrogen and progesterone level. The well-known selective serotonin reuptake inhibitors (SSRIs) Fluoxetine, Paroxetine, Citalopram and Sertraline, have been shown to be extremely efficacious in treating severe PMS and PMDD [6]. This gives additional, albeit indirect, support to theory of involvement of serotonin in PMS aetiology.

Vitamin B6 (pyridoxine) is a cofactor in the final step in the synthesis of serotonin and dopamine from dietary tryptophan. However, no data have yet demonstrated consistent abnormalities either of brain amine synthesis or deficiency of cofactors such as vitamin B6.

Low activity of gamma aminobutyric acid (GABA) has been reported in patients with depression, PMDD and PMS. Oestrogen increases binding of GABA agonists and the upregulation of GABA receptors. In addition to the effect of SSRIs on the serotonergic system, they have been shown to enhance GABA function, hence improving depressive symptoms. Investigations of the metabolites of progesterone have shown that women with PMS had lower levels of allopregnanolone in the luteal phase

[7]. This provides another plausible theory, as allopregnanolone has GABA-ergic activities and its deficiency can induce symptoms similar to those experienced in PMS (Fig. 41.2).

Treatment

Non–medical therapies

Claims, mainly unsubstantiated, have been made for the supplementation of calcium, vitamin E, magnesium, dietary change, vitamin B6, evening primrose oil, exercise, yoga, acupuncture, psychotherapy and many more. There is very little evidence that any of these treatments for PMS are effective with the exception of exercise and cognitive behavioural therapy.

Medical therapies

The management of PMS has, over the past few years, become increasingly easy if somewhat more invasive than these measures. First, it should be stated that there is overwhelming evidence that progesterone pessaries and oral progestagens are entirely ineffective [8]. Ironically, these are the only drugs in the United Kingdom and Europe which have a pharmaceutical licence for PMS. Remember that the proposed aetiology of PMS is that normal post-ovulatory progesterone gives rise to symptoms only in women who have increased sensitivity to progesterone and this is likely to be due to serotonin 'deficiency'. Broadly speaking, then, treatment should be achievable either by suppressing ovulation and the endocrine cycle either pharmacologically or by surgery or it may be achieved by altering the sensitivity to progesterone by elevating serotonin levels.

SSRIs

The latter can be achieved using SSRIs [6]. Increasing serotonin levels with SSRIs is clearly beneficial though none of these drugs now has pharmaceutical license for the management of PMS or PMDD. Fluoxetine 20 mg daily is usually sufficient to improve symptoms in most women. Side effects such as loss of libido may be partially avoided by administering the drug only during the luteal phase. Surprisingly the effect of the SSRIs is more instantaneous for PMS symptoms than is the case for depression. SSRIs are not licensed in the UK or Europe for PMS or PMDD. In the US Fluoxetine is licensed for PMDD under the name SARAFEM possibly to avoid the stigma of the name Prozac.

Cycle suppression

Suppression of the cycle can be achieved with Oestrogen [9] Danazol [10], GnRH agonist analogues [11] or bilateral oophorectomy [12]. Danazol, even at doses of 200 mg, is particularly effective for most symptoms of PMS but is limited by (anxieties of) masculinizing side effects. Side effects are minimal during luteal phase only administration but it is then effective only for breast symptoms [10].

GnRH agonist analogues (with and without add back)

GnRH agonist analogues are extremely effective [11]. These are best administered by injected depot preparations (goserelin or leuprorelin) as compliance is virtually guaranteed. Remember that as these are *agonist analogues* missed nasal doses will result in incomplete suppression and even re-stimulation of cycles. Without add back there will usually be the distressing symptoms of menopause. With add back therapy (particularly tibolone) the analogues remain equally effective but menopause symptoms are eliminated [11]. It is difficult to know whether long-term use of this combination is justified either medically or economically. It is probably reasonable to use it in those women approaching the menopause and in the medium term in younger women.

Oophorectomy

Bilateral oophorectomy usually with hysterectomy is almost always too invasive though is the only effective *cure* for premenstrual syndrome [12]. When removal of the ovaries is considered appropriate, it can be followed by oestrogen replacement without of course the need for cyclical progestagens. There is no logic why endometrial ablation should be effective; the studies which claim that ablation is beneficial in PMS were designed for the treatment of menorrhagia and so are not valid for PMS.

Any technique where the uterus is retained and oestrogen replacement is used will require progestagen to protect any remaining endometrium which may cause the PMS to return in many women.

Oestradiol

Transdermal oestradiol (as patches or implants) suppresses the ovarian cycle effectively without inducing the negative consequences of surgical or 'medical oophorectomy' [9]. In the presence of an intact uterus it is necessary to give progestogen to prevent endometrial hyperplasia – this, which we have seen, reintroduces 'PMS' [13].

Methods to avoid gestagen-induced PMS

Oestradiol treatment alone with regular endometrial biopsy. This is more likely to be used in the United States but it is rarely recommended in the United Kingdom – it is likely to be associated with bleeding problems.

Continuous combined hormone replacement therapy. Standard preparations would not suppress ovulation and would also increase the incidence of uterine bleeding. The use of the continuous combined oral contraceptive ought to be effective but this has not been adequately researched.

Oestradiol in doses sufficient to suppress ovulation with various other regimens

- Administering oestrogen and cyclical progesterone combined with SSRI.
- The use of less androgenic progestogens.

- Administration of the progesterone at less frequent intervals.
- Administer the progestogen by the intrauterine route using levonorgestrel intrauterine system.

In this approach, oestrogen suppresses ovulation and avoids menopausal symptoms. The intrauterine progestogen provides endometrial protection without achieving systemic levels that would act on the central nervous system reintroducing the PMS symptoms. This combination would have the added benefit of improving any menstrual problems and would provide contraception. There is only limited evidence that exists for this combination – suppression of ovarian function with oestrogen has clearly been shown to eliminate the symptoms. The Mirena intrauterine system reduces the incidence of endometrial hyperplasia. Large-scale studies

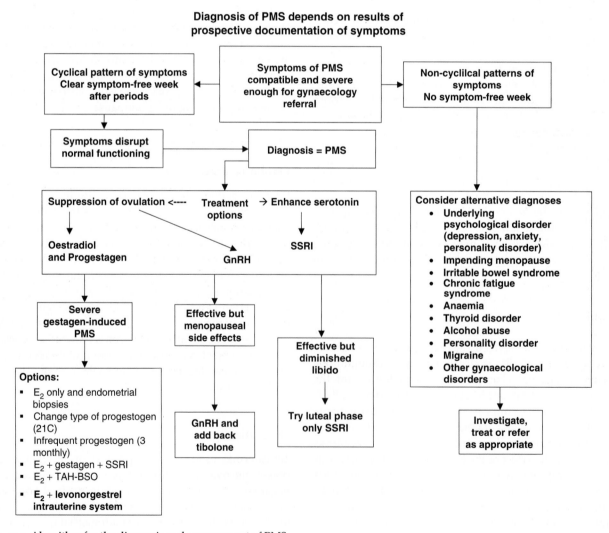

Fig. 41.2 Algorithm for the diagnosis and management of PMS.

are required to demonstrate the efficacy of this combination as it has the potential to achieve all that hysterectomy and bilateral oophorectomy achieve without major surgery.

Conclusion

Suppression of the ovarian cycle eliminates PMS effectively. This can be achieved by GnRH analogues with add back tibolone. The scope for long-term therapy is, however, limited. Oestrogen also suppresses ovulation and eliminates PMS without menopausal side effects. Intrauterine progestagen (as levonorgestrel IUS) avoids re-stimulation of premenstrual syndrome at the same time that it protects the endometrium; it reduces periods and provides contraception.

SSRIs are the simplest and most effective non-hormonal approach to treatment. Some consider them to be first line medical therapy. Some patients consider this form of therapy to be stigmatized.

St John's Wort has been shown to be effective as an antidepressant and could possibly be tried as a self-help measure in PMS though there is no valid evidence (it must not be taken with SSRIs).

Cognitive behavioural therapy is effective but access to clinical psychologists is extremely limited in the United Kingdom.

Non-medical treatments are of doubted efficacy but usually are harmless. They can be tried before resorting to medical therapy as there is no risk, except in severe cases where patients may be delaying therapy.

Correct diagnosis is all important and those patients without a symptom-free week probably have a continuous underlying psychological problem. They should be referred back to the general practitioner or, in severe cases, referred on to a psychiatrist.

The majority of patients can be treated simply by general practitioners or by self-help (NAPS www.pms.org.uk).

Only the most severe patients with clear-cut PMS requiring medical or surgical intervention should be referred for secondary care management. Those with complex psychological problems ought to be assessed by the psychiatrist. Gynaecologists, preferably those with an interest and expertise in the problem, should only be asked to manage PMS patients when symptoms are severe enough to justify endocrine or surgical intervention.

References

1. American Psychiatric Association (1994) Diagnostic and statistical manual of mental disorders: DSM-IV. 4th ed. Washington, D.C.
2. World Health Organization (1996) Mental, behavioral and developmental disorders.
3. Ismail KMK, Crome I, O'Brien PMS (2006) Psychological disorders in obstetrics and gynaecology for the MRCOG and beyond, pp 29–40. London: RCOG press.
4. Rapkin AJ 1992 The role of serotonin in premenstrual syndrome. *Clin Obstet Gynecol* **35**, 629–636.
5. Backstrom T, Andreen L, Birzniece V, *et al.* (2003) The role of hormones and hormonal treatments in the premenstrual syndrome. *CNS Drugs* **17**, 325–42.
6. Dimmock P, Wyatt K, Jones P, O' Brien PMS (2000) Efficacy of selective serotonin re-uptake inhibitors in premenstrual syndrome: a systematic review. *Lancet* **356**, 1131–6.
7. Rapkin AJ, Morgan M, Goldman L *et al.* (1997) Progesterone metabolite allopregnanolone in women with premenstrual syndrome. *Obstet Gynecol* **90**, 709–714.
8. Wyatt K, Dimmock P, Jones P, Obhrai M, O'Brien PMS (2001) Efficacy of progesterone and progestogens in management of premenstrual syndrome: systematic review. *BMJ* **323**, 776–80.
9. Watson NR, Studd JW, Savvas M *et al.* (1989) Treatment of severe premenstrual syndrome with oestradiol patches and cyclical oral norethisterone. *Lancet* **2**, 30–732.
10. O' Brien PMS, Abukhalil IEH (1999) Randomised controlled trial of the management of premenstrual syndrome and premenstrual mastalgia using luteal phase only danazol. *Am J Obstet Gynecol* **180**, 18–23.
11. Wyatt KM, Dimmock PW, Ismail KMK, *et al.* (2004) The effectiveness of GnRHa with or without 'addback' therapy in treating premenstrual syndrome: a meta analysis. *BJOG* **111**, 585–93.
12. Casson P, Hahn PM, Van Vugt DA *et al.* (1990) Lasting response to ovariectomy in severe intractable premenstrual syndrome. *Am J Obstet Gynecol* **162**, 99–105.
13. Hammarback S, Backstrom T, Holst J, *et al.* (1985) Cyclical mood changes as in the premenstrual tension syndrome during sequential estrogen-progestogen postmenopausal replacement treatment. *Acta Obstet Gynecol Scand* **64**, 393–7.

Chapter 42: Pelvic infection

Jonathan D.C. Ross and Peter Stewart

Pelvic infection is common and usually results from sexually transmitted pathogens ascending from the lower to upper genital tract. Infection can also occur following pelvic surgery, in the puerperium and after instrumenting the uterus.

Epidemiology and risk factors

How common is pelvic inflammatory disease?

Pelvic inflammatory disease (PID) is a major cause of morbidity in young women and it is becoming more common. About 2% of young women in the UK give a history of PID if asked, and about 1 in 50 consultations with general practitioners made by young women relate to PID [1]. The number of women in the UK with gonorrhoea and chlamydia, both recognized as major causes of PID, have recently increased dramatically and this is already reflected in a rising prevalence of PID.

Who gets pelvic inflammatory disease?

The risk factors for PID strongly reflect those of any sexually transmitted infection – young age, multiple sexual partners, lack of condom use, lower socio-economic status and Black Caribbean/Black African ethnicity. What is less certain is why some women with lower genital tract infection go on to develop upper genital tract disease – what factors encourage infection to spread from the vagina or cervix to the endometrium and fallopian tubes?

Cervical mucous provides an important barrier to ascending infection. Young women, with anovulatory cycles, have thinner cervical mucous and this, combined with higher rates of cervical ectopy and riskier sexual behaviour, may account for their high rates of PID. The ability of the immune response to control and contain infection will also determine the risk of upper genital tract involvement. Part of that immune response is genetically determined and an increased risk of PID is observed in women of HLA sub-type A31, while women with HLA DQA 0501 and DQB 0402 have lower rates of infertility following a diagnosis of PID. It is also possible that certain strains of bacteria are more likely to cause PID than others but the evidence for this is limited, for example, serogroup A *Neisseria gonorrhoeae*, serovar F *Chlamydia trachomatis*.

Differences in behaviour have been linked to the risk of PID. A clear association can be seen between vaginal douching and PID but more recent longitudinal studies suggest that douching does not cause PID – rather it would appear that the vaginal discharge and menstrual irregularities associated with PID may themselves lead to more douching [2]. Women who smoke are at higher risk of PID but it is unclear whether this is a marker for sexual high-risk behaviour or a direct effect of smoking itself.

Many women with PID also have bacterial vaginosis with an overgrowth of the normal commensual bacteria in the vagina and loss of vaginal lactobacilli. These same vaginal commensual bacteria are often isolated from the upper genital tract raising the possibility that bacterial vaginosis may lead to PID. Longitudinal studies do not support a direct causal association, although women who catch gonorrhoea or chlamydia infection are at higher risk of PID if they also have pre-existing bacterial vaginosis suggesting some synergy between the different infections [3].

The cost of treating PID

The psychological and fiscal costs of pelvic inflammatory disease are substantial. The uncertainty of the diagnosis and difficulty in predicting the subsequent risk of infertility, chronic pelvic pain or ectopic pregnancy add to the anxiety associated with PID, and are in addition to the feelings of blame, guilt and isolation that the diagnosis of a sexually transmitted infection may instil. Most of the monetary costs of PID arise from surgical interventions to diagnose and treat the consequences of tubal damage, and have been estimated at between £650 and £2000 per case [4]. These costs will rise substantially with improved availability of infertility treatments in the future.

Table 42.1 Organisms associated with pelvic inflammatory disease

Aerobic	Anaerobic	Viruses
Neisseria gonorrhoeae	Bacteroides sp.	Herpes simplex
Chlamydia trachomatis	Peptostreptococcus sp.	Echovirus
Ureaplasma urealyticum	*Clostridium bifermentans*	Coxsackie
Mycoplasma genitalium	Fusobacterium sp.	
Gardnerella vaginalis		
Strep. pyogenes		
Coagulase negative staphylococci		
Escherichia coli		
Haemophilus influenzae		
Mycoplasma hominis		
Strep. pneumoniae		
Mycobacterium tuberculosis		

Microbiology

Pelvic inflammatory disease is a polymicrobial infection. Gonorrhoea and chlamydia are the most frequently recognized pathogens but a wide variety of other bacteria and viruses can also be isolated from the fallopian tubes of women with PID (Table 42.1).

NEISSERIA GONORRHOEAE

Neisseria gonorrhoeae is a gram negative diplococcus which means that when a sample of cervical discharge is spread and fixed on a slide the bacteria can be seen on microscopy as pairs of red kidney-shaped organisms, mostly sitting within polymorphs. Gonorrhoea causes about 5% of PID in the UK [5,6].

N. gonorrhoeae initially infects the cervix but ascends to the upper genital tract in 10–20% of untreated cases. Around half of women with gonorrhoea are asymptomatic, but when symptoms are present the vaginal discharge tends to be thick and purulent. Although isolating gonorrhoea from the cervix supports a diagnosis of PID, its absence in the lower genital tract cannot exclude infection in the fallopian tubes or ovaries.

CHLAMYDIA TRACHOMATIS

Chlamydia trachomatis is an unusual bacterium as it requires a host cell to grow (obligate intracellular organism), behaving in some ways more like a virus. To detect the organism therefore, the optimal specimen needs to contain cells and should be collected by gently rubbing against the endocervix with a swab. The use of sensitive nucleic acid amplification tests (NAAT) also allows the use of other more accessible samples to detect chlamydia, for example, vulval swabs (which the patient can take herself after appropriate instruction) or first pass urine. Light microscopy is not useful since *C. trachomatis* is too small to be seen.

Chlamydia, like gonorrhoea, initially infects the cervix and sometimes also the urethra. It is the commonest identified cause of PID in the UK accounting for 30% of cases [5] and causes a more chronic low-grade infection than gonorrhoea. Over two thirds of women with chlamydial infection are asymptomatic.

MYCOPLASMA GENITALIUM

Evidence for the role of *Mycoplasma genitalium* in causing PID is growing. It has been isolated from the cervix, endometrium and, in a single case, from the fallopian tubes of women with PID [7]. Tubal factor infertility is strongly associated with past infection with *M. genitalium* and inoculation of the lower genital tract with mycoplasma causes PID in female monkeys [8]. Unfortunately no reliable routine test for *M. genitalium* is currently available.

ANAEROBES

Anaerobic bacteria are of particular importance in women with severe PID, and can often be isolated from tubo-ovarian abscesses. Their role in mild to moderate PID is less clear. *Bacteroides fragilis, peptostreptococci* and *peptococci* can all be isolated from the genital tract of women with PID and the production of mucinases and sialidases by anaerobic bacteria may break down cervical mucous, thus facilitating the passage of other bacteria into the upper genital tract.

ACTINOMYCES

Actinomyces israeli is occasionally detected in women with an intrauterine contraceptive device (IUCD) *in situ*. If there are no symptoms of vaginal discharge, intermenstrual bleeding or pelvic pain then the woman should be advised that neither treatment nor removal of the IUCD is required, but she should be reviewed in 6 months or earlier if symptoms develop. If symptoms are present then at least a 2-weeks therapy with a penicillin, tetracycline or macrolide antibiotic is indicated and the IUCD should be removed.

MYCOBACTERIUM TUBERCULOSIS

Tuberculous PID is largely limited to patients from developing countries. Pelvic infection usually occurs secondary to haematogenous spread from an extra genital source but occasionally *Mycobacterium tuberculosis* can be transmitted sexually [9]. Usually it is not possible to detect the organism in the lower genital tract and samples should be obtained by uterine curettage or from the fallopian tubes at laparoscopy to be sent for culture or nucleic acid testing. Standard quadruple anti-tuberculous therapy with isoniazid, rifampicin, ethambutol and pyrazinamide is effective but surgical intervention may be required for extensive disease.

VIRUSES

A number of viruses have been isolated from the upper genital tract in women with PID (Table 42.1) but their role in pathogenesis is unclear.

Clinical presentation

CLINICAL FEATURES

The clinical diagnosis of PID is based on the presence of lower abdominal pain, usually bilateral, combined with either adnexal tenderness or cervical excitation on vaginal examination (Fig. 42.1). A comprehensive medical history and examination including an accurate menstrual and sexual history may help to reach a diagnosis. A pelvic examination is essential and a speculum examination is necessary both to enable appropriate swabs to be taken and also to exclude foreign bodies in the vagina such as retained tampons. The poor specificity and associated low positive predicative value of this approach (65–90%) is justified because a delay in antibiotic therapy of even a few days leads to a large increase in the risk of impaired fertility [10]. The risks of giving antibiotics to a woman who turns out not to have PID are low, although important differential diagnoses first need to be excluded.

Essential features
Lower abdominal pain (usually bilateral)
or
Adnexal tenderness
or
Cervical motion tenderness

Supporting features
Intermenstrual/abnormal bleeding
Postcoital bleeding
Increased/abnormal vaginal discharge
Deep dyspareunia
Vaginal discharge
Fever
Nausea/vomiting
Right upper abdominal pain and tenderness
Generalized peritonitis

Fig. 42.1 Clinical features of PID.

Other clinical features can support a diagnosis of PID but are not essential before starting empirical therapy:
• intermenstrual or post coital bleeding – resulting from endometritis and cervicitis
• deep dyspareunia
• abnormal vaginal discharge – indicating lower genital tract infection
• fever – non-specific and usually only present in moderate to severe PID
• nausea/vomiting – may occur in severe PID but is more commonly associated with appendicitis.
PID caused by gonorrhoea presents more acutely and is more severe compared to chlamydial PID [11]. It is worth remembering that for every woman presenting with clinical features of PID there are two others who are asymptomatic.

Fitz-Hugh Curtis syndrome

Inflammation and infection of the liver capsule (perihepatitis) affects 10–20% of women with gonococcal or chlamydial PID and occasionally dominates the clinical presentation. Patients complain of right upper abdominal pain and have tenderness at the liver edge, occasionally accompanied by a hepatic friction rub.

Differential diagnosis

The main differential diagnoses are given in Table 42.2. The features which classically lead towards a diagnosis of PID are the typical 'G string' distribution of the

Table 42.2 Differential diagnosis of pelvic inflammatory disease

Differential diagnosis	Significant features
Ectopic pregnancy	Menstrual history, initially unilateral pain
Ovarian 'accident'	Initially unilateral pain, often mid-cycle
Appendicitis	Gastrointestinal symptoms, right sided pain
Irritable bowel syndrome	Central or left sided pain, no cervical excitation
Inflammatory bowel disease, e.g. Crohns, ulcerative colitis, diverticular disease	Colicky central or left sided abdominal pain, bowel symptoms
Urinary tract infection	Urinary symptoms +/− loin pain (chlamydial infections can present with urinary symptoms)
Bowel torsion	Central pain
Psychosomatic pain	Usually inconsistent symptoms

pain and bilateral tenderness on pelvic examination. In bowel-related disorders the pain tends to be higher in the abdomen and more central or to the left. Other conditions tend to give unilateral pain, at least at their onset. The main diagnoses to exclude are ectopic pregnancy and causes of an acute abdomen which may require surgical intervention, such as appendicitis and an ovarian 'accident' (e.g. torsion or persistent bleeding from a ruptured cyst). If the diagnosis is not clear then empirical treatment with antibiotics should be commenced, but the patient kept under close observation to ensure that an alternative diagnosis has not been missed.

Investigation

Rather like signs and symptoms, the investigations available to diagnose acute pelvic inflammatory disease lack sensitivity. Blood tests such as a white cell count, erythrocyte sedimentation rate and C-reactive protein are all relatively non-specific. They may be elevated in pelvic inflammatory disease but in mild cases can be normal. In particular a leukocytosis is often not seen in non-pyogenic infections.

A pregnancy test, preferably measuring serum beta HCG, is mandatory to exclude an ectopic pregnancy and also the possibility of an ovarian accident associated with a very early intrauterine pregnancy. This should always be performed before commencing empirical antibiotic treatment. In most hospitals this is available as an emergency investigation. If it is not, a simple urinary pregnancy test is almost as accurate.

Microbiological tests

The following microbiology tests should be offered to all women presenting with possible PID (Fig. 42.2):
• endocervical swab for gonorrhoea culture – this should be placed in transport medium (either Stuarts or Amies)

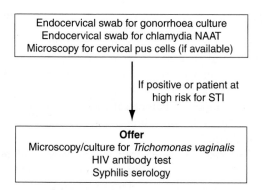

Fig. 42.2 Microbiological testing in women with suspected PID. (Abbreviations: NAAT, nucleic acid amplification test; STI, sexually transmitted infections).

and arrive at the laboratory preferably within 6 h but certainly within 24 h, otherwise viability is rapidly lost.
• endocervical swab for chlamydia nucleic acid amplification testing (NAAT) – the alternative chlamydia culture or enzyme linked immunosorbent assays (EIA) tests lack sensitivity, although EIA is still in widespread use.

The detection of gonorrhoea or chlamydia at the cervix greatly increases the likelihood of PID as the cause of lower abdominal pain, but many women with PID also have a negative infection screen from the lower genital tract.

A lack of polymorphs on a gram stained smear of cervical discharge makes PID unlikely but their presence is non-specific, that is, the absence of polymorphs has a good negative predictive value but their presence has a poor positive predictive value for PID [12].

Screening for other sexually transmitted infections should be offered to women who test positive for gonorrhoea or chlamydia, and to those who are at higher risk of infection, for example, two or more partners within the past year, lack of condom use or previous history of a sexually transmitted infection. An appropriate screen would include:
• microscopy and/or culture for *Trichomonas vaginalis* – the sample should be taken from the posterior fornix and transported in Amies or Stuarts media arriving at the laboratory within 6 h
• HIV antibody test
• syphilis serology.

If laparoscopy or laparotomy is performed then specimens from the fallopian tube should also be sent requesting bacterial culture, including gonorrhoea. Chlamydia nucleic acid amplification tests are not licensed for use for fallopian tube samples and therefore require cautious interpretation. Chlamydial culture can also be performed on this sample but is less sensitive, requires specific transport media and is not widely available.

Radiology investigations

Transvaginal ultrasound of the pelvis may be useful where there is diagnostic difficulty. There are no features, however, which are pathognomonic of acute PID. Free fluid in the Pouch of Douglas is a common normal finding and is therefore not helpful. Scanning may help to exclude ectopic pregnancy, ovarian cysts or appendicitis and can also identify dilated fallopian tubes or a tubal abscess. More recent work with power Doppler has suggested that inflamed and dilated tubes and tubal ovarian masses can be diagnosed reasonably accurately. This investigation, however, requires considerable expertise and may not be readily available in an emergency setting. It therefore has very little benefit to the routine diagnosis of PID. Magnetic resonance imaging can assist in making the diagnosis where there is difficulty, but is also not widely available and certainly has not yet entered routine management. Computerized tomography (CT) scanning in acute PID may show obscuring of the pelvic fascial planes, thickening of the uterosacral ligaments and accumulation of fluid in the tubes and endometrial canal. In the upper abdomen it can provide evidence of peri-hepatitis. Enhancement of the hepatic and splenic capsules on abdominal CT scan has been suggested as characteristic of the Fitz-Hugh-Curtis syndrome but is of little value as a routine investigation.

Surgical investigation

For many years the definitive diagnostic procedure for PID was considered to be laparoscopy and it probably remains more sensitive than any other investigation currently available. In many cases there will be clear evidence of dilated, hyperaemic tubes with an inflammatory, fibrinous exudate covering the tubes and the fundus of the uterus. In mild cases, however, intraluminal inflammation of the tubes may be missed and significant inter- and intra-observer variation in reporting the appearance of salpingitis at laparoscopy has been reported [13]. It does enable swabs to be taken from the fimbrial ends of the tubes, which may be more accurate than endocervical swabs, but the principal benefit of laparoscopy is to exclude other diagnoses. As an invasive procedure it should be reserved for those cases where there is an element of doubt as to the diagnosis of acute PID or in cases where the patient fails to respond to antibiotics within 48–72 h.

There is no evidence to support the routine use of hysteroscopy or endometrial biopsy in the routine diagnosis of acute PID. More invasive endoscopic techniques, such as fallaposcopy, may be potentially dangerous and have no place in management.

Histology and pathology

The spread of infection from the cervix to the endometrium leads to an acute, predominately polymorph mediated endometritis [14]. Transcervical suction biopsy of the endometrium allows assessment of the endometrial inflammation which correlates well with salpingitis [14]. Unfortunately the usefulness of this approach to diagnose PID is limited by the risk of introducing infection during the procedure, the time delay in fixing and staining the sample, and the uncertain significance of isolated endometritis.

The inflammatory response seen in the fallopian tubes depends on the underlying pathogen. Gonorrhoea infects the non-ciliated epithelial cells but production of tumour

necrosis factor and gamma interferon soon lead to collateral damage to the surrounding tissue and invasion of the submucosa. The tissue damage associated with chlamydia is mediated primarily by the immune response to the infection occurring as a result of a delayed type hypersensitivity reaction to one of the chlamydial heat shock proteins. This is characterized by a low-grade lymphocytic response compared with the acute neutrophil response of gonococcal salpingitis.

Recurrent infection with chlamydia causes further immune stimulation possibly mediated by a cross reaction between chlamydial and human heat shock proteins 60 [15]. This exaggerated immune response following re-exposure to chlamydia may explain the exponential increase in the risk of tubal damage which occurs with repeated infection.

Severe inflammation is associated with tubal occlusion and the production of a tubo-ovarian abscess or hydrosalpinx. Healing following acute inflammation may produce chronic fibrosis with associated damage to the ciliated epithelium, tubal blockage and pelvic adhesions. Histologically this chronic damage produces lymphoid follicles and a mononuclear cell infiltrate.

Treatment

Patients who are systemically unwell should be advised to rest and be prescribed adequate analgesia. Regular review to assess progress is required. If no improvement is observed after 3 days of antibiotic therapy then alternative diagnoses should be considered. Most patients can be managed as outpatients but those with severe symptoms, such as an acute abdomen, will require inpatient care. If the diagnosis is in doubt or if i.v. antibiotics are considered to be necessary then the patient should be admitted to hospital.

ANTIMICROBIALS

Broad spectrum antibiotic cover to include gonorrhoea, chlamydia and anaerobes is required. The optimal choice of antibiotics may be affected by knowledge of local bacterial resistance patterns, severity of disease, cost and patient convenience. Parenteral therapy should be continued until 24 h after clinical improvement and then switched to oral.

Randomized controlled trail evidence is available to support the use of the antibiotic regimens in Table 42.3 for outpatients and Table 42.4 for inpatients.

Quinolone resistance in gonorrhoea is common in many areas of the world and is rising in the UK. Ofloxacin should therefore be avoided if there is clinical suspicion

Table 42.3 Outpatient antibiotic regimens

Regimen 1*	Regimen 2*	Regimen 3
Ofloxacin 400 mg BD *plus* Metronidazole 400 mg BD	Ceftriaxone 250 mg i.m. stat (or cefoxitin 2 g i.m. stat plus probenecid 1 g orally stat) *plus* Doxycycline 100 mg BD *plus* Metronidazole 400 mg BD	Moxifloxacin 400 mg OD

BD, twice daily; i.m., intramuscularly; OD, once daily.
* To complete 14 days of therapy.

Table 42.4 Inpatient antibiotic regimens

Regimen 1	Regimen 2
i.v. cefoxitin 2 g QID (or cefotetan 2 g BD) *plus* i.v. or oral doxycycline 100 mg BD *followed by** oral doxycycline 100 mg BD *plus* metronidazole 400 mg BD	i.v. clindamycin 900 mg TID *plus* i.v. gentamycin 2 mg/kg loading dose followed by 1.5 mg/kg TID (a single daily dose may also be used) *followed by** oral doxycycline 100 mg BD *plus* metronidazole 400 mg BD

Regimen 3	Regimen 4
i.v. ofloxacin 400 mg BD *plus* i.v. metronidazole 500 mg TID *followed by** oral ofloxacin 400 mg BD *plus* oral metronidazole 400 mg BD	i.v. ciprofloxacin 200 mg BD *plus* i.v. or oral doxycycline 100 mg BD *plus* i.v. metronidazole 500 mg TID *followed by** oral doxycycline 100 mg BD *plus* Metronidazole 400 mg BD

BD, twice daily; TID, three times daily; QID, four times daily; i.m., intramuscularly; i.v., intravenously.
* Parenteral therapy should be continued until 24 h after clinical improvement.
Oral therapy to continue to complete 14 days of antibiotics in total.

of gonococcal PID, for example, clinically severe disease, history of partner with gonorrhoea, sexual contact abroad. Oral metronidazole can be discontinued in those with mild to moderate PID if the patient is unable to tolerate it.

MANAGEMENT OF PARTNERS

PID is usually secondary to a sexually acquired infection so, unless the male partners are identified and either screened for infection or treated empirically, the woman with PID is at high risk of a recurrence. Current male partners should be offered screening for gonorrhoea and chlamydia, and attempts made to contact other partners within the past 6 months, although the exact time period will be influenced by the sexual history. If screening for sexually acquired infections is not possible then antibiotic therapy effective against gonorrhoea and chlamydia should be given empirically to the male partners (Fig. 42.3; see British Association for Sexual Health and HIV guidelines for up to date treatment recommendations – www.bashh.org). The patient and their partners should be advised to avoid intercourse until they have completed the treatment course.

Surgical interventions

Surgical intervention is rarely required as a treatment for acute pelvic inflammatory disease. Most patients present at an early enough stage of the disease for antibiotic treatment to be fully effective. There may, however, be an indication for laparoscopy or laparotomy to drain a pelvic abscess if this is diagnosed on ultrasound scanning, and does not appear to be resolving with conservative antibiotic treatment. In these circumstances most surgeons would prefer to perform a laparotomy which would allow digital division of all adhesions and access to any loculated areas of abscess formation. The decision as to whether or not to carry out a salpingo oophorectomy in the presence of a large tubo-ovarian abscess will obviously depend on the patient's age and her reproductive history. In most circumstances, however, if the patient's condition warrants a laparotomy, then removal of the damaged organs may well be the preferred option. If at least one ovary is retained then *in vitro* fertilization (IVF) treatment remains a possibility if the patient wishes to achieve a pregnancy.

In cases of small abscesses or fluid collections in the Pouch of Douglas ultrasound-guided aspiration is less invasive and there is some evidence that it is as effective as laparoscopy or laparotomy. The usual technique is to aspirate the fluid transvaginally using transvaginal scanning. Occasionally a surgeon may consider draining an abscess in the Pouch of Douglas via the rectum, although this may lead to chronic sinus formation.

On the rare occasion when pelvic actinomyces is suspected, surgery should be avoided. The history is likely to be more chronic than in acute pelvic inflammatory disease, there is usually clear clinical evidence of a pelvic mass which does not appear to be an abscess on ultrasound

Test for gonorrhoea and chlamydia
Give empirical therapy for gonorrhoea and chlamydia if testing is not available (see www.bashh.org for current recommended therapies)
Advise to avoid intercourse until index patient and male partner have both completed antibiotic therapy

Fig. 42.3 Management of male contacts of women with PID.

scanning. There is also usually a history of recent use of an IUCD. If surgery is performed, then there is a significant risk of bowel damage.

Prognosis

The evidence quantifying the sequelae of PID is complicated by the variable definitions and diagnostic criteria used to identify the index episode of infection.

CHRONIC PELVIC PAIN

It is generally accepted that episodes of acute PID can lead on to symptoms of chronic pelvic pain. The cause of the chronic pelvic pain, however, remains controversial. It may be that damaged tubes act as a nidus for recurrent infections or it may be due to adhesions tethering or encapsulating the pelvic organs. It is even possible that the pain is due to altered behaviour of pelvic nerves damaged by infection. There is also little evidence as to the incidence of chronic pelvic pain resulting from single or multiple episodes of acute PID. It can be as high as 33% after recurrent episodes [16] and may have a significant effect on a patient's future quality of life [17]. The precautionary use of condoms after an episode of pelvic infection has been found to reduce the risk of chronic pelvic pain developing.

SUBFERTILITY AND ECTOPIC PREGNANCY

There is clear, population based, epidemiological evidence of the relationship between a finding of *Chlamydia trachomatis* specific IgG antibodies and subsequent tubal subfertility [18].

Some cohort studies have shown a rate of subsequent involuntary infertility of up to 40% after a single episode of PID [19]. Case controlled studies of patients who had laparoscopically verified acute PID show a relative risk of subsequent tubal subfertility of 7 for a single episode of PID rising to 28.3 after three episodes. There is also a relationship between the risk of subfertility and the severity of infection with a relative risk of 5.6 for severe infection compared to mild infection [20].

More recent prospective studies (in clinically mild/moderate disease) have suggested that with effective treatment infertility rates are not increased [16]. A delay in antibiotic therapy, however, of even a few days may lead to a large increase in the risk of impaired fertility [10].

There is also clear epidemiological evidence of a relationship between the risk of ectopic pregnancy and a previous episode of PID. In laparoscopically proven cases of PID the risk of an ectopic in the next index pregnancy is six times greater than in controls [20]. The absolute risk of ectopic pregnancy remains low, however, at 0.5–1%, at least in women with mild to moderate disease [16].

Special circumstances

Pregnancy.   Pelvic inflammatory disease associated with an intrauterine pregnancy is extremely rare except in cases of septic abortion. Cervicitis is commoner and associated with increased fetal and maternal morbidity. Treatment regimes will depend upon the organisms isolated while avoiding those antibiotics which are contraindicated in pregnancy, for example, tetracycline. Erythromycin and amoxycillin are not known to be harmful in pregnancy. In cases of septic abortion the organisms are more likely to be pyogenic than sexually transmitted. The use of broad-spectrum antibiotics such as a third generation cephalosporin together with metronidazole to treat anaerobic infections would be the regimen of choice.

Mild endometritis following surgical termination of pregnancy is relatively common ($\approx$ 1–2%) and needs to be treated aggressively to ensure future fertility. If pretreatment screening for sexually transmitted infection has been employed, it is very unusual to find a positive result on repeat swabs. It is, however, prudent to treat with a broad spectrum of antibiotics effective against both Chlamydia and anaerobes, for example, ofloxacin plus metronidazole, or moxifloxacin.

POST PELVIC SURGERY

Pelvic surgery such as hysterectomy is invariably associated with a significant risk of post-operative infection because it is virtually impossible to render the vagina totally aseptic. Prophylactic antibiotics are usually used during surgery, but post-operative pelvic infections, usually secondary to haematoma formation, are not uncommon. Most infections are due to anaerobes and should be treated with a regime which includes metronidazole or co-amoxyclav.

PELVIC INFECTION AND INTRAUTERINE CONTRACEPTIVE DEVICES

An IUCD only increases the risk of developing PID in the first few weeks after insertion and except for sub-acute infections with actinomyces, there appears to be no evidence of increased risk with the continuing use of an IUCD. Routine screening for chlamydia, gonorrhoea and bacterial vaginosis before insertion will therefore reduce the risk of PID in those women requiring an IUCD. The use of progesterone IUCDs has been associated with very low rates of PID.

The randomized controlled trial evidence for whether an IUCD should be left in situ or removed in women presenting with PID is limited [21,22]. Removal of the IUCD should be considered and may be associated with better short-term clinical outcomes [21] but the decision to remove the IUCD needs to be balanced against the risk of pregnancy in those who have had otherwise unprotected intercourse in the preceding 7 days. Hormonal emergency contraception may be appropriate for some women in this situation.

HIV

Women with HIV may have a more severe clinical presentation of PID, particularly in late stage HIV disease associated with severe immunosuppression. No alteration in therapy is required although caution is required to check for any interactions between the PID treatment and anti-retroviral medication.

Prevention

Chlamydia screening programme

Chlamydia is the commonest identified pathogen causing PID in the UK. Initial infection with chlamydia is usually asymptomatic but, if identified, can be treated simply and cheaply with antibiotics such as doxycycline or azithromycin thus preventing the development of PID. Screening young women for chlamydia is both feasible and cost-effective [23], and a national screening programme is now being rolled out across the UK targeting men and women under the age of 25 (further information is available at www.dh.gov.uk/PolicyAndGuidance/HealthAndSocialCareTopics/SexualHealth).

Instrumentation of the uterus

There is a significant risk of introducing infection into the upper genital tract when instrumenting the uterus, particularly in women at high risk of a sub-clinical cervical chlamydial infection (e.g. under 25-year olds). The most common indications for instrumenting the uterus are therapeutic surgical termination of pregnancy, insertion of an IUCD and investigations for subfertility. It is now considered mandatory to offer either a 'screen and treat' policy or routine prophylaxis for all women undergoing such management. In cases where a 'screen and treat' policy is inappropriate, for example, insertion of an IUCD for emergency contraception, it is essential to ensure adequate prophylaxis and a single 1 g dose of azithromycin is recommended.

Particular care needs to be taken in patients who are on immunosuppressant treatment (e.g. renal transplant patients) or in those who are immunocompromised because of chemotherapy or HIV.

Contraception

Consistent use of barrier methods has been shown to reduce the risk of recurrent episodes of pelvic infection and also the chronic sequelae of pelvic infection by between 30 and 60%.

All forms of hormonal contraception (e.g. combined oral contraceptive pill, progesterone-only pill, progesterone injections and implants and *Mirena* IUS) have been shown to reduce the incidence of symptomatic pelvic inflammatory disease compared to either the use of a standard IUCD or unprotected intercourse. This is presumed to be due to the protective effect of the progestogens which decreases the permeability of the cervical mucus both to sperm and pathogens.

It may also have an effect through endometrial suppression or a direct steroidal induced effect on the inflammatory response in the tubes. The beneficial effect of the oral contraceptive pill (OCP) may, however, be limited to PID which is symptomatic and caused by *C. trachomatis* [24] and it has been suggested that hormonal contraception may in fact simply be masking infection rather than preventing it [24]. A very recent cohort study which appeared to suggest that injectable progesterone contraception increased the risk of PID was methodologically flawed and hence may not be valid [25]. The true relationship between hormonal contraception and PID therefore still needs to be elucidated.

References

1. Simms I, Rogers P & Charlett A (1999) The rate of diagnosis and demography of pelvic inflammatory disease in general practice: England and Wales. *Int J STD AIDS* **10**, 448–51.
2. Ness RB, Hillier SL, Richter HE, Soper DE, Stamm C, Bass DC *et al.* (2003) Why women douche and why they may or may not stop. *Sex Transm Dis* **30**(1), 71–4.
3. Ness RB (2004) Bacterial vaginosis as a cause of PID. BASHH Conference, Bath.

4. Yeh JM, Hook III EW & Goldie SJ (2003) A refined estimate of the average lifetime cost of pelvic inflammatory disease. *Sex Transm Dis* **30**(5), 369–78.

5. Bevan CD, Ridgway GL & Rothermel CD (2003) Efficacy and safety of azithromycin as monotherapy or combined with metronidazole compared with two standard multidrug regimens for the treatment of acute pelvic inflammatory disease. *J Int Med Res* **31**(1), 45–54.

6. Eschenbach DA (1976) Acute pelvic inflammatory disease: etiology, risk factors and pathogenesis. *Clin Obstet Gynecol* **19**, 147–69.

7. Cohen CR, Manhart LE, Bukusi EA, Astete S, Brunham RC, Holmes KK *et al.* (2002) Association between Mycoplasma genitalium and acute endometritis. *Lancet* **359**(9308), 765–6.

8. Taylor-Robinson D, Furr PM, Tully JG, Barile MF & Moller BR (1987) Animal models of Mycoplasma genitalium urogenital infection. *Isr J Med Sci* **23**(6), 561–4.

9. Mardh PA (1980) An overview of infectious agents of salpingitis, their biology, and recent advances in methods of detection. *Am J Obstet Gynecol* **138**(7 Pt 2), 933–51.

10. Hillis SD, Joesoef R, Marchbanks PA *et al.* (1993) Delayed care of pelvic inflammatory disease as a risk factor for impaired fertility. *Am J Obstet Gynecol* **168**(5), 1503–9.

11. Svensson L, Westrom L, Ripa KT & Mardh PA (1980) Differences in some clinical and laboratory parameters in acute salpingitis related to culture and serologic findings. *Am J Obstet Gynecol* **138**(7 Pt 2), 1017–21.

12. Peipert JF, Ness RB, Soper DE & Bass D (2000) Association of lower genital tract inflammation with objective evidence of endometritis. *Infect Dis Obstet Gynecol* **8**(2), 83–7.

13. Molander P, Finne P, Sjoberg J, Sellors J & Paavonen J (2003) Observer agreement with laparoscopic diagnosis of pelvic inflammatory disease using photographs. *Obstet Gynecol* **101**, 875–80.

14. Kiviat NB, Wolner-Hanssen P, Eschenbach DA *et al.* (1990) Endometrial histopathology in patients with culture-proved upper genital tract infection and laparoscopically diagnosed acute salpingitis. *Am J Surg Pathol* **14**(2), 167–75.

15. Domeika M, Domeika K, Paavonen J, Mardh PA & Witkin SS (1998) Humoral immune response to conserved epitopes of *Chlamydia trachomatis* and human 60-kDa heat-shock protein in women with pelvic inflammatory disease. *J Infect Dis* **177**(3), 714–9.

16. Ness RB, Soper DE, Holley RL *et al.* (2002) Effectiveness of inpatient and outpatient treatment strategies for women with pelvic inflammatory disease: results from the Pelvic Inflammatory Disease Evaluation and Clinical Health (PEACH) Randomized Trial. *Am J Obstet Gynecol* **186**(5), 929–37.

17. Haggerty CL, Schulz R & Ness RB (2003) Lower quality of life among women with chronic pelvic pain after pelvic inflammatory disease. *Obstet Gynecol* **102**(5), 934–9.

18. Karinen L, Pouta A, Hartikainen A-K & Bloiga A (2004) Association between Chlamydia trachomatis antibodies and subfertility in the Northern Finland Birth Cohort 1966 at the age of 31 years. *Epidemiol Infect* **132**, 977–84.

19. Pavletic A, Wolner-Hanssen PK, Paavonen JA, Hawes SE & Eschenbach DA (1999) Infertility following pelvic inflammatory disease. *Infect Dis Obstet Gynecol* **7**, 145–50.

20. Westrom L & Eschenbach D (1999) Pelvic inflammatory disease. In: Holmes KK, Mardh P-A, Sparling PF, Stamm WE, Piot P & Wasserheit JN (eds) *Sexually Transmitted Diseases*. New York: McGraw Hill, 783–810.

21. Altunyurt S, Demir N & Posaci C (2003) A randomized controlled trial of coil removal prior to treatment of pelvic inflammatory disease. *Eur J Obstet Gynecol Reprod Biol* **107**, 81–4.

22. Soderberg G & Lindgren S (1981) Influence of an intrauterine device on the course of an acute salpingitis. *Contraception* **24**(2), 137–43.

23. Scholes D, Stergachis A, Heidrich FE, Andrilla H, Holmes KK & Stamm WE (1996) Prevention of pelvic inflammatory disease by screening for cervical chlamydial infection. *N Engl J Med* **334**(21), 1362–1366.

24. Washington AE, Gove S, Schachter J & Sweet RL (1985) Oral contraceptives, *Chlamydia trachomatis* infection, and pelvic inflammatory disease. A word of caution about protection. *JAMA* **253**(15), 2246–50.

25. Morrison CS, Bright P, Wong EL *et al.* (2004) Hormonal contraceptive use, cervical ectopy, and the acquisition of cervical infections. *Sex Transm Dis* **31**(9), 561–7.

26. Templeton A (1996) Recommendations arising from the 31st Study Group: The Prevention of Pelvic Infection. In: Templeton A, (ed.) *The Prevention of Pelvic Infection*. London: RCOG Press, 267–270.

Further reading

Some useful internet sites are listed as follows:

PID Treatment Guidelines – Royal College of Obstetrics and Gynaecologists (www.rcog.org)

PID Treatment Guidelines – British Association for Sexual Health and HIV (www.bashh.org)

Patient Information Leaflet for PID – Royal College of Obstetrics and Gynaecologists (www.rcog.org)

UK Chlamydia Screening Programme – Department of Health (www.dh.gov.uk)

Guideline on Screening and Testing for Sexually Transmitted Infections – British Association for Sexual Health and HIV (www.bashh.org)

Other relevant further reading includes:

Royal College of Obstetrics and Gynaecology guideline on the Management of Acute Pelvic Inflammatory Disease (www.rcog.org.uk)

PEACH study – one of the largest high quality PID treatment studies [16]

The Prevention of Pelvic Infection – Allan Templeton [26]

Clinical Evidence – Pelvic Inflammatory Disease (www.clinicalevidence.com)

Chlamydia trachomatis: summary and conclusions of CMO's Expert Advisory Group (http://www.dh.gov.uk/)

Chapter 43: Chronic pelvic pain

R. William Stones

Epidemiology of chronic pelvic pain

Initial reports relied on estimates from hospital series, naturally unrepresentative of the general population. Some population sample survey data are available: a US study reported the responses of women interviewed by telephone [1]. The age range of respondents was 18–50. 17,927 households were contacted, 5325 women agreed to participate and of these 925 reported pelvic pain of at least 6 months' duration, including pain within the past 3 months. Having excluded those pregnant or postmenopausal and those with only cycle related pain, 773 out of 5263 (14.7%) were identified as suffering from chronic pelvic pain (CPP). A British population survey used a postal sample of 2016 women randomly selected from the Oxfordshire Health Authority register of 141,400 women aged 18–49 [2]. Chronic pelvic pain was defined as recurrent pain of at least 6 months' duration, unrelated to periods, intercourse or pregnancy. For the survey, a 'case' was defined as a woman with CPP in the previous 3 months and on this basis the prevalence was 483 out of 2016 (24.0%). In this survey CPP was statistically associated both with dysmenorrhoea and dyspareunia.

Moving from the general population to those seen in general practice, a picture of consulting patterns was obtained using a national database study of UK general practices [3]. Data relating to 284,162 women aged 12–70 who had a general practice contact in 1991 were analysed to identify subsequent contacts over the following 5 years. The monthly prevalence rate was 21.5 per 1000 and the monthly incidence rate was 1.58 per 1000. These prevalence rates are comparable to those for migraine, back pain and asthma in primary care. Older women had higher monthly prevalence rates: for example, the rate was 18.2 per 1000 in the 15–20 year age group and 27.6 per 1000 in women over 60 years of age. This association was thought to be due to persistence of symptoms in older women, the median duration of symptoms being 13.7 months in 13–20 year olds and 20.2 months in women over the age of 60 [4]. It is clear that future population-based studies need to include older women.

It is clear that many women with symptoms do not seek care: among 483 women with CPP participating in the Oxfordshire population study discussed above, 195 (40.4%) had not sought a medical consultation, 127 (26.3%) reported a past consultation and 139 (28.8%) reported a recent consultation for pain [5]. The US population-based study discussed above also drew attention to the large numbers of women who have troublesome symptoms but do not seek medical attention: 75% of this sample had not seen a health-care provider in the previous 3 months. It might be thought that not seeking care would be an indicator of milder symptoms and indeed in the US study those who did seek medical attention had higher pain and lower general health scores than those who did not. However, among those not seeking help questionnaire scores for pain and functional impairment were still substantial, tending to suggest that there are barriers to care seeking, whether organizational or socio-cultural.

Clinical assessment

For patients presenting with CPP the gynaecological history needs be sufficiently broad as to enable understanding of the impact of symptoms. It is also useful to ascertain at an early stage whether the patient is primarily in search of symptom control, or of diagnosis, advice and explanation. Sometimes those with long standing and disabling symptoms are found to be reluctant to consider symptomatic treatments out of fear that some damaging disease process will be masked and overlooked. Table 43.1 presents a classification of causes of CPP that can be borne in mind while undertaking the clinical assessment.

Pain history

The history needs to include the onset and duration of symptoms, the location and radiation of pain, factors associated with exacerbation and relief and the relationship of pain to the menstrual cycle. Dysmenorrhoea may be a separate or related symptom. Dyspareunia may include

Table 43.1 Classification of causes of chronic pelvic pain

Inflammatory, infective: Chronic salpingitis
Inflammatory, non-infective: Endometriosis, Vulvodynia
  with dermatosis
Mechanical: Uterine retroversion, Adhesions
Functional: Pelvic congestion, Irritable bowel syndrome
Neuropathic: Postsurgical, Dysesthetic vulvodynia, Vulval
  vestibulodynia
Musculoskeletal: Pelvic floor myalgia, Abdominal and
  pelvic trigger points, Postural muscle strain

---

pain during intercourse, but for many women a particularly unpleasant symptom is post-coital pain and specific enquiry should be made about this.

A number of validated pain assessment measures are available for use in research and clinical practice, the most convenient of which are the 10 cm visual analogue scale, the Brief Pain Inventory (BPI), widely used in British pain clinics, and the McGill Short Form Pain Questionnaire. The McGill questionnaire is included in the International Pelvic Pain Society's assessment form, available for downloading at www.pelvicpain.org and the BPI may be downloaded at www.mdanderson.org where details of non-English versions may also be obtained. Patient's recall of pain symptoms over the previous month seems to be adequate and it is probably unnecessary to ask for a daily pain diary: 10 cm visual analogue scales for 'usual' and 'most severe' intensity of pain recalled over the past 4 weeks correlated very well with mean and maximal diary records [6].

Mood and impact on quality of life

It is important to identify coexisting mood disturbance. While it is unlikely that depression is the cause of CPP, the presence of disturbed mood makes it difficult for patients to engage fully with pain management initiatives and tackle associated lifestyle factors. The absence of laparoscopically visible pathology was not associated with a higher probability of depression [7,8]. In these studies no differences in mood-related symptoms were identified in women with CPP with and without endometriosis. Antidepressant therapy may be indicated to alleviate depression, but sertraline was not effective for relief of pelvic pain in a small but well-conducted randomized trial [9].

With regard to symptom impact, while a validated illness-specific instrument is not currently available, enquiry about the effect of the pain on work, leisure, sleep and sexual relationships is appropriate. This can shed further light on the patient's priorities for treatment. A generic quality of life measure such as the SF-36 may be used

for monitoring outcomes but may be too cumbersome for routine clinical use.

Sexual and physical abuse

Child sexual or physical abuse may be an antecedent for CPP but many individuals have suffered such abuse without this or other consequence in later life and the research literature is beset with the problem of appropriate comparison groups. Individual judgement is needed about whether to ask directly about sexual or physical abuse during a gynaecological consultation. Important considerations are the setting and plans for follow-up and support that are available to women following such disclosure. Sometimes such a history may be volunteered by the patient unprompted, especially so during a follow-up consultation when rapport has been established. Some women may even find it easier to raise the subject with an unfamiliar hospital specialist than with a general practitioner with whom they have regular consultations for other matters. It may be useful to incorporate questions on abuse into a self-completion questionnaire, such as that provided by the International Pelvic Pain Society, or in a multidisciplinary clinic to address the topic during a consultation with the nurse or psychologist. We have found it appropriate not to include those items in the package of questionnaires sent to patients for self-completion before the initial consultation.

In a study from a tertiary referral multidisciplinary pain clinic, 40% of those with CPP reported sexual abuse compared to 5(17%) in each of two comparison groups. In women with pelvic pain, abuse histories were evenly distributed among those with and without identified pelvic pathology such as endometriosis, but somatization scores were higher among those with identified pathology [10]. It has been suggested that the potential link between sexual abuse and pelvic pain might be that abuse is an observable marker for childhood neglect in general [11] and this might explain the association in some studies with physical rather than sexual abuse [12].

Systems review

Many women with chronic abdominal or pelvic pain will turn out to have irritable bowel syndrome (IBS) as their primary problem. These patients do not have good outcomes following (inappropriate) gynaecological referral and investigation [13]. Therefore it is particularly important that a detailed history is taken of bowel symptoms. The 'Rome II' criteria for the clinical diagnosis of IBS in those with chronic pain include at least two of:
• relief of pain with defecation
• change in the frequency of stool
• change in the appearance or form of stool.

Abdominal bloating in association with acute exacerbations of pain is indicative, but needs to be distinguished from menstrual cycle-related bloating. While dyspareunia is not likely to be due solely to IBS, bowel spasm may account for the experience of those patients who describe an interval between the end of intercourse and the onset of acute pain associated with the urge to defecate and abdominal distension [14].

Bladder symptoms also form an important part of the systems review. Urinary frequency and urgency, but most importantly exacerbation of pain associated with a full bladder may indicate the presence of interstitial cystitis, a neurogenic inflammatory condition of the bladder associated with chronic pain. As with IBS, it has been suggested that a proportion of cases of CPP seen by gynaecologists are in fact suffering from unrecognized interstitial cystitis on the basis of potassium chloride sensitivity testing [15].

Physical examination

Observing the patient as she walks may give an indication of a musculoskeletal problem and examination of the back is relevant in those giving a history of pain radiating or originating there. The abdominal examination should focus on distinguishing visceral from abdominal wall tenderness. 'Trigger point' tenderness elicited by palpation with one finger will suggest a nerve entrapment, often involving the ilioinguinal or iliohypogastric nerves. The ilioinguinal nerve runs in relation to abdominal muscle layers, initially superficial to transversus abdominus and deep to internal oblique. It penetrates the belly of the internal oblique muscle to lie deep to the external oblique at a point typically two centimetres medial to the iliac crest, at which point it is susceptible to entrapment. A trigger point is then evident at that site. As well as spontaneous entrapment previous surgery such as appendicectomy or a wide Pfannensteil incision may be responsible. The diagnosis is confirmed after obtaining appropriate consent by infiltration of local anaesthetic such as bupivicaine into the tender area. Interestingly the duration of relief is often much longer than the action of the local anaesthetic, perhaps because surrounding muscles are made to relax and are no longer pulling on the sensitive area.

'Ovarian point' tenderness has been described as a feature of pelvic congestion syndrome [16] but this sign is problematic in patients with IBS who often have similar abdominal tenderness. A general neurological examination is appropriate to exclude a systemic neuropathy or demyelination and if abnormalities are present a neurology opinion should be sought.

Vaginal examination should commence with a careful inspection of the vulva and introitus, paying particular attention to presence of erythema which might suggest primary vulval vestibulitis [17]. More frequently, no erythema is evident but a gentle touch with a cotton-tipped swab in the area just external to the hymeneal ring elicits intense sharp pain, even in patients who do not complain of dyspareunia. This allodynia in the absence of visible erythema probably represents referred sensation from painful areas higher in the pelvis but for some women represents the primary problem and can be termed 'vestibulodynia'. Vulval varices may indicate incompetence of valves in the pelvic venous circulation; this subgroup of patients may benefit from radiological assessment and treatment.

A gentle one finger digital examination commences with palpation of the pelvic floor muscles. Focal tenderness may be present, indicating a primary musculoskeletal problem that should prompt referral to a pelvic floor physiotherapist for further assessment. As with vestibulodynia pelvic muscle tenderness may be a residual secondary response to pain from other parts of the pelvis, for example, a previous episode of pelvic infection. Further digital examination may reveal nodularity in the pouch of Douglas or restricted uterine mobility suggestive of endometriosis. Adenomyosis may be suggested by a bulky tender uterus. Uterine retroversion should be noted although its relevance to dyspareunia is debatable. Adnexal rather than uterine tenderness may point to pelvic congestion syndrome. In the UK clinic setting pelvic tenderness alone is unlikely to be specific for chronic pelvic inflammatory disease although this diagnosis will be part of the differential among populations where early and appropriate antibiotic treatment for acute pelvic sepsis is less readily available.

Investigations

Excluding the possibility of ongoing pelvic infection such as Chlamydia by taking endocervical swabs is often useful to allay anxiety. Ultrasound examination may be useful in identifying uterine or adnexal pathology and has been shown to be an effective means of providing reassurance [18]. The presence of dilated veins may indicate pelvic congestion [19] but a recent study using power Doppler suggested that the primary value of sonography was to identify the characteristic multicystic ovarian morphology seen in this condition [20]. Transuterine venography is of limited value in routine clinical practice but is technically simpler than selective catheterization of the ovarian vein. MRI provides the opportunity to identify adenomyosis but is not routinely indicated.

Laparoscopy is commonly undertaken as the primary investigation for CPP. The aims are to give a diagnosis but also to provide 'one-stop' treatment for endometriosis and adhesions where these are identified. This approach is cost-effective for endometriosis treatment, as the expense of a second procedure or hormonal treatment is obviated [21]. The outcomes of this approach are not as good as might be expected: confusion can arise from a 'negative' laparoscopy [22] and where pathology is identified it may be coincidental rather than causal, especially in the case of adhesions. There is a lack of evidence for laparoscopy as a factor improving outcome in hospital referral populations with at least 6 months' history of pain [23,24]. It is therefore sensible to consider deferring laparoscopy and focus on symptomatic treatment in the first instance.

Pain mapping by laparoscopy under conscious sedation can be a useful procedure, particularly where the site of pain is unilateral, allowing comparison with a 'control' area, to assess the significance of adhesions, to identify unrecognized occult inguinal or femoral hernias and, in the negative sense, to identify individuals with a generalized hyperalgesic chronic pain state for whom further surgical intervention would be hazardous. The role of this procedure remains to be clarified in the overall context of pain assessment and management but reports of experience are now available in the literature [25]. Typical operative technique includes sedation with midazolam and fentanyl, infiltration of puncture sites with bupivicaine, use of a 5-mm laparoscope via a subumbilical puncture together with a fine suprapubic port for a probe. The maximum gas pressure is reduced to around 10 mmHg to minimize discomfort in the upper abdomen. Tenderness at specific sites is recorded on a 0–10 verbal rating scale. In this writer's practice its application is limited to the small subgroup of patients whose main priority is to obtain a definitive explanation for their problem, rather than symptom relief. Overall, after gaining initial experience following early positive reports, many clinicians no longer consider pain mapping to be useful.

Specific treatments for CPP: evidence from randomized trials

Limited randomized controlled trial (RCT) evidence is available to guide treatment decisions in CPP. It is important to be clear as to whether treatment is directed towards an underlying condition such as adhesions or whether pain itself is the main focus. While hormonal therapy aims to achieve benefit in a non-specific manner by inhibiting ovarian activity, based on the observation that many patients with CPP experience resolution at the time of the menopause, psychological approaches aim to enhance coping skills and reduce pain-associated distress. Many proven treatments for chronic neuropathic pain such as low-dose tricyclic antidepressants and gabapentin are equally relevant in CPP where there are neuropathic

features. With regard to specific approaches, systematic review identified 14 randomized controlled trials relevant to the management of CPP, the interventions in 12 of which are of practical applicability [26].

Medical therapy

Progestogen (medroxy progesterone acetate (MPA)) was effective after 4 months' treatment as reflected in pain scores (OR 2.64, 95% CI 1.33–5.25, $n = 146$) and a self-rating scale (OR 6.81, 95% CI 1.83–25.3, $n = 44$), but benefit was not sustained 9 months post-treatment [27,28]. MPA plus psychotherapy was effective in terms of pain scores (OR 3.94, 95% CI 1.2–12.96, $n = 43$) but not the self-rating scale at the end of treatment. Benefit was not sustained post-treatment. Venography scores, symptom and examination scores, mood and sexual function were improved to a greater extent 1 year after treatment with goserelin compared to progestogen [29].

No improvement in pain scores was seen in women taking sertraline compared to placebo. The SF-36 subscale 'Health perception' showed a small improvement in the sertraline arm, while the 'Role functioning-emotional' subscale showed a large fall in the sertraline arm [9].

Multidisciplinary management

Counselling supported by ultrasound scanning [18] was effective both in terms of pain scores (OR 6.77, 95% CI 2.83–16.19, $n = 90$) and mood. The use of a multidisciplinary approach [23] led to a positive outcome in a self-rating scale (OR 4.15, 95% CI 1.91–8.99, $n = 106$) and daily activity but not in pain scores. In British pain clinics, women with CPP rated the intensity of their pain similarly to those with other types of chronic pain. The pattern of interventions used for this group showed less recourse to nerve blocks among those with CPP. Access to clinical psychology input was sadly lacking among all groups of patients (Fig. 43.1, [30]).

Surgical treatment

The outcome in women undergoing adhesiolysis was not different to that in women who did not undergo surgery on any outcome measure (OR 1.54, 95% CI 0.81–2.93, $n = 148$). However, the small subgroup with severe adhesions did show a significant benefit for surgery (OR for self-rating scale 16.59, 95% CI 2.16–127.2, $n = 15$). Adhesiolysis was performed via laparotomy in one study [31] in contrast with a laparoscopic approach [32]. The latter study also included some men. Thus, there is still uncertainty about the place of adhesiolysis among patients presenting to gynaecologists and conclusion of this review

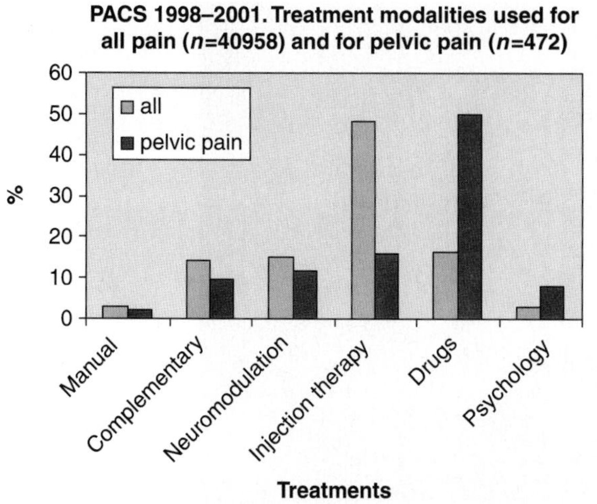

Fig. 43.1 Treatments used in UK pain clinics for patients with chronic pain (all causes) and women with CPP (from [30] reproduced with permission).

is that there is 'no evidence of benefit' rather than 'evidence of no benefit'.

Static magnetic therapy

The effects of wearing small magnets as therapy for CPP versus placebo were assessed [33]. No difference was seen following 2 weeks' treatment but some significant differences appeared at 4 weeks as assessed by the Pain Disability Index and the Clinical Global Impression Scale but not the McGill Pain Questionnaire. Analysed in terms of weighted mean differences the differences were nonsignificant and there was a substantial dropout rate. It is not clear whether this modality justifies further exploration. A clear mechanistic basis appears to be lacking, but another substantial study did show benefit for magnetic therapy in diabetic neuropathic foot pain, which may indicate some detectable actions of magnetic fields at the neuronal cellular level, such as modifying the abnormal discharge of damaged C fibre afferents [34].

Photographic reinforcement

Photographic reinforcement after surgery, that is, showing patients pictures of the findings, does not appear to have any beneficial effect [35]. Unfortunately the intervention group had a trend for greater pain intensity compared to controls at baseline which may have confounded a possible beneficial effect of photographic reinforcement. Moreover, 233 women were entered into the trial compared to the target of 450, so the final comparisons were somewhat different to those originally planned. This study is important in demonstrating how a well-intentioned intervention

reinforcing patient's knowledge of their condition may not have the intended beneficial impact.

Writing therapy

The aim of this intervention was to allow patients to identify and express through writing the thoughts and feelings associated with their pain, as a means of reducing their impact [36]. The main effects of writing about the stress of pelvic pain were limited: weighted mean differences (95% CI) on the various sub-categories of McGill pain questionnaire were: sensory pain 0.07 (−0.31 to 0.45), affective pain −0.12 (−0.42 to 0.18) and evaluation pain −1.16 (−1.96 to −0.36). Women with higher baseline ambivalence about emotional expression appeared to respond more positively to this intervention, thus showing a subgroup who may benefit specifically from this type of psychological approach.

Treatment dilemmas

Women may seek hysterectomy and oophorectomy as a solution to long-standing CPP. The evidence from observational studies is encouraging [37] but this is naturally a treatment of last resort. Where the underlying condition is neuropathic then there is a real possibility of making things worse. It is unclear whether a previous response to Gonadotrophin–releasing hormone (GnRH) agonist therapy fully predicts a positive response to oophorectomy, given the complexities of the influences of ovarian hormones on nociception.

Recently there has been a resurgence of interest in pelvic congestion as a cause of CPP pain owing to increased experience in North America of radiological embolization of pelvic 'varices'. There are issues of case definition and most studies have incomplete clinical documentation [38] but a recent comparative study indicates that this approach may have potential [39]. Radiological appearances of the ovarian veins before and after treatment are shown in Fig. 43.2a and b.

Many women seek complementary or alternative therapies for CPP. At present there is limited research evidence on which to base recommendations for specific treatments. Acupuncture has a place in the management of chronic pain in general, and there is supportive evidence for benefit in dysmenorrhoea [40]. Most importantly in this writer's view, many patients will appreciate a broad consideration of physical conditions, lifestyle factors, psychological stresses and advice on means of dealing with thoughts and feelings as part of a consultation for CPP, whether in 'conventional' or 'complementary' clinic settings.

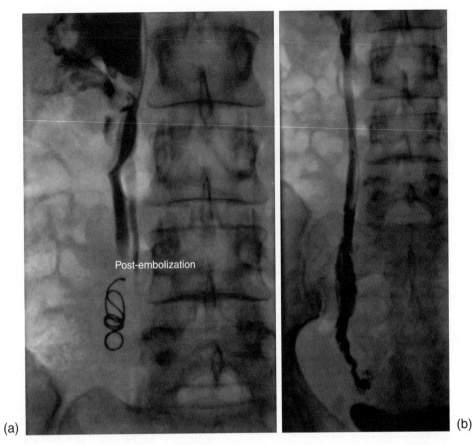

(a)   (b)

Fig. 43.2 (a) Right ovarian venogram showing parallel veins and venules over the sacral wing. (b) Post-embolization with several distal coils (not shown) and a single mid-vein embolization coil. A local sclerosant 0.5% Sodium Tetradecyl sulphate (Fibrovein) is mixed with air to form a mousse and injected through the catheter to reflux into small parallel venules and occlude these as well. Images courtesy of Dr Nigel Hacking.

Conclusion

To provide useful advice to women with CPP emphasis on careful clinical method is critical: a full history including details of symptoms from all relevant organs, a physical examination that aims to localize tenderness so as to narrow down the diagnostic options and deployment of relevant investigations. Not all patients require laparoscopy, the findings of which can sometimes confuse rather than aid diagnosis through the presence of coincidental findings. There are some therapeutic interventions backed up by randomized trial evidence, but most importantly clinicians need to match their advice to the aspirations and circumstances of each patient.

References

1. Mathias SD, Kuppermann M, Liberman RF, Lipschutz RC & Steege JF (1996) Chronic pelvic pain: prevalence, health-related quality of life, and economic correlates. *Obstet Gynecol* **87**, 321–7.

2. Zondervan KT, Yudkin PL, Vessey MP *et al.* (2001) Chronic pelvic pain in the community – symptoms, investigations, and diagnoses. *Am J Obstet Gynecol* **184**(6), 1149–55.

3. Zondervan KT, Yudkin PL, Vessey MP, Dawes MG, Barlow DH & Kennedy SH (1999) Patterns of diagnosis and referral in women consulting for chronic pelvic pain in UK primary care. *Br J Obstet Gynaecol* **106**, 1156–61.

4. Zondervan KT, Yudkin PL, Vessey MP, Dawes MG, Barlow DH & Kennedy SH (1999) Prevalence and incidence of chronic pelvic pain in primary care: evidence from a national general practice database. *Br J Obstet Gynaecol* **106**, 1149–1155.

5. Zondervan KT, Yudkin PL, Vessey MP, *et al.* (2001) The community prevalence of chronic pelvic pain in women and associated illness behaviour. *Br J Gen Pract* **51**(468), 541–7.

6. Stones RW, Bradbury L & Anderson D (2001) Randomized placebo controlled trial of lofexidine hydrochloride for chronic pelvic pain in women. *Hum Reprod* **16**(8), 1719–21.

7. Peveler R, Edwards J, Daddow J & Thomas EJ (1995) Psychosocial factors and chronic pelvic pain: a comparison of women with endometriosis and with unexplained pain. *J Psychosom Res* **40**, 305–15.

8. Waller KG & Shaw RW (1995) Endometriosis, pelvic pain, and psychological functioning. *Fertil Steril* **63**, 796–800.

9. Engel CC, Walker EA, Engel AL, Bullis J & Armstrong A (1998) A randomized, double-blind crossover trial of sertraline in women with chronic pelvic pain. *J Psychosomatic Res* **44**, 203–7.

10. Collett BJ, Cordle CJ, Stewart CR & Jagger C (1998) A comparative study of women with chronic pelvic pain, chronic nonpelvic pain and those with no history of pain attending general practitioners. *Br J Obstet Gynaecol* **105**, 87–92.

11. Fry RPW, Beard RW, Crisp AH & Mcguigan S (1997) Sociopsychological factors in women with chronic pelvic pain with and without pelvic venous congestion. *J Psychosom Res* **42**, 71–85.

12. Rapkin AJ, Kames LD, Darke LL, Stampler FM & Naliboff BD (1990) History of physical and sexual abuse in women with chronic pelvic pain. *Obstet Gynecol* **76**, 92–6.

13. Prior A & Whorwell PJ (1989) Gynaecological consultation in patients with the irritable bowel syndrome. *Gut* **30**, 996–8.

14. Whorwell P (1995) The gender influence. *Women & IBS* **2**, 2–3.

15. Parsons CL, Dell J, Stanford EJ, Bullen M, Kahn BS & Willems JJ (2002) The prevalence of interstitial cystitis in gynecologic patients with pelvic pain, as detected by intravesical potassium sensitivity. *Am J Obstet Gynocol* **187**, 1395–400.

16. Beard RW, Reginald PW & Wadsworth J (1988) Clinical features of women with chronic lower abdominal pain and pelvic congestion. *Br J Obstet Gynaecol* **95**, 153–61.

17. Gibbons JM (1998) Vulvar vestibulitis. In: Steage JF, Metzger DA & Levy BS (eds) Chronic Pelvic Pain: An Integrated Approach. Philadelphia: WB Saunders, 181–7.

18. Ghaly AFF (1994) The psychological and physical benefits of pelvic ultrasonography in patients with chronic pelvic pain and negative laparoscopy. A random allocation trial. *J Obstet Gynaecol* **14**, 269–71.

19. Stones RW, Rae T, Rogers V, Fry R & Beard RW (1990) Pelvic congestion in women: evaluation with transvaginal ultrasound and observation of venous pharmacology. *Br J Radiol* **63**, 710–1.

20. Halligan S, Campbell D, Bartram CI et al. (2000) Transvaginal ultrasound examination of women with and without pelvic venous congestion. *Clin Radiol* **55**(12), 954–8.

21. Stones RW & Thomas EJ (1995) Cost-effectve medical treatment of endometriosis. In Bonnar J (ed.) *Recent Advances in Obstetrics and Gnaecology no.19*. Edinburgh: Churchill Livingstone, 139–52.

22. Howard FM (1996) The role of laparoscopy in the evaluation of chronic pelvic pain: pitfalls with a negative laparoscopy. *J Am Assoc Gynecol Laparosc* **4**(1), 85–94.

23. Peters AA, van Dorst E, Jellis B, van Zuuren E, Hermans J & Trimbos JB (1991) A randomized clinical trial to compare two different approaches in women with chronic pelvic pain. *Obstet Gynecol* **77**, 740–4.

24. Selfe SA, Matthews Z & Stones RW (1998) Factors influencing outcome in consultations for chronic pelvic pain. *J Womens Health* **7**, 1041–8.

25. Howard FM (1999) Pelvic pain. In: Thomas EJ & Stones RW (eds) *Gynaecology Highlights 1998–99*. Oxford: Health Press, 53–63.

26. Stones W, Cheong Y & Howard FM (2005) Interventions for treating chronic pelvic pain in women. *The Cochrane Database Syst Rev* **3**, CD000387. DOI: 10.1002/14651858.CD000387.

27. Farquhar CM, Rogers V, Franks S, Pearce S, Wadsworth J & Beard RW (1989) A randomized controlled trial of medroxyprogesterone acetate and psychotherapy for the treatment of pelvic congestion. *Br J Obstet Gynaecol* **96**, 1153–62.

28. Walton SM & Batra HK (1992) The use of medroxyprogesterone acetate 50mg in the treatment of painful pelvic conditions: preliminary results from a multicentre trial. *J Obstet Gynaecol* **12**(Suppl 2), s50–3.

29. Soysal ME, Soysal S, Vicdan K & Ozer S (2001) A randomized controlled trial of goserelin and medroxyprogesterone acetate in the treatment of pelvic congestion. *Hum Reprod* **16**, 931–9.

30. Stones RW & Price C (2002) Health services for women with chronic pelvic pain. *J Royal Soc Med* **95**, 531–5.

31. Peters AAW, Trimbos-Kemper GCM, Admiraal C & Trimbos JB (1992) A randomized clinical trial on the benefit of adhesiolysis in patients with intraperitoneal adhesions and chronic pelvic pain. *Br J Obstet Gynaecol* **99**, 59–62.

32. Swank DJ, Swank-Bordewijk SC, Hop WC et al. (2003) Laparoscopic adhesiolysis in patients with chronic abdominal pain: a blinded randomised controlled multi-centre trial. *Lancet* **361**(9365), 1247–51.

33. Brown C, Pharm D, Ling F, Wan J & Pills A (2002) Efficacy of static magnetic field therapy in chronic pelvic pain: a double-blind study. *Am J Obstet Gynecol* **187**, 1581–7.

34. Weintraub MI, Wolfe GI, Barohn RA et al. (2003) Static magnetic field therapy for symptomatic diabetic neuropathy: a randomized, double-blind, placebo-controlled trial. *Arch Phys Med Rehab* **84**, 736–46.

35. Onwude L, Thornton J, Morley S, Lilleyman J, Currie I & Lilford R (2004) A randomised trial of photographic reinforcement during postoperative counselling after diagnostic laparoscopy for pelvic pain. *Eur J Obstet Gynecol Reprod Biol* **112**, 89–94.

36. Norman S, Lumley M, Dooley J & Diamond M (2004) For whom does it work? Moderators of the effects of written emotional disclosure in a randomised trial among women with chronic pelvic pain. *Psychosom Med* **66**, 174–83.

37. Beard RW, Kennedy RG, Gangar KF et al. (1991) Bilateral oophorectomy and hysterectomy in the treatment of intractable pelvic pain associated with pelvic congestion. *Br J Obstet Gynaecol* **98**, 988–92.

38. Stones RW (2003) Pelvic vascular congestion: half a century later. *Clin Obstet Gynecol* **46**, 831–6.

39. Chung M-H & Huh C-Y (2003) Comparison of treatments for pelvic congestion syndrome. *Tohoku J Exp Med* **201**, 131–8.

40. Proctor ML, Smith CA, Farquhar CM & Stones RW (2002) Transcutaneous electrical nerve stimulation and acupuncture for primary dysmenorrhoea. *Cochrane Database Syst Rev* **1**, CD002123. DOI: 10.1002/14651858.CD002123.

Chapter 44: Endometriosis

Stephen Kennedy and Philippe Koninckx

Endometriosis is usually defined as the presence of endometrial-like tissue, that is, glands and stroma, outside the uterus. The most commonly affected sites are the pelvic organs and peritoneum, although other parts of the body such as the lungs are occasionally affected. The disease varies from a few, small lesions on otherwise normal pelvic organs to solid infiltrating masses and ovarian endometriotic cysts (endometriomas) – often with extensive fibrosis and adhesion formation causing marked distortion of pelvic anatomy. Endometriosis should be suspected in women with subfertility, severe dysmenorrhoea, deep dyspareunia and chronic pelvic pain. However, many affected women are asymptomatic in which case the diagnosis is only made when the pelvis is inspected for an unrelated reason, for example sterilization.

Prevalence

The prevalence is estimated to be 8–10% in women in the reproductive years [1], although the precise rate in the general population is unknown because the pelvis has to be inspected at surgery to make a definitive diagnosis. In symptomatic women, the reported rates vary from 2 to 100% (Table 44.1) for which several explanations exist: (1) 'subtle' (e.g. small, non-coloured) peritoneal lesions were not recognized before 1985, leading to an apparent increased prevalence since then; (2) recognition increases with the surgeon's experience and interest in endometriosis; (3) the indication for laparoscopy influences how meticulously the pelvis is inspected, and (4) histological confirmation (close to 100% for deep lesions and at best 60% for subtle lesions) is not always obtained or reported. Whatever the true prevalence, it remains possible that the most common manifestation – subtle endometriosis – may not be a disease entity at all [2].

Classification systems

Several systems have been devised to classify disease severity. The most widely used is one developed by the American Society for Reproductive Medicine (ASRM), in which points are allocated for endometriotic lesions, periovarian adhesions and pouch of Douglas obliteration (Fig. 44.1) [3]. The total score is then used to describe the disease as minimal (Stage 1), mild (Stage 2), moderate (Stage 3) or severe (Stage 4). This system was designed to assist in the prognosis and management of patients undergoing surgery for subfertility. Deeply infiltrating endometriosis (DIE), a major cause of pelvic pain and dyspareunia, is typically assigned a low score (Stage 1 or 2) because only visible lesions contribute; this partly explains why there is little correlation between the total score and pain severity. Clearly, a better, more validated method to classify disease severity is needed, which can differentiate between typical lesions and DIE.

Aetiology

Implantation of viable endometrial cells and metaplasia of one tissue type into another are both reasonable explanations for the occurrence of endometriosis. However, neither theory can account for all aspects of the disease, which could mean that several mechanisms are involved or simply that the theories are inadequate. Both assume that endometriotic tissue consists of 'normal' cells but they fail to explain why development and progression occur only in some women. In contrast, the endometriotic disease theory [4] considers subtle lesions due to intermittent implantation to be a normal, physiological event. If these cells are transformed because of a genetic insult, they progress to typical, cystic and deep lesions, consisting of 'abnormal' cells. An alternative explanation is that endometriosis is a heterogeneous not a single disease and the different types, which are considered here, result from different disease processes each with their own aetiology [5].

Peritoneal endometriosis

Peritoneal endometriosis comprises superficial lesions scattered over the peritoneal, serosal and ovarian surfaces.

Table 44.1 Prevalence rates at laparoscopy for different indications

	Number of studies	Number of patients	Number with disease	% with disease (range)	% with Stage I-II disease (range)
Pelvic pain	15	2400	688	24.5 (4.5–62.0)	69.9 (61.0–100)
Infertility	32	14,971	2812	19.6 (2.1–78.0)	65.6 (16.3–95.0)
Sterilisation	13	10,634	499	4.1 (0.7–43.0)	91.7 (20.0–100)

From [1].

American Society for Reproductive Medicine: revised classification of endometriosis

Patient's name _____ Date _____

Stage I (minimal)   1–5
Stage II (mild)   6–15
Stage III (moderate) 16–40   Laparoscopy _____ Laparotomy _____ Photography _____
Stage IV (severe)   >40   Recommended treatment _____
Total _____   _____
                                Prognosis _____

Peritoneum	Endometriosis	<3 cm	1–3 cm	>3 cm
	Superficial	1	2	4
	Deep	2	4	6

Ovary		<3 cm	1–3 cm	>3 cm
	R Superficial	1	2	6
	Deep	4	10	20
	L Superficial	1	2	4
	Deep	4	16	20

	Posterior culdesac obliteration	Partial		Complete
		4		40

Ovary	Adhesions	<1/3 enclosure	1/3–2/3 enclosure	>2/3 enclosure
	R Filmy	1	2	4
	Dense	4	8	16
	L Filmy	1	2	4
	Dense	4	8	16

Tube	Adhesions	<1/3 enclosure	1/3–2/3 enclosure	>2/3 enclosure
	R Filmy	1	2	4
	Dense	4	8*	16
	L Filmy	1	2	4
	Dense	4	8*	16

*If the fimbriated end of the fallopian tube is completely enclosed change the point assignment to 16.
Denote appearance of superficial implant types as red [(R), red, mid-pink, flamelike, vesicular blobs, clear vesicles], white [(W) specifications, peritoneal defects, yellow-brown], or black [(B) black, hemosiderm deposits, black]. Denote percent of total described as R____% and B____%. Total should equal 100%.

Fig. 44.1 ASRM classification system [3].

These were typically described as 'powder-burn' or 'gun-shot' deposits until atypical or subtle lesions were recognized, including red implants, polypoid lesions, and serous or clear vesicles. It remains unclear, however, whether these subtle lesions are functionally active forms of early disease, or whether they are transient physiological events without any clinical significance. Subtle lesions can easily be explained by Sampson's theory of retrograde menstruation. Menstrual effluent containing viable cells is transported into the peritoneal cavity in a retrograde direction along the fallopian tubes and the refluxed endometrium then implants onto the surface of exposed tissues, principally the peritoneum. However, most women do not develop endometriosis even though retrograde menstruation occurs commonly, for which there are several explanations. First, the amount of menstrual effluent transported may be important as higher prevalence rates occur in women with increased menstrual exposure due to: (1) obstructed outflow associated with Müllerian anomalies and (2) short menstrual cycles, increased duration of bleeding and decreased parity [1]. Second, the expression of factors such as cell adhesion molecules, proteolytic enzymes and cytokines affecting the adherence, implantation and proliferation of tissue within the peritoneal cavity may differ between women, as may clearance of endometrial cells from the pelvis. Thus, defects in the immunological mechanisms responsible for the clearance of menstrual effluent from the peritoneal cavity (e.g. natural killer cell activity) may increase the likelihood of endometrial cells implanting. However, it is unclear whether such abnormalities are truly a cause or a result of the disease. Last, changes in systemic humoral immunity (altered B cell function and antibody production) have been implicated, and women with endometriosis have a higher prevalence of autoimmune diseases, for example, rheumatoid arthritis and systemic lupus erythematosus (SLE).

Ovarian endometriomas

Several variants on the implantation and metaplasia theories have been proposed to account for ovarian endometriomas. It has been suggested that superficial lesions on the ovarian cortex become inverted and invaginated, and that endometriomas are derived from functional ovarian cysts or metaplasia of the coelomic epithelium covering the ovary. Endometriomas have features in common with neoplasia such as clonal proliferation, which is consistent with the endometriosis disease theory, and they are associated with sub-types of ovarian malignancy, such as endometrioid and clear cell carcinoma. Genetic alterations in endometriotic tissue are reported in loss of heterozygosity (LOH) studies, particularly involving chromosomal regions containing known or putative tumour suppressor genes (TSGs) implicated in ovarian cancer. These data suggest that endometriomas are benign tumours although recently researchers have questioned whether endometriomas are truly monoclonal and whether they demonstrate LOH at TSG loci.

Deeply infiltrating disease

Several hypotheses explain the aetiology of DIE nodules which extend >5 mm beneath the peritoneum and may involve the uterosacral ligaments, vagina, bowel, bladder and ureters. Donnez *et al.* suggested these are a form of adenomyosis arising in Müllerian rests in the rectovaginal septum [6]. Koninckx and Martin described three macroscopic types [7]. Type I (conical lesions with the largest

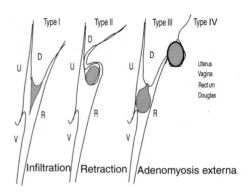

Fig. 44.2 Types of deeply infiltrating endometriosis [7].

area exposed to the peritoneal cavity) result from infiltration of superficial disease; they should be considered a form of typical endometriosis (Fig. 44.2). However, Type II infiltrating lesions with bowel retracted around and over the nodule and Type III lesions, which often occur in an otherwise normal pelvis, are morphologically like adenomyosis with mainly fibromuscular and little glandular tissue. The same applies to infiltrating lesions of the sigmoid (Type IV). Type I lesions, like typical ones, can be multifocal, but Type II and III are invariably singular: in a series of over 1000 cases, fewer than 50 women had nodules infiltrating both the rectum and sigmoid.

Disease risk factors

Risk factors include age, increased peripheral body fat, and greater exposure to menstruation (i.e. short cycles, long duration of flow and reduced parity), whereas smoking, exercise, and oral contraceptive use (current and recent) may be protective [1]. There is no evidence, however, that the natural history of the disease can be influenced by controlling these factors. Genetic predisposition is likely as endometriosis occurs 6–9 times more commonly in the 1st degree relatives of affected women than in controls, and in an analysis of >3000 Australian twin pairs, 51% of the variance of the latent liability to the disease was attributable to additive genetic influences [8]. Disease heritability is also apparent in non-human primates, which develop the disease spontaneously. These data imply that endometriosis is inherited as a complex genetic trait like diabetes or asthma, which means that a number of genes interact with each other to confer disease susceptibility but the phenotype probably emerges only in the presence of environmental risk factors. Recently, a genome-wide linkage study in 1176 affected sister pair families has identified a significant susceptibility locus for endometriosis on chromosome 10q26 and another region of suggestive linkage on chromosome 20p13 [9].

Endometriosis-associated pain symptoms

Severe dysmenorrhoea, deep dyspareunia, chronic pelvic pain, ovulation pain, cyclical or perimenstrual symptoms – often bowel or bladder related, causing dyschezia or dysuria – with or without abnormal bleeding, and chronic fatigue have all been associated with endometriosis. However, the predictive value of any one symptom or set of symptoms is uncertain as each can have other causes, and many affected women are asymptomatic. There is little correlation between disease stage and the type, nature and severity of pain symptoms, perhaps because the current classification systems are inadequate. However, endometriomas and DIE are clearly associated with severe pain, although some affected women are pain free; in the case of DIE, symptom severity is related to the depth of infiltration. Typical peritoneal lesions probably cause pain as symptoms are relieved by surgery; whether this applies to subtle lesions remains unclear. The suggested causes for the pain include peritoneal inflammation, activation of nociceptors, tissue damage and nerve irritation with deep infiltration. Pain symptoms are usually assessed in clinical trials using a four-point Verbal Rating Scale for three symptoms (dysmenorrhoea, dyspareunia and pelvic pain), and two signs (pelvic tenderness and induration). Increasingly, however, health-related quality of life is also being measured as traditional outcome measures may not adequately assess what the patient considers important. The only patient-generated, disease-specific tool is the Endometriosis Health Profile-30 (EHP-30), a 30-item questionnaire which covers five dimensions: pain, control and powerlessness, emotional well-being, social support and self-image [10].

Endometriosis-associated subfertility

Whether endometriosis causes subfertility or not is also controversial. It is generally accepted that endometriomas cause infertility because severe anatomical distortion must interfere with oocyte pick up. A causal relationship with minimal–mild disease (particularly subtle lesions) is much less certain. Numerous mechanisms have been proposed, including abnormal folliculogenesis, anovulation, luteal insufficiency, luteinized unruptured follicle syndrome, recurrent miscarriage, decreased sperm survival, altered immunity, intraperitoneal inflammation and endometrial dysfunction. However, all these functional disturbances can occur in subfertile women without endometriosis, which suggests that finding disease during investigation for subfertility may be coincidental.

Diagnosis

History and clinical examination

Making a diagnosis on the basis of symptoms alone is difficult as the presentation is so variable and other conditions such as irritable bowel syndrome and pelvic inflammatory mimic the disease. Consequently, there is often a delay of several years between symptom onset and a definitive diagnosis at laparoscopy. Finding pelvic tenderness, a fixed retroverted uterus, tender uterosacral ligaments or enlarged ovaries on examination is suggestive of endometriosis, although the findings can be normal. The diagnosis is likely if deeply infiltrating nodules are found on the uterosacral ligaments or in the pouch of Douglas, and is confirmed if visible lesions are seen in the vagina or on the cervix. Such nodules are most reliably detected when the examination is performed during menstruation [11].

Non-invasive tests

Compared to laparoscopy, trans-vaginal ultrasound is a useful tool to diagnose and exclude ovarian endometriomas but it has no value for peritoneal disease [12]. Although, it has been claimed that MRI has >90% sensitivity and specificity for endometriomas, a recent systematic review failed to find the supporting evidence (unpublished data). CA-125 measurement has no value as a diagnostic tool for minimal–mild endometriosis [13]. Serum levels are generally elevated in women with DIE and endometriomas but the test is rarely used in practice because clinical examination and ultrasound usually suffice.

Laparoscopy

Laparoscopy is the gold standard for diagnostic purposes, unless disease is visible in the vagina or elsewhere. Histological confirmation of at least one peritoneal lesion is ideal, and mandatory if DIE or a >3 cm diameter endometrioma is present. The entire pelvis should be inspected systematically, and good practice is to document in detail the type, location and extent of all lesions and adhesions. Ideally, the findings should be recorded on video or DVD. Depending upon the severity of disease found, best practice is to remove/ablate endometriosis at the same time, provided that adequate consent has been obtained.

General treatment issues

Patient participation in the decision-making process is essential as multiple options exist and endometriosis is

Table 44.2 Factors influencing
choice of treatment

Woman's age
Fertility status
Nature of symptoms
Severity of disease
Previous treatments
Priorities and attitudes
Resource implications
Costs + side-effect profile
Risks of treatment
Other subfertility factors
Intended duration of treatment
Best available evidence

Table 44.3 Treatment aims

What are you treating (disease, symptoms or both)?
Why are you treating?
Possible reasons to treat
    Improve natural fertility
    Enhance chances of success at ART
    Pain relief as an alternative to surgery
    Pain relief while awaiting surgery
    Adjunct to surgery
    Prophylaxis against disease occurrence
    Symptom recurrence

potentially a chronic problem. Choosing which treatment to have will depend upon a number of factors (Table 44.2).

Summarizing how these factors influence decision making is difficult because each patient is different and the decisions are often complex. However, some general principles apply. For example, a woman in her late 40s with debilitating pain and severe disease who has completed her family can be offered a hysterectomy and bilateral salpingo-oophorectomy provided that all the endometriotic tissue is removed at the same time. On the other hand, a young nulliparous woman with a similar presentation will want as much normal tissue as possible conserved if she opts for surgery.

Treatment aims

The treatment aims should be agreed with the patient (Table 44.3). For surgery, the intended benefits and the major risks and complications should be explained and documented on the consent form. When medical treatment is initiated, ideal practice would be to document in the notes, or in a letter to the patient, what options were discussed; why the decision to treat was made, as well as the treatment aims and side effects or risks.

Non-hormonal treatment for pain relief

Clinicians and self-help groups recognize that some women control their symptoms with analgesics or alternative therapies including Chinese herbal remedies, dietary manipulation, acupuncture and vitamin or mineral supplements. Although these measures can improve quality of life and relieve symptoms, it is inadvisable to make specific recommendations in the absence of evidence to support their effectiveness.

Hormonal treatments

Hormonal treatments have traditionally attempted to mimic pregnancy or the menopause, based upon the clinical impression that the disease regresses during these physiological states. The treatments currently available – combined oral contraceptives (COCs), progestagens, danazol, gestrinone and gonadotrophin-releasing hormone (GnRH) agonists – have been extensively reviewed. Despite different modes of action, they all appear to induce atrophy and decidualization of peritoneal deposits by suppressing ovarian function. Peritoneal lesions decrease in size during therapy but reappear rapidly following therapy; DIE responds in a similar manner (unpublished data). Endometriomas rarely decrease in size and adhesions will be unaffected.

Pain relief

All the hormonal treatments above (with the exception of dydrogesterone given in the luteal phase) relieve endometriosis-associated pain. However, using the total amount of pain (dysmenorrhoea, non-menstrual pain and dyspareunia) as the primary outcome measure inevitably produces a favourable result as all hormonal treatments abolish menstruation; the effects on non-menstrual pain and dyspareunia are variable. When taken for 6 months, the drugs are equally effective [14–17], but their side effect (Table 44.4) and cost profiles differ. These analyses include one RCT comparing a COC taken conventionally against a GnRH agonist: the COC was less effective in relieving dysmenorrhoea but there were no significant differences between the treatments in the relief of dyspareunia or non-menstrual pain [18]. It is important to emphasize that a 30% placebo effect is common in endometriosis studies; hence the need for placebo-controlled randomized controlled trials (RCTs).

The duration of GnRH agonist use is limited by the associated loss in bone density – up to 6% in the first 6 months, although the loss is restored almost completely 2 years after stopping treatment. The hypo-oestrogenic symptoms can be alleviated and bone loss prevented, without

Table 44.4 Side effects and complications of danazol and GnRH agonists

	Danazol	GnRH agonists
Side effects	Weight gain (1–5 kg)	Hot flushes
	Bloating	Night sweats
	Increased body hair	Headaches
	Acne and oily skin	Vaginal dryness
	Deep voice (irreversible)	Irritability
	Decreased breast size	Insomnia
	Muscle cramps	Decreased libido
	Headaches	Palpitations
	Hot flushes	Joint stiffness
	Limb tingling	
	Decreased libido	
	Menstrual spotting	
Complications	Liver tumours (long-term use)	Bone loss
	Adverse effect on lipids	'Flare' effect (starting treatment in follicular phase)

loss of efficacy, by using 'add-back therapy' in the form of oestrogens, progestagens or tibolone. How long this regimen can safely be continued is unclear, but there is evidence to suggest that bone density can be maintained over 2 years with add-back [19]. However, careful consideration should be given to the use of GnRH agonists with add-back in women who may not have reached their maximum bone density [20]. It has also been suggested that the local release of progestagens may be beneficial: in a recently published RCT comparing a GnRH agonist and the levonorgestrel-releasing intrauterine system (IUS), both treatments were equally effective at relieving endometriosis-associated pain [21].

Subfertility

Hormonal treatment for subfertility associated with minimal–mild endometriosis does not improve the chances of natural conception [22]. The odds ratio for pregnancy following ovulation suppression for 6 months with danazol, medroxyprogesterone acetate, or GnRH agonists versus placebo or no treatment was 0.74 (95% CI 0.48–1.15) (Fig. 44.3). Clearly treatment can do more harm than good because of the lost opportunity to conceive. In more advanced disease, there is no evidence of an effect on natural conception, but there may be a role for hormonal treatment as an adjunct to assisted conception. There are a few studies suggesting that prolonged down-regulation with a GnRH agonist prior to IVF in women with moderate–severe disease might improve pregnancy rates. There are no systematic reviews on this topic, but

it is nevertheless recommended that such treatment be discussed with patients [20].

Surgical treatment

The goal of surgery is to eliminate all visible peritoneal lesions, endometriomas, DIE and associated adhesions and to restore normal anatomy. Since depth of infiltration is difficult to judge, excision or vaporization is preferable for typical lesions. Excision is the preferred method for endometriomas since recurrence rates following marsupialization and focal treatment are much higher. It is controversial whether conservative discoid resection or resection anastamosis of larger DIE lesions should be offered. Laparoscopy should be used as it decreases morbidity and the duration of hospitalization, and therefore cost, compared to laparotomy. Whether laparoscopy also reduces post-operative adhesions is less clear. If local expertise is lacking, then referral to a specialized centre with the necessary expertise to offer all available treatments in a multidisciplinary context, including advanced laparoscopic surgery and laparotomy, is strongly recommended. This particularly applies if DIE or severe endometriosis is suspected or has been diagnosed. Lesions can be removed by surgical excision with scissors, ultracision or laser – CO_2 or potassium-titanyl-phosphate (KTP).

Pain relief

Ablation of lesions plus laparoscopic uterine nerve ablation (LUNA) in minimal–moderate disease reduces endometriosis-associated pain at 6 months compared to diagnostic laparoscopy; the smallest effect is seen in patients with minimal disease [23]. However, there is no evidence that LUNA is a necessary component, as LUNA by itself has no effect on dysmenorrhoea associated with endometriosis [24]. No RCTs have been conducted to assess the value of surgery for endometriomas or DIE since these would be difficult studies to conduct ethically. However, a number of retrospective studies demonstrate that approximately 80% of women with severe symptoms are pain free following surgery – a figure that clearly exceeds any likely placebo effect.

Subfertility

A recent Cochrane review concluded that ablation of lesions plus adhesiolysis in minimal–mild endometriosis enhances fertility significantly better than diagnostic laparoscopy alone (OR 1.64, 95% CI 1.05–2.57) [25]. Two relevant RCTs were identified (Fig. 44.4): the larger showed an increased chance of pregnancy and ongoing pregnancy rate after 20 weeks but the smaller one failed

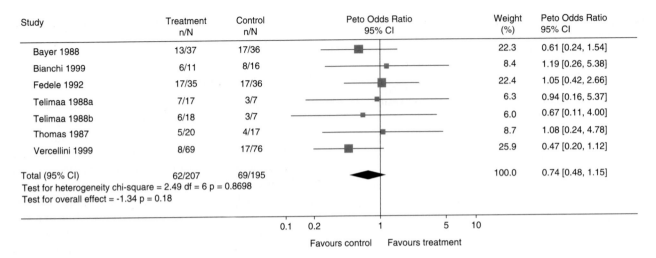

Study	Treatment n/N	Control n/N	Peto Odds Ratio 95% CI	Weight (%)	Peto Odds Ratio 95% CI
Bayer 1988	13/37	17/36		22.3	0.61 [0.24, 1.54]
Bianchi 1999	6/11	8/16		8.4	1.19 [0.26, 5.38]
Fedele 1992	17/35	17/36		22.4	1.05 [0.42, 2.66]
Telimaa 1988a	7/17	3/7		6.3	0.94 [0.16, 5.37]
Telimaa 1988b	6/18	3/7		6.0	0.67 [0.11, 4.00]
Thomas 1987	5/20	4/17		8.7	1.08 [0.24, 4.78]
Vercellini 1999	8/69	17/76		25.9	0.47 [0.20, 1.12]
Total (95% CI)	62/207	69/195		100.0	0.74 [0.48, 1.15]

Test for heterogeneity chi-square = 2.49 df = 6 p = 0.8698
Test for overall effect = -1.34 p = 0.18

Fig. 44.3 Cochrane review showing clinical pregnancy rates in studies comparing ovulation suppression and placebo [22].

to show benefit. The findings are nevertheless controversial because the patients were seemingly not blinded to whether they were treated or not in the larger study. Moreover, the cumulative pregnancy rate of approximately 30% in the treated group is comparable to previously reported rates in women with typical endometriosis treated expectantly.

No RCTs have been conducted to determine whether surgery for moderate–severe disease improves pregnancy rates. However, three studies show an apparent inverse correlation between endometriosis stage and the spontaneous cumulative pregnancy rate after surgery, although statistical significance was only reached in one study [20].

Ovarian endometriomas

Laparoscopic cystectomy for endometriomas is preferable to coagulation or laser vaporization with regard to recurrence of cysts and symptoms and subsequent spontaneous pregnancy in women who were previously subfertile [26]. If an endometrioma ≥4 cm in diameter is present before IVF, cystectomy is specifically recommended to confirm the diagnosis histologically; reduce the risk of infection following egg retrieval; improve access to follicles and possibly improve the ovarian response to gonadotrophins [20]. When the endometrioma is large, the remaining ovarian capsule is so thin that excision and coagulation will almost invariably remove or destroy a large part of the normal ovarian tissue. Therefore, a two-step procedure (marsupialization and rinsing followed by 3 months GnRH agonist therapy and then repeat surgery) should be considered if fertility is to be conserved; otherwise an oophorectomy should be considered as it is technically easier. Fertility patients should be counselled about the risks

of reduced ovarian function after endometrioma excision and the loss of an ovary.

Surgery for DIE

If there is clinical evidence of DIE, the possibility of ureteric, bladder and bowel involvement should be considered pre-operatively to determine the best management. Surgery needs to be performed as safely as possible and by the most appropriate surgeons because it may be necessary to resect part of the bladder or ureter, as well as bowel wall. Occasionally, more extensive bowel resection (e.g. the rectum and/or sigmoid) is needed. Such operations require a team of experienced surgeons rather than a single surgeon. Therefore, pre-operative assessment is important as it aims to predict as accurately as possible which specialities should be available to avoid leaving disease behind and unnecessary complications. The ideal work-up should comprise an intravenous pyelogram (IVP) to detect ureteric strictures and hydronephrosis and a contrast enema to diagnose extensive narrowing at the level of the rectum or sigmoid (an indication for bowel resection). Pre-operative ureteric stenting is advisable if a patient with bladder symptoms is found to have a vesico-uterine nodule on ultrasound. Whether ultrasound/CT/MR imaging should be routinely performed is unclear, although in less experienced centres the findings will influence the decision to refer to a tertiary centre. How radical surgery should be performed is also controversial. If a general principle of removing all endometriosis is adopted, then bowel resection with 2 cm safety margins should be considered as small endometriotic foci can be found up to 2 cm from a bowel lesion. A conservative discoid resection, however, is preferable for most patients as it

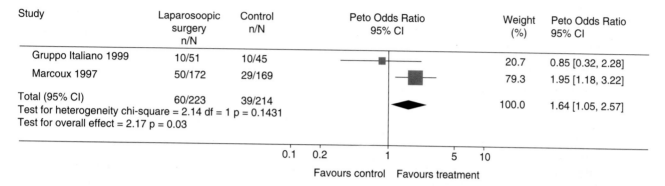

Fig. 44.4 Cochrane review showing ongoing pregnancy or live birth rates in controls and women undergoing laparoscopic surgery [25].

is associated with fewer complications. Moreover, a recurrence rate of only 1% casts doubt on the need to remove large segments of bowel.

Post-operative hormonal treatment

Compared to surgery alone or surgery plus placebo, postoperative hormonal treatment does not produce a significant reduction in pain recurrence at 12 or 24 months, and has no effect on disease recurrence; similarly, it has no effect on pregnancy rates [27]. Prescribing hormone replacement therapy (HRT) after bilateral oophorectomy is advisable in young women but the ideal regimen is unclear. Adding a progestagen after hysterectomy is unnecessary but should theoretically protect against the unopposed action of oestrogen on any residual disease – causing reactivation or, in rare circumstances, malignant transformation. This theoretical benefit must be balanced against the risk of recurrent disease which is remarkably small and the increase in breast cancer risk reported to be associated with both tibolone and combined oestrogen and progestagen HRT.

Assisted reproduction

In women with minimal–mild endometriosis and patent fallopian tubes, treatment with intrauterine insemination (IUI) along with ovarian stimulation improves fertility, but it is uncertain whether unstimulated IUI is effective. *In vitro* fertilization (IVF) is appropriate treatment for all disease severities, especially if tubal function is compromised or there are other problems such as male factor subfertility [20]. However, a systematic review (Fig. 44.5) showed that IVF pregnancy rates are lower in patients with endometriosis than in those with tubal subfertility [28], even though endometriosis does not appear adversely to affect pregnancy rates in some large databases (e.g.

Society of Assisted Reproductive Technologies (SART) and Human Fertilization and Embryo Authority (HFEA)). A poorly addressed issue is whether surgery should be considered before IVF in women with endometriomas to prevent complications (see p. 436). In the case of DIE, surgery beforehand is advisable as oocyte retrieval can be very painful and there is an increased risk of bowel perforation because of associated adhesions.

Alternative management protocols

Is it necessary to perform a laparoscopy in all cases of suspected endometriosis? The recommendation in the RCOG Guideline is 'If a woman is not trying to conceive and there is no evidence of a pelvic mass on examination, there may be a role for a therapeutic trial of a COC (monthly or tricycling) or a progestagen to treat pain symptoms suggestive of endometriosis without performing a diagnostic laparoscopy first'. Although, the recommendation reflects the common practice of using a COC in this way, or even continuously, there is no evidence that one method is better than any other, or that any COCs are better than others.

Subsequently, two management protocols along similar lines have been produced by North American authors [29,30]. Olive and Pritts [30] recommend the use of a non-steroidal anti-inflammatory drug (NSAID) or COC in the first instance and, if unsuccessful, operative laparoscopy or a therapeutic trial of a GnRH agonist plus add-back can be offered. Operative laparoscopy can also be performed if the GnRH agonist fails to relieve symptoms. The recommendations of Gambone *et al.* [29] are similar: first-line treatment with a NSAID or COC, or both, based upon the nature of the pain, any contraindications and the need for contraception. If first-line treatment fails, the options are operative laparoscopy or a therapeutic trial of danazol, a progestagen or a GnRH agonist with add-back

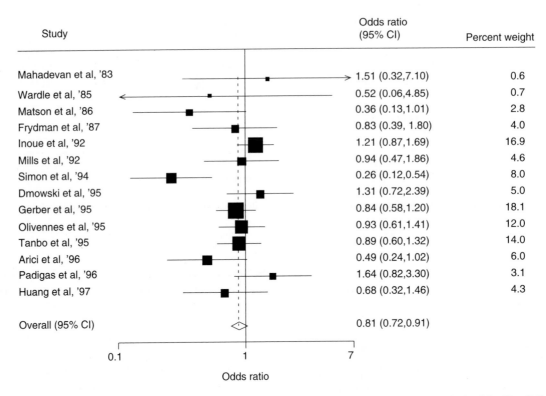

Fig. 44.5 Unadjusted meta-analysis of odds of pregnancy in endometriosis patients vs controls with tubal subfertility [28].

for 2 months, continuing for 6 months if successful. Both protocols acknowledge the value of continuing on maintenance therapy if adequate pain relief is achieved with one or a combination of drugs. It should be acknowledged, however, that these protocols have been at least partially inspired by cost considerations and, perhaps, by the realization that not all women with endometriosis-associated pain have access to adequate surgical treatment.

Chronic pelvic pain

The role of endometriosis in chronic pelvic pain remains controversial and difficult to quantify. In this chapter the management protocols for chronic pelvic pain are outlined and it is extremely important that patients who have endometriosis-related chronic pelvic pain are recognized as suffering with irritable bowel syndrome. The use of the holistic approach to these patients can be extremely effective in relieving some of their pelvic pain and improving their quality of life. This relates to improved diet, fluid intake, avoidance of constipation and exercise. There is also increasing evidence that self-management courses can be very effective in helping these women cope with their long-term problems of pain.

References

1. Eskenazi B & Warner ML (1997) Epidemiology of endometriosis. *Obstet Gynecol Clin North Am* **24**, 235–58.
2. Koninckx PR (1994) Is mild endometriosis a condition occurring intermittently in all women? *Hum Reprod* **9**, 2202–5.
3. Revised American Society for Reproductive Medicine classification of endometriosis. (1996) *Fertil Steril* **67**, 817–21.
4. Koninckx PR, Barlow D & Kennedy S (1999) Implantation versus infiltration: the Sampson versus the endometriotic disease theory. *Gynecol Obstet Invest* **47**, 3–9.
5. Nisolle M & Donnez J (1997) Peritoneal endometriosis, ovarian endometriosis, and adenomyotic nodules of the rectovaginal septum are three different entities. *Fertil Steril* **68**, 585–96.
6. Donnez J, Nisolle M, Gillerot S, Smets M, Bassil S & Casanas RF (1997) Rectovaginal septum adenomyotic nodules: a series of 500 cases. *Br J Obstet Gynaecol* **104**, 1014–8.
7. Koninckx PR & Martin DC (1992) Deep endometriosis: a consequence of infiltration or retraction or possibly adenomyosis externa? *Fertil Steril* **58**, 924–8.
8. Zondervan KT, Cardon LR & Kennedy SH (2001) The genetic basis of endometriosis. *Curr Opin Obstet Gynecol* **13**, 309–14.
9. Treloar SA, Wicks J, Nyholt DR *et al.* (2005) Genomewide linkage study in 1,176 affected sister pair families identifies a significant susceptibility locus for endometriosis on chromosome 10q26. *Am J Hum Genet* **77**, 365–77.

10. Jones G, Kennedy S, Barnard A, Wong J & Jenkinson C (2001) Development of an endometriosis quality-of-life instrument: The Endometriosis Health Profile-30. *Obstet Gynecol* **98**, 2–64.

11. Koninckx PR, Meuleman C, Oosterlynck D & Cornillie FJ (1996) Diagnosis of deep endometriosis by clinical examination during menstruation and plasma CA-125 concentration. *Fertil Steril* **65**, 280–7.

12. Moore J, Copley S, Morris J, Lindsell D, Golding S & Kennedy S (2002) A systematic review of the accuracy of ultrasound in the diagnosis of endometriosis. *Ultrasound Obstet Gynecol* **20**, 630–4.

13. Mol BW, Bayram N, Lijmer JG *et al.* (1998) The performance of CA-125 measurement in the detection of endometriosis: a meta-analysis. *Fertil Steril* **70**, 1101–8.

14. Moore J, Kennedy SH & Prentice A (2004) Modern combined oral contraceptives for pain associated with endometriosis (Cochrane Review). *The Cochrane Library*, Issue 3. Chichester, UK: John Wiley & Sons, Ltd.

15. Prentice A, Deary AJ, Goldbeck WS, Farquhar C & Smith SK (2004) Gonadotrophin-releasing hormone analogues for pain associated with endometriosis. *The Cochrane Library*, Issue 3. Chichester, UK: John Wiley & Sons, Ltd.

16. Prentice A, Deary AJ & Bland E (2004) Progestagens and anti-progestagens for pain associated with endometriosis. *The Cochrane Library*, Issue 3. Chichester, UK: John Wiley & Sons, Ltd.

17. Selak V, Farquhar C, Prentice A & Singla A (2004) Danazol for pelvic pain associated with endometriosis (Cochrane Review). *The Cochrane Library*, Issue 3. Chichester, UK: John Wiley & Sons, Ltd.

18. Vercellini P, Trespidi L, Colombo A, Vendola N, Marchini M & Crosignani PG (1993) A gonadotropin-releasing hormone agonist versus a low-dose oral contraceptive for pelvic pain associated with endometriosis. *Fertil Steril* **60**, 75–9.

19. Surrey ES & Hornstein MD (2002) Prolonged GnRH agonist and add-back therapy for symptomatic endometriosis: long-term follow-up. *Obstet Gynecol* **99**, 709–19.

20. Kennedy S, Bergqvist A, Chapron C *et al.* (2005) ESHRE Guideline for the diagnosis and treatment of endometriosis. *Hum Reprod* **20**, 2698–704.

21. Petta CA, Ferriani RA, Abrao MS *et al.* (2005) Randomized clinical trial of a levonorgestrel-releasing intrauterine system and a depot GnRH analogue for the treatment of chronic pelvic pain in women with endometriosis. *Hum Reprod* **20**, 1993–8.

22. Hughes E, Fedorkow D, Collins J & Vandekerckhove P (2004) Ovulation suppression for endometriosis (Cochrane Review). *The Cochrane Library*, Issue 3. Chichester, UK: John Wiley & Sons, Ltd.

23. Jacobson TZ, Barlow DH, Garry R & Koninckx P (2004) Laparoscopic surgery for pelvic pain associated with endometriosis (Cochrane Review). *The Cochrane Library*, Issue 3. Chichester, UK: John Wiley & Sons, Ltd.

24. Vercellini P, Aimi G, Busacca M, Apolone G, Uglietti A & Crosignani PG (2003) Laparoscopic uterosacral ligament resection for dysmenorrhea associated with endometriosis: results of a randomized, controlled trial. *Fertil Steril* **80**, 310–9.

25. Jacobson TZ, Barlow DH, Koninckx PR, Olive D & Farquhar C (2004) Laparoscopic surgery for subfertility associated with endometriosis (Cochrane Review). *The Cochrane Library*, Issue 3 Chichester, UK: John Wiley & Sons, Ltd.

26. Hart R, Hickey M, Maouris P, Buckett W & Garry R (2005) Excisional surgery versus ablative surgery for ovarian endometriomata. *Cochrane Database Syst Rev* **3**, CD004992.

27. Yap C, Furness S & Farquhar C (2004) Pre and post operative medical therapy for endometriosis surgery. *Cochrane Database Syst Rev* **3**, CD003678.

28. Barnhart K, Dunsmoor-Su R & Coutifaris C (2002) Effect of endometriosis on *in vitro* fertilization. *Fertil Steril* **77**, 1148–55.

29. Gambone JC, Mittman BS, Munro MG, Scialli AR, Winkel CA & The Chronic Pelvic Pain/Endometriosis Working Group (2002) Consensus statement for the management of chronic pelvic pain and endometriosis: proceedings of an expert-panel consensus. *Fertil Steril* **78**, 961–72.

30. Olive DL & Pritts EA (2002) The treatment of endometriosis: a review of the evidence. *Ann N Y Acad Sci* **955**, 360–72.

Further reading

Giudice LC & Kao LC (2004) Endometriosis. *Lancet* **364**, 1789–99.

Berkley KJ, Rapkin AJ & Papka RE (2005) The pains of endometriosis. *Science* **308**, 1587–9.

Dinulescu DM, Ince TA, Quade BJ, Shafer SA, Crowley D & Jacks T (2005) Role of K-ras and Pten in the development of mouse models of endometriosis and endometrioid ovarian cancer. *Nat Med* **11**, 63–70.

Chapter 45: Infertility

Siladitya Bhattacharya

Introduction

Infertility causes great distress to many couples, causing-increasing numbers of them to seek specialist fertility care. Most of those presenting with childlessness have reduced fertility, rather than absolute sterility, and many are likely to conceive spontaneously. In the absence of a robust evidence base, treatment has been largely intuitive, often dictated by tradition and personal preference. In addition, rapid progress in assisted reproduction has encouraged the incorporation of novel techniques into routine clinical practice without rigorous prior evaluation.

Epidemiology

In the general population, conception is expected to occur in 84% of women within 12 months and in 92% within 24 months (te Velde et al. 2000). Infertility is defined as the inability to conceive after one to two years of unprotected intercourse (Hull et al. 1985). Data from population-based studies suggest that 10–15% of couples in the Western world experience infertility (Templeton et al. 1990; Evers, 2003). Half of them (8%) will subsequently conceive without the need for specialist advice and treatment. Of the remaining 8% who require input from fertility clinics, half (4%) comprise couples with primary infertility (no history of a previous pregnancy) while the other half have secondary infertility (difficulties in conceiving after an initial pregnancy).

By convention, infertility is commonly divided into five major categories (Table 45.1) on the basis of aetiopathology, results of investigations and prognosis. The proportion of couples in each group varies from population to population depending on environmental factors and referral patterns. In general terms, the likelihood of spontaneous live birth in infertile couples is strongly influenced by female age, duration of infertility, previous pregnancies, and cause of infertility (Table 45.2). Unexplained infertility has the best outcome. A couple with primary unexplained infertility of 2 years duration where

Table 45.1 Diagnostic categories in infertility

	Primary (%)	Secondary (%)
Anovulation	20	15
Male	25	20
Tubal	15	40
Endometriosis	10	5
Unexplained	30	20

Adapted from: Templeton et al. Management of infertility for the MRCOG and beyond, 2000.

Table 45.2 Factors affecting the chance of live birth in infertile couples

Variable	Relative hazard of live birth (95% confidence interval)
Previous pregnancy	1.83 (1.24–2.69)
Infertility <3 years	1.68 (1.14–2.48)
Female age <30 years	1.50 (1.05–2.16)
Male factor	0.47 (0.27–0.81)
Endometriosis	0.39 (0.18–0.85)
Tubal defect	0.50 (0.40–0.63)

* $P < 0.01$
Adapted from: Collins et al. 1995.

the female partner is aged 28 years can expect a cumulative live-birth rate of 36% over the next 12 months (Collins et al. 1995). Previous pregnancy, shorter duration of infertility and age below 30 years all enhance a woman's chances of live birth, while male factor problems, tubal disease and endometriosis halve them.

Diagnostic categories in infertility

Although single aetiologies may occur, some of these categories (e.g. anovulation and male factor) may coexist, and this will need to be taken into account when planning investigations or treatment.

Table 45.3 Classification of disorders of ovulation *

Group	Site of lesion	Hormone concentration
Hypogonadotrophic Hypo-oestrogenic Normoprolactinaemic WHO type I	Central	Low FSH* Normal prolactin Low oestradiol
Normogonadotrophic	Hypothalamic pituitary	Normal FSH
Normo-oestrogenic Normoprolactinaemic WHO type II	Ovarian axis	Normal oestradiol Normal prolactin
Hypergonadotrophic Hyper-oestrogenic Normoprolactinaemic WHO type III	Ovarian failure	High FSH Low oestradiol Normal prolactin
Hyperprolactinaemic	Central	Low FSH Low oestradiol High prolactin

* FSH, follicle stimulating hormone.
Adapted from: Templeton *et al.* (2000) Management of infertility for the MRCOG and beyond. *RCOG*, Press London ISBN 1-900364-29-8.

Ovulatory disorders

Absence of ovulation (anovulation) or infrequent ovulation (oligo-ovulation) is seen in a fifth of all women presenting with infertility. Types of anovulatory infertility can be further classified as shown in Table 45.3.

HYPOTHALAMUS AND PITUITARY (HYPOGONADOTROPHIC HYPOGONADISM) (WHO TYPE I)

Abnormalities of gonadotrophin releasing hormone (GnRH) agonist secretion are associated with very low levels of oestradiol, follicle stimulating hormone (FSH) and luteinizing hormone (LH). Kallman's Syndrome is a congenital cause of anovulation characterized by isolated gonadotrophin deficiency and anosmia. Acquired causes include pituitary tumours, pituitary necrosis (Sheehan's syndrome), stress and excessive weight loss or exercise. Clinical examination of the visual fields and imaging of the pituitary fossa are indicated when a space occupying pituitary lesion is suspected.

NORMOGONADOTROPHIC HYPOGONADISM

The majority of women with normogodatotrophic anovulation have polycystic ovary syndrome (PCOS). Other causes include congenital adrenal hyperplasia, adrenal tumours and androgen producing ovarian tumours. The last three conditions present with coexistent hirsutism and require more detailed investigations including

Table 45.4 PCOS – the revised 2003 diagnostic criteria

Diagnosis of PCOS includes the presence of two out of the three listed below:
1. Oligo- and/or anovulation
2. Clinical and/or biochemical signs of hyperandrogenism*
3. Polycystic ovaries[†]
And the absence of other endocrine causes:
   Congenital adrenal hyperplasia
   Androgen secreting tumours
   Cushings syndrome
   Hyperprolactinaemia
   Thyroid dysfunction

* Clinical indicators of *hyperandrogenism* are hirsutism, acne and androgenic alopecia. The elevation of free testosterone and/or free testosterone (free androgen) index (FAI) are the biochemical indicators of PCOS. Some women with PCOS may have isolated elevations in dehydroepiandrosteronesulphate (DHEAS).
[†] The definition of polycystic appearing ovaries on scan includes the presence of 12 or more follicles in each ovary measuring 2–9 mm in diameter, and increased ovarian volume (>10 ml). The ovarian volume is calculated using the formula (0.5 × length × width × thickness). The distribution of follicles is not included in the definition and only one ovary fitting the description is sufficient for the diagnosis.

Adapted from: The Rotterdam ESHRE/ASRM-sponsored PCOS Consensus Workshop Group, 2004.

serum testosterone, dehydroepiandrostenedione sulphate (DHEAS) and 17 hydroxy progesterone.

Polycystic ovary syndrome

Polycystic ovary syndrome (PCOS) accounts for over 75% of all women with anovulation (Adams *et al.* 1986). Clinical features are heterogeneous and can vary in the same individual over time. Women with PCOS may present with anovulatory infertility, menstrual irregularities (usually oligoamenorrhoea/amenorrhoea), hirsutism and obesity. The currently accepted criteria for the diagnosis of PCOS are shown in Table 45.4 (see Chapter 39).

HYPERGONADOTROPHIC HYPOGONADISM (WHO TYPE III)

Amenorrhoea with elevated serum FSH and low or undetectable oestrogen levels signify ovarian failure. Known causes include Turners Syndrome (XO), Turner mosaic (XO, XX, XX) gonadal dysgenesis, autoimmune disorders, irradiation or chemotherapy. In many cases the cause is unknown. Turner's syndrome is characterized by a karyotype of 45 (XO) and phenotypic abnormalities including short stature, webbing of the neck, shield chest and cubitus valgus. By puberty the gonads can be identified as 'streak' ovaries with no functioning follicles by the age of puberty. In Turner mosaics, (45X/46XX) spontaneous ovulation and menstruation may occur.

HYPERPROLACTINAEMIA

Increased levels of prolactin interfere with normal pulsatile secretion of GnRH, resulting in anovulation, amenorrhoea and occasionally galactorrhoea associated with low FSH and oestradiol levels. Hyperprolactinaemia is a feature of prolactin producing pituitary adenomas or tumours blocking inhibitory control of the hypothalamus. Other causes include primary hypothyroidism, chronic renal failure, and drugs such as the combined oral pill, dopamine depleting agents (reserpine, methyldopa) and dopamine receptor inhibiting agents (metoclopramide and phenothiazines).

Male factor infertility

The male partner is directly responsible for 25% of cases of infertility and is thought to play a contributory role in another 25%. Male factor infertility implies a lack of sufficient numbers of competent sperm, resulting in failure to fertilize the normal ovum. The World Health Organization (WHO) has proposed a set of criteria for normal semen parameters (Table 45.5). This is useful as a point of reference for results from different laboratories. A list of underlying factors responsible for male infertility compiled by the WHO is shown in Table 45.6. This classification needs to be updated in the light of recent scientific advances, especially in the genetic causes of defective spermatogenesis. Some of the common causes are discussed below.

Table 45.5 Reference values for semen analysis

Parameter	Normal value
Volume	2.0 ml or more
PH	7.2–7.8
Sperm concentration	20×10^6/ml or more
Motility	50% or more with progressive motility (Grade a or b)*
Morphology	15–30%†
Viability	75% or more live
White blood cells	Fewer than 1×10^6/ml

* Grade a: rapid progressive motility; Grade b: slow or sluggish motility.
† Currently being reassessed by WHO. In the interim the proportion of normal forms accepted by laboratories in the UK is either the earlier WHO limit of 30 or 15% based on strict morphological criteria.

Adapted from: World Health Organization, 1999.

IDIOPATHIC IMPAIRMENT OF SEMEN QUALITY

In the majority of cases of male infertility the cause of impaired semen parameters is unknown. Azoospermia (absence of sperm) or significant oligozoospermia (sperm concentration <20 million per ml) may be associated with small soft testes and raised FSH levels. Histological changes within the tubules, such as the absence or reduced number of germ cells may be patchy and non-specific.

Asthenozoospermia implies impaired motility (less than 50%). Absent or very poor motility in sperm may be caused by structural abnormalities such as the absence of dynein arms, radial spokes or nexin bridges and dysplasia of the fibrous sheath. Similar defects are seen within respiratory cilia in the Immotile Cilia Syndrome comprising respiratory infection, sinusitis and bronchiectasis. The presence of situs inversus in these men leads to a diagnosis of Kartgener's Syndrome.

Teratozoospermia is the term used to describe abnormal sperm morphology on microscopy. Although the assessment is inevitably subjective, observance of strict criteria can lead to a degree of consistency of reporting, at least within each laboratory. Morphology is believed to reflect maturity and functional integrity of sperm and has been related to acrosomal defects and sperm motility.

Table 45.6 Causes of male infertility

Cause	Prevalence (%)
No demonstrable cause	12.6
Varicocoele	11.2
Idiopathic oligozoospermia	11.2
Accessory gland infection	6.9
Idiopathic teratozoospermia	5.9
Idiopathic asthenozoospermia	3.9
Isolated seminal plasma abnormalities	3.5
Suspected immunological infertility	3.0
Congenital abnormalities	1.7
Systemic diseases	1.4
Sexual inadequacy	1.3
Obstructive azoospermia	0.9
Idiopathic necrozoospermia	0.8
Ejaculatory inadequacy	0.7
Hyperprolactinaemia	0.6
Iatrogenic causes	0.5
Karyotype abnormalities	0.1
Partial obstruction to ejaculatory duct	0.1
Retrograde ejaculation	0.1
Immotile cilia syndrome	<0.1
Pituitary lesions	<0.1
Gonadotrophin deficiency	<0.1

Adapted from: Rowe *et al.* 1993.

VARICOCELE

A varicocele is a group of dilated veins in the pampiniform plexus of the spermatic cord. On examination, it is visible as a tangle of distended blood vessels in the scrotum. Usually left sided, varicoceles develop at puberty and affect 15% of otherwise healthy men (Evers and Collins, 2003). Observational data (WHO, 1992) have suggested that clinically detectable varicoceles are present in 12% of normal men and 25% of men with semen abnormalities. Spermatogenesis is believed to be prejudiced by impaired vascular drainage from the testis due to increased scrotal temperature, hypoxia, raised testicular pressure and reflux of adrenal metabolites (Evers and Collins, 2003). However, the presence of varicoceles in fertile men with normal sperm counts has led some workers to question the presence of a causal association.

GENETIC CAUSES

Chromosomal abnormalities have been detected in 2.1–8.9% of men attending infertility clinics and are related to the severity of the male factor problem. Azoospermia is associated with karyotypic abnormalities in 15% of cases, of which 90% are 47XXY (Klinefelter's Syndrome). Structural abnormalities of the Y chromosome, such as deletion of the distal fluorescent heterochromatin, may also be responsible for impaired spermatogenesis. Deletions affecting a family of genes on the Y chromosome have been found in 10% cases of non-obstructive azoospermia and some cases of severe oligozoospermia. Microdeletions have been found in three non-overlapping regions of the Y chromosome, AZF a-b-c. The commonest abnormality reported in the literature is a microdeletion in the AZFc region encompassing the DAZ gene (Hargreave, 2000).

CRYPTORCHIDISM

Undescended testes which remain untreated at 2 years of birth are likely to be histologically abnormal. Delay in surgical correction is associated with reduced fertility and a 4 to 10-fold increase in the risk of testicular cancer.

ORCHITIS

Symptomatic orchitis complicates 27–30% of cases of mumps in males. In 17% orchitis is bilateral and causes atrophy of the seminiferous tubules. Fertility is affected if bilateral orchitis occurs after puberty.

OCCUPATIONAL AND ENVIRONMENTAL FACTORS

Toxic effects of radiation, drugs, and chemicals can affect the rapidly dividing germ cells which are the precursors of spermatozoa. A number of heavy metals, chemicals and

Table 45.7 Therapeutic drugs interfering with male infertility

Drug	Action
Cancer chemotherapy	Alkylating agents cause irreversible damage
Hormone treatment	High-dose corticosteroids, androgens, anti-androgens, oestrogens and LHRH agonist
Cimetidine	May competitively inhibit androgen effect on the receptor
Sulphasalazine	Can cause impairment of sperm quality by direct toxicity
Spironolactone	Antagonizes the action of androgen in some tissues
Nitrofurantoin	May cause impairment of sperm quality by direct toxicity
Niradozole	May cause temporary depression of spermatogenesis
Colchicine	Cause depression of fertility by direct toxicity to spermatogenesis

Adapted from: Rowe *et al.* 1993.

pesticides have been associated with deranged spermatogenesis. Tobacco, cannabis, alcohol and lifestyle factors such as wearing tight underwear have also been linked with male infertility. Evidence regarding some of these associations is conflicting.

IATROGENIC

A number of commonly used drugs can impair semen quality. They are listed in Table 45.7, along with their mechanisms of action.

GENITAL TRACT OBSTRUCTION

Azoospermia in the presence of normal testicular volume and normal FSH suggests the possibility of genital tract obstruction. Previous vasectomy and congenital abnormalities are the principal causes, although infections such as tuberculosis and gonorrhoea predominate in some parts of the world. Congenital causes of obstruction of the male genital tract include agenesis or malformations of the Wolfian ducts affecting the epididymis and seminal vesicles. Congenital bilateral absence of the vas deferens (CBAVD) occurs in 2% of cases of obstructive azoospermia and is commonly associated with cystic fibrosis (Hargreave 2000). Young's Syndrome is characterized by obstruction at the junction of the caput and the body of the epididymis, chronic lung infection and bronchiectasis.

MALE ACCESSORY GLAND INFECTION

Infections caused by gram negative enterococci, chlamydia, and gonococcus can present with urethral discharge, painful ejaculation, dysuria, haematospermia, tenderness of the epididymis and prostate. Confirmation is by semen culture, urethral swabs and the presence of more than 1 million polymorphonuclear leucocytes per ml of semen. The role of subclinical infection in the genesis of male infertility is unclear and there is little consensus on appropriate criteria for diagnosis.

HYPOGONADOTROPHIC HYPOGONADISM

Hypogonadotrophic hypogonadism is a rare condition caused by congenital or acquired hypothalamic and pituitary failure. Where the condition is congenital, evidence of androgen deficiency usually leads to a diagnosis at puberty. A complete absence of GnRH results in absence of secondary sexual characteristics and total testicular failure. Many affected men have anosmia (Kallman's syndrome). Manifestations are less profound in men with partial deficiency. A diagnosis of hypogonadotrophic hypogonadism is confirmed by low or undetectable levels of gonadotrophins (LH and FSH) and testosterone. Trauma, tumours or chronic inflammation can cause adult onset hypothalamic hypogonadism presenting with infertility.

COITAL DYSFUNCTION

Infertility in the male can be due to problems with intercourse. Causes of coital dysfunction in men are shown in Table 45.8.

Table 45.8 Coital dysfunction

Problem	Cause
Ejaculatory failure	Spinal cord injury
	Medical disorders:
	Diabetes mellitus
	Multiple sclerosis
	Chronic renal failure
Erectile or ejaculatory problems	Depression
	Alcohol abuse
	Medication:
	Adrenergic blocking agents
	Antihypertensives
	Psychotropic agents
	Psychosexual
Loss of libido	Hyperprolactinaemia
Retrograde ejaculation	Transurethral prostatectomy
	Retroperitoneal lymph node dissection
	Neuropathy:
	Diabetic
	Injury to lumbar sympathetic nerves
	Damage to bladder neck

Adapted from: Templeton *et al.* Management of infertility for the MRCOG and beyond RCOG, 2000.

IMMUNOLOGICAL CAUSES

Antisperm antibodies are detected in one in six men attending infertility clinics. They are IgG or IgA isotypes and may be present in serum, seminal fluid or bound to various sites on the spermatozoa. Risk factors for the development of antisperm antibodies include reversal of vasectomy, prior infection such as epididymitis, sexually transmitted diseases and orchitis. Their effect on infertility is unclear. It is believed that antisperm antibodies can affect with sperm motility, cause acrosomal reaction abnormalities and inhibit zona pellucida binding. Antisperm antibodies are also present in fertile men and current techniques do not allow a meaningful way of separating different epitopes (Paradisi *et al.* 1995).

Tubal factor infertility

Tubal disease accounts for 15–20% of cases of primary infertility and approximately 40% of secondary infertility. It represents the aftermath of pelvic infection or surgery resulting in tissue damage, scarring and adhesion formation. This can affect tubal function and result in either partial or total tubal occlusion. As the distal portion of the tube is commonly affected, fluid can accumulate within the tubes causing a hydrosalpinx. Functional competence of the fallopian tubes implies not just patency but also the integrity of the mucosal lining or the endosalpinx. As any damage to the fallopian tubes tends to be irreversible correction can be difficult. Due to current limitations in investigating tubal function it is only possible to assess the macroscopic appearance and patency of the fallopian tubes.

INFECTION

The principal cause of tubal disease is pelvic inflammatory disease (PID) which may occur spontaneously or as a complication of miscarriage, puerperium, intrauterine instrumentation and pelvic surgery. A single episode of PID carries up to 10% risk of future tubal factor infertility. The risk is aggravated by further infections due to *Chlamydia trachomatis* or *Neisseria gonorrhoeae*. Chlamydia is now the most common sexually transmitted disease (STD) in Europe and responsible for at least 50% of identifiable cases of PID. Due to its silent nature, most affected women give no prior history of chlamydia infection, although three quarters of them have anti-chlamydial antibodies in their serum. Factors associated with chlamydia infection contribute to an increased risk of tubal disease. These include multiple sexual partners, young age at first intercourse, poor socio-economic status, heavy alcohol consumption and cigarette smoking. Opinion on previous termination of pregnancy is divided; some recent publications claim that there is no added increase in risk once other factors had been adjusted for.

SURGERY

Lower abdominal surgery is a risk factor for tubal infertility. Most abdominal and pelvic surgery causes adhesions. Gynaecological surgery, appendicectomy, bowel resection and urological operations are all thought to increase the risk of subsequent tubal disease.

OTHER CAUSES

The role of intrauterine contraceptive devices (IUCDs) in the aetiology of tubal disease is controversial. In the 1980s a number of studies reported an increased risk of PID in women who used IUCDs as compared to non-users. More recent data suggest that IUCD users, who are at low risk of sexually transmitted infections, face no added risks of PID. Congenital abnormalities are uncommon causes of tubal pathology and are associated with developmental anomalies of the urinary system. Endometriosis, cornual fibroids or polyps can cause cornual block or tubal distortion. Another relatively rare cause, salpingitis isthmica nodosa, described as nodular thickening of the proximal part of the fallopian tube is of unknown aetiology.

Endometriosis

Endometriosis is characterized by the presence of uterine endometrial tissue outside the cavity of the uterus. The common sites are the pelvic peritoneum, ovaries and rectovaginal septum. The prevalence of pelvic endometriosis in women with infertility has been shown to be 21% (Mahmood and Templeton, 1991).

The link between endometriosis and infertility has been demonstrated in some, but not all studies on this subject. Women with endometriosis undergoing assisted reproduction face a relatively poor outcome. A systematic review suggests that pregnancy rates are halved in comparison with women with tubal infertility (Barhart *et al.* 2002.). Data from *in vitro* fertilization (IVF) programmes also suggest diminished ovarian reserve, poor oocyte and embryo quality and impaired implantation in advanced endometriosis (Brosens, 2004). Peritoneal fluid from women with endometriosis containing high levels of cytokines, growth factors and activated macrophages has been shown to be toxic to sperm function and embryo survival (Guidice and Kao, 2004). In addition, there is increasing evidence to support the theory that abnormal eutopic endometrium may contribute to implantation failure (Guidice and Kao, 2004), see Table 45.9.

Table 45.9 Theories on the pathogenesis of endometriosis

Retrograde menstruation/transplantation
Coelomic metaplasia
Altered cellular immunity
Metastasis
Genetic basis
Environmental basis
Multifactorial mode of inheritance with interactions between specific genes and the environment

Adapted from: [Guidice and Kao, 2004.].

Unexplained infertility

Unexplained infertility is diagnosed where routine investigations including semen analyses, tubal evaluation and tests of ovulation yield normal results. Intrinsic differences within populations and variations in investigation protocols have led to a wide range in the reported prevalence of unexplained infertility, but most clinics now report incidences of 20–30%. Failure of routine tests to detect any obvious contributory factors has led clinicians to speculate about numerous factors contributing to a diagnosis of unexplained infertility (Table 45.10). Although of interest to researchers, their practical relevance has been diminished by the growing role of assisted reproduction, which bypasses most of the possible contributory factors.

Investigations of infertility

When to investigate

Couples should be seen when a fertility problem is perceived to exist. This first consultation can be in primary care and does not necessarily require referral to a specialist clinic. Exclusion of any obvious medical factors, explanation about normal patterns of conception and advice about lifestyle measures may be sufficient in many cases. Referral to a fertility clinic should take into account the age of the female partner and duration of infertility. In the absence of any known reproductive pathology, couples who have been trying for 1–2 years should be investigated and seen in a dedicated fertility clinic. Earlier intervention is indicated in the presence of specific high-risk factors in either partner. In the male, this could be a history of azoospermia, testicular surgery, vasectomy or coital failure. Reasons for early referral in a woman include oligoamenorrhoea, known endocrine conditions affecting ovulation, history of tubal disease, endometriosis or salpingectomy. Accessing fertility care is a joint decision for couples who should be encouraged to attend together. Proposed investigations and treatment should be explained by adequate verbal and written information. At all times, consideration should be given to the social and psychological needs of couples.

Table 45.10 Contributory factors to unexplained infertility

Luteal phase deficiency	Presumed defects in folliculogenesis and luteal function due to abnormalities of gonadotrophin secretion, defects of endometrial steroid receptors and abnormalities of luteal rescue
Luteinized unruptured follicle (LUF) syndrome	Diagnosed by serial ultrasound scans. There is a lack of uniformity of ultrasonic criteria for defining this syndrome
Hyperprolactinaemia	High levels of prolactin may be associated with deficient luteal function
Endometriosis	Mild endometriosis without gross distortion of pelvic anatomy has traditionally been linked to unexplained infertility and treated in a similar way
Subclinical pregnancy loss	The prevalence of this condition has been shown to be no different from that in the general population
Anatomical abnormalities	Tubocornual polyps and other subtle anatomical aberrations are of little relevance in the causation of unexplained infertility and their treatment seems to have minimal effect
Occult infection	Impaired tubal function due to previous infection has been suggested as a factor. There is no evidence to support the empirical use of antibiotics in unexplained infertility
Sperm dysfunction	It is likely that cases of unexplained infertility are associated with subtle disorders of sperm function as well as sperm–mucus and sperm–oocyte interaction which can only be exposed by IVF
Immunological causes	Antiphospholipid antibodies, including antibodies to any one of five to seven phospholipid antigens have been linked with infertility
Psychological factors	Proof of a direct correlation between objectively defined stress levels and unexplained infertility is unavailable

Adapted from: Templeton *et al.* Management of infertility for the MRCOG and beyond, 2000.

History

A detailed history should be elicited from both partners. This should include questions about the duration of infertility, general health, past medical and surgical history and specific questions about sexual history (Table 45.10). Both partners should be examined as shown in Table 45.11.

Investigations

Diagnostic tests in infertility act as screening tools to detect those who need further investigations, to identify the cause of infertility and to make a prognosis. When planning investigations it is important to question the relevance of the proposed test to subsequent clinical decision making. It is also important to be aware of the limitations of some of the commonly used tests and balance the risks versus potential benefits. Figure 45.1 summarizes the approach to the investigations for an infertile couple.

Initial investigations

MALE

Semen analysis remains the most commonly performed investigation in the male. To adjust for fluctuations in semen parameters, a minimum of two samples 4 weeks apart should be analysed. Samples should be collected after a period of 2–7 days of abstinence. There is some debate about the predictive value of the routine semen analysis. WHO reference values for semen quality have been based on populations of fertile men and can act as a guide (WHO, 2000). Large laboratories may have their own population-based normal ranges (Table 45.12). The standard semen analysis has a sensitivity of 89.6%, that is, it is able to detect 9 out of 10 men with a genuine problem. It is not, however, a particularly specific test and a single sample analysis will falsely identify 10% of men as abnormal. Repeating the test reduces this chance to 2%.

FEMALE

A normal menstrual cycle is suggestive of ovulation. Confirmation of ovulation is usually obtained by means of a mid-luteal serum progesterone level in excess of 30 nmol/l 7 days before the onset of menstruation (day 21 of a 28 day cycle). In addition to tests of ovulation, a rubella screen should be performed on each woman. There is little evidence that routine use of temperature charts and LH detection kits improves clinical outcome. There is no justification for routine assessment of FSH, LH, prolactin and thyroid function in ovulatory women.

Further investigations of female infertility

INVESTIGATIONS FOR ANOVULATION

Where the cycle length is either longer or shorter than 28 days a single day-21 progesterone level may be insufficient to pinpoint ovulation and serial progesterone checks may be needed (progesterone tracking). For example, in a 28–35 day cycle progesterone tracking could be started

Table 45.11 History taking in an infertile couple

General information	Duration of infertility
	Nature of infertility (primary or secondary)

Male

Fertility history	Evidence of previous fertility with past partners
	Previous investigations or treatment for infertility
Medical	Sexually transmitted diseases
	Epidydimitis
	Mumps orchiditis
	Testicular maldescent
	Chronic disease or medication
	Drug/alcohol abuse
	Recurrent urinary tract infection (UTI)
	Surgical
	Testicular torsion
	Orchidopexy
	Testicular injury
	Vasectomy and vasectomy reversal
Occupational	Exposure to toxins
Sexual	Decreased libido
	Impotence
	Anejaculation, premature ejaculation

Female

Fertility	Fertility in previous relationships
	Time to previous conceptions
	Previous fertility investigations or treatments
	Length and type of previous contraceptive use
Menstrual history	Cyclicity
	Amenorrhoea
	Dysmenorrhoea
	Heavy menstrual bleeding
	Intermenstrual bleeding
Obstetric history	Previous pregnancy
	Miscarriage, termination of pregnancy, ectopic pregnancy
Medical history	Chronic illnesses (diabetes, hypertension, renal disease)
	Known endocrine disorders, e.g. hypothyroidism, PCOS
	Previous STD's, e.g. Chlamydia
	Known endometriosis
	Galactorrhoea
	Cervical smear history
	Current medication including folate supplements
Surgical history	Tubal surgery including salpingectomy and salpingostomy
	Ovarian surgery
	Pelvic surgery for endometriosis
	Previous laparoscopy
	Appendicectomy
Sexual history	Coital frequency and timing

from day 21 and continued weekly until the next period begins. Where periods are either very irregular or absent it may be impractical (and irrelevant) to estimate progesterone levels. Instead, additional biochemical investigations are indicated to establish a possible endocrine cause of oligo/anovulation (Fig. 45.2). These include early follicular phase FSH and LH, prolactin, TSH, and where PCOS is suspected, serum testosterone androstenedione and SHBG. Where an adrenal cause is to be excluded, DHEA and DHEAS, 17–OH progesterone need to be checked. FSH and LH levels should be checked in the early follicular phase (days 1–3) in order to avoid the normal midcycle surge which can lead to abnormally high values. Where accurate timing of the test is impossible (as in amenorrhoeic women), a serum sample can be obtained at any time and the results interpreted with reference to the following period.

TUBAL PATENCY TESTING

Once preliminary investigations suggest that a woman is ovulating and semen parameters are satisfactory, the next step should be assessment of tubal status. Tubal disease implies tubal block and pelvic adhesions due to infection, endometriosis or previous surgery. Laparoscopy and chromotubation (lap and dye) is the investigation of choice as it is able to demonstrate tubal patency as

Table 45.12 Examination of the infertile couple

	Female	Male
General examination	Height, weight, body mass index (BMI)	Height, weight, BMI
	Blood pressure	Blood pressure
	Fat and hair distribution	
	Acne and galactorrhoea	
Local examination	*Abdominal examination*	*Groin*
	Scars	Hernia
	Abdominal masses	
	Pelvic	*Genitalia*
	Inspection of external genitalia	Presence, location and volume of testes
	Speculum examination: vaginal assessment – vaginal septa, infections	Epididymitis
		Vasa deferentia
	Cervix – ectopy, polyps	Varicocoele
	Accessibility of cervix for insemination	Penis for any structural abnormalities, e.g. hypospadias
	Bimanual palpation of uterus: size, shape, position, mobility. Presence of adnexal masses and tenderness	

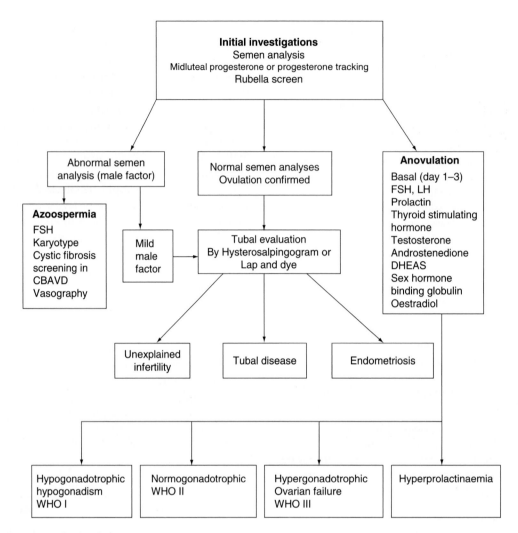

Fig. 45.1 Investigation of infertility.

well as assess the pelvis for the presence of endometriosis and adhesions. Hysterosalpingogram (HSG) which involves a pelvic X-ray following the injection of a radio opaque iodine-based dye through the cervix is less invasive and can be helpful in cases where laparoscopy is contraindicated/hazardous or in women at low risk of pelvic pathology (Evers, 2002).

As a test of tubal obstruction, HSG has a sensitivity of 0.65 (95% CI 0.50–0.78) and a specificity of 0.83 (95% CI of 0.77–0.88) (Swart *et al.* 1995). This suggests that it is a reliable indicator of tubal patency but poor at identifying cases of tubal occlusion. A meta-analysis of 23 studies has found that the discriminative capacity of chlamydial antibody testing using enzyme-linked immunofluorescent assay is comparable to HSG in the diagnosis of tubal pathology (Mol *et al.* 1997). The use of ultrasound along with injection of a sonoreflective contrast medium through the cervix (HyCosy) has been described, but is yet to become part of standard care in most centres. Preliminary

studies comparing it with lap and dye or HSG have shown good concordance (Dijkman *et al.* 2000). Further research is needed to ascertain the value of endoscopic tests such as fertiloscopy and falloposcopy. Routine assessment of tubal status is debatable in situations where knowledge of tubal patency is unlikely to change the proposed management plan – such as severe male factor infertility where intracytoplasmic sperm injection is indicated.

HYSTEROSCOPY AND PELVIC ULTRASOUND SCAN

Uterine pathology such as adhesions, polyps and submucous leiomyomas and septae have been found in 10–15% of women seeking fertility treatment. It is unclear whether hysteroscopy should be considered a routine investigation in infertile couples in addition to laparoscopy or HSG. While a causal relationship between uterine fibroids and infertility has been established (Donnez and Jadoul, 2002),

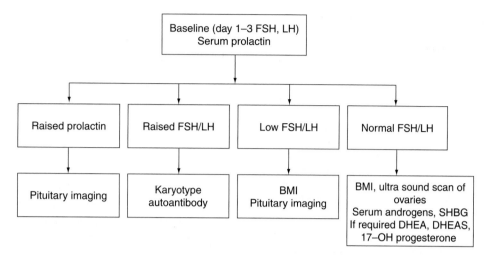

Fig. 45.2 Investigations for anovulation.

the effectiveness of surgical treatment of uterine abnormalities to enhance pregnancy rate is unproven. Transvaginal pelvic ultrasound (TVS) enables pelvic structures to be visualized and provides more information than a bimanual examination. It can identify endometrioma, ovarian cysts, polycystic ovaries, fibroids and hydrosalpinges. However, the routine use of this investigation in women without a history of pelvic pathology has yet to be established.

POST-COITAL TEST

The role of the post-coital test (PCT) to detect the presence of motile sperm is the subject of ongoing debate. It is useful in predicting spontaneous conception in couples with a short duration of infertility (<3 years) where female causes of infertility have been excluded (Glazener *et al.* 2000). A systematic review of observational studies has failed to confirm the predictive power of this test. A randomized trial on 444 women has failed to demonstrate any advantages of routine PCT in terms of cumulative pregnancy rates. Intervention rates were higher in women subjected to the investigation (Oei *et al.* 1998).

OVARIAN RESERVE

Women have a finite number of primordial ovarian follicles, which show an age related decline. Tests for ovarian reserve have been used to predict ovarian response to stimulation as part of fertility treatment. Observational studies have demonstrated an association between factors such as day-3 FSH, serum inhibin and antral follicle count, and subsequent ovarian response to stimulation. Currently available tests of ovarian reserve do not possess

adequate levels of sensitivity or specificity to justify their routine use in all women with infertility.

ENDOMETRIAL BIOPSY

The role of endometrial biopsy is not established in routine practice. While useful in cases where endometrial pathology is suspected on the basis of menstrual dysfunction, women should not be offered an endometrial biopsy to evaluate the luteal phase. There is no evidence that medical treatment of luteal phase defects improves pregnancy rates (Balasch *et al.* 1992).

SCREENING FOR CHLAMYDIA

Screening for chlamydia *trachomatis* can reduce the incidence of PID in women at increased risk of chlamydia (Scholes *et al.* 1996). Uterine instrumentation undertaken as part of investigation or treatment may reactivate upper genital tract infection. Hence women scheduled to undergo uterine instrumentation should be offered screening for chlamydia *trachomatis*.

Further investigations of male infertility

Other tests may be considered if the semen analysis is abnormal or if the history and clinical examination are suggestive.

ENDOCRINE TESTS

In men with azoospermia serum FSH levels help to differentiate between obstructive and non-obstructive causes. Normal levels are indicative of obstructive azoospermia

Table 45.13 Methods for sperm retrieval

Procedure	Type of azoospermia	Comments
Percutaneous epididymal sperm aspiration (PESA)	Obstructive	Outpatient, under local anaesthetic
Testicular sperm aspiration (TESA)	Non-obstructive	Outpatient, under local anaesthetic
Testicular sperm extraction (TESE)	Non-obstructive	Under general anaesthetic
Microsurgical sperm extraction (MESA)	Obstructive	Under general anaesthetic

where surgical sperm retrieval may be considered while elevated levels are suggestive of failure of spermatogenesis (Table 45.13). In rare cases undetectable levels of FSH can be suggestive of hypogonadotrophic hypogonadism where treatment with exogenous FSH may be effective. Testosterone and LH measurements are helpful in the assessment of men where androgen deficiency is suspected or where there is a need to exclude sex steroid abuse or steroid secreting tumours of the testes or adrenals. As men with hyperprolactinaemia have sexual dysfunction, it is necessary to exclude elevated prolactin levels in men with loss of libido and impotence. Persistently elevated prolactin levels warrant further investigations such as imaging of the pituitary gland.

CHROMOSOMAL AND GENETIC STUDIES

Men with azoospermia or severe oligozoospermia should undergo chromosomal analysis. A cystic fibrosis screen should be performed for men with CBAVD which is associated with defects in the cystic fibrosis transmembrane conductance regulator (CFTR) gene.

MICROBIOLOGY OF SEMEN

The significance of asymptomatic infection of the male genital tract as demonstrated by white blood cells in the ejaculate is unclear. Semen culture is indicated in men with microscopic evidence of infection. Male partners of women with chlamydia infection should be screened.

IMAGING OF THE MALE GENITAL TRACT

A number of techniques have been used for imaging varicoceles. Doubts about the justification of routine treatment for varicoceles have diminished the enthusiasm for these investigations. Although expensive, retrograde venography is the gold standard. Other tests include ultrasound and Doppler, radionucleotide angiography and thermography. Scrotal ultrasound scans are helpful if testicular tumours are suspected. In obstructive lesions of the male genital tract, vasography can be used to detect the site of obstruction. This is of limited clinical use with the advent of surgical sperm extraction and intracytoplasmic sperm injection.

IN VITRO TESTS OF SPERM FUNCTION

Introduction of assisted reproduction techniques such as IVF and ICSI has reduced the significance and clinical relevance of *in vitro* tests of sperm function including tests of acrosome reaction, zona binding and the zona free hamster egg penetration test (Table 45.14).

TESTICULAR BIOPSY

Testicular biopsy has been used in the past as a diagnostic tool to differentiate between obstructive and non-obstructive azoospermia. There is limited scope for the use of this invasive technique whose benefits are outweighed by potential risks such as reduction of testicular mass, devascularization, fibrosis and autoimmune response.

ANTISPERM ANTIBODIES

Tests for antisperm antibodies are not routine. The presence of sperm agglutination should alert the laboratory to the potential presence of antisperm antibodies. Subsequent tests to be done on a fresh sample should include MAR (mixed agglutinin reaction) and the immunobead test.

MAR involves incubating semen with red blood cells coated with non-specific antibody to IgA or IgG (anti-IgA or anti-IgG). Sperm with antisperm antibodies will adhere to treated red blood cells.

The immunobead test relies on micron-sized polyacrylic beads with covalently bound albumin IgA and IgG antibodies. Binding of sperm with antisperm antibodies to the beads allows detection of the presence as well as the site of antibodies.

Treatment of infertility

All couples trying for a pregnancy will benefit from some general advice such as cessation of smoking and limiting alcohol intake. Pre-treatment counselling should include advice about general lifestyle measures including the need to achieve an optimum BMI. This will involve weight loss in women with a BMI of over 30, but may require some

Table 45.14 Techniques used in assisted reproduction and their outcomes

Technique	Major indications	Outcome
Intrauterine insemination (IUI)	Unexplained infertility Mild male factor infertility	SO/IUI : 13% pregnancy rate per cycle[*] IUI alone: pregnancy rate per woman 24%[†]
In vitro fertilization or intracytoplasmic sperm injection (IVF or ICSI)	Prolonged infertility (see below)	Live-birth rate per cycle started 22%[‡] Live-birth rate per cycle started 28%[§]
In vitro fertilization (IVF)	Tubal disease Intractable pathology Failed primary treatment	Pregnancy rate per oocyte recovery 25%[*] Live-birth rate per oocyte recovery 34%[§]
Intracytoplasmic sperm injection (ICSI)	Severe oligozoospermia in the male Failed fertilization with IVF	Pregnancy rate per oocyte recovery 26%[*] Live-birth rate per oocyte recovery 32%[§]
Donor insemination (DI)	Azoospermia Infectious disease in the male partner Prevent transmission of genetic conditions	Pregnancy rate per cycle 16%[*] Live-birth rate per cycle 11%[‡]
Oocyte donation (OD)	Absent or non-functioning ovaries Prevent transmission of genetic conditions Repeated poor response with IVF treatment	Live-birth rate per transfer 50%[§]

[*] Nyboe Anderson *et al.* 2005.
[†] Goverde *et al.* 2000.
[‡] Human Fertilization and Embryology Authority, 2005.
[§] US Department of health and Human Services, Centres for Disease Control and Prevention, 2004.

women with weight-related amenorrhoea and anovulation to gain weight. Periconceptual dietary supplementation of folate has been shown to reduce the risk of neural tube defects (OR 0.28, 95% CI 0.13–0.58) and a daily dose of 0.4 mg is recommended for all women (National Collaborating Centre for Women's and Children's Health (NICE) guideline, 2004). The investigation of couples with infertility will result in a number of diagnostic categories – each with its own management pathway (Fig. 45.3). Details of management for each group are discussed below. Regardless of the diagnosis, prolonged infertility refractory to conventional treatment is treated by *in vitro* fertilization.

Anovulation

Women should be made aware of potential risks of multiple pregnancy and ovarian hyperstimulation. Male factor problems and tubal pathology should be excluded. In the absence of a history suggestive of tubal disease it may be reasonable to defer formal tubal patency tests for three cycles to allow less invasive treatment options such as clomifene to be used.

WHO TYPE I

In women with weight loss associated amenorrhoea, treatment should be deferred until a target BMI of 20 kg/m^2 is reached. The most physiological treatment of WHO type I anovulation or hypothalamic amenorrhoea is with pulsatile administration of GnRH agonists administered through a portable battery-operated pump (Filicori *et al.* 1994). Observational studies suggest that cumulative pregnancy rates of 80–90% over 12 cycles of treatment can be achieved by means of GnRHa at a dose of 15–20 μg subcutaneously or 2.5–5 μg intravenously. The intravenous route requires lower doses of GnRH, maintains a better physiological hormonal profile and provides higher rates of ovulation. Monitoring is performed by means of serum oestrogen and pelvic ultrasound. Luteal phase support is provided by means of human chorionic gonadotriphin (hCG) injections. Despite high success rates and a reduced risk of multiples, GnRH pumps may be unpopular with some women due to concerns about inconvenience and pump failure.

WHO TYPE II (PCOS)

Weight loss and dietary measures

Weight loss should be the first line of treatment in obese women with anovulation due to PCOS. Central obesity and high BMI are important predisposing factors for insulin resistance, hyperinsulinaemia and hyperandrogenaemia. Effective treatment of obesity can reverse these

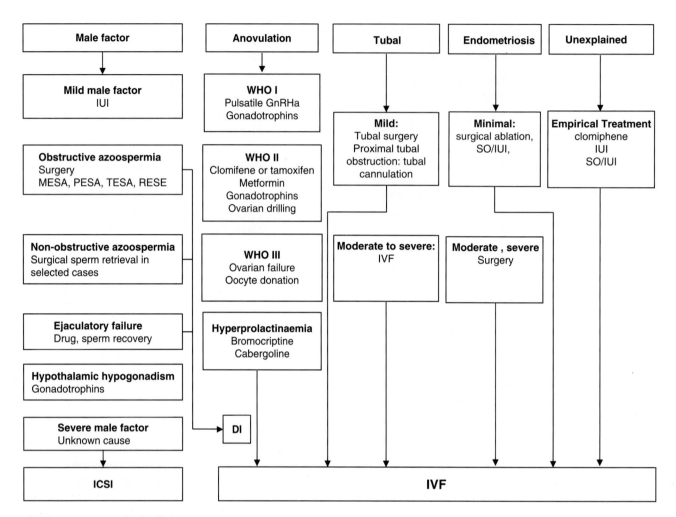

Fig. 45.3 Treatment of infertility.

effects and facilitate the effects of ovulation induction agents. In obese women with PCOS a loss of 5–10% of body weight may be enough to restore reproductive function in 55–100% women within 6 months (Clark *et al.* 1995).

Clomifene citrate

Clomifene citrate is an orally active synthetic non-steroidal compound with oestrogenic as well as anti-oestrogenic properties, which has traditionally been the treatment of choice in women with anovulatory PCOS. It displaces oestrogen from its receptors in the hypothalamic-pituitary axis, reduces the negative feedback effect of oestrogen and encourages GnRH secretion. It is administered in an initial daily dose of 50 mg on days 2–6 of a spontaneous or induced menstrual period. The dose can be increased by 50 mg per day till ovulation is achieved, up to a maximum of 150 mg per day. Couples are advised to have intercourse every other day from day 9 of the cycle for at

least one week. A course of 6 to 12 cycles can be used in women who respond to the drug. It is necessary to monitor follicular response, at least in the first cycle of treatment, with TV scans to minimize the risk of multiple pregnancy. Mid-luteal progesterone levels are checked in each cycle. Ovulation is expected to occur in 80% and pregnancy in 35–40% women on clomifene (Imani *et al.* 2002). Approximately 20–25% of women show no response to clomifene citrate and are considered to be resistant.

Adverse reactions

Anti-oestrogenic effects include thickening of cervical mucus and hot flushes in 10% of women. Other side effects include abdominal distension (2%), abdominal pain, nausea, vomiting, headache, breast tenderness and reversible hair loss. Clomifene has a mydriatic action that can result in blurred vision and scotomas in 1.5% of women. These changes are reversible. Significant ovarian enlargement

Table 45.15 Classification of OHSS

Severity	Clinical findings	Ultrasound picture
Mild	Abdominal bloating with some pain	Ovaries less than 8 cm
Moderate	Nausea, vomiting and increased abdominal discomfort Evidence of ascites	Ovarian size 8–12 cm
Severe	Clinical ascites ± hydrothorax with hypovolemia, oliguria (with normal serum creatinine), haemoconcentration (>45%), leucocytosis (>15,000/ml) and liver dysfunction	Ovaries over 12 cm Ascites
Critical	Tense ascites, haematocrit >55%, leucocytosis > 25,000/ml, oliguria (with raised serum creatinine), renal failure, thromboembolic complications Adult Respiratory Distress Syndrome may be seen	Ovaries over 12 cm Gross ascites

Adapted from: RCOG Guideline no 5, 1995.

Table 45.16 Risk factors for OHSS

Women under 30 years
Low BMI
PCOS
Use of GnRH agonists in combination with gonadotrophins
Use of exogenous hCG either as ovulatory trigger or luteal support
Endogenous surge of hCG due to pregnancy
Many small and intermediate follicles (<14 mm)
High E2 level (>9000 pmol/l)
Rapid increase in oestradiol levels (more than 75% increase from previous day)
Large number of oocytes (>20) collected in IVF/ICSI cycles

Adapted from: Whelan and Vlahos, 2000.

occurs in 5% but ovarian hyperstimulation syndrome (OHSS) is rare (<1%). The multiple pregnancy rate associated with clomifene is 7–10%. Most multiples are twins. A putative link with ovarian cancer has been described in women receiving more than 12 cycles of clomifene.

Tamoxifen

Tamoxifen has a structure similar to clomifene. The recommended dose is 20–40 mg per day from day 3, for 5 days. Pregnancy rates with tamoxifen are similar to those obtained with clomifene (OR 1.00 95% CI 0.48, 2.09) (Beck *et al.* 2005) and it may have a less potent anti-oestrogenic action on cervical mucus.

Gonadotrophins

Treatment with gonadotrophins is contemplated when women either do not respond to clomifene or fail to conceive after 6–12 ovulatory cycles. Preparations in common use include recombinant FSH or purified urinary human menopausal gonadotrophin which contains FSH as well as LH. Gonadotrophin regimens include a standard step-up protocol, chronic low-dose step-up protocol and step-down protocol. Acceptable cumulative conception rates have been achieved with standard step-up treatment starting with a dose of 150 IU/day. Due to the increased sensitivity of the PCO to gonadotrophins, this regimen carries a 34% risk of multiple pregnancy and 4.6% risk of OHSS (Homburg, 2003). Therefore a low-dose FSH

regimen is usually used to reduce the risk of multiple follicular development (Homburg, 2003). A low starting dose of 75 IU is administered for 14 days, followed by small incremental dose increases, when necessary, at intervals of not less than 7 days, until follicular development is initiated (Homburg, 2003). This dose is then continued until 1–2 leading follicles >17–18 mm are identified. Compared to the conventional regimen, the low-dose step-up regimen has been shown to yield slightly better pregnancy rates (40 versus 24%) while reducing the incidence of OHSS and multiple pregnancies. Unifollicular ovulation occurs in 74% of cases (Homburg, 2003). A systematic review (Nugent *et al.* 2005) found no significant difference between human menopausal gonadotrophin (HMG) and urinary FSH in terms of pregnancy rate per cycle (0.89, 95% CI 0.53–1.49). Similarly no differences in pregnancy rates have been found between the use of recombinant FSH and urinary FSH (Homburg, 2003). In women with PCOS treatment with gonadotrophins results in cumulative pregnancy rates of 40–50%, a miscarriage rate of between 25% and 30% and a 1–2% risk of serious OHSS (Tables 45.15 and 45.16).

GnRH analogues in ovulation induction

GnRH agonists have been used in conjunction with gonadotrophins to achieve pituitary downregulation and to facilitate cycle control. There are few data to support the routine use of this practice. A systematic review of three randomized controlled trials (RCTs) failed to reveal any added benefit associated with the use of GnRH agonists along with gonadotrophins in terms of pregnancy rates (OR 1.50; 95% CI 0.72–3.12) (Hughes *et al.* 2000).

Metformin

The strong association between anovulation and insulin resistance/hyperinsulinaemia has led to speculation that lowering insulin levels would lead to improvement in the clinical and metabolic profile of women with PCOS. While this could be achieved by weight loss alone, an insulin sensitizing agent like metformin was felt to be particularly suitable. Metformin is an oral biguanide, which has been used for the treatment of hyperglycaemia in maturity onset diabetics but which does not lower glucose levels in euglycaemic subjects. Its actions include decrease in insulin levels, lowering of circulating total and free androgen levels and improvement in the clinical sequelae of hyperandrogenism. A systematic review (Lord *et al.* 2003) has shown that metformin is more effective in achieving ovulation in women with PCOS in comparison with a placebo (OR 3.88, 95% CI 2.25–6.69). In combination with clomifene, it is more effective than clomifene alone in achieving ovulation (OR 4.41, 95% CI 2.37–8.22) as well as pregnancy (OR 4.40, 95% CI 1.96–9.85). Metformin has been shown to have a beneficial effect on fasting insulin, blood pressure, low-density lipoprotein cholesterol but evidence of any effect on body mass ratio or waist/hip ratio is lacking. It is associated with a higher incidence of nausea, vomiting and other gastrointestinal disturbances and can cause lactic acidosis in patients with deranged renal function. The evidence regarding the safety and efficacy of metformin has been encouraging so far (Homburg 2003). It remains to be proven whether metformin will emerge as the drug of choice in all infertile women with PCOS. Metformin is currently unlicensed for use in PCOS and although preliminary data suggest that the drug is safe in pregnancy (and may even decrease miscarriage rates), (Homburg, 2003) more data on efficacy and safety from randomized trials are awaited. Other serum insulin lowering compounds, like the glitazones (rosiglitazone and pioglitazone) and d-chiro-inositol are currently under investigation.

Laparoscopic ovarian drilling

Laparoscopic ovarian drilling (LOD) by diathermy or laser is a further treatment option for women with anovulation associated with PCOS. The procedure appears to be more successful in women who are slim and have high LH levels; the mechanism for its effect is unknown. A unipolar coagulating current is used to deliver four punctures to a depth of 4 mm in each ovary. A Cochrane review (Farquhar *et al.* 2000) showed that ongoing cumulative pregnancy rates following LOD were similar to those obtained with 3–6 cycles of gonadotrophins (OR 1.27, 95% CI 0.77, 1.98). Multiple pregnancies were reduced in women treated by ovarian drilling (OR 0.16, 95% CI 0.03, 0.98). The principal advantages of ovarian drilling include monofollicular ovulation resulting in fewer multiple pregnancy rates.

Aromatase inhibitors

Aromatase inhibitors have been used as alternatives to clomifene in view of their lack of anti-oestrogenic effects. They suppress oestrogen production and mimic the central reduction of negative feedback by ovarian oestrogen. Data from early trials confirm the effectiveness of Letrozole, the most commonly used agent (Homburg 2003). Evidence from larger trials is awaited.

WHO TYPE III

Egg donation may be the only option for patients with ovarian failure. This is discussed in greater detail later in the chapter on assisted reproduction (Chapter 46).

HYPERPROLACTINAEMIA

Prolactin secretion is regulated by the tonic inhibitory control of dopamine. Bromocriptine, which has a dopamine like action, is effective in hyperprolactinaemia. It shrinks 80% of macroadenomas, and can help to normalize prolactin values in 80–90% and restore ovulation in 70–80% of women. Long-term treatment with bromocriptine results in pregnancy rates of 35–70% per woman. Due to its short half-life, bromocriptine needs to be administered two to three times a day. Side effects including nausea, headache, vertigo, postural hypotension, fatigue and drowsiness can be minimized by initiating treatment with a low dose of bromocriptine (1.25 mg) at bedtime with a snack, and gradually increasing up to 2.5 mg three times a day with food over 2 to 3 weeks. Cabergoline and *Quinogolide* are newer dopamine agonists which have recently been licensed for treatment of hyperprolactinaemia. Fewer side effects and longer half-lives allow a once daily dose for quinogolide and a twice weekly dose for Cabergoline. Data from two randomized controlled trials have shown cabergoline to be more effective than bromocriptine in restoring normoprolactinaemia and ovulation.

Treatment of hyperprolactinaemia is mainly medical. In rare cases surgery may be considered in women with pituitary tumours who despite normalization of prolactin levels do not show adequate tumour shrinkage. Alternatively it may be considered in patients with large macroadenomas who are intolerant or resistant to drug treatment. Despite the invasive nature of surgery, its effects are modest. Post surgery, prolactin values return to normal in 50% of microadenomas and 10–15% of macroadenomas.

Management of male factor infertility

General measures should include advice about stopping smoking and reducing alcohol consumption. Where a specific cause is identified, targeted treatment should be considered. In the majority of cases no cause for abnormal semen parameters can be identified, and assisted reproduction offers the only option for men to have their own genetic offspring.

INTRAUTERINE INSEMINATION

Intrauterine insemination (IUI) using washed sperm may be considered in cases where semen parameters show mild or moderate abnormalities. A systematic review (Cohlen *et al.* 2000) found that compared with timed intercourse, IUI resulted in increased pregnancy rates, both in natural cycles (OR 2.5, 95% CI 1.6– 3.9) and stimulated cycles (OR 2.2, 95% CI 1.4–3.6). No difference was found between stimulated and unstimulated cycles (OR 1.8, 95% CI 0.98–3.3). As stimulated cycles are associated with a risk of multiple pregnancy, it may be prudent to consider IUI in a natural cycle in these cases. The evidence in favour of IUI has to be interpreted in the context of the overall prognosis for male infertility, which is poor, in the absence of assisted reproduction. Thus, although that IUI increases the relative odds of pregnancy, the absolute chances of conception remain low.

IVF/ICSI

Where semen parameters are poor, it may be appropriate to consider IVF treatment straightaway. In men with grossly reduced sperm concentrations (below 5 million/ml) ICSI is the treatment of choice. Obstructive azoospermia, in the presence of normal testicular volume and FSH levels can be treated by surgical sperm retrieval followed by ICSI. The prognosis for non-obstructive azoospermia associated with small atrophied testes and high FSH levels in poor and donor insemination (DI) may need to be considered.

DONOR INSEMINATION

Where surgical sperm retrieval is not possible, or when ICSI is not feasible, insemination of thawed frozen donor sperm may be considered. Donors are screened for hereditary conditions and blood-borne viruses. Tubal patency will need to be documented in the female partner and ovulation induction considered where cycles are irregular. Where ovulation has been demonstrated, monitoring of LH in blood or urine is carried out to time insemination approximately hours after ovulation. IUI has been shown to be more effective than intra-cervical insemination (ICI) in terms of pregnancy rates (OR 2.4, 95% CI 1.5–3.8) (Goldberg *et al.* 1999). Use of controlled ovarian stimulation has been used in women undergoing donor insemination leading to a higher incidence of multiple birth

and should be avoided. Data from national donor insemination programmes suggest that the live-birth rate per cycle of DI is 10.3–11.6%. Cumulative pregnancy rates show little increase after the sixth cycle of treatment and women should therefore be offered other treatment such as IVF using donor sperm thereafter.

Conventional treatment for male infertility

GONADOTROPHINS

Hypogonadotrophic hypogonadism responds to gonadotrophin treatment although this has yet to be evaluated in the context of RCTs. Data from uncontrolled observational studies report that administration of FSH and hCG is well tolerated and effective in achieving an acceptable sperm count in 80% of men. Pulsatile GnRH may be as effective as hCG and hMG in improving sperm production in these situations.

SURGICAL TREATMENT

Data on success rates after surgical procedures for post-infective block, including epididymovasotomy, are limited. Observational studies have described a post-surgical patency rate of 52% and a pregnancy rate of 38%. A systematic review based on seven RCTs found no evidence that surgical repair of varicoceles improved pregnancy rates in couples with male or unexplained infertility (RR 1.01 95% CI 0.73–1.40) (Evers, 2002).

EJACULATORY FAILURE

Sildenafil is an effective treatment in men with erectile dysfunction (Burls *et al.* 2001). Medical treatment of an ejaculation has included the use of alpha-agonists like imipramine and pseudoephedrine or parasympathomimetic drugs such as neostigmine. The former are less successful than the latter (19 versus 51%) (Kamischke and Nieschlag, 1999). Medical treatment of retrograde ejaculation has relied on measures to increase sympathetic stimulation of the bladder and decrease parasympathetic stimulation, but no clear difference in effectiveness has been found between alpha-agonists and anticholinergic drugs in this context. Sperm recovery from urine has been used successfully in some cases of retrograde ejaculation. Electro ejaculation may be considered in others, especially in men with neurological impairment. In the absence of other options, surgical sperm retrieval followed by IVF/ICSI may be considered.

Other interventions in male factor infertility

Gonadotrophins have no role in enhancing pregnancy rates in men with idiopathic oligozoospermia. Other interventions which have been shown to be ineffective include anti-oestrogens (clomifene and tamoxifen), androgens, bromocriptine and kinin enhancing drugs. Antioxidants (Vitamins C and E and glutathione) can improve semen parameters in men, but in the absence of data on more definitive outcomes such as pregnancy or live-birth rates, their use cannot yet be recommended. Mast cell blockers have shown some initial promise in men with severe oligizoospermia (National Collaborating Centre for Women's and Children's Health (NICE) guideline, 2004).

Treatment of tubal factor infertility

The majority of women with moderate to severe tubal damage are unlikely to conceive spontaneously and IVF is generally accepted as the treatment of choice in these cases. In the absence of randomized trials, evidence to support this strategy is mainly derived from observational studies.

A number of techniques for surgical reconstruction of damaged or occluded tubes have been described. Higher pregnancy rates have been reported in women who underwent tubal surgery than in those who did not (29 versus 12%) over a period of 3 years (Wu and Gocial, 1988). The success of surgical treatment depends on the extent of tubal damage, age of the woman, experience and training of the operator and availability of suitable equipment. Surgery has been shown to be effective in minor or moderate tubal damage, but of no benefit to women with severe tubal disease (Akande *et al.* 2004). Data from a case series have suggested that pregnancy rates following surgical treatment of proximal occlusion, mild distal block and flimsy adhesions are comparable to those after IVF. However, greater access to assisted reproduction in recent years has significantly reduced the role of tubal surgery in these cases.

Uncontrolled data indicate that approximately 50% of women with proximal tubal block can achieve a term pregnancy after microsurgical tubocornual anastomosis (Maranna and Quagliarello, 1988). Proximal tubal obstruction can be treated by tubal catheterization or cannulation under radiological or hysteroscopic guidance. In the absence of any direct comparisons between the two approaches, data from observational studies suggest a higher pregnancy rate (49 versus 21%) with the latter. Tubal cannulation can lead to tubal perforation in 2–5% of cases and ectopic pregnancy is 3–9% (Honore *et al.* 1999).

Endometriosis

In the absence of sufficient evidence from randomized trials, the treatment of endometriosis is mainly reliant on results of observational studies. The options are expectant management, medical treatment, surgical treatment, conventional fertility and assisted reproduction.

EXPECTANT MANAGEMENT (NO TREATMENT)

The presence of endometriosis has been shown to compromise the chance of spontaneous pregnancy (Collins *et al.* 1995). The prognosis is also related to the severity of the disease as staged by the revised American Fertility Society Guidelines. As with unexplained infertility, initial treatment of minimal and mild endometriosis may involve a period of expectant management.

MEDICAL TREATMENT

Pharmacological agents used for the treatment of endometriosis include the following: combined oral contraceptives, progestogens, danazol, gestrinone and GnRH analogues. Treatment with ovulation suppression agents has not been shown to improve pregnancy rates in comparison with either no treatment (OR 0.74 95% CI 0.48–1.15) (Hughes *et al.* 2003), or danazol (OR 1.3, 95% CI 0.97–1.76) (Harrison and Barry-Kinsella, 2000). A subsequent trial comparing medroxyprogesterone acetate with placebo failed to show any benefits associated with the drug. Many of the drugs used to suppress ovulation have undesirable side effects such as weight gain, hot flushes and bone loss. Thus, current evidence does not support the use of medical treatment in infertility associated endometriosis. The role of medical treatment as an adjunct to surgery is uncertain. Two RCTs compared the use of post-operative GnRH with expectant treatment and found no differences in pregnancy rates. Similar outcomes were found following the use of post-operative danazol or naferelin nasal spray in comparison with expectant treatment or placebo (National Collaborating Centre for Women's and Children's Health (NICE) guideline, 2004), see Chapter 44.

SURGICAL TREATMENT

Despite the association between early stage endometriosis and infertility, it is unclear whether there is a causal relation. A meta-analysis of two RCTs (Jacobson *et al.* 2002) showed that laparoscopic surgical treatment of minimal and mild endometriosis increased ongoing pregnancy/live-birth rates (OR 1.64, 95% CI 1.05–2.57). Although the individual trials have conflicting outcomes, the results are dominated by the larger trial (Marcoux *et al.* 1997) whose results suggest that eight women would need to undergo laparoscopic surgery to achieve one pregnancy. The potential benefit of this intervention has to be balanced against the added risks and costs of surgery in these women.

Anatomical distortion of the pelvis secondary to moderate and severe endometriosis can be corrected by surgery. A systematic review of observational studies of surgical treatment (Adamson *et al.* 1993) supports the role of surgery. The effectiveness of alternative routes (*laparotomy versus laparoscopy*), nature of surgery (*excision versus ablation of endometriotic deposits*) and the role of co-interventions in the form of assisted reproduction remain to be explored further. Data from an observational study (Paulson *et al.* 1991) suggest pregnancy rates of 81% after laparoscopy, 84% after laparotomy and 54% following medical treatment. Any benefits should be balanced against the risks of anaesthesia and surgical complications. Cohort studies of women with moderate and severe endometriosis indicate that pregnancy rates are better following laparoscopic surgery (54–66%) as opposed to laparotomy (36–45%) (National Collaborating Centre for Women's and Children's Health (NICE) guideline, 2004).

Routine use of post-operative medical treatment with GnRH agonists (naferelin, goserelin, luprolide) or danazol is not recommended (National Collaborating Centre for Women's and Children's Health (NICE) guideline, 2004). There is some uncertainty about the best treatment for endometrioma; a single trial has reported higher cumulative pregnancy rates at 2 years following laparoscopic cystectomy in comparison with drainage and coagulation (Beretta *et al.* 1998). More clinical trials are needed to evaluate existing and new surgical interventions in terms of effectiveness and safety. There are concerns that widespread excision or ablation of endometriotic tissue could damage healthy ovarian cortex and lead to diminished ovarian reserve (Guidice and Kao, 2004).

INTRAUTERINE INSEMINATION

Controlled ovarian hyperstimulation along with IUI has been used to treat women with minimal or mild endometriosis where the fallopian tubes are patent. A meta-analysis of results from two trials shows that stimulated IUI improved live-birth rates (RR 2.3 95% CI 1.1–4.6) (National Collaborating Centre for Women's and Children's Health (NICE) guideline, 2004).

IN VITRO FERTILIZATION

Although widely used in this context, the role of IVF in endometriosis has not been subjected to any form of rigorous evaluation. See Chapter 46 on assisted reproduction.

Unexplained infertility

In the absence of a specific diagnosis, any form of treatment for unexplained infertility is speculative. While planning treatment, the likelihood of a spontaneous pregnancy must be taken into account, as even relatively invasive assisted reproduction techniques offer fairly modest pregnancy rates. A period of 3 years of unexplained infertility is generally accepted as a minimum duration before active intervention is considered. The decision to initiate treatment also needs to take the woman's age into consideration. Successful communication with the couple is vital at this point and the importance of detailed discussion, supported, where necessary, by written information sheets, cannot be overstated. Many couples feel frustrated by the apparent refusal to accede to their request for early treatment and need careful counselling.

EMPIRICAL CLOMIFENE

Clomifene citrate has been shown to increase the number of follicles produced per cycle, thus increasing the odds of a fertilized embryo reaching the uterine cavity. Its use in unexplained infertility is still open to debate. A meta-analysis has demonstrated a statistically significant benefit following the use of clomifene in unexplained infertility (Hughes *et al.* 2000). The combined odds ratio (OR) for clinical pregnancy per patient was 2.37 (CI 1.43–3.94). The small sample sizes of the trials included in this review inevitably means that the present conclusions are likely to be affected by the outcome of future studies. Traditionally, clomifene has been viewed as an inexpensive and relatively innocuous drug and its empirical use preferred by many to the more invasive assisted reproduction techniques. Concerns about clomifene induced multiple pregnancy and inability to rule out a potential link with ovarian cancer underline the need to weigh the risk–benefit ratio carefully. The approach to the use of clomifene in unexplained infertility differs from that in anovulatory women. A starting dose of 50 mg is used and a day-12 scan performed to assess ovarian follicular response. If the ovarian response is very brisk, the dose should be cut down to 25 mg. The aim is to achieve no more than two preovulatory follicles over 17 mm.

INTRAUTERINE INSEMINATION WITH OR WITHOUT SUPEROVULATION

Intrauterine insemination in natural (unstimulated) cycles as well as in combination with superovulation (SO/IUI) have been used to treat unexplained infertility. Neither treatment has been evaluated in comparison with expectant management. IUI with SO is the more commonly used intervention. Data to support its effectiveness come from a systematic review showing that gonadotrophins along with IUI led to higher pregnancy rates compared to gonadotrophins along with timed intercourse (OR 2.37,

95% CI 1.43–3.90) (Hughes 1997). A single randomized trial (Goverde *et al.* 2000) showed that pregnancy rates in women treated by IUI alone were comparable to those in women treated by SO/IUI or IVF. A much larger multicentre American trial (Guzick *et al.* 1999) found SO/IUI to be more effective than IUI alone in terms of live-birth rates (OR 1.7, 95% CI 1.2–2.6) but associated with an appreciably higher risk of multiple pregnancy. IUI in an unstimulated cycle thus offers the safer option, while SO/IUI may enhance success rates at the cost of a higher multiple pregnancy rate.

Conclusion

The key to effective management of infertility is an appreciation of the likelihood of spontaneous pregnancy in a couple. This is done by means of a systematic diagnostic workup which can identify the nature of infertility and allow the merits of individual treatments to be balanced against potential risks. Adoption of an evidence-based approach in fertility care has led to a re-evaluation of many of the traditional practices and identified evidence of potential benefit as well as harm. Where there is insufficient evidence of effect, an individualized treatment strategy based on the best available evidence and the preferences of the couple is necessary. The availability of assisted reproduction techniques has revolutionized the outlook for many couples with refractory infertility. The challenge now is to improve treatment success while minimizing risks. In the face of rapidly evolving new technology, it is important to ensure that new techniques are subjected to adequate evaluation before being absorbed into routine clinical practice.

References

1. Adams J, Polson DW, & Franks S (1986) Prevalence of polycystic ovaries in women with anovulation and idiopathic hirsutism. *Br Med J* **293**, 355–9.
2. Adamson GD, Hurd SJ, Pasta, DJ, & Rodriguez BD (1993) Laparoscopic endometriosis treatment: is it better? Fertil Steril **59**, 35–44.
3. Akande V, Hunt LP, Cahill DJ, Caul EO, Ford WCL & Jenkins JM (2003) Tubal damage in infertile women: prediction using Chlamydia serology. *Hum Reprod* **18**[9], 1841–7.
4. Akande V, Cahill DJ, Wardle PG, Rutherford AJ & Jenkins JM (2004) The predictive value of the "Hull and Rutherford" classification for tubal damage. *Br J Obstet Gynaecol* **111**, 1236–41.
5. Andersen AN, Gianaroli L, Felberbaum R, de Mouzon J & Nygren KG (2005) Assisted reproductive technology in Europe, 2001. Results generated from European registers by

ESHRE. The European IVF-monitoring programme (EIM), Europea
6. Balasch J, Fabregues F, Creus M & Vanrell JA (1992) The usefulness of endometrial biopsy for luteal phase evaluation in infertility. *Hum Reprod* **7**, 973–9.
7. Barhart KT, Dunsmoor SR & Coutifaris C (2002) Effect of endometriosis on *in vitro* fertilisation. *Fertil Steril* **77**, 1148–55.
8. Beck JI, Boothroyd C, Proctor M, Farquhar C & Hughes E (2005) Oral anti-oestrogens and medical adjuncts for sub-fertility associated with anovulation. *Cochrane Database Syst Rev* **1**, CD002249.
9. Beretta P, Franchi M, Ghezzi F, Busacca M, Zupi E, & Bolis P (1998) Randomized clinical trial of two laparoscopic treatments of endometriomas: cystectomy versus drainage and coagulation. *Fertil Steril* **70**, 1176–80.
10. Brosens I (2004) Endometriosis and the outcome of *in-vitro* fertilisation. *Fertil Steril* **81**, 1198–2000.
11. Burls A, Gold L & Clark W (2001) Systematic review of randomised controlled trials of sildenafil (Viagra) in the treatment of male erectile dysfunction. *Br J Gen Pract* **51**, 1004–12.
12. CDC, American Society for Reproductive Medicine, and Society for Assisted Reproductive Technology. 2002 assisted reproductive technology success rates. Atlanta, GA: US Department of Health and Human Services, CDC, National Center for Chronic Disease Prevention and Health Promotion; 2004.
13. Clark AM, Ledger W, Galletly C *et al.* (1995) Weight loss results in significant improvement in pregnancy and ovulation rates in anovulatory obese women. *Hum Reprod* **10**, 2705–12.
14. Cohlen BJ, Vandekerckhove P, te Velde ER & Habbema JD (2000) Timed intercourse versus intra-uterine insemination with or without ovarian hyperstimulation for subfertility in men. *Cochrane Database Syst Rev* **2**, CD000360.
15. Collins JA, Burrows EA & Wilan AR (1995) The prognosis for live birth among untreated infertile couples. *Fertil. Steril* **64**, 1, 22–28.
16. Dijkman B, Mol BW, van der Veen F, Bossuyt PM & Hogerzeil HV (2000) Can hysterosalpingocontrast-sonography replace hysterosalpingography in the assessment of tubal subfertility? *Eur J Radiol* **35**, 44–8.
17. Donnez J & Jadoul P (2002) What are the implications of myomas on fertility? A need for a debate? *Hum Reprod* **17**, 1424–30.
18. Evers JLH (2002) Female subfertility. *Lancet* **2**, 151.
19. Evers JLH & Collins JA (2003) Assessment of efficacy of varicocoele repair for male subfertility: a systematic review. *Lancet* **361**, 1849–52.
20. Farquhar C, Vandekerckhove P, Arnot M & Lilford R (2000) Laparoscopic "drilling" by diathermy or laser for ovulation induction in anovulatory polycystic ovary syndrome. *Cochrane Database Syst Rev* **2**, CD001122.
21. Filicori M, Flamigni C, Dellai P, Cognigni G, Michelacci L, Arnone R, Sambataro M & Falbo A. J. Clin (1994) Treatment of anovulation with pulsatile gonadotropin-releasing hormone: prognostic factors and clinical results in 600 cycles. *Endocrinol. Metab.* 1994, **79**, 4, 1215–1220.

22. Glazener C, Ford WC & Hull MG (2000) The prognostic power of the post-coital test for natural conception depends on duration of infertility. *Hum Reprod* **15**, 1953–7.

23. Goldberg JM, Mascha E, Falcone T & Attaran M (1999) Comparison of intra-uterine and intra-cervical insemination with frozen donor semen: a meta-analysis. *Fertil Steril* **72**, 792–5.

24. Goverede AJ, McDonell J, Vermeiden JP, Schatz R, Rutten FF & Schoemaker J (2000) Intrauterine insemination or *in-vitro* fertilisation in idiopathic subfertility and male subfertility: a randomised trial and cost effectiveness analysis. *Lancet* **355**, 13–8.

25. Guidice LC & Kao LC (2004) Endometriosis. *Lancet* **364**, 1890–799.

26. Guzick DS, Carson SA, Coutifaris C *et al.* (1999) Efficacy of superovulation and intrauterine insemination in the treatment of infertility. *N Engl J Med* **340**, 177–83.

27. Hargreave TB (2000) Genetic basis of male infertility. *Br Med Bull* **56**, 650–71.

28. Harrison RF & Barry-Kinsella C (2000) Efficacy of medroxyprogesterone treatment in infertile women with endometriosis: a prospective randomised placebo controlled study. *Fertil Steril* **74**, 24–30.

29. Homburg R (2003) The management of infertility associated with polycystic ovary syndrome. *Reprod Biol Endocrinol* **14**(1), 109–20

30. Honore GM, Holden AE & Schenken RS (1999) Pathophysiology and management of proximal tubal blockage. *Fertil Steril* **71**, 785–95.

31. Hughes,E.G (1997) The effectiveness of ovulation induction and intrauterine insemination in the treatment of persistent infertility: a meta-analysis. Hum.Reprod., 1997, 12, 9, 1865-1872.

32. Hughes E, Collins J & Vanderkerckhove P (2000) Gonadotrophin-releasing hormone analogue as an adjunct to gonadotropin therapy for clomiphene-resistant polycystic ovarian syndrome. *Cochrane Database Syst Rev* **2**, CD000097.

33. Hughes E, Collins J & Vandekerckhove P (2000) Clomiphene citrate for unexplained subfertility in women. *Cochrane Database Syst Rev* **3**, CD000057.

34. Hughes E, Fedorkow DM, Collins J & Vanderkerckhove P (2003) Ovulation suppression for endometriosis. *Cochrane Database Syst Rev* **3**, CD000155.

35. Hull MG, Glazener CM, Kelly HJ, Conway D I, Foster PA, Hinton RA, *et al.* (1985) Population study of causes, treatment, and outcome of infertility. *Br Med J* **291**, 1693–97.

36. Human Fertilisation and Embryology Authority (2005) IVF National Data Statistics. London: The Stationery Office.

37. Imani B, Eijkemans MJ & te Velde ER (2002) A nomogram to predict the probability of live birth after clomiphene citrate induction of ovulation in normogonadotropic oligomenorrheic infertility. *Fertil Steril* **77**, 91–7.

38. Jaccobson TZ, Barlow DH, Konickx PR Ollive D & Farquhar C (2002) Laparoscopic surgery for subfertility associated with endometriosis. *Cochrane Database of Syst Rev* **4**, CD001398.

39. Kamischke A & Nieschlag E (1999) Treatment of retrograde ejaculation and anejaculation. *World J Urol* **11**, 89–95.

40. Lord JM, Flight IHK & Norman RJ (2003) Metformin in polycystic ovarian syndrome: a systematic review and meta-analysis. *Br Med J* **327**, 1–6.

41. Mahmood TA & Templeton A (1991) Prevalence and genesis of endometriosis. *Hum Reprod* **6**, 544–549.

42. Marana R & Quagliarello J (1988) Proximal tubal occlusion: microsurgery versus IVF – a review. *Int J Fertil* **33**, 338–40.

43. Marcoux S, Maheux R & Canadian Collaborative Group on Endometriosis (1997) Berube S Laparoscopic surgery in infertile women with minimal or mild endometriosis. *N Engl J Med* **337**, 217–22.

44. Mol BW, Dijkman B, Wertheim P, Lijmer J, van der Veen F & Bossuyt PM (1997) The accuracy of serum chlamydial antibodies in the diagnosis of tubal pathology: a meta-analysis. *Fertil Steril* **12**, 1031–7.

45. National Collaborating Centre for Women's and Children's Health (2004) Fertility: assessment and treatment of people with fertility problems. Clinical guideline. London: RCOG Press.

46. Nugent D, Vanderkerckhove P, Hughes E, Arnot M & Lilford R (2005) Gonadotrophin therapy for ovulation induction in subfertility associated with polycystic ovary syndrome. *Cochrane Database Syst Rev* **3**, CD000410.

47. Oei SG, Helmerhorst FM, Bloemenkamp KW, Hollants FA, Meerpoel DE & Keirse MJ (1998) Effectiveness of the postcoital test: randomised controlled trial. *Br Med J* **317**, 502–5.

48. Opsahl MS, Dixon NG, Robins ER & Cunningham DS (2000) *Single vs. multiple semen specimens in screening for male infertility factors. A comparison.* Cambridge: Cambridge University Press.

49. Pandian Z, Bhattacharya S, Nikolaou N, Vale L & Templeton A (2002) *In-vitro* fertilisation for unexplained infertility. *Cochrane Database Syst Rev* **2**, CD003357.

50. Paradisi R, Pession A, Ballavia E, Foccacci M & Flamingni C (1995) Characterisation of human sperm antigens reacting with antisperm antibodies from autologous sera and seminal plasma in a fertile population. *J Reproductive Immunol* **28**, 61–73.

51. Paulson JD, Asmar P & Saffan DS (1991) Mild and moderate endometriosis. Comparison of treatment modalities for infertile couples. *J Reprod Med* **36**, 151–5.

52. The Rotterdam ESHRE/ASRM-Sponsored PCOS consensus workshop group. Revised 2003 consensus on diagnostic criteria and long-term health risks related to polycystic ovary syndrome (PCOS). Hum Reprod 2004;19:41–7.

53. RCOG (1999) The management of menorrhagia in secondary care. Evidence-based clinical guidelines No. 5. Royal College of Obstetricians & Gynaecologists.

54. Rowe PJ, Comhaire FH, Hargreave TB & Mellows HJ (eds) (1993): WHO manual for the standardized investigation and diagnosis of the infertile couple. Cambridge University Press, Cambridge.

55. Scholes D, Stergachis A, Heidrich FE, Andrilla H, Holmes KK & Stamm WE (1996) Prevention of pelvic inflammatory disease by screening for cervical chlamydial infection. *N Engl J Med* **334**, 1362–6.

56. Swart P, Mol BW, van Beurden M, van der Veen F, Redekop WK & Bossuyt PM (1995) The accuracy of

hysterosalpingography in the diagnosis of tubal pathology: a meta-analysis. *Fertil Steril* **64**, 486–91.

57. te Velde ER, Eijkemans R & Habbema HDF (2000) Variation in couple fecundity and time to pregnancy, an essential concept in human reproduction. *Lancet* **355**, 1928–9.

58. Templeton A, Fraser C & Thompson B (1990) The epidemiology of infertility in Aberdeen. *Br Med J* **301**, 148–52.

59. Templeton A & Shetty A, Ashok P, Bhattacharya S, Gazvani R, Hamilton M, S Macmillan (2000) The management of infertility for the MRCOG and beyond. RCOG Press, London ISBN 1-900364-29-8

60. Whelan JG III and Vlahos NF (2000) The ovarian hyperstimulation syndrome. *Fertil. Steril.* **73**, 883–896.

61. World Health Organisation (1992) The influence of variocoele on parameters of fertility in a large group of men presenting to infertility clinics. *Fertil Steril* **57**, 1289–93.

62. World Health Organisation (2000) WHO Laboratory Manual for the Examination of Human Semen and Sperm-Cervical Mucus Interaction. Cambridge: Cambridge University Press.

63. Wu CH & Gocial B (1988) A pelvic scoring system for infertility surgery. *Int J Fertil* **33**, 341–6.

Chapter 46: Assisted reproduction

Geoffrey Trew

Introduction

Assisted conception is the facilitation of natural conception by some form of scientific intervention. It has been available for many years, but one of the first recorded and possibly best known instances of assisted conception was that performed by the eminent surgeon, John Hunter, in London in 1785. The husband, in this infertile couple, had hypospadias and artificial insemination of ejaculated sperm was performed on the wife. This resulted in a successful pregnancy and subsequent birth. This basic assisted conception continued until scientific techniques improved in the middle of the twentieth century. The advent of improved techniques, particularly in the form of ovulation induction and controlled ovarian stimulation, has allowed the successful treatment of the anovulatory female. The purification and use of human menopausal gonadotrophins (hMG's) in the 1960s led to multiple follicular development allowing *in vitro* fertilization (IVF). Over the last 40 years there have been dramatic improvements in the treatment of both the infertile female as well as the male. There is now a full panoply of techniques with acronyms ranging from the more well known such as IUI, IVF, ICSI and PGD, through to ones that have now become more esoteric due to lack of success rates such as DOT, PROST and even DIPI (Table 46.1). With these advances it is possible to treat the vast majority of subfertile men and women successfully and give them the child they so desire.

Investigations prior to assisted conception

Even though the diagnosis may have been made and the most appropriate form of treatment decided upon there are a few essential investigations that should be performed prior to any form of assisted conception. These will not only ensure the best results when the assisted conception is performed, but also reduce the chance of any diagnosis being missed before multiple cycles are embarked upon with the subsequent emotional and financial cost to the patient if they are unsuccessful.

Table 46.1

Acronym	Definition
IVF	*In vitro* fertilization
IUI	Intrauterine insemination
ICSI	Intra-cytoplasmic sperm injection
PGD	Preimplantation genetic diagnosis
PGS	Preimplantation genetic screening
DOT	Direct oocyte transfer
PROST	Pro-nuclear stage transfer
DIPI	Direct intraperitoneal insemination
MESA	Microepididymal sperm aspiration
PESA	Percutaneous epididymal sperm aspiration
TESE	Testicular sperm extraction
GIFT	Gamete intrafallopian transfer

Female

An early follicular phase follicle- stimulating hormone (FSH) level is essential in all forms of assisted conception to ensure the patient has normal ovarian reserve. Most forms of assisted conception, excluding egg donation, require normal FSH levels to have any significant chance of success. Some forms of assisted conception, particularly IUI or IVF, can be used in circumstances of reduced ovarian function, but subsequent live birth rates are correspondingly reduced. If the patient has irregular periods, then prolactin, thyroid function and, if appropriate, testosterone and sex hormone binding globulin (SHBG) levels should also be performed.

If the patient is undergoing a licensed form of assisted conception under the 1990 Human Fertilisation and Embryology Act, then both the male and female partner have to be screened for Hepatitis B, Hepatitis C and HIV. It is generally thought to be good practice that even in forms of assisted conception, such as IUI, which is not covered by the 1990 Act, both partners are also similarly screened. If either partner is positive for the above conditions this does not preclude them from being treated but unless specific embryo cryopreservation facilities are available embryo freezing of surplus embryos cannot be performed. This is due to the theoretical risk of cross infectivity between the patients' embryos and unaffected embryos from other patients.

ULTRASOUND

Virtually all ultrasound scanning in assisted conception is performed transvaginally. The initial scan assesses several areas: (1) The ovarian morphology: if there are underlying polycystic ovaries, they may be hyper-responsive to stimulation with gonadotrophins (see p.461); (2) The presence of ovarian cysts: and if present suitable treatment arranged; (3) Many centres now also measure the ovarian volumes as well as the antral follicle count as these are also used in the dose calculation of FSH for the stimulation phase of IVF; (4) The ovaries are assessed for accessibility, not just for the monitoring itself but also if transvaginal oocyte retrieval (TVOR) is planned, to ensure that this can be performed without undue difficulty. Sometimes in patients who have abdominal adhesions (either from iatrogenic causes, previous pelvic inflammatory disease (PID) or endometriosis) then gentle abdominal pressure can be applied during the screening ultrasound to ensure that the ovary can be moved down to a more accessible position for egg collection; (5) The uterus is also assessed for the presence of abnormalities such as uterine fibroids, to make sure the endometrium appears normal and there are no other abnormalities; (6) The rest of the pelvis is also screened in a systematic fashion to exclude other pathology.

UTERINE CAVITY AND TUBAL PATENCY

Both the uterine cavity and the fallopian tubes should be examined prior to all forms of assisted conception. For techniques such as IUI, where either one or both fallopian tubes are required to be patent, it is obvious why both the cavity and the tubes should be checked. Less obviously, the fallopian tubes require inspection for techniques such as IVF, even though they are not required for the actual procedure. We know from grade A evidence [1] that the presence of hydrosalpinges can significantly reduce the implantation rate due to reflux of the hydrosalpingeal fluid into the uterine cavity (see p.461). The integrity of the uterine cavity should be evaluated as various forms of pathology ranging from intrauterine adhesions, congenital abnormalities such as large septate uterus, submucus fibroids and intrauterine polyps can all significantly reduce the implantation rate and hence the subsequent live birth rate, from all forms of assisted conception. If a significant problem is noted in the uterine cavity, this would normally be corrected prior to the assisted conception cycles being

performed. The uterine cavity and the fallopian tubes can be investigated by the following means.

HYSTEROSALPINGOGRAPHY

Hysterosalpingography (HSG) has been used for many decades but had a reputation for being painful. With newer techniques and in particular the advent of suction caps and small balloon catheters, the need for unnecessary trauma is obviated. It allows assessment of both the uterine cavity and the fallopian tubes and it is an extremely useful screening test that can be performed with a high degree of accuracy without the need for a general anaesthetic. It is recommended that chlamydial screening should be performed beforehand, preferably as part of the initial work up of the female partner, and antibiotic cover for the procedure should be used.

HYSTERO-CONTRAST SONOGRAPHY

There have been several ultrasound techniques developed to try and assess tubal patency, the most commonly used one being Echovist. This is an echogenic fluid instilled inside the uterine cavity and down the fallopian tubes, which can be tracked by ultrasound. This can be a good method for assessing tubal patency, but due to the high echogenicity of the fluid, it can sometimes miss the uterine cavity lesions such as intrauterine adhesions and subtle distortions by submucus fibroids [2].

LAPAROSCOPY AND HYSTEROSCOPY

These are commonly performed infertility investigations particularly if the patient has other presenting complaints, particularly pelvic pain.

If the screening test such as hysterosalpingogram has been performed and an intrauterine lesion found, then hysteroscopy would also be performed and if the diagnosis confirmed the lesion then removed. For example if there are intrauterine adhesions, these can be divided hysteroscopically, or a submucus fibroid can be resected by transcervical resection of this fibroid.

Male partner

A comprehensive semen analysis should be performed on all males referred for assisted conception to ascertain the most appropriate technique suitable for the patient. Most assisted conception units not only look at the normal WHO sperm criteria, but also do some form of sperm function test to assess the best way to use the sperm – generally IVF if the parameters are good and intra-cytoplasmic sperm injection (ICSI) if there is a severe problem. The presence of other problems such as anti-sperm antibodies within the ejaculate are also ascertained and if present further samples can be obtained with the patient ejaculating directly into culture medium to try and lessen the impact of these antibodies on sperm function. This can sometimes mean that a sample severely affected by anti-sperm antibodies only deemed suitable for IVF, can sometimes be 'upgraded' to techniques such as IUI if ejaculation into medium is performed.

Important coexistent pathologies

There are several other coexistent pathologies that can significantly reduce the successful outcome of assisted conception or increase the complication rate from it.

UTERINE FIBROIDS

Uterine fibroids are very commonly picked up by transvaginal scanning of the infertile woman. It has always been difficult to ascertain the causality of these fibroids pertaining to the patient's infertile status. The presence of fibroids does not necessarily mean there is a direct causative link between the fibroids and infertility. On the other hand there are a number of reported case series where removal of fibroids resulted in subsequent improved conception rates between 30 and 80% [3]. It was previously thought that fibroids only significantly reduced implantation rates if the uterine cavity was distorted. There are two series looking at the affect on implantation in IVF cycles of fibroids in other locations. In the first of these, Eldar-Geva [4] showed that intramural fibroids significantly reduced implantation rates and this was then also confirmed by Hart *et al.* [5]. Both of these studies confirmed the impact of fibroids that do not distort the uterine cavity but this appears to be only for fibroids above 3 cm in size. Therefore, any patient who has fibroids larger than 3 cm, and in particular who have recurrent implantation failures, should be considered for myomectomy prior to further assisted conception. Although there does appear to be an impact on the presence of these fibroids with implantation rates, Surrey *et al.* [3] in a randomized trial have failed to demonstrate improved live birth rates.

HYDROSALPINGES

There have been several studies that have shown the adverse effect of hydrosalpinges on IVF outcome. Indeed three randomized controlled trials were included in the Cochrane review [6] to see if salpingectomy would be useful for patients with hydrosalpinges prior to undergoing IVF. Surgical treatment of these hydrosalpinges versus non-surgical treatment increased the odds of live birth plus ongoing pregnancy (OR 2.13, 95% CI 1.24–3.65) and

of pregnancy (OR 1.75, 95% CI 1.07–2.86). It has now been shown that removal of these diseased tubes by salpingectomy prior to IVF leads to implantation rates as would be expected in patients unaffected with hydrosalpinges. Whether these hydrosalpinges should be removed or drained by distal salpingostomy will depend on several factors including the degree of tubal damage. Whether they are to be removed prior to a first cycle of IVF, before the ovarian response is known, or after a first cycle is also unknown. Most practitioners would individualize the treatment of hydrosalpinges and take all other variable parameters into consideration ranging from any male factor present through to degree of tubal disease, as well as the known ovarian function of the patient prior to removing them.

POLYCYSTIC OVARIES

Polycystic ovaries as seen by ultrasound are an extremely common finding in women of child bearing age and can occur in ~20% of patients. Patients with polycystic ovaries can be more difficult to stimulate with gonadotrophins either for IUI or IVF. Initially there can be a degree of resistance at lower doses but then a very narrow therapeutic window before the patient overstimulates and this can quite often lead to cycle cancellation. In view of the severe complications resulting from ovarian hyperstimulation syndrome (OHSS), one should always start on a low dose and then build it up in small increments until the appropriate therapeutic window is achieved. Some have advocated the use of laparoscopic ovarian drilling to try and improve this therapeutic window, as well as the pre-cycle treatment of all insulin sensitizing agents such as Metformin. The use of both of these modalities is yet to be fully assessed in prospective randomized controlled studies with IVF patients.

ENDOMETRIOTIC CYSTS

Endometriosis is a common coexistent pathology in patients undergoing assisted conception. Whereas there has been no suggestion in improvement of assisted conception cycles by treating peritoneal endometriosis, there can be a benefit to treating large endometrioma prior to the IVF. It is thought this may benefit the cycle in several ways including the ovarian response itself and overall number of eggs obtained (particularly in the ovary containing the endometrioma). The second concern with ovarian endometriomas is that these can be inadvertently punctured during TVOR and there is a significant increase in ovarian abscess formation if this occurs. Pre-cycle drainage by needle aspiration can also give a significant rate of ovarian abscesses and this is generally not advised. If the ovarian endometrioma is felt to be a significant size that may adversely affect the cycle outcome or the chance of inadvertent needling then it is better that these are surgically treated prior to the initiation of the cycle itself. Prolonged down-regulation with gonadotrophin-releasing hormone (GnRH) analogues can shrink the cysts but can also make it harder to stimulate the ovaries as well.

SMOKING

Patients should be advised to stop smoking as smoking significantly reduces the effectiveness of all forms of assisted conception.

OBESITY

It is recommended that a patient should have a (Body Mass Index) BMI of between 19 and 30, as outside this range success rates of assisted conception are reduced. We also know that if the BMI is above 30, not only are success rates lower, but miscarriage rates higher and complications such as OHSS are also increased. It is therefore recommended that the female partner should be encouraged to lose weight.

Types of assisted conception

There are many types of assisted conception available in the modern unit. These range from less invasive procedures such as IUI through to the widely known IVF, with or without ICSI. The use of other procedures such as gamete intra fallopian transfer (GIFT) has reduced due to the improving success rates of IVF. Other techniques associated with assisted conception cycles such as preimplantation genetic diagnosis (PGD) and preimplantation genetic screening (PGS) are also performed in a few specialized centres.

Intrauterine insemination

Intrauterine insemination (IUI) is where a prepared sample of sperm (normally produced by masturbation) is inseminated into the uterine cavity at the appropriate time of the patient's menstrual cycle. Approximately two weeks later a pregnancy test is performed to see if the cycle has been successful.

PROTOCOLS

IUI can be performed in a natural cycle, with Clomid alone, with Clomid and then FSH injection or purely with FSH. If any form of ovulation induction has been used it is also quite common to use a single human chorionic gonadotrophin (hCG) injection approximately 36 hours prior to the insemination to ensure optimal timing with ovulation.

MONITORING

Although for unstimulated cycles it is possible just to do urinary LH monitoring by home dipstick methods, this does not to give the best success rates. If any form of ovulation induction has been used, then it is recommended that more accurate monitoring is performed. This is normally performed by transvaginal ultrasound and has benefits of not only deciding the best time to give the dose of hCG and hence the timing of the insemination, but also to ensure the ovulation induction is having the desired effect; that is, one (or at most two) developing follicle over 18mm. If there is over response from the ovaries, then this can be detected by the ultrasound, the cycle cancelled and the patient advised against having unprotected intercourse due to the increased risk of higher order multiple pregnancies.

Success rates increase from unstimulated IUI through to stimulation with Clomid and FSH. The overall success rate, as with any subfertile couple, depend on multiple factors, most importantly female age and with IUI the quality of the sperm. Though IUI can be used for mild male factor problems, it is not recommended for anything more severe. Success rates of around 5% per cycle have been quoted for unstimulated IUI going up to 8 to 10% for stimulation with Clomid and then generally accepted levels of between 12 and 18% per cycle when FSH is used in the protocol. Although success rates of 35% have been quoted in literature, these tend to be highly selective series and not necessarily representative of a general case mix of patients across a wider age range [7].

COMPLICATIONS

The main complication of IUI occurs when FSH has been used and this is higher order multiple births. Most centres would expect a twinning rate of between 10 and 15% and a triplet rate of less than 1%. If the triplet rate is higher than 1%, and in particular if there are even higher numbers than this, then this is normally due to inadequate monitoring and inadequate numbers of cycles being cancelled when an over response of the ovaries has been seen.

Although ovarian hyperstimulation can occur, particularly in the protocols where FSH is used, this would normally be mild to moderate at most, and it is very unusual to get a case of severe hyperstimulation in IUI cycles. If this happens it tends to be when an inappropriate starting dose of FSH has been used and again when inadequate monitoring has been performed.

The patient should also be warned about the possibility of ectopic pregnancies, and most clinics would offer an early ultrasound scan in the patients who have had a positive pregnancy test, at between 6 to 7 weeks gestation.

ADVANTAGES

IUI is relatively a simple technique that is cost-effective and can be offered by both secondary and tertiary fertility centres. It is not as invasive as IVF and allows fertilization to occur within the fallopian tubes and therefore is generally acceptable to most religious groups.

DISADVANTAGES

The success rates are lower than those with IVF and if the cycle fails less information is obtained than with an IVF cycle – particularly pertaining to possible egg or subsequent embryo quality. It also requires at least one healthy fallopian tube and reasonable sperm parameters. If monitoring is suboptimal then there can be a significant increase in higher order multiple birth with the expected sequelae of these.

INDICATIONS

- Unexplained infertility
- Mild male Factor
- Ejaculatory problems
- Cervical problems
- Ovulatory disorders
- Mild endometriosis
- To optimize the use of donor sperm

In vitro fertilization

IVF is where the mature oocyte is surgically removed from the ovary and then fertilized with sperm in the laboratory. The world's first successful IVF baby was delivered by Patrick Steptoe in 1978 after a number of years collaborating with Robert Edwards. Over the last 25 years the success rates and types of IVF have greatly improved and at present there are well over 2 million babies born throughout the world by this technique.

INDICATIONS

- Severe tubal disease – tubal blockages
- Severe endometriosis
- Moderate male factor
- Unexplained infertility
- Unsuccessful IUI

PROTOCOLS

Initially simple forms of ovulation induction using Clomid and human menopausal gonadotrophins (hMG's) were used. Over the last 20 years protocols have been refined and these are now broken down into three main categories.
1 Natural Cycle
2 Long protocol – Agonist cycles
3 Short protocol – Antagonist cycles
Although there are other short protocols using agonists, these are now less used due to poorer success rates.

AGONIST CYCLES

Long protocols are still at present the most widely used protocols throughout the world. They involve the use of a GnRH agonist which can be taken either on a daily basis nasally (e.g. Buserelin, Nafarelin) or daily subcutaneous injection (e.g. Buserelin, Leuprorelin) or in a depo preparation (Goserelin Leuprorelin). The agonist is given continuously and initially increases the production of gonadotrophins (FSH and LH) from the pituitary gland. If this continuous administration is maintained then the so-called down-regulation effect on the GnRH receptors is achieved. This causes a fall of LH and FSH levels and with this a reduction in stimulation of the ovary, folliculogenesis is suppressed and blood oestradiol levels fall to menopausal levels within 3 weeks. As long as the agonists are continued then the ovary is suppressed unless exogenous gonadotrophins are given.

The start of agonist administration can either be on day 2 of the menstrual cycle or, more commonly, day 21.

The rationale behind using these long protocols is to create a temporary menopause from which the ovaries can then be stimulated by the daily use of FSH/hMG injections.

In a mid-luteal start, (normally around day 21) the patient is reviewed when her period starts approximately 7–10 days after the agonist is initiated. A scan and often a blood oestradiol level are performed to ensure the patient is adequately suppressed. If this is the case then the gonadotrophins are started the following day and continued until an adequate ovarian response is gained.

Early follicular, or day 2, can also be used and the patient bought back for their scan and blood test to see if they are suppressed on average 2 weeks later. As in the luteal start, if adequate suppression is obtained, then exogenous gonadotrophins are started and then continued until satisfactory ovarian response is obtained.

ANTAGONIST PROTOCOLS

Antagonists (Ganirelix and Cetrorelix) have been in use for the last 5 years. The antagonist has an almost immediate effect on the pituitary and does not need the several days to achieve menopausal levels of the pituitary derived gonadotrophins that agonists do. Therefore the patient is prevented from having a premature LH surge and ovulating spontaneously within an hour of the start of the antagonist. A daily dose of 0.25 mg is normally given and there is also a 3 mg dose of Cetrorelix which can last for several days. The drugs are given subcutaneously and are started either on a fixed day of FSH stimulation (normally on the 5th day) or when the lead follicle is a certain size by ultrasound monitoring (normally 14mm). The antagonists are continued alongside the gonadotrophin stimulation until an adequate response is achieved and then stopped prior to the hCG injection.

The benefits of antagonists versus agonists are:
- No menopausal side effects
- No cyst formation from the initial gonadotrophin surge
- Shorter cycle duration
- Less gonadotrophin required per cycle – therefore lower drug costs

MONITORING

It is essential that adequate monitoring is performed during stimulation of the ovaries with exogenous gonadotrophins. Serial transvaginal ultrasounds to assess the follicular growth should be used and a decreasing amount of units continue to use serial oestradiol levels to add to the information obtained from the ultrasound. The use of serial oestradiol can be useful is some patient groups, particularly if a under or over response is anticipated. An under response can sometimes be anticipated in the older patient or the patient with previously raised FSH levels. An over response can sometimes be anticipated if there has been a previous over response or if the patient has got a polycystic ovarian morphology on her initial diagnostic ultrasound. There seems to be no value in routine oestradiol monitoring.

Monitoring during the stimulatory phase allows the dose to be increased or decreased, if appropriate, as well as to allow for the timing of the hCG injection.

hCG INJECTION

This is used to induce final maturation of the oocytes prior to the oocyte retrieval. 10,000 units of urinary hCG is generally used although in patients with an over response this can be decreased down to 5000 units. With the recent introduction of recombinant hCG given, the usual dose is 150 μg given subcutaneously.

hCG should be given when either one or two lead follicles have reached 18mm. The injection is normally given around midnight to allow for oocyte retrieval approximately 34 hours later prior to physiological ovulation occurring. If the hCG injection is incorrectly administered

then either very few or no eggs are obtained at the egg collection itself.

OOCYTE RETRIEVAL

Originally, this was done laparoscopically but with the advent of real-time ultrasound this allowed a less invasive oocyte retrieval by ultrasound directed needling of the ovaries. Smaller and better quality ultrasound probes, particularly with the advent of transvaginal (TV) scanning, has allowed both the monitoring of the ovary during stimulation and the actual retrieval itself to be done transvaginally. Virtually all oocyte retrievals at present are performed by this TV ultrasound directed route. The laparoscopic route is still occasionally used if the ovaries are inaccessible transvaginally. This can occasionally occur in frozen pelvises or when the ovaries have been moved out of the pelvis prior to pelvic irradiation.

Transvaginal egg (oocyte) retrievals (TVORs) can be performed under general anaesthesia or, more commonly these days, local anaesthesia and some form of intravenous sedation. The procedure generally takes 20–30 min, depending on how many follicles are present. A single use disposable needle is inserted under ultrasound control directly into the follicles of one ovary and the fluid aspirated and given directly to the embryologist. If the egg is not found after all the fluid has been aspirated, then the follicle is flushed and re-aspirated to try and find the egg, as well as using gentle needle agitation (Fig. 46.1). After all the follicles have been exhausted from one ovary, the needle is then withdrawn and re-inserted under ultrasound control into the other ovary and the process repeated. After the ultrasound probe is removed, the vaginal vault is checked for bleeding and although bleeding is usually not a problem, occasionally an absorbable suture has to be inserted under direct vision for a specific bleeding point. Most patients go home a few hours after the procedure has finished.

EMBRYO TRANSFER

Eggs are fertilized either by routine insemination with a concentration of approximately 100,000 normally motile sperm per ml or by ICSI (see p.467). They are incubated in a commercially prepared culture medium under strict laboratory conditions. Not only is the temperature carefully controlled within the incubators but also the gas content and pH.

Most embryos are transferred at day 2 post egg collection. More embryos are now being transferred on day 5, at the blastocyst stage. Approximately 55 to 60% of all mature eggs fertilize normally and then these are graded by the

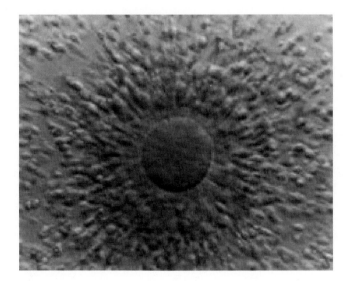

Fig. 46.1 Human oocyte with cumulus cells.

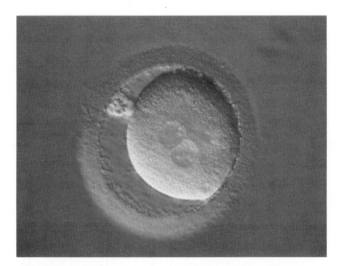

Fig. 46.2 Human Embryo 2 pro-nuclear (PN) stage day 1 – normal fertilization.

embryologist on day 2, prior to transfer (Fig. 46.2). At present the guidelines from the Humam Fertilization and Embryology Authority (HFEA) state that only 2 embryos should be transferred in people under the age of 40, unless exceptional circumstances are present, but over the age of 40 then three embryos can be transferred. In other countries in the world there is less regulation; in the USA, it would not be unusual for between 3 up to 5 embryos to be transferred, depending on the age of the patient. On the other hand in some Scandinavian countries, if the patient is 35 years old or younger, then they are moving towards elective single embryo transfer to reduce the incidence of twins or triplets. Although this would have a slight effect on success rates, the other normal embryos are

frozen and hence if a cycle is unsuccessful, then the patient can undergo repeated single embryo transfers from frozen embryo replacement cycles.

The benefits of a day 2 transfer are that a single stage culture medium can be used and also that the majority of normal embryos survive to this stage. After two or three embryos have been replaced, there may be surplus embryos of a satisfactory quality that are suitable for cryopreservation. The potential downside of a day 2 transfer is that in a normal menstrual cycle, the day 2 embryo is still in the fallopian tube and not in the uterine cavity. The grading system utilized by the embryologist is not totally accurate and therefore it can sometimes be difficult to judge the best two embryos out of potentially 6 or 7 to transfer fresh. The benefit for a day 5, or blastocyst, transfer is that the embryo has been replaced when it would physiologically be in the uterine cavity and this may have some benefits regarding certain growth factors which can improve embryo development. Blastocyst transfer also allows better selection of the embryos as the majority of abnormal embryos perish between day 2 and day 5 (Figs 46.3–46.6). However, even in the best cycles there are quite often only 2 or sometimes 3 blastocysts left after 5 days of culture. The downside of blastocyst transfer is that it requires a 2 stage culture medium as the blastocyst metabolic requirements change after day 2 and that there are generally no embryos left over that would be suitable for freezing. The other potential downside is in some patients all of the embryos may perish before day 5 and hence the patient may have nothing to transfer at all. It is for this last reason that the majority of centres will only do a blastocyst transfer if the patient has five or more good quality embryos. Embryo transfer is performed without any anaesthetic and a Cuscoe's speculum is generally used to visualize the cervix. The cervix is cleaned carefully and a sterile, single use, embryo transfer catheter carefully inserted through the cervical canal. Where in the uterine cavity the embryos are replaced is a topic of great debate, but it is not uncommon for people to place them in the mid-cavity portion and generally to stop insertion of the catheter before it hits the fundus where it could potentially cause some slight trauma and bleeding. Embryo transfer should be performed under ultrasound guidance as this allows more accurate placement of the embryos in the uterine cavity and has been shown to significantly improve success rates [8]. After the outer sheath has been inserted in the correct location, an inner catheter containing the embryos is inserted into the outer sheath. When it is in the correct position a very small aliquot of fluid is used to emit the embryos from the end of the catheter. The inner catheter is then removed and handed back to the embryologists who check to make sure there are no retained embryos in this inner catheter. If the catheter is clear then

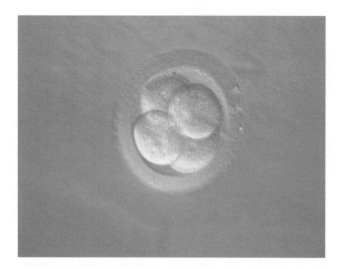

Fig. 46.3 4 cell stage – day 2.

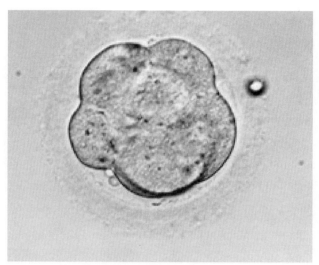

Fig. 46.5 Morula – day 4.

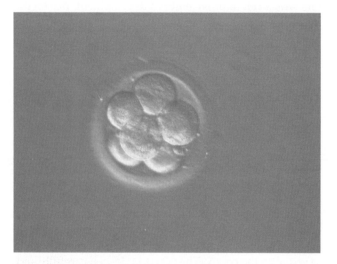

Fig. 46.4 8 cell stage – day 3.

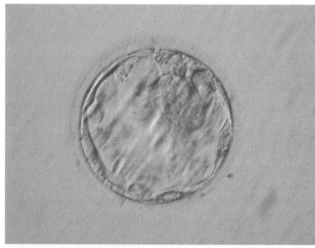

Fig. 46.6 Blastocyst – day 5.

the outer sheath is gently withdrawn and the speculum removed.

Although there is no chance that the embryos can 'fall out', many patients are not surprisingly very cautious at this stage and quite often are allowed to rest in a supine position for anywhere up to 2 hours before being allowed to leave the hospital. There has been no evidence that has shown that leaving the patients in a supine position increases pregnancy rates, but it certainly does help the patients psychologically.

LUTEAL PHASE SUPPORT

With modern assisted conception utilizing either agonist or antagonist protocols some form of luteal phase support

(LPS) is generally thought necessary. Although natural cycle IVF does not need this, supraovulation may impair normal corpus luteal function and the use of LPS has been shown to improve success rates [9]. The use of LPS with antagonist cycles is more debatable, but pregnancy rates without it are generally thought to be significantly lower [10]. LPS is broadly divided into two types, first the use of luteolytic preparations, such as hCG and second, the use of progestogens or progesterone. hCG is given by a subcuticular injection in small aliquots that stimulates the patient's own ovaries to produce more progesterone. It has been shown to be equally efficacious as progesterone but does require an injection and also increases the risk of ovarian hyperstimulation syndrome in some patients.

The use of progesterones is more common and these can be given as tablets, injections or vaginal pessaries/rectal suppositories. Intravaginal or rectal use of progesterone achieves extremely good tissue levels very rapidly. It is known that LPS should be given for a minimum of 2 weeks, but some clinics routinely use up to 12 weeks or even later but there is no evidence that continuing it beyond 2 weeks significantly improves pregnancy rates. The minimum dose required is 200 mg of the cyclogest a day but the most commonly prescribed dose is 400–800 mg a day.

PREGNANCY TEST

The wait between the embryos being replaced and the pregnancy test is the most psychologically stressful time for the majority of patients. Some patients start bleeding prior to the pregnancy test, (although it is not unusual for the progesterone to delay this bleeding) even if they are not pregnant. Generally pregnancy tests are performed around 12 days from the embryo transfer and can either be performed at home with a urinary pregnancy test or at the clinic with a serum pregnancy test. A home pregnancy test is obviously more convenient, but unfortunately only has sensitivity down to 50 IU. If the pregnancy test is positive and in the normal range, then it is usual to offer the patient a transvaginal scan 2 to 3 weeks later to ensure that the pregnancy is intrauterine and also to assess its viability. If the initial hCG level is low, then this is often repeated 48 h later to assess the rise, and it if it is suboptimal, then the possibility of an ectopic pregnancy or miscarriage has to be considered.

RESULTS

The most important factor by far when assessing the pregnancy outcomes of IVF cycles is female age (see Table 46.2 with most recent data from The Centre for Disease Control, USA). Male age in comparison has very little impact. The aetiology of the infertility also has a significant effect as can be seen from Table 46.3. The 2 factors that patients have under their own control that can adversely affect pregnancy results are smoking and obesity (see NICE guidelines). Laboratory conditions have gradually improved along with transfer techniques which have resulted in an increase in overall results over the last 6 years (Table 46.4).

Intra-cytoplasmic sperm injection

Intra-cytoplasmic sperm injection (ICSI) is where individual morphologically normal sperm are immobilized and injected into a mature oocyte that has had its surrounded cumulus and corona cells removed. An inverted microscope with a heated stage and micromanipulating equipment (Fig. 46.7) is used. The oocyte is carefully positioned using a holding pipette under gentle suction, a very sharp glass injecting pipette is slowly inserted to rupture the oolemma and the immobilized sperm injected into the oocyte with a very small volume of the medium. The injecting pipette is then carefully removed and the oocyte incubated under the usual stringent laboratory conditions.

INDICATIONS

• Severe male factor including azoospermia and subsequent surgical sperm retrieval, either by MESA, TESE, PESA etc.
• Severe oligo-asthenoterato-zoospermia.
• Poor or total non-fertilization from previous IVF cycles.
• Preimplantation Genetic diagnosis cycles.

Most IVF units would have approximately 40 to 60% of their total IVF cycles using ICSI. Studies have been performed to see whether ICSI improves pregnancy rates with normal sperm parameters but there has not been any improvement shown by the routine use of ICSI [11].

RESULTS

Pregnancy rates of 36.5% per transfer are reported [12] with live birth rates of 30.4% per transfer based on over 28,800 cycles.

SAFETY

ICSI has been in clinical use since 1991 and all the results of the follow-up studies are generally reassuring. The current recommendations are that any male who has sperm parameters that require ICSI should be offered screening for karyotype as well as cystic fibrosis screening. Some centres also advocate the use of Y chromosome microdeletion screening, although this is not routinely offered. Cystic fibrosis screening is essential in cases of azoospermia, particularly if it is related to the condition of congenital bilateral absence of the vas deferens, as a significant proportion of these patients will be carriers of the cystic fibrosis mutations. Being a carrier does not preclude them being treated as a couple, but the female partner is then offered screening, and if she also is found to be a carrier, then they should be referred for consideration of IVF–ICSI with PGS.

If all the above results are normal, then the patients should be counselled carefully that there is a slight increase in genetic abnormalities of the offspring. Most of these abnormalities are thought to be minor and the major

Table 46.2 (a) Live births per transfer and singleton live births per transfer for assisted reproductive technology procedures performed among women who used freshly fertilized embryos from their own eggs, by patient's age — United States, 2002. (b) Live Births per Transfer for ART Cycles Using Fresh Embryos from Own and Donor Eggs, by ART Patient's Age, 2002

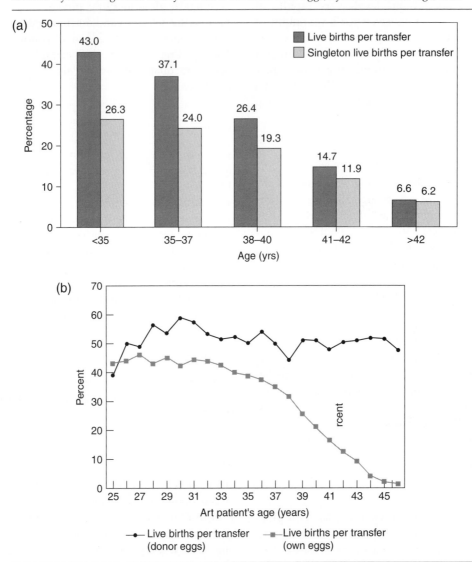

congenital malformation rate is generally thought to be similar to that of the general population.

Gamete intrafallopian tube transfer

Gamete intrafallopian tube transfer (GIFT) was first used around 1984 and here the eggs are collected laparoscopically, identified by the embryologist and then placed back in the fallopian tube, again laparoscopically, with a small aliquot of specially prepared highly motile sperm. The use of GIFT reached a peak in the early 1990s and has been diminishing since then.

ADVANTAGES

GIFT was initially developed to increase the availability of assisted conception due to the scarcity of suitable laboratory facilities and embryological skills. Since the eggs did not have to be cultured outside the body then few of the usual laboratory facilities were needed. Also it appears to be very physiologically sound as both the egg and sperm are in the appropriate place at the appropriate time. The embryo travels physiologically down into the uterine cavity and hence there is no disruption of the endometrial environment – as there is with normal embryo transfer from IVF.

Table 46.3 Live birth rates for assisted reproductive technology (ART) transfer procedures performed among patients who used freshly fertilized embryos from their own eggs, by patient age and selected patient ad treatment factors—United States, 2002

	Patient age (yrs)				
	<35 Live births per transfer procedure (%)	35–37 Live births per transfer procedure (%)	38–40 Live births per transfer procedure (%)	41–42 Live births per transfer procedure (%)	>42 Live births per transfer procedure (%)
Total	43.0	37.1	26.4	14.7	6.6
Patient factors					
Diagnosis					
Tubal factor	43.4*	37.2	28.3	14.5*	6.4
Ovulatory dysfunction	45.0	40.5	27.3	15.3	6.3
Diminished ovarian reserve	35.7	29.2	21.7	16.5	7.1
Endometriosis	43.9	37.4	31.6	20.3	7.0
Uterine factor	37.2	30.0	24.7	19.4	6.7
Male factor	45.2	39.2	28.2	15.4	4.4
Other causes	40.9	40.1	28.3	16.9	6.3
Unexplained cause	43.1	39.6	28.6	15.3	8.6
Multiple factors, female only	41.0	32.7	23.5	12.7	6.7
Multiple factors, female and male	40.9	35.7	23.9	12.1	5.9
Number of previous ART procedures					
0	45.2*	39.2*	28.1*	15.1	6.1
≥1	39.4	34.8	24.9	14.3	7.0
Number of previous births					
0	41.6*	35.6*	25.2*	14.0	6.4
≥1	48.5	40.3	28.7	15.9	7.0
Treatment factors					
Method of embryo fertilization and transfer[†]					
IVF-ET without ICSI	45.3*	39.9*	28.2*	17.2*	8.2*
IVF-ET with ICSI among couples diagnosed with male factor infertility	43.2	37.1	25.9	12.6	5.1
IVF-ET with ICSI among couples not diagnosed with male factor infertility	39.5	33.6	24.5	13.6	5.5
Number of days of embryo culture[§]					
3	41.9*	36.8*	25.7*	14.5*	6.3*
5	49.7	42.7	35.1	20.9	14.8
Number of embryos transferred					
1	20.8*	14.6*	10.4*	3.5*	1.0*
2	46.3	37.7	23.3	10.4	5.0
3	43.6	39.6	28.9	13.5	5.9
4	39.0	38.4	29.9	16.6	8.4
≥5	39.2	38.1	28.1	21.8	10.2
Extra embryo(s) available and cryopreserved					
Yes	50.4*	46.7*	38.1*	24.4*	15.3*
No	37.5	32.9	23.8	13.7	6.2
Use of gestational carrier					
Yes	49.2	43.7	27.8	24.2*	11.1
No	42.9	37.0	26.4	14.6	6.6

*$P < 0.05$; chi-square to test for variations in live birth rates across patient and treatment factor categories within each age group.

[†]IVF-ET = *in vitro* fertilization with transcervical embryo transfer, and ICSI = intra-cytoplasmic sperm injection. ART procedures including GIFT, ZIFT, and a combination of IVF with or without ICSI and either GIFT or ZIFT were not included because each of these accounted for a limited proportion of procedures.

[§]Limited to 3 and 5 days to embryo culture. ART procedures including 1, 2, 4 and 6 days to embryo culture were not included because each of these accounted for a limited proportion of procedures.

Table 46.4 Live births per Transfer, by Type of ART Procedure, 1996, 2001, and 2002

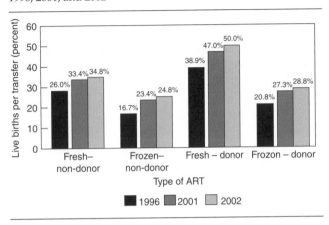

DISADVANTAGES

It is more invasive than IVF as a laparoscope is used to replace the embryos and sperm through the fimbrial end of the fallopian tube. The eggs are generally collected by transvaginal egg collection as it has been shown that more eggs are obtained by this route. As part of good clinical practice, only a limited number of eggs are replaced, even though it is not known whether these will fertilize normally by the sperm that is added. Therefore less information is obtained than with an IVF cycle. At least one fallopian tube should be healthy. Normal sperm parameters are also optimal, although GIFT can be used in cases of mild male factor disease.

The place of GIFT in the third millennium is often debated and its routine use is now very limited. Most

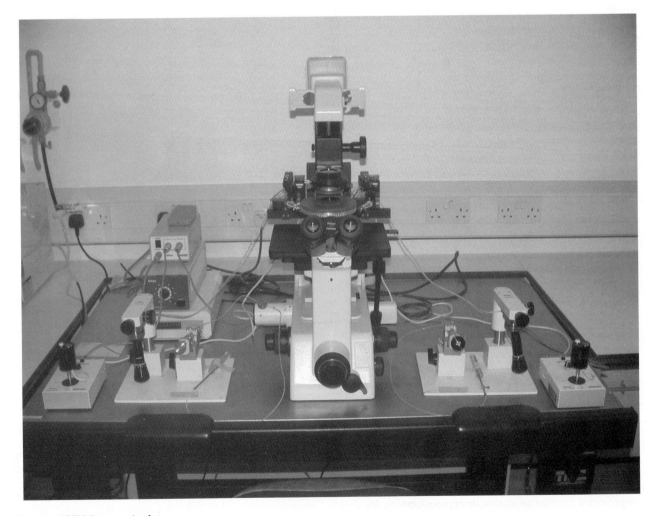

Fig. 46.7 ICSI Micromanipulator.

European centres would only use it in cases where IVF is not allowed for religious reasons. Since conception occurs within the body, GIFT is often acceptable even though IVF is not. In some cases of totally unexplained infertility, where there has been repeated IUI and IVF failures, GIFT may also have a small place.

SUCCESS RATES

These vary enormously depending on patient selection, but success rates in appropriate circumstances can be 30% live birth per transfer [12]. Apart from a few advocates the use of GIFT in most large clinics accounts for less than 0.5% of all their assisted reproductive technology (ART) cycles.

Frozen embryo replacement cycle

The first pregnancy resulting from a frozen human embryo was in 1985 and since then the use of frozen cycles has increased dramatically. Freezing surplus morphologically normal embryos allows the use of those embryos which otherwise may have been wasted. It therefore gives double benefit from one fresh cycle and significantly adds the cumulative conception rate per cycle when surplus embryos are frozen. Normally embryos are frozen on day 2 after the selected ones have been replaced fresh, but can be frozen anytime from day 1 through to day 5 if excess blastocysts are obtained. The use of day 1 freezing is normally confined to elective freezing of all embryos when there is a high risk of ovarian hyperstimulation syndrome occurring. At day 2 any morphologically normal embryos of suitable quality are selected and through specific cryopreservation protocols are frozen and stored in liquid nitrogen in specially monitored tanks. The success rates of day 1 and day 2 embryos are cited as 20.4% live birth rate per transfer [12]. The success rates of frozen blastocyst cycles are still suboptimal although a lot of work is going on at present to try and improve the cryoprotectants used as well as the actual programmes for preserving them.

TRANSFER OF FROZEN EMBRYOS

There are 2 main ways to transfer frozen embryos; first, replace them in a spontaneous menstrual cycle or, second, suppress the patient's own menstrual cycle with GnRH agonists and then supplement with oestrogen to thicken the endometrium prior to embryo replacement.

NATURAL CYCLE

The patient has to have regular menstrual cycles for this to be a feasible option and the patient's cycle is then monitored by serial ultrasound scan as well as hormone profiling, including oestradiol and LH measurement. As long as there are no adverse factors noted on these measurements, the embryos are thawed and replaced approximately 3 days after the LH surge has been detected. Approximately two thirds of all frozen embryos survive the thaw process, and depending on the age of the patient, two or three embryos are replaced. No luteal phase support is required as the ovaries are not down-regulated, and sufficient natural progesterone is produced from the patient's own corpus luteum.

SUPPRESSED CYCLES

The majority of FERCs are with suppressed cycles as this gives better control and better results. A GnRH agonist is used to suppress the patient's menstrual cycle and is normally started on day 21. If the patient is menopausal then this is not required and only oestrogen supplementation is used. After adequate suppression has been achieved then hormone supplementation in the form of oestrogen is used. This is generally an increasing regime with either tablets or patches until sufficient endometrial thickness has been achieved. The embryos are replaced in a similar fashion to IVF and, due to ovarian suppression, LPS is required. If the patient is pregnant this is continued up to approximately 12 weeks of pregnancy.

Virtually all IVF units should have a frozen embryo replacement programme and it is not only generally accepted as a safe and effective means of treatment but also one that is cost beneficial, maximizing the use of the patient's fresh cycle.

Egg donation

Oocyte donation is where a donor oocyte obtained from a fresh IVF cycle from a suitable screened donor is fertilized with the recipient's partner's sperm and the fertilized embryo replaced in the patient, the recipient. The first successful pregnancy from an egg donation cycle was in 1983.

PROCEDURE

Unfertilized mature oocytes are obtained from a donor who in the UK should be a maximum of 35 years old, healthy and preferably of known fertility. The donor is screened for Hepatitis B, C and HIV as well as for appropriate genetic diseases. It is generally recommended that both the donor and recipient undergo counselling with regard to the implications of egg donation and the possible outcome. A routine IVF cycle is then performed and depending on the sperm parameters of the male partner of the recipient, the eggs fertilized either routinely or with

ICSI. The resultant embryos can be replaced fresh or in a frozen cycle.

The recipient is prepared in a similar way to FERCs – if the menstrual cycle is regular the embryos can be replaced in a natural cycle (although this is unusual as recipients rarely have normal menstrual cycles). More often than not, they are replaced as in a suppressed FERC with the use of oestrogen to get an optimum endometrium for implantation.

INDICATIONS

• Ovarian failure – either premature or physiological.
• Patients with very poor ovarian function where previous IVF has repeatedly failed.
• Patients over the age of 45 and with severe male factor disease necessitating ICSI.
• Patients with hereditary genetic disease where using the patients own gametes is not advisable.

BENEFITS

The recipient adopts the success rate corresponding to the age of the donor. Therefore success rates with egg donation are generally high. Any resultant offspring have the aneuploidy rates of the age of the donor as well. Therefore for a patient who is over the age of 40, the success rates are far greater and the risks of genetic disease, such as Downs Syndrome, significantly lower.

PROBLEMS

The main problem with oocyte donation is obtaining eggs. In the UK it is illegal at present to pay donors for their eggs and they are only allowed to be compensated minimally for their time and inconvenience. Since 1 April 2005 anonymity for the donors has also been repealed and any resultant offspring can trace their genetic mother from the age of 18. Not surprisingly, there is therefore a great paucity of suitable egg donors in the UK and most programmes at present rely on altruistic donors bought in by the recipients themselves. These are generally either family members or friends.

Egg share programmes can be used where a person requiring IVF for their own personal reasons agrees to donate half their eggs to an unknown recipient in lieu of having a reduced cost for their own IVF cycle. The use of egg share programmes has diminished since 1 April 2005, again because of this lack of anonymity to the donor.

Elsewhere in the world, particularly in the United States, donors are paid and therefore there tends not to be a lack of donors, but cycle costs are considerably higher.

Surrogacy

Surrogacy is used when a patient's uterus is either absent or unable to maintain a pregnancy, and a surrogate uterus is used to carry the pregnancy. Generally this procedure is used where a young patient has lost her uterus to cancer or to uncontrollable bleeding, e.g. post-partum haemorrhage or following a difficult myomectomy. The patient's own eggs are obtained as in an IVF cycle, fertilized by her partner's sperm and the resultant embryos replaced within the surrogate.

Counselling is obligatory for both the patients and the surrogate, and generally surrogates are women who have already had children themselves and are recruited either by the patients or through an organization such as COTS (Childlessness Overcome Through Surrogacy).

Surrogacy is legal in the UK and the surrogate can be compensated for time lost away from employment during the pregnancy. However, the child's legal mother is the woman who delivers the child and therefore the patient and the husband have to undergo formal adoption procedures to become the legal parents of their genetic offspring which the surrogate has delivered.

Egg freezing

Egg freezing is where eggs are obtained from an IVF cycle, but rather than being fertilized with sperm, are left unfertilized and then frozen for future use. Unfortunately, unfertilized eggs do not survive the freeze/thaw process anywhere near as well as an embryo due to the large size of the unfertilized eggs and the high water content. This causes problems during the freezing process as ice crystals can form within the egg, disrupting the delicate structures which can result in its demise when thawed. (Once an oocyte is fertilized the resultant cells are considerably smaller and therefore the problem of ice formation within these cells is significantly lower.) Success rates of egg freezing programmes at the moment give a per cycle pregnancy rate of approximately 2%. This will hopefully be significantly improved as cryoprotectants and protocols for freezing and thawing improve as research progresses in this difficult field.

INDICATIONS

• Fertility preservation, prior to chemotherapy or radiotherapy where the patient has not got a male partner.

- 'Social' egg freezing in professional women to try and preserve fertility, related to age related decreases in ovarian function.

Preimplantation genetic diagnosis

Preimplantation genetic diagnosis (PGD) is where one or two cells (blastomeres) are removed from the embryo prior to replacement in an IVF cycle. These are tested for specific genetic diseases and only unaffected embryos replaced. This was first used to try and diagnose either single gene defects or sex related disease. The first successful pregnancy was in 1990 in a couple who were both carriers of the Delta F508 Cystic Fibrosis gene, who already had an affected child [13]. This technique can now been used whenever there is a suitable probe for a single gene defect, or indeed any technique which could identify the gene sequence that gives rise to the particular disease.

INDICATIONS

- Single gene defects such as Cystic Fibrosis, Lesch-Nyham or Familial Polyposis Coli
- Sex linked disorders such as haemophilia or Duchenne muscular dystrophy

PROCEDURE

The embryos are obtained as with any routine IVF procedure, although generally ICSI is now used to minimize the potential for genetic contamination. The zona pellucida of the embryo is then opened either by using acid-tyrodes or using special lasers, and one or two blastomeres gently teased out of the embryo for the specific test itself. If it is a specific single gene defect, the embryos are tested by some form of polymerase chain reaction (PCR) whereas if it is for sexing the embryo, this is normally done by fluorescent in situ hybridization (FISH). Depending on the method of testing, the unaffected (or specific sex) embryos are then replaced either on day 2 or day 3 post collection.

Preimplantation genetic screening

Preimplantation genetic screening (PGS) is used to screen embryos for common aneuploidies by techniques such as FISH. Initially five chromosomes were screened (13, 18, 21, x and y) and now more commonly seven and colour FISH is used (13, 16, 18, 21, 22, x and y). As techniques progress then more chromosomes can be looked at, although there can be a problem with error rates, as you have to rehybridize the blastomere. The way forward is likely to be techniques that can look at the whole 23 pairs of chromosomes, such as whole genomic amplification and the use of gene chip technology.

INDICATIONS

At present the recommended indications for PGS are:
- Recurrent miscarriages
- Recurrent IVF failures
- Patients over the age of 37 undergoing IVF
- Previous aneuploid pregnancy

BENEFITS

If these techniques are shown to be clinically successful, then the obvious benefits would be improvement in overall IVF success rates, reduction in miscarriage rates and a reduction in terminations of pregnancies for aneuploidies such as Downs Syndrome.

PROBLEMS

At present there is not a robust enough evidence base to recommend PGS and more research needs to be done. Most importantly the use of techniques that can screen more of the chromosomes will be developed to make PGS more likely to be clinically beneficial. Surprisingly, the safety aspects so far appear to be very reassuring and even though potentially a quarter of the embryo is removed this does not seem to impact on the overall implantation rate and health of the offspring. Again, longer-term follow-up is required to prove conclusively the safety of these techniques.

They are also relatively expensive and require dedicated laboratory facilities, particularly if specific gene defects are looked for.

Surgical sperm retrieval

In cases where there is either azoospermia or necro-zoospermia surgical sperm retrieval can be performed to obtain sperm directly from either the epididymus (microepididymal sperm aspiration – MESA) or directly from the testis (Testicular Sperm Extraction – TESE) or (Percutaneous Epididymal Sperm Aspiration – PESA). A biopsy should always be taken from each testis and sent off to histopathology, as carcinoma in situ can be found in approximately 1% of subfertile men.

These techniques can be performed either under local anaesthetic or under a light general anaesthetic. The patient should be screened for cystic fibrosis and karyotyping prior to the procedure. There are major chromosomal abnormalities in just over 2% of infertile men, which is 3 times the normal instance. In the case of azoospermia this rises to over 15%. If semen results are in the normal range, then chromosomal abnormalities are significantly lower. An FSH level is also beneficial in so far as if this is in the normal range, then the chance of getting usable spermatozoa is much higher (around 90% if the testicular volumes are normal) whereas if the FSH is markedly raised then the chance is significantly lower. (Less than 10% if the testicular volumes are reduced.)

Any sperm obtained through these techniques is then cryopreserved for future use. The sperm can be used fresh if the operation is timed to coincide with the oocyte retrieval on the female side. ICSI has to be used in all cases of surgical sperm retrieval as there is not enough motile sperm for normal fertilization.

Donor sperm

If there is no usable sperm obtained either from surgical sperm retrieval or from ejaculation, then the use of donor sperm is generally offered. Donor sperm is obtained by masturbation from healthy screened donors. All donor sperm in the UK has to be stored for 6 months, and then the donor screened again. Sperm can then only be released for use after both sets of screening have been found to be negative.

INDICATIONS

- Azoospermia
- Carriers of Severe Genetic Disease
- Lesbian/single women

USE

Donor sperm used to be inseminated around the cervix using an unprepared specimen around what was thought to be the fertile time. Now a prepared sample of sperm is used and inseminated directly into the uterine cavity as part of an intrauterine insemination (IUI) programme. The patient has the usual screening tests including a test of tubal patency, and then as long as the menstrual cycle is regular, the cycle is monitored and then at the appropriate time, around ovulation, the prepared sample is inseminated directly into the cavity. If the patient has irregular cycles or unstimulated IUI has been unsuccessful, then stimulated IUI can be performed and success rates are generally higher. If the fallopian tubes are severely damaged or blocked, then the donor sperm has to be utilized with techniques such as IVF. Success rates are almost entirely dependant on the age of the patient herself.

Complications of assisted conception

Multiple births

The most common complication of assisted conception is that of multiple births. Of all the patients that have become pregnant through IVF programmes, approximately 25% have twins when 2 or 3 embryos are transferred. Triplet rates vary depending on the percentage of embryo transfers that are three embryos or more. In the UK the maximum of 3 embryos can be transferred, but only under exceptional circumstances or if the patient is 40 years old or greater. The majority of embryo transfers in the UK at present are two embryo transfers. Even with a twin pregnancy, the risk of cerebral palsy is up to 8 times greater than that of a singleton pregnancy. In triplet pregnancies, the rate can be as high as 47 times greater. The offspring also are at risk of all the other multiple sequelae of prematurity [14].

To try and reduce the rate of multiple births, the HFEA has made strong recommendations that only 2 embryos are transferred. As success rates across the world improve, then there is more of a move towards single embryo transfers, which will reduce the twin rate to monozygotic twins only. Indeed in some Scandinavian countries, if the patient is 35 years old or under then elective single embryo transfer is the only route allowed. One embryo is transferred fresh and all the other embryos are frozen, and then the patient undergoes repeated single embryo transfer until she gets the desired outcome, or all the embryos are used up. This is certainly the way forward, but to persuade patients themselves that this is suitable is more difficult as at present many patients see the desired outcome as being twins.

Ovarian hyperstimulation syndrome

Ovarian hyperstimulation syndrome (OHHS) can occur in any IVF cycle, but usually is only mild to moderate. Severe OHHS can be life threatening and should happen in less than 2% of cases. It generally occurs in specific at-risk groups, in particular in young patients who have polycystic ovaries. In these situations the starting dose of gonadotrophins should be lowered to take account of the increased sensitivity of the polycystic ovaries. Even in the best centres with the adequate monitoring there can be a surprisingly brisk ovarian response and the ovaries can hyperstimulate. In these situations several options are available. The cycle can be abandoned and then re-started at a lower dose or the eggs collected, fertilized and then all the embryos electively frozen as severe hyperstimulation tends to be most severe in patients who become pregnant from a fresh transfer. Lastly, if the risks have been fully considered and thought still acceptable, then the embryos can be transferred and the patient very carefully monitored. If she then goes on to develop severe hyperstimulation, she has to be admitted to hospital, her fluid balance managed very carefully and in particular her plasma protein levels monitored and human albumin solution given if they drop significantly. If the patient develops tense ascites then these can be drained on a daily basis, but not more than 1 litre should be drained in multiple aliquots as this often gives great relief, increases urinary output but does not drop the patient's protein levels too abruptly. If the patient develops pleural effusions, these also can be tapped, although generally draining the ascites helps these as well. Due to the increased risk of thrombo-embolitic disease, patients also should be given thrombo-prophylaxis in the form of antithrombotic stockings and low molecular weight heparin daily. Generally the condition is self-limiting but the patient should be kept in hospital and closely monitored until the OHSS has resolved. The condition does not appear to adversely effect the fetus and generally they go on to have successful pregnancies. In rare occasions where the situation is deteriorating and the patient's life is at risk, the pregnancy may need to be terminated, although fortunately this is rarely needed.

Ectopic pregnancies

Ectopic pregnancies can occur with any of the assisted reproductive techniques. This is not only in patients with tubal disease, but any patient undergoing any form of assisted conception is at a greater risk. In IVF programmes the generally accepted rate is between 2 and 5%, even though the embryos are transferred directly into the uterine cavity. This may be due to uterine contractions and it is probable that embryos move into the fallopian tubes at some stage but return to the uterine cavity in the majority of cases. Tubal contractions also facilitate transfer of the embryo towards the uterine cavity as it would in any physiological situation. It is for these reasons that all patients who have become pregnant by assisted conception, should be followed up by quantitative Beta hCG levels, and then most importantly offered an early scan to ensure that the pregnancy is intrauterine. If the pregnancy is found to be extra-uterine, then the full range of treatment options should be discussed with the patient.

With the increasing amount of salpingectomies performed for hydrosalpinges, it is hoped that the incidence of ectopic pregnancies with IVF will reduce.

TVOR complications

There are always accepted risks of complications from ultrasound-guided oocyte retrievals, and these can range from infection of the ovaries causing ovarian abscess, through to damage to the bowel. These are generally quoted at 1% or less, and all patients should be counselled about them prior to starting their treatment.

References

1. Strandell A, Bourne T, Bergh C, Granberg S, Asztely M & Thorburn J (1999) The assessment of endometrial pathology and tubal patency: a comparison between the use of ultrasonography and X-ray hysterosalpingography for the investigation of infertility patients. *Ultrasound Obstet Gynecol* **14**, 200–4.
2. Strandell A, Lindhard A, Waldenstrom U & Thorburn J (2001) Hydrosalpinx and IVF outcome: cumulative results after salpingectomy in a randomized controlled trial. *Hum Reprod* **16**, 2403–10.
3. Surrey ES, Minjarez DA, Stevens JM & Schoolcraft WB (2005) Effect of myomectomy on the outcome of assisted reproductive technologies. *Fertil Steril* **83**, 1473–9.
4. Eldar-Geva T, Meagher S, Healy DL, MacLachlan V, Breheny S & Wood C (1998) Effect of intramural, subserosal and submucosal intrauterine fibroids on the outcome of assisted reproductive technology treatment. *Fertil Steril* **70**, 687–91.
5. Hart R, Khalaf Y, Yeong CT, Seed P, Taylor A & Braude P (2001) A post prospective control study on the effect of intramural fibroids on the outcome of assisted conception. *Hum Reprod* **60**, 2411–7.
6. Johnson NP, Mak W & Sowter MC (2004) Surgical treatment for tubal disease in women due to undergo *in vitro* fertilisation. *Cochrane Databse Syst Rev* **3**, CD002125.
7. Cohlen BJ, Vandekerckhove P, te Velde ER & Habbma JD (2000) Timed intercourse versus intra-uterine insemination with or without ovarian hyperstimulation for subfertility in men. *Cochrane Database Syst Rev* **2**, CD000360.
8. Buckett WM (2003) A meta-analysis of ultrasound-guided versus clinical touch embryo transfer. *Fertil Steril* **80**, 1037–41.
9. Nosarka S, Kruger T, Siebert I, Grove D (2005) Luteal phase support in IVF: meta-analysis of randomised trials *Gynecol Obstet Invest* **60**, 67–74.
10. Daya S & Gunby J (2004) Luteal phase support in assisted reproduction cycles. *Cochrane Database Syst Rev* **3**, CD004830.
11. Devroey P (1998) Clinical application of new micromanipulative technologies to treat the male. *Hum Reprod* **13**(Suppl 3), 112–22.
12. Society for Assisted Reproductive Technologies (2004) Assisted reproductive technologies in the united states: 2000 results *Fertil Steril* **81**, 1207–20.
13. Ao A, Ray P, Harper J et al. (1996) Clinical experience with preimplantation genetic diagnosis of cystic fibrosis (delta F508). *Prenat Diagn* **16**, 137–42.

14. Pharoah PO (2005) Risk of cerebral palsy in multiple pregnancies. *Obstet Gynecol Clin North Am* **32**, 55–67.

Further reading

Brinsden P (ed.) (1999) *A Textbook of In Vitro Fertilisation and Assisted Reproduction: the Bourn Hall Guide to Clinical and Laboratory Practice*, 2nd edn. London: Parthenon Publishing.

Gardner DK, Weissman A, Howles CM & Shoham Z (eds) (2004) *Textbook of Assisted Reproductive Techniques – Laboratory & Clinical perspectives*. London: Taylor & Francis, A Martin Dunitz Book.

Report on Fertility Clinical Guidelines at: www.nice.org.uk

CDC report on ART in the USA 2002: www.cdc.gov/reproductivehealth

Chapter 47: Menopause and the postmenopausal woman

Nick Panay

Introduction

We live in an era when the population is ageing; at the time of writing more than 30% of women are aged 50 years of age or over. Maintenance of peri- and postmenopausal health is therefore of paramount importance if we are to minimize the economic impact on society in this and future millennia. The recent adverse media on hormone replacement therapy (HRT), still the most effective treatment available for the alleviation of menopausal symptoms, could therefore not have come at a worse time. The controversy surrounding the pros and cons of HRT has left menopausal women, health professionals and society in general, confused as to how best to deal with both the short- and long-term sequelae of the menopause. The immediate symptoms, often debilitating and the long-term sequelae such as osteoporosis, still need to be dealt with, and will take on ever increasing importance because of our ageing society.

Menopause demographics

Two hundred years ago only 30% of women lived through a menopause; now, more than 90% will. Thus, the menopause transition and postmenopause is very much a condition of the 20th and 21st centuries. Life expectancy is now 82 years of age for a woman living in the UK. The majority of women can therefore expect to live over a third of their lives in a menopausal state (Fig. 47.1).

Unfortunately, many of these postmenopausal women will have a progressively declining quality of life. Optimization of menopause health care should produce a rectangularization of society where postmenopausal women remain at the peak of health.

Menopause physiology

The menopause, from the Greek 'Menos' (month) and 'Pausis' (cessation) is defined as the last menstrual period. The diagnosis can only be made retrospectively after

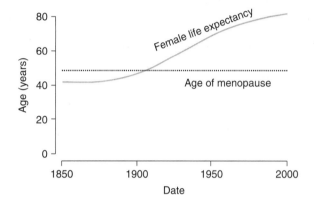

Fig. 47.1 Female life expectancy. From Cope 1976.

a minimum of 1 year's amenorrhoea. Although the menopause occurs at an average age of 51, the physiological changes which result in the final menstrual period (FMP) can start 10 years prior to this. Hormonal changes continue long after the FMP. This episode of dynamic neuroendocrine change is characterized by 'the climacteric' from the Greek 'Klimax' ladder, that is, the climb to the menopause. It may be associated with distressing clinical problems such as reduced fertility, menstrual irregularity and vasomotor symptoms. The intermediate sequelae of these changes are typically seen in the skin and urogenital tract and in the long term, in skeletal and cardiovascular pathology.

The declining oocyte pool

A newborn female infant has over a million oocytes; the oocyte cohort shrinks throughout life such that there are only a few thousand oocytes left as a woman enters her forties and few or none in the postmenopause. It is the depletion of oocytes which eventually leads to the cessation of menstruation, the cardinal sign of the menopause. There are two landmarks in the ovarian failure process. First, there is a marked decline in fertility with no cycle dysfunction. Subsequently, cycle changes become noticeable as the follicular phase shortens and luteal phase dysfunction occurs.

Compensated and decompensated failure

Initially, the ovarian failure is compensated by gonadotrophin levels starting to rise, in some women from the age of 30 years. During this time there is evidence for a reduced number of gonadotrophin receptors in perimenopausal ovaries and Inhibin production from granulosa cells falls leading to a reduced Inhibin : FSH ratio. Decompensated failure then occurs due to the critical decline in the oocyte pool leading to further rises in follicle stimulating hormone (FSH) (10 to 20-fold); Luteinizing hormone (LH) rises only three fold due to its shorter half-life. Oestrogen levels drop due to a reduction in follicle number and qualitative effect on granulosa cell ageing. There is permanent cessation of progesterone production. Studies have shown that the decline in Inhibin B is progressive and not superior to FSH as a predictor of the FMP [1]. However, the early follicular phase drop is more readily detectable than FSH as an initial predictor of reduced ovarian reserve and menstrual irregularity.

Other hormonal changes

Both adrenal and ovarian androgen levels start to decline, from as early as 20 years of age through to the perimenopause stabilizing by the time of the FMP. Some testosterone continues to be produced by ovarian theca cells. The drop in androgen levels is particularly profound in premature ovarian failure, spontaneous or iatrogenic. Oestrogen therapy can increase sex hormone binding globulin levels which leads to further falls in free androgen levels. The main postmenopausal oestrogen is oestrone which is produced mainly in peripheral adipose tissue and the postmenopausal ovary by aromatization of adrenal androstenedione. The somatotrophic axis becomes less active with ageing leading to insulin resistance and a rise in central adiposity. This in turn leads to the change in body shape from the female gynaecoid shape to the male android shape, itself an independent risk factor for coronary heart disease. There are a number of factors involved in perimenopausal weight gain including genetic predisposition, socio-economic influences, reduction in caloric need and expenditure, reduced lean body mass and a reduction in resting basal metabolic rate.

The menstrual cycle

Anovulatory cycles become progressively common. If three or more menstruations are missed within a 12-month period it is likely that the menopause transition will be completed within 4 years. There can be continued oestrogen production in the absence of progesterone leading to endometrial proliferation, hyperplasia and at its extreme carcinoma. As a result, menstruation can become heavy, prolonged and unpredictable with intermenstrual bleeding (Fig. 47.2).

Prediction of ovarian reserve

The classic study of the Hutterite population who do not use contraception showed that fertility rates rapidly decrease over the age of 35 years due to reduced oocyte numbers, poor oocyte quality, reduced fertilization and implantation rates, reduced coital frequency and increased chromosomal anomalies. The success of oocyte donation in *in vitro* fertilization (IVF) treatment suggests that the endometrium remains healthy and receptive. Ovarian reserve and response to gonadotrophin stimulation can now be predicted by two methods; first, by estimation of early follicular phase FSH levels or Inhibin B and second by ultrasonographic measurement of ovarian volume.

An FSH level of >30 is regarded as being diagnostic of the menopause but can be misleading as levels can fluctuate if ovarian activity resumes as often does in the climacteric. Work is currently being conducted to develop an accurate predictive model for the menopause by combining FSH and Inhibin with anti-Mullerian hormone (AMH). There has been a great deal of publicity recently that follicular reserve can be predicted by measurement of ovarian volume [2]. The original work in fact took place over 10 years ago; a nomogram was produced from measurement in over 2000 normally cycling women where the mean volume was estimated to be 3.57 cm^3 [3]. Further work is required to confirm the predictive value of this model but it is conceivable that a model could be developed which would combine both hormonal and sonographic measurements.

Premature ovarian failure

Premature ovarian failure is said to have occurred when menstruation ceases before the age of 40 years and early menopause before the age of 45 years. Although there are many causes of early ovarian failure, the main cause is spontaneous or idiopathic. The main identified genetic causes are Turner's syndrome and Fragile X. Recently, forkhead genes (FOX03A defect) have been discovered which lead to early follicular activation and thus premature depletion of the follicle pool. Other causes include FSH receptor polymorphisms, where follicles are present but unable to respond due to the loss of the FSH receptor.

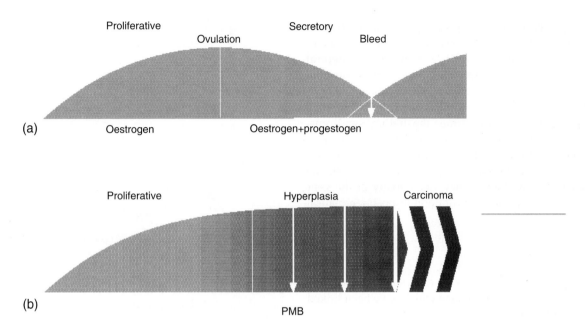

Fig. 47.2 Endometrial effects of perimenopause: (a) Normal cycle; (b) Unopposed oestrogen effect. From Kumar RJ (ed.) (2002) Blaustein's pathology of the female genital tract, 5th edn. New York: Springer.

The proportion of women with iatrogenic premature ovarian failure is growing as increasing numbers of women survive leukaemias, lymphomas and gynaecological cancers due to improved surgical techniques, radiotherapy and chemotherapeutic regimens.

Consequences of the menopause

Immediate

Seventy percent of Caucasians and Afro-Caribbeans suffer from hot flushes and sweats, the commonest menopausal symptoms. This compares to 10–20% of Japanese and Chinese women and may reflect cultural differences or may be diet related (e.g. isoflavone consumption in Asia). Hot flushes are thought to arise due to loss of oestrogenic induced opioid activity in the hypothalamus leading to thermo-dysregulation. It is thought that noradrenaline and serotonin mediate this activity; hence the rationale for using the alpha agonist clonidine and the selective serotonin and noradrenaline reuptake inhibitor (SNRI) venlafaxine as alternatives to HRT. Obese women are protected from these symptoms due to their production of large amounts of oestrone and their low sex hormone binding globulin levels which leaves more of the free active hormone.

Other typical immediate menopausal symptoms include insomnia, anxiety, irritability, memory loss, tiredness and poor concentration. Mood disturbances can occur due to fluctuation in hormone levels leading to perimenopausal depression. Falling oestrogen levels are thought to lead to similar falls in neurotransmitter levels such as serotonin which trigger these symptoms [4,5]. Women who have suffered from post-natal depression and premenstrual syndrome appear to be particularly predisposed to depression in the perimenopause. Stabilization of hormone levels, for example, with transedermal oestradiol appears to be particularly effective in ameliorating these symptoms. The effect of menopause on cognitive function is unclear; some studies suggest a reduction in cognitive ability during the menopause transition, for example mathematical or visuo-spatial tasks which can be improved with oestrogen replacement but larger randomized studies are required to confirm these findings.

The menopause transition can also be associated with a significant reduction in sexuality and libido. This is not only because of decreased vaginal lubrication leading to dyspareunia but also due to the reduction in androgen levels discussed earlier. In fact, there are more androgen receptors in the female forebrain than in the male which modulate for psychosexual parameters. The drop in androgens is particularly profound in women who have undergone early menopause or premature ovarian failure either spontaneously or due to iatrogenic intervention.

Intermediate

Oestrogen deficiency leads to the rapid loss of collagen which contributes to the generalized atrophy that occurs after the menopause. In the genital tract this is manifested by dyspareunia and vaginal bleeding from fragile atrophic skin. There is loss of rugations and occasionally stenosis. In the lower urinary tract, atrophy of the urethral epithelium occurs with decreased sensitivity of urethral smooth muscle and decreased amount of collagen in periurethral collagen. All this results in dysuria, urgency and frequency, commonly termed the urethral syndrome. More generalized changes are seen in the older woman as increased bruising and thin translucent skin which is vulnerable to trauma and infection. A similar loss of collagen from ligaments and joints may cause many of the generalized aches and pains so common in postmenopausal women.

Long term

Osteoporosis, cardiovascular disease and dementia are three long-term health problems which have been linked to the menopause.

OSTEOPOROSIS

Osteoporosis, or osteopenia, is a disorder of the bone matrix resulting in a reduction of bone strength to the extent that there is a significant increased risk of fracture. These fractures cause considerable morbidity in the elderly requiring prolonged hospital care and difficulties in remobilization. The economic consequences are also considerable: in the UK osteoporosis causes more than 150,000 fractures each year with an estimated cost of £1.75 billion per annum in the UK and $5 billion in the USA. With an ageing population and a real increase in the incidence of osteoporosis, this figure will rapidly rise.

Osteoporosis is predominantly a disease of women who achieve a lower peak bone mass than men and are then subjected to an accelerated loss of bone density following the menopause. The hypoestrogenic state leads to activation of the bone remodelling units with an excess of bone resorption relative to formation (Fig. 47.3) [6]. Women lose 50% of their skeleton by the age of 70 years, but men only lose 25% by the age of 90 years. The strength of bone is decreased to such an extent that by 70 years of age, 50% of women will have sustained at least one osteoporotic fracture.

Although the process of bone remodelling or its control has not yet been fully elucidated there is, at present, sufficient information available to conclude that ovarian steroids (oestrogens, androgens, progesterone) play an essential role in skeletal homeostasis. The mechanism of action of sex steroids on the skeleton is still not entirely clear, but it has traditionally included indirect effects on systemic hormones that regulate calcium balance and a direct receptor-mediated action. More recently, changes

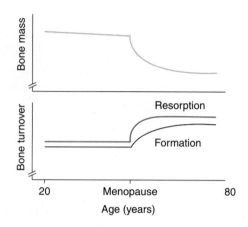

Fig. 47.3 Bone mass and turnover. From [6].

in cytokine production within the bone marrow, as well as pro-apoptotic and anti-apoptotic effects in the osteoblastic cells, have been proposed as new perspectives on the cellular and molecular mechanisms by which sex steroids influence adult bone homeostasis. Other factors influencing the predisposition to osteoporosis include genetic and racial predisposition, for example, Afro-Caribbean women are less susceptible to osteoporosis, use of corticosteroids and any factor which predisposes to a hypoestrogenic state including premenopausal amenorrhoea, low weight, smoking and premature ovarian failure. There are several genetic polymorphisms which may predispose to osteoporosis including the vitamin D and oestrogen receptor genes, the collagen 1A1 gene and genes for various cytokines including interleukin 6 and tumour growth factor-β.

CARDIOVASCULAR

Women are protected against cardiovascular disease before the menopause, after which the incidence rapidly increases reaching a similar frequency to men by the age of 70 years [7]. Surveys of menopausal women have shown that their perceived risk is that 4% will develop heart disease and 46% breast cancer whereas in reality 50% will develop heart disease and 4% breast cancer.

The protective effect of oestrogen in premenopausal women is thought to be mediated by an increase in high density lipoprotein (HDL) and a decrease in low density lipoprotein (LDL), nitric oxide mediated vasodilatation leading to increased myocardial blood flow, an antioxidant effect on endothelial cells and a direct effect on the aorta decreasing atheroma. Cross-sectional and prospective observational studies have shown that women going through the menopause transition have elevation of cholesterol, triglyceride and LDL levels and a reduction in HDL2 levels. A 9-year prospective study of 438 Australian women looked at the risk factors for women aged 45–55 years having a coronary event. Significant risk factors included a high body mass index (BMI) ($p < 0.001$) and a decrease in oestradiol levels ($p < 0.001$) [8]. A recent study showed that oestrogen status was an independent predictor of atherosclerotic plaque area after controlling for age, hypertension, diabetes, etc. [9]. Even normally cycling premenopausal women appear to have an increased cardiovascular disease risk if they have reduced ovarian reserve. Women with a day 3 FSH > 7 IU/l compared to those with a day 3 FSH < 7 IU/l were found to have significantly higher lipid levels, for example cholesterol ($p < 0.001$) and LDL ($p < 0.019$) [10].

CNS

Oestrogen also appears to have a direct effect on the vasculature of the central nervous system and promotes neuronal growth and neurotransmission. Studies have demonstrated that oestrogen may improve cerebral perfusion and cognition in women. In the long term this may prevent diseases with a vascular aetiology such as vascular dementia and Alzheimer's as the vasculature is clearly involved in this. In addition to the effect on vasculature in Alzheimer's disease, oestrogen may also intervene at the level of amyloid precursor protein. The failure to show benefit for dementia in older populations, and possibly an increased risk with HRT in some studies (Women's Health Initiative Memory Study [11]), may reflect the predominance of the pro-thrombotic effect of oestrogen in this age group (see 'HRT').

Patient assessment

The diagnosis of the menopause can usually be ascertained from a characteristic history of the vasomotor symptoms of hot flushes and night sweats and prolonged episodes of amenorrhoea. Measurement of plasma hormone levels in patients with classical symptoms are unnecessary, expensive, time consuming and of little clinical significance. However, in the young patient or in a woman after hysterectomy, where the diagnosis is more difficult and the metabolic implications are serious, measurement of FSH levels may be helpful, in which case repeated measurements of 15 IU/L or above may be regarded as climacteric. In patients still menstruating, persistent hot flushes and night sweats are suggestive of the climacteric, but in those patients with psychological symptoms the diagnosis may be more difficult even with an elaborate psychiatric history. In such cases it may be justified to give a trial of oestrogen therapy and monitor the response before discounting a hormonal aetiology.

After the diagnosis has been established, investigations should be no more than the annual screening which is normally applicable to middle-aged women. This should include assessment of weight, blood pressure and routine cervical cytology. Fasting lipid profile estimation may be useful in women with risk factors not only from a general screening point but also if the patient is contemplating starting HRT. A reanalysis of the data from the Women's Health Initiative (WHI) study (see 'HRT controversy') in which women with abnormal baseline lipids were excluded found no excess risk of cardiovascular disease [12]. If abnormal lipids are detected these should be corrected by diet and statins, if appropriate on an individual basis, before HRT is commenced.

Routine breast palpation and pelvic examination is unnecessary; these need only be performed if clinically indicated. Mammography should be performed as part of the national screening programme every 3 years unless more frequent examinations are clinically indicated. However, if a woman chooses to use HRT beyond the current age of breast screening cessation (65 years), mammographic screening should also continue. In women over 45 years of age it is best to arrange screening before starting oestrogen therapy to identify patients with sub-clinical disease. Endometrial biopsy is not a necessary prerequisite to treatment with HRT unless there are symptoms of postmenopausal bleeding or irregular perimenopausal bleeding. In the few cases where an underlying malignancy is present, bleeding will be irregular after starting treatment, indicating the need for immediate further investigation.

The best currently available measurement of osteoporosis risk is dual energy X-ray absorptiometry (DEXA) measurement of the lumbar spine and hip. Other assessment techniques such as peripheral X-ray screening, for example, proximal phalanx and calcaneal and ultrasound screening are improving in terms of their sensitivity and correlation with DEXA but the latter still remains the gold standard. Markers of bone formation and breakdown can be useful in that changes occur more rapidly than with bone density but their use is largely confined to research.

There has been some enthusiasm for the implementation of a national osteoporosis screening programme by measurement of bone density, because prediction of osteoporosis from clinical risk factors and the intensity of short-term symptoms is unreliable. This judgement is premature as no studies have yet demonstrated that bone densitometry is suitable for mass screening. The Royal College of Physicians (RCP) has therefore issued guidelines as to which high-risk patients should be targeted for DEXA screening (see 'useful websites'). The RCP advises that DEXAs are performed no more frequently than every 2 years because changes in bone mineral density are so small that they often do not exceed the margin of error of the equipment and assessor.

Therapeutic options

HRT

OESTROGEN

Dosage

There is general agreement now that patients should be started on the minimum effective dose of oestradiol, increasing the dose only if needed to alleviate symptoms. Although there is no direct evidence that higher doses of exogenous oestrogen are associated with increased risk of breast cancer or heart disease there is a link with venous thromboembolic risk. Importantly, lower doses of oestrogen are less likely to produce breast tenderness and bleeding problems which will reduce continuance of therapy.

The minimum dosages of currently available systemic oestrogen are as follows:
- 0.3–0.625 mg oral conjugated equine oestrogens
- 1 mg of oral micronized oestradiol or oestradiol valerate
- 25–50 mcg transdermal oestradiol
- 25–50 mg of implanted oestradiol
- 150 mcg transnasal oestradiol
- 50 mcg oestradiol silicone ring

Data suggest that the benefits of a 2 mg dose of oestradiol for symptoms and bone protection can be maintained by a 1 mg dose and similarly the benefits of a 50 mg oestradiol implant are maintained by a 25 mg implant [13]. Studies are currently ongoing to facilitate the licensing of a 0.5 mg oestradiol containing preparation which appears to adequately relieve symptoms. Exceptions to this 'low dose rule' are women who suffer premature ovarian failure who need higher doses of oestrogen to reproduce the physiological hormone levels which would have been present if the ovaries had not failed early. The optimum route of administration or dosage in this group of young women has yet to be determined.

Route of administration

If we adhere to the principle that we should try to reproduce the most physiological state possible with a 2:1 oestradiol: oestrone ratio then we should avoid the oral route altogether. Oral oestradiol preparations are partially metabolized to oestrone by hepatic first pass metabolism and therefore do not fully restore this ratio. There are twice weekly or once weekly changed transdermal systems containing either oestradiol alone or both oestradiol and progestogen. The combined patches are available in either sequential or continuous regimens. The hormone is adsorbed onto the adhesive matrix which avoids the skin reactions caused by the old alcohol reservoir patches.

Oestradiol can also be used transnasally in a 'pulsed' fashion which is thought to maintain the benefits while minimizing the side effects of chronically elevated oestrogen, for example, breast tenderness. It is also available as a low-volume daily transdermal gel or even as a silicone vaginal ring delivering oestradiol systemically for 3 months. The nasal, gel and ring preparations are oestrogen alone and should be combined with progestogen in women with a uterus (see 'Progestogens').

Local (vaginal) oestrogen [14]

Recently developed vaginal HRT regimens have managed to avoid the problem of endometrial stimulation. Creams using oestriol do not produce endometrial hyperplasia and the 17β oestradiol vaginal tablet and silicone vaginal ring also provide effective relief of local symptoms without any significant endometrial effects. These preparations can be used without progestogenic opposition but are only licensed for 3 months use in the UK and 1 year in Europe. Options for local vaginal oestrogen are as follows:
- 0.01% Oestriol cream and pessaries
- 0.1% Oestriol cream
- 25 mcg/24 h Oestradiol vaginal tablets
- 7.5 mcg/24 h Oestradiol releasing silicone ring
- Premarin cream – this preparation can potentially cause endometrial hyperplasia and should not be used without progestogenic opposition for more than 3 months.

PROGESTOGEN/PROGESTERONE

Regimens

Oestrogen was originally used unopposed in non-hysterectomized women. It was noted that this led to endometrial hyperplasia in up to 30% of cases. Progestogen has therefore been added to oestrogen therapy for the last 30 years to avoid hyperplasia and carcinoma. It is generally accepted that women commencing HRT should start on a sequential regimen, that is, continuous oestrogen with progestogen for 12 to 14 days per month. The typical dosages of the more commonly used progestogens are shown in Table 47.1.

Bleeding problems

If bleeding is heavy or erratic the dose of progestogen can be doubled or duration increased to 21 days. Persistent bleeding problems beyond 6 months warrant investigation with ultrasound scan and endometrial biopsy. After 1 year of therapy women can switch to a continuous combined regimen which aims to give a bleed free HRT regimen which will also minimize the risk of endometrial hyperplasia. Alternatively, women can be switched to the

Table 47.1 Minimum doses of progestogen given orally in HRT as endometrial protection

Progestogen type	Sequential combined daily dosage	Continuous combined daily dosage
C19 – testosterone derived progestogens		
Norethisterone	5 mg	0.5 mg
Levonorgestrel	75 mcg	n/a
Levonorgestrel (IUS)	n/a	20 mcg (10 mcg in development)
Norgestrel	150 mcg	50 mcg
C21- progesterone derived progestogens		
Dydrogesterone	10 mg	5 mg
Cyproterone	2 mg	1 mg
Medroxyprogesterone acetate	5 mg	2.5 mg
Micronized Progesterone	200 mg	100 mg
Cyclogest pessaries	400 mg	200 mg
Crinone gel (4 or 8 %)	Alternate day/12 days of cycle	Twice weekly

IUS, Intrauterine system.

tissue selective agent tibolone. With both these regimens there may be some erratic bleeding to begin with but 90% of those that persist with this regimens will eventually be completely bleed free. If starting HRT de novo a bleed free regimen can be used from the outset if the last menstrual period was over a year ago.

Progestogenic side effects

It is vital that we maximize compliance if patients are to receive the full benefits from hormone replacement therapy (HRT). One of the main factors for reduced compliance is that of progestogen intolerance. Progestogens have a variety of effects apart from the one for which their use was intended, that of secretory transformation of the endometrium. Symptoms of fluid retention are produced by the sodium retaining effect of the renin-aldosterone system which is triggered by stimulation of the mineralocorticoid receptor. Androgenic side effects such as acne and hirsuitism are a problem of the testosterone derived progestogens due to stimulation of the androgen receptors. Mood swings and PMS-like side effects result from stimulation of the central nervous system progesterone receptors [15].

Minimizing progestogen intolerance

The dose can be halved and duration of progestogen can be reduced to 7–10 days. However, this may result in bleeding problems and hyperplasia in a few cases (5–10%) so there should be a low threshold for performing ultrasound scans and endometrial sampling in these women. Natural progesterone has less side effects due to progesterone receptor specificity but is only available in a vaginal form in the UK (200–400 mg pessaries or 4–8% progesterone gel) though micronized oral progesterone is available in France. The levonorgestrel intrauterine system, recently granted a 4 year license in the UK for progestogenic opposition, also minimizes systemic progestogenic side effects by releasing the progestogen directly into the endometrium with low systemic levels. However, in severely progestogen intolerant women, even the low systemic levels of the 20 mcg levonorgestrel intrauterine system can still produce side effects. A smaller, lower dose, 10 mcg system is in phase III clinical trial stage of development and should be ideal for the severely progestogen intolerant woman [16]. A new progestogen, drospirenone, a spironolactone analogue, has recently been incorporated with low dose oestrogen in a continuous combined formulation. It is not only progesterone receptor specific but also has anti-androgenic and anti-mineralocorticoid properties, the former making it useful for hirsuitism and the latter for fluid retention. Also, it may have anti-hypertensive benefits.

Progestogenic risks

The Women's Health Inititiative (WHI) [17] and Million Women Study (MWS) [18] studies showed clearly that there is an excess risk of breast cancer using oestrogen and progestogen HRT compared to oestrogen alone. It has therefore been mooted that even non-hysterectomized women should be treated with oestrogen-only containing preparations. According to the MWS data, after 10 years of oestrogen and progestogen HRT there would be an extra 19 per 1000 cases of breast cancer and no cases of endometrial cancer; after 10 years of oestrogen alone in non-hystectomized women, there would be an extra 5 cases per 1000 of breast cancer and 10 cases per 1000 of endometrial cancer (total 15:1000). From this simplistic point of view, it would seem reasonable that all women (even with a uterus) should receive oestrogen alone. However, this does not take into account the excess cases of endometrial hyperplasia and bleeding problems. This would generate excessive investigations such as endometrial sampling, hysteroscopies and even hysterectomies which would not be without their own morbidity and mortality.

Current advice remains that progestogenic opposition should still be used. However, it is imperative that we continue to seek improved ways of administering the progestogens which are important in protecting the endometrium to avoid progestogenic side effects and minimize effects on breast tissue, for example, vaginal and intrauterine progestogens and natural progesterone. However, there is a lack of data as to the risk of breast cancer in women using oestrogen with a levonorgestrel intrauterine system.

TESTOSTERONE

Preparations/regimens

Unfortunately, only 100 mg/6 months implanted testosterone pellets are licensed for use in women; 25 mg pellets exist but must be ordered on a named patient basis. The realization that there is currently an unfilled market for female androgen replacement has led to the development of the 300 mcg per day testosterone transdermal system to treat 'hypoactive sexual desire disorder'. While the license for this product is awaited it is necessary to continue improvising if one wishes to use preparations other than implants.

One option is to use testosterone gel which comes in 50 mg, 5 ml sachets at a dose of 0.5–1.0 ml/day. If the free androgen index is kept within the physiological range there are rarely any side effects such as hirsuitism. Levels should be checked at baseline and repeated at 4–6 weeks. Research so far has suggested at worst a neutral effect on the cardiovascular system, for example, arterial compliance and lipid effects. Alternatives to this include scaled down dosages of testosterone injections and oral preparations though many avoid the latter route because of hepatic concerns.

THE HRT CONTROVERSY

Over the last few years, health professionals and their patients have been inundated with information regarding the potential benefits and risks of hormone replacement therapy. Information is available from a variety of sources; some are more reliable than others. The popular press subeditors, responsible for the headlines, often sensationalize the risks of HRT. This has left the average health professional in a very difficult position as to what to advise their patients and has left patients bemused as to where they should turn to obtain reliable advice.

Breast

Recent prospective randomized data from the WHI combined HRT study have confirmed the previous observational data from the Imperial Cancer Research Fund [19] (now 'Cancer Research UK') regarding the risks of breast cancer with HRT. The WHI study was stopped prematurely by the data safety monitoring board after running a

mean of 5.2 rather than 8.5 years. This was because it was deemed that the risk versus benefit statistic was exceeded due to an excess of breast cancer and coronary heart disease cases in the treatment arm (continuous combined conjugated equine oestrogens 0.625 mg and medroxyprogesterone acetate 2.5 mg). The data from the WHI study suggested an excess risk of breast cancer with combined hormone therapy of 4 cases per 1000 women after 5 years. A further analysis of the data this year detected a hazards ratio for breast cancer of 1.24 ($p > 0.001$) for an average of 5.6 year's exposure to HRT [20].

The MWS, a large questionnaire survey by Cancer Research UK of women attending the NHS breast screening programme, reported an increased risk of breast cancer diagnosis with all HRT regimens (Relative Risk [RR] 1.66 95% CI 1.58–1.75); there was a statistically higher risk with oestrogen/progestogen HRT (RR 2.00 [1.91–2.09]) than that seen with oestrogen alone (RR 1.30 [1.22–1.38]) or tibolone (RR 1.45 [1.25–1.67]). This was alarmingly reported by the press as a doubling of risk of breast cancer with HRT, failing to mention the absolute risk in terms of actual numbers of cases. For oestrogen alone it represented an additional 1.5 per 1000 cases after 5 years of use and for oestrogen/progestogen, an additional 6 per 1000 cases after 5 years of HRT. In women aged 50–64, whose baseline risk is 32:1000 anyway, this translated to 33.5 per 1000 and 38 per 1000 cases, respectively.

The higher risk estimates from the MWS compared to WHI were probably due to the observational nature of the MWS which underestimated duration of usage of HRT as it did not count years of HRT exposure from baseline to breast cancer reporting on the UK cancer registry. Also, bearing in mind the natural biology of breast cancer development, it is unlikely that the cancers diagnosed after 1 year had developed de novo – it is more likely that these cancers were missed by mammography at baseline and that HRT had acted as a promoter rather than an initiator. Although the MWS reported on there being an increase in mortality, this was of borderline significance RR 1.22 (CI 1.00–1.48) ($p = 0.05$); the absence of tumour details also made it difficult to draw any definitive conclusions on this issue. Numerous authors have expressed their reservations regarding the limitations of both the MWS and WHI data [21,22]. On the positive side, a second WHI study in hysterectomized women using unopposed oestrogen reported that the rate of invasive breast cancer diagnosed was 23% lower in the conjugated oestrogen group compared to the placebo and this comparison narrowly missed statistical significance ($p = 0.06$). This result was unanticipated and appears to suggest that it is the addition of progestogen to oestrogen which leads to the increased risk of breast cancer, not oestrogen alone [23].

Cardiovascular (coronary heart disease and stroke)

Initial cardiovascular data from observational studies suggested up to a 50% reduction in risk of coronary heart disease in HRT users and a neutral effect on stroke. The Heart Estrogen Replacement Study (HERS), however, did not confirm these data in women started on HRT for secondary prevention of coronary heart disease and the WHI did not show any benefit in a primary prevention setting [24]. In fact, WHI suggested that after a mean usage of 5 years there was an excess of heart disease cases in the active treatment arm of the study compared to placebo. The study also found an excess of stroke. The cardiovascular risks in WHI were small, equating to an extra 7–8 cases per 10,000 women per year. These were largely accounted for by an excess of cases in the first couple of years of use, probably due to an initial pro-thrombotic effect of the preparation used. The increase in risk for stroke was clearly age related (age 50–59, 4 cases, 60–69, 9 cases and 70–79 years, 13 cases per 10,000 women per year).

Encouragingly, results from the conjugated oestrogen only arm of the WHI study showed that there was no significant effect on Coronary heart disease (CHD) (primary outcome) compared with placebo (hazard ratio 0.91; 95% CI 0.72–1.15). This latest result again suggests that progestogen may be the problem with HRT. In view of the data from HERS and WHI, guidelines were issued from the American Heart Association and Medicines and Health Care Products Regulatory Agency (MHRA) that HRT should not be used for primary or secondary prevention of CHD.

Future work should now focus on new preparations in younger populations of women. A randomized pilot study from the National Heart and Lung Institute in women using another type of HRT (1 mg oestradiol 0.5 mg norethisterone) after myocardial infarction showed a reduction in risk of re-infarction in the active arm of the study. A larger study, funded by the MRC, is planned as a result of these data [25]. A recent meta-analysis of randomized controlled trials in women using HRT in over 26,000 women showed that in those who started HRT before the age of 60 years there was a 39% lower mortality compared to those on placebo RR 0.61 (CI 0.39–0.95) [26].

Dementia

Observational and case control data suggested a protective effect for oestrogen for the prevention of Alzheimer's disease. These data have not been supported by the recent randomized controlled data from the WHI memory study (WHIMS) which showed that there was a two fold increase risk of all-cause dementia [11]. However, the WHIMS data were from an older age group of women (average 67 years)

and it may be that the 'window' for Alzheimer's prevention may be in a much younger age group. There is growing evidence that the chief mechanism of action in all types of dementia is infarction secondary to cerebral micro-emboli. This is much more likely to happen if HRT is started in older age group women due to the predominance of pro-thrombotic events in the first few years. In a younger age group, the beneficial physiological effects of oestrogen on blood flow and lipids could potentially lead to long-term benefits [27].

Endometrial cancer

Some authors suggest that sequential combined HRT appears to slightly increase endometrial cancer risk with long-term use [28]. However, continuous combined HRT appears to confer a small protective effect as witnessed by the trend towards protection in the WHI RR 0.83 (0.47–1.47) and other studies [16,29].

The MWS Investigators recently published the analysis of the endometrial cancer data [30]. Non-HRT users had a risk of 3 cases per 1000 women after 5 years. Encouragingly, sequential combined HRT appeared to have a neutral effect overall on the endometrium. The study confirmed that continuous combined HRT had a protective effect (2/1000 after 5 years) and that women using oestrogen alone had an increased risk (5/1000 after 5 years). Surprisingly, there were also a larger number of endometrial cancers reported in the users of the tissue selective agent tibolone (6/1000 after 5 years). This can possibly be explained by the fact that higher risk women, for example, with a family history of endometrial cancer or with previous bleeding problems, have preferentially been started on tibolone because it has been viewed as a lower-risk product. The results of a large (>3000 women) two year prospective randomized trial (THEBES) comparing the effect of tibolone to placebo showed no evidence of endometrial hyperplasia or carcinoma with tibolone [31]. The safety monitoring board has encouragingly allowed the study to continue unchanged.

Venous thromboembolism

It is clear from studies including HERS and WHI that there is a two to three fold increase in risk of venous thromboembolism (VTE) with oral HRT with the greatest risk occurring in the first year of use. However, recent data suggest that transdermal therapy may not increase the risk of VTE [32]. There is biological plausibility for this; avoidance of hepatic first pass metabolism minimizes adverse effects on clotting factors and the fibrinolytic system.

Osteoporosis

For many years bone marker and bone density data suggested that HRT had a beneficial effect on the skeleton. The data from the WHI study finally provided strong grade A (randomized placebo controlled) evidence for the gold standard outcome measure, that is, prevention of fractures of the hip and spine (5 less cases per 10,000 women per year).

Colorectal cancer

The WHI study confirmed previous observational studies for the beneficial effect of combined HRT in reducing the incidence of colorectal cancer (6 less cases per 10,000 women per year) although interestingly not with oestrogen alone. As yet, there is still uncertainty as to the mechanism of action of HRT in reducing the risk of colorectal cancer.

CONTRAINDICATIONS TO HRT

Coronary heart disease, stroke and venous thromboembolism were considered in the previous section.

Natural oestrogens when given to normotensive or hypertensive women do not cause an elevation in blood pressure, and when given in combination with oral progesterone may actually lower blood pressure; therefore, there is no justification for withholding HRT from hypertensive women.

Fibroids are responsive to oestrogens, and involute after the menopause. HRT may continue to stimulate these benign gynaecological tumours causing some to increase in size. This can cause an increase in menstrual blood loss, but in practice this does not usually represent a problem as treatment can easily be discontinued. However, in patients with a good indication who wish to continue therapy, fibroid resection, embolization, myomectomy or hysterectomy are all options available.

Patients who have suffered with endometriosis and become menopausal, are usually 'cured' of their symptoms. Some may wish to consider HRT and recurrence rates of 4% on HRT can be expected. Recurrence of symptoms is alleviated by stopping HRT.

Treatment of patients with a past history of endometrial cancer is controversial, but there are reports of oestrogen use without any detrimental effects in stage I to III disease [33]. Squamous cervical cancer is not oestrogen sensitive. There are no adverse data in ovarian cancer survivors although there may be a very small increased risk of ovarian cancer with long-term unopposed oestrogen use in healthy women. There are no data for adenocarcinoma of the cervix, vaginal or vulval cancer.

Breast cancer must be regarded as the principal contraindication to oestrogen treatment, but high-risk women with a strong family history of breast malignancy or those with benign breast disease should not necessarily be denied treatment. It is unclear what the precise risk of breast cancer recurrence is with HRT use. A study in breast cancer survivors using HRT was terminated because of an apparent excess risk. Unfortunately, this led to the premature termination of two other studies running concomitantly in which no excess risk had been detected [34]. A large tibolone study (LIBERATE) in breast cancer survivors is still in progress and encouragingly has been allowed to continue by the data monitoring board.

DURATION OF THERAPY

According to WHI, the risk of breast cancer appears to increase after 4 years. The MWS has shown a significantly increased risk after only 1 year. However, cancers appearing at 1 year must have been present at baseline with HRT acting as a promoter rather than an initiator. An editorial lead in *The Lancet* written by an epidemiologist [35] unrealistically suggested that the duration of therapy should be limited to 3–6 months. Unfortunately, it is recognized that symptoms often return when HRT is ceased, even after many years of use. If the underpinning principle of HRT is that it should be used to improve and maintain a good quality of life, in women in whom this principle is maintained, it is difficult to argue that they should have arbitrary deadlines imposed on them. Thus, duration of therapy requires careful judgement of benefits and risks on an individual basis. If therapy is to be discontinued, the dose should be reduced in a stepwise fashion over a minimum of 6 months to reduce the risk of immediate severe symptom resurgence.

OFFICIAL PRESCRIBING ADVICE

How are health professionals supposed to react to these data and advise their patients? Guidance from the Medicine's and Healthcare Products Regulatory Agency (MHRA) (see 'useful websites') has advised that HRT should not be recommended for primary or secondary prevention of heart disease. It is recommended that HRT be used merely for symptom relief in the short term at the lowest effective dose and alternatives should be considered in the long term for prevention of osteoporosis. Annual reappraisal of HRT use should be carried out with weighing up of the pros and cons on an individual basis. However, the British Menopause Society (see 'useful websites') consensus statement advises that prescribing habits need not be changed by the recent studies because HRT use in the UK was primarily for symptom relief rather than primary or secondary prevention.

Alternatives to HRT [36,37]

FOR SYMPTOMS

There is little scientific evidence that complementary and alternative therapies can help menopausal symptoms or provide the same benefits as conventional therapies. Yet many women use them, believing them to be safer and 'more natural' especially following the current controversies regarding HRT. The choice of treatments is confusing and unlike conventional medicines, little is known about their active ingredients, safety or side effects or how they may interact with other therapies. They can interfere with warfarin, antidepressants and anti-epileptics with potentially fatal consequences. Some herbal preparations may contain oestrogenic compounds and this is of concern for women with hormone dependent disease such as breast cancer. There is also concern about contaminants such as mercury, arsenic, lead and pesticides. Legislation is soon to be introduced which will make it mandatory for herbal preparations to at least be registered with the MHRA. This will at least allow some control over products which may be completely ineffective or dangerous and it is essential that alternatives to licensed preparations should be judged by similar standards.

Why not HRT?

There are a number of reasons why alternatives to HRT may be sought. The main reason is that an individual does not wish to use hormone therapy because they are concerned about the potential side effects and risks. There may be clinician concerns because of the personal or family history of the women, for example, cardiovascular disease, venous thromboembolism or breast cancer. It may be deemed that an alternative preparation is actually a better choice than traditional HRT. While many more exist (over 200!) focus here is on those preparations for which some trial evidence exists. The increasing use of complementary therapies has been confirmed by recent studies; 68% of women attending a menopause clinic in London had ever tried an alternative treatment for symptoms and that 62% of these women were satisfied with the results [38].

Lifestyle measures

There is some evidence that women who are more active tend to suffer less from the symptoms of the menopause but not all types of activity lead to an improvement in symptoms. High-impact infrequent exercise can actually make symptoms worse; the best activity is aerobic sustained regular exercise [39]. Avoidance or reduction of intake of alcohol and caffeine can reduce the severity and frequency of vasomotor symptoms.

Non-pharmacological alternatives

GELS FOR VAGINAL SYMPTOMS, E.G. REPLENS

This vaginal bioadhesive moisturizer is a more physiological way of replacing vaginal secretions than with lubricant vaginal gels such as KY jelly. It actually rehydrates the tissues and provides a reasonable alternative to systemic or vaginal HRT.

Pharmacological alternatives

PROGESTOGENS

Progestogens have traditionally been a popular alternative to combined HRT in women with intractable vasomotor symptoms who have contraindications to oestrogen [40]. However, recent studies, for example, WHI/MWS, have questioned the safety of progestogens because of concerns that the increase in risk of breast cancer with HRT is due to the combination of oestrogen and progestogen (rather than oestrogen alone). Thus, caution should be exercised in treating women with progestogens who have an increased risk of breast cancer. The potential risk to the breast also needs to be taken into account when using progestogens as an alternative in those at risk of thromboembolism.

ALPHA 2 AGONISTS

Clonidine, a centrally active alpha2 agonist, has been one of the most popular alternative preparations for the treatment of vasomotor symptoms. Unfortunately it is also one of the preparations for which the least evidence exists for efficacy – at best the trial data show a weak benefit [41].

BETA BLOCKERS

Beta blockers have been postulated as a possible option for treating vasomotor symptoms but the small trials which have been conducted have been disappointing.

SELECTIVE SEROTONIN REUPTAKE INHIBITORS SSRIS/SELECTIVE NORADRENALINE REUPTAKE INHIBITORS SNRIS

A significant amount of evidence exists for the efficacy of SSRIs and SNRIs in the treatment of vasomotor symptoms. Although there are some data for SSRIs such as fluoxetine and paroxetine, the most convincing data are for the

SNRI (venlafaxine) at a dose of 37.5 mg bd [42]. The key effect with these preparations appears to be stimulation of the noradrenergic as opposed to the serotonergic pathways, hence the preferential effect of SNRIs. The trials demonstrate a 50–60% reduction in hot flush frequency and severity. This compares with an 80–90% symptom reduction with traditional hormone therapy. The main drawback with these preparations (especially the SNRIs) is the high incidence of nausea which often leads to withdrawal from therapy before maximum symptom relief efficacy has been achieved. Trials in this area are ongoing.

GABAPENTIN

Recent work with the antiepileptic drug Gabapentin has shown efficacy for hot flush reduction compared to placebo. Gabapentin at a dose of 900 mg per day has been shown to reduce hot flush frequency by 45% and symptom severity by 54%. Further work is being conducted to confirm the efficacy and safety of this preparation.

Complementary therapies

Among the largest group of users of complementary therapies, middle age women, up to 33% of the population have used these preparations at any one time (European Menopause Survey 2005 [43]). It is estimated that the cost of complementary therapies amounts to 17 billion US dollars per annum. The majority of the costs are borne by the consumer as these are unlicensed preparations. These preparations are often used by women as they are perceived to be a safe alternative to traditional hormone therapies. However, the safety of a number of these preparations has been called into question. The current regulation of complementary and alternative medicine is inadequate and fragmented with only osteopaths and chiropractors currently regulated professions.

PHYTOESTROGENS

Phytoestrogens are plant substances that have effects similar to those of oestrogens. Since the first discovery of the oestrogenic activity of plant compounds, over 300 plants have been found to have phytoestrogenic activity. Preparations vary from enriched foods such as bread or drinks (soy milk) to more concentrated tablets. The most important groups are called isoflavones and lignans. The major isoflavones are genistein and daidzein. The major lignans are enterolactone and enterodiol. Isoflavones are found in soybeans, chick peas, red clover and probably other legumes (beans and peas). Oilseeds such as flaxseed are rich in lignans, and they are also found in cereal bran, whole cereals, vegetables, legumes and fruit. The role of phytoestrogens has stimulated considerable interest since populations consuming a diet high in isoflavones such as the Japanese appear to have lower rates of menopausal vasomotor symptoms, cardiovascular disease, osteoporosis; breast, colon, endometrial and ovarian cancers. The evidence from randomized placebo-controlled trials in Western populations is conflicting for both soy and derivatives from red clover. Similarly, there are also debates about the effects on lipoproteins, endothelial function and blood pressure. Currently other studies are underway to assess these products.

Soy

Twelve randomized controlled trials have been published comparing various preparations of soy with placebo. Only four out of the nine studies with a treatment phase lasting more than 6 weeks showed a significant improvement in symptoms compared to placebo. The most important of these trials includes a study of 102 women treated for 12 weeks which showed a 45% reduction in hot flushes in comparison to a 30% reduction in the placebo group [44]. Mammographic density, a risk marker for breast cancer, does not appear to be affected by soy preparations even after 2 year usage. However, long-term treatment with soy has raised some concerns with regard to a low risk of endometrial hyperplasia [45].

Red clover

Red clover has a high content of the isoflavones biochanin A and formononetin, while soy contains predominantly genistein, daidzein and glycitein. Soy isoflavones and red clover isoflavones display different affinities for the steroid receptors which may produce differential effects on symptoms though this requires confirmation. Five placebo-controlled studies evaluating the use of red clover isoflavones in the treatment of vasomotor symptoms have been conducted. While the doses of red clover isoflavones (40–160 mg) and the duration of treatment (12–16 weeks) varied in these studies, all showed a numerical reduction in the number of hot flushes compared to placebo [46]. However, the differences only reached statistical significance in two out of the five studies [47]. There were no serious safety concerns associated with short-term administration of red clover isoflavones in any of these studies. Breast density does not appear to be adversely affected by red clover although long-term randomized studies of breast cancer incidence are lacking. Endometrial biopsy data are also lacking though ultrasound scans of endometrial thickness have been reassuring.

Black cohosh

Black cohosh is a herbaceous perennial plant native to North America, widely used to alleviate menopausal symptoms. There are four randomized controlled trials using black cohosh but only one of these was placebo controlled. Three trials have shown benefit for vasomotor symptoms including one where black cohosh was compared to conjugated oestrogens but further efficacy data are required [48]. There have been seven serious adverse events reported recently due to hepatotoxicity; one case requiring liver transplantation [49]. There does not appear to be an endometrial effect and there are no clinical trials assessing the effects of black cohosh on the breast.

Evening primrose oil

Evening primrose oil is rich in gamma linolenic acid. Even though widely used by women, there is no evidence for efficacy in the menopause [50].

Dong quai

Dong quai is a perennial plant native to southwest China, commonly used in traditional Chinese medicine. It has not been found to be superior to placebo for menopausal symptoms in one randomized trial. Interaction with warfarin and photosensitization has been reported due to the presence of coumarins.

Ginkgo biloba

Use is widespread but there is little evidence to show that it improves menopausal symptoms. Some studies have shown a benefit for relief of anxiety and depression. There are claims for cognitive benefits from recent studies in postmenopausal women but these require confirmation from large long-term studies [51].

St John's Wort

St John's Wort has been shown to be efficacious in mild to moderate depression both in peri- and premenopausal women due to its SSRI type effect [52], but its efficacy for vasomotor symptoms has not been proven. It has potential interactions with various drugs including warfarin and the pill due to induction of the cytochrome P450 enzymes.

STEROIDS

DHEA (dehydroepiandrosterone)

Blood levels of DHEA drop dramatically with age. This had led to suggestions that the effects of ageing can be counteracted by DHEA 'replacement therapy'. DHEA is increasingly being used in the USA, where it is classed as a food supplement, for its supposed anti-ageing effects. Some studies have shown benefits on the skeleton, cognition, well-being, libido and the vagina. There is no evidence that DHEA has any effect on hot flushes. The short-term effects of taking DHEA are still controversial and possible harmful effects of long-term use are, as yet, unknown.

Progesterone transdermal creams

Progesterone creams derived from wild yam have been advocated for the treatment of menopausal symptoms and skeletal protection. Claims have been made that steroids (diosgenein) in yams (dioscorea villosa) can be converted in the body to progesterone, but this is biochemically impossible. Progesterone creams have recently been the subject of clinical trials, and no benefit on vasomotor symptoms was demonstrated [53]. Despite previous claims, there was no effect on bone mineral density.

VITAMINS AND MINERALS

Vitamins such as E [54] and C, and minerals such as selenium are present in various supplements. The evidence that they are of any benefit to postmenopausal women is lacking.

HOMEOPATHY

Data from case histories, observational studies and a small number of randomized trials are encouraging but clearly more research is needed. A recent paper reported on an investigation of the homeopathic approach to the management of symptoms of oestrogen withdrawal in women with breast cancer. Significant improvements in mean symptom scores were seen over the study period and for the primary end-point 'the effect on daily living' scores. Symptoms other than hot flushes such as fatigue and mood disturbance also appear to be helped [55].

ACUPUNCTURE

A recent small randomized controlled trial of 45 postmenopausal women undergoing shallow acupuncture, electro-acupuncture or oral oestrogen administration showed a significant reduction in hot flush frequency in all three groups. The degree of symptom reduction was greatest in the oestrogen group [56]. Although no adverse effects were demonstrated in this study, rare adverse effects such as cardiac tamponade, pneumothorax and hepatitis have been described. Further data are required to establish the precise benefits of acupuncture for the menopause.

REFLEXOLOGY

Reflexology aims to relieve stress or treat health conditions through the application of pressure to specific points or areas of the feet. While it has been used for various conditions such as pain, anxiety and premenstrual syndrome there have been few studies for menopausal complaints. One randomized trial has been published so far where 67 women with vasomotor symptoms aged 45–60 years were randomized to receive reflexology or non-specific foot massage. There was a reduction in symptoms in both groups but there was no significant difference between the groups [57].

Alternatives to HRT

SKELETAL PROTECTION

In December 2004, the European Medicines Agency ruled that HRT should no longer be used as a first line treatment for osteoporosis. This advice was mirrored by the MHRA in the UK who proclaimed that the long-term risks of HRT outweighed the benefits and that alternative preparations should be used for osteoporosis prophylaxis and treatment. The National Institute for Clinical Excellence (NICE) has recently carried out a technology appraisal for three of the main alternatives to HRT, bisphosphonates, raloxifene and parathyroid hormone. Treatment guidelines have been issued (Jan 2005 NICE website) but there is a delay in the advice regarding prophylaxis as it was only agreed to issue the latter advice after protests from the National Osteoporosis and British Menopause Societies. The most commonly employed alternatives to HRT for bone protection will now be considered.

Lifestyle measures

Every woman should be encouraged to take plenty of regular exercise in addition to having a well-balanced diet and avoiding smoking. There are studies which show that women who take regular weight-bearing exercise have higher bone mineral densities compared to sedentary controls. Exercise appears to reduce bone loss rather than reverse osteoporosis. It also improves muscle tone thus reducing falls. There is also evidence for reduction in bone loss by the daily use of calcium ($\approx$ 1500 mg elemental calcium) and vitamin D (4–600 IU) supplements.

Bisphosphonates

Bisphosphonates are pyrophosphate analogues which interfere with osteoclastic resorption. Etidronate was the first bisphosphonate to be licensed but alendronate and risedronate are much more commonly used now due to their significantly higher antiresorptive power. Both these products have grade A randomized controlled trial data for both prevention and treatment of spine and hip fractures (up to 50% reduction), now with 10 year efficacy data for alendronate [58]. There is also good evidence of bone preservation in women who discontinue alendronate though not to the same extent as those who continue therapy. The main side effects of these products are gastro-oesophageal irritation and ulceration although the once weekly preparations have made them more tolerable. To improve compliance, a once a month (ibandronate) and a once a year (zolendronate) formulation are in development.

Raloxifene

Raloxifene belongs to the group of compounds called SERMS (Selective Estrogen Receptor Modulators) which are agonistic in the skeleton and cardiovascular system and antagonistic in the breast and endometrium. Raloxifene is the first of these products to be licensed – it produces modest increases in bone mineral density (BMD) (2–3% per annum) and is licensed for fracture reduction in the spine [59]. However, as it lacks grade A evidence for fracture prevention in the hip, NICE have declared it a second line preparation after bisphosphonates (raloxifene).

Strontium ranelate

Strontium ranelate is also antiresorptive and anabolic in its action (dual action bone agent). It has recently been licensed for fracture treatment in both hip and spine (3 year efficacy data with 41% reduction in spine fractures). It has the advantage over bisphosphonates that it does not produce gastrointestinal side effects [60].

Parathyroid hormone (teriparatide)

The parathyroid hormone analogue teriparatide is both antiresorptive and anabolic and is licensed for treatment of spine fractures. Due to its mode of administration (daily injection) and its expense NICE have advised that it should be used as third line treatment in elderly women with previous fractures with the severest osteoporosis.

Statins

There are limited data for an effect of statins on the skeleton but benefits have not been confirmed by randomized trials in human subjects.

Conclusion

We must not underestimate women's desire for a high quality of life in the menopause. Women will continue to demand HRT or a safe, effective alternative for their symptoms. It is, therefore, our duty to strive to provide the best therapy for women to achieve this goal. With every new study there appears to be a change in advice given by the regulatory agencies as to how we should advise our patients, leading to a great deal of confusion.

Best practice should involve the following:

1 Discussion of lifestyle measures, HRT and alternatives should take place from the outset.

2 Management should be individualized taking into account risks and benefits.

3 The main indication for use of HRT should be for symptom relief rather than for prevention of long-term problems.

4 Low-dose HRT should usually be commenced, except in premature ovarian failure, and increased, if necessary, to achieve effective symptom relief.

5 Rigid cut off's in duration of therapy should be avoided with regular reappraisal (at least annual) of the benefits and risks for each individual.

6 Delivery of services should be from a multidisciplinary team if possible with close liaison with allied specialties and experts.

References

1. Landgren B-M *et al.* (2004) Menopause transition: annual changes in serum hormonal patterns over the menstrual cycle in women during a 9 year period prior to menopause. *J Clin Endocrinol Metab* **89**(6), 2763–9.
2. Wallace WH & Kelsey TW (2004) Ovarian reserve and reproductive age may be determined from measurement of ovarian volume by transvaginal sonography. *Hum Reprod* **19**(7), 1612–7.
3. Goswamy RK, Campbell S & Royston JP *et al.* (1988) Ovarian size in postmenopausal women. *BJOG* **95**(8), 795–801.
4. Panay N & Studd JWW (1998) The psychotherapeutic effects of estrogens. *Gynaecol Endocrinol* **12**(5), 353–65.
5. Studd JWW & Panay N (2004) Hormones and depression in women. *Climacteric* **7**(4), 338–46.
6. Bjarnason NH (1998) Postmenopausal bone remodelling and hormone replacement. *Climacteric* **1**(1), 72–9.
7. Tunstall-Pedoe H (1998) Myth and paradox of coronary risk and the menopause. *Lancet* **351**(9113), 1425–7.
8. Guthrie JR (2004) *et al.* (2004) Association between hormonal changes at menopause and the risk of a coronary event: a longitudinal study. *Menopause* **11**(3), 315–22.
9. Christian RC, Harrington S, Edwards WD, Oberg AL & Fitzpatrick LA (2002) Estrogen status correlates with the calcium content of coronary atherosclerotic plaques in women. *J Clin Endocrinol Metab* **87**(3), 1062–7.
10. Chu MC, Rath KM, Huie J & Taylor HS (2003) Elevated basal FSH in normal cycling women is associated with unfavourable lipid levels and increased cardiovascular risk. *Hum Reprod* **18**(8), 1570–3.
11. Shumaker SA, Legault C, Rapp SR *et al.* (2003) Estrogen plus progestin and the incidence of dementia and mild cognitive impairment in postmenopausal women: the Women's Health Initiative Memory Study: a randomized controlled study. *J Am Med Assoc* **289**, 2651–62.
12. Jackson G (2003) Royal College of Physicians of Edinburgh Consensus Statement on HRT.
13. Panay N, Versi E & Savvas MA (2000) comparison of 25 mg and 50 mg oestradiol implants in the control of climacteric symptoms following hysterectomy and bilateral salpingo-oophorectomy. *Br J Obstet Gynaecol* **107**(8), 1012–6.
14. Kalentzi T & Panay N (2005) The safety of vaginal estrogen in postmenopausal women. *TOG* **7**(4), 241–4.
15. Panay N & Studd JWW (1997) Progestogen intolerance and compliance with hormone replacement therapy in menopausal women. *Hum Reprod Update* **3**(2), 159–71.
16. Raudaskoski T, Tapanainen J & Tomas *et al.* (2002) Intrauterine 10 microg and 20 microg levonorgestrel systems in postmenopausal women receiving oral oestrogen replacement therapy: clinical, endometrial and metabolic response. *Br J Obstet Gynaecol* **109**(2), 136–44.
17. Writing Group for the Women's Health Initiative Investigators (2002) Risks and benefits of estrogen plus progestin in healthy postmenopausal women: principal results From Women's Health Initiative randomized controlled trial. *J Am Med Assoc* **288**(3), 321–33.
18. Million Women Study Collaborators (2003) Breast cancer and HRT in the Million Women Study. *Lancet* **362**, 419–27.
19. Collaborative Group on Hormonal Factors in Breast Cancer (1997) Breast cancer and hormone replacement therapy: collaborative reanalysis of data from 51 epidemiological studies of 52,705 women with breast cancer and 108,411 women without breast cancer. *Lancet* **350**(9084), 1047–59.
20. Chlebowski RT, Hendrix SL, Langer RD *et al.* (2003) Influence of estrogen plus progestin on breast cancer and mammography in healthy postmenopausal women. The women's health initiative randomised trial. *J Am Med Assoc* **289**, 3243–53.
21. Gambacciani M & Genazzani AR (2003) The study with a million women (and hopefully fewer mistakes). *Gynecol Endocrinol* **17**, 359–62.
22. (2003) Breast Cancer and hormone replacement therapy: the Million Women Study (Letters). *Lancet* **362**, 1328–32.
23. The Women's Health Initiative Steering Committee (2004) Effects of conjugated equine estrogen in postmenopausal women with hysterectomy: the women's health initiative randomized controlled trial. *J Am Med Assoc* **291**(14), 1701–12.
24. Hulley S, Grady D, Bush T *et al.*, Heart and Estrogen/progestin Replacement Study (HERS) Research Group. (1998) Randomized trial of estrogen plus progestin for secondary prevention of coronary heart disease in postmenopausal women. *J Am Med Assoc* **280**(7), 605–13.
25. Stevenson J (2003) Long term effects of hormone replacement therapy. *Lancet* **361**(9353), 253–4.

26. Salpeter SR, Walsh JM, Greyber E, Ormiston TM & Salpeter EE (2004) Mortality associated with hormone replacement therapy in younger and older women: a meta-analysis. *J Gen Intern Med* **19**(7), 791–804.

27. Kalantaridou *et al.* (2004) Impaired endothelial function in young women with premature ovarian failure: normalization with hormone therapy. *J Clin Endocrinol Metab* **89**(8), 3907–13.

28. Weiderpass E, Adami HO, Baron JA (1999) Risk of endometrial cancer following estrogen replacement with and without progestins. *J Natl Cancer Inst* **91**, 1131–7.

29. Sturdee DW, Ulrich LG *et al.* (2000) The endometrial response to sequential and continuous combined oestrogen-progestogen replacement therapy. *BJOG* **197**, 1392–400.

30. Million Women Study Collaborators (2005) Endometrial Cancer and hormone-replacement therapy in the Million Women Study. *Lancet* **365**, 1543–51.

31. Ferenczy A. Abstracts of the 7th European Congress on Menopause, 3–7 June, 2006, Istanbul, Turkey. Maturity. 2006; 54 suppl. 1:S1–122.

32. Scarabin PY, Olger E, Plu-Bureau G (2003) Differential association of oral and transdermal oestrogen replacement therapy with venous thromboembolism risk. *Lancet* **362**, 428–32.

33. Suriano KA, McHale M, McLaren CE, Li KT, Re A & DiSaia PJ (2001) Estrogen replacement therapy in endometrial cancer patients: a matched control study. *Obstet Gynecol* **97**(4), 555–60.

34. von Schoultz E & Rutqvist LE (2005) Menopause hormone therapy after breast cancer: the Stockholm randomized trial. *J Natl Cancer Inst* **97**(7), 471–2.

35. Lagro–Janssen T, Rosser W & Van Weel C (2003) Breast cancer and hormone replacement therapy: up to general practice to pick up the pieces. *Lancet* **362**, 414–5.

36. Nachtigall LE, Barber RJ, Barentsen R, Durand N, Panay N, Pitkin J, van de Weijer P & Wysoki S (2006) Complementary and Hormonal Therapy for Vasomotor Symptom Relief: A Conservative Clinical Approach. *J Obstet Gynaecol Can* **28**(4), 279–89.

37. Panay N & Rees M (2006) The use of alternatives to HRT for the Management of menopause symptoms *RCOG Scientific Advisory Committee* Opinion Paper no 6.

38. Vashisht A, Domoney CL, Cronje W & Studd JW (2001) Prevalence of and satisfaction with complementary therapies and hormone replacement therapy in a specialist menopause clinic. *Climacteric* **4**(3), 250–6.

39. Lindh-Astrand L, Nedstrand E, Wyon Y & Hammar M (2004) Vasomotor symptoms and quality of life in previously sedentary postmenopausal women randomised to physical activity or estrogen therapy. *Maturitas* **48**, 97–105.

40. Loprinzi CL, Michalak JC, Quella SK *et al.* (1994) Megestrol acetate for the prevention of hot flashes. *N Engl J Med* **331**(6), 347–52.

41. Nelson HD, Vesco KK, Haney E *et al.* (2006) Nonhormonal therapies for menopausal hot flashes: systemic review and meta-analysis. *JAMA* **295**(17), 2057–71.

42. Loprinzi CL, Kugler JW, Sloan JA *et al.* (2000) Venlafaxine in the management of hot flashes in survivors of breast cancer: a randomised controlled trial. *Lancet* **356**(9247), 2059–63.

43. Genazzani AR, Schneider HR, Panay N & Nijland EA (2006) The European Menopause Survey 2005: women's perceptions on the menopause and postmenopausal hormone therapy. *Gynecol Endocrinol* **22**(7), 369–75.

44. Huntley AL & Ernst E (2004) Soy for the treatment of perimenopausal symptoms – a systematic review. *Maturitas* **47**, 1–9.

45. Unfer V, Casini ML, Castabile L, Mignosa M, Gerli S & Di Renzo GC (2004) Endometrial effects of long-term treatment with phytoestrogens: a randomized, double-blind, placebo-controlled study. *Fertil Steril* **82**, 145–8.

46. Tice JA, Ettinger B, Ensrud K, Wallace R, Blackwell T & Cummings SR (2003) Phytoestrogen Supplements for the Treatment of Hot Flashes: The Isoflavone Clover Extract (ICE) Study. *JAMA* **290**(2), 207–14.

47. Van de Weijer P & Barentsen R (2002) Isoflavones from red clover (Promensil) significantly reduce menopausal hot flush symptoms compared with placebo. *Maturitas* **42**, 187–93.

48. Huntley A & Ernst E (2003) A systematic review of the safety of black cohosh. *Menopause* **10**(1), 58–64.

49. Medicines and Healthcare products Regulatory Agency. Black cohosh (cimicifuga racemosa) and hepatotoxicity. (2004) The Current Problems in Pharmacovigilence Oct:10th.

50. Chenoy R, Hussain S, O'Brien PM, Moss MY & Morse PF (1994) Effect of oral gamolenic acid from evening primrose oil on menopausal flushing. *Br Med J* **308**(6927), 501–3.

51. Elsabagh S, Hartley DE & File SE (2005) Limited cognitive benefits in Stage +2 postmenopausal women after six weeks of treatment with Gingko biloba. *J Psychopharmacol* **19**(2), 173–81.

52. Linde K, Ramirez G, Mulrow CD, Pauls A, Weidenhammer W & Melchart D (1996) St John's Wort for depression – an overview and meta-analysis of randomised clinical trials. *Br Med J* **313**(7052), 253–8.

53. Leonetti HB, Longo S & Anasti JN (1999) Transdermal progesterone cream for vasomotor symptoms and postmenopausal bone loss. *Obstet Gynecol* **94**(2), 225–8.

54. Miller ER 3rd, Pastor-Barriuso R, Dalal D, Riemersma RA, Appel LJ & Guallar E (2005) Meta-analysis: high-dosage vitamin E supplementation may increase all-cause mortality. *Ann Intern Med* **142**(1), 37–46.

55. Thomson EA & Reilly D (2003) The homeopathic approach to the treatment of symptoms of oestrogen withdrawal in breast cancer patients. A prospective observational study. *Homeopathy* **92**(3), 131–4.

56. Wyon Y, Wijma K, Nedstrand E & Hammar M (2004) A comparison of acupuncture and oral estradiol treatment of vasomotor symptoms in postmenopausal women. *Climacteric* **7**(2), 153–64.

57. Williamson J, White A, Hart A & Ernst E (2002) Randomised controlled trial of reflexology for menopausal symptoms. *Br J Obstet Gynaecol* **109**(9), 1050–5.

58. Bone HG, Hosking D, Devogelaer JP *et al.* (2004) Ten years' experience with alendronate for osteoporosis in postmenopausal women. *N Engl J Med* **350**(12), 1189–99.

59. Delmas PD, Ensrud KE, Adachi *et al.* (2002) Efficacy of raloxifene on vertebral fracture risk reduction in postmenopausal women with osteoporosis: four-year

results from a randomized clinical trial. *J Clin Endocrinol Metab* **87**(8), 3609–17.

60. Meunier PJ, Roux C & Seeman E *et al.* (2004) The effects of strontium ranelate on the risk of vertebral fracture in women with postmenopausal osteoporosis. *N Engl J Med* **350**(5), 459–68.

Further reading

Badawy SZA (ed.) (1999) *Clinical Management of the Perimenopause*. London: Arnold Press.

Ernst E, Pittler MH, Stevinson C & White AR (2001) *The Desktop Guide to Complementary and Alternative Medicine*. Edinburgh: Mosby.

Panay N, Dutta R, Ryan A & Broadbent M (2004) *Crash Course in Obstetrics & Gynaecology* (Revision textbook). Edinburgh: Mosby.

Rees M & Keith L (2004) *The Year in Postmenopausal Health*. Oxford: Clinical Publishing.

Rees M & Mander A (2004) *Managing the Menopause Without Oestrogen*. London: Royal Society of Medicine Press.

Studd J. (2000) The management of the menopause, 3rd edn. Parthenon Publishing.

Zollman C & Vickers A (1999) ABC of complementary medicine. Complementary medicine in conventional practice. *Br Med J* **319**, 901–4.

Useful web sites

www.the-bms.org (the British Menopause Society site)
www.mhra.gov.uk (the medical and Healthcare Products Regulatory Agency)
www.menopausematters.co.uk
www.pms.org.uk (the Premenstrual Syndrome website)
www.nos.org.uk (the National Osteoporosis Society)
www.menopause.org (the North American society)
http://emas.obgyn.net/ European Menopause Society
http://www.emea.eu.int/ European Medicines Agency
www.imsociety.org (the International Menopause Society)
http://nccam.nih.gov/health/alerts/menopause/ National Centre for Complementary and Alternative Medicine. Alternative therapies for managing menopausal symptoms.
www.phytohealth.org (The PHYTOHEALTH Network aims to establish a pan-European network of institutions dealing with safety and health effect of phytoestrogens, identification of optimal sources and processing technologies).
http://dietary-supplements.info.nih.gov The NIH Office of Dietary Supplements
http://dietarysupplements.info.nih.gov/Health_Information/IBIDS.aspx Office of dietary supplements. IBIDS database.
www.whi.org WHI Website
http://www.rcplondon.ac.uk/pubs/wp_osteo_update.htm Royal College of Physicians Guidelines on Osteoporosis
http://medicines.mhra.gov.uk/ourwork/ monitorsafe-qualmed/currentproblems/currentproblems_oct04.pdf Current Problems in Pharmacovigilance Oct 2004: Review of the Evidence regarding Long term Safety of HRT
http://www.organon.com/news/2005_03_08_women_believe_menopausal_symptoms_require_treatment_with_64_percent_experiencing_severe_problems.asp). (European Menopause Survey 2005, Organon International Website)

Chapter 48: Pelvic floor dysfunction I: uterovaginal prolapse

Anthony R.B. Smith

Introduction

Up to half of the normal female population will develop uterovaginal prolapse during their lifetime. Twenty percent of these women will be symptomatic and need treatment [1]. A North American actuarial analysis revealed that a woman up to the age of 80 years has an 11% risk of needing surgery for pelvic floor weakness. Furthermore, if she has an operation, she has a 29% risk of requiring further surgery [2]. These figures suggest that the current management of pelvic floor dysfunction is less than ideal. As the population of the world continues to increase in age, the prevalence of pelvic floor dysfunction is likely to increase. Gynaecologists need to improve their understanding of pelvic floor dysfunction and its sequelae to improve the outcomes from treatment.

Structure and function of the pelvic floor

The pelvic floor functions to support the pelvic and abdominal viscera and help maintain control of their contents. It has two major components which are interdependent: the muscle and facia.

Muscle

Levator ani muscles consist of pubococcygeus, coccygeus and ileococcygeus muscles on each side which together form a muscular floor to the pelvis. The striated muscle of levator ani is under voluntary control but is a unique striated muscle in having a resting tone. As with other striated muscles its strength can be increased by exercise as with pelvic floor physiotherapy. Contraction of the muscles results in a forward elevation of the pelvic floor which is important in their role in continence. This forward elevation helps to increase the angulation between bladder and urethra anteriorly and rectum and anal canal posteriorly. Increase in this angulation is one of the fundamental mechanisms which aid continence. Thus, the healthy pelvic floor muscle will, at rest, provide support

and assistance with continence. When the intra-abdominal pressure rises levator ani muscles contract and provide additional support and outlet resistance to the bladder and rectum. This reflex response to intra-abdominal pressure rises also requires an intact innervation. Damage to the pelvic floor muscle innervation is likely to impair the pelvic floor muscle responses.

Fascia

Fascia envelopes levator ani, attaches it to bone at its origin and holds the two muscles together in the midline. The urethra, vagina and rectum perforate this midline fascia. Thus, the pelvic viscera are supported both by the levator ani muscle below and the fascial attachments which are condensed in some areas and are often referred to as ligaments – the uterosacral, cardinal and round ligaments being examples. There has been much debate for over a century about the structure and function of the pelvic fascia. It is generally accepted that the pelvic floor has evolved as man has assumed the upright stature and this evolution has involved replacement of some of the muscular component of the pelvic floor with fascia to provide additional supportive strength to cope with the effect of gravity. Thus, any factor that influences the strength or integrity of pelvic floor fascia will influence the function of the pelvic floor. These factors may be congenital (such as hyperelasticity of the collagenous component of fascia) or environmental, such as stretching or tearing of fascia during childbirth or heavy lifting.

Weakness of the pelvic floor, which may result from impairment of function of either muscle or fascia, can result in uterovaginal prolapse. Prolapse is largely a result of loss of support from the pelvic floor but the pelvic floor dysfunction may produce other accompanying symptoms than those due to the displacement of the pelvic viscera. An understanding of the pathophysiology of pelvic floor dysfunction will help to develop an appropriate management strategy.

Pathophysiology of pelvic floor dysfunction

Muscle

The striated muscle of the pelvic floor, in common with other striated muscles throughout the body, undergoes a gradual denervation with age [3]. This denervation will result in a gradual weakening of the muscle over time. While some of the aging effect can be counteracted by muscle training, the impact of denervation will be to diminish the number of neurones which can stimulate muscle fibres to contract. Pelvic floor muscle denervation is increased by vaginal delivery, particularly if the active second stage of labour is prolonged [4].

Caesarean section may offer some protection from this injury. Following childbirth some reinnervation will occur which will result in rehabilitation of the muscle at least to some degree. Reinnervation results in more muscle fibres being innervated by each remaining nerve fibre. This results in the pelvic floor muscle being more vulnerable to age-related denervation since further nerve loss with age will result in a more marked loss of muscle fibre activity. Thus, the damage to the pelvic floor muscle during childbirth often only becomes evident when age-related changes are superimposed. The site of pelvic floor muscle denervation during childbirth is unclear. It has been proposed that stretching of the pudendal nerve distal to Alcock's canal at the ischial spine results in nerve injury but crushing injury at the neuromuscular junction in the muscle must also be possible.

In neurological diseases like multiple sclerosis, pelvic floor muscle may behave unpredictably ranging from inappropriate relaxation causing incontinence to spasm resulting in voiding dysfunction.

Women with ectopia vesicae have incomplete development of the pelvic floor anteriorly. This predisposes them to uterovaginal prolapse which is an additional surgical challenge to treat partly because of previous surgical procedures and partly because of anatomical distortion from the absence of a normally formed anterior pelvis (bony and soft tissue).

Fascia

Fascia is composed of a number of components including collagen, elastin and smooth muscle embedded in a connective tissue matrix. Each of the components may influence the overall biomechanical properties of the fascia. The following factors have a significant influence on pelvic floor support.

CONGENITAL

Congenital differences in collagen behaviour are clinically evident in women who have increased joint elasticity.

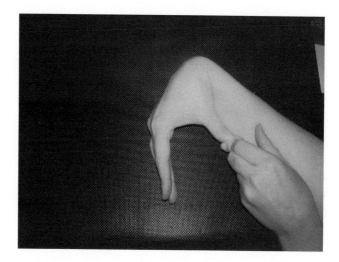

Fig. 48.1 Joint hyperextensibility as an index of fascial stretchiness.

Women with hyperextensible joints will also have additional pelvic fascia stretchiness which may be manifested in the development of uterovaginal prolapse at an earlier age. Such women often excel at sports requiring increased joint elasticity (such as gymnastics) and they develop fewer striae gravidarum during pregnancy because of increased skin elasticity. Labour may be rapid because of reduced obstruction from the pelvic floor fascia. Extreme forms of this are seen in Ehrlers Danos syndrome but much more commonly seen are milder forms (see picture of joint hyperextension). It is important for gynaecologists to recognize women who have such problems because their treatment may need to be different. Recurrence after surgery is more likely and use of prosthetic support materials may be advisable (see Fig. 48.1). Some forms of collagen disorder are also associated with clotting problems.

AGE

With increasing age fascial tissues become stiffer and more liable to rupture. The young child is invariably stiffer in movement than the elderly adult. The fascia of the pelvic floor will provide weaker support with advancing years. Gynaecologists repairing the pelvic floor often recognize that the tissues used for building a repair are of poor quality and are poorly vascularized. The repair after surgery will heal with less strength and more slowly. The recurrence of prolapse seen after surgery in one out of three cases must in some part be due to a deterioration of fascial strength with age. This is supported by the fact that the longer the follow-up period after surgical treatment the higher the risk of recurrence.

CHILDBIRTH INJURY

Most women recognize that their pelvic floor is different after vaginal delivery. Furthermore, regaining the tone and shape of their anterior abdominal wall is also often a difficult challenge. These changes are due to a combination of muscle and fascial changes. There has been much unresolved debate as to whether pelvic floor fascia stretches or tears during pregnancy and childbirth. Some believe that stretching occurs and therefore repair of the pelvic floor during prolapse surgery should involve fascial plication. Others believe that fascia can only tear and does not stretch and therefore repair should involve determining the site of the tears and repairing them (site specific repair - see p. 500).

ENDOCRINE

The menstrual cycle, pregnancy and the menopause are the most significant endocrine events which may influence pelvic floor fascia. Women often declare that prolapse symptoms are worse around the time of menstruation. This is thought to be secondary to higher progesterone levels increasing fascial elasticity. Recent studies have shown that women examined at the time of menstruation will have a higher stage of prolapse than at other times of the cycle. This has important implications when deciding on treatment. During pregnancy, prolapse symptoms will be more evident in the first trimester but diminish as the pregnant uterus enlarges out of the pelvis. During pregnancy many women develop stress incontinence of urine for the first time. Research has shown that fascial elasticity increases in pregnancy [5] and this probably results in diminished pelvic floor support and a tendency to stress incontinence. Women who develop stress incontinence of urine during pregnancy are more likely to experience the same symptom after childbirth. The prevalence of uterovaginal prolapse increases after the menopause. How much this is secondary to the endocrine changes rather than age-related changes is not known.

Uterovaginal prolapse

Description

Prolapse is normally divided into anterior, uterine/vault and posterior compartments. Although anterior vaginal wall prolapse is still commonly called a cystocoele and posterior prolapse a rectocoele or enterocoele the difficulty in providing reproducible descriptions for the purpose of research has led to the development of scoring systems. The most frequently used validated method in current literature is a system called the POPQ (Pelvic Organ Prolapse

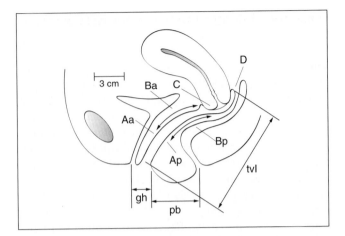

Fig. 48.2 Abbreviations: Aa, anterior wall; Ap, posterior wall; Ba, anterior wall; Bp, posterior wall; C, cervix or cuff; D, posterior fornix; gh, genital hiatus; pb, perineal body; tvl, total vaginal length.

Quantification [6]. The system is shown diagrammatically in Fig. 48.2.

Symptoms

Prolapse classically produces a sensation of fullness in the vagina or a visible or palpable lump at the introitus. This sensation is always posture dependant as are many prolapse symptoms. If the symptoms do not resolve when lying down an alternative aetiology should be considered. Low backache is a common symptom but is also commonly experienced by women who do not have prolapse. Vaginal atrophy, if present, will exacerbate many prolapse symptoms and should be treated as a first priority with topical oestrogens unless clinically contraindicated.

URINARY SYMPTOMS

Anterior vaginal wall prolapse may result in a range of urinary symptoms. While women who have anterior prolapse may have stress incontinence, particularly if the urethra is not well supported, they may also have voiding dysfunction secondary to kinking of the urethra. Voiding dysfunction may result in frequency (due to incomplete bladder emptying), hesitancy and a poor urinary stream. Incomplete bladder emptying may in turn result in recurrent urinary infection with accompanying frequency, urgency and urge incontinence. It is important to realize that anterior vaginal wall prolapse does not of itself produce detrusor overactivity which may have an independent pathology. Thus, repair of anterior vaginal wall prolapse may not resolve urinary symptoms if this is the case. Furthermore, if the anterior prolapse is kinking the urethra, it may be preventing stress incontinence of urine. Surgical repair may then result in the development of stress incontinence *de novo* which will not please the patient. Occasionally posterior vaginal wall prolapse if associated with obstructed defaecation may result in urinary voiding dysfunction.

BOWEL SYMPTOMS

Posterior vaginal wall prolapse may be associated with a range of bowel symptoms. It is often difficult to know whether the bowel symptoms are caused by the prolapse or associated with a fascial weakness which may also be affecting the bowel. Slow transit constipation and diverticular disease are bowel disorders more prevalent in women with fascial weakness. Constipation is a common symptom in women and may contribute to obstructed defaecation. The presence of posterior vaginal wall prolapse may not be the cause of the obstructed defaecation but more a symptom of it. Posterior vaginal wall prolapse does not normally result in ano-rectal incontinence.

COITAL SYMPTOMS

Uterovaginal prolapse in all but the most severe cases regresses when a woman is lying in bed. Prolapse often does not interfere with normal sexual activity. However, many women feel unhappy with the vaginal discomfort experienced through the day and the presence of the prolapse can inhibit couples from continuing normal sexual activity for mainly aesthetic reasons but also from concern about causing harm. Additionally, concern about continence or other urinary and bowel symptoms may be inhibiting. Some couples find that the loss of tone in the vagina leads to sexual dissatisfaction for both parties. The growth in interest in cosmetic vaginal surgery and drugs for male impotence may be influencing this area.

Investigation of prolapse symptoms

EXAMINATION

General examination should include fitness for surgery. Abdominal examination should be performed to exclude an intra-abdominal mass. A bimanual pelvic examination or ultrasound should exclude a pelvic mass and delineate the size of the uterus and ovaries if present.

The patient should be examined in the horizontal position, conventionally in the left lateral position with a Sims speculum. If prolapse is not evident, even with a Valsalva manoeuvre, the patient should be examined in the upright position. It is important to reproduce the symptoms and signs with which the patient presents. If this is not possible a further examination may be required. Many women are only aware of their symptoms after a long period in the upright position. An early morning clinic appointment may preclude detection of the prolapse. Some clinicians examine women in the lithotomy position. This enables closer inspection of vaginal supports, particularly if looking for site-specific defects in the endopelvic fascia. A second retracting instrument will be required to do this to visualize the lateral sulci.

The POPQ examination (see p. 498) gives an objective record of the prolapse stage.

URODYNAMICS STUDIES

If there are no urinary symptoms urodynamic studies are not justified outside the research setting. If a woman has significant urinary symptoms urodynamics may help define the cause of the symptoms which will enable the gynaecologist to give some prognosis for treatment. Hence, if urodynamics indicate obstructed voiding there is a good prognosis for surgical repair of the cystocoele resolving the voiding dysfunction while if the urodynamics suggest the bladder is atonic the prognosis is less favourable. If urodynamics indicate that the bladder is overactive then it is unlikely that surgery will improve the urinary symptoms. This may influence a woman's decision on whether to proceed with surgery.

The development of stress incontinence is an irritating sequel to anterior vaginal wall repair in some women. Some clinicians perform a urinary stress test with the prolapse reduced either digitally with a sponge forceps or a ring pessary. There is no evidence that this technique reliably predicts which women will develop stress incontinence after surgery.

PROCTOGRAPHY

An anterior rectocoele may result in obstructed defaecation. Rectal mucosal prolapse may also result in obstructed defaecation and will not be apparent on vaginal examination. Proctography can give some insight into factors which may be contributing to difficulty with defaecation and may help avoid unnecessary, unhelpful vaginal operations.

MAGNETIC RESONANCE IMAGING

Magnetic resonance imaging has been used as a research tool to try to identify prolapse not clinically evident. It has not been proved to aid or improve treatment outcome to date.

Treatment

CONSERVATIVE

Some women elect for non-surgical treatment of their prolapse either because:

1 the prognosis offered for treatment is not sufficiently attractive

2 they are unfit for surgery

3 they wish to delay surgical treatment for other reasons.

Conservative treatment may involve:

Lifestyle advice. This may include advice on diet and weight loss including avoidance of caffeine containing drinks, water intake, fibre content, laxative use and modification of drug regimes, e.g. diuretics. Avoidance of high-impact exercise and lifting may improve symptoms.

Pelvic floor physiotherapy. There have been no studies on the value of pelvic floor physiotherapy on vaginal prolapse symptoms. While it is unlikely that advanced prolapse will be helped by pelvic floor exercises, earlier stage prolapse may be improved sufficiently to avoid further intervention.

Vaginal pessary. Vaginal pessaries have been available in some form for 4000 years. The first pessaries described were pomegranate skins. Currently in the UK the most frequently used pessary is the polypropylene ring pessary (Fig. 48.3). The most appropriate anatomical configuration for the ring pessary has not been defined but if there is little or no posterior perineal support the ring pessary will often not be retained. The optimal size is usually determined by trial and error. The optimal time interval for changing pessaries has also not been defined, nor has the role of topical oestrogens. In North America a wider range of vaginal pessaries is available (www.milexproducts.com). Companies advise regular washing of the pessary by the patient without any evidence for the value of so doing.

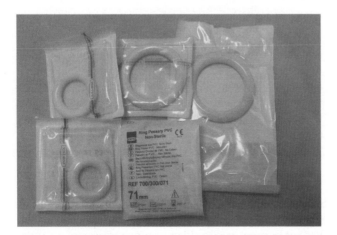

Fig. 48.3 Ring

Pessaries such as the ring can normally allow sexual intercourse without problems although a few women prefer to remove the pessary. Space occupying pessaries such as the shelf pessary preclude normal sexual relations and are therefore unsuitable for sexually active women. The shelf pessary may be particularly helpful for uterine or vaginal vault prolapse. The shelf pessary may be quite difficult to change and can become embedded in the vaginal wall. Careful examination, at least every 6 months is advisable and topical oestrogens may reduce the risk of ulceration and erosion.

SURGICAL

Over the last 100 years surgery has been considered to be the treatment of choice for uterovaginal prolapse. The surgical techniques employed until recently have differed little from those described by the surgical icons of a century ago. Increasingly it is being acknowledged that a desirable outcome should include more than a satisfactory anatomical result. Functional outcome may be more important to the patient. There have been very few robust studies of prolapse surgery performed which define both the anatomical and functional outcome with some measure of the impact on the patient's quality of life. Further research is urgently needed in this field.

Surgically the key issues are:

1 which technique produces the best, long-lasting anatomical result?

2 is the use of a synthetic support material helpful?

3 is the abdominal approach superior to the vaginal approach?

Anterior vaginal wall prolapse

In 1909, White [7] described the vaginal paravaginal repair to repair a cystocoele (see Fig. 48.4). Four years later Kelly [8] described the anterior vaginal repair with a central plication of the pubocervical fascia (see Fig. 48.4). The Kelly operation became the treatment of choice for anterior prolapse partly because of the simplicity of the procedure and partly because of Kelly's high standing in the surgical community.

Debate about the relative merits of the Kelly type repair and the paravaginal repair continue to this day. A literature review of over 90 articles between 1966 and 1995 by Weber and Walters [9] illustrated the deficiencies of the literature and found that there was no significant difference in success rate between the paravaginal repair (failure rate 3–14%), whether performed vaginally or abdominally, and the central plication repair (failure rate 0–20%). Beck [1] reviewed 246 anterior repairs and noted that 5% women developed *de novo* stress

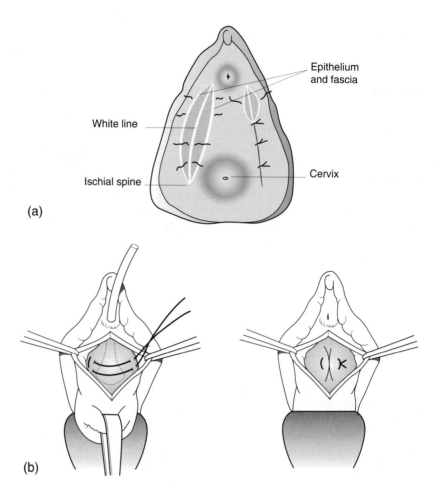

(a)

(b)

Fig. 48.4

incontinence and 5% *de novo* detrusor overactivity post-operatively. Long-standing voiding problems occurred in less than 1%. Post-operative pyrexia developed in 10% of women but the overall morbidity can be described as low.

There have been a few trials published on the use of additional support materials such as polypropylene mesh to strengthen the anterior vaginal repair. The results suggest that a reduction in the risk of recurrence is accompanied by a significant risk of mesh erosion. It would appear that the optimal mesh material has not yet been developed. The use of support materials in primary repairs would certainly not appear to be justified.

Posterior vaginal wall prolapse

The classical posterior vaginal repair involves not only plication of the fascia underlying the vaginal skin but also a central plication of the fascia overlying the pubo-coccygeus muscle even including the muscle itself. There can be little doubt that inclusion of the pubococcygeus fascia and muscle will create a more solid repair with accompanying intra- and post-operative morbidity but it

is unclear whether the functional outcome is better. Kahn and Stanton [10] performed a 2-year follow-up of their posterior vaginal repairs performed in the conventional manner (including levator plication). They noted that in addition to one in four of the women having posterior prolapse on examination more women volunteered functional problems with respect to bowel and dyspareunia than pre-operatively. Some have suggested that a transanal approach to rectocoele repair should be more effective for treatment of defaecation difficulty but the limited robust literature available does not support this [11]. Although the site-specific fascial defect repair has been found to be more effective by some surgeons [12] it has not been studied in a robust, systematic manner.

Similarly, there have been few studies reported to assess the value of adding support materials to a posterior vaginal wall repair. The risk of mesh erosion must be weighed against the potential benefit of reduced risk of recurrence.

Perineal descent is commonly seen with posterior vaginal wall prolapse. Its clinical relevance is not clear but in anatomical terms it indicates either that the perineum is no longer supported by the pelvic floor or that there is weakness of the pelvic floor as a whole. This may be an index of the support of the vaginal vault or the uterus and vaginal apex.

Uterine prolapse

The current conventional approach to uterine prolapse when a woman no longer wishes to have children is a vaginal hysterectomy with any additional repair to the vaginal walls as appropriate. The vaginal vault is then supported by reattaching the uterosacral/cardinal ligaments to the vagina. These ligaments can also be plicated together in the midline to try to prevent the development of enterocoele. The Manchester repair is now less popular but also employed the cardinal ligaments brought together anterior to the cervix which was amputated as part of the operation. The use of the uterosacral/cardinal ligaments has the fundamental problem that it is the weakness of these ligaments that has contributed to the development of the prolapse. Use of such weak tissues must make the risk of recurrence a concern. There is no evidence that uterine conservation, either by abdominal sacrohysteropexy or sacrospinous hysteropexy provides a lower risk of prolapse recurrence. Nor is there evidence that routine use of sacrospinous colpopexy performed at the time of hysterectomy reduces the risk of vault prolapse though the morbidity of the procedure is likely to be higher.

This would suggest that, in the absence of evidence to the contrary, for uterine prolapse the gynaecologist should perform a vaginal hysterectomy with the provision of support to the vaginal vault from the uterosacral ligaments. In the absence of defined support tissue a sacrospinous colpopexy or sacrocolpopexy may be required.

Vaginal vault prolapse

Vaginal vault prolapse occurs in approximately 5% of women after hysterectomy. Most studies indicate that an equal proportion of women have had an abdominal or a vaginal hysterectomy which, given that abdominal hysterectomy is performed more frequently than vaginal, suggests that vaginal hysterectomy predisposes to vault prolapse. Vault prolapse is always accompanied by some degree of upper anterior and posterior vaginal prolapse, the latter usually being the predominant component. Frequently extensive vaginal epithelial stretching occurs and this is usually of the posterior vaginal wall (see Fig. 48.5). Failure to treat extensive vault prolapse may lead to ulceration and less commonly bowel extrusion.

Vaginal vault prolapse may be treated surgically by a vaginal sacrospinous colpopexy or an abdominal (or laparoscopic) sacrocolpopexy. A Cochrane review [11] has reported that the sacrocolpopexy has a higher cure rate and recurrence, when it occurs, will occur sooner with

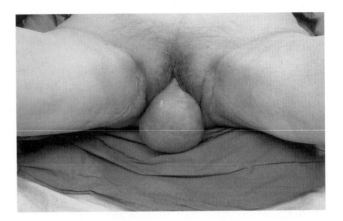

Fig. 48.5

a sacrospinous colpopexy. Dyspareunia appears to occur more frequently after sacrospinous colpopexy. The two procedures do not appear to produce any difference in urinary and bowel symptoms post-operatively. Sacrocolpopexy is associated with a longer recovery (when performed as an open procedure) and is therefore more expensive. Adverse events appear to occur with similar frequency and patient satisfaction rates are similar. Both procedures have the potential to cause large volume haemorrhage (sacrum for sacrocolpopexy and pudendal vessels for sacospinous colpopexy). There is conflicting evidence on which procedure produces a more correct anatomical result.

Mesh erosion is a significant problem after sacrocolpopexy and infrequently may lead to the need for complete mesh removal. Colpocleisis, whereby the vaginal lumen is completely occluded, may be used rarely in women who are unfit for major surgery and in whom conservative measures have failed. Strips of vaginal skin are removed from anterior and posterior vaginal walls and the two are sutured together.

Conclusions

Pelvic floor weakness can result in prolapse with accompanying mechanical and functional symptoms. Improving our understanding of the aetiology of prolapse should help direct the treatment including non-surgical and surgical methods. More research is required into treatment and outcome measures from treatment if gynaecologists are to make significant progress in this field.

References

1. Beck RP, McCormick S & Nordstrom L (1991) A 25-year experience with 519 anterior colporrhaphy procedures. *Obstet Gynecol* **78**(6), 1011–8.

2. Olsen AL, Smith VJ, Bergstrom JO, Colling JC & Clark AL (1997) Epidemiology of surgically managed pelvic organ prolapse and urinary incontinence. *Obstet Gynecol* **89**(4), 501–6.

3. Smith AR, Hosker GL & Warrell DW (1989) The role of partial denervation of the pelvic floor in the aetiology of genitourinary prolapse and stress incontinence of urine. A neurophysiological study. *Br J Obstet Gynaecol* **96**(1), 24–8.

4. Allen RE *et al.* (1990) Pelvic floor damage and childbirth: a neurophysiological study. *Br J Obstet Gynaecol* **97**(9), 770–9.

5. Landon CR, Smith ARB, Crofts CD & Trowbridge EA (1990) Mechanical properties of fascia in pregnancy: its possible relationship to the later development of stress incontinence of urine. *Contemp Rev Obstet Gynaecol* **2**, 40–6.

6. Bump RC *et al.*, The Continence Program for Women Research Group (1996) Randomized prospective comparison of needle colposuspension versus endopelvic fascia plication for potential stress incontinence prophylaxis in women undergoing vaginal reconstruction for stage III or IV pelvic organ prolapse. *Am J Obstet Gynecol* **175**(2), 326–33; discussion 333–5.

7. White GR (1909) Cystocele. *J Am Med Assoc* **21**, 1707–10.

8. Kelly HA (1913) Incontinence of urine in women. *Urol Cutan Rev* **17**, 291–3.

9. Weber AM & Walters MD (1997) Anterior vaginal prolapse: review of anatomy and techniques of surgical repair. *Obstet Gynecol* **89**(2), 311–8.

10. Kahn MA & Stanton SL (1997) Posterior Colporrhaphy: its effects on bowel and sexual function. *Br J Obstet Gynaecol* **104**(1), 82–6.

11. Maher C, Baessler K, Glazener CMA, Adams EJ & Hagen S (2004) Surgical management of pelvic organ prolapse in women (Review). Cochrane Collaboration 2005 **4**, CD004014.

12. Shull BL (1991) Urologic surgical techniques. *Curr Opin Obstet Gynecol* **3**(4), 534–40.

Chapter 49: Urinary incontinence

D. Robinson and L. Cardozo

Urinary incontinence is a distressing condition that, although rarely life threatening, severely affects all aspects of a woman's quality of life. Through ignorance, embarrassment and a belief that loss of bladder control is a 'normal' result of child birth and ageing, many women suffer for years before seeking help [1]. This is unfortunate because with appropriate investigations an accurate diagnosis can be made and many women can be cured, most improved and all helped by various different management strategies.

Urinary incontinence is defined as the complaint of any involuntary loss of urine [2]. Conversely, continence is the ability to hold urine within the bladder at all times except during micturition. Both continence and micturition depend upon a lower urinary tract, consisting of the bladder and urethra, which is structurally and functionally normal. In order to understand urinary incontinence in women it is necessary to have a basic knowledge of the embryology, anatomy and physiology of the lower urinary tract.

Structure of the lower urinary tract

Embryology

In women the lower urinary and genital tracts develop in close proximity. The gut is formed by an invagination of the yolk sac and the most caudal part (hindgut) develops a diverticulum, the allantois (Fig. 49.1a). That part of the hindgut connected to the allantois is the cloaca. At about 28 days after fertilization a mesenchymal wedge of tissue, the urorectal septum, starts to migrate caudally and divides the cloaca into a ventral part, the urogenital sinus and a dorsal part, which will become the anorectal canal (Fig. 49.1b). The two are eventually separated from one another when the septum fuses with the cloacal membrane some 10 days later.

At the same time the pronephros develops within the mesoderm but this undergoes early degeneration. The mesonephros initially forms a primitive kidney draining into the mesonephric duct on each side. The tubules undergo degeneration but the ducts remain and grow caudally to enter the anterior part of the cloaca on each side. This divides the urogenital sinus into two parts: the area lying between the mesonephric ducts and allantois is the vesicourethral canal and the area below the mesonephric ducts is the urogenital sinus (Fig. 49.1c). The ureteric bud develops as an outgrowth from the mesonephric duct by proliferation of cells. It grows towards the caudal end of the nephrogenic ridge and initiates the development of the metanephros (later to become the kidney) between 30 and 37 days after fertilization.

Dilatation of the cranial portion of the vesicourethral canal leads to the development of the bladder. The area of the bladder bounded by the ureteric orifices cranially and the termination of the mesonephric ducts caudally gives rise to the trigone. The caudal part of the vesicourethral canal narrows to form the upper urethra. The urogenital sinus gives rise to the distal part of the urethra and part of the vagina. These developments occur by 42 days after fertilization (Fig. 49.1d).

Anatomy

The bladder is a hollow muscular organ normally situated behind the pubic symphysis and covered superiorly and anteriorly by peritoneum. It is composed of a syncytium of smooth muscle fibres known as the detrusor. Contraction of this meshwork of fibres results in simultaneous reduction of the bladder in all its diameters. The smooth muscle cells within the detrusor contain significant amounts of acetylcholinesterase, representing their cholinergic parasympathetic nerve supply.

The trigone is easily distinguishable from the rest of the smooth muscle of the bladder as it is divided into two layers. The deep trigonal muscle is similar to that of the detrusor, whereas the superficial muscle of the trigone is thin with small muscle bundles; the cells are devoid of acetylcholinesterase and have a reduced cholinergic nerve

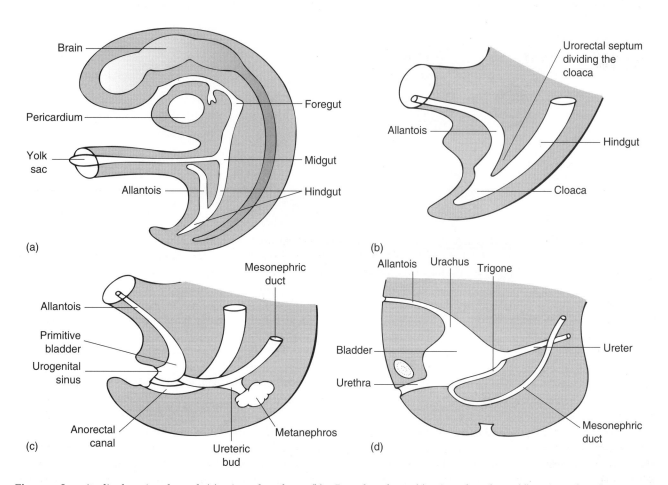

Fig. 49.1 Longitudinal section through (a) a 4-week embryo; (b) a 5-week embryo; (c) a 6-week embryo; (d) an 8-week embryo.

supply. This superficial trigonal muscle merges into the proximal urethra and into the ureteric smooth muscle. In women the smooth muscle of the bladder neck is also different from that of the detrusor with orientation of the muscle bundles obliquely or longitudinally; they do not form a sphincter in women. The smooth muscle fibres of the detrusor, trigone and urethra have been shown embryonically to be distinct from one another. The urothelium lining the bladder is composed of two or three layers of transitional cells.

The normal adult female urethra is between 3 and 5 cm in length (Fig. 49.2). It is a hollow tubular structure joining the bladder to the exterior and is located under the pubic symphysis, piercing the pelvic diaphragm anterior to the vagina. It is lined with pseudo-stratified transitional cell epithelium in its proximal half and distally by non-keratinized stratified squamous epithelium. Beneath this is a rich vascular plexus which contributes up to one-third of the urethral pressure and which decreases with age. Beneath this there is longitudinally orientated smooth muscle which is continuous morphologically with

the detrusor, but histochemically distinct. Contraction of this muscle layer leads to shortening and opening of the urethra. The main bulk of striated muscle is located in the middle third of the urethra and is orientated in bundles of circularly arranged fibres, thickest anteriorly, thinning laterally and almost totally deficient posteriorly. This is the rhabdosphincter urethrae, and has also been called the external sphincter or the intrinsic sphincter mechanism. The muscle fibres of the rhabdosphincter consist of small diameter slow twitch fibres which are rich in acid-stable myosin adenosine triphosphatase (ATPase) and possess a number of mitochondria. This muscle mass is responsible for urethral closure at rest.

The extrinsic sphincter mechanism consists of striated periurethral muscle (levator ani) which has no direct connection with the urethra and is situated at the junction of the middle and lower thirds of the urethra. This muscle consists of large diameter fibres, most of which are rich in alkaline-stable myosin ATPase characteristic of fast twitch muscle fibres. This extrinsic sphincter mechanism contributes an additional closure force at times of physical

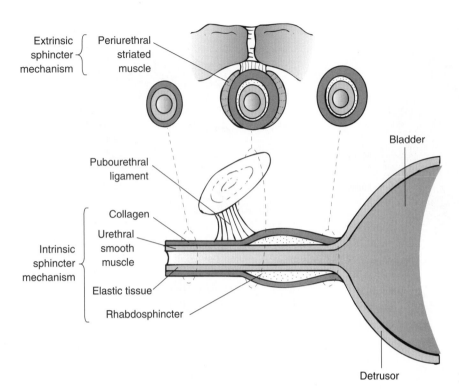

Extrinsic sphincter mechanism { Periurethral striated muscle

Bladder

Pubourethral ligament

Collagen
Urethral smooth muscle
Intrinsic sphincter mechanism {
Elastic tissue
Rhabdosphincter

Detrusor

Fig. 49.2 The adult female urethra.

effort. Together the intrinsic and extrinsic sphincter mechanisms of the urethra produce a greater pressure within the urethra than in the bladder. This is known as the positive closure pressure and is partly responsible for the maintenance of continence.

The proximal urethra is supported by the pubourethral ligaments which attach the proximal urethra to the posterior aspect of the pubic symphysis. These were originally described by Zacharin [3]) as consisting of parallel collagen bundles and elastic connective tissue. However, his histological examinations were of cadaveric specimens and Wilson *et al.* [4] have shown in operative specimens that these ligaments contain large numbers of smooth muscle bundles. Gosling *et al.* [5] reported that the pubourethral suspensory ligaments are histochemically identical to the detrusor with an abundant supply of cholinergic nerve fibres. But Wilson *et al.* [4] failed to demonstrate acetylcholinesterase activity in these fibres, thus their origin remains unclear. DeLancey [6] has described two distinct entities: the pubourethral ligament composed of collagen and a pubovesical ligament containing muscle fibres.

Innervation

The detrusor muscle is innervated primarily by the parasympathetic nerves S2–4 and receives a rich efferent supply (Fig. 49.3). Adrenergic receptors have also been shown to be present in the lower urinary tract, with β receptors in the dome of the bladder and bladder neck, and α receptors in the bladder neck and urethra [7]. Sympathetic outflow is from T10 to L2 but it is unclear whether it acts directly on β receptors in the bladder, causing relaxation, or indirectly via parasympathetic ganglia, causing inhibition of the excitatory parasympathetic supply. Visceral afferent fibres travel with the thoracolumbar and sacral efferent nerves conveying the sensation of bladder distension.

Urethral smooth muscle is innervated by sympathetic efferent fibres; cholinergic stimulation of these produces contraction. The rhabdosphincter urethrae is supplied via sacral nerve roots (S2–4) which travel with the pelvic splanchnics to the intrinsic smooth muscle of the urethra. The levator ani is also innervated by motor fibres of S2–4 origin, but these fibres travel via the pudendal nerve. This explains why electromyographic activity of the pelvic floor and urethral sphincter are not necessarily the same.

The central nervous control of micturition is complex and requires a sacral spinal reflex arc controlled by the cerebral cortex, the cerebellum and subcortical areas, including the thalamus, basal ganglia, limbic system, hypothalamus and pontine reticular formation. There are parasympathetic, sympathetic and somatic afferent and efferent connections from the brainstem. Stretch receptors within the bladder wall pass impulses through the pelvic plexus and via the visceral afferent fibres travelling

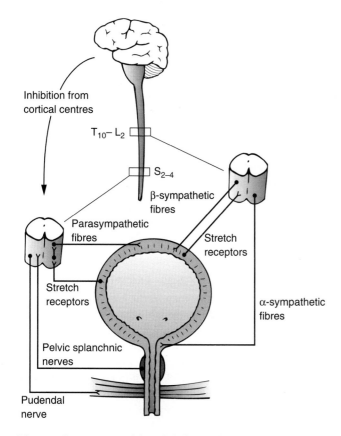

Fig. 49.3 Innervation of the adult female lower urinary tract.

with the pelvic splanchnic nerves, ending in S2–4 of the spinal cord. This visceral reflex arc is controlled by both the excitatory and inhibitory centres which, under normal circumstances, prevent detrusor contractions and maintain urethral sphincter control, thereby inhibiting micturition.

Functioning of the lower urinary tract

Physiology

The main role of the bladder is to store the urine which continuously enters it, in order to achieve convenient intermittent voiding. Thus the bladder must act as an efficient low pressure continent reservoir. Urine from the kidneys enters the bladder via the ureters at a rate of 0.5–5 ml/min. Normally, the first sensation of bladder filling is noted at between 150 and 250 ml and there is a strong desire to void at approximately 400–600 ml (bladder capacity). During filling the bladder pressure should not normally rise by more than 10 cm of water to 300 ml, or 15 cm of water to 500 ml. In order to maintain continence the maximum urethral pressure must exceed the bladder pressure at all times except during micturition. Thus, for continence to exist it is not only essential that the intravesical pressure remains low but also that the urethral

lumen should seal completely. Three essential components of urethral function are required to achieve hermetic closure: (1) urethral inner wall softness; (2) inner urethral compression; and (3) outer wall tension. These three functions are dependent on an intact urothelium, together with a major component from the submucosal vascular plexus as well as the collagen and elastic tissue within the urethra and the striated and smooth muscle.

STORAGE PHASE

During this time the urethra remains closed as previously described. Proprioceptive afferent impulses from the stretch receptors within the bladder wall pass via the pelvic nerves to the sacral roots S2–4. These impulses ascend the cord via the lateral spinothalamic tracts and the detrusor motor response is subconsciously inhibited by descending impulses from the basal ganglia. Gradually, as the bladder volume increases, further afferent impulses are sent to the cerebral cortex and the first sensation of desire to void is usually appreciated at about half the functional bladder capacity. Inhibition of detrusor contraction becomes cortically mediated. As the bladder fills further, these afferent impulses reinforce the desire to void and conscious inhibition of micturition occurs until a suitable time. When functional capacity is reached, voluntary pelvic floor contraction is initiated to aid urethral closure. This may result in marked variations in urethral pressure as the sensation of urgency develops.

VOIDING PHASE

At a suitable time and place, cortical inhibition is released and relaxation of the pelvic floor occurs, together with relaxation of the intrinsic striated muscle of the urethra. This results in a fall in urethral pressure which occurs a few seconds prior to the increase in bladder pressure. A few seconds later, a rapid discharge of efferent parasympathetic impulses via the pelvic nerve causes the detrusor to contract and also possibly to open the bladder neck and shorten the urethra. The detrusor pressure rises by a variable amount, normally less than 60 cm of water in women. However, it may not need to rise at all if the fall in urethral resistance is adequate for the urethral pressure to be lower than the intravesical pressure, so that urine is voided.

Once micturition has been initiated the intravesical pressure normally remains constant. The efficiency of detrusor contraction increases as the muscle fibres of the detrusor shorten, therefore decreasing the forces which are required to maintain micturition.

Interruption of micturition is usually achieved by contraction of the extrinsic striated muscle of the pelvic floor, associated with a rise in urethral pressure to exceed the intravesical pressure and thus stop the flow of urine. Since the detrusor is composed of smooth muscle, it is much slower to relax and therefore continues to contract against the closed sphincter; this causes an isometric detrusor contraction which will eventually die away to the premicturition detrusor pressure.

When the bladder empties at the end of micturition, the urinary flow stops, the pelvic floor and intrinsic striated muscle of the urethra contract and any urine which is left in the proximal urethra will be milked back into the bladder. As the urethra closes off, subconscious inhibition of the sacral micturition centre is reinstituted and the bladder storage phase begins again.

Pathophysiology of urinary incontinence

Under normal circumstances, in a woman with a healthy lower urinary tract, urine will only leave the bladder via the urethra when the intravesical pressure exceeds the maximum urethral pressure. In general terms and in the majority of cases of urinary incontinence, the bladder pressure exceeds the urethral pressure because the urethral sphincter mechanism is weak (urodynamic stress incontinence) or because the detrusor pressure is excessively high (detrusor overactivity; neurogenic detrusor overactivity).

In urodynamic stress incontinence the factors which maintain positive urethral closure pressure at rest may be inadequate when there is an increase in intra-abdominal pressure. This is particularly likely to occur if the bladder neck and proximal urethra are poorly supported or have descended through the pelvic floor, as in cases of concomitant cystourethrocele.

An abnormally high detrusor pressure may occur in detrusor overactivity when there is inability to inhibit detrusor contractions. In cases of a low compliance, incontinence may occur when there is a failure of the bladder to accommodate a large volume of urine for a small rise in pressure.

Epidemiology

Prevalence of urinary incontinence

Urinary incontinence is common. Table 49.1 shows the prevalence of urinary incontinence in women living at home according to a report published by the Royal College of Physicians [8]. Thomas *et al.* [9] have shown that urinary incontinence occurs twice or more per month in at least a third of the female population over the age of 35 years and, although there is a small rise with increasing age, it is a very common problem in women of all ages. The situation is worst amongst the elderly and in psychogeriatric hospital wards, where up to 90% of female

Table 49.1 Prevalence of urinary incontinence

	Age (years)	Incontinence (%)
Women living at home	15–44	5–7
	45–64	8–5
	65+	10–20
Men living at home	15–64	3
	65+	7–10
Both sexes living in institutions		
Residential homes	25	
Nursing homes	40	
Hospital	50–70	

Data from Royal College of Physicians (1995).

patients are incontinent of urine. A MORI poll [10] showed that at last 3.5 million women in the UK suffer from urinary incontinence and it is possible that the number is far greater [11]. More recently a large epidemiological study of urinary incontinence has been reported in 27,936 women from Norway [12]. Overall 25% of women reported urinary incontinence of which 7% felt it to be significant and the prevalence of incontinence was found to increase with age. When considering the type of incontinence 50% of women complained of stress, 11% urge and 36% mixed incontinence. Further analysis has also investigated the effect of age and parity. The prevalence of urinary incontinence among nulliparous women ranged from 8% to 32% and increased with age. In general parity was associated with incontinence and the first delivery was the most significant. When considering stress incontinence in the age group 20–34 years the relative risk was 2.7 (95%CI: 2.0–3.5) for primiparous women and 4.0 (95%CI: 2.5–6.4) for multiparous women. There was a similar association for mixed incontinence although not for urge incontinence [13].

In a large study of patients assessed after tertiary referral 60% of women were found to have delayed seeking treatment for more than one year from the time their symptoms became severe. Of these women 50% claimed that this was because they were too embarrassed to discuss the problem with their doctor, and 17% said that they thought the problem was normal for their age [1].

The financial burden of incontinence is also considerable. In 1998 the annual economic cost was projected to be approximately £354 million [14]. Of this total £22.7 million is spent on drugs, £58.6 million on appliances and £69 million on containment products such as pads and pants. Surgery only accounts for £13.3 million whilst the largest amount is spent on staff costs, this amounting to £189.9 million [15]. Worldwide the situation is similar with $26 billion being spent per annum in the United States alone [16].

Age

The incidence of urinary incontinence increases with increasing age. Elderly women have been found to have a reduced flow rate, increased urinary residuals, higher filling pressures, reduced bladder capacity and lower maximum voiding pressures. In a large study of 842 women aged 17–64 years the prevalence rates of urinary incontinence increased progressively over seven birth cohorts (1900–1940) from 12% to 25%. These findings agree with those of a large telephone survey in the United States of America which reported a prevalence of urge incontinence of 5% in the 18–44 age rising to 19% in women over 65 years of age [17]. Conversely, as mobility and physical exercise decrease with advancing age so does the prevalence of stress urinary incontinence.

Race

Several studies have been performed examining the impact of racial differences on the prevalence of urinary incontinence in women. In general there is evidence that there is a lower incidence of both urinary incontinence and urogenital prolapse in black women and North American studies have found a larger proportion of white than African American women reported symptoms of stress incontinence (31% versus 7%) and a larger proportion were found to have demonstrable stress incontinence on objective assessment (61% versus 27%). Overall white women had a prevalence of urodynamic stress incontinence 2.3 times higher than African American women [18]. Whilst most studies confirm these findings there is little evidence regarding the prevalence of urge incontinence or mixed incontinence.

Pregnancy

Pregnancy is responsible for marked changes in the urinary tract and consequently lower urinary tract symptoms are more common and many are simply a reflection of normal physiological change. Urine production increases in pregnancy due to increasing cardiac output and a 25% increase in renal perfusion and glomerular filtration rate.

Frequency of micturition is one of the earliest symptoms of pregnancy affecting approximately 60% in the first- and mid-trimester and 81% in the final trimester. Nocturia is also a common symptom although it was only thought to be a nuisance in 4% of cases. Overall frequency occurs in over 90% of women in pregnancy.

Urgency and urge incontinence have also been shown to increase in pregnancy. Urge incontinence has been shown to have a peak incidence of 19% in multiparous women whilst other authors have reported a rate of urge incontinence of 10% and urgency of 60%. The incidence of detrusor overactivity and low compliance in pregnancy has been reported as 24% and 31%, respectively. The cause of the former may be due to high progesterone levels whilst the latter is probably a consequence of pressure from the gravid uterus.

Stress incontinence has also been reported to be more common in pregnancy, with 28% of women complaining of symptoms although only 12% remained symptomatic following delivery. The long-term prognosis for this group of women remains guarded. Continent women delivered vaginally have been compared to those who had a caesarean section. Whilst there was initially a difference in favour of caesarean section this effect was insignificant by three months following delivery [19].

Childbirth

Childbirth may result in damage to the pelvic floor musculature as well as injury to the pudendal and pelvic nerves. The association between increasing parity and urinary incontinence has been reported in several studies. Some authorities have found this relationship to be linear whilst others have demonstrated a threshold at the first delivery and some have shown that increasing age at first delivery is significant. A large Australian study has demonstrated a strong relationship between urinary incontinence and parity in young women (18–23 years) although in middle age (45–50 years) there was only a modest association and this was lost in older women (70–75 years) [20].

Obstetric factors themselves may also have a direct effect on continence following delivery. The risk of incontinence increases by 5.7-fold in women who have had a previous vaginal delivery although a previous caesarean section did not increase the risk [21]. In addition, an increased risk of urinary incontinence has been associated with increased exposure to oxytocic drugs, vacuum extraction, forceps delivery and fetal macrosomia.

Menopause

The urogenital tract and lower urinary tract are sensitive to the effects of oestrogen and progesterone throughout adult life. Epidemiological studies have implicated oestrogen deficiency in the aetiology of lower urinary tract symptoms occurring following the menopause with 70% of women relating the onset of urinary incontinence to their final menstrual period. Lower urinary tract symptoms have been shown to be common in postmenopausal women attending a menopause clinic with 20% complaining of severe urgency and almost 50% complaining of stress incontinence. Urge incontinence in particular is more prevalent following the menopause and the prevalence would appear to rise with increasing years of oestrogen deficiency. Some studies have shown a peak incidence in perimenopausal women whilst other evidence suggests that many women develop incontinence at least 10 years prior to the cessation of menstruation with significantly more premenopausal women than postmenopausal women being affected.

Quality of life

Urinary incontinence is a common and distressing condition known to adversely affect quality of life [22]. Research has often concentrated on the prevalence, aetiology, diagnosis and management of urinary incontinence with little work being performed on the effects of this chronic condition, or its treatment, on quality of life (QoL). Over the last few decades interest in the incorporation of patient assessed health status or QoL measures into the evaluation of the management of urinary incontinence has increased [23].

The views of clinicians and patients regarding QoL and the effects of treatments differ considerably. Consequently there is increased recognition of the patients' perception when assessing new interventions in the management of lower urinary tract dysfunction. The measurement of QoL allows the quantification of morbidity, the evaluation of treatment efficacy and also acts as a measure of how lives are affected and coping strategies adopted. It is estimated that 20% of adult women suffer some degree of life disruption secondary to lower urinary tract dysfunction [24].

The World Health Organisation has defined health as 'not merely the absence of disease, but complete physical, mental and social well-being' [25]. Quality of life has been used to mean a combination of patient assessed measures of health including physical function, role function, social function, emotional or mental state, burden of symptoms and sense of well-being [26]. QoL has been defined as including 'those attributes valued by patients including their resultant comfort or sense of well-being; the extent to which they were able to maintain reasonable physical, emotional, and intellectual function; the degree to which they retain their ability to participate in valued activities within the family and the community' [27]. This helps to emphasize the multidimensional nature of QoL and the importance of considering patients perception of their own situation with regard to non-health related aspects of their life [28].

Whilst quality of life is highly subjective it has now been acknowledged that it is as important as physical disease state in the management of women with lower urinary tract dysfunction [29]. Consequently the success of treatment can no longer be judged on clinical parameters alone and quality of life needs to be considered in both clinical and research settings [30].

Quality of life assessment

There are many validated questionnaires available although all have the same structure, consisting of a series of sections (domains) designed to gather information regarding particular aspects of health (Table 49.2). There are two types of QoL questionnaires, generic and disease, or condition-specific.

More recently the International Consultation on Incontinence (ICI) has published levels of recommendation for both generic and disease-specific questionnaires [31] (Table 49.3).

Generic QoL questionnaires

Generic questionnaires are designed as general measures of QoL and are therefore applicable to a wide range of populations and clinical conditions. Many different validated

Table 49.2 Quality of life domains

Domains of quality of life
Physical function, e.g. mobility, self-care, exercise
Emotional function, e.g. depression, anxiety, worry
Social function, e.g. intimacy, social support, social contact leisure activities
Role performance, e.g. work, housework, shopping
Pain
Sleep/nausea
Disease-specific symptoms
Severity measures

Table 49.3 Criteria for the recommendation of questionnaires

Grade of recommendation	Evidence required
Grade A Highly recommended	Published data indicating that it is valid, reliable and responsive to change on psychometric testing
Grade B Recommended	Published data indicating that it is valid and reliable on psychometric testing
Grade C With potential	Published data (including abstracts) indicating that it is valid or reliable or responsive on psychometric testing

Table 49.4 Generic quality of life questionnaires

Generic quality of life questionnaires (Grade A)
Short form 36 (SF-36) [32]

Generic quality of life questionnaires (Grade B)
Sickness impact profile [33]
Nottingham health profile [34]
Goteborg quality of life [35]

Table 49.5 Disease-specific quality of life questionnaires

Disease-specific quality of life questionnaires (Grade A)
Urogenital distress inventory (UDI) [36]
Urogenital distress inventory – 6 (UDI-6) [37]
Urge UDI [38]
Incontinence severity index [39]
Quality of life in persons with urinary incontinence
  (I-QoL) [40]
King's health questionnaire [22]
Incontinence impact questionnaire (IIQ) [41]

Table 49.6 Causes of urinary incontinence in women

Urodynamic stress incontinence (urethral sphincter
  incompetence)
Detrusor overactivity (neurogenic detrusor overactivity)
Overactive bladder
Retention with overflow
Fistulae – vesicovaginal, ureterovaginal, urethrovaginal,
  complex
Congenital abnormalities, e.g. epispadias, ectopic ureter,
  spina bifida occulta
Urethral diverticulum
Temporary, for example, urinary tract infection, faecal
  impaction
Functional, for example, immobility

Table 49.7 Causes of incontinence in the
elderly – many of which may be transient

Infection (e.g. urinary tract infection)
Confusional states (e.g. dementia)
Faecal impaction
Oestrogen deficiency
Restricted mobility
Depression
Drug therapy (e.g. diuretics)
Endocrine disorder (e.g. diabetes)
Limited independence

generic questionnaires have been developed although not all are suitable for the assessment of lower urinary tract problems Table 49.4. They are not specific to a particular disease, treatment or age group and hence allow broad comparisons to be made. Consequently they lack sensitivity when applied to women with lower urinary tract symptoms and may be unable to detect clinically important improvement.

Disease-specific QoL questionnaires

To improve the sensitivity of QoL questionnaires disease-specific tools have been developed to assess particular medical conditions more accurately and in greater detail (Table 49.5). The questions are designed to focus on key aspects associated with lower urinary tract symptoms whilst scoring is performed so that clinically important changes can be detected.

In general, perhaps the best solution when assessing women with urinary incontinence is to use a generic and a disease-specific questionnaire in combination, both of which have been validated and used previously.

Classification

Urinary incontinence is best classified according to aetiology as shown in Table 49.6. There are a number of additional causes of urinary incontinence in elderly woman (Table 49.7), many of which can be reversed by appropriate intervention.

More recently the term Overactive Bladder (OAB) has been introduced to describe the symptom complex of urgency with, or without urge incontinence, usually with frequency and nocturia [2]. Recent epidemiological studies have reported the overall prevalence of OAB in women to be 16.9% suggesting that there could be 17.5 million women in the United States of America who suffer from the condition. The prevalence increases with age, being 4.8% in women under 25 years to 30.9% in those over the age of 65 years [17]. This is supported by recent prevalence data from Europe in which 16,776 interviews were conducted in a population based survey [42]. The overall prevalence of overactive bladder in individuals 40 years and above was 16.6% and increased with age. Frequency was the most commonly reported symptom (85%) whilst 54% complained of urgency and 36% urge incontinence. When considering management 60% had consulted a physician although only 27% were currently receiving treatment.

Clinical presentation of urinary incontinence

Symptoms of lower urinary tract dysfunction fall into three main groups: (1) incontinence; (2) overactive bladder symptoms; and (3) voiding difficulties.

Stress incontinence is the most common complaint. It may be a symptom or a sign but it is not a diagnosis. Apart from stress incontinence, women may complain of urge incontinence, dribble or giggle incontinence or incontinence during sexual intercourse. Nocturnal enuresis (bed wetting) may occur on its own or in conjunction with other complaints. Symptoms of voiding difficulty include hesitancy, a poor stream, straining to void and incomplete bladder emptying.

Apart from the symptoms of lower urinary tract dysfunction, it is important to take a full history from all women who present with urinary incontinence. Other gynaecological symptoms such as prolapse or menstrual disturbances may be relevant. A fibroid uterus may compress the bladder and can cause urinary frequency and urgency. There is an increased incidence of stress incontinence amongst women who have had large babies, particularly following instrumental vaginal delivery, so an obstetric history may be helpful. Information regarding other urological problems such as recurrent urinary tract infections, episodes of acute urinary retention or childhood enuresis should be sought.

Urinary incontinence is sometimes the first manifestation of a neurological problem (notable multiple sclerosis) so it is important to enquire about neurological symptoms. Endocrine disorders such as diabetes may be responsible for symptoms of lower urinary tract dysfunction and should therefore be recorded.

Some drugs affect urinary tract function, especially diuretics, which increase urine output. In older people they may cause urinary incontinence where only urgency existed previously. Other drugs which affect detrusor function include tricyclic antidepressants, major tranquillizers and α adrenergic blockers.

Unfortunately, clinical examination is usually unhelpful in cases of female urinary incontinence. General examination should include the subject's mental state and mobility as well as the appearance of local tissues. Excoriation of the vulva will indicate the severity of the problem and atrophic changes may reveal long-standing hormone deficiency. A gynaecological/urological examination should be carried out and, although stress incontinence may be demonstrated, this will only confirm the patient's story; it will not actually indicate the cause. If a neurological lesion is suspected then the cranial nerves and sacral nerve roots S2–4 should be examined.

The bladder has been described as an 'unreliable witness'. The correlation between clinical diagnosis and urodynamic diagnosis is poor and therefore it is unusual to be able to make an accurate diagnosis based on history and examination alone. Urodynamic stress incontinence is the commonest cause of urinary incontinence in women and detrusor overactivity is the second most common cause. These two diagnoses account for over 90% of cases of female urinary incontinence. As their treatment differs it is important to make an accurate initial diagnosis. Jarvis *et al.* [43] studied 41 women with urodynamic stress incontinence and 34 women with detrusor overactivity. They found that, although 98% of women with urodynamic stress incontinence complained of the symptom of stress incontinence, so did 25% of those with detrusor overactivity. In addition, 89% of women with detrusor overactivity complained of the symptom of urge incontinence, but so did 37% of those with urodynamic stress incontinence. Thus, it is difficult to separate these two common conditions on history alone. In fact, comparing the initial clinical diagnosis with the accurate urodynamic diagnosis, Jarvis *et al.* [43] found that 68% of those with urodynamic stress incontinence were correctly diagnosed, whereas only 51% of those with detrusor overactivity would have been correctly allocated.

Investigations

Investigations range from the very simple to the highly sophisticated and complex and are outlined in Table 49.8.

MID-STREAM URINE (MSU) SAMPLE

A mid-stream specimen of urine should always be sent for culture and sensitivity prior to further investigation. Although the patient's symptoms are unlikely to be caused by a urinary tract infection, they can be altered by one, and catheterization in the presence of an infection could result in septicaemia. In addition, the results of the investigations themselves may be inaccurate in the presence of an infection.

Table 49.8 Investigations of female urinary incontinence

General practitioner/outpatient
Mid-stream specimen of urine
Frequency/volume chart
Pad test

Basic urodynamics
Uroflowmetry
Cystometry
Videocystourethrography

Specialized
Urethral pressure profilometry
Cystourethroscopy
Ultrasound
Cystourethrography
Intravenous urography
Electromyography
Ambulatory urodynamics

Time	Day 1 In	Out	W	Day 2 In	Out	W	Day 3 In	Out	W	Day 4 In	Out	W	Day 5 In	Out	W
6 am															
7 am							200	150						300	
8 am 8.30	200 200	350		200	250		200				350		200		
9 am										400	50		200	150	
10 am 10.45	200	50			75										
11 am								50		200					
12 pm				200	60		200				50			50	
1 pm	200	100						25					200		
2 pm				200	60					200	100			175	
3 pm	100				100					100					
4 pm		75					200	100							
5 pm .30	100			50	150			300		100					
6 pm .15		150									100		40		
7 pm		100			50									100	
8 pm							200	175		200	150				
9 pm		250			100						150		50	100	
10 pm	200				50		200				100				
11 pm .30		200 100						325			100			150	
12 am							100								
1 am .30		100		100	50						100				
2 am								50							
3 am		75													
4 am					150										
5 am											150			200	

Fig. 49.4 King's College Hospital frequency–volume chart. Example of a frequency–volume chart showing frequent small voided volumes.

FREQUENCY–VOLUME CHARTS

It is often helpful to ask women to complete a frequency–volume chart or urinary diary (Fig. 49.4). This is informative for the doctor as well as the patient and may indicate excessive drinking or bad habit as the cause of lower urinary tract symptoms. There is a tendency for patients to exaggerate their urinary symptoms when giving a history [44] and their recall of incontinent episodes may not be reliable. The frequency–volume chart (urinary or bladder diary) provides an objective assessment of a patient's fluid input and urine output.

As well as the number of voids and incontinence episodes, the mean volume voided over a 24-h period can also be calculated as well as the diurnal and nocturnal volumes. Frequency–volume charts have the advantage of assessing symptom severity in the everyday situation.

Self-monitoring techniques may themselves modify the behaviour they are assessing [45]. However, reported micturition frequency and the number of incontinent episodes have been found to be highly reproducible on test–retest analysis [44, 46]. There is ongoing discussion regarding the optimum duration that the charts should be completed

for. Clearly there needs to be a balance between asking the patient to complete a diary for a long period of time and thus increasing the reliability and the inconvenience this causes. Current practice is to use a five-day chart although some authorities would suggest only three days. The results obtained in each week of a two week diary have been compared [44] and there is a strong correlation between the two weeks suggesting that seven days is an acceptable alternative to fourteen. A short urinary diary of only two days has also been assessed in 151 asymptomatic women aged 19–81 years [46]. Of these women only 8% had a micturition frequency of eight times or more in 24 h with a tendency for the number of nocturnal micturitions to increase with age. Unfortunately, in symptomatic women it is not possible to reliably distinguish patients with urodynamic stress incontinence from those with other urodynamic diagnoses using a frequency–volume chart alone [47].

PAD TEST

Incontinence can be confirmed (without diagnosing the cause) by performing a pad weighing test. Many different types of pad test have been described. The following is just an example. The subject is asked to drink 500 ml of water. She then applies a preweighed perineal pad (sanitary towel) to her perineum and spends the next hour walking around, performing normal household duties. She performs a series of exercises, including coughing and deep knee bending and washes her hands under running water before the pad is reweighed. A weight gain of more than 1 g in 1 h normally represents urinary incontinence. The 24- and 48-h home pad tests have been described and, although they may be more representative, they require greater patient compliance and motivation to perform.

Urodynamics

The term urodynamic studies describes several investigations which are employed to determine bladder function.

UROFLOWMETRY

Uroflowmetry, the measurement of urine flow rate, is a simple test which can exclude the presence of outflow obstruction, or a hypotonic detrusor, but on its own will not differentiate between the two. Various different types of flowmeter are available and utilize a strain gauge weighing transducer, an electronic dipstick, a rotating disc or ultrasound. In order to obtain a flow rate, the patient is asked to void on to the flowmeter, in private, when her bladder is comfortably full. The maximum flow rate

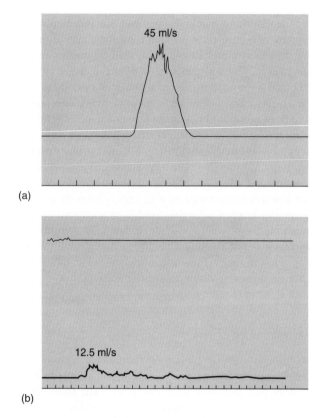

(a)

(b)

Fig. 49.5 (a) Normal uroflowmetry (maximum flow 45 ml/s, voided volume 330 ml); (b) reduced flow rate (maximum flow rate 12.5 ml/s, voided volume 225 ml).

and volume voided are recorded. In women, the normal recording is a bell-shaped curve with a peak flow rate of at least 15 ml/s for a volume of 150 ml of urine voided (Fig. 49.5a). A reduced flow rate in an asymptomatic woman may be important if she is to undergo incontinence surgery as she is more likely to develop voiding difficulties in the postoperative period (Fig. 49.5b).

CYSTOMETRY

Cystometry, which measures the pressure–volume relationship within the bladder, can differentiate between urodynamic stress incontinence and detrusor overactivity in the majority of cases (Fig. 49.6). Simple cystometry is easy to perform and can be carried out in all district general hospitals. The bladder is filled with physiological saline via a blood-giving set and urethral catheter (Fig. 49.7). During bladder filling the intravesical (total bladder) pressure is measured using a central venous pressure line water manometer. This type of simple cystometry is subject to two major sources of error. First, the intravesical pressure cannot be measured continuously during bladder filling so sequential bladder filling must be employed.

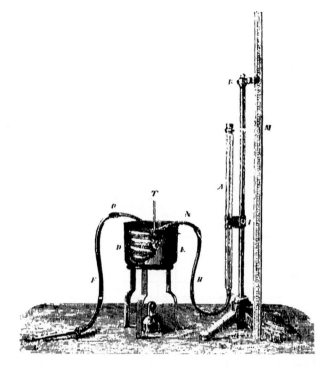

Fig. 49.6 The first cystometer. From Mosso and Pellacani (1882).

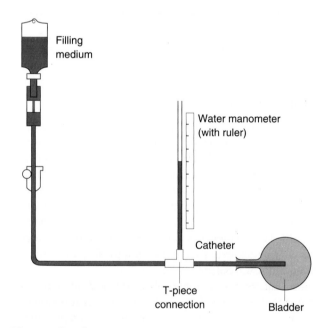

Fig. 49.7 Simple cystometry.

Second, measurement of the intravesical pressure does not always accurately represent changes in detrusor pressure. As the bladder is an intra-abdominal organ the detrusor is subject to changes in intra-abdominal pressure and therefore subtracted cystometry, which involves measurement

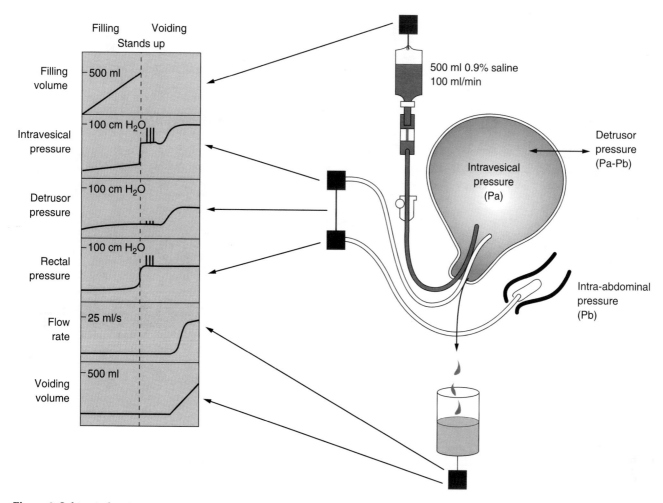

Fig. 49.8 Subtracted cystometry.

of both the intravesical and the intra-abdominal pressure simultaneously, is more accurate.

SUBTRACTED CYSTOMETRY

A subtracted cystometrogram can be performed in many different ways, but in the UK the bladder is normally filled with physiological saline at body temperature and the pressure is measured via a narrow fluid-filled catheter using a large external pressure transducer. The rectal (or vaginal) pressure is recorded to represent intra-abdominal pressure and this is subtracted from the bladder (intravesical) pressure to give the detrusor pressure (Fig. 49.8). Catheter-mounted solid state microtip pressure transducers are becoming increasingly popular for bladder and rectal pressure measurements. They are more expensive and less durable than the large external pressure transducers but have the advantage of reducing the bulk of the urodynamic equipment.

The information which can be obtained from a subtracted cystometrogram includes sensation, capacity, contractility and compliance (Fig. 49.9). The urinary residual volume is normally less than 50 ml, the first sensation of desire to void is normally 150–250 ml and the cystometric bladder capacity is normally 400–600 ml. Under normal circumstances, the detrusor pressure does not rise more than 10 cm of water for a volume of 300 ml, or 15 cm of water for a volume of 500 ml, and there are no detrusor contractions during bladder filling. When the bladder has been filled to capacity the woman is stood up and the filling catheter removed. She is asked to cough several times and to heel bounce and any rise in detrusor pressure or leakage per urethram is recorded. She is then asked to pass urine and the detrusor pressure is measured. At some point during voiding she is told to interrupt her urinary stream. The striated urethral sphincter and pelvic floor will contract immediately, but the smooth muscle of the detrusor will not relax instantaneously and

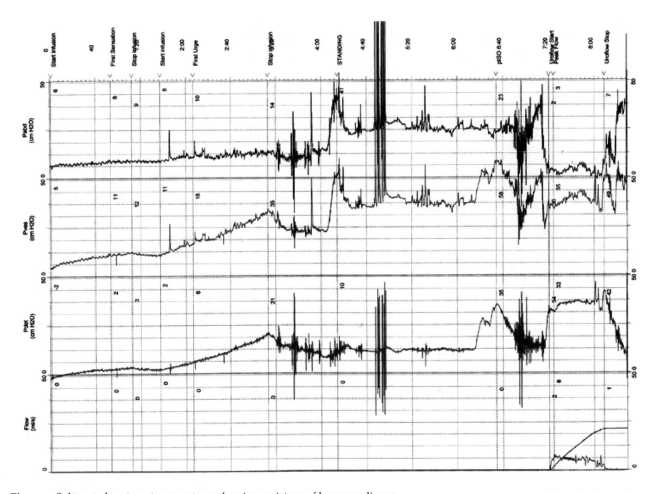

Fig. 49.9 Subtracted cystometrogram trace showing a picture of low compliance.

the resulting rise in detrusor pressure is known as the isometric detrusor contraction. When the detrusor pressure has fallen to its premicturition level, the subject is asked to empty her bladder completely and any urinary residual volume can be noted. The normal maximum voiding pressure is not more than 60 cm of water in women (Fig. 49.10).

VIDEOCYSTOURETHROGRAPHY

Videocystourethrography with pressure and flow studies, which combines cystometry, uroflowmetry and radiological screening of the bladder and urethra, is the single most informative investigation (Fig. 49.11). It is relatively expensive and time consuming and is only available in tertiary referral centres. A radiological contrast medium such as Urografin is used to fill the bladder instead of saline and a subtracted provocative cystometrogram is performed in the normal way. After bladder filling the patient is tilted erect on the X-ray screening table and the image intensifier is used to visualize her bladder and urethra. She is asked to cough with a full bladder and the extent of bladder base descent and any leakage of contrast medium are recorded. During voiding abnormal bladder morphology can be assessed as well as the presence of vesicoureteric reflux, trabeculation or diverticula. Occasionally a urethral diverticulum or vesicovaginal fistula may be identified (Fig. 49.12). In addition, bony abnormalities of the pelvis may occasionally be seen. The whole investigation can be recorded on video tape or computer with a sound commentary for immediate and later replay, in order to facilitate diagnosis, audit, data storage, research and education. Although videocystourethrography has no advantage over subtracted cystometry when differentiating between urodynamic stress incontinence and detrusor overactivity, there are some occasions when videocystourethrography is particularly useful. These include patients in whom previous incontinence surgery has failed, mixed or unusual symptoms and neurological disorders (Fig. 49.13).

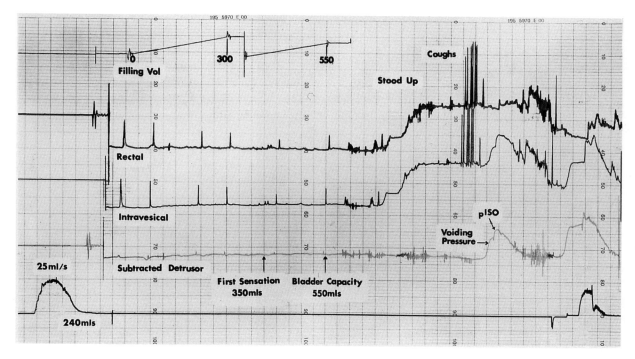

Fig. 49.10 A normal cystometrogram trace (the bottom line represents the flow rate, which is normal).

VOIDING CYSTOMETRY

Following the completion of filling cystometry the filling catheter is removed prior to voiding to prevent any unnecessary urethral obstruction. The intravesical and rectal pressure recording lines are left in situ, allowing simultaneous measurement of detrusor pressure along with the urine flow rate (Fig. 49.14). As with uroflowmetry, the patient is asked to void while sitting on a flowmeter in private.

During normal voiding there is a coordinated contraction of the bladder and at the same time relaxation of the urethra which is sustained until the bladder is empty. Women normally void with a detrusor pressure of less than 60 cm H_2O and a peak flow of >15 ml/s for a voided volume of at least 150 ml (Benness 1997). Some women have an excellent flow of urine with little or no rise in detrusor pressure which is simply a reflection that the contraction has occurred in the presence of low outlet resistance. However, if the detrusor pressure during voiding is reduced with low flow rates and a significant postmicturition residual the patient is classified as having voiding difficulty. In women, voiding problems are rarely due to bladder outflow obstruction and much more likely to be secondary to impaired detrusor contractility. Bladder outflow obstruction is characterized by a low flow rate and raised detrusor pressure during voiding. The patient may also be seen to use additional abdominal straining to try and improve the intravesical pressure.

The situation is further complicated by the fact that in some women with outflow obstruction the detrusor decompensates with time, resulting in both low detrusor pressure and low flow rate [48]. In some women, and particularly those with overt neurological disease, pathological contraction of the external sphincter occurs during a bladder contraction. This is called detrusor sphincter dyssynergia (DSD). Characteristically there is a high detrusor pressure during voiding associated with a poor flow rate. In some women urinary retention may occur and catheterization is therefore necessary.

Both relaxation of the urethral sphincter and initiation of voiding are subject to cortical influence, so the results of urodynamic investigation may be confounded by embarrassment or an unfamiliar testing environment. Most patients are able to pass urine at the end of the investigation but their inability to do so does not necessarily indicate a functional abnormality. Some women will subsequently have free flow rates and residual urine assessments which indicate normality.

Special investigations

Urethral pressure profilometry

The resting urethral pressure profile (UPP) is a graphical record of pressure within the urethra at successive points along its length. A number of measurements can be

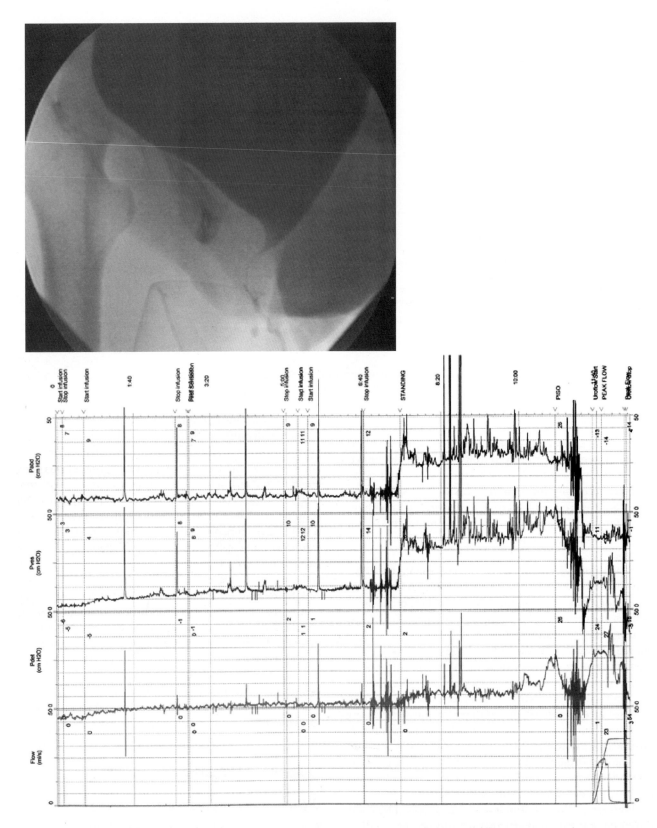

Fig. 49.11 Videocystourethrography demonstrating urodynamic stress incontinence. Subtracted filling cystometry showing no evidence of detrusor overactivity and synchronous screening demonstrating urethral sphincter incompetence on coughing.

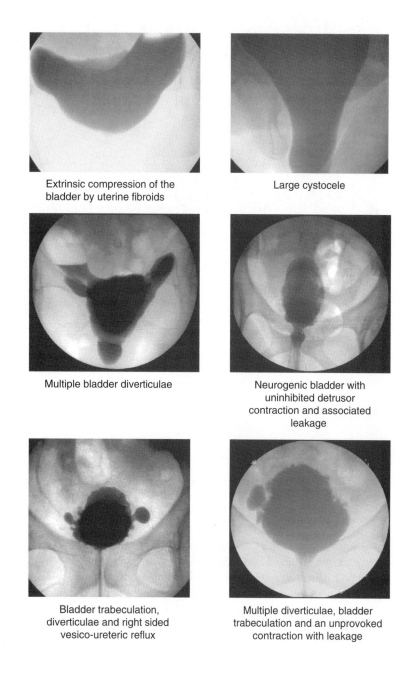

Extrinsic compression of the bladder by uterine fibroids

Large cystocele

Multiple bladder diverticulae

Neurogenic bladder with uninhibited detrusor contraction and associated leakage

Bladder trabeculation, diverticulae and right sided vesico-ureteric reflux

Multiple diverticulae, bladder trabeculation and an unprovoked contraction with leakage

Fig. 49.12 Videocrystourethrography: Images.

taken allowing an objective comparison of urethral function between patients and also before and after treatment. Although the concept of measuring the urethral pressure profile appears physiological there is considerable uncertainty regarding its use as a measure of urethral function and also as a prognostic tool.

Urethral pressure profilometry has been performed for at least 50 years, initially using balloon catheters and subsequently fluid perfusion. However, both these methods were unsatisfactory as they only enabled urethral pressure profile measurements to be made at rest and not under stress. Solid state microtransducer catheters are now employed. Two micro transducers are sited 6 cm apart on a 7 French silicone-coated solid catheter. They are gradually withdrawn at a constant rate along the length of the urethra, enabling the intraurethral and intravesical pressure to be recorded simultaneously. Many different parameters can be measured [49]; of particular interest are the maximum urethral closure pressure and functional urethral length (Figs 49.15 and 49.16). In addition, stress pressure

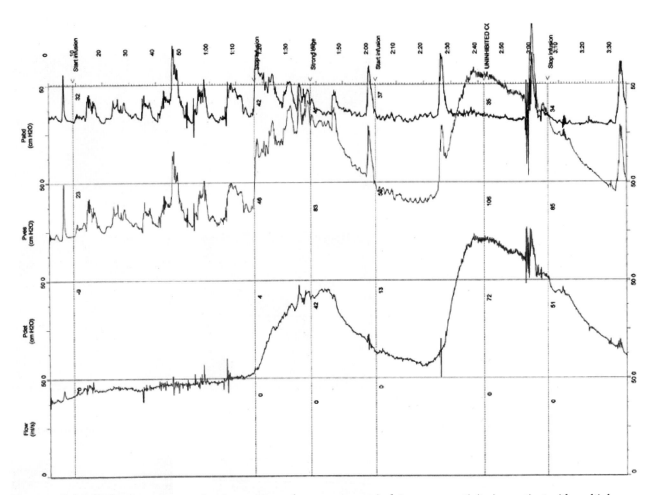

Fig. 49.13 Subtracted cystometrogram showing a picture of severe neurogenic detrusor overactivity in a patient with multiple sclerosis.

profiles can be performed if the patient coughs repeatedly during the procedure. This enables the pressure transmission ratio (the increment in urethral pressure, on stress, as a percentage of the simultaneously recorded increment in intravesical pressure) to be calculated. Urethral instability or relaxation can also be identified. Although urethral pressure profilometry is not useful in the diagnosis of urodynamic stress incontinence [50, 51], it is helpful in women whose incontinence operations have failed and also in those with voiding difficulties.

CYSTOURETHROSCOPY

Cystourethroscopy is normally carried out under general anaesthesia, but local anaesthesia is adequate if a flexible cystoscope is employed. Cystoscopy is particularly useful when there is a history of haematuria or recurrent urinary tract infections, or when no underlying cause can be found for sensory urgency or the symptoms

of frequency, urgency or dysuria with normal urodynamic results. Cystoscopy may reveal abnormalities of the bladder epithelium, such as inflammation suggestive of infection, petechial haemorrhages or shallow ulcers due to interstitial cystitis. Papillomas or other tumours may be seen. Biopsies can be taken to confirm the underlying diagnosis, for example, mast cell infiltration in interstitial cystitis or a possible transitional cell carcinoma.

IMAGING OF THE LOWER URINARY TRACT

Imaging of the lower urinary tract can be informative and, although videocystourethrography and cystoscopy are still the most commonly employed techniques, other forms of radiology, ultrasound and, most recently, magnetic resonance imaging (MRI) are being employed increasingly frequently.

Micturition cystography has largely been replaced by videocystourethrography, as the morphological

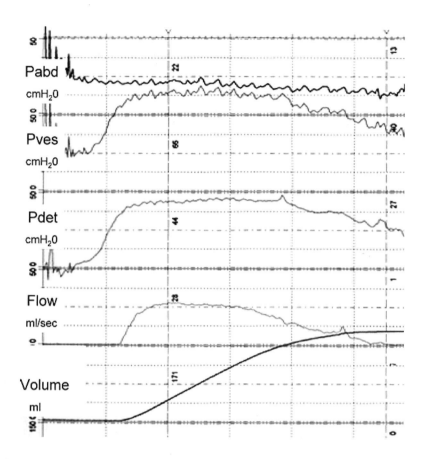

Fig. 49.14 Voiding cystometry.

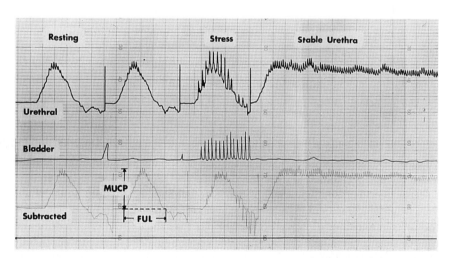

Fig. 49.15 Urethral pressure profilometry – normal trace.

information it provides is similar. However, it can be used to diagnose an anatomical abnormality such as a fistula or a urethral diverticulum when lower urinary tract dysfunction is not suspected.

Intravenous urography has now largely been replaced by ultrasound of the upper urinary tract. However, it is important to perform an intravenous urogram in cases

of haematuria, recurrent urinary tract infections, voiding difficulties or vesicoureteric reflux (Fig. 49.17). Additional pathology may be diagnosed, such as the presence of a ureteric fistula, a transitional cell carcinoma or calculi.

Ultrasound is now routinely used for assessing bladder volumes [52]. Abdominal, vaginal, rectal, perineal and introital ultrasound have all been employed and are

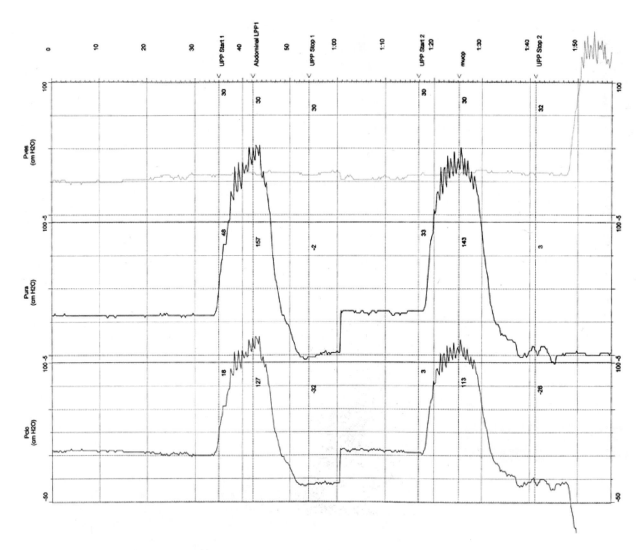

Fig. 49.16 Normal urethral pressure profile trace.

useful for estimating bladder capacity, urinary residual volume and assessing the upper urinary tracts. However, the role of ultrasound in the diagnosis of lower urinary tract dysfunction is still undergoing evaluation. Transvaginal ultrasound does allow clear visualization of the urethra and urethral diverticula. Bladder wall thickness of an empty bladder can be measured transvaginally giving a reproducible, sensitive method of screening for detrusor overactivity (a mean bladder wall thickness of >5 mm gave a predictive value of 94% in the diagnosis of detrusor overactivity) [53]. Measurement of bladder wall thickness has also been shown to have a role as an adjunctive test in those women whose lower urinary tract symptoms are not explained by conventional urodynamic investigations [54].

Rectal ultrasound [55] and perineal ultrasound [56] have been employed to examine the anatomy and mobility of the bladder neck and urethra, but it is important to appreciate that ultrasound cannot be used instead of urodynamic investigations which assesses the function rather than the morphology of the lower urinary tract.

Three-dimensional ultrasound is currently being employed mainly as a research tool. It can be used to estimate the volume of irregularly shaped organs such as the rhabdosphincter urethrae, which has been shown to be smaller in women with urodynamic stress incontinence than those with detrusor overactivity [57] and has also been shown to correlate with maximum urethral closure pressure [58]. Three-dimensional ultrasound has also been used to measure the levator ani hiatus which is significantly larger in women with prolapse than those with urodynamic stress incontinence or asymptomatic women [59].

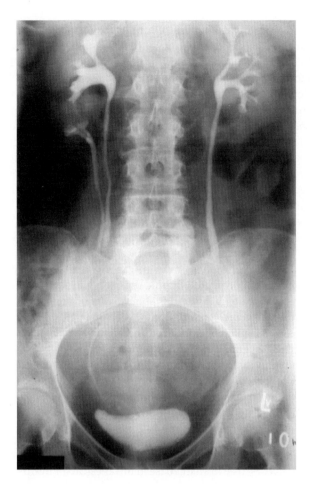

Fig. 49.17 Intravenous urogram showing a right duplex ureter.

MRI is non-invasive and non-ionizing and allows tissues to be visualized in great detail. The urethra, bladder neck and pelvic floor have been examined [60] and fast MRI scan has been used to study prolapse [61]. Recently an erect MRI scan has been described but its applications have not yet been identified [62]. The use of this type of technology in clinical practice is contentious as it is expensive for limited information.

ELECTROMYOGRAPHY

Electromyography can be employed to assess the integrity of the nerve supply to a muscle. The electrical impulses to a muscle fibre are measured following nervous stimulation. Two main types of electromyography are employed in the assessment of lower urinary tract dysfunction. Surface electrodes can be placed on the perineum, vagina or anal canal as an anal plug. The pudendal nerve is stimulated and potentials measured via the electrode. This is inaccurate as the muscular activity of the levator ani is not necessarily representative of that of the rhabdosphincter urethrae. Single fibre electromyography is more accurate

as it assesses the nerve latency within individual muscle fibres of the rhabdosphincter. In this way denervation of motor units can be assessed. Research from Manchester has suggested that the occurrence of urodynamic stress incontinence postpartum is due to partial denervation of the pelvic floor musculature and rhabdosphincter urethrae and is characterized by increased motor latencies [63].

Electromyography is not useful in the routine clinical evaluation of patients with uncomplicated urinary incontinence. However, it may be useful in the assessment of women with neurological abnormalities or those with voiding difficulties and retention of urine. However, work from our own unit showed no difference in urethral sphincter electromyography parameters when women with urodynamically proven urodynamic stress incontinence ($n = 33$) and a continent control group ($n = 35$) were compared. Our findings suggested that denervation and reinnervation of the striated urethral sphincter may not be a major aetiological factor in the development of urodynamic stress incontinence [64].

Urethral electric conductance has not gained wide acceptance in the routine urodynamic assessment of women with urinary incontinence [65, 66]. A 7 French flexible probe with two ring electrodes 1 mm apart is withdrawn along the urethra. It measures the passage of urine along the urethra by registering the change in conductivity. This technique can be employed at the bladder neck to assess bladder neck opening, or in the distal urethra to detect urine loss. Different conductivity patterns are associated with different urodynamic diagnoses, and distal urethral electrical conductance has been recommended as a screening test for detrusor overactivity [67, 68]. It is now seldom used in clinical practice.

AMBULATORY URODYNAMICS

All urodynamic tests are unphysiological and most are invasive. Various authors have suggested that long-term ambulatory monitoring may be more physiological as the assessment takes place over a prolonged period of time and during normal daily activities [69].

Ambulatory urodynamic studies are defined as a functional test of the lower urinary tract utilizing natural filling and reproducing the subjects everyday activities [2].

There are three main components to an ambulatory urodynamic system; the transducers, the recording unit and the analysing system (Fig. 49.18). The transducers are solid state and are mounted on 5 french and 7 french bladder and rectal catheters. It is our practice to use two bladder transducers in order to reduce artefact. The recording system should be portable in order to allow freedom of movement with a digital memory aiding compression and expansion of the traces which are obtained. An event marker is attached to the recording unit allowing the patient to mark episodes of urgency and also to document voids. In addition the recording unit is attached to an electronic (urilos) pad to document episodes of leakage during the study and should have the facility to attach to a flowmeter so as to record pressure flow voiding studies. The ambulatory protocol at Kings College Hospital consists of a 4-h period during which time the patient is asked to drink 200 ml of fluid every 30 min and also to keep a diary of events and symptoms (Fig. 49.19). On completion of the test the trace is then analysed with the patient using a personal computer and the urinary diary. Detrusor overactivity should only be diagnosed if there is a detrusor contraction noted in both bladder lines in the presence of symptoms (Fig. 49.20).

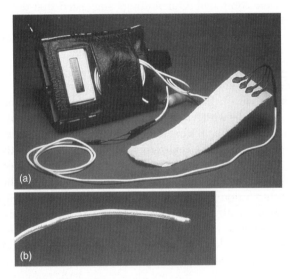

Fig. 49.18 Ambulatory urodynamic equipment demonstrating the (a) digital recording unit, and urilos pad and (b) microtip pressure transducer.

The clinical usefulness of ambulatory urodynamics is limited by the high prevalence of abnormal detrusor (38–69%) contractions in asymptomatic volunteers [70,71]. However the diagnosis of detrusor overactivity is highly dependent on interpretation of the results; in a prospective study of 26 asymptomatic women the incidence of detrusor overactivity varied from 11.5% to 76.9% depending on the criteria used [72]. However, if the criteria for defining abnormal detrusor contractions are a simultaneous pressure rise on both bladder lines in addition to patient reported symptoms of urgency or urge incontinence the findings are normal in 90% of women which is similar to that reported in laboratory urodynamics.

Although ambulatory urodynamics is still considered to be mainly a research tool there is no doubt that it is often exceedingly helpful in cases where the clinical and conventional urodynamic diagnoses differ, or when no abnormality is found on laboratory urodynamics [73]. Ambulatory urodynamics have been shown to be more sensitive than laboratory urodynamics in the diagnosis of detrusor overactivity but less sensitive in the diagnosis of urodynamic stress incontinence [74] although their role in clinical practice remains controversial [75].

Causes of urinary incontinence

Urethral incontinence will occur whenever the intravesical pressure involuntarily exceeds the intraurethral pressure. This may be due to an increase in intravesical (or detrusor) pressure or a reduction in urethral pressure or a combination of the two. Thus the fault which leads to incontinence may lie in the urethra or the bladder or both.

Urodynamic stress incontinence

Urodynamic stress incontinence is defined as the involuntary leakage of urine during increased abdominal pressure

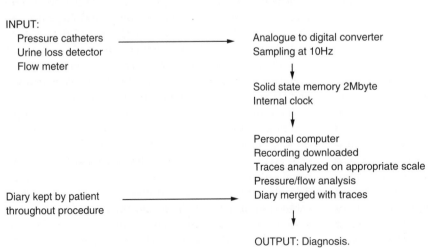

INPUT:
    Pressure catheters ——————————→ Analogue to digital converter
    Urine loss detector   Sampling at 10Hz
    Flow meter

Solid state memory 2Mbyte
Internal clock

Personal computer
Recording downloaded
Traces analyzed on appropriate scale
Pressure/flow analysis

Diary kept by patient ——————————→ Diary merged with traces
throughout procedure

OUTPUT: Diagnosis.

Fig. 49.19 Schematic flow diagram representing ambulatory urodynamics: 4-h test, standardized fluid intake, instruction sheet.

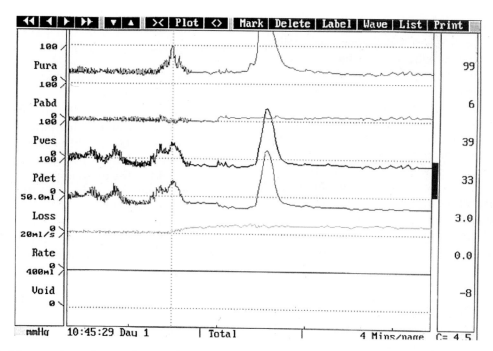

Fig. 49.20 Ambulatory urodynamic trace showing detrusor overactivity which is associated with urine loss into the urilos pad.

Table 49.9 Causes of urodynamic stress incontinence

Urethral hypermobility
Urogenital prolapse

Pelvic floor damage or denervation
Parturition
Pelvic surgery
Menopause

Urethral scarring
Vaginal (urethral) surgery
Incontinence surgery
Urethral dilatation or urethrotomy
Recurrent urinary tract infections
Radiotherapy

Raised intra-abdominal pressure
Pregnancy
Chronic cough (bronchitis)
Abdominal/pelvic mass
Faecal impaction
Ascites
(Obesity)

in the absence of a detrusor contraction [2]. There are various different underlying causes which result in weakness of one or more of the components of the urethral sphincter mechanism (Table 49.9).

The bladder neck and proximal urethra are normally situated in an intra-abdominal position above the pelvic floor and are supported by the pubourethral ligaments.

Damage to either the pelvic floor musculature (levator ani) or pubourethral ligaments may result in descent of the proximal urethra such that it is no longer an intra-abdominal organ and this results in leakage of urine per urethram during stress.

It has been postulated that vaginal delivery results in denervation of the urethral sphincter mechanism [63]. Snooks *et al.* [76] employed electromyography to reveal evidence of pelvic floor denervation in women who had delivered vaginally but not those who had undergone caesarean section. They later compared antenatal with postpartum women and confirmed that vaginal delivery results in pelvic floor denervation [77]. In a study of 96 nulliparous women who delivered vaginally, Allen *et al.* [78] have reported electromyographic evidence of denervation of the pelvic floor in postpartum women with urinary incontinence. A long active second stage of labour was the only factor associated with severe damage.

Although pudendal function has been shown to recover with time [76, 79] it has also been shown to deteriorate progressively with ageing and subsequent vaginal deliveries [80]. Because of the increased incidence of pelvic floor trauma with vaginal delivery, especially instrumental delivery, it has been proposed that elective caesarean section should be offered to women who are at increased risk [81].

More recently the 'mid-urethral theory' or 'integral theory' has been described by Petros and Ulmsten [82]. This concept is based on earlier studies suggesting that the distal and mid-urethra play an important role in the continence mechanism [83] and that the maximal urethral closure pressure is at the mid urethral point [84]. This theory proposes that damage to the pubourethral ligaments supporting the urethra, impaired support of the anterior vaginal wall to the mid urethra, and weakened function of part of the pubococcygeal muscles which insert adjacent to the urethra are responsible for causing stress incontinence.

Urodynamic stress incontinence is the commonest cause of urinary incontinence in women and represents over half of those referred for a gynaecological opinion. Women usually complain of the symptom of stress incontinence with or without frequency, urgency, urge incontinence or prolapse [85]. Stress incontinence may be demonstrated on clinical examination, but this will only verify the patient's history and will not diagnose the cause of the incontinence. Usually the diagnosis of urodynamic stress incontinence is made by negative findings rather than positive ones. If cystometry is normal and stress incontinence is observed, a diagnosis of urodynamic stress incontinence can be made. If a woman complains of stress incontinence as her sole symptom and stress incontinence can be demonstrated on coughing, there is a 95% chance that the diagnosis is urodynamic stress incontinence. However, Haylen *et al.* [86] have shown that only 2% of women who present for urodynamic assessment fall into this category.

CONSERVATIVE TREATMENT

Types of conservative treatment for urodynamic stress incontinence are listed in Table 49.10. Conservative treatment is indicated when the incontinence is mild, the patient is medically unfit for surgery or does not wish to undergo an operation, or in women who have not yet completed their families. It may also be useful prior to surgery when the patient's name is on a long waiting list. However, it is unusual for anything more than mild urodynamic stress incontinence to be completely cured by these conservative measures and most women require surgery eventually [87].

Table 49.10 Conservative treatment for urodynamic stress incontinence

Kegel (pelvic floor) exercises
Perineometry
Vaginal cones
Faradism
Interferential therapy
Maximum electrical stimulation
Duloxetine

Pelvic floor muscle training

Pelvic floor muscle training (PFMT) and pelvic floor physiotherapy remain the first line conservative measure since their introduction in 1948 [88]. PFMT appear to work in a number of different ways:
1 Women learn to consciously pre-contract the pelvic floor muscles before and during increases in abdominal pressure to prevent leakage ('the knack').
2 Strength training builds up long-lasting muscle volume and thus provides structural support.
3 Abdominal muscle training indirectly strengthens the pelvic floor muscles [89].
In addition during a contraction the urethra may also be pressed against the posterior aspect of the symphysis pubis producing a mechanical rise in urethral pressure [90]. Since up to 30% of women with stress incontinence are unable to contract their pelvic floor correctly at presentation [91], some patients may simply need to be re-taught the 'knack' of squeezing the appropriate muscles at the correct time [92]. Cure rates varying between 21% and 84% have been reported [88, 93, 94]. Success appears to depend upon the type and severity of incontinence treated, the instruction and follow-up given, the compliance of the patient and the outcome measures used. However, the evidence would suggest that PFMT is more effective if patients are given a structured programme to follow rather than simple verbal instructions [95].

The success of PFMT may be further enhanced by the use of biofeedback [96]. This technique allows patients to receive visual or audio feedback relating to contraction of their pelvic floor. The most commonly used device in clinical practice is the perineometer which may give women an improved idea of a pelvic floor contraction and provide an effective stimulus to encourage greater and continued effort.

Perineometry

A perineometer is a cylindrical vaginal device which can be used to assess the strength of pelvic floor contractions. It can be used to help an individual to contract her pelvic floor muscles appropriately and is also useful in detecting improvement following pelvic floor exercises. Perineometers are available for both hospital and home use.

Weighted vaginal cones

These are currently available as sets of five or three [97], all of the same shape and size but of increasing weight (20–90 g). When inserted into the vagina a cone stimulates the pelvic floor to contract to prevent it from falling out and this provides 'vaginal weight training'. A 60–70%

improvement rate has been reported using this technique [98] and two studies have shown that cones are as effective as more conventional forms of pelvic floor re-education and require less supervision [99, 100]. However, longer term studies suggest that initial improvement may not be maintained [101] and their effectiveness in the treatment of urodynamic stress incontinence is limited with a randomized controlled study of conservative treatments showing that only 7.5% of women felt they no longer had a continence problem after using vaginal cones for six months. In addition there was no difference in pelvic muscle strength when compared with the control group [93]. Furthermore there have been some reports that vaginal cones may produce prolonged isometric contraction of the pelvic floor muscles and muscle injury if overused [102].

Maximal electrical stimulation

This can be carried out using a home device which utilizes a vaginal electrode through which a variable current is passed. The woman is able to adjust the strength of the stimulus herself and is instructed to use the device for 20 min daily initially for 1 month. Maximum electrical stimulation has been employed in both the management of urodynamic stress incontinence and detrusor overactivity although it has not gained popularity. In a multicentre trial Sand *et al.* (1995) have shown that this type of electrical stimulator is more effective both subjectively and objectively (pad weighing test) than a sham device in the treatment of urodynamic stress incontinence. In addition a more recent meta-analysis has shown that electrical stimulation is as effective as PFMT for the treatment of urodynamic stress incontinence [103].

Vaginal devices

There are many women who for various reasons are not suitable for or do not wish to undergo active treatment of their incontinence. They do, however, require some sort of 'containment' of their leakage and vaginal devices may be useful for use during exercise on a short term basis.

Sanitary tampons are easily available and reduce urinary leakage by elevating the bladder neck and causing a degree of outflow obstruction. However, they are irritant to the vagina when used frequently and sponge tampons are now available which can be soaked in water prior to use and therefore remain moist whilst *in situ*. The Conveen Continence Guard is a specially shaped vaginal tampon which has been assessed in a multicentre trial of 85 women with urodynamic stress incontinence aged 31–65 years. It was used daily for 4 weeks and assessed both subjectively and objectively using a pad weight test [104]. Overall 75% of the women were objectively improved whilst the device was *in situ*. More recently the Conveen Continence Guard (CCG) has been compared with the Contrelle Continence Tampon (CCT) (Fig. 49.21) in a prospective study of 94 women with urodynamic stress incontinence [105]. Overall both devices were found to significantly reduce the amount of urinary leakage but this was significantly greater in the CCT group. In addition two-thirds of women preferred the CCT to the CCG. There were no serious

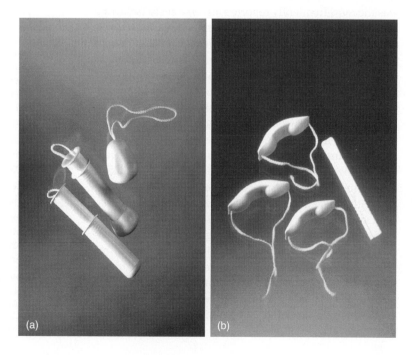

Fig. 49.21 Vaginal continence devices.
(a) Contrelle (CCT) and (b) Conveen (CCG).

adverse events and no association with vaginal or lower urinary tract infections.

Medical therapy

Whilst various agents such as α_1-adrenoceptor agonists, oestrogens and tricyclic antidepressants have all been used anecdotally in the past for the treatment of stress incontinence duloxetine is the first drug to be specifically developed and licensed for this indication.

Duloxetine is a potent and balanced serotonin (5-Hydroxytryptamine) and noradrenaline reuptake inhibitor (SNRI) which enhances urethral striated sphincter activity via a centrally mediated pathway [106]. The efficacy and safety of duloxetine (20 mg, 40 mg, 80 mg) has been evaluated in a double-blind randomized parallel group placebo controlled phase II dose finding study in 48 centres in the United States involving 553 women with stress incontinence [107]. Duloxetine was associated with significant and dose dependent decreases in incontinence episode frequency. Reductions were 41% for placebo and 54%, 59% and 64% for the 20, 40 and 80 mg, groups respectively. Discontinuation rates were also dose dependent; 5% for placebo and 9%, 12% and 15% of 20 mg, 40 mg and 80 mg respectively, the most frequently reported adverse event being nausea.

A further global phase III study of 458 women has also recently been reported [108]. There was a significant decrease in incontinence episode frequency and improvement in quality of life in those women taking duloxetine 40 mg od. when compared to placebo. Once again nausea was the most frequently reported adverse event occurring in 25.1% of women receiving duloxetine compared to a rate of 3.9% in those taking placebo. However, 60% of nausea resolved by 7 days and 86% by 1 month. These findings are supported by a further double-blind, placebo controlled study of 109 women awaiting surgery for stress incontinence [109]. Overall there was a significant improvement in incontinence episode frequency and quality of life in those women taking duloxetine when compared to placebo. Furthermore, 20% of women who were awaiting continence surgery changed their mind whilst taking duloxetine. More recently the role of synergistic therapy with pelvic floor muscle training and duloxetine has been examined in a prospective study of 201 women with stress incontinence. Women were randomized to one of four treatment combinations; duloxetine 40 mg bd, PFMT, combination therapy or placebo. Overall duloxetine, with or without PFMT was found to be superior to placebo or PFMT alone whilst pad test results and quality of life analysis favoured combination therapy to single treatment [110].

Surgery

Surgery is usually the most effective way of curing urodynamic stress incontinence and a 90% cure rate can be expected for an appropriate, properly performed primary procedure. Surgery for urodynamic stress incontinence aims to elevate the bladder neck and proximal urethra into an intra-abdominal position, to support the bladder neck and align it to the posterosuperior aspect of the pubic symphysis, and in some cases to increase the outflow resistance. Undoubtedly the results of suprapubic operations such as the Burch colposuspension or Marshall–Marchetti–Krantz procedure are better than those for the traditional, anterior colporrhaphy with bladder neck buttress [111]. Numerous operations have been described and many are still performed today. Common operations for urodynamic stress incontinence are listed in Table 49.11.

A systematic review of the effectiveness of surgery for stress incontinence in women [112] revealed only 11 randomized controlled trials, 20 non-randomized trials and 45 retrospective studies. This review showed that evidence as to the effectiveness of surgery for stress incontinence is weak, but that colposuspension is more effective and long lasting than anterior colporrhaphy or needle suspension. Reliable data on the frequency of complications following surgery were lacking but repeat operations were noted to be less successful than first procedures.

Table 49.11 Operations for urodynamic stress incontinence

Vaginal
Anterior colporrhaphy +/− Kelly/Pacey
  suture
Urethrocliesis
Urethral bulking agents
Retropubic tape procedures
Transobturator tape procedures

Abdominal
Marshall–Marchetti–Krantz procedure
Burch colposuspension

Laparoscopic
Colposuspension

Combined
Sling
Endoscopic bladder neck suspension,
  for example, Stamey, Raz

Complex
Neourethra
Artificial sphincter
Urinary diversion

ANTERIOR COLPORRHAPHY

Anterior colporrhaphy is still performed for stress incontinence. Although it is usually the best operation for a cystourethrocele, the cure rates for urodynamic stress incontinence are poor compared to suprapubic procedures [113]. Since prolapse is relatively easier to cure than stress incontinence, it is appropriate to perform the best operation for incontinence when the two conditions coexist.

MARSHALL–MARCHETTI–KRANTZ

The Marshall–Marchetti–Krantz procedure is a suprapubic operation in which the paraurethral tissue at the level of the bladder neck is sutured to the periostium and/or perichondrium of the posterior aspect of the pubic symphysis. This procedure elevates the bladder neck but will not correct any concomitant cystocele. It has been largely superseded by the Burch colposuspension because its complications include osteitis pubis in 2–7% of cases.

COLPOSUSPENSION

The Burch colposuspension has been modified by many authors, since its original description [114]. Until recently colposuspension has been the operation of choice in primary urodynamic stress incontinence as it corrects both stress incontinence and a cystocele. It may not be suitable if the vagina is scarred or narrowed by previous surgery. The operation is performed via a low transverse suprapubic incision. The bladder, bladder neck and proximal urethra are dissected medially off the underlying paravaginal fascia and three or four pairs of non-absorbable or long-term absorbable sutures are inserted between the fascia and the ipsilateral iliopectineal ligament. Haemostasis is secured and the sutures are tied, thus elevating the bladder neck and bladder base (Fig. 49.22). Simultaneous hysterectomy does not improve results but if there is uterine pathology (menorrhagia or uterovaginal prolapse) then a total abdominal hysterectomy should be performed at the same time. Postoperatively a suction drain is left in the retropubic space and a suprapubic catheter is inserted into the bladder. Perioperative antibiotics and/or subcutaneous heparin may be employed. In virtually all reported series comparing results of a Burch colposuspension with any other procedure to cure urodynamic stress incontinence, the results of the colposuspension have been the best.

Whilst the colposuspension is now well recognized as an effective procedure for stress incontinence it is not without complications. Detrusor overactivity may occur *de novo* or may be unmasked by the procedure [115] which may lead to long-term urinary symptoms. Voiding difficulties are common postoperatively and although they usually

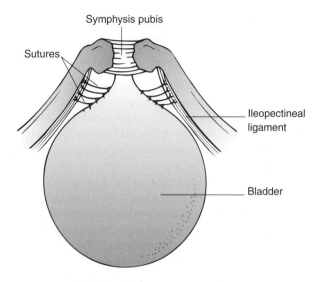

Fig. 49.22 Modified Burch colposuspension.

resolve within a short time after the operation, long-term voiding dysfunction may result. In addition, a rectoenterocele may be exacerbated by repositioning the vagina [116]. However, the colposuspension is the only incontinence operation for which long-term data are available. Alcalay *et al.* [117] have reported a series of 109 women with an overall cure rate of 69% at a mean of 13.8 years.

LAPAROSCOPIC COLPOSUSPENSION

Minimally invasive surgery is attractive and this trend has extended to surgery for stress incontinence. Although many authors have reported excellent short-term subjective results from laparoscopic colposuspension [118], early studies have shown inferior results to the open procedure [119, 120].

More recently two large prospective randomized controlled trials have been reported from Australia and the United Kingdom comparing laparoscopic and open colposuspension. In the Australian study 200 women with urodynamic stress incontinence were randomized to either laparoscopic or open colposuspension [121]. Overall there were no significant differences in objective and subjective measures of cure or in patient satisfaction at 6 months, 24 months or 3–5 years. Whilst the laparoscopic approach took longer (87 versus 42 min; $p < 0.0001$) it was associated with less blood loss ($p = 0.03$) and a quicker return to normal activities ($p = 0.01$).

These findings are supported by the UK multicentre randomized controlled trial of 291 women with urodynamic stress incontinence comparing laparoscopic to open colposuspension [122]. At 24 months intention to treat analysis showed no significant difference in cure rates between the procedures. Objective cure rates for open and laparoscopic colposuspension were 70.1% and 79.7% respectively whilst subjective cure rates were 54.6% and 54.9%, respectively.

These studies have confirmed that the clinical effectiveness of the two operations is comparable although the cost effectiveness of laparoscopic colposuspension remains unproven. A cost analysis comparing laparoscopic to open colposuspension was also performed alongside the UK study [123]. Healthcare resource use over the first six month follow-up period translated into costs of £1805 for the laparoscopic group versus £1433 for the open group.

It is important that this information is made available to women who are undergoing incontinence surgery as most would prefer their stress incontinence to be cured rather than a reduced hospital stay. In addition it has been well established that the first operation is the one most likely to succeed and therefore it is unfortunate if a good outcome is prejudiced by an inferior operation.

SLING PROCEDURES

Sling procedures are normally performed as secondary operations where there is scarring and narrowing of the vagina. The sling material can either be organic (rectus fascia, porcine dermis) or inorganic (Mersilene, Marlex, Gore-tex or Silastic). The sling may be inserted either abdominally, vaginally or by a combination of both. Normally the sling is used to elevate and support the bladder neck and proximal urethra, but not intentionally to obstruct it. Sling procedures are associated with a high incidence of side effects and complications. It is often difficult to decide how tight to make the sling. If it is too loose, incontinence will persist and if it is too tight, voiding difficulties may be permanent. Women who are going to undergo insertion of a sling must be prepared to perform clean intermittent self-catheterization postoperatively. In addition, there is a risk of infection, especially if inorganic material is used. The sling may erode into the urethra or vagina, in which case it must be removed and this can be exceedingly difficult. Early reports of the use of needle suspension patch slings using fascia or Gore-tex suggests a reduced complication rate with similar efficacy but long-term series have been published to date.

RETRO-PUBIC TAPE PROCEDURES

Tension free vaginal tape

The tension free vaginal tape (TVT, Gynaecare), first described by Ulmsten in 1996 [124], is now the most commonly performed procedure for stress urinary incontinence in the UK and more than one million procedures

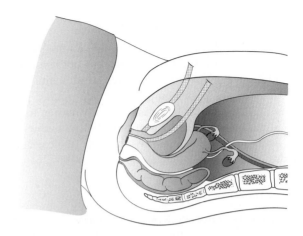

Fig. 49.23 Tension free vaginal (TVT).

have been performed worldwide. A knitted 11 mm × 40 cm polypropylene mesh tape is inserted trans-vaginally at the level of the mid-urethra, using two 5 mm trochars (Fig. 49.23). The procedure may be performed under local, spinal or general anaesthesia. Most women can go home the same day, although some do require catheterization for short term voiding difficulties (2.5–19.7%). Other complications include bladder perforation (2.7–5.8%), *de novo* urgency (0.2–15%) and bleeding (0.9–2.3%) [125].

A multicentre study carried out in six centres in Sweden has reported a 90% cure rate at one year in women undergoing their first operation for urodynamic stress incontinence, without any major complications [126]. Long term results would confirm durability of the technique with success rates of 86% at 3 years [127], 84.7% at 5 years [128] and 81.3% at 7 years [129].

The tension free vaginal tape has also been compared to open colposuspension in a multicentre prospective randomized trial of 344 women with urodynamic stress incontinence [130]. Overall there was no significant difference in terms of objective cure; 66% in the tension free vaginal tape group and 57% in the colposuspension group. However, operation time, postoperative stay and return to normal activity were all longer in the colposuspension arm. Analysis of the long-term results at 24 months using a pad test, quality of life assessment and symptom questionnaires showed an objective cure rate of 63% in the tension free vaginal tape arm and 51% in the colposuspension arm [131]. At 5 years there were no differences in subjective cure (63% in the tension free vaginal tape group and 70% in the colposuspension group), patient satisfaction and quality of life assessment. However, whilst there was a significant reduction in cystocele in both groups there was a higher incidence of enterocele, rectocele and apical prolapse in the colposuspension group [132]. Furthermore, cost utility analysis has also shown that at six months follow up tension free vaginal tape resulted in a mean cost saving of £243 when compared to colposuspension [133].

A smaller randomized study has also compared tension free vaginal tape to laparoscopic colposuspension in 72 women with urodynamic stress incontinence. At a mean follow-up of 20 months objective cure rates were higher in the tension free vaginal tape group when compared to the laparoscopic colposuspension group; 96.8% versus 71.2% respectively ($p = 0.056$) [134].

SPARC-mid urethral sling suspension system

The SPARC sling system (American Medical Systems) is a minimally invasive sling procedure using a knitted 10 mm wide polypropylene mesh which is placed at the level of the mid-urethra by passing the needle via a suprapubic to vaginal approach [135] Fig. 49.24. The procedure may be performed under local, regional or general anaesthetic. A prospective multicentre study of 104 women with urodynamic stress incontinence has been reported from France [136]. At a mean follow up of 11.9 months the objective cure rate was 90.4% and subjective cure 72%. There was a 10.5% incidence of bladder perforation and 11.5% of women complained of de novo urgency following the procedure. More recently SPARC has been compared to tension free vaginal tape in a prospective randomized trial of 301 women [137]. At short-term follow-up there were no significant differences in cure rates, bladder perforation rates and de novo urgency. There was, however, a higher incidence of voiding difficulties and vaginal erosions in the SPARC group.

TRANSOBTURATOR SLING PROCEDURES

The transobturator route for the placement of synthetic mid-urethral slings was first described in 2001 [138]. As with the retro-pubic sling procedures transobturator tapes may be performed under local, regional or general anaesthetic and have the theoretical advantage of eliminating some of the complications associated with the retropubic route. However, the transobturator route may be associated with damage to the obturator nerve and vessels; in an anatomical dissection model the tape passes 3.4–4.8 cm from the anterior and posterior branches of the obturator nerve respectively and 1.1 cm from the most medial branch of the obturator vessels [139]. Consequently nerve and vessel injury in addition to bladder injury and vaginal erosion remain a potential complication of the procedure.

The transobturator approach may be used as an 'inside–out' (TVT-O, Gynaecare) (Fig. 49.25) or alternatively an 'outside–in' (Obtape, Mentor; Monarc, American Medical Systems; Obtryx, Boston Scientific) technique. To date there have been several studies documenting the short-term efficacy of transobturator procedures but less long-term evidence. Initial studies have reported cure and improved rates of 80.5% and 7.5% respectively at 7 months [140] and 90.6% and 9.4% respectively at 17 months [141].

More recently the transobturator approach (TVT-O) has been compared to the retropubic approach (TVT) in an Italian prospective multicentre randomized study of 231 women with urodynamic stress incontinence [142]. At a mean of 9 months subjectively 92% of women in the TVT group were cured compared to 87% in the TVT-O group. Objectively, on pad test testing, cure rates were 92% and 89% respectively. There were no differences in voiding difficulties and length of stay although there were more bladder perforations in the TVT group; 4% versus

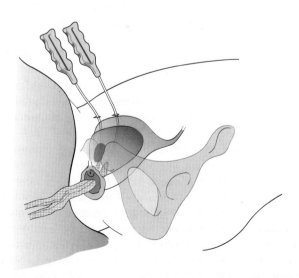

Fig. 49.24 SPARC-mid urethral sling suspension system.

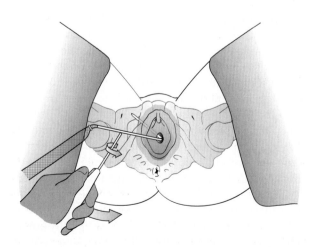

Fig. 49.25 Transobturator tape-'inside–out' procedure.

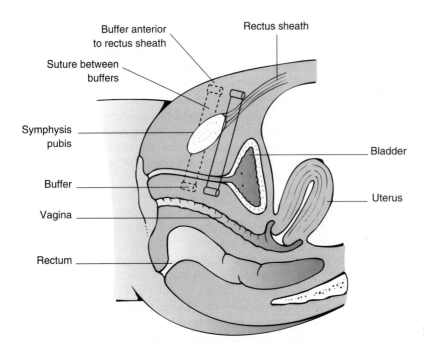

Buffer anterior
to rectus sheath

Rectus sheath

Suture between
buffers

Symphysis
pubis

Bladder

Buffer

Uterus

Vagina

Rectum

Fig. 49.26 Stamey procedure.

none in the TVT-O group. A further multicentre prospective randomized trial comparing TVT and TVT-O has also recently been reported from Finland in 267 women complaining of stress urinary incontinence [143]. Objective cure rates at 9 weeks were 98.5% in the TVT group and 95.4% in the TVT-O group ($p = 0.1362$). Whilst complication rates were low and similar in both arms of the study there was a higher incidence of groin pain in the TVT-O group (21 versus 2; $p = 0.0001$).

BLADDER NECK SUSPENSION PROCEDURES

Endoscopically guided bladder neck suspensions [144–146] are simple to perform but may be less effective than open suprapubic procedures and are now seldom used. In all these operations a long needle is used to insert a loop of nylon on each side of the bladder neck; this is tied over the rectus sheath to elevate the urethrovesical junction (Fig. 49.26). Cystoscopy is employed to ensure accurate placement of the sutures and to detect any damage to the bladder caused by the needle or the suture. In the Stamey procedure buffers are used to avoid the sutures cutting through the tissues, and in the Raz procedure a helical suture of Prolene is inserted deep into the endopelvic fascia lateral to the bladder neck to avoid cutting through. The main problem with all these operations is that they rely on two sutures and these may break or pull through the tissues. However, endoscopically guided bladder neck suspensions are quick and easy to perform. They can be carried out under regional blockade and postoperative recovery is fast. Temporary voiding difficulties are common after long needle suspensions but these usually resolve and there are few other complications.

URETHRAL BULKING AGENTS

Urethral bulking agents are a minimally invasive surgical procedure for the treatment of urodynamic stress incontinence and may be useful in the elderly and those women who have undergone previous operations and have a fixed, scarred fibrosed urethra.

Although the actual substance which is injected may differ the principle is the same. It is injected either periurethrally or transurethrally on either side of the bladder neck under cystoscopic control and is intended to 'bulk' the bladder neck, in order to stop premature bladder neck opening, without causing out-flow obstruction. They may be performed under local, regional or general anaesthesia. There are now several different products available (Table 49.12). The use of minimally invasive implantation systems (Fig. 49.27) has also allowed some of these procedures to be performed in the office setting without the need for cystoscopy.

In the first reported series 81% of 68 women were dry following two injections with collagen [147]. There have been longer term follow-up studies most of which give a less than 50% objective cure rate at 2 years but a subjective improvement rate of about 70% [148–150]. Macroplastique has recently been compared to Contigen in a recent North American study of 248 women with urodynamic stress incontinence. Outcome was assessed objectively using

Table 49.12 Urethral bulking agents

Urethral bulking agent	Application technique
Gluteraldehyde cross linked bovine collagen **(Contigen)**	Cystoscopic
Polydimethylsiloxane **(Macroplastique)**	Cystoscopic MIS implantation system
Pyrolytic carbon coated zirconium oxide beads in β glucan gel **(Durasphere)**	Cystoscopic
Ethylene vinyl co-polymer in dimethyl sulfoxide (DMSO) gel **(Tegress, Uryx)**	Cystoscopic
Calcium hydroxylapatite in carboxymethylcellulose gel **(Coaptite)**	Cystoscopic
Copolymer of hyaluronic acid and dextranomer **(Zuidex)**	Cystoscopic Implacer system
Polyacrylamide hydrogel **(Bulkamid)**	Cystoscopic

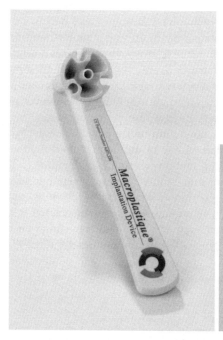
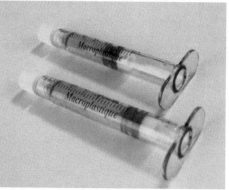

Fig. 49.27 Macroplastique urethral bulking agent and implantation device.

pad tests and subjectively at 12 months. Overall objective cure and improvement rates favoured Macroplastique over Contigen (74% versus 65%; $p = 0.13$). Whilst this difference was not significant subjective cure rates were higher in the Macroplastique group (41% versus 29%; $p = 0.07$) [151]. A 12 month open label European study of 142 women with urodynamic stress incontinence treated with Zuidex has reported cure and improvement rates of 78% at 12 weeks and 77% at 12 months [152].

Whilst success rates with urethral bulking agents are generally lower than those with conventional continence surgery they are minimally invasive and have lower complication rates meaning that they remain a useful alternative in selected women.

ARTIFICIAL URINARY SPHINCTER

An artificial sphincter is an ingenious device which may be employed when conventional surgery fails [153]. This is implantable and consists of a fluid-filled inflatable cuff which is surgically placed around the bladder neck. A reservoir, containing fluid, is sited in the peritoneal cavity and a small finger-operated pump is situated in the left labium majus. The three major components are connected via a control valve. Under normal circumstances the cuff is inflated, thus obstructing the urethra. When voiding is desired the pump is utilized to empty the fluid in the cuff back into the balloon reservoir so that voiding may occur. The cuff then gradually refills over the next few minutes. Artificial sphincters are associated with many problems. They are expensive, the surgery required to insert them is complicated and the tissues around the bladder neck following previous failed operations may be unsuitable for the implantation of the cuff. In addition, mechanical failure may occur, necessitating further surgery. However, there is a place for these devices and their technology is likely to improve in the future.

There are a few unfortunate women in whom neither conventional nor even the newer forms of incontinence surgery produce an effective cure. For them a urinary diversion may be a more satisfactory long-term solution than the continued use of incontinence aids.

It is important to remember that the first operation for stress incontinence is the most likely to succeed. Most suprapubic operations in current use produce a cure rate in excess of 85–90% in patients undergoing their first operation for correctly diagnosed urodynamic stress incontinence. The Burch type of colposuspension has long been recognized as the 'best' first operation although tension free vaginal tape (TVT) is now the most commonly performed continence procedure. Whilst transobturator tapes are becoming increasingly popular at present there is little long term data to support their use over the retropubic approach. Subsequent surgery may have to be performed on a vagina which is less mobile and where there is fibrosis of the urethra. In such cases, a urethral bulking agent may be easier to perform and more effective. Ultimately it is important that the operative procedure performed is tailored to suit the needs of the individual.

Detrusor overactivity

Detrusor overactivity is defined as a urodynamic observation characterized by involuntary contractions during the filling phase which may be spontaneous or provoked [2]. It is the second commonest cause of urinary incontinence in women and accounts for 30–40% of cases. The incidence is higher in the elderly and after failed incontinence surgery. The actual cause of detrusor overactivity is unknown and in the majority of cases it is idiopathic, occurring when there is a failure of adequate bladder training in childhood or when the bladder escapes voluntary control in adult life. Often emotional or other psychosomatic factors are involved. In some cases detrusor overactivity may be secondary to an upper motor neurone lesion, especially multiple sclerosis. In such cases it is known as neurogenic detrusor overactivity. In men detrusor overactivity may be secondary to outflow obstruction and will be cured when the obstruction is relieved. However, outflow obstruction in women is rare.

Low compliance is said to exist when there is a sustained rise in detrusor pressure without actual detrusor contractions during bladder filling. There are a variety of causes, including radical pelvic surgery, radiotherapy, recurrent urinary tract infections and interstitial cystitis; but the symptoms associated with phasic detrusor overactivity and with low compliance may be indistinguishable without cystometry (Figs 49.28 and 49.29).

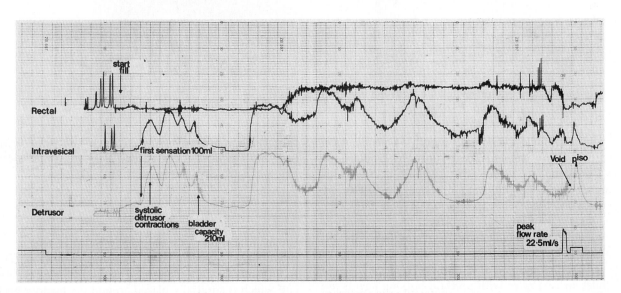

Fig. 49.28 Cystometrogram recording showing phasic detrusor instability.

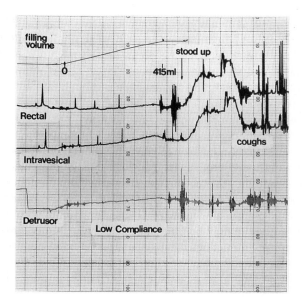

Fig. 49.29 Cystometrogram recording showing low compliance.

PATHOPHYSIOLOGY OF DETRUSOR OVERACTIVITY

The pathophysiology of detrusor overactivity remains elusive. *In vitro* studies have shown that the detrusor muscle in cases of idiopathic detrusor overactivity contracts more than normal detrusor muscle. These detrusor contractions are not nerve mediated and can be inhibited by the neuropeptide vasoactive intestinal polypeptide [154]. Other studies have shown that increased α-adrenergic activity causes increased detrusor contractility [155]. There is evidence to suggest that the pathophysiology of idiopathic and obstructive detrusor overactivity is different. From animal and human studies on obstructive overactivity it would seem that the detrusor develops postjunctional supersensitivity possibly due to partial denervation [156], with reduced sensitivity to electrical stimulation of its nerve supply but a greater sensitivity to stimulation with acetylcholine [157]. If outflow obstruction is relieved the detrusor can return to normal behaviour and reinnervation may occur [158].

Relaxation of the urethra is known to precede contraction of the detrusor in a proportion of women with detrusor overactivity [159]. This may represent primary pathology in the urethra which triggers a detrusor contraction, or may merely be part of a complex sequence of events which originate elsewhere. It has been postulated that incompetence of the bladder neck, allowing passage of urine into the proximal urethra, may result in an uninhibited contraction of the detrusor. However, Sutherst and Brown [160] were unable to provoke a detrusor contraction in 50 women by rapidly infusing saline into the posterior urethra using modified urodynamic equipment.

More recently Brading and Turner [161] have suggested that the common feature in all cases of detrusor overactivity is a change in the properties of the smooth muscle of the detrusor which predisposes it to overactive contractions. They hypothesize that partial denervation of the detrusor may be responsible for altering the properties of the smooth muscle leading to increased excitability and increased ability of activity to spread between cells, resulting in coordinated myogenic contractions of the whole detrusor [162]. They dispute the concept of neurogenic detrusor overactivity, that is, increased motor activity to the detrusor, as the underlying mechanism in detrusor overactivity proposing that there is a fundamental abnormality at the level of the bladder wall with evidence of altered spontaneous contractile activity consistent with increased electrical coupling of cells, a patchy denervation of the detrusor and a supersensitivity to potassium [163]. Other authorities suggest that the primary defect in the idiopathic and neurogenic bladders is a loss of nerves accompanied by hypertrophy of the cells and an increased production of elastin and collagen within the muscle fascicles [164].

CLINICAL SYMPTOMS

Most women with an overactive bladder exhibit a multiplicity of symptoms, including urgency, urgency incontinence, stress incontinence, enuresis, frequency and especially nocturia and sometimes incontinence during sexual intercourse. There are no specific clinical signs and the diagnosis can only be made urodynamically when there is a failure to inhibit detrusor contractions during cystometry.

Treatment for detrusor overactivity aims to re-establish central control or to alter peripheral control via bladder innervation (Table 49.13). The fact that so many different types of treatment are available for this condition shows that none is universally successful. Various behavioural interventions (habit retraining) have been successfully used to treat idiopathic detrusor overactivity and have been shown to improve symptoms in up to 80% of women [165, 166]. Unfortunately, these types of therapy are time consuming and require the patient to be fairly intelligent and highly motivated. In addition, there is a high relapse rate and patients do not seem to respond as well on a second occasion. However, it is always appropriate to instruct patients with detrusor overactivity regarding the use of bladder drill, often as an adjunct to drug therapy. The regimen suggested by [167] is commonly employed and is described as follows.

1 Exclude pathology.
2 Explain rationale to the patient.

Table 49.13 Treatment of detrusor overactivity

Psychotherapy
Bladder drill
Biofeedback
Hypnotherapy
Acupuncture

Drug therapy
Inhibit bladder contractions
anticholinergic agents
musculotrophic relaxants
tricyclic antidepressants
Improve local tissues
Oestrogens
Reduce urine production
DDAVP (synthetic vasopressin)

Intravesical therapy
Capsaicin
Resiniferatoxin
Botulinum toxin

Neuromodulation
Cystoplasty
Clam ileocystoplasty
Detrusor myectomy

Other
Maximum electrical stimulation
Acupuncture
Transcutaneous electrical neuromuscular stimulation (TENS)

3 Instruct to void every 1.5 h during the day; she must not void between these times, she must wait or be incontinent.
4 Increase voiding interval by half an hour when initial goal achieved, and continue with 2-hourly voiding and so on.
5 Give normal volume of fluids.
6 Keep fluid balance chart.
7 Give encouragement.

Drug therapy

Drug therapy is the most widely employed treatment for detrusor overactivity Table 49.14. From the number of preparations studied it is clear that there are no ideal drugs and very often the clinical results have been disappointing, this being partly due to poor efficacy and side effects [168]. The symptoms of OAB are due to involuntary contractions of the detrusor muscle during the filling phase of the micturition cycle. These involuntary contractions are mediated by acetylcholine-induced stimulation of bladder muscarinic receptors [169].

MUSCARINIC RECEPTORS

Molecular cloning studies have revealed five distinct genes for muscarinic acetylcholine receptors in rats and humans and it has been shown that five receptor subtypes (M_1–M_5) correspond to these gene products [170]. In the human bladder the occurrence of mRNA encoding M_2 and M_3 subtypes has been demonstrated although not for M_1 [171]. The M_3 receptor is thought to cause a direct smooth muscle contraction [172]. Whilst the role of the M_2 receptor has not yet been clarified it may oppose sympathetically mediated smooth muscle relaxation [173] or result in the activation of a non-specific cationic channel and inactivation of potassium channels [174]. In general it is thought that the M_3 receptor is responsible for the normal micturition contraction although in certain disease states, such as neurogenic bladder dysfunction, the M_2 receptors may become more important in mediating detrusor contractions [175].

(A) Drugs that have a mixed action

Oxybutynin Oxybutynin is a tertiary amine that undergoes extensive first-pass metabolism to an active metabolite, N-desmethyl oxybutynin [176] which occurs in high concentrations [177] and is thought to be responsible for a significant part of the action of the parent drug. It has a mixed action consisting of both an antimuscarinic and a direct muscle relaxant effect in addition to local anaesthetic properties. The later is important when given intravesically but probably has no effect when given systemically. Oxybutynin has been shown to have a high affinity for muscarinic receptors in the bladder [178] and has a higher affinity for M_1 and M_3 receptors over M_2 [179].

The effectiveness of oxybutynin in the management of patients with detrusor overactivity is well documented. A double-blind placebo controlled trial found oxybutynin to be significantly better than placebo in improving lower urinary tract symptoms although 80% of patients complained of significant adverse effects, principally dry mouth or dry skin [180]. Similar results have also been demonstrated in further placebo-controlled trials [181, 182].

The antimuscarinic adverse effects of oxybutynin are well documented and are often dose limiting [183]. Using an intravesical route of administration higher local levels of oxybutynin can be achieved whilst limiting the systemic adverse effects. Using this method oxybutynin has been shown to increase bladder capacity and lead to a significant clinical improvement [184]. Rectal administration has also been shown to be associated with fewer adverse effects when compared to oral administration [185].

More recently a controlled release oxybutynin preparation using an osmotic system (OROS) have been developed which have been shown to have comparable efficacy when compared with immediate release oxybutynin although are associated with fewer adverse effects [186].

Table 49.14 Drugs used in the management of detrusor overactivity

	Level of evidence	Grade of recommendation
Antimuscarinic drugs		
Tolterodine	1	A
Trospium	1	A
Solifenacin	1	A
Darifenacin	1	A
Propantheline	2	B
Atropine, hyoscamine	2	D
Drugs acting on membrane channels		
Calcium channel antagonists	Under investigation	
Potassium channel openers	Under investigation	
Drugs with mixed actions		
Oxybutynin	1	A
Propiverine	1	A
Dicyclomine	4	C
Flavoxate	4	D
Alpha-blockers		
Alfuzosin	4	D
Doxazosin	4	D
Prazosin	4	D
Terazosin	4	D
Tamsulosin	4	D
Beta agonists		
Terbutaline	4	D
Clenbuterol	4	D
Salbutamol	4	D
Antidepressants		
Imipramine	2	C
Amitriptylline	3	(with caution)
Prostaglandin synthesis inhibitors		
Indomethacin	4	C
Flurbiprofen	4	C
Vasopressin analogues		
Desmopressin	1	A
Other drugs		
Baclofen	2*	C*
Capsaicin	3	C
Resiniferatoxin	Under investigation	

Levels of evidence and assessment with recommendations (see Appendix).
* Intrathecal.

These findings are in agreement with a further study of controlled release oxybutynin (Lyrinel XL®) which reported the incidence of moderate to severe dry mouth to be 23% and only 1.6% of participants discontinuing the medication due to adverse effects [187].

In order to maximize efficacy and minimize adverse effects alternative delivery systems are currently under evaluation. An oxybutynin transdermal delivery system (Kentera)® has recently been developed and compared with extended release tolterodine in 361 patients with mixed urinary incontinence. Both agents significantly reduced incontinence episodes, increased volume voided and lead to an improvement in quality of life when compared to placebo. The most common adverse event in the oxybutynin patch arm was application site pruritis in 14%

although the incidence of dry mouth was reduced to 4.1% compared to 7.3% in the tolterodine arm [188].

Propiverine Propiverine has been shown to combine anticholinergic and calcium channel blocking actions [189] and is the most popular drug for detrusor overactivity in Germany, Austria and Japan. Open studies in patients with detrusor overactivity have demonstrated a beneficial effect [190] and in a double-blind placebo-controlled trial of its use in neurogenic detrusor overactivity it has been shown to significantly increase bladder capacity and compliance in comparison to placebo. Dry mouth was experienced by 37% in the treatment group as opposed to 8% in the placebo group with dropout rates being 7% and 4.5% respectively [191].

(B) Antimuscarinic drugs

Tolterodine Tolterodine is a competitive muscarinic receptor antagonist with relative functional selectivity for bladder muscarinic receptors [192] and whilst it shows no specificity for receptor subtypes it does appear to target the bladder over the salivary glands [193]. The drug is metabolized in the liver to the 5-hydroxymethyl derivative which is an active metabolite having a similar pharmacokinetic profile and is thought to significantly contribute to the therapeutic effect [194].

Several randomized, double-blind, placebo controlled trials both on patients with idiopathic detrusor overactivity and neurogenic detrusor overactivity have demonstrated a significant reduction in incontinent episodes and micturition frequency [195–197]. Further studies have confirmed the safety of tolterodine and at the recommended daily dosage the incidence of adverse events was no different to that in patients taking placebo [198].

A pooled analysis of the safety, efficacy and acceptability of tolterodine in 1,120 patients in four randomized, double-blind, parallel, multicentre trials found that both tolterodine and oxybutynin significantly decreased incontinent episodes although tolterodine was associated with fewer adverse events, dose reductions and patients withdrawals than oxybutynin [199].

Tolterodine has also been developed as an extended release once daily preparation, Detrusitol XL®. A recent double blind multicentre trail of 1,235 women has compared extended release tolterodine to immediate release tolterodine and placebo. Whilst both formulations were found to reduce the mean number of urge incontinence episodes per week the extended release preparation was found to be significantly more effective [200]. In addition to increased efficacy extended release tolterodine has been shown to have better tolerability. In a double blind, multicentre, randomized placebo controlled trial of 1,529 patients extended release tolterodine was found to be 18% more effective in the reduction of episodes of urge incontinence whilst having a 23% lower incidence of dry mouth [201].

Extended release oxybutynin (ER) and extended release tolterodine (ER) have also been compared. In the OPERA (Overactive bladder: Performance of Extended Release Agents) study, which involved 71 centres in the United States, improvements in episodes of urge incontinence were similar for the two drugs although oxybutynin ER was significantly more effective than tolterodine ER in reducing frequency of micturition. Significantly more women taking oxybutynin were also completely dry (23% versus 16.8%; $p = 0.03$) although dry mouth was significantly more common in the oxybutynin group [202].

Trospium Trospium chloride is a quaternary ammonium compound which is non selective for muscarinic receptor subtypes, shows low biological availability [203]. It crosses the blood brain barrier to a limited extent and hence would appear to have few cognitive effects [204]. In a recent placebo-controlled, randomized, double-blind, multicentre trial trospium chloride produced significant improvements in maximum cystometric capacity and bladder volume at first unstable contraction. Clinical improvement was significantly greater in the group receiving trospium and the frequency of adverse events was similar in both groups [205]. Trospium chloride has also been compared to oxybutynin in a randomized, double-blind, multicentre trial. With both agents there was a significant increase in bladder capacity, a decrease in maximum voiding detrusor pressure and a significant increase in compliance although there were no statistically significant differences between the two treatment groups. Those taking trospium had a lower incidence of dry mouth (4% versus 23%) and were also less likely to withdraw (6% versus 16%) when compared to the group receiving oxybutynin [206].

Solifenacin Solifenacin is a potent M_3 receptor antagonist that has selectivity for the M_3 receptors over M_2 receptors and has much higher potency against M_3 receptors in smooth muscle than it does against M_3 receptors in salivary glands.

The clinical efficacy of solifenacin has been assessed in a multicentre, randomized, double-blind, parallel group, placebo controlled study of solifenacin 5 and 10 mg once daily in patients with overactive bladder [207]. The primary efficacy analysis showed a statistically significant reduction of the micturition frequency following treatment with both 5 and 10 mg doses when compared with placebo although the largest effect was with the higher dose. In addition solifenacin was found to be superior to placebo with respect to the secondary efficacy variables of mean volume voided per micturition, episodes of urgency per 24 h, number of incontinence episodes and episodes of urge incontinence. The most frequently reported adverse events leading to discontinuation were dry mouth and constipation. These were also found to be dose related. In order to assess the long-term safety and efficacy of solifenacin (5 and 10 mg once daily) a multicentre open label long-term follow up study has recently been completed. This was essentially an extension of two previous double-blind placebo controlled studies in 1,637 patients [208]. Overall the efficacy of solifenacin was maintained in the extension study with a sustained improvement in symptoms of urgency, urge incontinence, frequency and nocturia over the 12-month study period. The most commonly reported adverse events were dry mouth (20.5%), constipation (9.2%) and blurred vision (6.6%) and were the primary reason for discontinuation in 4.7% of patients.

More recently solifenacin 5 and 10 mg od have been compared with tolterodine ER 4 mg od in the Solifenacin (flexible dosing) od and Tolterodine ER 4 mg od as an Active comparator in a Randomized trial (STAR) [209]. This was a prospective double-blind, double dummy, two-arm, parallel-group, 12-week study of 1,200 patients with the primary aim of demonstrating non-inferiority of solifenacin to tolterodine ER. Solifenacin was non inferior to tolterodine ER with respect to change from baseline in the mean number of micturitions per 24 h (reduction of 2.45 micturitions/24 h versus 2.24 micturitions/24 h; $p = 0.004$). In addition solifenacin resulted in a statistically significant improvement in urgency ($p = 0.035$), urge incontinence ($p = 0.001$) and overall incontinence when compared with tolterodine ER. In addition 59% of solifenacin treated patients who were incontinent at baseline became continent by the study endpoint compared with 49% of those on tolterodine ER ($p = 0.006$). The most commonly reported adverse events were dry mouth constipation and blurred vision and were mostly mild to moderate in severity. The number of patients discontinuing medication was similar in both treatment arms (3.5% in the solifenacin arm versus 3.0% in the tolterodine arm).

Darifenacin Darifenacin is a tertiary amine with moderate lipophilicity and is a highly selective M_3 receptor antagonist which has been found to have a 5-fold higher affinity for the human M_3 receptor relative to the M_1 receptor [210].

A review of the pooled darifenacin data from the three phase III, multi-centre, double-blind clinical trials in patients with OAB has recently been reported in 1059 patients [211]. Darifenacin resulted in a dose-related significant reduction in median number of incontinence episodes per week. Significant decreases in the frequency and severity of urgency, micturition frequency, and number of incontinence episodes resulting in a change of clothing or pads were also apparent, along with an increase in bladder capacity. Darifenacin was well tolerated. The most common treatment-related adverse events were dry mouth and constipation, although together these resulted in few discontinuations. The incidence of CNS and cardiovascular adverse events were comparable to placebo.

(C) Antidepressants

Imipramine Imipramine has been shown to have systemic anticholinergic effects [212] and blocks the re-uptake of serotonin. Some authorities have found a significant effect in the treatment of patients with detrusor overactivity [213] although others report little effect [214]. In light of this evidence and the serious adverse effects associated with tricyclic antidepressants their role in detrusor overactivity remains of uncertain benefit although they are often useful in patients complaining of nocturia or bladder pain.

(D) Prostaglandin synthetase inhibitors

Bladder mucosa has been shown to have the ability to synthesize eicosanoids [215] although it is uncertain whether they contribute to the pathogenesis of uninhibited detrusor contractions. However, they may have a role in sensitizing sensory afferent nerves increasing the afferent input produced by a given bladder volume. A double-blind controlled study of flurbiprofen in women with detrusor overactivity was shown to have an effect although it was associated with a high incidence of adverse effects (43%) including nausea, vomiting, headache and gastrointestinal symptoms [216]. Indomethacin has also been reported to give symptomatic relief although the incidence of adverse effects was also high (59%) [217]. At present this evidence does not support their use in detrusor overactivity.

(E) Antidiuretic agents

Desmopressin Desmopressin (1-desamino-8-D-arginine vasopressin; DDAVP) is a synthetic vasopressin analogue. It has strong antidiuretic effects without altering blood pressure. The drug has been used primarily in the treatment of nocturia and nocturnal enuresis in children [218] and adults [219]. More recently nasal desmopressin has been reported as a 'designer drug' for the treatment of daytime urinary incontinence [220]. Desmopressin is safe for long-term use, however the drug should be used with care in the elderly due to the risk of hyponatraemia.

(F) Intravesical therapy

Capsaicin This is the pungent ingredient found in red chillies and is a neurotoxin of substance P containing (C) nerve fibres. Patients with neurogenic detrusor overactivity secondary to multiple sclerosis appear to have abnormal C fibre sensory innervation of the detrusor, which leads to premature activation of the holding reflex arc during bladder filling [221]. Intravesical application of capsaicin dissolved in 30% alcohol solution appears to be effective for up to 6 months. The effects are variable [222] and the clinical effectiveness remains undefined.

Resiniferatoxin This is a phorbol related diterpene isolated from the cactus and is a potent analogue of capsaicin that appears to have a similar efficacy but with fewer side effects of pain and burning during intavesical instillation [223]. It is 1,000 times more potent than capsaicin at stimulating bladder activity [224]. As with capsaicin the currently available evidence does not support the routine clinical use of the agents although they may prove to have a role as an intravesical preparation in neurological patients with neurogenic detrusor overactivity.

Botulinum toxin   In 1817 an illness caused by Clostridium botulinum toxin was first recorded, when Justinus Kerner described a link between a sausage, and a paralytic illness that affected 230 people. He was a district health officer and made botulism (Latin 'botulus' meaning sausage) a notifiable disease [225]. In 1897, the microbiologist Emile-Pierre van Ermengen identified a gram-positive, spore-forming, anaerobic bacterium in a ham that caused 23 cases of botulism in a Belgian nightclub. He termed the bacterium *Bacillus botulinus*; it was later re-termed *Clostridium Botulinum* [226].

The bacterium produces its effect by production of a neurotoxin – different strains produce seven distinct serotypes designated A–G. All seven have a similar structure and molecular weight, consisting of a heavy (H) and a light (L) chain, joined by a disulphide bond [227]. They interfere with neural transmission by blocking the calcium-dependent release of neurotransmitter, acetylcholine, causing the affected muscle to become weak and atrophic. The affected nerves do not degenerate, but as the blockage is irreversible, only the development of new nerve terminals and synaptic contacts allows recovery of function.

The use of intravesical Botulinum toxin was first described in the treatment of intractable neurogenic detrusor overactivity in 31 patients with traumatic spinal cord injury [228]. Subsequently a larger European study has reported on 231 patients with neurogenic detrusor overactivity [229]. All were treated with 300 units of Botulinum-A toxin which was injected cystoscopically into the detrusor muscle at 30 different sites sparing the trigone. At 12 and 36 week follow up there was a significant increase in cystometric capacity and bladder compliance. Patient satisfaction was high, the majority stopped taking antimuscarinic medication and there were no significant complications. More recently the first randomized placebo controlled trial has been reported in 59 patients with neurogenic detrusor overactivity [230]. At 6 months there was a significant reduction in incontinence episodes in the botox group compared to placebo and a corresponding improvement in quality of life evaluation.

Whilst the role of Botulinum toxin has been established in the treatment of neurogenic detrusor overactivity the data regarding its use in intractable idiopathic detrusor overactivity is less robust. A prospective open label study has recently been reported assessing the use of Botulinum-A toxin in both neurogenic (300 units) and idiopathic (200 units) detrusor overactivity in 75 patients [231]. When considering urodynamic outcome parameters in both groups there was a significant increase in cystometric capacity and decrease in maximum detrusor pressure during filling in both groups. Clinically there was also a significant reduction in frequency and episodes of urge incontinence. Interestingly however 69% of patients with neurogenic detrusor overactivity required self-catheterization following treatment compared to 19.3% of those with idiopathic detrusor overactivity.

At present the evidence would suggest that intravesical administration of Botulinum toxin may offer an alternative to surgery in those women with intractable detrusor overactivity although the effect is only temporary and at present there is little long term data regarding the efficacy and complications associated with repeat injections [232].

Neuromodulation

Stimulation of the dorsal sacral nerve root using a permanent implantable device in the S3 sacral foramen has been developed for use in patients with both idiopathic and neurogenic detrusor overactivity. The sacral nerves contain nerve fibres of the parasympathetic and sympathetic systems providing innervation to the bladder as well as somatic fibres providing innervation to the muscles of the pelvic floor. The latter are larger in diameter and hence have a lower threshold of activation meaning that the pelvic floor may be stimulated selectively without causing bladder activity. Prior to implantation, temporary cutaneous sacral nerve stimulation is performed to check for a response, and if successful, a permanent implant is inserted under general anaesthesia. Initial studies in patients with detrusor overactivity refractory to medical and behavioural therapy have demonstrated that after 3 years, 59% of 41 urinary urge incontinent patients showed greater than 50% reduction in incontinence episodes with 46% of patients being completely dry [233]. Whilst neuromodulation remains an invasive and expensive procedure in the future, it offers a useful alternative to medical and surgical therapies in patients with severe, intractable detrusor overactivity.

Surgery

For those women with severe detrusor overactivity which is not amenable to simple types of treatment, surgery may be employed.

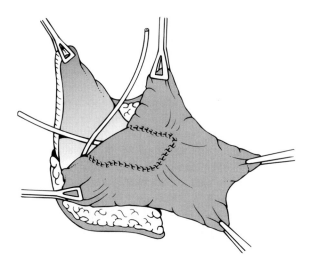

Fig. 49.30 Clam ileocystoplasty.

CLAM CYSTOPLASTY

In the clam cystoplasty [234, 235] the bladder is bisected almost completely and a patch of gut (usually ileum) equal in length to the circumference of the bisected bladder (about 25 cm) is sewn in place (Fig. 49.30). This often cures the symptoms of detrusor overactivity [236] by converting a high-pressure system into a low-pressure system although inefficient voiding may result. Patients have to learn to strain to void, or may have to resort to clean intermittent self-catheterization, sometimes permanently. In addition, mucus retention in the bladder may be a problem, but this can be partially overcome by ingestion of 200 ml of cranberry juice each day [237] in addition to intravesical mucolytics such as acetylcysteine. The chronic exposure of the ileal mucosa to urine may lead to malignant change [238]. There is a 5% risk of adenocarcinoma arising in ureterosigmoidostomies, where colonic mucosa is exposed to N-nitrosamines found in both urine and faeces, and a similar risk may apply to enterocystoplasty. Biopsies of the ileal segment taken from patients with 'clam' cystoplasties show evidence of chronic inflammation of villous atrophy, and diarrhoea due to disruption of the bile acid cycle is common [239]. This may be treated using cholestyramine. In addition, metabolic disturbances such as hyperchoraemic acidosis, B_{12} deficiency and occasionally osteoporosis secondary to decreased bone mineralization may occur.

DETRUSOR MYECTOMY

Detrusor myectomy offers an alternative to clam cystoplasty by increasing functional bladder capacity without the complications of bowel interposition. In this procedure, the whole thickness of the detrusor muscle is excised from the dome of the bladder thereby creating a large bladder diverticulum with no intrinsic contractility [240]. Whilst there is a reduction in episodes of incontinence, there is little improvement in functional capacity, and thus frequency remains problematic [241, 242].

URINARY DIVERSION

As a last resort for those women with severe detrusor overactivity or neurogenic detrusor overactivity who cannot manage clean intermittent catheterization, it may be more appropriate to perform a urinary diversion. Usually this will utilize an ileal conduit to create an abdominal stoma for urinary diversion. An alternative is to form a continent diversion using the appendix (Mitrofanoff) or ileum (Koch pouch) which may then be drained using self-catheterization.

Mixed incontinence

Although a large proportion of women complain of both stress and urge incontinence, only about 5% suffer from mixed detrusor overactivity and urethral sphincter incompetence. They pose a difficult management problem. A study comparing medical and surgical treatment has shown that of the 27 women who underwent a Burch colposuspension, 59% were cured and 22% improved; whereas of the 25 who received drug therapy (oxybutynin, imipramine and oestrogen) 32% were cured and 28% improved. The authors concluded that combined stress incontinence and detrusor overactivity should be managed medically initially as this will reduce the need for surgical intervention [243]. In such cases, it is our practice to treat the detrusor overactivity with antimuscarinic agents and to repeat the urodynamic assessment while the patient is taking her medication. If she still leaks without significant detrusor activity and her main complaint is stress incontinence, we would undertake conventional bladder neck surgery. However, if urge incontinence still predominates, surgery may aggravate her symptoms.

Retention with overflow

In women, chronic retention with resultant overflow incontinence is uncommon and often no cause can be found. It is one manifestation of the wide range of voiding difficulties which may occur, the major causes of which are shown in Table 49.15.

Women with overflow incontinence present in a variety of ways. They may complain of dribbling urine or of voiding small amounts at frequent intervals, or of stress incontinence. Alternatively, they may notice recurrent urinary tract infections. The diagnosis is usually made by the

Table 49.15 Causes of voiding difficulties leading to overflow incontinence in women

Neurological
Lower motor neurone lesion
Upper motor neurone lesion

Inflammation
Urethritis, e.g. 'honeymoon cystitis'
Vulvitis, e.g. herpes
Vaginitis, e.g. candidiasis

Drugs
Tricyclic antidepressants
Antimuscarinic agents
Ganglion blockers
Epidural anaesthesia
Patient-controlled analgesia

Obstruction
Urethral stenosis/stricture
Oedema following surgery or parturition
Fibrosis due to repeated dilatation or irradiation
Pelvic mass, e.g. fibroids, retroverted uterus, ovarian cyst, faeces
Urethral distorsion due to large cystocele

Myogenic
Atonic detrusor secondary to over distension

Functional
Anxiety

discovery of a large bladder on clinical examination. This can be confirmed by a postmicturition ultrasound scan to assess the residual urine volume or by catheterization, which will reveal a residual volume greater than 50% of her bladder capacity. There may, in addition, be a reduced peak flow rate of less than 15 ml/s.

Clinical examination will rule out many of the causes, such as a pelvic mass or a cystocele. It is important to investigate cases of urinary retention thoroughly in order to exclude any treatable underlying pathology. A midstream specimen of urine should be sent for culture and sensitivity, and the appropriate swabs (urethral, vaginal and cervical) should be sent. Radiological investigations should include intravenous urography, an X-ray of the lumbosacral spine and an MRI where indicated. It is particularly important to identify diabetes so that treatment can be undertaken before permanent damage occurs.

Treatment for overflow incontinence will depend upon the underlying pathology. If the detrusor is hypotonic, cholinergic agents such as bethanechol 25 mg three times a day may be helpful. If there is outflow obstruction, urethral dilatation or urethrotomy may be required. In cases where no cause can be found, clean intermittent self-catheterization is the best long-term method of management for these patients.

If it is possible, it is far better to avoid urinary retention by implementing prophylactic measures. The human female bladder, once overdistended, may never contract normally again [244]. When bladder neck surgery for urinary incontinence or radical pelvic surgery for malignant disease is undertaken, adequate postoperative bladder drainage (preferably with a suprapubic catheter) should be employed until normal voiding per urethram has resumed. When epidural anaesthesia is used for surgical procedures or childbirth, an indwelling Foley catheter should be left *in situ* for at least 6 and probably 12 h after normal sensation to the lower limbs is present. Those women who are known to have inefficient voiding (a low flow rate together with a low maximum voiding pressure) should be taught clean intermittent self-catheterization prior to any surgical intervention for urodynamic stress incontinence.

Acute urinary retention needs to be dealt with as an emergency. A catheter, either indwelling urethral or suprapubic, should be inserted immediately and left on free drainage. There is no need for intermittent clamping of the catheter as this can lead to further overdistension and there is no evidence to suggest that sudden decompression of the bladder is harmful. The volume of urine which drains should be recorded and if it is over a litre the catheter should be left *in situ* on free drainage for a week or two before initiating a trial of voiding per urethram. It is, of course, easier to do this is if a suprapubic catheter has been inserted. The urinary residuals should be checked regularly once spontaneous micturition has been resumed to ensure that the bladder is emptying adequately. This can be achieved by 'in–out' catheterization, or less invasively by transabdominal ultrasound. Unless there is an obvious cause for the episode of acute retention, investigations should be undertaken. If further episodes of retention occur, it is prudent to teach the woman clean intermittent self-catheterization to avoid damage to the bladder by overdistension should she find herself in the same position again.

Oestrogens in the management of incontinence

Oestrogen preparations have been used for many years in the treatment of urinary incontinence [245, 246] although their precise role remains controversial.

In order to clarify the situation a meta-analysis from the Hormones and Urogenital Therapy (HUT) Committee has been reported [247]. Of 166 articles identified which were published in English between 1969 and 1992 only 6 were controlled trials and 17 were uncontrolled series. Meta-analysis found an overall significant effect of oestrogen therapy on subjective improvement in all subjects and for subjects with urodynamic stress incontinence alone.

Subjective improvement rates with oestrogen therapy in randomized controlled trials ranged from 64% to 75% although placebo groups also reported an improvement of 10–56%. In uncontrolled series, subjective improvement rates were 8–89% with subjects with urodynamic stress incontinence showing improvement of 34–73%. However, when assessing objective fluid loss there was no significant effect.

A further meta-analysis performed in Italy has analysed the results of randomized controlled clinical trials on the efficacy of oestrogen treatment in postmenopausal women with urinary incontinence [248]. A search of the literature (1965–1996) revealed 72 articles of which only four were considered to meet the meta-analysis criteria. There was a statistically significant difference in subjective outcome between oestrogen and placebo although there was no such difference in objective or urodynamic outcome.

The most recent meta-analysis of the effect of oestrogen therapy on the lower urinary tract has been performed by the Cochrane group [249]. Overall 28 trials were identified, including 2,926 women. In the 15 trials comparing oestrogen to placebo there was a higher subjective impression of improvement rate in those women taking oestrogen, and this was the case for all types of incontinence (RR for cure 1.61; 95% CI 1.04–2.49). Equally, when subjective cure and improvement were taken together there was a statistically higher cure and improvement rate for both urge (57% versus 28%) and stress (43% versus 27%) incontinence. In those women with urge incontinence, the chance of improvement was 25% higher than in women with stress incontinence and, overall about 50% of women treated with oestrogen were cured or improved compared to 25% on placebo. The authors conclude that oestrogens can improve or cure incontinence and that the effect may be most useful in women complaining of urge incontinence.

SYSTEMIC HRT AND URINARY INCONTINENCE

Several large scale systemic HRT studies have recently been reported which have led to greater controversy regarding the role of oral oestrogens on the lower urinary tract.

The role of oestrogen replacement therapy in the prevention of ischaemic heart disease has been assessed in a 4-year randomized trial, the Heart and Estrogen/progestin Replacement Study (HERS) [250] involving 2,763 postmenopausal women younger than 80 years. Overall combined hormone replacement therapy was associated with worsening stress and urge urinary incontinence, although there was no significant difference in daytime frequency, nocturia or number of urinary tract infections.

These findings have also been confirmed in the Nurse's Health Study which followed 39,436 postmenopausal women aged 50–75 years over a four year period. The risk of incontinence was found to be elevated in those women taking HRT when compared to those who had never taken HRT [251]. The most recent paper to be reported by the Women's Health Initiative (WHI) writing group has also studied the effect of oestrogens, with and without progestogens, on urinary incontinence [252]. In this study, 27,347 postmenopausal women aged 50–79 years were assessed in a multicentre, double blind placebo controlled trial. Of these, 23,296 were known to complain of lower urinary tract symptoms at baseline and one year follow-up. Overall, hormone replacement therapy was found to increase the incidence of all types of urinary incontinence at one year in those women continent at baseline. The risk was highest for stress incontinence followed by mixed incontinence whilst the effect on urge urinary incontinence was not uniform.

These results, whilst supportive of the previously reported HERS study and Nurse Health study, would certainly seem to contradict much of the previous work assessing the use of oestrogens in the management of lower urinary tract symptoms. The current evidence from all trials suggests that oestrogen replacement therapy may have a minor role in lower urinary tract dysfunction and the findings of the WHI studies should not prevent its usage in women who complain of troublesome menopausal symptoms after appropriate counselling and discussion.

Fistulas

Urinary fistulas may be ureterovaginal, vesicovaginal, urethrovaginal or complex, and can occur following pelvic surgery or in cases of advanced pelvic malignancy, especially when there has been radiotherapy. The most common varieties in the UK are lower ureteric or bladder fistulas occurring after an abdominal hysterectomy. In developing countries, poor obstetrics with obstructed labour resulting in ischaemic necrosis of the bladder base is more likely to be the cause of a vesico- or urethrovaginal fistula.

Fistulas give rise to incontinence which is continuous, occurring both day and night. They are usually visible on speculum examination but cystoscopy and intravenous urography may be required to confirm the diagnosis.

Treatment is surgical. Ureterovaginal fistulas should be repaired as quickly as possible to prevent upper urinary tract damage. Vesicovaginal fistulas are usually treated conservatively initially with bladder drainage and antibiotics, during which time some will close spontaneously. Abdominal or vaginal repair is normally performed 2 or

3 months after the initial injury, although there is now a trend towards earlier repair; if a fistula is detected within a very short period of time after the initial operation, it can often be closed immediately.

Congenital abnormalities

Congenital abnormalities are uncommon and are usually diagnosed at birth or in childhood. The most gross abnormality is ectopia vesicae, which requires surgical reconstruction during the neonatal period. Other less obvious congenital abnormalities include epispadias, which can be diagnosed by the bifid clitoris. This abnormality is difficult to treat and may require reconstruction in the form of a neourethra. An ectopic ureter may open into the vagina and cause urinary incontinence which is not diagnosed until childhood, and spina bifida occulta may present with urinary symptoms during the prepubertal growth spurt.

Urethral diverticulum

Urethral diverticula are becoming more common, presumably because of the increased incidence of sexually transmitted diseases. They are found in women of any age and lead to various complaints including pain, particularly after micturition, postmicturition dribble and dyspareunia. Diagnosis can be made either radiologically on a micturating cystogram or videocystourethrogram, or by urethroscopy. Urethral diverticula should be managed conservatively initially with intermittent courses of antibiotics if necessary; but if there are severe symptoms, then surgical excision of the diverticulum may be required. It is usual to perform a subtotal diverticulectomy in order to avoid urethral stricture formation.

Temporary causes of urinary incontinence

Lower urinary tract infections (cystitis or urethritis) may uncommonly cause incontinence of urine which is temporary and will resolve once treatment with the appropriate antibiotics has been employed. Diuretics, especially in the elderly, may also be responsible for urgency, frequency and incontinence. In older people, anything which limits their independence may cause urge incontinence where only urgency existed before. This applies particularly to immobility, and if an older person is unable to reach the toilet in a short space of time, she may become incontinent. Thus, the provision of appropriate facilities and adequate lighting can alleviate the problem. Faecal impaction may cause urinary incontinence or retention of urine which will resolve once suitable laxatives or enemas have been effective.

Functional incontinence

In a small proportion of women, no organic cause can be found for incontinence. Some of them have anxiety states which respond well to physiotherapy or to psychotropic drugs such as diazepam. Immobility may prevent a woman from reaching the lavatory in time and for her simple remedies such as a toilet downstairs or the use of a commode may prevent urinary leakage.

General therapeutic measures

All incontinent women benefit from simple measures such as the provision of suitable incontinence pads and pants. Those with a high fluid intake should be advised to restrict their drinking to a litre a day, particularly if frequency of micturition is a problem. Caffeine-containing drinks (such as teas, coffee and cola) and alcohol are irritant to the bladder and act as diuretics, so should be avoided, if possible. Anything which increases intra-abdominal pressure will aggravate incontinence, so patients with a chronic cough should be advised to give up smoking, and constipation should be treated appropriately. Pelvic floor exercises may be particularly helpful in the puerperium or after pelvic surgery. For younger, more active women who have not yet completed their family, a device or sponge tampon may be used during strenuous activity such as sport. Oestrogen replacement therapy for postmenopausal women is often beneficial as it improves quality of life as well as helps with the overactive bladder symptoms. Diuretics, which are often given to older people for fluid retention or mild hypertension, may make their urinary symptoms worse and should be stopped if possible.

Women with long-standing severe incontinence, especially the elderly, may be more comfortable and easier to manage with a regularly changed indwelling suprapubic catheter; and for the young disabled, urinary diversion should be considered earlier rather than later. It is not always possible to cure urinary incontinence but it is usually possible to help the sufferer and thus improve her quality of life.

Other lower urinary tract disorders

Urethral lesions

URETHRAL CARUNCLE

A urethral caruncle is a benign red polyp or lesion covered by transitional epithelium usually found on the posterior aspect of the urethral meatus. It is commonly seen in postmenopausal women and although usually asymptomatic it may cause pain, bleeding and dysuria. The cause is unknown. Treatment is by excision biopsy followed by local or systemic oestrogens.

URETHRAL MUCOSAL PROLAPSE

Prolapse of the urethral mucosa also occurs in the post-menopausal woman but in addition, is sometimes seen in girls (usually black) between the ages of 5 and 10 years. It is a reddish lesion which encompasses the whole circumference of the external urethral meatus, thus differentiating it from the urethral caruncle. Urethral mucosal prolapse is not painful but may cause bleeding, dysuria or urethral discharge. It may be treated by excision or cautery.

URETHRAL STENOSIS ·OR STRICTURE

Outflow obstruction due to urethral stenosis or a stricture is rare in women. Such lesions usually present after the menopause and are found in the distal urethra. They are often the result of chronic urethritis or may follow fibrosis from repeated urethral dilatations or other surgery to the urethra. The most common symptoms are of voiding difficulties, but recurrent urinary tract infections may occur. Diagnosis can be made using uroflowmetry in conjunction with cystometry or by videocystourethrography. Urethral pressure profilometry or cystourethroscopy will help to localize the lesion. Urethrotomy, either Otis or open, is the treatment of choice, and local oestrogen therapy may be helpful in postmenopausal women.

CARCINOMA OF THE URETHRA

Urethral carcinoma is rare and is usually a transitional cell carcinoma located in the proximal urethra. Secondary deposits may arise from adenocarcinoma of the endometrium, transitional cell carcinoma of the bladder or squamous carcinoma of the vulva or vagina. Symptoms include haematuria, vaginal bleeding and discharge, frequency of micturition, dysuria and recurrent urinary tract infections. A mass may be palpable or may be seen on speculum examination. The diagnosis can be confirmed by taking urethroscopically directed biopsies. Treatment consists of radical surgery, usually cystourethrectomy and lymph node dissection followed by radiotherapy.

Urinary frequency and urgency

DEFINITIONS [2]

1 *Diurnal frequency*. The complaint by the patient who considers that she voids too often by day.
2 *Nocturia*. The complaint that the individual has to wake one or more times at night to void.

3 *Urgency*. The complaint of a sudden compelling desire to pass urine which is difficult to defer.
4 *Urge incontinence*. The complaint of involuntary leakage accompanied by or immediately preceded by urgency.

PREVALENCE

Frequency and urgency are common symptoms in women of all ages which often coexist and may occur in conjunction with other symptoms such as urinary incontinence or dysuria. It is unusual for urgency to occur alone because once it is present it almost invariably leads to frequency to avoid urge incontinence and to relieve the unpleasant painful sensation. Bungay *et al.* [253] found that approximately 20% of a group of 1120 women aged between 30 and 65 years admitted to frequency of micturition and 15% of women from the same series reported urgency. In this study there was no specific increase in the prevalence of frequency or urgency with age or in relation to the menopause.

Over the age of about 60 years it is common for women to develop 'nocturia'. This increases once per decade of life so that it is not unusual for a woman in her eighties to have to rise four times during the night to void. This represents a relative impairment in cardiovascular function rather than a urological abnormality.

CAUSES AND ASSESSMENT

There are many different causes of frequency and urgency of micturition; the more common ones are shown in Table 49.16.

Clinical examination will exclude many of the causes. This is important before expensive time-consuming investigations are undertaken. As one of the commonest causes of frequency of micturition is a lower urinary tract infection it is important to send a mid-stream specimen of urine for culture and sensitivity. If difficulty is encountered obtaining an uncontaminated mid-stream specimen of urine suprapubic aspiration should be employed. When urine culture is repeatedly negative in a woman with urgency, frequency and dysuria where no other cause can be found, urine should be sent for culture of fastidious organisms such as *Mycoplasma hominis* and *Ureaplasma urealyticum*, which are being seen with increasing frequency in symptomatic women.

Those women who have an abnormal vaginal discharge, history of sexually transmitted diseases or obvious vulval excoriation should have vaginal, cervical and urethral swabs sent for culture. *Chlamydia* may be a causative organism which requires a special culture medium for its detection. If there is a history of haematuria, loin or groin pain, and a urinary tract infection cannot be

Table 49.16 Causes of urgency and frequency in women

Urological	Urinary tract infection
	Urethral syndrome
	Detrusor overactivity
	Bladder tumour
	Bladder calculus
	Small capacity bladder
	Interstitial cystitis
	Radiation cystitis/fibrosis
	Chronic retention/residual
	Urethral diverticulum
Gynaecological	Cystocele
	Pelvic mass, e.g. fibroids, ovarian cyst
	Previous pelvic surgery
Genital	Urethritis ('honeymoon cystitis')
	Vulvovaginitis
	Urethral caruncle
	Herpes
	Warts
	Sexually transmitted diseases
	Atrophy (hypo-oestrogenism)
Medical	Upper motor neurone lesion
	Impaired renal function
	Diabetes mellitus
	Diabetes insipidus
	Hypothyroidism
	Congestive cardiac failure
	Diuretic therapy
	Faecal impaction
General	Excessive drinking habit
	Anxiety
	Pregnancy

identified, intravenous urography and cystoscopy should be performed and the patient referred to a urologist. In cases of impaired renal function serum urine electrolyte concentration and urine osmolarity should be estimated. A plain radiograph of the abdomen (kidneys, ureter and bladder) is useful in the diagnosis of a calculus and if a significant urinary residual volume is discovered then an X-ray of the lumbar sacral spine should be obtained.

The investigations performed should be organized around the patient's precise symptomatology. However, a frequency-volume chart is often useful as it may identify excessive drinking as the cause of urinary frequency. In addition cystourethroscopy may reveal underlying pathology within the bladder or urethra. For women with incontinence in addition to frequency with or without urgency it is best to organize urodynamic studies prior to cystoscopy as the latter is usually unrewarding. Subtracted cystometry detects detrusor overactivity, which is a major cause of urgency and frequency and also reveals chronic retention of urine with an atonic bladder which

may lead to frequency or recurrent urinary tract infections. For women with frequency, urgency and dysuria without incontinence a cystourethroscopy may be more helpful than urodynamic assessment.

Urethral pressure profilometry may reveal urethral relaxation which will cause incontinence [254, 255]. Unfortunately the clinical significance of urethral relaxation is poorly understood. In a series of 107 healthy female volunteers from a gynaecology clinic none of whom had previous urological complaints 16% had pressure variations greater than one-third of their maximum urethral pressures [256] but there was no association with symptoms of lower urinary tract dysfunction.

In a large proportion of cases no obvious cause will be found for the symptoms of frequency and urgency. Some patients with negative findings void frequently from habit which usually develops following an acute urinary tract infection or an episode of incontinence. Alternatively bad habits may have been present since childhood, especially if one parent voids frequently. It is interesting that often several members of the same family suffer from similar urinary complaints.

TREATMENT

This should be directed towards the underlying cause if one has been identified. Those women who drink excessively should be advised to limit their fluid intake to between 1 and 1.5 l/day and to avoid drinking at times when their frequency causes the most embarrassment. Certain drinks such as tea, coffee and cola (all of which contain caffeine) and alcohol precipitate frequency especially nocturia in some individuals and should therefore be avoided.

Habit retraining (bladder drill) is useful for women without organic disease and can be undertaken by patients at home [166]. Inpatient bladder drill is more effective but often impossible to organize, and the regimen described by Jarvis and Millar [165] is easy to follow and effectively improves symptoms in up to 80% of women initially. Unfortunately the relapse rate is high [257]. This is mainly due to the underlying factors in the patient's home environment which exacerbate her symptoms.

Sometimes antimuscarinic drug therapy may be helpful. If anxiety or nocturia is a problem then imipramine or amitriptyline 50 mg *nocte* can be tried. Desmopressin nasal spray or tablets may also be useful in patients who complain of nocturia alone.

Urethral pain syndrome

This is defined as the occurrence of recurrent episodic urethral pain usually on voiding with daytime frequency and nocturia in the absence of infection or other obvious pathology [2]. The urethral pain syndrome can occur at any age. There are believed to be two basic causative factors – a bacterial and a urethral element. The bacterial element is thought to be due to migration of *Escherichia coli* across the perineum and up the urethra for which Smith [258] has recommended perineal hygiene, especially after sexual intercourse. In the case of an acute attack many authorities suggest a high fluid intake combined with bicarbonate of soda to alter the pH of the urine and short courses of antibiotics such as co-trimoxazole, nitrofurantoin or, more recently, norfloxacin. Prolonged low dose chemotherapy is sometimes necessary for relapsing and chronic cases. Norfloxacin 400 mg *nocte* taken for 3 months can be employed. *Chlamydia trachomatis* is a possible causative organism [259] in which case doxycycline 100 mg *nocte* for 3 months is an effective antibiotic.

Various surgical manoeuvres have been tried for resistant cases of urethral pain syndrome. Urethral dilatation has been employed but there is no rationale behind its use since it is rare to find outflow obstruction in these women. Similarly urethrotomy is sometimes performed. However, it is not indicated and may cause incontinence or a urethral stricture. Rees *et al.* [260] found that less than 8% of 156 women with the urethral syndrome had outflow obstruction and that the results of urethral dilatation or internal urethrotomy were no better than medication alone.

Interstitial cystitis

Painful bladder syndrome is the compliant of suprapubic pain related to bladder filling accompanied by other symptoms such as increased daytime and night time frequency, in the absence of proven urinary infection or other obvious pathology [2]. A cause of painful bladder syndrome in women is interstitial cystitis.

Interstitial cystitis produces severe symptoms which include frequency, dysuria, lower abdominal and urethral pain. It affects individuals of both sexes although only about 10% of sufferers are men. Although the peak age is 30–50 years [261] it has also been found in children [262]. The aetiology remains obscure but the absence of any detectable bacterial or fungal agent is a prerequisite for the diagnosis [263]. There is growing evidence that interstitial cystitis is an autoimmune disease. Histological changes in bladder wall biopsies are consistent with a connective tissue disorder. The most common marker is mast cell infiltration of the muscularis layer of the bladder. This was first recognized in 1958 by Simmons and Bruce and, although there is no consensus on the role of mast cells and their usefulness as a diagnostic criterion, two papers have investigated degranulation of mast cells [264, 265] both showing increased degranulation in patients

suffering from interstitial cystitis. Parsons *et al.* [266] proposed that there is a failure of the protective function of the mucosal glycosaminoglycan layer of the bladder thus allowing infective agents to attack the underlying epithelium and subsequently they postulated that patients with interstitial cystitis have an abnormal sensitivity to intravesical potassium [267].

The diagnosis of interstitial cystitis can be difficult to make. Pain is the most common presenting complaint and occurs in 70% of sufferers. This is usually suprapubic although urethritis, loin pain and dyspareunia are also frequently encountered. A long history of a combination of overactive urinary symptoms (frequency, urgency and dysuria) in the absence of proven infection is often present. Other urinary complaints may coexist. Many of the women have previously undergone hysterectomy although it is difficult to know if this represents a true relationship or just reflects desperate attempts on the part of the doctor to relieve the patient's symptoms.

Clinical examination is usually unrewarding and the diagnosis is often based on the finding of sensory urgency (painful catheterization, urgency and the absence of a rise in detrusor pressure and a bladder capacity of less than 300 ml) at dual-channel subtracted cystometry. Cystoscopy needs to be undertaken preferably under general anaesthesia in order to obtain a good-sized bladder base biopsy. Terminal haematuria at either urodynamic investigation or cystoscopy is suggestive of interstitial cystitis (Fig. 49.31). Characteristically the cystoscopic findings include petechial haemorrhages on distension, especially second fill, reduced bladder capacity and classically, although uncommonly, ulceration. There is still confusion due to the lack of conformity in diagnostic parameters commonly used. Bladder capacity in particular is a contentious issue. Hanno [268] states that the bladder capacity must not exceed 350 ml whereas Messing and Stamey [269] demonstrated that the bladder capacity differed significantly between cystoscopies performed under local or no anaesthetic and those performed under general anaesthesia concluding that bladder volumes were not a useful guide to diagnosis. Gillespie [270] states that restricting the maximum bladder capacity excludes patients who may have early interstitial cystitis and may benefit from treatment before an accepted diagnosis can be established. Table 49.17 lists the criteria for excluding a diagnosis of interstitial cystitis.

It is likely that the condition we call interstitial cystitis is the final common pathway of a multifactorial disease process and it is therefore not surprising that many different types of treatment have been proposed (none of which has proved to be completely satisfactory). Both non-steroidal and steroidal anti-inflammatory agents such as azathioprine, sodium chromoglycate and chloroquine

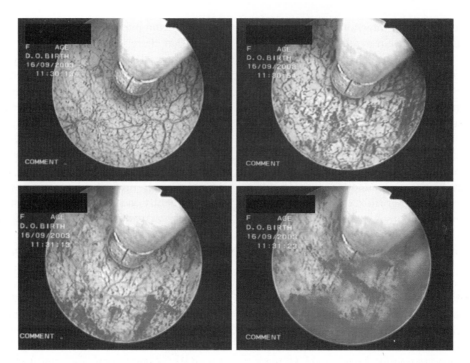

Fig. 49.31 Series of cystoscopic images showing gradual cystodistension with haemorrahage in a young woman with interstitial cystitis.

Table 49.17 Criteria for the exclusion of a diagnosis of interstitial cystitis

Bladder capacity of >350 ml on awake cystometry
Absence of an intense desire to void at 150 ml during medium fill cystometry (30–100 ml/min)
Demonstration of phasic involuntary bladder contractions on cystometry
Symptomatology of <9 months duration
Absence of nocturia
Symptoms relieved by antimicrobials, urinary antiseptics, antimuscarinics or antispasmodics
Urinary diurnal frequency <9 times
A diagnosis of bacterial cystitis within last 3 months
Bladder calculi
Active genital herpes
Gynaecological malignancy
Urethral diverticulum
Chemical cystitis
Tuberculosis
Radiation cystitis
Bladder tumours
Vaginitis
Age <18 years

have been tried [271]. Sodium pentosanpolysulphate is believed to decrease the bladder wall permeability and variable success rates have been quoted from 27% [272] to 83% [273]. It appears to be effective when administered intravesically [274]. Heparin, which is thought to reduce the available cations and have a similar effect to sodium pentosanpolysulphate, has also been employed [267].

Those who prefer an infective hypothesis of causation have employed long-term antibiotics. Norfloxacin can be given 400 mg *nocte* for 3 months or alternatively a bladder antiseptic such as hexamine hipurate may be used.

Dimethylsulphone (DMSO) has been instilled into the bladder with some success [275]. Many clinicians believe that this gives good symptomatic relief even if only in the short term although there are concerns that it may be carcinogenic. Other treatments which have been tried include local anaesthetics, calcium channel blockers and tricyclic antidepressants which should probably be used as an adjunct to treatment to help to relive pain [268].

Although bladder distension has been used for the treatment of sensory bladder disorders there is no evidence to support use of this technique in interstitial cystitis. Short-term benefit may be reported but repeated distensions can lead to an exacerbation of symptoms. Denervation procedures using surgical techniques or phenol have largely been abolished although recently Gillespie [276] has described laser ablation of the vesicoureteric plexus with impressive results. There is still a place for either substitution cystoplasty or urinary diversion in severely affected patients but augmentation cystoplasty is rarely effective as pain continues to be a problem.

Many patients benefit from simple self-help measures [270], and the avoidance of caffeine-containing compounds (tea, coffee and cola). Gillespie [277] has written extensively about the role of diet in the management of interstitial cystitis.

The majority of women who suffer with interstitial cystitis do so for many years until they either find ways of coping with their symptoms or eventually undergo surgery. Fortunately the symptoms tend to wax and wane and it is often possible to provide support and intermittent therapy until a remission occurs [278].

Sexual problems

Many women develop an urgent desire to pass urine during or immediately after sexual intercourse. This is thought to be caused by the rigid nulliparous perineum which allows irritation of the posterior bladder wall to occur during repeated penile thrusting [279]. Postcoital dysuria, commonly known as 'honeymoon cystitis', may be followed by a urinary tract infection. The use of the contraceptive diaphragm may lead to bouts of frequency, urgency and dysuria as well as recurrent urinary tract infections [280]. An alternative method of contraception should be employed. Symptoms of urgency and frequency following sexual intercourse can be helped by simple measures such as perineal hygiene, change of coital technique and voiding a fairly full bladder after sexual intercourse.

For postmenopausal women, failure of adequate lubrication during sexual intercourse may be a problem so a lubricant gel or preferably oestrogen replacement should be prescribed [281]. For those women with a uterus who do not wish to suffer the recurrence of monthly withdrawal bleeds local oestrogen therapy using oestriol pessaries, low dose sustained released 17β oestradiol tablets (Vagifem) or a sustained release oestradiol impregnated ring (Estring) may be employed.

Occasionally women who associate attacks of the urethral syndrome with sexual intercourse have a urethral meatus which is situated far back along the anterior vaginal wall where it is vulnerable to trauma during coitus. Symptoms in such women may be relieved by urethrovaginoplasty with freeing and advancement of the urethra or urethrolysis.

For premenopausal women who develop recurrent urinary tract infections associated with sexual intercourse, postcoital antibiotic prophylaxis has been shown to be highly effective. Trimethoprim, nitrofurantoin or cephalexin have all been employed and a more recent highly satisfactory addition is norfloxacin 400 mg taken at around the time of sexual intercourse.

Conclusion

Urinary incontinence is common and, whilst not life threatening, is known to have a significant effect on quality of life. Appropriate investigation and management allows an accurate diagnosis and avoids inappropriate treatment. Whilst many forms of conservative therapy may be initiated in primary care continence surgery, and the investigation of more complex and recurrent cases of incontinence, should be performed in specialist secondary and tertiary referral units. Ultimately, an integrated pathway utilizing a multidisciplinary team approach including specialist nurses, continence advisors, physiotherapists, urologists and colorectal surgeons will ensure the best possible outcomes in terms of 'cure' and patient satisfaction.

Appendix: Levels of evidence [282, 283]

I   Systematic review of all relevant RCTs
IIA One randomized controlled trial (RCT) – low probability of bias and high probability of causal relationship
IIB One randomized controlled trial (RCT)
IIIA Well designed controlled trials (no randomization)
IIIB Cohort or case-control studies
IIIC Multiple time series or dramatic results in uncontrolled experiments
IV   Expert opinion (traditional use)

Grades of recommendations

A   A systematic review of RCTs or a body of evidence consisting principally of studies rated as 1 directly applicable to the target population and demonstrating overall consistency of results.
B   A body of evidence including studies rated as 2A directly applicable to the target population and demonstrating overall consistency of results *or* Extrapolated evidence from studies rated as 1.
C   A body of evidence including studies rated as 2B directly applicable to the target population and demonstrating overall consistency of results *or* Extrapolated evidence from studies rated as 2.
D   Evidence level 3 or 4 *or* Extrapolated evidence from studies rated as 2.

References

1. Norton P, MacDonald L, Sedgwick P & Stanton SL (1988) Distress and delay associated with urinary incontinence, frequency and urgency in women. *Br Med J* **297**, 1187–9.
2. Abrams P, Cardozo L, Fall M, Griffiths D, Rosier P, Ulmsten U *et al.* (2002) The standardisation of terminology of lower urinary tract function. Report from the standardisation committee of the International Continence Society. *Neurourol Urodynam* **21**, 167–78.
3. Zacharin R (1963) The suspensory mechanism of the female urethra. *J Anat* **97**, 423–7.
4. Wilson PD, Dixon JS, Brown ADG & Gosling JA (1979) A study of the pubo-urethral ligament in normal and incontinent women. In: *Proceedings of the 9th International Continence Society Meeting.* Rome.
5. Gosling JA, Dixon JS & Humpherson JR (1983) *Functional Anatomy of the Lower Urinary Tract.* London: Churchill Livingstone.
6. DeLancey JOL (1989) Pubovesical ligament: a separate structure from the urethral supports ('pubo-urethral ligaments'). *Neurourol Urodyn* **8**, 53–61.
7. Khanna OMP (1986) Disorders of micturition: neurophysiological basis and results of drug therapy. *Urology* **8**, 316–28.
8. Royal College of Physicians (1995) Incontinence: Causes, management and provision of services.
9. Thomas TM, Plymat KR, Blannin J & Meade TW (1980) Prevalence of urinary incontinence. *Br Med J* **281**, 1243–5.
10. MORI (1991) *Health Survey Questionnaire.* Topline results. 6040.
11. Brocklehurst JC (1993) Urinary incontinence in the community – analysis of a MORI poll. *Br Med J* **306**, 832–4.
12. Hannestad YS, Rortveit G, Sandvik H & Hunskar S (2000). A community-based epidemiological survey of female urinary incontinence: The Norwegian EPINCONT Study. *J Clin Epidem* **53** 1150–7.
13. Rortveit G, Hannnestad YS, Daltveit AK & Hunskaar S (2001) Age and type dependent effects of parity on urinary incontinence: the Norwegian EPINCONT study. *Obstet Gynaecol* **98**, 1004–10.
14. Department of Health (1998) Modernising Health and Social Services; National Priorities Guidance 1999/2000-2001/2002.
15. Continence Foundation, 1998.
16. Smith CP & Chancellor MB (2001) Genitourinary tract patent update. *Exp Opin Ther Patents* **11**, 17–31.
17. Stewart WF, Corey R, Herzog AR *et al.* (2001) Prevalence of overactive bladder in women: results from the NOBLE program. *Int Urogynaecol J* **12**(3), S66.
18. Bump RC (1993) Racial comparisons and contrasts in urinary incontinence and pelvic organ prolapse. *Obstet Gynaecol* **81**, 421.
19. Viktrup L, Lose G, Rolff M & Farfoed K (1992) The symptom of stress incontinence caused by pregnancy or delivery in primiparas. *Obstet Gynaecol* **79**, 945.
20. Chairelli P, Brown W & Mcelduff P (1999) Leaking urine: prevalence and associated factors in Australian women. *Neurourol Urodyn* **18**, 567.
21. Hojerberg KE, Salvig JD, Winslow NA, Lose G & Secher NJ (1999) Urinary incontinence; prevalence and risk factors at 16 weeks of gestation. *Br J Obstet Gynaecol* **106**, 842.
22. Kelleher CJ, Cardozo LD, Khullar V & Salvatore S (1997) A new questionnaire to assess the quality of life of urinary incontinent women. *Br J Obstet Gynaecol* **104**, 1374–9.
23. Fitzpatrick R, Fletcher A, Gore S, Jones D, Spiegelhalter D & Cox D (1992) Quality of life measures in healthcare. 1: Applications and issues in assessment. *Br Med J* **305**, 1075–7.
24. Burgio KL, Matthews KA & Engel BT (1991) Prevalence, incidence and correlates of urinary incontinence in healthy, middle-aged women. *J Urol* **146**, 1255–9.
25. World Health Organisation (1978) Definition of health from preamble to the constitution of the WHO basic documents, 28th edn. Geneva: WHO, p. 1.
26. Coulter A (1993). Measuring quality of life. In: Kinmouth AL & Jones R (eds) *Critical Reading in General Practice.* Oxford: Oxford University Press.
27. Naughton MJ & Shumaker SA (1996) Assessment of health related quality of life. In : Furberg CD & DeMets DL, eds. *Fundamentals of Clinical Trials*, 3rd edn. St Louis: Mosby Press, p. 185.
28. Gill TM & Feinstein AR (1974) A critical appraisal of the quality of life measurements. *JAMA* **272**(8), 619–26.
29. Murawaski BJ (1978) Social support in health and illness; the concept and it's measurement. *Ca Nurs* **1**, 365–71.
30. Blavis JG, Appell RA, Fantl JA *et al.* (1997) Standards of efficacy for evaluation of treatment outcomes in urinary incontinence: recommendations of the urodynamics society. *Neurourol Urodynam* **16**, 145–7.
31. Donovan JL, Badia X, Corcos J, Gotoh M, Kelleher CJ, Naughton M & Shaw C. Symptom and Quality of life assessment. In Abrams P, Cardozo L, Khoury S & Wein A (eds) *Intontinence*, 2nd edn. Health Publication Ltd, Plymouth, UK, pp. 267–316.
32. Lyons RA, Perry HM & Littlepage BNC (1994). Evidence for the validity of the short form 36 questionnaire (SF-36) in an elderly population. *Age Ageing* **23**, 182–4.
33. Hunskaar S & Vinsnes A (1991) The quality of life in women with urinary incontinence as measured by the sickness impact profile. *J Am Geriatric Soc* **39**, 378–2.
34. Grimby A, Milsom I, Molander U, Wiklund I & Ekelund P (1993) The influence of urinary incontinence on the quality of life of elderly women. *Age Aging* **22**, 82–9.
35. Sullivan M, Karlsson J, Bengtsson C, Furunes B, Lapidus L & Lissner L (1993) The Goteberg Quality of life instrument – A psychometric evaluation of assessments of symptoms and well being among women in a general population. *Scand J Prim Health Care* **11**, 267–75.
36. Shumaker SA, Wyman JF, Uebersax JS, McClish D & Fantl JA (1994) Health related quality of life measures for women with urinary incontinence: the Incontinence Impact Questionnaire and the urogenital distress inventory. *Qual Life Res* **3**, 291–306.
37. Uebersax JS, Wyman JF, Shumaker SA, McClish DK & Fantl AJ (1995) Short forms to assess life quality and symptom distress for urinary incontinence in women;

The incontinence impact questionnaire and the urogenital distress inventory. *Neuourol Urodynam* **14**, 131–9.

38. Lubeck DP, Prebil LA, Peebles P & Brown JS (1999) A health related quality of life measure for use in patients with urge urinary incontinence: a validation study. *Qual Life Res* **8**, 337–44.

39. Sandvik H, Hunskaar S, Seim A, Hermstad R, Vanik A & Bratt H (1993). Validation of a severity index in female urinary incontinence and its implementation in an epidemiological survey. *J Epidemio Commun Health Med* **47**, 497–9.

40. Wagner TH, Patrick DL, Bavendam TG, Martin ML & Buesching DP (1996) Quality of life of persons with urinary incontinence: development of a new measure. *Urology* **47**, 67–72.

41. Wyman JF, Harkins SW, Taylor JR & Fantl JA (1987) Psychosocial impact of urinary incontinence in women. *Obstet Gynaecol* **70**, 378–81.

42. Milsom I, Abrams P, Cardozo L, Roberts RG, Thuroff J & Wein AJ (2001) How widespread are the symptoms of overactive bladder and how are they managed? A population-based prevalence study. *BJU Int* **87**(9), 760–6.

43. Jarvis GJ, Hall S, Stamp S, Miller DR & Johnson A (1980) An assessment of urodynamic examination in incontinent women. *Br J Obstet Gynaecol* **87**, 893–6.

44. Wyman JF, Sung CC, Harkins SW, Wilson MS & Fantl JA (1988) The urinary diary in the evaluation of incontinent women: a test-retest analysis. *Obstet Gynaecol* **71**, 812–17.

45. Verbrugge LM (1980) Health diaries. *Med Care* **18**, 73.

46. Larsson G & Victor A (1988) Micturition patterns in a healthy female population studied with a frequency volume chart. *Scan J Urol Nephrol Suppl* **4**, 53–7.

47. Barnick C (1997). Frequency/Volume Charts. In: Cardozo L (ed.) *Urogynaecology*. London: Churchill Livingstone, pp. 101–7.

48. Cutner A (1997) Uroflowmetry. In Cardozo L (ed) *Urogynaecology*. London: Churchill Livingstone, pp. 109–16.

49. Hilton P & Stanton SL (1983) Urethral pressure measurement by microtransducer: the results in symptom free women and in those with genuine stress incontinence. *Br J Obstet Gynaecol* **90**, 919–33.

50. Versi E & Cardozo LD (1988) Symptoms and urethral pressure profilometry for the diagnosis of genuine stress incontinence. *J Obstet Gynaecol* **9**, 168–9.

51. Versi E (1990) Discriminant analysis of urethral pressure profilometry data for the diagnosis of genuine stress incontinence. *Br J Obstet Gynaecol* **97**, 251–9.

52. Haylen BT (1989) Residual urine volumes in a normal female population: application of transvaginal ultrasound. *Br J Urol* **64**, 347–9.

53. Khullar V, Salvatore S, Cardozo LD, Hill S & Kelleher CJ (1994) Ultrasound bladder wall measurement: a non-invasive sensitive screening test for detrusor instability. *Neurourol Urodyn* **13**, 461–2.

54. Robinson D, Anders K, Cardozo L, Bidmead J, Toozs-Hobson P & Khullar V (2002) Can Ultrasound replace ambulatory urodynamics when investigating women with irritative urinary symptoms? *Br J Obstet Gynaecol* **109**(2), 145–8.

55. Richmond DH & Sutherst JR (1989) Clinical application of transrectal ultrasound for the investigation of the incontinent patient. *Br J Urol* **63**, 605–9.

56. Gordon D, Pearce M, Norton P & Stanton SL (1989) Comparison of ultrasound and lateral chain urethrocystography in the determination of bladder neck descent. *Am J Obstet Gynecol* **160**, 182–5.

57. Khullar V, Salvatore S, Cardozo LD, Hill S & Kelleher CJ (1994a) Three dimensional ultrasound of the urethra and urethral sphincter: a new diagnostic technique. *Neurourol Urodyn* **13**, 352–4.

58. Robinson D, Toozs-Hobson P, Cardozo L & Digesu A (2004) Correlating structure and function; three-dimensional ultrasound of the urethral sphincter. *Ultrasound Obstet Gynaecol* **23**, 272–6.

59. Athanasiou S, Hill S, Cardozo LD, Khullar V & Anders K (1995) Three dimensional ultrasound of the urethra, peri-urethral tissues and pelvic floor. *Int Urogynecol J* **6**, 239.

60. Klukte C, Golomb J, Barbaric Z & Raz S (1990) The anatomy of stress incontinence; magnetic resonance imaging of the female bladder neck and urethra. *J Urol* **143**, 563–6.

61. Yang A, Mostwin JL, Rosenheim NB & Zerhouni EA (1991) Pelvic floor descent in women: dynamic evaluation with fast magnetic resonance imaging and cinematic display. *Radiology* **179**, 25–33.

62. Versi E, Griffiths DJ, Fielding J, Mulkern R, Lehner M & Jolesz F (1996) Erect position magnetic resonance imaging of the pelvic floor. *Neurourol Urodyn* **15**, 332–3.

63. Smith ARB, Hosker GL & Warrell DW (1989) The role of pudendal nerve damage in the aetiology of genuine stress incontinence in women. *Br J Obstet Gynaecol* **96**, 29–32.

64. Barnick CGW & Cardozo LD (1993) Denervation and re-inervation of the urethral sphincter in the aetiology of genuine stress incontinence: an electromyographic study. *Br J Obstet Gynaecol* **100**, 750–3.

65. Plevnik S, Vrtacnik P & Janez P (1983) Detection of fluid entry into the urethra by electrical impedence measurement: electric fluid bridge test. *Clin Phys Physiol Meas* **4**, 309–13.

66. Plevnik S, Holmes DM, James J, Mundy AR & Vrtacnik P (1985) Urethral electric conductance (UEC) – a new parameter for evaluation of urethral and bladder function: methodology of the assessment of this clinical potential. In: *Proceedings of the 15th Annual Meeting of the International Continence Society.* London: pp. 90–1.

67. Peattie AB, Plevnik S & Stanton SL (1988a) Distal urethral electric conductance test: a screening test for female urinary stress incontinence? *Neurourol Urodyn* **7**, 173–4.

68. Creighton SM, Plevnik S & Stanton SL (1991) Distal urethral electric conductance (DUEC) – a preliminary assessment of its role as a quick screening test for incontinent women. *Br J Obstet Gynaecol* **98**, 69–72.

69. van Waalwijk van Doorn ESC, Zwiers W, Wetzels LLRH & Debruyne FMJ (1987) A comparative study between standard and ambulatory urodynamics. *Neurourol Urodyn* **6**, 159–60.

70. Heslington K & Hilton P (1996) Ambulatory urodynamic monitoring. *Br J Obstet Gynaecol* **103**, 393–9.

71. Robertson AS, Griffiths CJ, Ramsden PD & Neal DE (1994) Bladder function in healthy volunteers: ambulatory monitoring and conventional urodynamic studies. *Br J Urol* **73**, 242–9.

72. Salvatore S, Khullar V, Cardozo L, Anders K, Zocchi G & Soligo M (2001) Evaluating ambulatory urodynamics: a prospective study in asymptomatic women. *Br J Obstet Gynaecol* **108**, 107–11.

73. Cardozo LD, Khullar V, Anders K & Hill S (1995) Ambulatory urodynamics: a useful urogynaecological service? *Proceedings of the 27th British Congress of Obstetrics and Gynaecology*. London: RCOG, p. 404.

74. Anders K, Khullar V, Cardozo L *et al.* (1997) Ambulatory urodynamic monitoring in clinical urogynaecological practice. *Neurourol Urodyn* **5**, 510–12.

75. Gorton E & Stanton S (2000) Ambulatory urodynamics: do they help clinical management? *Br J Obstet Gynaecol* **107**, 316–19.

76. Snooks SJ, Swash M, Setchell M & Henry MM (1984) Injury to innervation of the pelvic floor sphincter musculature in childbirth. *Lancet* **ii**, 546–60.

77. Snooks SJ, Swash M, Henry MM & Setchell M (1986) Risk factors in childbirth causing damage to the pelvic floor innervation. *Int J Colorect Dis* **1**, 20–4.

78. Allen RE, Hosker GL, Smith ARB & Warrell DW (1990) Pelvic floor damage and childbirth: a neurophysiological study. *Br J Obstet Gynaecol* **97**, 770–9.

79. Tetzschuer T, Sorensen M, Lose G & Christiansen J (1996) Pudendal nerve recovery after a non-instrumental vaginal delivery. *Int Urogynecol J* **7**, 102–4.

80. Snooks SJ, Swash M, Mathers SE & Henry MM (1990) Effects of vaginal delivery on the pelvic floor: a five year follow-up. *Br J Surg* **77**, 1358–60.

81. Sultan A & Stanton SL (1996) Preserving the pelvic floor and perineum during childbirth – elective caesarean section? *Br J Obstet Gynaecol* **103**, 731–4.

82. Petros P & Ulmsten U (1990) An integral theory of female urinary incontinence. Experimental and clinical considerations. *Acta Obstet Gynaecol Scand* **153** (Suppl), 7–31.

83. Ingelman-Sundberg A (1953) Urinary incontinence in women, excluding fistulas. *Acta Obstet Gynaecol Scand* **31**, 266–95.

84. Westbury M, Asmussen M & Ulmsten U (1982) Location of maximal intraurethral pressure related to urogenital diaphragm in the female subject as studied by simultaneous urethra-cystometry and voiding urethrocystography. *Am J Obstet Gynaecol* **144**, 408–12.

85. Cardozo LD & Stanton SL (1980) Genuine stress incontinence and detrusor instability – a review of 200 cases. *Br J Obstet Gynaecol* **87**, 184–90.

86. Haylen BT, Sutherst JR & Frazer MI (1989) Is the investigation of most stress incontinence really necessary? *Br J Urol* **64**, 147–9.

87. Tapp A, Cardozo LD, Hills B & Barnick C (1988) Who benefits from physiotherapy? *Neurourol Urodyn* **7**, 259–61.

88. Kegel AH (1948) Progressive resistance exercise in the functional restoration of the perineal muscles. *Am J Obstet Gynaecol* **56**, 238–49.

89. Bo K (2004) Pelvic floor muscle training is effective in treatment of female stress urinary incontinence, but how does it work? *Int Urogynaecol J Pelvic Floor Dysfunct* **15**, 76–84.

90. DeLancey JOL (1988) Anatomy and mechanics of structures around the vesical neck: how vesical position may affect its closure. *Neurourol Urodyn* **7**, 161–2.

91. Bo K, Larsen S, Oseid S, Kvarstein B & Hagen RH (1988) Knowledge about and ability to correct pelvic floor muscle exercises in women wit urinary stress incontinence. *Neurourol Urodyn* **7**, 261–2.

92. Miller JM, Ashton Miller JA & DeLancey JOL (1998) A pelvic muscle precontraction can reduce cough-related urine loss in selected women with mild SUI. *J Am Geriatric Soc* **46**, 870–4.

93. Bo K, Talseth T & Holme I (1999) Single blind, randomised controlled trial of pelvic floor muscles exercises, electrical stimulation, vaginal cones and no treatment in management of genuine stress incontinence in women. *Br Med J* **318**, 487–93.

94. Bernstein IT (1997) The pelvic floor muscles: muscle thickness in healthy and urinary incontinent women measured by perineal ultrasonography with reference to the effect of pelvic floor training. Oestrogen receptor studies. *Neurourol Urodyn* **16** 237–75.

95. Bo K, Hagen RH, Kvarstein B, Jorgensen J & Larsen S (1990) Pelvic floor muscle exercise for the treatment of female stress urinary incontinence. III: Effects of two different degrees of pelvic floor muscle exercise. *Neurourol Urodyn* **9**, 489–502.

96. Burgio KL, Robinson JC & Engel BT (1986) The role of biofeedback in Kegel exercise training for stress urinary incontinence. *Am J Obstet Gynacol* **154**, 58–63.

97. Plevnik S (1985) New methods for testing and strengthening the pelvic floor muscles. In: *Proceedings of the 15th Annual Meeting of the International Continence Society*. London: pp. 267–8.

98. Peattie AB, Plevnik S & Stanton SL (1988b) Vaginal cones: a conservative method of treating genuine stress incontinence. *Br J Obstet Gynaecol* **95**, 1049–53.

99. Olah KS, Bridges N, Denning J & Farrar D (1990) The conservative management of patients with symptoms of stress incontinence: a randomised prospective study comparing weighted vaginal cones and interferential therapy. *Am J Obstet Gynecol* **162**, 87–92.

100. Haken J, Benness CJ, Cardozo LD & Cutner A (1991) A randomised trial of vaginal cones and pelvic floor exercises in the management of genuine stress incontinence. *Neurourol Urodyn* **10**, 393–4.

101. Kato K, Kondo A, Hasegalera S *et al.* (1992) Pelvic floor muscle training as treatment of stress incontinence. The effectiveness of vaginal cones. *Jpn J Urol* **83**, 498–504.

102. Bo K (1995) Vaginal weighted cones. Theoretical framework, effect on pelvic floor muscle strength and female stress urinary incontinence. *Acta Obstet Gynaecol Scand* **74**, 87–92.

103. Berghmans LC, Hendricks HJ, Bo K, Hay-Smith EJ, de Bie RA & van Waalwijk van Doorn ES (1998) Conservative treatment of stress incontinence in women. A systematic

review of randomised review of randomised clinical trials. *Br J Urol* **82**, 181–91.

104. Thyssen H & Lose G (1996) Long term efficacy and safety of a vaginal device in the treatment of stress incontinence. *Neurourol Urodyn* **15**, 394–5.

105. Thyssen H, Bidmead J, Lose G, Moller Bek K, Dwyer P & Cardozo L (2001) A new intravaginal device for stress incontinence in women. *BJU Int* **88**, 889–92.

106. Thor KB & Katofiasc MA (1995) Effects of Duloxetine, a combined serotonin and norepineephrine reuptake inhibitor, on central neural control of lower urinary tract function in the chloralose-anesthetised female cat. *J Pharmacol Exp Ther* **74**, 1014–24.

107. Norton PA, Zinner NR, Yalcin I, Bump RC & Duloxetine Urinary Incontinence Study Group (2002) Duloxetine versus placebo in the treatment of stress urinary incontinence. *Am J Obstet Gynaecol* **187**(1), 40–8.

108. Millard R, Moore K, Yalcin I & Bump R (2003) Duloxetine vs. placebo in the treatment of stress urinary incontinence: a global phase III study. *Neurourol Urodynam* **22**, 482–3.

109. Cardozo L, Drutz HP, Baygani SK & Bump RC (2004) Pharmacological treatment of women awaiting surgery for stress urinary incontinence. *Obstet Gynaecol* **104**, 511–19.

110. Ghoniem GM, Van Leeuwen JS, Elser DM, Freeman RM, Zhao YD, Yalcin I, Bump RC & Duloxetine/Pelvic Floor Muscle Training Clinical Trail Group (2005) A randomised controlled trial of duloxetine alone, pelvic floor muscle training alone, combined treatment and no active treatment in women with stress urinary incontinence. *J Urol* **173**, 1453–4.

111. Stanton SL & Tanagho E (1986) *Surgery of Female Incontinence*, 2nd edn. Berlin: Springer-Verlag.

112. Black NA & Downs SH (1996) The effectiveness of surgery for stress incontinence in women: a systematic review. *Br J Urol* **78**, 497–510.

113. Hilton P (1990) Which operation for which patient? In: Drife J, Hilton P & Stanton SL (eds) *Micturition*. Berlin: Springer-Verlag.

114. Burch J (1961) Urethrovaginal fixation to Cooper's ligament for correction of stress incontinence, cystocele and prolapse. *Am J Obstet Gynaecol* **81**, 281.

115. Cardozo LD, Stanton SL & Williams JE (1979) Detrusor instability following surgery for stress incontinence. *Br J Urol* **58**, 138–42.

116. Wiskind AK, Creighton SM & Stanton SL (1991) The incidence of genital prolapse following the Burch colposuspension operation. *Neurourol Urodyn* **10**, 453–4.

117. Alcalay M, Monga A & Stanton SL (1995) Burch colposuspension: 10–20 year follow-up. *Br J Obstet Gynaecol* **102**, 740–5.

118. Liu CY (1993) Laparoscopic retropubic colposuspension (Burch procedure): a review of 58 cases. *J Reprod Med* **38**, 526–30.

119. Burton G (1994) A randomised comparison of laparoscopic and open colposuspension. *Neurourol Urodyn* **13**, 497–8.

120. Su T, Wang K, Hsu C, Wei H & Hong B (1997) Prospective comparison of laparoscopic and traditional colposuspension in the treatment of genuine stress incontinence. *Acta Obstet Gynecol Scand* **76**, 576–82.

121. Carey MP, Goh JT, Rosamilia A, Cornish A, Gordon I, Hawthorne G, Maher CF, Dwyer PL, Moran P & Gilmour DT (2006) Laparoscopic versus open Burch colposuspension: a randomised controlled trial. *BJOG* **113**, 999–1006.

122. Kitchener HC, Dunn G, Lawton V, Reid F, Nelson L & Smith ARB on behalf of the COLPO study group (2006) Laparoscopic versus open colposuspension- results of a prospective randomised controlled trial. *BJOG* **113**, 1007–13.

123. Dumville JC, Manca A, Kitchener HC, Smith ARB, Nelson L & Torgerson DJ, on behalf of the COLPO study group (2006) Cost effectiveness analysis of open colposuspension versus laparoscopic colposuspension in the treatment of urodynamic stress incontinence. *BJOG* **113**, 1014–22.

124. Ulmsten U, Henriksson L, Johnson P & Varhos G (1996) An ambulatory surgical procedure under local anesthetic for treatment of female urinary incontinence. *Int Urogynaecol J* **7**, 81–6.

125. Nilsson CG Tension free vaginal tape procedure for treatment of female urinary stress incontinence. In: Cardozo L & Staskin D. (eds) *Textbook of Female Urology and Urogynaecology.* Infroma Healthcare: Abingdon, UK, pp. 917–23.

126. Ulmsten U, Falconer C, Johnson P, Jones M *et al.* (1998) A multicentre study of Tension Free Vaginal Tape (TVT) for surgical treatment of stress urinary incontinence. *Int Urogynecol J* **9**, 210–13.

127. Ulmsten U, Johnson P & Rezapour M (1999) A three year follow up of tension free vaginal tape for surgical treatment of female stress urinary incontinence. *BJOG* **106**, 345–50.

128. Nilsson CG, Kuuva N, Falconer C *et al.* (2001) Long term results of the tension free vaginal tape (TVT) procedure for surgical treatment of female stress urinary incontinence. *Int Urogynaecol J* **12**(Suppl), 5–8.

129. Nilsson CG, Falconer C & Rezapour M (2004) Seven year follow up of the tension free vaginal tape procedure for the treatment of urinary incontinence. *Obstet Gynaecol* **104**, 1259–62.

130. Ward K, Hilton P & United Kingdom and Ireland Tension Free Vaginal Tape Trial Group (2002) Prospective multicentre randomised trial of tension free vaginal tape and colposuspension as primary treatment for stress incontinence. *BMJ* **325**, 67.

131. Ward KL, Hilton P & UK and Ireland TVT Trial Group (2004) A prospective multicentre randomised trial of tension free vaginal tape and colposuspension for primary urodynamic stress incontinence: two-year follow up. *Am J Obstet Gyanecol* **190**, 324–31.

132. Ward K & Hilton P (2006) Multicentre randomised trial of tension free vaginal tape and colposuspension for primary urodynamic stress incontinence: five year follow up. *Neurourol Urodynam* **6**, 568–9.

133. Manca A, Sculpher MJ, Ward K & Hilton P (2003) A cost utility analysis of tension free vaginal tape versus colposuspension for primary urodynamic stress incontinence. *BJOG* **110**, 255–62.

134. Paraiso MF, Walters MD, Karram MM & Barber MD (2004) Laparoscopic Burch colposuspension versus tension free

vaginal tape: a randomised trial. *Obstet Gyanecol* **104**, 1249–58.

135. Staskin DR & Tyagi R (2004) The SPARC sling system. *Atlas Urol Clinic* **12**, 185–95.

136. Deval B, Levardon M, Samain E, Rafii A, Cortesse A, Amarenco G, Ciofu C & Haab F (2003) A French multicentre clinical trial of SPARC for stress urinary incontinence. *Eur Urol* **44**, 254–8.

137. Lord HE, Taylor JD, Finn JC, Tsokos N, Jeffery JT, Atherton MJ, Evans SF, Bremner AP, Elder GO & Holman CD (2006) A randomised controlled equivalence trial of short term complications and efficacy of tension free vaginal tape and suprapubic urethral support sling for treating stress incontinence. *BJU Int* **98**, 367–6.

138. Delorme E (2001) [Transobturator urethral suspension: mini-invasive procedure in the treatment of stress urinary incontinence in women.] *Prog Urol* **11**, 1306–13.

139. Whiteside JL & Walters MD (2004) Anatomy of the obturator region: relations to a transobturator sling. *Int Urogynaecol J Pelvic Floor Dysfunct* **15**, 223–6.

140. Costa P, Grise P, Droupy S *et al.* (2004) Surgical treatment of female stress urinary incontinence with a transobturator tape (TOT). Uratape: short term results of a prospective multicentric study. *Eur Urol* **46**, 102–6.

141. Delorme E, Droupy S, De Tayrac R *et al.* (2004) Transobturator tape (Uratape): a new minimally invasive procedure to treat female urinary incontinence. *Eur Urol* **45**, 203–7.

142. Meschia M, Pifarotti P, Bernasconi F, Baccichet R, Magatti F, Cortese P, Caria M & Bertozzi R (2006) Multicentre randomised trial of tension free vaginal tape (TVT) and transobturator tape in out technique (TVT-O) for the treatment of stress urinary incontinence. *Int Urogynaecol J Pelvic Floor Dysfunct* **17**, S92–3.

143. Laurikainen EH, Valpas A, Kiiholma P, Takala T, Kivela A, Aukee P, Kalliola T, Rinne K & Nilsson CG (2006) A prospective randomised trial comparing TVT and TVT-O procedures for treatment of SUI: immediate outcome and complications. *Int Urogynaecol J Pelvic Floor Dysfunct* **17**, S104–5.

144. Pereyra A (1959) A simplified surgical procedure for the correction of stress incontinence in women. *West J Surg* **67**, 223.

145. Stamey T (1973) Endoscopic suspension of the vesical neck for urinary incontinence. *Surg Gynecol Obstet* **136**, 547–54.

146. Raz S (1981) Modified bladder neck suspension for female stress incontinence. *Urology* **17**, 82.

147. Appell RA (1990) New developments: injectables for urethral incompetence in women. *Int Urogynaecol* **1**, 117–19.

148. Harris DR, Iacovou JW & Lemberger RJ (1996) Peri-urethral silicone micro implants (Macroplastiqie) for the treatment of genuine stress incontinence. *Br J Urol* **78**, 722–8.

149. Khullar V, Cardozo LD, Abbot D & Anders K (1997) GAX collagen in the treatment of urinary incontinence in elderly women: a 2 year follow-up. *Br J Obstet Gynaecol* **104**.

150. Stanton SL & Monga AK (1997) Incontinence in elderly women: is periurethral collagen an advance? *Br J Obstet Gynaecol* **104**, 154–7.

151. Ghoniem G, Bernhard P, Corcos J, Comiter C, Tomera K, Westney O, Herschorn S, Lucente V, Smith J, Wahle G & Mulcahy J (2005) Multicentre randomised controlled trial to evaluate Macroplastique urethral bulking agent for the treatment of female stress urinary incontinence. *Int Urogynaecol J* **16**(2), S129–30.

152. Chapple CR, Haab F, Cervigni M, Dannecker C, Fianu-Jonasson A & Sultan AH (2005) An open, multicentre study of NASHA/Dx Gel (Zuidex) for the treatment of stress urinary incontinence. *Eur Urol* **48**, 488–94.

153. Scott FB, Bradley WE & Tim G (1973) Treatment of urinary incontinence by implantable prosthetic sphincter. *Urology* **1**, 252.

154. Kinder RB & Mundy AR (1987) Pathophysiology of idiopathic detrusor instability and detrusor hyperreflexia – an *in vitro* study of human detrusor muscle. *Br J Urol* **60**, 509–15.

155. Eaton AC & Bates CP (1982) An *in vitro* physiological, study of normal and unstable human detrusor muscle. *Br J Urol* **54**, 653–7.

156. Sibley GN (1997) Developments in our understanding of detrusor instability. *Br J Urol* **80**, 54–61.

157. Sibley GNA (1985) An experimental model of detrusor instability in the obstructed pig. *Br J Urol* **57**, 292–8.

158. Speakman MJ, Brading AF, Gilpin CJ, Dixon JS, Gilpin SA & Gosling JA (1987) Bladder outflow obstruction – cause of denervation supersensitivity. *J Urol* **183**, 1461–6.

159. Wise BG, Cardozo LD, Cutner A, Benness CJ & Burton G (1993) The prevalence and significance of urethral instability in women with detrusor instability. *Br J Urol* **72**, 26–9.

160. Sutherst JR & Brown M (1978) The effect on the bladder pressure of sudden entry of fluid into the posterior urethra. *Br J Urol* **50**, 406–9.

161. Brading AF & Turner WH (1994) The unstable bladder: towards a common mechanism. *Br J Urol* **73**, 3–8.

162. Brading AF (1997) A myogenic basis for the overactive bladder. *Urology* **50**, 57–67.

163. Mills IW, Greenland JE, McMurray G, McRoy R, Ho KM, Noble JG & Brading AF (2000) Studies of the pathophysiology of idiopathic detrusor instability: the physiological properties of the detrusor smooth muscle and it's pattern of innervation. *J Urol* **163**(2), 646–51.

164. Charlton RG, Morley AR, Chambers P & Gillespie JI (1999) Focal changes in nerve, muscle and connective tissue in normal and unstable human bladder. *BJU Int* **84**(9), 953–60.

165. Jarvis GJ & Millar DR (1980) Controlled trial of bladder drill for detrusor instability. *Br Med J* **281**, 1322–3.

166. Frewen WK (1982) Bladder training in general practice. *Practitioner* **266**, 1874–9.

167. Jarvis GJ (1981) The management of urinary incontinence due to vesical sensory urgency by bladder drill. In: *Proceedings of the 11th Annual Meeting of the International Continence Society.* Lund, pp. 123–4.

168. Kelleher CJ, Cardozo LD, Khullar V & Salvatore S (1997) A medium-term analysis of the subjective efficency of treatment for women with detrusor instability and low bladder compliance. *Br J Obstet Gynaecol* **104**, 988–93.

169. Andersson K-E (1997) The overactive bladder: Pharmacologic basis of drug treatment. *Urology* **50**(6A Suppl.), 74–84.

170. Caulfield MP & Birdsall NJ (1998) International Union of Pharmacology XVII. Classification of muscarinic acetylcholine receptors. *Pharmacol Rev* **50**, 279.

171. Yamaguchi O, Shisida K, Tamura K *et al.* (1996) Evaluation of mRNAs encoding muscarinic receptor subtypes in human detrusor muscle. *J Urol* **156**, 1208.

172. Harris DR, Marsh KA, Birmingham AT *et al.* (1995) Expression of muscarinic M₃ receptors coupled to inositol phospholipid hydrolysis in human detrusor cultured smooth muscle cells. *J Urol* **154**, 1241.

173. Hedge SS, Chopin A, Bonhaus D *et al.* (1997) Functional role of M₂ and M₃ muscarinic receptors in the urinary bladder of rats in vitro and in vivo. *Br J Pharmacol* **120**, 1409.

174. Hedge SS & Eglen RM (1999) Muscarinic receptor subtypes modulating smooth muscle contractility in the urinary bladder. *Life Sci* **64**, 419.

175. Braverman AS & Ruggieri MR (1998) The M₂ receptor contributes to contraction of the denervated rat urinary bladder. *Am J Physiol* **275**, 1654.

176. Waldeck K, Larsson B & Andersson KE (1997) Comparison of oxybutynin and it's active metabolite, N-desmethyl-oxybutynin, in the human detrusor and parotid gland. *J Urol* **157** 1093–7.

177. Hughes KM, Lang JCT, Lazare R *et al.* (1992) Measurement of oxybutynin and its N-desethyl meatbolite in plasma, and its application to pharmacokinetic studies in young, elderly and frail elderly volunteers. *Xenobiotica* **22**, 859–69.

178. Nilvebrant L, Andersson KE & Mattiasson A (1985) Characterization of the muscarinic cholinoreceptors in the human detrusor. *J Urol* **134**, 418–23.

179. Nilvebrant L & Sparf B (1986) Dicyclomine, benzhexol and oxybutynin distingush between subclasses of muscarinic binding sites. *Eur J Pharmacol* **123**, 133–43.

180. Cardozo LD, Cooper D & Versi E (1987) Oxybutynin chloride in the management of idiopathic detrusor instability. *Neurourol Urodyn* **6**, 256–7.

181. Moore KH, Hay DM, Imrie AE, Watson A & Goldstein M (1990) Oxybutynin hydrochloride (3 mg) in the treatment of women with idiopathic detrusor instability. *Br J Urol* **66**, 479–85.

182. Tapp AJS, Cardozo LD, Versi E & Cooper D (1990). The treatment of detrusor instability in post menopausal women with oxybutynin chloride: a double blind placebo-controlled study. *Br J Obstet Gynaecol* **97**, 479–85.

183. Baigrie RJ, Kelleher JP, Fawcett DP & Pengelly AW (1988) Oxybutynin: is it safe? *Br J Urol* **62**, 319–22.

184. Weese DL, Roskamp DA, Leach GE & Zimmern PE (1993) Intravesical oxybutynin chloride: experience with 42 patients. *Urology* **41**, 527–30.

185. Collas D & Malone-Lee JG (1997). The pharmacokinetic properties of rectal oxybutynin – a possible alternative to intravesical administration. *Neurourol Urodyn* **16**, 533–42.

186. Anderson RU, Mobley D, Blank B, Saltzstein D, Susset J & Brown JS (1999) Once daily controlled versus immeadiate release oxybutynin chloride for urge urinary incontinence. OROS Oxybutynin Study Group. *J Urol* **161**(6), 1809–12.

187. Gleason DM, Susset J, White C, Munoz DR & Sand PK (1999) Evaluation of a new once-daily formulation of oxybutynin for the treatment of urinary urge incontinence. Ditropan XL Study Group. *Urology* **54**(3), 420–3.

188. Dmochowski RR, Sand PK, Zinner NR, Gittelman MC, Davila GW, Sanders SW & Transdermal Oxybutynin Study Group (2003) Comparative efficacy and safety of transdermal oxybutynin and oral tolterodine versus placebo in previously treated patients with urge and mixed urinary incontinence. *Urology* **62**(2), 237–42.

189. Haruno A, Yamasaki Y, Miyoshi K *et al.* (1989) Effects of propiverine hydrochloride and its metabolites on isolated guinea pig urinary bladder. *Folia Pharmacol Jpn* **94**, 145–50.

190. Mazur D, Wehnert J, Dorschner W, Schubert G, Herfurth G & Alken RG (1995) Clinical and urodynamic effects of propiverine in patients suffering from urgency and urge incontinence. *Scand J Urol Nephrol* **29**, 289–94.

191. Stoher M, Madersbacher H, Richter R, Wehnert J & Dreikorn K (1999) Efficacy and safety of propiverine in SCI-patients suffering from detrusor hyperreflexia: a double-blind, placebo-controlled clinical trial. *Spinal Cord* **37**(3), 196–200.

192. Ruscin JM & Morgenstern NE (1999) Tolterodine use for symptoms of overactive bladder. *Ann Pharmacother* **33**(10), 1073–82.

193. Nilvebrant L, Andersson K-E, Gillberg P-G, Stahl M & Sparf B (1997) Tolterodine - a new bladder selective antimuscarinic agent. *Eur J Pharmacol* **327**, 195–207.

194. Nilvebrant L, Hallen B & Larsson G (1997) Tolterodine – a new bladder selective muscarinic receptor antagonist: preclinical pharmacological and clinical data. *Life Sci* **60**(13–14), 1129–36.

195. Hills CJ, Winter SA & Balfour JA. Tolterodine (1998) *Drugs* **55**, 813–20.

196. Jonas U, Hofner K, Madesbacher H & Holmdahl TH (1997) Efficacy and safety of two doses of tolterodine versus placebo in patients with detrusor overactivity and symptoms of frequency, urge incontinence, and urgency: urodynamic evaluation. *World J Urol* **15**, 144–51.

197. Millard R, Tuttle J, Moore K *et al.* (1999) Clinical efficacy and safety of tolterodine compared to placebo in detrusor overactivity. *J Urol* **161**(5), 1551–5.

198. Rentzhog L. Stanton SL, Cardozo LD, Nelson E, Fall M & Abrams P (1998) Efficacy and safety of tolterodine in patients with detrusor instability: a dose ranging study. *Br J Urol* **81**(1), 42–8.

199. Appell RA (1997) Clinical efficacy and safety of tolterodine in the treatment of overactive bladder: a poled analysis. *Urology* **50**, 90–6.

200. Swift S, Garely A, Dimpfl T, Payne C & Tolterodine Study Group (2003) A new once daily formulation of tolterodine provides superior efficacy an is well tolerated in women with overactive bladder. *Int J Pelvic Floor Dysfunct* **14**(1), 50–4.

201. Van Kerrebroeck P, Kreder K, Jonas U, Zinner N, Wein A & Tolterodine Study Group (2001) Tolterodine once-daily: superior efficacy and tolerability in the treatment of overactive bladder. *Urology* **57**(3), 414–21.

202. Diokno AC, Appell RA, Sand PK, Dmochowski RR, Gburek BM, Klimberg IW, Kell SH & OPERA Stuy Group (2003) Prospective, randomised, double blind study of the efficacy and tolerability of the extended-release formulations of oxybutynin and tolterodine for overactive bladder: results of the OPERA trial. *Mayo Clin Proc* **78**(6), 687–95.

203. Schladitz-Keil G, Spahn H & Mutschler E (1986) Determination of bioavailability of the quaternary ammonium compound trospium chloride in man from urinary excretion data. *Arzneimittel Forsch/Drug Res* **36**, 984–7.

204. Fusgen I & Hauri D (2000) Trospium chloride: an effective option for medical treatment of bladder overactivity. *Int J Clin Pharmacol Ther* **38**(5), 223–34.

205. Cardozo LD, Chapple CR, Toozs-Hobson P *et al.* (2000) Efficacy of trospium chloride in patients with detrusor instability: a placebo-controlled, randomized, double-blind, multicentre clinical trial. *BJU Int* **85**(6), 659–64.

206. Madersbacher H, Stoher M, Richter R, Burgdorfer H, Hachen HJ & Murtz G (1995) Trospium choride versus oxybutynin: a randomized, double-blind, multicentre trial in the treatment of detrusor hyperreflexia. *Br J Urol* **75**(4), 452–6.

207. Cardozo L, Lisec M, Millard R, van Vierssen Trip O, Kuzmin I, Drogendijk TE, Huang M & Ridder AM (2004). Randomised, double blind placebo controlled trial of the once daily antimuscarinic agent solifenacin succinate in patients with overactive bladder. *J Urol* **172**, 1919–24.

208. Haab F, Cardozo L, Chapple C, Ridder AM & Solifenacin Study Group (2005) Long-term open label solifenacin treatment associated with persistence with therapy in patients with overactive bladder syndrome. *Eur Urol* **47**, 376–84.

209. Chapple CR, Martinez-Garcia R, Selvaggi L, Toozs-Hobson P, Warnack W, Drogendijk T, Wright DM, Bolodeoku J & for the STAR study group (2005). A comparison of the efficacy and tolerability of solifenacin succinate and extended release tolterodine at treating overactive bladder syndrome: results of the STAR trial. *Eur Urol* **48**, 464–70.

210. Alabaster VA (1997) Discovery and development of selective M3 antagonists for clinical use. *Life Sci* **60**(13–14), 1053–60.

211. Chapple CR (2004) Darifenacin is well tolerated and provides significant improvement in the symptoms of overactive bladder: a pooled analysis of phase III studies. *J Urol* **171 Suppl**, 130 (abstract 487).

212. Baldessarini KJ (1985) Drugs in the treatment of psychiatric disorders. In: Gilman *et al.* (eds) *The Pharmacological Basis of Therapeutics*, 7th edn. McMillan Publishing Co., pp. 387–445.

213. Castleden CM, Duffin HM & Gulati RS (1986) Double-blind study of imipramine and placebo for incontinence due to bladder instability. *Age Aging* **15**, 299–303.

214. Diokno Ac, Hyndman CW, Hardy DA & Lapides J (1972) Comparison of action of imipramine (Tofranil) and propantheline (Probanthine) on detrusor contraction. *J Urol* **107**, 42–3.

215. Jeremy JY, Tsang V, Mikhailidis DP, Rogers H, Morgan RJ & Dandona P (1987) Eicosanoid synthesis by human urinary bladder mucosa: pathological implications. *Br J Urol* **59**, 36–9.

216. Cardozo LD, Stanton SL, Robinson H & Hole D (1980) Evaluation on flurbiprofen in detrusor instability. *Br Med J* 1980; 280: 281–2.

217. Cardozo LD & Stanton SL (1980) A comparison between bromocriptine and indomethacin in the treatment of detrusor instability. *J Urol* **123**, 399–401.

218. Norgaard JP, Rillig S & Djurhuus JC (1989) Nocturnal enuresis: an approach to treatment based on pathogenesis. *J Pediatr* **114**, 705–9.

219. Mattiasson A, Abrams P, Van Kerrebroeck P, Walter S & Weiss J (2002) Efficacy of Desmopressin in the treatment of nocturia: a double blind placebo controlled studying men. *BJU Int* **89**, 855–62.

220. Robinson D, Cardozo L, Akeson M, Hvistendahl G, Riis A & Norgaard J (2004) Anti-diuresis – a new concept in the management of daytime urinary incontinence. *BJU Int* **93**, 996–1000.

221. Fowler CJ, Jewkes D, McDonald WI, Lynn B & DeGroat WC (1992) Intravesical capsaicin for neurogenic bladder dysfunction. *Lancet* **339**, 1239.

222. Chandiramani VA, Peterson T, Beck RO & Fowler CJ (1994) Lessons learnt from 44 intravestial instillations of capsaicin. *Neurourol Urodynam* **13**, 348—9.

223. Kim DY & Chancellor MB (2000) Intravesical neuromodulatory drugs: capsaicin and resiniferatoxin to treat the overactive bladder. *J Endourol* **14**, 97–103.

224. Ishizuka O, Mattiasson A & Andersson K-E (1995) Urodynamic effects of intravesical resiniferatoxin and capsaicin in conscious rats wth and without outflow obstruction. *J Urol* **154**, 611–16.

225. Kerner J (1817) Vergiftung durch verdobene Würste. *Tübinger Blätt Naturwißenschaften Arzenykunde* **3**, 1–25.

226. van Ermenegen E (1897). Über einen neuen anaeroben Bacillus und seine Beziehungen zum Botulismus. *Z Hyg Infektionskrankh* **26**, 1–56.

227. Dolly JO (1997) Therapeutic and research exploitation of Botulinum neurotoxins. *Eur J Neurol* **4**(Suppl. 2), S5–10.

228. Schurch B, Stohrer M, Kramer G, Schmid DM, Gaul G & Hauri D (2000) Botulinum-A toxin for treating detrusor hyperreflexia in spinal cord injured pateints: a new alternative to anticholinergic drugs? Preliminary results. *J Urol* **164**, 692–7.

229. Reitz A, Stroher M, Kramer G, Del Popolo G, Chartier-Kastler E, Pannek J, Burgdorfer H, Gocking K, Madersbacher H, Schumacher S, Richter R, von Tobel J & Schurch B (2004). European experience of 200 cases treated with botulinum-A toxin injections into the detrusor muscle for urinary incontinence due to neurogenic detrusor overactivity. *Eur Urol* **45**, 510–15.

230. Schurch B, de Seze M, Denys P, Chartier-Kastler E, Haab F, Everaert K, Plante P, Perrouin-Verbe B, Kumar C, Fracek S, Brin MF & Botox Detrusor Hyperreflexia Study Team (2005) *J Urol* **174**, 196–200.

231. Popat R, Apostolidis A, Kalsi V, Gonzales G, Fowler CJ & Dasgupta P (2005) A comparison between the response of patients with idiopathic detrusor overactivity and

neurogenic detrusor overactivity to the first intradetrusor injection of Botulinum-A toxin. *J Urol* **174**, 984–9.

232. Grosse J, Kramer G & Stoher M (2005) Success of repeat detrusor injections of Botulinum-A toxin in patients with severe neurogenic detrusor overactivity and incontinence. *Eur Urol* **47**, 653–9.

233. Seigel SW, Cantanzaro F, Dijkema he *et al.* (2000) Long term results of a multicentre study on sacral nerve stimulation for treatment of urinary urge incontinence, urgency-frequency and retention. *Urology* **56**, 87–91.

234. Mast P, Hoebeke, Wyndale JJ, Oosterlinck W & Everaert K (1995) Experience with clam cystoplasty. A review. *Paraplegia* **33**, 560–4.

235. Bramble FJ (1990) The clam cystoplasty. *Br J Urol* **66**, 337–41.

236. McRae P, Murray KH, Nurse DE, Stephenson JP & Mundy AR (1987) Clam entero-cystoplasty in the neuropathic bladder. *Br J Urol* **60**, 523–5.

237. Rosenbaum TP, Shah PJR, Rose GA & Lloyd-Davies RW (1989) Cranberry juice helps the problem of mucus production in enterouroplastics. *Neurourol Urodynam* **8**, 344–5.

238. Harzmann R & Weckerman D (1992) Problem of secondary malignancy after urinary diversion and enterocystoplasty. *Scand J Urol Nephrol* **142**(Suppl), 56.

239. Barrington JW, Fern Davies H, Adams RJ, Evans WD, Woodcock JP & Stephenson TP (1995) Bile acid dysfunction after clam enterocystoplasty. *Br J Urol* **76**, 169–71.

240. Cartwright PC & Snow BW (1989) Bladder autoaugmentation: partial detrusor excision to augment the bladder without use of bowel. *J Urol* **142**, 1050–3.

241. Snow BW & Cartwright PC (1996) Bladder autoaugmentation. *Urol Clin N Am* **23**, 323–31.

242. Kennelly MJ, Gormley EA & McGuire EJ (1994) Early clinical experience with adult bladder autoaugmentation. *J Urol* **152**, 303–6.

243. Karram MM & Bhatia NN (1989) Management of co-existant stress and urge incontinence. *Br J Urol* **57**, 641–6.

244. Shah PJR (1990) Pathophysiology of voiding disorders. In: Drife J, Hilton P & Stanton S (eds) *Micturition*. London: Springer-Verlag.

245. Salmon UL, Walter RI & Gast SH (1941) The use of oestrogen in the treatment of dysuria and incontinence in postmenopausal women. *Am J Obstet Gynaecol* **14**, 23–31.

246. Youngblood VH, Tomlin EM & Davis JB (1957) Senile urethritis in women. *J Urol* **78**, 150–2.

247. Fantl JA, Cardozo LD, McClish DK & the Hormones and Urogenital Therapy Committee (1994) Oestrogen therapy in the management of incontinence in postmenopausal women: a meta-analysis. First report of the Hormones and Urogenital Therapy Committee. *Obstet Gynaecol* **83**, 12–18.

248. Zullo MA, Oliva C, Falconi G, Paparella P & Mancuso S (1998) Efficacy of oestrogen therapy in urinary incontinence. A meta-analytic study. *Minerva Ginecol* **50**(5), 199–205.

249. Moehrer B, Hextall A & Jackson S (2003) Oestrogens for urinary incontinence in women. Cochrane database of systematic reviews.

250. Grady D, Brown JS, Vittinghoff E, Applegate W, Varner E & Synder T (2001) Postmenopausal hormones and incontinence: the Heart and Estrogen/progestin Replacement Study. *Obstet Gynaecol* **97**, 116–20.

251. Grodstein F, Lifford K, Resnick NM & Curhan GC (2004) Postmenopausal hormone therapy and risk of developing urinary incontinence. *Obstet Gynaecol* **103**, 254–60.

252. Hendrix SL, Cochrane BR, Nygaard IE, Handa VL, Barnabei VM, Iglesia C, Aragaki A, Naughton MJ, Wallace RB & Mc Neeley SG (2005) Effects of estrogen with and without progestin on urinary incontinence. *JAMA* **293**(8), 935–48.

253. Bungay G, Vessey MP & McPherson CK (1980) Study of symptoms in middle life with special reference to the menopause. *Br Med J* **281**, 181–3.

254. Kulseng-Hanssen S (1983) Prevalence and pattern of unstable urethral pressure in 174 gynecologic patients referred for urodynamic investigation. *Am J Obstet Gynecol* **146**, 895–900.

255. Sand PK, Bowen LW & Ostergard DR (1986) Uninhibited urethral relaxation: an unusual cause of incontinence. *Obstet Gynecol* **68**, 645–8.

256. Tapp A, Cardozo LD, Versi E & Studd JWW (1988) The prevalence of variation of resting urethral pressure in women and its association with lower urinary tract function. *Br J Urol* **61**, 314–17.

257. Holmes DM, Stone AR, Barry PR, Richards CJ & Stephenson TP (1983) Bladder training – 3 years on. *Br J Urol* **55**, 660–4.

258. Smith PJ (1981) The urethral syndrome. In: Fisher AM & Gordon H (eds) *Gynaecological Enigmata*. Clin Obstet Gynaecol WB Saunders, London, pp. 161–72.

259. Stamm WE, Running K, McKevitt M, Counts GW, Turck M & Holmes KK (1981) Treatment of the acute urethral syndrome. *N Engl J Med* **304**, 956–8.

260. Rees DL, Whitfield HN & Islam AK (1975) Urodynamic findings in the adult female with frequency and dysuria. *Br J Urol* **47**, 853–60.

261. Oravisto KJ (1980) Interstitial cystitis as an autoimmune disease. *Eur Urol* **6**, 10–13.

262. Geist RW & Antolak SJ (1970) Interstitial cystitis in children. *J Urol* **138**, 508–12.

263. Parivar F & Bradbrook RA (1986) Interstitial cystitis. *Br J Urol* **58**, 239–44.

264. Lynes WL, Flynn LD, Shortliffe ML, Zipser R, Roberts J & Stamey TA (1987) Mast cell involvement in interstitial cystitis. *J Urol* **138**, 746–52.

265. Christmas TJ & Rode J (1991) Characteristics of mast cells in normal bladder, bacterial cystitis and interstitial cystitis. *Br J Urol* **68**, 473–8.

266. Parsons CL, Stanffer C & Schmidt JD (1980) Bladder surface glycosaminoglycans. An efficient mechanism of environmental adaptation. **208**, 605–9.

267. Parsons CL, Stein PC, Bidair M & Lebow D (1994) Abnormal sensitivity to intravesical potassium in interstitial cystitis. *Neurourol Urodyn* **13**, 515–20.

268. Hanno PM (1994) Amitriptyline in the treatment of interstitial cystitis. *Urol Clin N Am* **21**, 89–91.

269. Messing ED & Staney TA (1978) Interstitial cystitis: early diagnosis, pathology and treatment. *Urology* **12**, 381–91.

270. Gillespie L (1986) *You Don't Have To Live With Cystitis!* New York: Avon Books.

271. Badenoch AW (1971) Chronic interstitial cystitis. *Br J Urol* **43**, 718–21.

272. Mulholland SG, Hanno P, Parsons CL, Sant GR & Staskin DR (1990) Pentosan polysulfate sodium for therapy of interstitial cystitis. A double blind placebo-controlled clinical study. *Urology* **35**, 552–8.

273. Parsons CL, Schmidt JD & Pollen JY (1983) Successful treatment of interstitial cystitis with sodium pentosanpolysulphate. *J Urol* **130**, 57–5.

274. Bade JJ, Laseur M, Nieuwenburg L, van der Weele Th & Mensink HJA (1997) A placebo-controlled study of intravesical pentosanpolysulphate for the treatment of interstitial cystitis. *Br J Urol* **79**, 168–71.

275. Childs SJ (1994) Dimethyl sulfone (DMSO) in the treatment of interstitial cystitis. *Urol Clin N Am* **21**, 85–8.

276. Gillespie L (1994) Destruction of the vesico-ureteric plexus for the treatment of hypersensitive bladder disorders. *Br J Urol* **74**, 40–3.

277. Gillespie L (1992) *My Body, My Diet*. California: American Foundation for Pain Research, Beverley Hills.

278. Whitmore KE (1994) Self care regimens for patients with interstitial cystitis. *Urol Clin N Am* **21**, 121–30.

279. Masters WH & Johnson VE (1966) *Human Sexual Response*. London: Churchill Livingstone.

280. Vessey MP, Metcalf MA, McPherson K & Yeates D (1987) Urinary tract infection in relation to diaphragm use and obesity. *Int J Epidemiol* **16**, 1–4.

281. Cardozo LD (1988) Sex and the bladder. *Br Med J* **296**, 587–8.

282. Hadorn DC, Baker D, Hodges JS & Hicks N (1996) Rating the quality of evidence for clinical practice guidelines. *J Clin Epidemiol* **49**(7), 749–54.

283. Harbour R & Miller J (2001) A new system for grading recommendations in evidence based guidelines. *BMJ* **323**, 334–6.

Further reading

Appell RA, Rackley RR & Dmochowski RR (1996) Vesila percutaneous bladder-neck stabilization. *J Endourol* **10**, 221–5.

Awad SA, Acker KL, Flood HD & Clarke JC (1987) Selective sacral cryourolysis in the treatment of patients with detrusor instability/hyperreflexia and hypersensitive bladder. *Neurourol Urodyn* **6**, 263–4.

Bates CP, Loose H & Stanton SLR (1973) The objective study of incontinence after repair operations. *Surg Gynecol Obstet* **136**, 12–22.

Bergman A, Koonings PP & Ballard CA (1989) Primary stress urinary incontinence and pelvic relaxation: prospective randomised comparison of three different operations. *Am J Obstet Gynecol* **161**, 97–100.

Bhatia NN & Bergman A (1985) Modified Burch retropubic urethropexy versus modified Pereyra procedure for stress urinary incontinence. *Obstet Gynecol* **66**, 255–61.

Blackford W, Murray K, Stephenson TP & Mundy AR (1984) Results of transvesical infiltration of the pelvic plexus with phenol in 116 patients. *Br J Urol* **56**, 647–9.

Bramble FJ (1982) The treatment of adult enuresis and urge incontinence by enterocystoplasty. *Br J Urol* **54**, 693–6.

Cardozo LD (1986) Urinary frequency and urgency. *Br Med J* **293**, 1419–23.

Cardozo LD (1989) Urinary frequency and urgency. Gynaecology clinical algorithms. *Br Med J (Suppl.)*, 17–21.

Delaere KPJ & Strijbos WEM (1987) Desmopressin in the management of nocturnal enuresis in young adults. *Neurourol Urodyn* **6**, 262.

Fantl JA, Wyman JF, Anderson RL, Matt DW & Bump RC (1988) Postmenopausal urinary incontinence comparison between non-estrogen supplemented and estrogen supplemented women. *Obstet Gynecol* **71**, 823–8.

Fantl JA, Cardozo LD & McClish DK (1994) Estrogen therapy in the management of urinary incontinence in postmenopausal women: a meta-analysis. *Obstet Gynecol* **83**, 12–18.

Foote AJ, Moore KH & King J (1996) A prospective study of the long term use of the bladder neck support prosthesis. *Neurourol Urodyn* **15**, 404–6.

Fowler JE (1981) Prospective study of intravesical dimethyl sulfoxide in the treatment of suspected early interstitial cystitis. *Urology* **18**, 21–6.

Fritjosson A, Fall M, Juhlin R, Person BE & Ruutu M (1987) Treatment of ulcer and non-ulcer interstitial cystitis with sodium pentosanpolysulfate: a multicentre trial. *J Urol* **138**, 508–12.

Hilton P (1989) Urinary incontinence in women. Gynaecology clinical algorithms. *Br Med J* 55–61.

Hilton P & Stanton SL (1982) The use of desmopressin (DDAVP) in nocturnal urinary frequency in the female. *Br J Urol* **54**, 252–5.

Hilton P, Tweedell AL & Mayne L (1990) Oral and intravaginal estrogens alone and in combination with alpha-adrenergic stimulation in genuine stress incontinence. *Int Urogynecol J* **1**, 80–6.

Jarvis GJ (1994) Surgery for stress incontinence. *Br J Obstet Gynaecol* **101**, 371–4.

Knudsen UB, Rittig S, Pederson JB, Norgaard JP & Djurhus JC (1989) Long-term treatment of nocturnal enuresis with desmopressin – influence on urinary output and haematological parameters. *Neurourol Urodyn* **8**, 348–9.

Langer R, Golan A, Neuman M, Schneider D, Bokovsky I & Capsi E (1990) The effect of large uterine fibroids on urinary bladder function and symptoms. *Am J Obstet Gynecol* **163**, 1139–41.

Lobel RW & Sand PK (1996) Long-term results of laparoscopic Burch colposuspension. *Neurourol Urodyn* **15**, 398–9.

Madersbacher H, Knoll M & Kiss G (1991) Intravesical application of oxybutynin: a mode of action in controlling detrusor hyperreflexia. *Neurourol Urodyn* **10**, 375–6.

Mantle J & Versi E (1991) Physiotherapy for stress urinary incontinence: a national survey. *Br Med J* **302**, 509–18.

Milani R, Maggioni A, Colombo M, Pisani G & Quinto M (1991) Burch colposuspension versus modified Marshall–Marchetti–Krantz for stress urinary incontinence: a controlled clinical study. *Neurourol Urodyn* **10**, 454–5.

Mosso A & Pellacani P (1882) Sur les fonctions de la vessie. Methode de recherche. *Arch Ital Biol* **1**, 97–128.

Mundy AR (1983) A trial comparing the Stamey bladder neck suspension procedure with colposuspension for the treatment of stress incontinence. *Br J Urol* **55**, 687–90.

Mundy AR & Stephenson TP (1985) 'Clam' ileocystoplasty for the treatment of refractory urge incontinence. *Br J Urol* **57**, 614–16.

Oravisto KJ & Alfthan OS (1976) Treatment of interstitial cystitis with immunosuppression and chloraquine derivatives. *Eur Urol* **2**, 82–4.

Osborne JL (1976) Post-menopausal changes in micturition habits and in urine flow and urethral pressure studies. In Campbell S (ed.) Lancaster: MTP Press, pp. 285–9.

Parsons CL (1986) Bladder surface glycosaminoglycan layer: efficient mechanism of environmental adaptation. *Urology* **27**, 9–14.

Parsons CL & Mulholland SG (1987) Successful therapy of interstitial cystitis with pentosanpolysulfate. *J Urol* **138**, 513–16.

Plevnik S, Janez J, Vrtacnik P, Trasinar B & Vodusek DB (1986) Short term electrical stimulation: home treatment for urinary incontinence. *World J Urol* **4**, 24–6.

Powell PH, George NJR, Smith PJB & Fenely RCL (1981) The hypersensitive female urethra – a cause of recurrent frequency and dysuria. In: *Proceedings of the 11th Annual Meeting of the International Continence Society.* Lund: pp. 81–2.

Quinn MJ (1990) Vaginal ultrasound and urinary stress incontinence. *Contemp Rev Obstet Gynecol* **2**, 104–10.

Rosenbaum TP (1990) The Autocath: a new concept to facilitate self catheterisation in the female. *Urogynecologia* **IV**, 134.

Rosenbaum TP, Shah PJR & Worth PHL (1988) Transtrigonal phenol: the end of an era? *Neurourol Urodyn* **7**, 294–5.

Sand PK, Richardson DA, Satskin DR *et al.* (1994) Pelvic floor stimulation in the treatment of genuine stress incontinence: a multi-centre placebo-controlled trial. *Neurourol Urodyn* **13**, 356–7.

Simmons JL & Bruce PL (1958) On the use of an antihistamine in the treatment of interstitial cystitis. *Am Surg* **24**, 664–7.

Smith PJ (1977) The menopause and the lower urinary tract – another case for hormonal replacement therapy. *Practitioner* **218**, 97–9.

Stanton SL & Cardozo LD (1979) A comparison of vaginal and suprapubic surgery in the correction of incontinence due to urethral sphincter incompetence. *Br J Urol* **51**, 497–9.

Stanton SL, Chamberlain G & Holmes D (1985) Anterior colporrhaphy versus colposuspension in the treatment of genuine stress incontinence. In: *Proceedings of the 25th British Congress of Obstetrics and Gynaecology.* London.

Staskin D, Sant G, Sand P *et al.* (1995) Use of an expandable urethral insert for GSI – long term results of multicenter trial. *Neurourol Urodyn* **14**, 420–2.

Stewart BH & Shirley SW (1976) Further experience with intravesical DMSO in the treatment of interstitial cystitis. *J Urol* **116**, 36–8.

Sultana CJ & Walters MD (1995) Estrogen and urinary incontinence in women. *Maturitas* **20**, 129–38.

Tapp A, Fall M, Norgaard J *et al.* (1987) A dose titrated multicentre study of terodiline in the treatment of detrusor instability. *Neurourol Urodyn* **6**, 254–5.

Turner-Warwick RT & Ashken MH (1967) The functional results of partial, sub-total and total cystoplasty with special reference to uretercystoplasty, selective sphincterotomy and cystocystoplasty. *Br J Urol* **39**, 3–12.

Ulmsten U, Henriksson L & Iosif S (1982) The unstable female urethra. *Am J Obstet Gynecol* **144**, 93–7.

Versi E & Cardozo LD (1985) Urethral instability in normal postmenopausal women. In: *Proceedings of the 15th Annual Meeting of the International Continence Society.* London: pp. 115–16.

Wall LL & Stanton SL (1989) Transvesical phenol injection of pelvic nerve plexuses in females with refractory urge incontinence. *Br J Urol* **63**, 465–8.

Walter S, Kjaergaard B, Lose G *et al.* (1990) Stress urinary incontinence in postmenopausal women treated with oral estrogen (estriol) and in alpha-andrenoreceptor-stimulating agent (phenylpropanolamine). A randomised double blind placebo controlled study. *Int Urogynecol J* **1**, 74–9.

Weil A, Reyes H, Bischoff P, Rottenberg RD & Kraurer F (1984) Modifications of the urethral resting and stress profiles after different types of surgery fro urinary stress incontinence. *Br J Obstet Gynaecol* **91**, 46–55.

Wise BG, Cardozo LD, Cutner A, Burton G & Abbott D (1992) The effect of a vaginal ultrasound probe on lower urinary tract function. *Br J Urol* **70**, 12–16.

Chapter 50: Hysteroscopy and laparoscopy

Adam Magos

If I were asked what has been the single most important change in gynaecological surgical practice over the last 20–30 years, I would have no hesitation in answering that it is endoscopic surgery. Thanks to pioneers such as Semm and Lindemann from Germany, Bruhat and Hamou from France, Sutton from England, and Reich, Neuwirth and Goldrath from the United States to name but a few, modern gynaecological surgery has undergone a revolution since the 1970s and 1980s, a revolution characterized by the realization that many patients formerly treated by laparotomy or hysterectomy could be managed by laparoscopic or hysteroscopic surgery.

In many ways, gynaecologists were the leaders in this change of practice; whereas laparoscopic procedures such as ovarian cystectomy, salpingo-oophorectomy and myomectomy were described by Semm as early as 1979, the first comparable general surgical procedure, laparoscopic cholecystectomy, was only described several years later. Indeed, it was Semm, the gynaecologist, who carried out the first laparoscopic appendicectomy in 1983 [1].

Since those early days, what has come to be known as 'Minimal Access Surgery' (MAS) has affected every area of gynaecology, from diagnosis to therapy, from reproductive medicine to urogynaecology to oncology. The advantages seemed obvious – less post-operative pain, shorter hospitalization and faster return to normal activities. While it has to be admitted that the widespread adoption of endoscopic surgery has not always been based on proof of its efficacy and safety compared with traditional surgery, and indeed many questions remain to be answered, it is equally true to say that MAS has introduced a scientific rigour into surgical practice which was rarely seen with the 'old' surgery. As a result, the medical literature on MAS across all surgical specialities is extensive and growing by the day, and randomized controlled trials, cost-benefit analysis, and quality adjusted life years have become common currency among surgeons just as they have been for many years for physicians.

Instruments and equipment for endoscopy

Much more than is the case with conventional surgery, endoscopic surgery relies heavily not only on the skill of the surgeon but also on technology. The vision of the early pioneers would have been but nothing without technical developments in optics, illumination, video technology and instrumentation. There has always been a close link between the endosopic surgeon and industry, and it is not an exaggeration to claim that the instruments and equipment for MAS is an inherent part of the surgery. It is therefore essential that the surgeon fully understands all aspects of their use if he or she is to be a safe and effective operator, from basic physical principles to how equipment is assembled and connected, from when and how to use a particular instrument to what to do when it appears to be malfunctioning.

Equipment common to hysteroscopy and laparoscopy

LIGHT SOURCE AND LIGHT LEAD

Without adequate illumination, endoscopic surgery becomes an impossibility. Illumination is primarily a function of the power of the light source and the light transmission properties of the light lead, but is also influenced by the size and tissue properties of what is being illuminated; for instance, laparoscopy requires a brighter light to sufficiently illuminate a larger cavity at a greater distance compared with hysteroscopy, and the same is true in the presence of bleeding as blood absorbs light.

Older tungsten and metal halide light sources have been superseded by more powerful xenon generators. When used with modern auto-aperture cameras they should be set to maximum illumination during surgery. Conversely, the light source should not be switched off between cases but merely put on standby to prolong the life of the bulb. Although modern light bulbs are guaranteed for several hundred hours use, a spare one should be available in the operating theatre in case the bulb fails in the middle of a procedure.

Light leads are of two types, fibre optic or liquid. The former are more common because they are cheaper, but the fibres are prone to breaking with gradual deterioration in light transmission. Rough handling (e.g. kinking, knotting or tight rolling) should be avoided as this will tend to damage the delicate light fibres. The state of the fibres is easily checked by aiming one end at a light and looking at the other end for dark areas. Liquid light cables do not suffer from this problem but can be irreversibly damaged if the outer casing is punctured.

Whatever the power of the light source or the type of light lead, and despite the common use of the term 'cold light fountain' to describe medical light systems, the light produced at the end of the light lead is very much 'hot' even in standby mode to the extent that it can burn drapes as well as the patient if inadvertently left in contact.

CAMERA AND MONITOR SYSTEM

There is little doubt that the introduction of video cameras and high resolution colour monitors in the 1980s played a major role in popularizing endoscopic surgery. Until then, only the surgeon could see the surgery, and it was difficult for assistants to play a useful role as they were blind to the procedure. An optical teaching aid could be attached to the telescope, but this merely limited movement of the endoscope and reduced illumination, and was not really a solution. Then, suddenly, after years of working in the dark as far as the rest of the operating theatre staff were concerned, everyone could see the operation! Assistants could assist, the surgeon could teach, and even the anaesthetist felt more involved.

Early tube cameras were superseded by single CCD (charged coupled device) chip cameras, which in turn have been superseded by current 3-chip cameras. Videolaparoscopes are now also available where the chips are built into the end of the optic, as are 3D camera systems, but these have not yet achieved popularity. Apart from focus, various other functions can usually be controlled through the camera itself (e.g. white balance, taking a still image), and it is useful to be able to have a zoom facility. Some cameras can be autoclaved, the alternative being to place the camera and lead in a sterile sleeve.

The camera is connected to a control unit and thence to a high-resolution colour monitor; an ordinary television, which has a relatively low resolution, would provide a far inferior image.

ELECTROSURGICAL GENERATOR

Electrosurgery, often referred to as 'diathermy', has been used in surgery for over 100 years for haemostasis or cutting, and has become a very important component of both hysteroscopic and laparoscopic surgery. The modern solid-state generator safely and reliably delivers a high-frequency current at low voltage and is a very different machine from the spark generators of years gone by. It can be used in one of three modalities: bipolar, monopolar cutting (including pure cut and blended cut) and monopolar coagulation (including desiccation, fulguration and spray). Bipolar coagulation, for instance, is often used in laparoscopy for haemostasis, whereas the resectoscope is traditionally a monopolar instrument.

There is insufficient space in this chapter to discuss the principles of electrosurgery fully, but the following are useful practical points for the endoscopic surgeon, which are not always appreciated:

1 The bipolar, monopolar cut and monopolar coagulation are three independent circuits within the generator. For instance, blending a monopolar cut waveform is not influenced at all by the setting on the monopolar coagulation circuit.

2 Bipolar electrosurgery is inherently safer than monopolar as the current only has to travel between the prongs of the electrodes and not between the electrode and the patient plate. It should therefore be used in preference to monopolar electrosurgery whenever possible.

3 The minimum power and voltage should be used which will achieve the desired end result. Remember that the current produced when activating the bipolar circuit has the lowest voltage while monopolar coagulation the highest, monopolar cut being intermediate. Voltage is what drives the current and also causes sparking. From this point of view as well, bipolar electrosurgery is the safest and monopolar coagulation the most dangerous when working in a confined space such as the pelvis.

4 As the bipolar electrodes are in effect made up of the active and return electrodes, a patient plate is not required for bipolar electrosurgery.

5 The terms 'cut' and 'coagulation' are in some respects a misnomer. Electrosurgical cutting depends on electrical arcing between the electrode and tissue resulting in vaporization and cell explosion, whereas coagulation is achieved with the electrode in contact with tissue causing heating and coagulation. As these effects are independent of the current waveform, it is possible to achieve both cutting and coagulation with a cutting current by simply altering the position of the electrode; keeping the electrode off the tissue will result in cutting while deliberately touching the tissue will produce coagulation. As the cutting current is at a lower voltage, coagulating with monopolar cut is inherently safer than using monopolar coagulation, although it may not be as effective.

6 Some other practical aspects of electrosurgery will be addressed later in the chapter. Electrosurgery is, however, such a useful and powerful tool that I urge the reader to study the subject in greater depth (see 'Further reading').

LASER

Lasers, an acronym for *l*ight *a*mplification by *s*timulated *e*mission of *r*adiation, have always had a mystique, perhaps because they are expensive and therefore available only to a few. Unlike electrosurgery, lasers are by no means essential for effective endoscopic surgery as there is no evidence that they produce a better end result. However, under certain conditions such as dissecting near vital structures, lasers may represent a safer surgical modality because thermal spread tends to be less (e.g. CO_2 laser) and distant burns, insulation failure and capacitive coupling cannot happen. Conversely, lasers tend to be less efficient at haemostasis than diathermy.

Several different lasers are available for endoscopy, but of these CO_2, Nd:YAG (neodymium:yttrium aluminium garnet), argon and KTP (potassium titanyl phosphate) lasers tend to be used for laparoscopy, and Nd:YAG for hysteroscopy. The CO_2 laser is an optical laser which is delivered through a tubular arm containing mirrors. It is almost completely absorbed by water, and is therefore suited to laparoscopy because it cuts accurately with minimal thermal spread. On the negative side, CO_2 lasers are poor haemostats, and the need for an optical arm makes it cumbersome to operate and prone to misalignment. The Nd:YAG laser is a fibre-optic laser which makes it easier to use, and as the energy is poorly absorbed by water, this type of laser is suitable for hysteroscopic procedures as well as laparoscopy. For the same reason, the thermal spread with Nd:YAG is greater making it more suited to tissue coagulation rather than vaporization. Tissue penetration can, however, be reduced and precision increased by using a sapphire tip at the end of the fibre-optic cable. The argon and KTP lasers are also fibre lasers with tissue effects intermediate between CO_2 and Nd:YAG.

PHOTO AND VIDEO DOCUMENTATION

The universal use of video cameras at endoscopic surgery lends itself to recording still images, short excerpts of procedures or even whole procedures. Photographs are useful clinical records which can be discussed with the patient as well as colleagues if a second opinion is sought. Video recordings are excellent for teaching, and can also be used for research, to measure performance and to assess instrumentation. We, for instance, record all our operations and keep the recordings for at least 2 weeks in case there is a post-operative complication; we can then review the surgery to determine any possible intraoperative cause.

Not surprisingly, the instrument manufacturers all sell equipment for photo and video recording. Digital systems have replaced analogue recording, and typically consist of a modified computer with a touch screen, DVD writer and colour printer. Although convenient, commercial systems are generally expensive and have limited continuous recording capabilities because they contain relatively little memory. It is possible to construct a digital recording system base around a standard personal computer whose recording capacity is hundreds of times greater, limited only by the size of the hard disk inside [2].

It must be remembered that local guidelines have to be followed when any visual recordings are made of patients. In the UK, for instance, the General Medical Council has issued guidelines which state that, in the case of laparoscopic images or images of internal organs, permission or consent is not required from patients provided the recording are effectively anonymized by removal of any identifying marks.

Equipment for hysteroscopy

HYSTEROSCOPES

Both rigid and flexible hysteroscopes are available, the majority of gynaecologists preferring the former because the image tends to be superior, the equipment is more robust, it can be used with a resectoscope, and not least, the purchase cost is significantly less. Rigid hysteroscopes generally have a Hopkins rod-lens optical system whereas flexible and very narrow rigid hysteroscopes contain optical fibres.

Rigid hysteroscopes come in different sizes in terms of their outer diameter, 4 and 2.9 mm being popular sizes. They are available at 0°, 12°, 15° or 30° angles of view, the oblique view ones being most suited to working within the uterine cavity. For any procedure other than contact hysteroscopy, at least a single sheath has to be fitted to the optic to allow uterine distension, while continuous flow sheaths permit simultaneous irrigation/suction and tend to be used for surgery (inner sheath for inflow, outer sheath for outflow).

UTERINE DISTENSION

The uterine cavity is a potential space and has to be distended at relatively high pressure to afford a panoramic view. To achieve this, gas (CO_2), low-viscosity fluids (e.g. N/saline, 5% dextrose, 1.5% glycine, 3% sorbitol, 5% mannitol) or high-viscosity fluid (e.g. Hyskon, which is 32% dextran 70 in dextrose) can be used. Diagnostic hysteroscopy is typically done using CO_2 or N/saline, operative hysteroscopy with mechanical instruments or laser

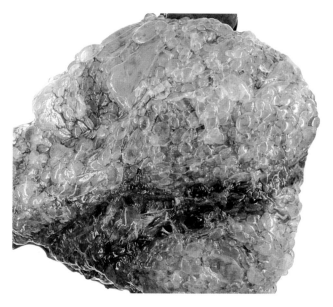

Plate 15.1 The typical macroscopic appearance of a complete mole.

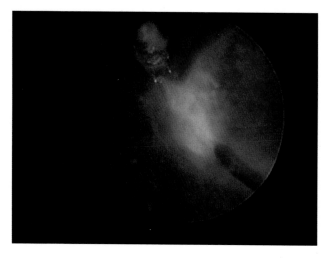

Plate 20.1 Endoscopic view of chorionic plate vasculature in twin–twin transfusion syndrome, showing laser ablation to anastomosis.

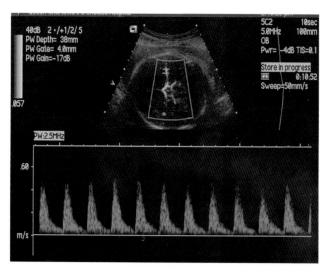

Plate 17.1 Colour Doppler flow pattern of the 'Circle of Willis' in the fetal brain. The callipers are put with a 0° angle on the middle cerebral artery and the pulse wave Doppler flow pattern demonstrated.

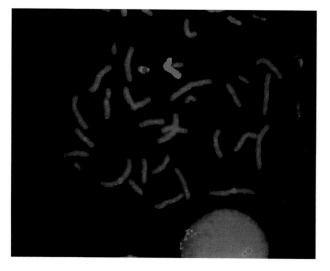

Plate 39.1 A case of premature ovarian failure in a 37-year-old woman who was found to have an XY genotype and, apart from short stature, was a phenotypically normal female. This patient exhibited features more typical of Turner's mosaicism than of a 'classical XY female'. Mosaicism was indeed found on examination of the ovarian tissue, although even then the mosaic was 45X/46XY. The figure represents dual colour fluorescence in situ hybridization (FISH) on interphase nuclei, using probes for the alpha satellite centromeric regions of the X and Y chromosome. Both single X and double XY signals were detected, with the majority of nuclei showing a single X signal, suggesting predominance of the 45X cell line. Mutation analysis of the SRY gene was performed and the SRY gene was found to be normal [60].

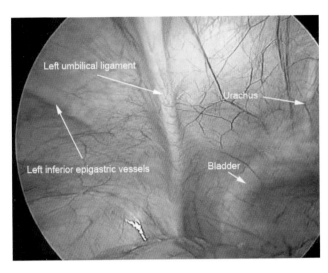

Plate 39.2 A polycystic ovary after laparoscopic ovarian diathermy. Reproduced from *Infertility in Practice*, 2nd edn., Balen & Jacobs, Churchill Livingstone 2003, with permission.

Plate 50.2 Laparoscopic view of the left inferior epigastric vessels lateral to the umbilical ligament (obliterated umbilical vessels).

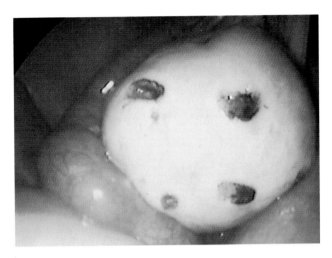

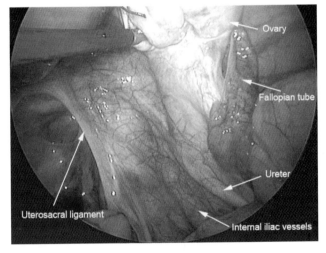

Plate 50.1 Laparoscopic view of the 'safe triangle'

Plate 50.3 View of the right lateral pelvic side wall after elevation and rotation of the ovary.

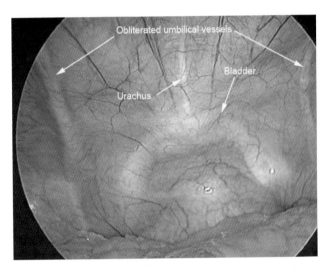

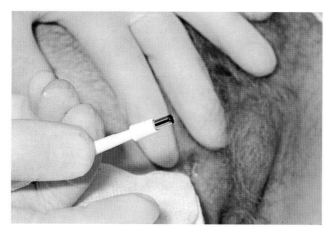

Plate 51.1 *4 mm Disposable punch biopsy* – with practice a vulval biopsy should be a minimally painful 10 min procedure, using a tiny bleb of lignocaine with adrenalin injected with an insulin syringe. Sutures are rarely required.

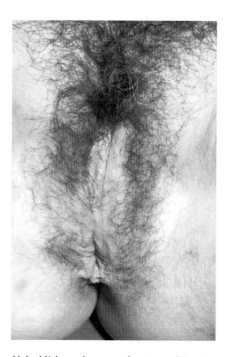

Plate 51.3 *Vulval lichen sclerosus* – showing whitening, ecchymoses, rubbery oedema and disturbance of normal architecture.

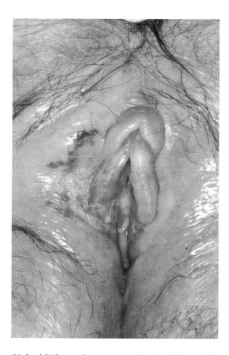

Plate 51.2 *Vulval lichen sclerosus* – early established disease showing rubbery oedema of labia minora and clitoral hood and stark whitening extending to perianal skin. Note currently healed fissure at 6 o'clock.

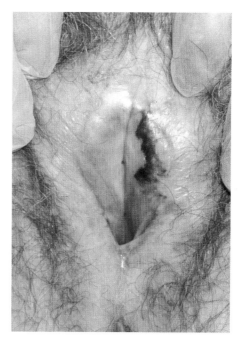

Plate 51.4 *'Advanced vulval lichen sclerosus'*. Stark whitening, complete burying of the clitoral and total replacement of architecture with 'plastering' down and resorption of labia. Gross ecchymoses and narrowing of vaginal introitus.

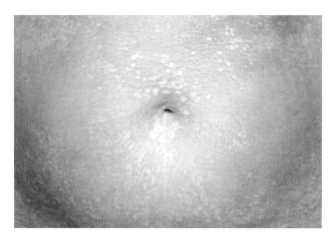

Plate 51.5 *Extra-genital lichen sclerosus – 'white spot disease'*. Stark white spots, above the umbilicus showing perifollicular situation and below coalescing to form a white scarred plaque. Stretching the skin would reveal follicular delling and/or hyperkeratotic plugs giving a nutmeg grater feel, hence differentiating from vitiligo.

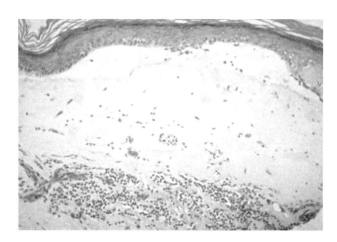

Plate 51.6 *History of lichen sclerosus* – (H&E × 40). The classical features are seen on atrophic epidermis with hyperkeratosis an effaced dermo-epidermal function with loss of melanocytes, a thick pale zone of hyaline scarring in the upper dermis, 'sandwiched' below the causative bearing band of attacking lymphocytes. Effective treatment must eliminate/neutralize these.

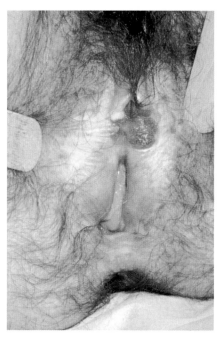

Plate 51.7 *Lichen sclerosus complicated by squamous carcinoma*. Note the classical cigarette-paper scarring and stark background whitening. Here the squamous cell carcinoma presents as a fleshy nodule, but persistent erosion should also prompt biopsy.

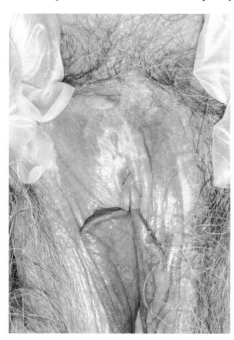

Plate 51.8 Lichen sclerosus with the overlying benign thickened epidermis (hypertrophic lichen sclerosus) seen in some 30% of patients. It is in such a setting that squamous cell carcinoma may arise and should arouse vigilance.

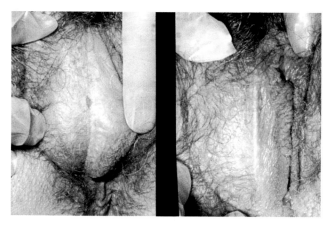

Plate 51.9 *Response of lichen sclerosus to 6 weeks of Grade I topical steroids*. The precise regimen detailed in the text should be adhered to. Non-responders may have an alternative more resistant condition such as lichen planus or cicatricial pemphigoid.

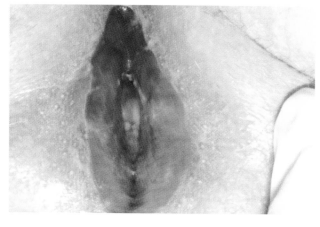

Plate 51.11 *Erosive lichen planus*. The vestibule is derided and scarred with loss of labia minora and Wickham's striae extending out into the perianal skin. Note the characteristic 'milky-line' (see Plate 51.12 for close up).

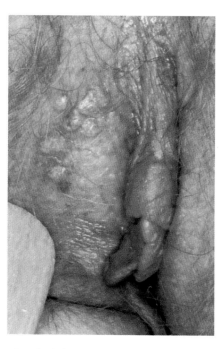

Plate 51.10 *Papular lichen planus*. Typical coalescing flat topped papules, showing white Wickham's striae. They are bluish colour and are usually also found on the inner wrists and elsewhere.

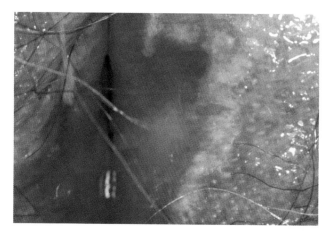

Plate 51.12 *Close-up of 'milky-line' of erosive lichen planus*. A biopsy either side of this line is liable to give 'burnt out' non-diagnostic findings – hence the line itself should be sampled.

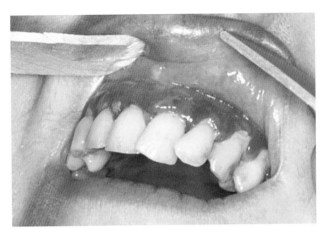

Plate 51.13 *Erosive lichen planus of the gums, accompanying vulval changes.* Despite the appearances such lesions characteristic of the vulvo-vaginal-gingival syndrome (of Hewitt and Pelisse) may be asymptomatic.

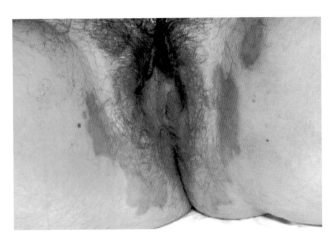

Plate 51.15 *Lichen simplex chronicus.* A well-demarcated patch of lichenification on the right interlabial sulcus is seen. The patient points to such a lesion as the site of her itch.

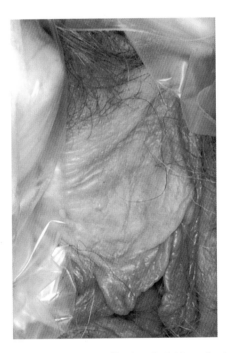

Plate 51.14 *Psoriasis.* Plaques affecting the labia and extending onto the genitocrural folds. Scaling is lost in this flexural occluded site. Lesions are asymptomatic but secondary vulvodynia not uncommonly complicates the clinical and therapeutic picture.

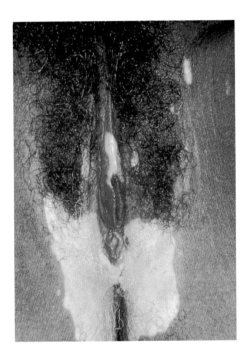

Plate 51.16 *Vitiligo.* Showing start of symmetrical depigmentation in this black patient.

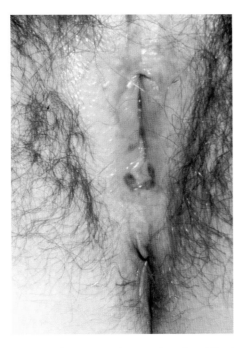

Plate 51.17 *Post-inflammatory pigmentation – here following lichen planus.* Such changes less commonly occur with lichen sclerosus.

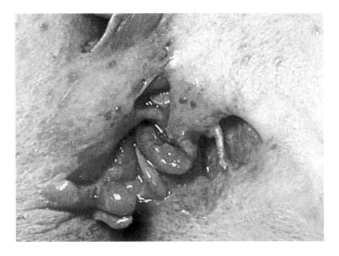

Plate 51.19 *Crohn's disease – severe perineal ulceration and fissure formation.* A spectre not easily forgotten.

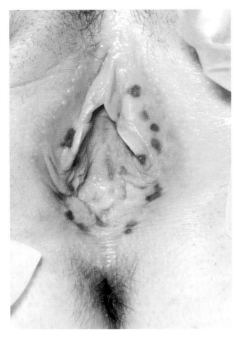

Plate 51.18 *Idiopathic pigmentation of Laugier.* There is no history of antecedent inflammation. Similar lesions can affect men.

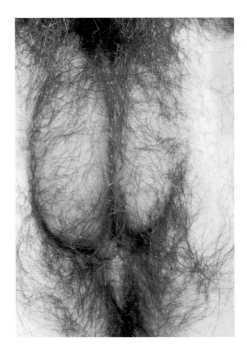

Plate 51.20 *Unilateral vulval oedema – Crohn's disease.* Sometimes vulval oedema, usually unilateral, can accompany Crohn's disease of gastrointestinal tract.

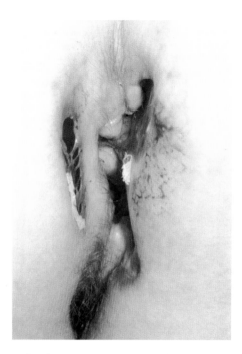

Plate 51.21 *Pyoderma gangrenosum*. Here destroying the perineum of a 36-year-old woman. Several surgical interventions with subsequent extension of disease preceded the clinical diagnosis.

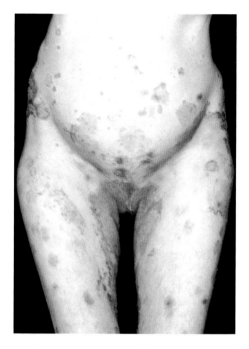

Plate 51.23 *Glucagonoma syndrome*. The characteristic picture of peri-orificial annular lesions of neurolytic migratory erythema in a patient with a pancreatic glucagonoma.

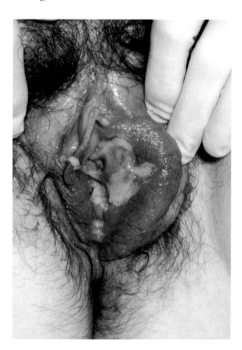

Plate 51.22 *Behçets syndrome*. Extensive deep ulcers, here penetrating the labia in a 45-year-old Turkish woman.

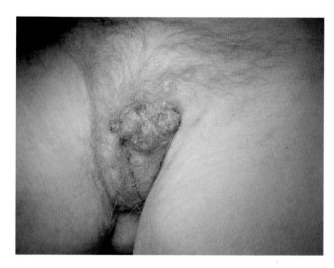

Plate 52.1 Large anterior vulval cancer with satellite skin deposits.

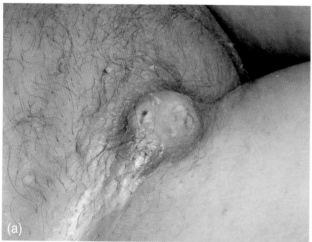

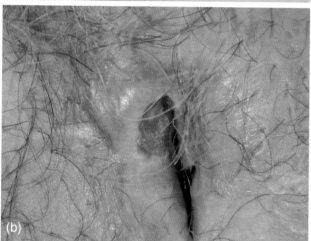

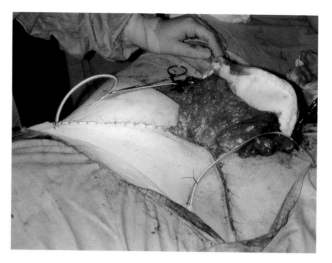

Plate 52.3 En-bloc dissection of the inguinofemoral lymph nodes.

Plate 52.2 (a) Recurrence in the right groin after previous simple vulvectomy. (b) Anterior local recurrence after radical vulvectomy.

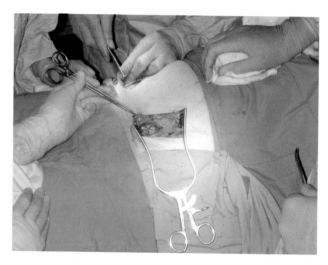

Plate 52.4 Separate groin incisions.

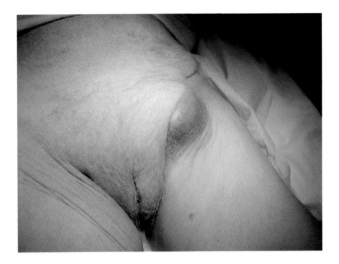

Plate 52.5 Clinically suspicious left groin nodes.

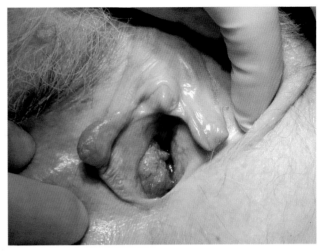

Plate 52.7 Vaginal cancer.

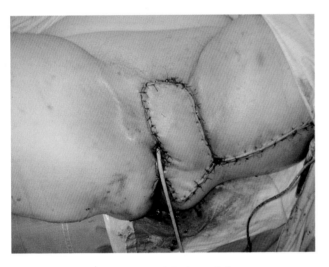

Plate 52.6 Rotation skin flap to fill a large defect.

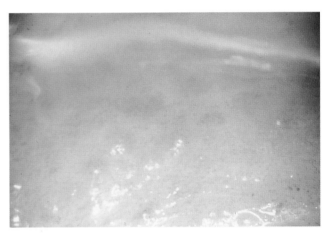

Plate 53.1 Trichomoniasis with 'strawberry' vaginitis.

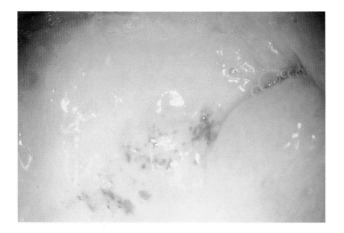

Plate 53.2 Bleeding and adhesions at the vaginal vault.

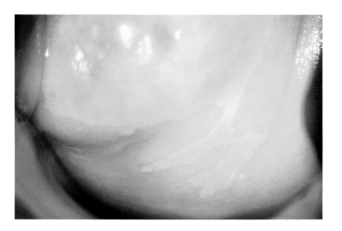

Plate 53.3 VAIN as an extension of a cervical lesion.

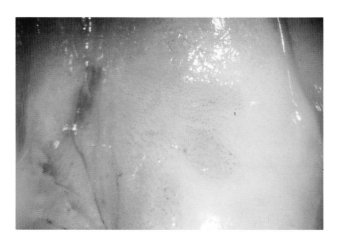

Plate 53.4 VAIN in a post-hysterectomy vaginal angle.

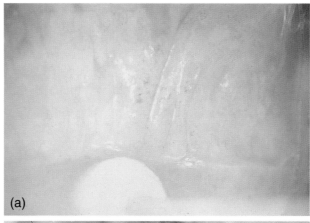

(a)

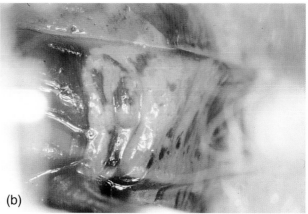

(b)

Plate 53.5 (a & b) Area of VAIN before and after the application of iodine solution.

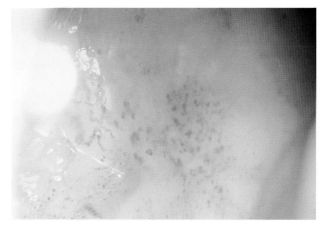

Plate 53.6 Appearances of the vaginal vault after radiotherapy.

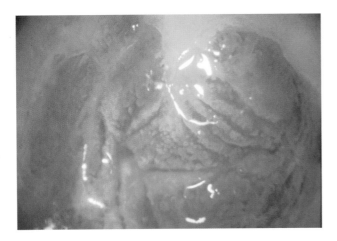

Plate 53.7 Eversion of the cervix during pregnancy.

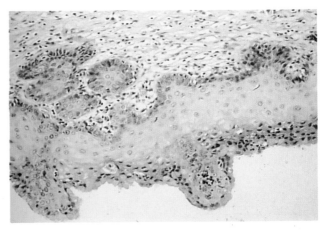

Plate 53.9 Photomicrograph of columnar and multilayered immature metaplastic epithelia.

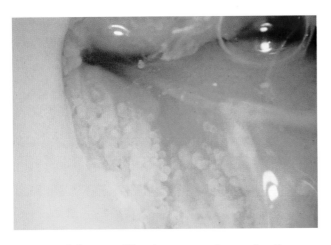

Plate 53.8 Columnar villi at the squamocolumnar junction.

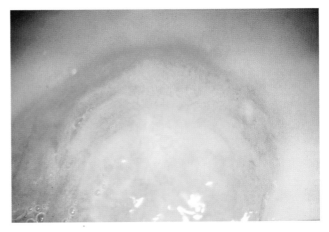

Plate 53.10 Squamous metaplasia of the cervix.

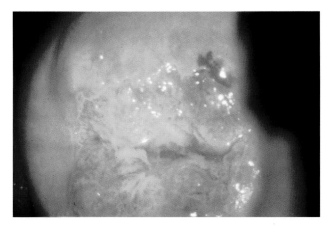

Plate 53.11 A typical transformation zone with a mucus-filled Nabothian follicle at 11 o'clock.

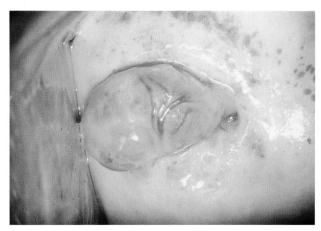

Plate 53.13 A large polyp with adjacent atrophic epithelium and ecchymoses.

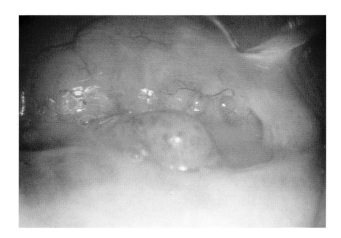

Plate 53.12 A small endocervical polyp.

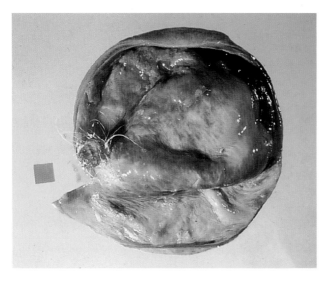

Plate 53.14 A benign cystic teratoma of the ovary showing hair and skin.

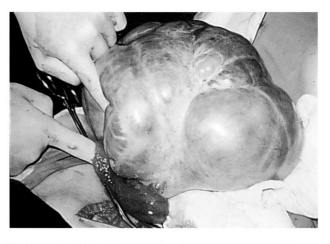

Plate 53.16 (right) A large multicystic ovarian tumour with venous congestion and infarction from torsion of the ovary and tube.

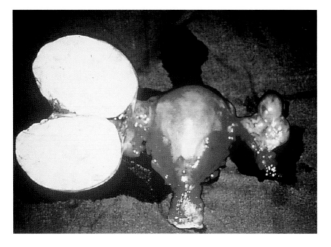

Plate 53.15 An ovarian fibroma.

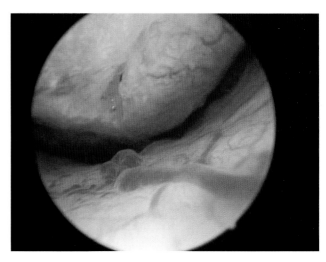

Plate 56.1 A hysteroscopic view of an intra-uterine polyp in a woman receiving tamoxifen. By kind permission of Dr Justine Clark, Consultant Gynaecologist, Birmingham Women's Hospital.

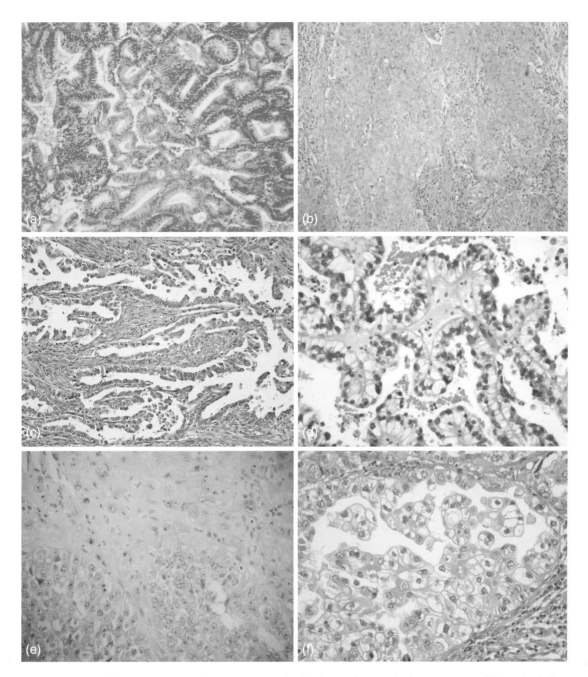

Plate 57.1 (a) H & E well differentiated glandular architecture of a Grade 1 endometrial adenocarcinoma. (b) Poorly differentiated Grade 3 endometrial adenocarcinoma showing solid architecture. (c) H & E section showing typical papillary pattern of uterine serous carcinoma. (d) H & E section showing typical hyalinised papillae covered by cells with prominent clear cytoplasm in an endometrial clear cell carcinoma. (e) Carcinosarcoma. (f) Clear Cell.

with N/saline, and resectoscopic surgery with electrolyte-free solutions such as glycine, sorbitol or mannitol.

The pressure required to provide an adequate view of the uterine cavity depends on a number of factors, but tends to be around 100 mmHg. An enlarged, non-compliant uterus, leakage of distension medium through the cervix or excessive suction when using a continuous flow system will mean that a higher inflow pressure is required. To achieve the desired distension, gravity, pressure bags or special hysteroscopic pumps are available. Modern pumps designed for low-viscosity fluids can not only control the intrauterine pressure with a press of a button, but also monitor fluid balance thereby reducing the risk of fluid overload. Pumps which control flow rather than pressure should not be used for hysteroscopy as they tend to over-distend and promote fluid overload.

Similarly, if using CO_2 for diagnostic hysteroscopy, a special hysteroscopic insufflator must be used as laparoscopic insufflators produce too high a pressure and too fast a flow rate of gas and risk cardiac arrhythmias or worse.

MECHANICAL INSTRUMENTS

Miniature flexible or semi-rigid mechanical instruments such as scissors, grasping and biopsy forceps and monopolar electrodes can be used with operating sheaths for minor procedures such as target biopsy or polypectomy. These instruments tend to be fragile because of their size, typically 7 or 5 Fr gauge (3 Fr = 1 mm), so replacements should be available should they break. On the plus side, they are very unlikely to injure the patient.

RESECTOSCOPE

The resectoscope was introduced into gynaecology by Robert Neuwirth in 1978 when he described its use to resect small submucous fibroids [3]. It has since proved itself to be a highly efficient and versatile operative tool for gynaecologists just as it has been for urologists earlier, not just for myomectomy, but for polypectomy, metroplasty, adhesiolysis and endometrial resection/ablation.

The modern resectoscope consists of five components, the optic, handle mechanism, inflow and outflow sheaths and an electrode (Fig. 50.1). The handle mechanism can be active or passive in design; for hysteroscopy, a passive handle is preferable as it maintains the electrode inside the sheathing system out of view and out of harms way. A typical resectoscope has an outer diameter of 26 or 27 Fr gauge (8.7–9 mm), uses a 4-mm oblique view optic, and is designed for use with electrolyte-free low-viscosity distension media. Smaller resectoscopes are also available, but the electrodes are less robust because of their size. As

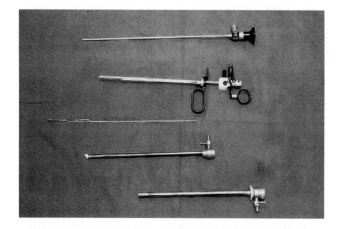

Fig. 50.1 A continuous flow resectoscope with a passive handle mechanism.

already noted, it is essential to connect the inflow tubing to the inner sheath and the outflow to the outer sheath.

Traditionally, the resectoscope uses monopolar electrosurgical energy to activate the electrode although bipolar resectoscopes are also now available. The electrodes themselves come in different design, but the cutting loop (for polypectomy, myomectomy and endometrial resection), rollerball or rollerbar (for endometrial ablation or tissue vaporization) and the knife electrode (for metroplasty) are the most popular. The power settings for monopolar electrosurgery depend on the characteristics of the electrosurgical generator, the resectoscope and the patient's tissues, so it is difficult to be prescriptive, but 100–120 W pure cut or blend 1 cut is usually sufficient to avoid too much drag or charring. As always, the lowest power setting should be used to minimize the risks of electrosurgical injury.

VERSAPOINT

Although bipolar resectoscopes are beginning to be introduced, the Versapoint (Gynecare, USA) is already available. Based around 5 Fr electrodes of different design (e.g. spring, twizzle, ball) and a dedicated electrosurgical generator, it can be used via a standard rigid hysteroscope or a dedicated Versascope for polypectomy, myomectomy of small intracavitary fibroids, and metroplasty [4]. As it is a bipolar instrument, physiological solutions such as N/saline and Hartman's solution can be used for uterine distension.

LASER HYSTEROSCOPE

The clinical application of laser for intrauterine surgery was first reported by Goldrath *et al.* [5]. The use of laser energy for hysteroscopic surgery also has the advantage over the monopolar resectoscope that distension media such as N/saline can be used. Nd:YAG is the preferred laser energy, the fibre being passed down the operating channel of a standard hysteroscope and used in contact or non-contact mode to vaporize or coagulate, respectively. Partly because of cost, longer operating time and higher rates of equipment failure, laser intrauterine surgery has lost much of its popularity [6].

Equipment for laparoscopy

LAPAROSCOPES

As with rigid hysteroscopes, most laparoscopes are built around a rod-lens system and come in a number of diameters (3–12 mm) and angles of view [0°–30°], with 10 mm 0° scopes being the most widely used; fibre-optic micro-laparoscopes are also available but are much more fragile and provide an inferior image. Operating laparoscopes have an additional operating channel for instruments or lasers but are less popular, most gynaecologists preferring to use a multipuncture approach with instruments inserted through ancillary ports. Videolaparoscopes, with CCD chips built into the tip of the instrument, are as yet too new and expensive for widespread use.

VERESS NEEDLE

Traditionally, gynaecologists use a Veress needle to insufflate the abdomen with gas at the start of laparoscopy. Veress was a Hungarian chest physician who, in the 1930s [7], invented the special needle which takes his name for draining chest empyemas; when used at laparoscopy, the Veress needle's design is meant to reduce the risk of intra-abdominal injury to bowel or major blood vessels. The Veress needle is usually inserted transabdominally, but in obese patients can be introduced through the uterine fundus [8,9]. It is available in reusable and disposable forms.

TROCARS AND CANNULAE

Trocars and cannulae act as a conduit for the laparoscope and other instruments. They come in a variety of sizes depending on the diameter of the instrumentation to be accommodated, with 5 mm and 10–12 mm ports being the most commonly required. Traditionally, trocars and cannulae are made of surgical steel and are non-disposable, but there is an ever growing array of disposable plastic designs incorporating safety shields, optical cannulae, expanding sleeves, various shaped tips and different methods of anchoring to name but a few of the options. Of the disposable instruments, pyramidal trocar-cannula systems require the least force for insertion, while blunt conical cannulae and those with expanding sleeves produce the smallest fascial defect [10,11,73]. Disposable instruments, of course, are more expensive, but if non-disposable trocars and cannulae are being used it is important that the trocar tips are regularly sharpened to avoid having to use too much force during insertion.

Non-disposable cannulae typically contain a flap or trumpet valve to prevent the leakage of gas. Such valves, however, can damage instruments and make laparoscopic suturing difficult, so modern disposable cannulae generally have a simple diaphragm valve.

LAPAROSCOPIC INSUFFLATOR

Although 'gasless' laparoscopy has its advocates [12], the overwhelming majority of gynaecologists operate within a CO_2 pneumoperitoneum. Most of the principles of safe abdominal insufflation were established by Kurt Semm in the 1970s, and modern fast flow insufflators are merely faster, computerized versions of his original design. As in the case of hysteroscopy, these pumps control intra-abdominal pressure rather than flow, and this should be set at 12–15 mmHg; a higher pressure of up to 25 mmHg is acceptable during the set-up phase as this has the effect of increasing the distance between any trocar being inserted and bowel or large blood vessels, thereby in theory at least, reducing the risk of injury [13]. Some insufflators allow the CO_2 to be warmed prior to insufflation and others have smoke traps built into them, useful when doing CO_2 laser surgery.

SUCTION/IRRIGATION PUMP

An absolute requirement for operative procedures is a suction/irrigation pump. Not only can this be used to aspirate blood and clean the pelvis, but ovarian cysts can be quickly deflated, ectopic pregnancies sucked out, and hydrodissection used in difficult cases. While a basic system using pressure bags and ordinary theatre suction unit is useable, any serious laparoscopic surgeon benefits from the convenience of a dedicated, high-pressure unit.

ANCILLARY INSTRUMENTS

There is an enormous range of disposable and non-disposable instruments available for laparoscopy of various designs and sizes. The usual starting points are 5-mm instruments, although some specialist instruments are only available in larger form (e.g. retrieval bags, morcellators, certain staplers).

If the laparoscope is the eye of the surgeon, grasping forceps are the surgeon's hands. A pair of atraumatic 5-mm grasping forceps is therefore indispensable, ideally ones

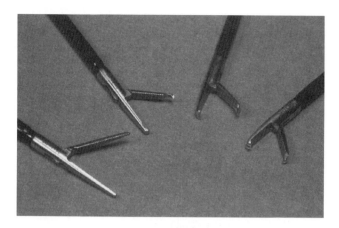

Fig. 50.2 5-mm laparoscopic grasping forceps.

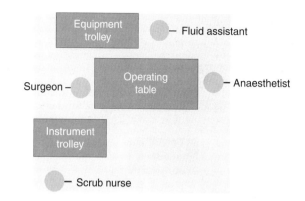

Fig. 50.3 Theatre set-up for hysteroscopic surgery.

which are easy to lock and unlock (Fig. 50.2). Sharp scissors is the other essential if surgery is to be done, and curved Mayo type are arguably the most versatile. Similarly, a suction/irrigation cannula is usually a basic requirement for surgery.

Bipolar forceps should always be available for haemostasis. While scissors can be used electrosurgically to cut or coagulate, and may be considered more convenient, they are generally monopolar instruments and therefore require greater care to avoid unintended burns; monopolar electrosurgery is insufficient for larger vessels (e.g. ovarian or uterine arteries). The argon beam coagulator can be used for fulguration. Clips and staples are also available for haemostasis. The harmonic scalpel and the Ligasure device (Valleylab, USA) are relatively new instruments which can be used both for dissection and haemostasis and may well have an increasingly important role in operative laparoscopy.

Pre-tied loop sutures, suture carriers and needle holders should be available for major procedures both for haemostasis and repair.

Retrieval bags are extremely useful and a better option than extending incisions for the removal of larger masses from the pelvis (e.g. intact ovarian cyst). Once the specimen is in the bag, it is sometimes easier to bring it out through a posterior colpotomy. The gynaecologist is fortunate that, unless the Pouch of Douglas is obliterated, all patients have this exit route. Powered morcellators are an alternative, but small diameter ones tend to be time consuming whereas large ones, although time efficient, leave a relatively large external scar.

Operating theatre organization

Hysteroscopy

While diagnostic hysteroscopy has become an outpatient procedure in most cases, and even minor operative procedures can be done under local anaesthesia, more major surgery (e.g. hysteroscopic myomectomy) usually requires a general anaesthetic. Wherever it is being done, there are a few basic principles to remember. It is best to have all the necessary equipment together on a surgical cart, with the monitor at a comfortable height and position for the operator (and patient if she is awake) (Fig. 50.3).

In the case of an operative procedure where fluid balance becomes an issue, a collecting drape should be placed under the buttocks to save any cervical leakage of irrigant. A member of staff should be appointed whose only duty is to control and monitor fluid balance; for instance, it is important to ensure that air bubbles do not get into the inflow tubing as this risks air embolism.

Laparoscopy

The set-up for laparoscopy is more varied than for hysteroscopy partly because there tends to be more equipment and partly because laparoscopy is not 'solo' surgery but, as is the case with laparotomy, requires the help of assistants. Where they stand, where the surgical carts are placed, where the scrub nurse is situated with the ancillary instruments, and so on, becomes largely a matter of personal preference.

As most laparoscopists prefer to use 0° optics, it is common for one of the assistants to stand on the contralateral side of the patient and control the laparoscope leaving the main surgeon free to operate with two hands. Some, including the author, prefer to use a 30° laparoscope as the ability to 'look around the corner' often affords a better view. On the negative side, the use of an oblique view optic is more difficult, and I therefore prefer to control the laparoscope myself and operate single-handedly (except for suturing and tissue stripping); the first assistant's role then is to hold and retract tissue (Fig. 50.4).

Scheme A

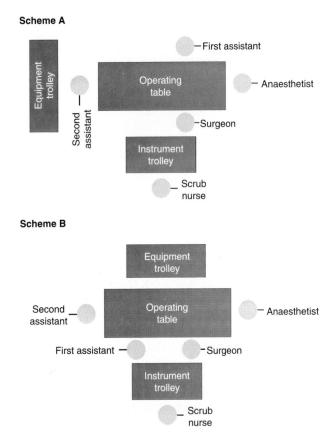

Scheme B

Fig. 50.4 Two schemes for theatre set-up for laparoscopic surgery.

Diagnostic hysteroscopy

Diagnostic hysteroscopy has become a basic investigation in modern gynaecology and has essentially replaced the time honoured D & C (dilation and curettage). It can be done as an outpatient procedure, and is an integral component of a One-Stop approach to the management of menstrual symptoms [14]. Hysteroscopy provides a virtually instant diagnosis, and is the logical precursor to operative hysteroscopy. The Royal College of Obstetricians and Gynaecologists (RCOG) has recognized the importance of diagnostic hysteroscopy and it is now part of core training in our speciality. The indications and contraindications, of which there are few, are summarized in Table 50.1. The hysteroscopic view is best in the immediate postmenstrual phase, but a diagnosis is usually possible at any time, even during menstruation. Liquid distension has several advantages over the use of CO_2 [15].

TECHNIQUE

The patient should be in the correct position, which means lithotomy with the hips well flexed and the buttocks

Table 50.1 Indications and contraindications to diagnostic hysteroscopy

Indications	Abnormal menstruation (age >40 years)
	Abnormal menstruation not responsive to medical treatment (age <40 years)
	Intermenstrual bleeding (IMB) despite normal cervical smear
	Post coital bleeding (PCB) despite normal cervical smear
	Post menopausal bleeding (PMB) (persistent or endometrial thickness ≥4 mm)
	Abnormal pelvic ultrasound findings (e.g. endometrial polyps, submucous fibroids)
	Subfertility
	Recurrent miscarriage
	Asherman's syndrome
	Congenital uterine anomaly
	Lost intrauterine contraceptive device (IUCD)
Contraindications	Pelvic infection
	Pregnancy
	Cervical cancer
	(Heavy uterine bleeding)

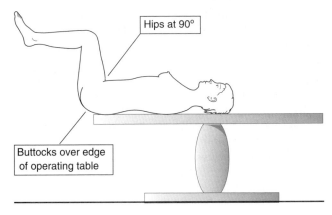

Fig. 50.5 Patient position for hysteroscopy.

slightly over the edge of the table to allow unimpeded access irrespective of uterine position (Fig. 50.5). The perineum and vagina are usually washed with a warmed antiseptic solution, although there are those who do not clean the vagina. Full draping of the perineum, legs and lower abdomen is rarely required. A gentle bimanual examination should be done to determine the size and position of the uterus.

CONVENTIONAL TECHNIQUE

The conventional approach to diagnostic hysteroscopy, and certainly the one that is quickest and easiest if the

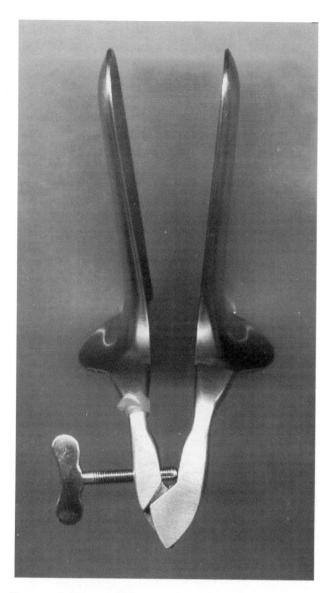

Fig. 50.6 Collin speculum.

Table 50.2
Anaesthesia for
hysteroscopy

Intracervical L.A.
L.A. spray
L.A. gel
Paracervical L.A.
Regional anaesthesia
General anaesthesia
Nothing

L.A. Local anaesthetic

Unlike in cystoscopy, it is better to guide the hysteroscope into the uterine cavity under direct vision rather than blindly by means of on obturator. When using an oblique-view optic, it is important to take account of this angulation by adjusting the approach accordingly (Fig. 50.7a–d). Once in the uterine cavity, it is simply a matter of systematically inspecting the fundus, tubal areas and the four walls of the uterus by a combination of rotating (if using an oblique-view hysteroscope) and moving the hysteroscope up/down and left/right. If the view is poor, it is usually because the intrauterine pressure is too low, either because the distending medium is at a relatively low pressure or pressure is lost through cervical leakage. Once the uterine cavity has been inspected, the hysteroscope is withdrawn which is the best time to inspect the endocervical canal. A biopsy can then be taken, if indicated, using a small curette or a device such as a Pipelle, or a change made to an operative sheath for a target biopsy.

'NO TOUCH' HYSTEROSCOPY AND 'NO TOUCH' BIOPSY

An alternative approach to the above is 'no touch' or vaginoscopic hysteroscopy [17]. This technique is ideally suited to the outpatient clinic as it minimizes patient discomfort by the simple fact that no additional instruments (e.g. speculum and tenaculum) need to be inserted into the vagina. Instead, the tip of the hysteroscope is introduced into the vaginal introitus, the low-viscosity distension medium is turned on, and the hysteroscope is guided under direct vision to the external cervical os, along the cervical canal and thence the uterine cavity. This method works in the majority of cases unless there is cervical stenosis, and it is uncommon to have to stop to give local anaesthetic. As a result, this is now our default approach to outpatient hysteroscopy.

It is now also possible to take an endometrial biopsy using a 'no touch' technique without the need to instrument the uterus. Based on the Pipelle, the H Pipelle (Laboratoire C.C.D., France) is approximately twice as

patient is asleep, is to insert a speculum into the vagina to visualize the cervix (a single-hinged Collin speculum is preferable to a Cuscoe as it can be removed once the hysteroscope has been inserted) (Fig. 50.6), hold the anterior lip with a tenaculum, sound the cervix and uterine cavity, and then insert the hysteroscope with or without prior cervical dilatation depending on the calibre of the cervical canal. A similar technique can also be used in the outpatient setting, with the option of giving a local anaesthetic if required (Table 50.2); the injection of 2–4 ml of 2.2% lignocaine with 1:80,000 adrenaline via a dental syringe and needle is arguably the easiest and safest. Pre-emptive analgesia with non-steroidals seems to make little difference to any discomfort [16].

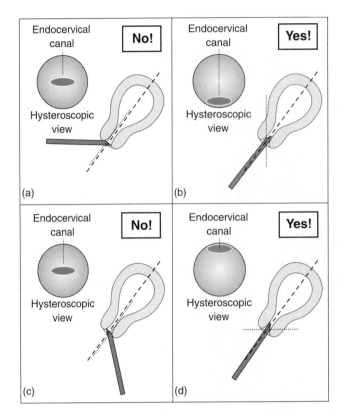

Fig. 50.7 How to insert an oblique view hysteroscope into the uterus. (a) Incorrect insertion hysteroscope looking upwards. (b) Correct insertion hysteroscope looking upwards. (c) Incorrect insertion hysteroscope looking downwards. (d) Correct insertion hysteroscope looking downwards.

long but narrow enough to be passed through even a narrow diagnostic sheath. At the end of the hysteroscopy, the hysteroscope is not fully withdrawn from the cervix. The diagnostic sheath is then unlocked and the optic removed to be replaced by the H Pipelle which is pushed through the sheath into the uterine cavity (Fig. 50.8). Once the uterine fundus is reached, the sheath is pulled out of the cervix and an endometrial biopsy taken in the usual fashion [18].

RESULTS

The medical literature is replete with studies of diagnostic hysteroscopy, and although arguments rage with those who favour ultrasound, it remains the gold standard technique for the assessment of the uterine cavity. Even outpatient hysteroscopy has been shown to have a success rate of well over 90% [19]. The pick-up rate of pathology depends on the indication, but about 40–50% of women with menstrual symptoms will have positive findings, chiefly fibroids and polyps [19], and figures as high as 60% have been reported in infertility [20,21].

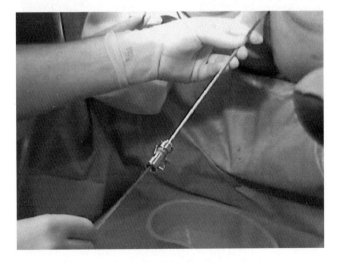

Fig. 50.8 The H Pipelle being used for biopsy after vaginoscopic or 'no touch' hysteroscopy.

COMPLICATIONS

Diagnostic hysteroscopy is a safe procedure, and complications are uncommon [19]. Perhaps the most frequently seen problem is pain when negotiating the cervix or distending the uterine cavity, and a vaso-vagal reaction to cervical dilatation. The simple act of stopping and giving local anaesthesia is usually enough to solve the problem, and it is rare to have to resort to giving atropine for a bradycardia. Uterine perforation should not happen if the hysteroscope is introduced under direct vision unless there is extreme cervical stenosis; in this situation, insertion of the hysteroscope under ultrasound guidance is a useful ploy, as may be prior priming with a prostaglandin [22]. Infection and excessive bleeding are rarely seen.

Operative hysteroscopy

Hysteroscopic surgery has a number of well-defined indications (Table 50.3), and is the treatment of choice for polypectomy, myomectomy for intracavitary or submucous fibroids, adhesiolysis and metroplasty. The various techniques of endometrial destruction have been superseded to some extent by the newer, second generation ablative techniques which are technically easier to perform [23]. Not listed in Table 50.3 is hysteroscopic sterilization which has become a reality with the introduction of the Essure device [24].

Any of the modalities already discussed can be used for surgery, but even now the resectoscope remains the most versatile of instruments and is a skill well worth learning. Pretreatment to thin the endometrium and make it less fluffy is often worthwhile for the more major procedures as it greatly facilitates the surgery [25]. The choice is between using GnRH analogues, danazol, a progestogen or the combined pill, usually for at least 6 weeks prior to surgery. The alternative is either to time the operation to just after menstruation, which can be difficult, or to curette the endometrium prior to hysteroscopy, but neither is as good as endometrial preparation.

Table 50.3 RCOG classification of operative hysteroscopy procedures

Level 1	Diagnostic hysteroscopy with target biopsy Removal of simple polyps Removal of intrauterine contraceptive device
Level 2	Proximal fallopian tube cannulation Minor Asherman's syndrome Removal of pedunculated fibroid (type 0) or large polyp
Level 3	Division/resection of uterine septum Major Asherman's syndrome Endometrial resection of ablation Resection of submucous fibroid (type 1 or type 2) Repeat endometrial ablation or resection

TECHNIQUES

Although minor procedures using mechanical instruments or the Versapoint can be done under local anaesthesia, more major cases are generally managed under general anaesthesia. However, even such cases can be carried out under local anaesthesia combined with light sedation. Our regimen, for instance, consists of a diclofenac and temazepam premed, followed by small doses of midazolam and fentanyl or alfentanyl in the operating theatre, finished with intracervical, paracervical and intrauterine local anaesthetic injections, the latter given via an injection needle option to our resectoscope [26].

There is insufficient space here to describe how to use all the various instruments available to the hysteroscopic surgeon or how to carry out specific procedures, but because of its versatility and usefulness, it is worthwhile discussing the principles of using the resectoscope safely and effectively.

Using a resectoscope

The resectoscope is a very powerful instrument which has to be used correctly to ensure the safety of the patient. The first step is to dilate the cervix sufficiently to allow easy insertion but not to over-dilate and risk excessive leakage of the uterine irrigant and poor distension; dilating to 1 mm above the diameter of the resectoscope is adequate for this. Once the resectoscope has been inserted and the decision made that hysteroscopic surgery can proceed, there are three cardinal rules to remember:

1 The electrode should only be activated as it is being moved into the resectoscope sheath, that is, towards the cervix; activating the electrode as it is being pushed out risks uterine perforation, a potentially life-threatening complication. The only exception to this rule is metroplasty when the cut has to be made towards the uterine fundus.

2 The myometrium should not be cut too deeply, particularly at the cornu and in the cervix; if cut ends of arterioles become visible, the resection is too deep. Cutting deeply does not only risk uterine perforation, but also major haemorrhage.

3 Fluid balance should be monitored continuously. Several methods of fluid monitoring have been suggested (e.g. assessment of central venous pressure, serial measurement of serum Na +, osmolality or tracer substances such as 1% ethanol, weighing the patient), but the simplest is to keep an inflow/outflow chart. In any event, surgery should be stopped if fluid absorption exceeds 1.5–2 l to avoid serious fluid overload and a transurethral resection of prostate (TURP)-like syndrome [27].

RESULTS

Provided the indication is appropriate, hysteroscopic surgery can be highly effective. The literature concerning polypectomy is not extensive but logically, removal of polyps under direct vision is likely to be superior to blind curettage [71,28]. In contrast, there are numerous series showing the efficacy of hysteroscopic myomectomy particularly when the uterus is not grossly enlarged and the fibroid(s) are mainly intracavitary [29,30]. Metroplasty should no longer be done by laparotomy [31], and the same applies to the treatment of Asherman's syndrome [32]. Hysteroscopic endometrial resection or ablation have been subjected to numerous randomized trials and cost–benefit analyses showing that they are effective and useful alternatives to hysterectomy (e.g. [33,34,72]), but are no more effective than the newer second generation techniques [23]. The Mirena IUS (Schering) is of course another effective alternative for such patients [35].

COMPLICATIONS

Although complications are uncommon with operative hysteroscopy [36], anyone carrying out hysteroscopic surgery should be aware of the risks, their prevention and management (Table 50.4). Uterine perforation is the most feared complication because if it occurs while the hysteroscope is being activated, major intra-abdominal trauma can result with haemorrhage and viscus injury. The first sign of perforation might be a sudden loss of uterine distension or rapid absorption of fluid. A laparoscopy and arguably a laparotomy is mandatory to check the abdominal contents; if there is no injury, hysteroscopic surgery can continue once the perforation has been sutured. Perforation is most likely when using the resectoscope, although proper technique can greatly reduce this risk [37].

Fluid overload with low-viscosity fluids, particularly those which are electrolyte free, is the second fear of the hysteroscopic surgeon. Fluid is absorbed throughout surgery by intravasation and transtubal loss. Apart from the cardiac and pulmonary effects, major electrolyte imbalance can result [38]. This complication is totally avoidable by proper monitoring during surgery and stopping the procedure before the patient is placed at risk. We also catheterize the bladder and give a low dose of frusemide once glycine absorption exceeds 1.5 l to induce a diuresis, monitoring recovery by regular assay of serum Na + 0.

Intraoperative haemorrhage can accompany uterine perforation but is more often a sign of surgery deep in the myometrium. Electrocoagulation (or laser coagulation) of the offending vessel can be one solution, but if the bleeding persists at the end of the procedure, tamponade for a few hours with a balloon catheter usually works [39].

Air embolism is a rare but devastating complication [40]. It usually happens if air is allowed to get into the distension tubing, typically when bags of irrigant are being changed. Air embolism therefore is largely preventable.

Infection is rare after hysteroscopic surgery. Although there is no evidence in its favour [41], I prescribe prophylactic antibiotics to women undergoing operative hysteroscopy (usually 1.2 g Augmentin® i.v).

Cervical priming with misoprostol has been proposed as a means of reducing the risk of cervical lacerations during dilatation [42], but in my experience this is a very rare complication.

The late adverse consequences of endometrial ablation are all relatively rare. Cervical stenosis in the presence of functional endometrial tissue can lead to the development of haematometra, and women who have been sterilized can develop painful swellings of the fallopian tubes secondary to retrograde menstruation [43]. Pregnancies have been reported, many with complications [44]. A handful of cases of endometrial cancer have been described after endometrial ablation, but the majority had risk factors [45].

Table 50.4 Complications of operative hysteroscopy

Early	Uterine perforation
	Fluid overload
	Haemorrhage
	Gas embolism
	Infection
	Cervical trauma
Late	Intrauterine adhesions
	Haematometra (after endometrial ablation)
	Postablation sterilization syndrome (after endometrial ablation)
	Pregnancy (after endometrial ablation)
	Cancer (after endometrial ablation)

Diagnostic laparoscopy

Having replaced culdoscopy in the 1960s and 1970s, diagnostic laparoscopy has been an accepted part of gynaecological care even longer than diagnostic hysteroscopy. It is usually done as an inpatient procedure under general anaesthesia, although microlaparoscopes have been used with some success [46]. The main indication for diagnostic laparoscopy is the investigation of pelvic pain and subfertility (Table 50.5). While the list of contraindications is relatively long, few patients fall into these categories.

Table 50.5 Indications and contraindications for diagnostic laparoscopy

Indications	Acute or chronic pelvic pain
	Ectopic pregnancy
	Pelvic inflammatory disease (including TB)
	Endometriosis
	Adnexal torsion
	Subfertility
	Congenital pelvic abnormality
	Abnormal pelvic scan
	Unexplained pelvic mass
	Staging for ovarian malignancy
Absolute and relative contraindications	Mechanical or paralytic bowel obstruction
	Generalized peritonitis
	Diaphragmatic hernia
	Major intraperitoneal haemorrhage (e.g. shock)
	Severe cardiorespiratory disease
	Massive obesity
	Inflammatory bowel disease
	Large abdominal mass
	Advanced pregnancy
	Multiple abdominal incisions
	Irreducible external hernia

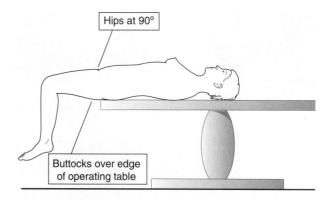

Fig. 50.9 Patient positioning during laparoscopy.

Table 50.6 Technique for subumbilical insufflation and insertion of the primary port

Palpate for aorta
Elevate anterior abdominal wall (to increase distance between needle and bowel/major vessels)
Aim Veress needle and trocar and cannula towards the hollow of the sacrum (away from major vessels)
Create a high-pressure pneumoperitoneum prior to inserting umbilical trocar and cannula (to increase distance between needle and bowel/major vessels)
Insert trocar and cannula no more than a few centimetres into the peritoneal cavity (to reduce risk of bowel or vascular injury)
Avoid Trendelenburg tilt (head down) until laparoscope has been inserted (to avoid bringing major vessels closer to umbilicus)
Avoid excessive force during insertion (to limit the distance the instruments advance into the peritoneal cavity)

TECHNIQUES

As with hysteroscopy, it is important to position the patient correctly on the operating table. Again, this means ensuring that the buttocks are over the edge of the table to allow full uterine anteversion. The legs are ideally placed in hydraulic leg supports with the thighs at about 45° to the horizontal while ensuring that the hips can be extended sufficiently to bring the thighs in line with the trunk should the need arise for any abdominal (cf. pelvic) surgery (Fig. 50.9).

After washing and draping, the bladder is checked and if full, emptied with a catheter. Bimanual examination will also confirm the size, position and mobility of the uterus as well as any adnexal pathology. The uterus is sounded and a uterine cannula inserted, firstly to permit effective uterine manipulation and secondly to allow for hydrotubation if required; should the uterus be retroverted, it is worthwhile attempting to forcibly antevert it by rotating the uterine cannula 180° as this will greatly improve access to the Pouch of Douglas at laparoscopy.

Subumbilical insufflation

Although open and gasless laparoscopy have their proponents, for most gynaecologists laparoscopy starts with insufflation of the peritoneal cavity with CO_2 using a Veress needle. The spring mechanism of the Veress needle should be checked as this is an essential safety feature. It is also useful to check the flow of gas through the needle, making a note of the pressure in the tubing as this information can be used later to confirm proper intraperitoneal placement. The usual insertion point for the Veress needle is the inferior border of the umbilicus, and we prefer to make a vertical midline incision long enough to accommodate the umbilical trocar and cannula.

The actual technique of inserting the Veress needle and subsequently the trocar and cannula for the laparoscope are summarized in Table 50.6. The aim is to instrument the peritoneal cavity without causing any unnecessary trauma; it should be remembered, for instance that the aortic bifurcation is inferior to the umbilicus in a significant proportion of women, and account should be taken of this with the umbilical instruments [47].

Once the Veress needle is in place, correct positioning can be checked using Palmer's test; the basis of the test is that saline in a syringe should be sucked into the peritoneal cavity because of its negative pressure. Alternatively, the gas tubing can be connected and the flow and pressure

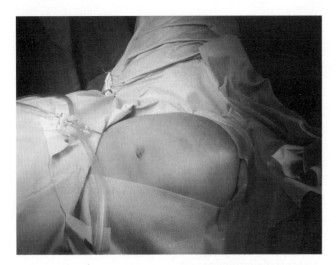

Fig. 50.10 CO$_2$ insufflation via Palmer's point.

of gas monitored; little flow at high pressure suggests some obstruction, often retroperitoneal placement, and the Veress should then be repositioned. It is reasonable to insufflate to a relatively high intra-abdominal pressure (e.g. 20–25 mmHg) to reduce the risk of viscus injury during insertion of the primary trocar and cannula [13].

Once the correct distension has been reached, the gas is switched off, the Veress needle removed and the trocar and cannula inserted, again taking care to aim towards the sacral hollow. Some gynaecologists manually elevate the lower abdominal wall at this time, others press the upper abdomen to increase the gas bubble in front of the oncoming trocar.

Insufflation via Palmer's point

A well-recognized alternative to subumbilical insufflation is the use of Palmer's point, which is situated in the left mid-clavicular line approximately 3 cm below the costal margin (Fig. 50.10). The left upper quadrant of the abdomen is the area least likely to be affected by adhesions, so Palmer's point is useful when there is a concern about possible lower abdominal or peri-umbilical adhesions (e.g. midline laparotomy incision, appendicitis). Palmer's point is also useful when dealing with a large pelvic mass. The technique of entry is similar to that already described.

Open laparoscopy

There is much debate about the relative safety of 'closed' and 'open' laparoscopy, which was in fact first described by Hasson, a gynaecologist, in 1970 (see for an update and description of the technique the article by Hasson

et al. [48]). While open laparoscopy is favoured by surgeons, and this approach is claimed to reduce the risk of vascular and bowel injury, this is by no means proven [49]. However, there have been no large-scale randomized comparisons and for now at least, the overwhelming majority of gynaecologists continue to use a Veress needle for insufflation [50,51].

INSERTION OF ANCILLARY PORT(S)

Once the laparoscope has been inserted, the patient can be placed head down to encourage the bowel out of the pelvis and lower abdomen; the greater the tilt, the better the view of the pelvis but the more difficult it is for the anaesthetist to ventilate the patient. A quick check is made of the abdominal cavity, and one or two ancillary ports are inserted in the lower abdomen. Injury by the ancillary ports can be minimized by inserting them under direct vision having identified the deep and superficial epigastric vessels and the bladder [52].

A useful concept here is that of the 'safe triangle' which is bounded by the umbilical ligaments (remnants of the umbilical vessels) laterally with the symphysis pubis as its base and the umbilicus as its apex (Plate 50.1, *facing p. 562*); although the position of the inferior epigastric vessels can be variable [53], their course is always lateral to the safe triangle (Plate 50.2, *facing p. 562*). Ports should therefore be placed either inside the safe triangle or lateral to the inferior epigastric vessels.

INSPECTING THE PELVIS AND ABDOMEN

It is not possible to inspect the pelvis properly without using at least one probe or grasper to manipulate the pelvic organs. Once the upper abdomen has been checked, bowel in the cul-de-sac should be gently pushed cephalad. The best way to inspect the adnexa and pelvic side wall is to grasp, lift and rotate the ovary towards the ipsilateral round ligament, a manoeuvre which also reveals the course of the ureter (Plate 50.3, *facing p. 562*). Don't forget to inspect the uterovesical fold which can be the sole site of endometriosis. Tubal patency can then be checked by hydrotubation with dilute methylene blue solution.

ENDING THE PROCEDURE

The ancillary ports should be removed under direct vision followed by deflation of the abdomen via the port used for the optic. By keeping the laparoscope inside the cannula as it is being withdrawn, it is possible to check that this port site is not bleeding and has not caught a loop of bowel or omentum. The fascia in lateral ports ≥ 10 mm should be formally closed to prevent herniation [54].

RESULTS

The rate of detection of pathology very much depends on the indication for the laparoscopy. Some abnormalities will be obvious from preoperative investigation, usually ultrasound, where laparoscopy is merely used to confirm or clarify the diagnosis. Although diagnostic laparoscopy is no longer recommended as a standard investigation for all infertile couples [55], the detection rate for unexpected conditions such as endometriosis and pelvic adhesions is about 20% [56]. In the case of chronic pelvic pain, one study reported positive findings in every one of the 141 patients laparoscoped [57].

COMPLICATIONS

Diagnostic laparoscopy is a safe procedure with published complication rates of 2–4 per 1000 [58,59]. By definition, as no laparoscopic surgery is being done, most complications occur during the set-up phase of the procedure when the abdomen is being instrumented (e.g. injury to the inferior epigastric vessels or major retroperitoneal vessels, bowel injury). Bleeding from the inferior epigastrics should be avoidable with good technique, but if does occur, a variety of instruments and techniques have been described to control the bleeding [60]. Injury to retroperitoneal vessels usually requires immediate laparotomy, whereas bowel injury can be managed laparoscopically provided the perforation is small and there is minimal faecal soiling [58].

Operative laparoscopy

The question these days is not so much what can be done laparoscopically, but what cannot? The answer is that most procedures done by laparotomy can be done laparoscopically provided there is no large pelvic mass or extensive malignancy (Table 50.7). This does not mean that laparoscopy is the best option or should be done in all these cases, and there is much debate about the more complex procedures in particular. In fact, only a few procedures have been subjected to prospective randomized comparisons (e.g. ectopic pregnancy, colposuspension, endometriosis, hysterectomy), so in many cases the decision about the route of surgery depends more on the particular skills of the gynaecologist, the presence of contraindications, and the relative risks of complications.

TECHNIQUES

There is insufficient space to describe individual procedures, but the following considerations and techniques are generally applicable to operative laparoscopy.

Table 50.7 RCOG classification of laparoscopic procedures

Level 1	Diagnostic laparoscopy
	Sterilization
	Aspiration of ovarian cyst
	Ovarian biopsy
Level 2	Division of filmy adhesions
	Linear salpingotomy or salpingectomy for ectopic pregnancy
	Salpingostomy for infertility
	Ovarian cystectomy
	Treatment of endometrioma
	Salpingo-oophorectomy
	Ovarian drilling with laser or diathermy for polycystic ovaries
	Treatment of American Fertility Society (AFS) Stage I and II endometriosis
	Myomectomy for pedunculated subserous fibroid
	Laparoscopic uterosacral nerve ablation (LUNA)
	Laparoscopically assisted vaginal hysterectomy (LAVH) without significant associated pathology
Level 3	Division of thick adhesions
	LAVH with significant associated pathology
	Total laparoscopic hysterectomy
	Myomectomy for intramural fibroids
	Treatment of AFS Stage III and IV endometriosis
	Pelvic and aortic lymphadenectomy
	Pelvic side wall and ureteric dissection
	Presacral neurectomy
	Incontinence procedures
	Prolapse procedures

WHERE TO PLACE THE ANCILLARY PORTS

Operative laparoscopy inevitably requires multiple ports, and 2–3 ancillary ports are the norm. The ports are most usefully placed well lateral to the inferior epigastric vessels, and should be inserted high enough so that any instrument can be used on both sides of the pelvis. If there is to be anything more than the occasional suturing, a 10-mm port will allow the insertion of curved needles without having to remove the ports with each suture [61]; a larger cannula will also accept larger diameter instruments (e.g. SEMM claw forceps).

TISSUE DISSECTION AND HYDRODISSECTION

The principles of dissection and adhesiolysis are the same as at laparotomy, that is traction and counter-traction. Dissection can be done with scissors, and if monopolar electrosurgery or CO_2 laser is used, additional care has to be taken to avoid thermal damage to nearby structures. High-pressure irrigation can sometimes facilitate dissection as well as protect underlying structures from thermal injury.

SAFE USE OF ELECTROSURGERY

Electrosurgery is widely used at laparoscopy for haemostasis as well as cutting. As electrosurgical injury is one of the most feared of complications, it is essential that every care is taken. Whatever instrument is used, it should only be activated when in view of the laparoscope, and the electrode(s) should be withdrawn fully into the cannula afterwards to avoid accidental injury. Electrosurgery should only be used close to bowel or other vital structures in short bursts, if at all. The surgeon should be aware of risks due to insulation failure, direct and capacitive coupling, and remember that the electrodes remain hot for a few seconds after activation.

LAPAROSCOPIC SUTURING

The ability to suture extra- and intracorporeally is an extremely useful skill and can mean the difference between a successful laparoscopy and laparotomy. Pre-tied loop sutures are the easiest to use and are ideal for procedures such as salpingectomy. Untied ties can be used to tie off adhesions or vascular pedicles (e.g. infundibulo-ligament at hysterectomy or salpingo-oophorectomy) and are secured with slip knots (e.g. Roeder, Weston or surgeon's knot) and a knot pusher. Needle sutures are used to repair incisions (e.g. uterine repair at myomectomy), and can be tied extra-corporeally or tied inside the body in the case of delicate tissue (e.g. ovarian repair after cystectomy).

RESULTS

Laparoscopic surgery, for whatever indication, is typically associated with less postoperative discomfort, shorter hospitalization and faster return to normal activities than laparotomy. On the down-side, the more complex procedures tend to take longer, and the operating time is less predictable [62]. Cost comparisons produce variable results, a longer operating time and the use disposable instruments often outweighing any advantages of shorter hospitalization.

COMPLICATIONS

Laparoscopic surgery appears to be inherently safer than conventional surgery [63]. However, although the overall complication rate is generally less, this is not inevitable (e.g. [64]) (Table 50.8). What is definitely true is that (1) major complications such as viscus injury and bleeding from retroperitoneal vessels are more common, and, unfortunately, (2) many of the injuries are not recognized during the procedure.

Table 50.8 Complications of laparoscopic surgery

Intraoperative	Bowel injury
	Vascular injury
	Bladder injury
	Ureteric injury
	Surgical emphysema
	Anaesthetic complications
Post operative	Unrecognized visceral or vascular injury
	Venous thromboembolism
	Infection
	Port site hernia

The reported rate of complications from major national surveys give an overall figure of 7–12.6 per 1000 procedures, with the more complex procedures having a greater risk of injury [59,65,66]. More specifically, the risk of intraoperative intestinal injury has been estimated as 1.6–2.4 per 1000, major vascular injuries as 0.3 per 1000, and damage to the urinary tract in 2–8.5 per 1000 cases. Laparoscopic hysterectomy, in particular, places the ureter at risk of injury [64,66,67]. About 1:3 complications occur during the set-up phase, and 1:4 are not recognized during the surgery, including more than half of bowel and ureteric injuries. Conversion to laparotomy is required, on average, in 2% of patients [68]. The mortality after gynaecological laparoscopy is 4.4 per 100,000, which compares with mortality of 150 per 100,000 for hysterectomy for benign indications [68,69].

Informed consent for endoscopy

There is a common misconception among patients that 'key hole' surgery converts a 'major' surgical procedure in to a 'minor' one, and not only is the cosmetic result better and recovery faster, but the risks are also lessened. The reality is that it is only the incision size which is different. It is not surprising therefore that if there is a problem, patients often assume there has been negligence. As a result, endoscopic surgery has become one of the major areas of medical litigation in gynaecology [70].

The Department of Health as well as the General Medical council have issued guidelines regarding informed consent for surgery, and there is also much useful information available on the internet on this topic. While appropriate indications for surgery and good surgical technique are basic requirements for effective patient care, the patients also have to be provided with sufficient information on which to base their decision to undergo a particular procedure. All patients should be told not only what and why they are undergoing a particular procedure, but also warned about the relative risks of MAS compared with conventional surgery. In particular, patients need to be aware that any endoscopic operation may have to be converted to laparotomy, that bowel, bladder and ureteric injury are accepted risks with laparoscopy, and uterine perforation and fluid overload with hysteroscopy.

Training in endoscopic surgery

One area which MAS has changed for ever is surgical training. Endoscopic surgery is very different to conventional surgery and it probably takes longer to acquire the necessary skills to operate without the benefits of direct vision and tissue handling.

As an acknowledgement of the importance of hysteroscopic and laparoscopic surgery to modern gynaecological care coupled to a wish to improve and structure training in this area, the Royal College of Obstetricians and Gynaecologists have made basic endoscopic surgery (Level 1 hysteroscopy and laparoscopy) a core curriculum subject for trainees. The College has appointed preceptors, and is currently introducing Special Skills Modules for advanced hysteroscopic and laparoscopic surgery as a means of accreditation for those wishing to extend their skills. This is the first time that surgical proficiency in a particular area has been so tested and these modules may yet prove to be models for other surgical procedures.

References

1. Semm K (1983) Endoscopic appendectomy. *Endoscopy* **15**, 59–64.
2. Magos A, Kosmas I, Taylor A, Sharma M & Buck L (2005) Digital recording of surgical procedures using a personal computer. *Eur J Obset Gynaecol* **120**, 206–9.
3. Neuwirth RS (1978) A new technique for and additional experience with hysteroscopic resection of submucous fibroids. *Am J Obstet Gynecol* **131**, 91–4.
4. Kung RC, Vilos GA, Thomas B, Penkin P, Zaltz AP & Stabinsky SA (1999) A new bipolar system for performing operative hysteroscopy in normal saline. *J Am Assoc Gynecol Laparosc* **6**, 331–6.
5. Goldrath MH, Fuller TA & Segal S (1981) Laser photovaporization of endometrium for the treatment of menorrhagia. *Am J Obstet Gynecol* **140**, 14–9.
6. Lethaby A & Hickey M (2002) Endometrial destruction techniques for heavy menstrual bleeding. *Cochrane Database Syst Rev* **2**, CD001501.
7. Gordon AG & Magos AL (1989) The development of laparoscopic surgery. *Baillieres Clin Obstet Gynaecol* **3**, 429–49.
8. Sanders RR & Filshie GM (1974) Transfundal induction of pneumoperitoneum prior to laparoscopy. *J Obstet Gynaecol Br Commonw* **81**, 829–30.
9. Santala M, Jarvela I & Kauppila A (1999) Transfundal insertion of a Veress needle in laparoscopy of obese subjects: a practical alternative. *Hum Reprod* **14**, 2277–8.
10. Tarnay CM, Glass KB & Munro MG (1999) Entry force and intra-abdominal pressure associated with six laparoscopic trocar-cannula systems: a randomized comparison. *Obstet Gynecol* **94**, 83–8.
11. Yim SF & Yuen PM (2001) Randomized double-masked comparison of radially expanding access device and conventional cutting tip trocar in laparoscopy. *Obstet Gynecol* **97**, 435–8.
12. Alijani A & Cuschieri A (2001) Abdominal wall lift systems in laparoscopic surgery: gasless and low-pressure systems. *Semin Laparosc Surg* **8**, 53–62.
13. Reich H, Ribeiro SC, Rasmussen C, Rosenberg J & Vidali A (1999) High-pressure trocar insertion technique. *JSLS* **3**, 45–8.
14. Baskett TF, O'Connor H & Magos AL (1996) A comprehensive one-stop menstrual problem clinic for the diagnosis and management of abnormal uterine bleeding. *Br J Obstet Gynaecol* **103**, 76–7.
15. Nagele F, Bournas N, O'Connor H, Broadbent M, Richardson R & Magos A (1996) Comparison of carbon dioxide and normal saline for uterine distension in outpatient hysteroscopy. *Fertil Steril* **62**, 305–9.
16. Nagele F, Lockwood G & Magos AL (1997) Randomised placebo controlled trial of mefenamic acid for premedication at outpatient hysteroscopy: a pilot study. *Br J Obstet Gynaecol* **104**, 842–4.
17. Cicinelli E, Parisi C, Galantino P, Pinto V, Barba B & Schonauer S (2003) Reliability, feasibility, and safety of minihysteroscopy with a vaginoscopic approach: experience with 6,000 cases. *Fertil Steril* **80**, 199–202.
18. Di Spiezio SA, Sharma M, Taylor A, Buck L & Magos A (2004) A new device for 'no touch' biopsy at 'no touch' hysteroscopy: the H Pipelle. *Am J Obstet Gynecol* **191**, 157–8.
19. Nagele F, O'Connor H, Davies A, Badawy A, Mohamed H & Magos A (1996) 2500 outpatient diagnostic hysteroscopies. *Obstet Gynecol* **88**, 87–92.
20. Valle RF (1980) Hysteroscopy in the evaluation of female infertility. *Am J Obstet Gynecol* **137**, 425–31.
21. Preutthipan S & Linasmita V (2003) A prospective comparative study between hysterosalpingography and hysteroscopy in the detection of intrauterine pathology in patients with infertility. *J Obstet Gynaecol Res* **29**, 33–7.
22. Preutthipan S & Herabutya Y (1999) A randomized controlled trial of vaginal misoprostol for cervical priming before hysteroscopy. *Obstet Gynecol* **94**, 427–30.
23. Bradley LD (2004) New endometrial ablation techniques for treatment of menorrhagia. *Surg Technol Int* **12**, 161–70.
24. Kerin JF, Carignan CS & Cher D (2001) The safety and effectiveness of a new hysteroscopic method for permanent birth control: results of the first Essure pbc clinical study. *Aust N Z J Obstet Gynaecol* **41**, 364–70.
25. Romer T (1998) Benefit of GnRH analogue pretreatment for hysteroscopic surgery in patients with bleeding disorders. *Gynecol Obstet Invest* **45**(Suppl 1), 12–20.
26. Lockwood GM, Baumann R, Turnbull AC & Magos AL (1992) Extensive hysteroscopic surgery under local anaesthesia. *Gynaecol Endosc* **1**, 15–21.
27. Baumann R, Magos AL, Kay JDS & Turnbull AC (1990) Absorption of glycine irrigating solution during transcervical resection of endometrium. *Br Med J* **300**, 304–5.

28. Cravello L, Stolla V, Bretelle F, Roger V & Blanc B (2000) Hysteroscopic resection of endometrial polyps. A study of 195 cases. *Eur J Obstet Gynecol Reprod Biol* **93**, 131–4.

29. Derman SG, Rehnstrom J & Neuwirth RS (1991) The long-term effectiveness of hysteroscopic treatment of menorrhagia and leiomyomas. *Obstet Gynecol* **77**, 591–4.

30. Hart R, Molnar BG & Magos A (1999) Long term follow up of hysteroscopic myomectomy assessed by survival analysis. *Br J Obstet Gynaecol* **106**, 700–5.

31. Homer HA, Li TC & Cooke ID (2000) The septate uterus: a review of management and reproductive outcome. *Fertil Steril* **73**, 1–14.

32. Magos A (2002) Hysteroscopic treatment of Asherman's syndrome. *Reprod Biomed Online* **4**(Suppl 3), 46–51.

33. Sculpher MJ, Dwyer N, Byford S & Stirrat GM (1996) Randomised trial comparing hysterectomy and transcervical endometrial resection: effect on health related quality of life and costs two years after surgery. *Br J Obstet Gynaecol* **103**, 142–9.

34. O'Connor H & Magos A (1996) Endometrial resection for the treatment of menorrhagia: evaluation of the results at 5 years. *N Engl J Med* **335**, 151–6.

35. Rauramo I, Elo I & Istre O (2004) Long-term treatment of menorrhagia with levonorgestrel intrauterine system versus endometrial resection. *Obstet Gynecol* **104**, 1314–21.

36. Aydeniz B, Gruber IV, Schauf B, Kurek R, Meyer A & Wallwiener D (2002) A multicenter survey of complications associated with 21,676 operative hysteroscopies. *Eur J Obstet Gynecol Reprod Biol* **104**, 160–4.

37. Overton C, Hargreaves J & Maresh M (1997) A national survey of the complications of endometrial destruction for menstrual disorders: the MISTLETOE study. Minimally Invasive Surgical Techniques-Laser, EndoThermal or Endoresection. *Br J Obstet Gynaecol* **104**, 1351–9.

38. Istre O, Bjoennes J, Naess R, Hornbaek K & Forman A (1994) Postoperative cerebral oedema after transcervical endometrial resection and uterine irrigation with 1.5% glycine. *Lancet* **344**, 1187–9.

39. Erian MM & Goh JT (1996) Transcervical endometrial resection. *J Am Assoc Gynecol Laparosc* **3**, 263–6.

40. Brooks PG (1997) Venous air embolism during operative hysteroscopy. *J Am Assoc Gynecol Laparosc* **4**, 399–402.

41. Bhattacharya S, Parkin DE, Reid TM, Abramovich DR, Mollison J & Kitchener HC (1995) A prospective randomised study of the effects of prophylactic antibiotics on the incidence of bacteraemia following hysteroscopic surgery. *Eur J Obstet Gynecol Reprod Biol* **63**, 37–40.

42. Preutthipan S & Herabutya Y (2000) Vaginal misoprostol for cervical priming before operative hysteroscopy: a randomized controlled trial. *Obstet Gynecol* **96**, 890–4.

43. Townsend DE, McCausland V, McCausland A, Fields G & Kauffman K (1993) Post-ablation–tubal sterilization syndrome. *Obstet Gynecol* **82**, 422–4.

44. Cook JR & Seman EI (2003) Pregnancy following endometrial ablation: case history and literature review. *Obstet Gynecol Surv* **58**, 551–6.

45. Valle RF & Baggish MS (1998) Endometrial carcinoma after endometrial ablation: high-risk factors predicting its occurrence. *Am J Obstet Gynecol* **179**, 569–72.

46. O'Donovan PJ & McGurgan P (1999) Microlaparoscopy. *Semin Laparosc Surg* **6**, 51–7.

47. Hurd WW, Bude RO, DeLancey JO & Pearl ML (1992) The relationship of the umbilicus to the aortic bifurcation: implications for laparoscopic technique. *Obstet Gynecol* **80**, 48–51.

48. Hasson HM, Rotman C, Rana N & Kumari NA (2000) Open laparoscopy: 29-year experience. *Obstet Gynecol* **96**, 763–6.

49. Chapron C, Cravello L, Chopin N, Kreiker G, Blanc B & Dubuisson JB (2003) Complications during set-up procedures for laparoscopy in gynecology: open laparoscopy does not reduce the risk of major complications. *Acta Obstet Gynecol Scand* **82**, 1125–9.

50. Garry R (1999) Towards evidence-based laparoscopic entry techniques: clinical problems and dilemmas. *Gynaecol Endosc* **8**, 315–26.

51. Jansen FW, Kolkman WMD, Bakkum EA, de Kroon CD, Trimbos-Kemper TCM & Trimbos JB (2004) Complications of laparoscopy: an inquiry about closed- versus open-entry technique. *Am J Gynecol Obstet* **190**, 634–8.

52. Hurd WW, Amesse LS, Gruber JS, Horowitz GM, Cha GM & Hurteau JA (2003) Visualization of the epigastric vessels and bladder before laparoscopic trocar placement. *Fertil Steril* **80**, 209–12.

53. Hurd WW, Bude RO, DeLancey JO & Newman JS (1994) The location of abdominal wall blood vessels in relationship to abdominal landmarks apparent at laparoscopy. *Am J Obstet Gynecol* **171**, 642–6.

54. Boike GM, Miller CE, Spirtos NM *et al.* (1995) Incisional bowel herniations after operative laparoscopy: a series of nineteen cases and review of the literature. *Am J Obstet Gynecol* **172**, 1726–31; discussion 1731–3.

55. NICE (2004) *Guideline No. 11, Fertility: Assessment and Treatment for People with Fertility Problems.* London: National Institute for Clinical Excellence.

56. Henig I, Prough SG, Cheatwood M & DeLong E (1991) Hysterosalpingography, laparoscopy and hysteroscopy in infertility. A comparative study. *J Reprod Med* **36**, 573–5.

57. Carter JE (1994) Combined hysteroscopic and laparoscopic findings in patients with chronic pelvic pain. *J Am Assoc Gynecol Laparosc* **2**, 43–7.

58. Chapron C, Pierre F, Harchaoui Y, Lacroix S, Beguin S & Querleu D *et al.* (1999) Gastrointestinal injuries during gynaecological laparoscopy. *Hum Reprod* **14**, 333–7.

59. Harkki-Siren P, Sjoberg J & Kurki T (1999) Major complications of laparoscopy: a follow-up. *Finnish Study Obstet Gynecol* **94**, 94–8.

60. Chatzipapas IK & Magos AL (1997) A simple technique of securing inferior epigastric vessels and repairing the rectus sheath at laparoscopic surgery. *Am J Obstet Gynecol* **90**, 304–6.

61. Reich H, Clarke HC & Sekel L (1992) A simple method for ligating with straight and curved needles in operative laparoscopy. *Obstet Gynecol* **79**, 143–7.

62. Shushan A, Mohamed H & Magos AL (1999) A case-control study to compare the variability of operating time in laparoscopic and open surgery. *Hum Reprod* **14**, 1467–9.

63. Chapron C, Fauconnier A, Goffinet F, Breart G & Dubuisson JB (2002) Laparoscopic surgery is not inherently dangerous for patients presenting with benign gynaecologic

pathology. Results of a meta-analysis. *Hum Reprod* **17**, 1334–42.

64. Garry R, Fountain J, Mason S *et al.* (2004) The eVALuate study: two parallel randomised trials, one comparing laparoscopic with abdominal hysterectomy, the other comparing laparoscopic with vaginal hysterectomy. *Br Med J* **328**, 129.

65. Jansen FW, Kapiteyn K & Trimbos-Kemper T *et al.* (1997) Complications of laparoscopy: a prospective, multicentre, observational study. *Br J Obstet Gynaecol* **104**, 595–600.

66. Chapron C, Querleu D & Bruhat MA *et al.* (1998) Surgical complications of diagnostic and operative gynecologic laparoscopy: a series of 29 966 cases. *Hum Reprod* **13**, 867–72.

67. Saidi MH, Sadler RK, Vancaillie TG, Akright BD, Farhart SA & White AJ (1996) Diagnosis and management of serious urinary complications after major operative laparoscopy. *Obstet Gynecol* **87**, 272–6.

68. Magrina JF (2002) Complications of laparoscopic surgery. *Clin Obstet Gynecol* **45**, 469–80.

69. Varol N, Healey M, Tang P, Sheehan P, Maher P & Hill D (2001) Ten-year review of hysterectomy morbidity and mortality: can we change direction? *Aust N Z J Obstet Gynaecol* **41**, 295–302.

70. Argent VP (2003) Medico-legal problems in gynaecology. *Curr Obstet Gynaecol* **13**, 294–9.

71. Nagele F, Mane S, Chandrasekaran P, Rubinger T & Magos AL (1996) How successful is hysteroscopic polypectomy. *Gynaecol Endosc* **5**, 137–40.

72. O'Connor H, Broadbent JA, Magos AL & McPherson K (1997) Medical Research Council randomised trial of endometrial resection versus hysterectomy in management of menorrhagia. *Lancet* **349**, 897–901.

73. Tarnay CM, Glass KB & Munro MG (1999) Incision characteristics associated with six laparoscopic trocar-cannula systems: a randomized, observer-blinded comparison. *Obstet Gynecol* **94**, 89–93.

Further reading

Chapron CM, Pierre F, Lacroix S, Querleu D, Lansac J & Dubuission J-B (1997) Major vascular injuries during gynecological laparoscopy. *J Am Coll Surg* **185**, 476–81.

Magos A, Chapman L (2004) Hysteroscopic tubal sterilization. *Obstet Gynecol Clin North Am* **31**, 705–19.

Merlin T, Maddern G, Jamieson G, Hiller J, Brown A & Kolbe A (2001) A systematic review of the methods used to establish laparoscopic pneumoperitoneum. ASERNIP-S Report no. 13. Adelaide, South Australia: ASERNIP-S. October 2001 (Available from The Royal Australasian College of Surgeons, PO Box688, North Adelaide, South Australia 5006, Australia).

Wu MP, Ou CS, Chen SL, Yen EY & Rowbotham R (2000) Complications and recommended practices for electrosurgery in laparoscopy. *Am J Surg* **179**, 67–73.

Sutton C, Diamond MP (eds) (1998) *Endoscopic Surgery for Gynaecologists*, 2nd Edition. London: WB Saunders Company Ltd.

Rock JA, JOnes HW III (eds) (2003) *Te Linde's Operative Gynaecology*, 9th edn. Philadelphia: Lippincott Williams & Wilkins.

Tulandi T (2004) Advances in laparoscopy and hysteroscopy techniques. *Obstet Gynecol Clin North Am* **31**.

Chapter 51: Benign disease of the vulva

Richard Staughton

Introduction

A large proportion of women with vulval symptomatology have neither gynaecological nor venereological problems, but a vulval *skin* complaint [1–3]. Hence, since many primary care physicians still refer such patients to gynaecological departments, it behoves all gynaecologists to acquire a working knowledge of vulval skin disease. This chapter is aimed squarely at them, with the encouragement that identifying common skin conditions accurately and using simple, safe, appropriate treatments is not only helpful to their patients but rewarding in itself.

At many hospitals combined clinics have been formed where patients with vulval symptomatology can be discussed and dealt with appropriately in a one-stop fashion, saving time and expense. Combined clinics act as important referral centres for other specialists.

In spite of the changes brought about by more open journalism many patients, not always the older ones, are embarrassed by vulval symptoms and are sometimes tragically late in presenting. Anything that can be done to mitigate this situation is desirable and an open, gentle and tactful approach is not only good professional behaviour but the essential first step towards helping them.

History taking

The embarrassment and delicacy of the situation can be lessened by enquiring first about past and background dermatological history – noting skin colour; sensitivity to soaps and irritants; past history of atopy (eczema in childhood, asthma and hay fever); allergies, e.g. nickel, the commonest marker of a tendency to contact dermatitis and more relevantly perfumes, creams and latex; a past and family history of psoriasis (scaly plaques on scalp, knees and elbows) and symptoms suggestive of seborrhoeic dermatitis (dandruff, para-nasal rash).

By this time the patient should be more relaxed and a more fluent exposure of the history of the present complaint can be obtained. Most importantly:
- What is the main symptom – itch or pain?
- What is its frequency?
- Have skin changes been seen or felt?
- Are there lesions elsewhere?
- Has there been any vaginal discharge and what is its nature?
- What medications or other remedies have been employed and what has been the response to these?

Examination

Good strong lighting, a trained chaperone and an appropriately positioned examination couch are essential; some authorities use a colposcope, but a 4× lens magnifying loop is equally effective.

A systematic approach is recommended and should start with a general view of the vulva, looking at the skin and hair of the mons pubis and labia majora.

1 General view
  (a) Hairs
    i. Distribution and extent (e.g. alopecia areata, evidence of virilization)
    ii. Quality and condition (e.g. colour, broken hairs from friction)
    iii. Infestation
  (b) Skin colour
    i. Pigmentary disturbance (e.g. vitiligo)
    ii. Inflammation present or absent
  (c) Skin texture
    i. Abnormal thickness (e.g. lichenification or atrophy)
  (d) Skin surface
    i. Integrity
    ii. Excoriation
    iii. Erosions
  (e) Palpation
    i. Tenderness or underlying masses (e.g. cysts)
2 Labia minora
  (a) Presence or absence
  (b) Development abnormality
3 Clitoral area
  (a) Hood
  (b) Clitoris – normal size and surface

4 Vestibule
  (a) Urethral opening
  (b) Vaginal aperture
  (c) Epithelial surface – colour, texture and palpation
  with cotton-tipped swab
5 Perianal area

An examination of the vulva is not complete without an inspection of the whole perineum including the perianal skin (embryologically derived from the cloaca)

Biopsy of the vulva

This is a simple procedure requiring a local anaesthetic and should be performed as an outpatient procedure, taking some 10 min. A punch biopsy is all that is usually needed, using either a 3 or 4 mm dermatopunch (Plate 51.1, *facing p. 562*). It is important to state the exact site that is biopsied in the vulva, as the histology will differ according to the area 4 sampled.

Indications for biopsy include:
1 Difficulty in establishing a clinical diagnosis.
2 All blistering disorders: separate punch biopsy for immunofluorescence should be taken and placed in special transport media.
3 All pigmented lesions.
4 Inflammatory lesions that do not respond as expected to anti-inflammatory drugs in order to exclude neoplasia.
5 Persistently erosive lesions.

Procedure

1 Ten minutes before the biopsy an application of local anaesthetic cream (e.g., lignocaine plus prilocaine or lignocaine gel) from the interlabial sulcus inwards will blunt the pain of injection of local anaesthetic.
2 The area is cleaned with diluted chlorhexidine antiseptic.
3 Plain lidocaine (1%), with or without adrenaline, is instilled with a fine needle.
4 Surgical procedure:
  Punch biopsy. A 3 or 4 mm punch will usually be adequate (Plate 51.1, *facing p. 562*). The punch is driven full thickness through the epithelial surface. The surrounding skin is pressed and the plug will pop outwards. This can be 'harpooned' with a fine needle. Taking care not to damage the overlying epithelium the plug is lifted and snipped off at its base with scissors.

Inflammatory skin diseases of the vulva

Lichen sclerosus

TERMINOLOGY

The old terms kraurosis vulvae, leukoplakia and leukoplastic vulvitis are no longer valid, but were undoubtedly

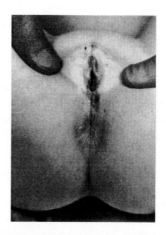

Fig. 51.1 *Pre-pubertal lichen sclerosus* – at the age of 5. Note the well demarcated whitening, rubbery oedema of labia minora and purpura. Such changes can be mistakenly taken as evidence of sexual abuse. Note fissuring around the anal canal. This causes painful defaecation and hence retention so that constipation is a frequent presenting symptom in girls.

applied to cases of lichen sclerosus, lichen planus and cicatricial pemphigoid in the past. Likewise vulval dystrophy and vulval squamous cell hyperplasia are unhelpful terms that should no longer be used.

DEFINITION

Lichen sclerosus is a destructive inflammatory condition with a predilection for genital skin [5] (Fig. 51.1), (Plates 51.2–51.9, *facing p. 562*).

AETIOLOGY

There is mounting evidence that lichen sclerosus is an autoimmune disorder occurring in genetically predisposed individuals. In one study 44% had significant auto-antibodies, 22% a family history and 21% a further autoimmune disease [7]. Vitiligo and alopecia areata are not uncommon in the vulval clinic, and myxoedema is not infrequently diagnosed in follow-up patients.

PATHOPHYSIOLOGY

The autoimmune attack is by lymphocytes in the upper dermis, and both the dermo-epidermal junction above and the dermis below suffer – there is liquefactive degeneration of the basal cell layer with destruction of melanocytes and stimulation of dermal fibroblasts to produce a vast sheet of homogenized collagen in the upper dermis [6,8] (Plate 51.6, *facing p. 562*). This produces the physical signs of bright whitening and scarring – the 'primary' lesion being a white spot often with follicular indentation (Plate 51.5, *facing p. 562*). The overlying epidermis sometimes responds with compensatory epidermal proliferation, causing thickening and hyperkeratosis (Plate 51.8, *facing p. 562*). This continuous 'wounding' process of the dermo-epidermal junction by the autoimmune lymphocyte attack, and the prolonged stimulation of repair processes is hypothesized by some to be the trigger for the increased incidence of squamous cell carcinoma arising in the setting of lichen sclerosus (and lichen planus) [9,10].

INCIDENCE

Lichen sclerosus is seen in both sexes, at any body site and in all races; but most commonly affects the genital skin of white women. The peak ages for presentation are childhood and around or after the menopause. The true incidence is unknown, prevalence has been estimated at between 1 in 300 and a 1:1000 of the population.

PRESENTATION IN CHILDHOOD

Phimosis due to lichen sclerosus is the chief reason for young boys to require medical circumcision [4]. Lichen sclerosus affects the perianal skin in females (but not males) and fissuring around the anal canal causes painful defaecation and hence retention. Constipation is a frequent presenting symptom in girls [1] (Fig. 51.1).

PRESENTATION IN ADULTS

Affected women present with pruritus and only rarely is pain or dyspareunia a prominent complaint [5]. The condition is commonly misdiagnosed as 'recurrent candidiasis', and many years may pass until the correct diagnosis is made. It is salutary that many of those newly referred have long histories as well as physical signs that must have been established over many years.

CLINICAL FINDINGS (PLATES 51.2–51.4, FACING P. 562)

The first changes occur on the labia minora and clitoral hood. Close examination shows the normal supple pink lips to become swollen with a rubbery oedema and take on a dull creamy colour. Similar changes may extend to the fourchette where small tears may be seen. If unchecked inflammation progresses destroying melanocytes and stimulating scarring. The whole perineum and genitocrural folds may become bright white with progressive shrinkage and resorption of normal vulval architecture. The labia minora become 'plastered down' and the clitoris buried as the hood tightens over it. The surface becomes wrinkled, there is 'cigarette-paper scarring' and the poorly supported blood vessels rupture easily causing purpura

and ecchymoses; such changes can be mistakenly taken as evidence of sexual abuse in young girls [12]. Continued resorption of the labia minora tightens the introitus, (Plate 51.4, *facing p. 562*) sometimes alarmingly; however, the vaginal mucosa is always spared and hence can be used in reconstruction operations when necessary.

Every time a patient with lichen sclerosus is reviewed the epidermis overlying the scarred white areas should be closely scrutinized – the search is for the squamous cell carcinoma that rarely supervenes (or approx. 3–4%) [10] – this may begin as a persistent erosion, hyperkeratotic papule or a firm fleshy nodule, which may ulcerate and infiltrate deeply – any suspicious area or persistent erosion should be biopsied [11] (Plate 51.7, *facing p. 562*). About a third of patients with lichen sclerosus have a thickened epidermis (hypertrophic lichen sclerosus) and although this mostly resolves with adequate topical cortico-steroid treatment it is in such a setting that a squamous cell carcinoma usually arises [10] (Plate 51.8, *facing p. 562*).

The histological pattern of lichen sclerosus associated with squamous cell carcinoma includes epidermal hyperplasia and differentiated intraepithelial neoplasia (dysplastic changes confined to the basal layers) [10].

TREATMENT

The current treatment of choice is a super-potent topical corticosteroid (e.g. clobetasol propionate ointment). The precise regimen is important – small (30 gm) tubes of *ointment* are preferred. The first tube should suffice for 3 months. A small 'pea-sized' amount is applied at night to the vulva. The frequency should be nightly for 4 weeks, alternate nights for four weeks and then twice weekly for 4 weeks (Plate 51.9, *facing p. 562*). On review at three months the patient is instructed to use the medication for 2–3 nights in succession if symptoms recur [1, 4]. Non-responders should be carefully reviewed as some may prove to have another more resistant condition, such as lichen planus or cicatricial pemphigoid.

Topical testosterone has no role [14]. The place of the newer non-steroidal anti-inflammatory immunomodulating topicals (e.g. tacrolimus and pimecrolimus) is debatable. The author feels that care should be exercised with agents that could theoretically accelerate cancerous change. The use of these agents should probably be confined to those rare patients not responding to super-potent topical corticosteroids [15].

EXTRA-GENITAL LESIONS

These are rare in men, but can be found in 5–10% of women (Plate 51.5, *facing p. 562*). Common sites include upper back, shoulders, hips and pressure sites (lichen sclerosus is one of the koebnerizing dermatoses, appearing at sites of previous skin damage, for example, scars, vaccination, radiation, etc.). Skin lesions may show follicular hyperkeratotic plugs giving a 'nutmeg grater' feel and after the plugs have dislodged prominent follicular 'delling' is characteristic. Such changes help differentiate lichen sclerosus from other white lesions such as morphoea, scleroderma, scars or vitiligo [1].

HISTOLOGY

The most obvious change is the pale zone of acellular hyaline scarring in the upper dermis. Beneath this is a heavy bluish band of infiltrating lymphocytes giving a 'sandwich effect'. The epidermis above is flattened with loss of rete ridges and melanocytes, 30% of patients have overlying epidermal hyperplasia [6] (Plate 51.6, *facing p. 562*).

LICHEN SCLEROSUS AND MALIGNANCY (PLATE 51.7, FACING P. 562)

There is a bimodal incidence of vulval squamous cell carcinoma, younger woman with vulval intraepithelial neoplasia (VIN) usually carrying oncogenic strains of human papilloma virus (HPV) and older without evidence of HPV infection [9, 10, 34]. Although there is undoubtedly an increased incidence of squamous cell carcinoma in patients with lichen sclerosus [11, 13], this has been exaggerated in the past and is certainly no justification for prophylactic mutilating surgery. In practice the incidence is well below 5%. When pathological specimens of squamous cell carcinoma are reviewed concomitant lichen sclerosus is found in over 50% [10, 11, 13].

Lichen planus

'The blue rash' – lichen planus is characterized by small purplish polygonal papules with shiny surfaces (Plate 51.10, *facing p. 562*). These are most frequently found on the inner wrists, axillary folds and genitalia [16]. Annular lesions and lesions appearing in recent scratch marks (koebner phenomenon) are further diagnostic pointers. Lesions are intensely itchy, almost as much as scabies. The inner cheeks should be searched for white lace-like areas and the tongue for asymmetrical 'bald' patches of papillary loss with a bluish hue [1].

AETIOLOGY

The cause is unknown but, like lichen sclerosus, it involves a lymphocyte mediated attack. In this case it is more closely focused on basal keratinocytes at the dermoepidermal junction and does *not* cause the hyaline band of dermal scarring [6]. A heavy band of lymphocytes lie beneath the basal keratinocytes, some of which die by apoptosis leaving their corpses as colloid bodies in a sea of liquefactive degeneration. There is pigmentary incontinence, with tattooing of the dermis by pigment laden macrophages. The overlying ridges are effaced in a 'saw-tooth' pattern. As in lichen sclerosus there may be overlying hyperkeratosis but without dysplasia.

PATHOPHYSIOLOGY

Though the cause is unknown lichen planus seems likely to be another autoimmune disease. T-lymphocytes mount the immunological attack against basal keratinocytes and the condition is associated in some patients with other autoimmune conditions such as Primary Biliary Sclerosis. Moreover, similar 'lichenoid' changes can be seen in bone marrow transplant patients with graft-versus-host disease. Lichen planus can be triggered by drugs (e.g. β blockers, gold). Familial cases have been described and there is some evidence for association with HLA-DR1.

1 Diagnostic check list
- Intensely itchy blue papules (check wrists) may appear in scratch marks, often annular lesions
- Check inner cheeks for lace-like pattern
- Primary lesion – flat topped shiny polygonal papule, may show Wickham's striae
- Nail changes can rarely occur
  — Age: 25–40 year olds, rare in childhood and old age

2 Clinical setting and evolution
- Good prognosis, natural history usually 9–18 months though some may have many years of disease
- Lesions leave pigmented tattoos which last 9–12 months

3 Management
- Punch biopsy for confirmation
- Raised active papules should respond well to (grade I) super-potent topical corticosteroid (e.g. clobetasol propionate)
- Second line treatment – topical immunomodulators (e.g. tacrolimus – 0.1%)

Erosive lichen planus

Vulvo-vaginal-gingival syndrome – (syndrome of Hewitt and Pelisse) [17, 18]. This rare condition presents with vulval *pain*, caused by erosions of the labia minora and vestibule (Plates 51.11 and 51.12, *facing p. 562*). The labia majora and remaining skin are unaffected but anal, oral (Plate 51.13, *facing p. 562*) and vaginal mucosa often are. The condition rapidly leads to scarring, often with synechiae, and causes alarming loss of normal architecture with atrophy, fusion, scarring and burying of the clitoris.

There may be characteristic milky striae at the margins (Plates 51.11 and 51.12, *facing p. 562*). Vaginal examination is often very painful and a virginal speculum should be used. Touch bleeding and erosions are seen with synechiae and stenosis. Shortening of the vagina can occur.

The aetiology is unknown but histology shows an aggressive form of lichen planus (though biopsies can show only non-specific ulceration if samples are not taken from the advancing edge of lesions) (Plate 51.12, *facing p. 562*).

AETIOLOGY

There is an association with HLA-DQB, 0201.
1 Diagnostic check list
  (a) Severely painful vulva
  (b) Bleeding dyspareunia
  (c) Vaginal discharge
  (d) Eroded inner lips of labia minora and introitus
  (e) Marginal milky striae
  (f) Vaginal erosions, touch bleeding ± synechiae
  (g) Gingivae denuded and ulcerated
  (h) (Conjuctivae spared, cf cicatricial pemphigoid)
2 Evolution
  (a) Poor prognosis, chronic relapsing condition
  (b) Poor response to treatment
  (c) Burnt-out cases leave considerable scarring

MANAGEMENT

This is exceedingly difficult. Swabs should be taken intermittently searching for treatable secondary infection, for example, β haemolytic streptococcus or candida. Antiseptic emollient soaks can soothe (e.g. Emulsiderm, Dermal.) Specific treatment is aimed at the lymphocyte attack, for example, topical steroids of super-potent strength (e.g. clobetasol propionate or diflucortosone 0.3% – Nerisone forte oily cream). These can be applied generously to dissolvable seaweed dressings (e.g. Sorbsan), applied directly to the vulva or wrapped around a tampon inserted into the introitus for 15–30 min. Daily attendance at a specialist dermatological nursing day care establishment for a week or so can be very helpful.

The newer non-steroidal remedies, for example, topical tacrolimus, can produce benefit in some, but irritate others, however theoretically these might provoke neoplastic change [15]. Delivery of steroid into the vagina is relatively easy. A steroid cream can be introduced with an applicator, steroid suppositories are available and steroid foams (used for proctitis and colitis) can be used (e.g. hydrocortisone acetate foam 10%).

Vaginal synechiae and stenosis can be managed by gynaecologists and dermatologists together as postoperative topical or sometimes oral steroids should be used together with dilators to try and arrest re-sealing [4].

SYSTEMIC TREATMENT

Oral steroids may be tried but often disappoint. Standard immunosuppressive regimes with azathioprine, ciclosporin and the like have not proved helpful.

Eczema

Eczema and dermatitis are terms used synonymously for conditions causing epidermal inflammation of a non-scarring and reversible nature. Whereas in urticaria sudden leakage of tissue fluid from dilated capillaries fills the dermis to form wheals under an unchanged epidermis (hives, nettle rash), in eczema/dermatitis the *epidermis* fills with fluid. Histologically this is termed spongiosis and in severe cases may ooze onto the surface ('wet eczema') or pool in vesicles (vesicular eczema). The epidermis and underlying dermis are infiltrated by inflammatory cells (lymphocytes, eosinophils, basophils, polymorphic leukocytes); epidermal macrophages (Langerhans cells) probably play a pivotal role in marshalling such inflammation. The affected epidermis becomes hyperproliferative and parakeratotic so that scaling is seen (which in moist vulval areas becomes a macerated greyish white 'dulling' of the normal pink colour) [1,4].

Vulval eczema is frequent and occurs in various clinical situations, for example, atopic skin disease, seborrhoeic eczema, irritant dermatitis, contact allergic dermatitis and frictional eczema, for example, lichen simplex chronicus.

SEBORRHEIC DERMATITIS

This is a common itchy, red, scaly eruption with a predilection for face and scalp skin. A long history of intermittent dandruff is usually forthcoming. Patients show poorly demarcated red scaly patches in the seborrheic areas – scalp, behind ears, sideburns and nasolabial gutters. The eyebrows and external auditory meati often show scaling on an erythematous base. A proportion of patients show similar changes in other moist areas – central chest, axillae, perineum and groins. Female patients may complain of vulval itching and may well be labelled chronic recurrent candidiasis although they will have no history of discharge. In subtle cases the diagnosis may be difficult and search beneath the hairs in the labium majorae for pink dry thickened scaly dermatitis should be made. More severe cases show extension onto the pubic mound and genitocrural folds.

Aetiology

A genetic tendency to seborrheic dermatitis probably exists in over 15% of the population and can occur at any age – with peaks in infancy (cradle cap) and early adulthood. Increasing evidence links the condition to an individual's reactivity to commensal lipophilic yeasts (malassezia furfur) whose population is greatest in greasy and occluded sites.

Treatment

Successful treatment involves first quelling the eczema by (1) the avoidance of irritants and (2) the use of anti-inflammatories (e.g. soap substitutes and topical corticosteroids, grade III or sometimes II) and then curtailing the yeast population with anti-fungals (e.g. Imidazole topicals).

Seborrheic dermatitis versus psoriasis

Text book examples of either condition give contrasting physical signs, but often, especially in flexural areas such as the vulva, a mixed picture is found. Chronic plaque psoriasis gives the familiar well-demarcated dry scaly meaty plaques over the extensor surfaces (e.g. elbows, knees, sacrum and scalp). In flexural areas the scales become macerated and less obvious, yet lesions are still well demarcated (Plate 51.14, *facing p. 562*). Such crisp demarcation is a diagnostic pointer to psoriasis whereas in seborrheic dermatitis lesions melt imperceptibly into surrounding normal skin. Pure seborrheic dermatitis itches whereas psoriasis is either asymptomatic or sometimes painful, especially when fissured. (Such fissures may extend up the natal cleft.)

When confronted with a red perineum the following may help differentiate:

	Seborrheic dermatitis	Psoriasis
Symptoms	Itch	Asymptomatic – (unless 2° vulvodynia, q.v.)
Signs	Vague margins	Well demarcated
		Extension up natal cleft
Scalp	Dandruff	Scaly thick plaques
Elbows and knees	Nil	Plaques
Nails	Nil	10% thimble pitted
Incidence	15% of population	2% of population

IRRITANT DERMATITIS

Vulval skin differs from skin elsewhere by being more porous, like its male counterpart the scrotum, both to transpiration and to easier penetration [19]. This leads to a susceptibility to primary irritant dermatitis from, for example, bubble bath, disinfectants, deodorants, infective vaginal discharges, faeces and medicines such as anti-wart remedies and topical cytotoxics.

The diagnosis may or may not be obvious as patients do not always readily recognize or volunteer the relevant history.

Management

Treatment involves identification and withdrawal of the irritant, the use of emollient soap substitutes, for example, aqueous cream BP or Emulsiderm and the use of a grade IV or sometimes III topical corticosteroid for 7–10 days.

CONTACT ALLERGIC ECZEMA

The possibility of contact allergic eczema is often overlooked, probably because it is so much more uncommon than in perianal skin [20]. However the skin over the pubic mound and labia majora can certainly manifest a contact dermatitis. Delayed (type IV) hypersensitivity is tested by patch tests read at 48 h. Possible culprit allergens include medicaments (e.g. neomycin, local anaesthetics, ethylene diamine and even some corticosteroid molecules such as hydrocortisone acetate or clobetasol propionate) rubber (e.g. in condoms) or other chemicals (e.g. spermicides and perfumes).

Management involves appropriate patch testing by specialist dermatological units and avoidance of the culprit allergen. Grade II or in severe cases grade I topical corticosteroids are needed, though in very severe cases systemic steroids are used (e.g. prednisolone 30 mg a day for 5 days). In acute weeping eczema potassium permanganate soaks for a few days are very helpful.

ALLERGIC CONTACT URTICARIA OF THE VULVA

Contact urticaria to latex is an increasing problem especially in regular wearers of rubber gloves such as health-care workers [21]. Patients usually make the diagnosis themselves and note lip swelling immediately after blowing up balloons. In such individuals latex condoms can cause immediate uncomfortable urticarial swelling of the labia [21]. Contact urticaria to seminal fluid has been described – either to the semen itself or to medication or other allergens (e.g. penicillin) carried in the seminal fluids [22]. Specific immunotherapy against semen has been described [23].

LICHEN SIMPLEX CHRONICUS

A vicious circle can be set up in which scratching (for whatever reason) leads to thickened itchy patches of skin. Further scratching worsens the situation and eventually a subconscious scratching habit can become established. It may be triggered by heat (e.g. in bed, after hot bathing), irritants (e.g. soaps, bubble baths, etc.) or psychological factors. The habit is difficult to break, especially because patients are largely unaware of their scratching behaviour.

Common sites for lichen simplex chronicus include areas easily accessible to the dominant hand, for example, right side of the back of neck, right calf, right labia majorum (and right side of the scrotum) [1].

The commonest clinical situation is of a patient complaining bitterly of pruritus vulvae who, on initial examination, seems to have a normal vulva. However, a search under the hairs on the labium majorum may reveal the typical lichenified thickened dark red scaly patch. If the patient is asked to point with one finger at the worst area she will usually pinpoint the lesion (Plate 51.15, *facing p. 562*).

Management involves reassurance and an explanation of the 'itch-scratch' cycle. This often heightens at times of stress and certainly a confrontational approach is seldom helpful. An emollient and short-term grade I or II topical cortico steroids can help break the habit. Behavioural therapy can be particularly successful at helping to extinguish the habit of scratching [24].

PSORIASIS

In both medical and lay minds psoriasis is rightly associated with scaly plaques on extensor surfaces of knees, elbows and scalp, rather than perineum. However, genital psoriasis is very common. The genetic tendency to psoriasis probably exists in some 5% of all populations with a point incidence of some 2%.

Body psoriasis is not generally itchy but patients with vulval lesions may complain of discomfort or pain. There is often a secondary vulvodynia (q.v.).

Lesions can cause difficulty in diagnosis because at this occluded site the usual silvery scales become macerated and the plaque appears as an inflamed 'beefy-red' lesion. The edge, however, remains crisply defined and plaques have a symmetrical appearance (Plate 51.15, *facing p. 562*).

Any area within the perineum can be affected but the vaginal mucosa is always spared. Perianal skin may well be affected extending up the natal cleft where painful fissures sometimes occur.

Corroborative lesions should be sought elsewhere. As in many patients with vulval symptomatology close inspection of the scalp can be very helpful – in this case revealing well-demarcated scaly plaques. The classical psoriatic areas of elbows, knees, sacrum and scalp should be checked. Nails show signs of psoriasis in some 10% of patients, with thimble pitting, sub-ungual hyperkeratosis and onycholysis. However, in some patients genital lesions may be the only manifestation of psoriasis.

The etiology is entirely unknown but there is a genetic predisposition and lesions can be precipitated (1) by streptococcal infection (usually guttate psoriasis) and (2) trauma (the Koebner phenomenon). Histopathology shows marked thickening of the epidermis (acanthosis), with the epidermal ridges projecting deep down into the dermis with rounded burgeoning tips. No nuclear atypia is seen. The thickened epidermis may show patches of spongiosis with neutrophil infiltration and overlying parakeratosis. The underlying blood vessels are often grossly dilated with surrounding chronic inflammatory cells.

Management

A full explanation and reassurance about the non-infectious nature of psoriasis is mandatory. A gentle explanation that scratching exacerbates and that the use of emollients and soap substitutes can soothe lesions at this occluded warm site is necessary. Rarely can secondary infection, for example, with candida albicans, be found.

Anti-psoriatic topical remedies, for example, dithranol and calcipotriol, helpful elsewhere, may prove too irritant at this occluded site. However, others can be very helpful including tar, tacalcitol, calcitriol and topical corticosteroids no stronger than grade II (e.g. 1:4 Betnovate ointment RD with or without 5% coal tar solution).

In patients with severe and extensive psoriasis systemic treatments are sometimes used (e.g. weekly oral methotrexate or retinoids or ciclosporin). Flexural sites can be confidently expected to respond equally well, such patients should be under the supervision of a specialist clinic for such prescriptions to be considered.

Certain medications can exacerbate psoriasis (e.g. lithium, chloroquine and betablockers).

Reiters's disease (circinate ulcerative vulvitis). The associated symptoms of uveitis and arthritis point to the diagnosis. Circinate balanitis is well recognized but the corresponding vulvitis is very much rarer [25]. Lesions may be eroded, ulcerative or scaly. Histologically the changes are similar to those seen in pustular psoriasis.

Pigmentary changes of vulval skin

White patches

Vitiligo is a common autoimmune disorder with strikingly symmetrical areas of bright white complete depigmentation, usually in peri-orificial sites especially around the genitalia (Plate 51.16, *facing p. 562*). It is often also found in the axillae and is cosmetically feared on the face and hands.

Lichen Sclerosus lesions can be bright white but are easily differentiated from vitiligo by scarring and purpura.

Dark patches

Post-inflammatory pigmentation is the commonest cause of dark patches on the vulva. This most often follows destructive inflammation such as caused by lichen planus and less often lichen sclerosus (Plate 51.17, *facing p. 562*). Pigment is collected in the dermis by macrophages which are slow to disperse. The larger asymmetrical patches that follow a fixed drug eruption last many months.

An idiopathic acquired pigmentation (of Laugier) [26] is well recognized, there is no history of antecedent inflammation (Plate 51.18, *facing p. 562*) and histology does not show melanocytic proliferation but increased pigmentation in the basal area and *pigmentary incontinence*. Such lesions are fixed and biopsy confirms their benign nature.

Ulcerating and blistering (bullous) disorders

Such lesions usually cause pain rather than itch and most of them are rare. It is important to examine other mucous membranes for evidence of disease. Biopsy with specialized immunofluorescent pathology is often required to establish the diagnosis and dermatological advice should be sought.

Aphthae

Although oral aphthae are common and well known, their vulval equivalent is often not recognized, or diagnosed as 'recurrent herpes'. The vulval ulcers are usually single, round with a yellowish floor and red rim.

Treatment of recurrent aphthae is notoriously difficult. Five percent Lignocaine Ointment can give symptomatic relief and some patients respond to topical tetracycline.

Erythema multiforme

This is an acute skin reaction pattern usually lasting approximately a fortnight and some cases are confined to the mucosae (oral, ocular and genital) but these are usually accompanied by small round areas of erythema on the hands and feet, which have a typical target-like morphology. In severe cases, extensive bullous lesions, sometimes leading to chronic scarring can occur (the Stevens-Johnson Syndrome). Severe cases are common in HIV disease.

Erythema multiforme can occur 8–10 days after an antigenic stimulation, such as a viral infection with herpes simplex or drug exposure; but in half the patients no cause is found.

MANAGEMENT

The trigger antigen should be sought, followed by putative drug avoidance or suppression of recurrent herpes simplex virus with long-term low-dose Aciclovir if necessary. Oral and ocular involvement should be evaluated and treated. Cutaneous lesions can be treated with a grade I topical corticosteroid for 1 to 2 weeks. Short courses of systemic steroids can reduce fever, toxicity and ease local pain, for example, prednisolone 40 mg per day reducing over 6 days.

Toxic epidermal necrolysis (TEN) (Lyell's syndrome)

This is a more severe form of superficial reactive infarction which can cause extensive, even fatal, skin loss [27]. Again such lesions are common in HIV disease. Hypersensitivity to drugs is the usual cause (non-steroidal anti-inflammatory agents, Carbamazepine, Phenytoin, Co-Trimoxazole, Dapsone and Sulpha drugs.)

Management requires early diagnosis and *rapid* cessation of the triggering drug, as well as early transfer of patients to a high-dependency treatment unit. Previously, high-dose systemic steroids were used but can be associated with increased mortality due to serious infections. Intravenous immunoglobulin has been proposed and is currently undergoing trials. Local treatment for both ocular and vulval skin lesions is required by experienced nurses to prevent synechiae and permanent scarring. The disease has a significant mortality.

A less severe and more superficial variant is seen in childhood, caused by staphylococcal exotoxin – the Staphylococcal Scalded Skin Syndrome [28].

Fixed drug eruption (FDE)

In this condition, asymmetrical patches of intense inflammation occur both on skin and mucosal surfaces each time the offending drug is taken. Patients rarely associate the eruption with the medication, which may be a proprietary one, for example, Codeine in an analgesic or a phenolphthalein laxative [29]. Other drugs imputed include paracetamol, non-steroid anti-inflammatory agents, tetracycline, griseofulvin and cytotoxics. A challenge results in reaction at exactly the same sites each time starting within 24 h. Healing often leaves darkly pigmented patches as evidence for many months.

MANAGEMENT

The history and physical signs should suggest the diagnosis but identifying the trigger drugs can take time. Hypersensitivity is lifelong.

Bullous pemphigoid

This is an uncommon autoimmune bullous disease affecting both skin and mucous membranes including the vulva. It is more common in older women, but sometimes occurs in children [30]. The condition is caused by a circulating antibody which reacts against the dermo-epidermal junction. This can be identified by indirect or direct immunofluorescent techniques. There is association with other autoimmune diseases including lichen sclerosus.

For management dermatological advice should always be obtained. Local super-potent topical steroids are a very considerable aid to treatment but systemic steroids are usually required with or without cytotoxic drugs.

Cicatricial pemphigoid

This is a rare variant of pemphigoid in which the mucous membrane involvement is the most prominent feature. This leads to scarring, particularly troublesome in the vulva and conjunctivae. Again older women are most often affected. Circulating antibodies are not always found but direct immunofluorescence of a biopsy is positive [31].

Pemphigus vulgaris

This is a rare severe immunologically mediated bullous eruption affecting the mucous membranes and the skin. Blisters are fragile and short lived leaving characteristic erosions. Most patients are young adults Indian and Semitic peoples are particularly affected. Dermatological advice should be sought and high-dose systemic steroids, cytotoxics or mycophenolate mofetil are usually required.

Benign familial pemphigus (Hailey-Hailey Disease)

This is a rare genetically determined disorder where friction causes erosions, most commonly of flexural skin, for example, neck, axillae and vulva. Histology is diagnostic.

Benign Tumours of vulval skin

Congenital tumours

VASCULAR BIRTHMARKS

These are not uncommon. Capillary naevi are present at birth and do not fade. They have no functional sequelae and treatment, for example, with laser, must depend on cosmetic considerations.

CAVERNOUS HAEMANGIOMA (STRAWBERRY NAEVUS)

Such lesions usually appear within the first 6 weeks, can grow rapidly, and can occur at genital sites. Occasionally they break down and can be a site of ingress of serious infection. In general, they gradually resolve spontaneously over a 10-year period but early assessment in specialized Dermatological Laser Units should be considered when lesions threaten functionally or cosmetically.

Angiokeratomata

These appear as tiny ectatic dark red/blue vascular proliferations with overlying hyperkeratosis. They occur in some 2% of women. Similar lesions are seen on scrotal skin [32].

Acrochordia (skin tags)

These are extremely common in all frictional and flexural sites such as axillae, eyelids and groins. They can achieve quite a large size and if they twist on their stalk thrombose painfully. Treatment is by scissor amputation.

VESTIBULAR/LABIAL PAPILLOMATOSIS

This is a variant of normal. Unusually prominent thickening and folding of the labial epithelium may be stimulated by puberty or pregnancy. Such changes are often mistaken for HPV infection, especially as both types of lesions demonstrate 'aceto-whitening' after application of 4% acetic acid. (Warts are focal, asymmetrical and scattered.) Biopsy results can also be confusing as the glycogen-rich pale cells of the hypertrophic vestibular epithelium stain pale and can be mistaken for viral koilocytes by an inexperienced pathologist.

KERATINOUS CYSTS

Closed and open comedones are common on the labia majora. Acniform inflammation or calcification can occur.

VENOUS VARICOSITIES

These are asymptomatic but may enlarge during and shrink after pregnancy.

VESTIBULAR MUCINOUS CYSTS

These are not uncommon in adults but are occasionally seen in adolescents and are harmless.

PAPILLARY HIDRADENOMATA

These are sweat gland adenomas with apocrine differentiation. They occur most commonly in the ano-genital region of middle-aged white women. A firm asymptomatic papule or nodule is found on the labia majora or any part of the perineum. Very occasionally multiple lesions occur. Excision is required for histological confirmation.

SYRINGOMATA [33]

These are uncommon eccrine duct tumours which are usually asymptomatic multiple, bilateral and symmetrical occurring on the labia majora. They can be destroyed by electro-desiccation under local anaesthesia.

GIANT VENOUS ECTASIA

This is a florid form of venous varicosity of the labia. These dilate further during pregnancy and can cause problems during delivery.

Vulval cutaneous manifestations of underlying systemic disease

1 Crohn's disease
2 Pyoderma gangrenosum
3 Behcet's Syndrome
4 Necrolytic migratory erythema (NME)
5 Acrodermatitis enteropathica
6 Acanthosis Nigricans

Crohn's disease

Once seen, the ulceration, fissuring, sinuses and fistulae of the perineum accompanying Crohn's disease are not easily forgotten (Plate 51.19, *facing p. 562*). Perineal involvement can indeed precede, sometimes by many years, the recognition of inflammatory bowel disease. Cutaneous lesions in the ano-genital area are the commonest lesions and are seen in up to 30% of Crohn's disease patients. If the lesions are clear of the anal margin they are often referred to as 'metastatic lesions'. Vulval lesions are often of this nature. The most usual presentation being with chronic unilateral labial oedema (Plate 51.20, *facing p. 562*), later the more familiar ulceration, fissuring and fistulae may occur [35].

Histology often shows granulomatous inflammation but is not specific and diagnosis can be difficult particularly in the absence of demonstrable bowel disease.

Hidradenitis suppurativa can be clinically differentiated by the presence of bridged comedones and typical axillary and retro-auricular lesions.

Treatment is problematic. Local measures with antiseptic soaks and topical anti-inflammatory steroids can assuage, but often systemic treatment is required. There is some evidence that suppression or removal of *inflammatory bowel* can help. Oral steroids with or without azathioprine or cyclosporin can help. Recently there have been encouraging anecdotal reports of benefit with Infliximab.

Pyoderma gangrenosum

In this condition violaceous purulent cutaneous ulceration most commonly occurs on the shins, but lesions can be seen on the vulva [36] (Plate 51.21, *facing p. 562*). The aetiology is unknown but lesions often Koebnerize and thus any attempt at surgical treatment is often followed by rapid extension of disease. An underlying inflammatory process is found in some 50% of cases, including rheumatoid arthritis, ulcerative colitis, Crohn's disease, myelo-proliferative disorders and paraproteinaemia. The histology is inflammatory but non-specific and diagnosis is usually clinical. The condition usually responds promptly to systemic steroids but sometimes other agents are required to halt the progression (e.g. dapsone, azathioprine, minocycline and cyclosporin).

Behçets syndrome

In the 1930s Behçet described a triad of oral and genital ulceration with ocular uveitis. The condition can in fact affect many other systems and the diagnostic criteria have been refined. Recurrent oral ulceration is obligatory and must be accompanied by two of the following: recurrent genital ulceration, eye lesions, cutaneous lesions and a positive pathergy test. The causative agent may be viral, and the pathogenesis of lesions is probably vascular. There is an association with HLA-B5 in some parts of the world.

Onset is usually before the age of fifty.

Oral ulcers are indistinguishable from recurrent aphthae. Vulval ulcers most commonly occur on the labia minora, are long lasting, recurrent, painful and heal with scarring (Plate 51.22, *facing p. 562*).

Cutaneous lesions include sterile pustules following trauma such as a needle prick (pathergy) or pyodermatous plaques and erythema nodosum.

The histology may show non-specific ulceration but sometimes thrombosed arterioles are seen beneath lesions.

The aim is to halt progression to blindness and neurological complications.

Vulval ulcers may respond to topical tetracycline and corticosteroids. Resistant severe ulceration usually heals with surprisingly low doses of Thalidomide but supplies are difficult to obtain and the drug is teratogenic. Treatment can be complicated by neuropathy and is best handled in experienced centres. Recently intralesional recombinant human granulocyte/macrophage colony-stimulating factor (rhGM-CSF) has been reported as healing large ulcers.

Necrolytic migratory erythema (glucagonoma syndrome)

This vanishingly rare syndrome comprises a distinctive peri-orificial migrating erosive eruption associated with pancreatic islet-cell glucagonoma [1, 4] (Plate 51.23, *facing p. 562*). The perineum is most severely affected but peri-oral lesions are seen. There is associated glossitis and often diabetes. Diagnosis is made by finding a raised glucagon level. Subjects are usually middle-aged women, but the link between pancreas and skin is still unexplained. Theories include a deficiency of amino acids, fatty acids and zinc.

Acrodermatitis enteropathica

This condition is usually seen in neonates or children and characteristic red, eroded vesiculo-pustular lesions particularly affect the genital area but also peri-oral skin [1, 4]. Zinc deficiency is the cause and lesions heal swiftly once this is administered. Deficiency can be caused by a recessively inherited defect or acquired, for example, with total parenteral nutrition, prematurity, gut bypass surgery or penicillamine treatment of Wilson's disease.

Acanthosis nigricans

Acanthosis nigricans can occur in obesity with or without insulin resistance and is thought to be due to a growth hormone-like effect. There is symmetrical velvety brown thickened skin spreading out from the labia majora onto the groins and extending peri-anally, often with similar lesions in the axillae. There may be accompanying skin tags. Rarely such changes are seen in thin individuals and are a reliable and ominous marker of underlying malignancy [4].

Vulvodynia and vestibulodynia [37–43]

The concept of the various pain syndromes has undergone considerable debate and scrutiny over the past decade.

General practitioners, specialists and patients alike have been perplexed by a history of disabling and significant symptoms of discomfort in the absence of visible or histological abnormality. Neurologists and pain physicians have helped greatly in the understanding of such pain syndromes. The names used depend on the anatomical site affected – glossodynia (mouth), anodynia (perianal), vulvodynia (vulva) and vestibulodynia (vulval vestibule).

The perception of touch/pain depends on complex neurological pathways from skin receptors, via sensory nerves and spinal ganglia, to central pain reception areas. Such pathways are also influenced by higher centers – fear of pain being a potent exacerbator.

The pain is very real – understanding its cause and alleviation more difficult.

Patients without overt pathology tend to fall into two groups. Older sexually inactive women tend to have severe intermittent symptoms – often using words such as 'burning' or 'aching' – and cannot tolerate hard chairs or prolonged sitting. Point tenderness is not a particular feature on examination with cotton buds. Dysaesthetic vulvodynia is used to describe this group. Younger women on the other hand often experience vulval pain with touch only. On examination tenderness can be elicited at 5 to 7 o'clock in the vulval vestibule. These patients complain of superficial dyspareunia and inability to tolerate tampons – hence the term Vestibulodynia [37,38]. A proportion of both groups of patients complain of urethral pain and dysuria. They may be thought to have recurrent urinary tract infections – cultures are always negative. The urethral symptoms are thought to be part of the same pain syndrome.

In addition it is now recognized by experienced vulvologists that vulvodynia can be precipitated by a previous inflammatory dermatosis, for example, lichen planus or psoriasis (secondary vulvodynia).

MANAGEMENT

Experience is required to help such patients. Careful and patient listening to symptoms and a gentle confident approach is required. Excessive investigation can undermine this and unnecessary biopsies or cystoscopies can themselves trigger further post-operative pain.

A 'neurological sensory' based explanation can help greatly. The use of topical local anaesthetics such as Lidocaine 5% ointment helps and can build confidence and allow continuing sexual relations.

The older fashioned tricyclic antidepressants and centrally acting drugs such as Gabapentin and Carbamazepine form the mainstay of the physician's armourmentarium. Amitriptyline (sedating), Imipramine and Nortriptyline are the agents of first choice [42,43]. It can help to explain that such drugs are used in higher dosages for the treatment of depression but that lower dosages may well prove adequate for suppression of vulval pain. Patients should be started on 10 mg nightly, increasing by 10 mg each week until pain relief is achieved. If at 90 mg there is no response this medication should be abandoned and another tried. The dosage at which pain relief is achieved should then be continued for a full 3–6 months before gradual withdrawal. Patients can be helped by learning that pain physicians use such drugs to help alleviate pain in other circumstances and indeed co-consultation with such colleagues can assist.

In general most young patients respond well to topical treatments alone and in time the medications can be stopped. Older women may require more prolonged periods of treatment.

References

1. Leibowitch M, Staughton RC, Neill SM, Barton S & Marwood R (1997) *An Atlas of Vulval Disease. A Combined Dermatological, Gynaecological and Venerological Approach.* Oxford: Dunitz.
2. Ridley CM & Neill SM (1999) *The Vulva.* Oxford: Blackwell Science.
3. Bunker CB & Staughton RC (2004) Genital Dermatology Atlas. In: Edwards L (ed.). Baltimore: Lippincott Williams and Wilkins.
4. Bunker CB & Neill SM (2004) The genial, perianal and umbilical regions. In: Burns A, Breathnach, S, Cox N & Griffiths C (eds) Rook's *Textbook of Dermatology*, 7th edn. Oxford: Blackwell Science.
5. Wallace HJ (1971) Lichen sclerosus et atrophicus. *Trans St John's Hosp Dermatol Soc* **57**, 9–30.
6. Fung MA & LeBoit PE (1998) Light microscopic criteria for the diagnosis of early vulvar lichen sclerosus: a comparison with lichen planus. *Am J Surg Pathol* **22**, 473–8.
7. Meyrick Thomas RH, Ridley CM, McGibbon DH *et al.* (1988) Lichen sclerosus et atrophicus and autoimmunity. *Br J Dermatol* **118**, 41–6.
8. Marren P, Dean D, Charnock M *et al.* (1997) Basement membrane zone in lichen sclerosus: an immunohistological study. *Br J Dermatol* **136**, 508–14.
9. Leibowitch M, Neill S, Pelisse M & Moyal-Barracco M (1990) The epithelial changes associated with squamous cell carcinoma of the vulva: a review of the clinical, histological and viral findings in 78 women. *Br J Obstet Gynaecol* **97**, 1135–9.
10. Vilmer C, Cavelier-Balloy B, Nogues C, Trassard M & Le Doussal V (1998) Analysis of alterations adjacent to invasive vulvar cancer and their relationship with the associated carcinoma: a study of 67 cases. *Eur J Gynecol Oncol* **19**, 25–31.
11. Carli P, Cattaneo A & de Magnis A *et al.* (1995) Squamous cell carcinoma arising in lichen sclerosus: a longitudinal cohort study. *Eur J Cancer Prev* **4**, 491–5.
12. Jenny C, Kirbu P & Furquay D (1989) Genital lichen sclerosus mistaken for child sexual abuse. *Pediatrics* **83**, 597–9.
13. Crum CP, McLachlin CM, Tate JE & Mutter GL (1997) Pathobiology of vulval squamous neoplasia. *Curr Opin Obstet Gynecol* **9**, 63–9.
14. Sideri M, Origini M, Spinachi L & Ferrari A (1994) Topical testosterone in the treatment of vulvar lichen sclerosus. *Int J Gynaecol Obstet* **46**, 53–56.
15. Bunker CB, Neill S & Staughton RC (2003) Topical tacrolimus, genital lichen sclerosus and risk of squamous cell carcinoma. *Arch Dermatol* **139**, 922–4.
16. Lewis FM, Shah M & Harrington CI (1996) Vulval involvement in lichen planus: a study of 37 women. *Br J Dermatol* **135**, 89–91.
17. Pelisse M, Leibowitch M, Sedel D *et al.* (1982) Un nouveau syndrome vulvo-vagino-gingival: lichen planus erosive plurimuqueux. *Am Dermatol Venereol* **109**, 797–8.
18. Pelisse M (1996) Erosive vulvar lichen planus and desquamativie vaginitis. *Semin Dematol* **15**, 47–50.
19. Elsner P, Wilhelm D & Maibach HI (1990) Physiological skin surface water loss dynamics of human vulvar and forearm skin. *Acta Derm Venereol (Stockh)* **70**, 141–4.
20. Goldsmith PC, Rycroft RJ, White IR *et al.* (1997) Contact sensitivity in women with anogenital dermatoses. *Contact Dermatitis* **36**, 174–5.
21. Schimkat H-G, Meynadier JM & Meynadier J (1993) Contact urticaria. In: Elsner P & Martius J (eds) *Vulvovaginitis.* New York: Marcel Dekker, 85–110.
22. Green RL, Green MA (1985) Post-coital urticaria in a penicillin-sensitive patient: possible seminal transfer of penicillin. *J Am Med Assoc* **254**, 531.
23. Boom BW, van Toorenenbergen AW, Nierop G *et al.* (1991) A case of seminal fluid allergy successfully treated with immunotherapy in a one day rush procedure. *J Dermatol* **18**, 206–10.
24. Bridgett CK, Noren P & Staughton RC (1996) *Atopic Skin Disease: A Manual for Practitioners.* Petersfield: Wrightson Biomedical.
25. Edwards L & Hansen RC (1992) Reiter's syndrome of the vulva. *Arch Dermatol* **128**, 811–4.
26. Dupre A & Viraben R (1990) Laugier's disease. *Dermatologica* **181**, 183–6.
27. Meneux E, Paniel BJ Pouget F *et al.* (1997) Vulvovaginal sequelae in toxic epidermal necrolysis. *J Reprod Med* **42**, 153–6.
28. O'Keefe, R, Dagg JH & Mackie RM (1987) The staphylococcal scalded skin syndrome in two elderly immunocompromised patients. *Br Med J* **295**, 179–80.
29. Ackroyd JF (1985) Fixed drug eruptions. *Br Med J* **290**, 1533–4.
30. Wakelin SH, Allen J & Wojnarowska F (1995) Childhood bullous pemphigoid. Report of a case with dermal fluorescence on salt split skin. *Br J Dermatol* **133**, 615–8.
31. Setterfield J, Bhogal B, Shirlaw P *et al.* (1996) A comprehensive study of the clinical immunopathological and immunogenetic findings in cicatricial pemphigoid. *Br J Dermatol* **136**(Suppl 47), 13.
32. Blair C (1970) Angiokeratoma of the vulva. *Br J Dermatol* **83**, 409–11.
33. Carter J & Elliott P (1990) Syringoma: an unusual cause of pruritus vulvae. *Aust N Z J Obstet Gynaecol* **30**, 382–3.

34. Trimble CL, Hildesheim A, Brinton LA, Shah KV & Kurman RJ (1996) Heterogeneous aetiology of squamous cell carcinoma of the vulva. *Obstet Gynecol* **87**, 59–64.

35. Urbanek M, McKee PH & Neill SM (1996) Vulval Crohn's: difficulties in diagnosis. *Clin Exp Dermatol* **21**, 211–4.

36. McCalmont CS, Leshin B, White W, Greiss FC Jr & Jorizzo JL (1991) Vulvar pyoderma gangrenosum. *Int J Gynaecol Obstet* **35**, 175–8.

37. Danielsson I, Sjoberg I & Wikman M (2000) Vulvar vestibulitis: medical, psycho- sexual and psychological aspects, a case-control study. *Acta Obstet Gynecol Scand* **79**, 872–8.

38. Bergeron S, Binik Y, Khalife S *et al.* (2001) A randomized comparison of group cognitive-behavioural therapy, surface electromyographic biofeedback, and vestibulectomy in the treatment of dyspareunia resulting from vulvar vestibulitis. *Pain* **91**, 297–306.

39. Bergeron S, Binik YM, Khalife S & Pagidas K (1997) Vulvar vestibulitis syndrome: A critical review. *Clin J Pain* **13**, 27–42.

40. de Jong JM, van Lunsen RHW, Robertson EA, Stam LNE & Lammes FB (1995) Focal vulvitis: a psychosexual problem for which surgery is not the answer. *J Psychosom Obstet Gynaecol* **16**, 85–91.

41. Jadresic D, Barton S, Neill S, Staughton R & Marwood R (1993) Psychiatric morbidity in women attending a clinic for vulval problems: is there a higher rate in vulvodynia? *Int J STD AIDS* **4**, 237–9.

42. Leijon G & Boivie J (1989) Central post stroke pain – a controlled trial of amitriptyline and Carbamazepine. *Pain* **36**, 27–36.

43. Volmink J, Lancaster T, Gray S & Silagy C (1996) Treatments of postherpetic neuralgia. A systemic review of randomised controlled trials. *Fam Pract* **13**, 84–91.

Chapter 52: Malignant disease of the vulva and the vagina

David M. Luesley

Background

Vulval cancer is rare accounting for 6% of gynaecological malignancies and 1% of all cancers in women with an incidence rate of 1.7/100,000. In 2000, 996 new cases were registered in the UK [1].

Most vulval cancers occur after the menopause with the peak incidence between 65 and 75 years (Fig. 52.1), but the incidence has increased in younger women with 15% cases occurring in women less than 40 years of age. These tumours appear to be more frequently associated with vulval intraepithelial neoplasia, human papilloma virus (HPV) infection, and immunosuppression. In older women they are more frequently associated with non-neoplastic epithelial disorders such as lichen sclerosus. This suggests that there may be at least two oncogenic pathways for the development of this cancer. The overall increase in vulval cancer might be explained by the rise in the average age of the female population and possibly because of an increase in HPV infection in younger women.

The most recent mortality figures (2002) recorded 364 deaths for all age groups, giving a death rate of 1.2 per 100,000 women ($0.6/10^5$ persons) ranking it the 19th most common cause of cancer death in women (23rd overall).

There are recognized risk factors for developing vulval cancer:
- Lichen sclerosus (4–7% risk of developing cancer) [2,3]
- Vulval intra epithelial neoplasia (VIN) and multifocal disease (5–90%) [4,5]
- Paget disease [6]
- Melanoma, *in situ* [7,8]
- Smoking
- Immunosuppression
- Advanced age
- History of cervical neoplasia [9].

Aetiology

The aetiology remains unknown. Oncogenic HPVs are, however, strongly associated with some vulvar cancers [10] and non-neoplastic epithelial disorders (lichen sclerosus) with others. Currently available data suggest two hypotheses. First, the classic de novo neoplasm in the elderly frequently seen in association with conditions such as lichen sclerosus (but no evidence of a direct cause as yet). The second type is more often associated with VIN, particularly multifocal disease and disease elsewhere in the lower genital tract. This 'infectious like' type is presumed to be HPV linked [11].

Histology

The majority of vulvar cancers are squamous in origin (Fig. 52.2). Non-squamous cancers of the vulva account for 10% of all vulval cancers. They include – Bartholin's gland cancer, malignant melanoma, Paget's disease, sarcomas, dermatofibrosarcoma protuberans, Kaposi's sarcoma, metastatic malignant disease and lymphomas. Verrucous cancer and basal cell cancer are variants of squamous cell carcinoma and account for the remainder. Histology does have a bearing on management largely because of the different risks of nodal metastases and the predilection for distant spread.

Presentation

Most squamous cancers involve primarily the medial aspects of the labia majora with the labia minora being involved only a third as often. Other sites of predilection include the clitoral and periurethral areas. Small lesions may be asymptomatic and go unnoticed by the patient although even now there would appear to be excessive delay in diagnosis in a small group of women. The intimate nature of the disease and the advanced age of many patients probably accounts for delays such as those cited by Monagham who found that 32 out of 335 patients delayed more than 24 months and only 35 out of 335 presented within 3 months in his series [12]. Similar delays ranging from 1 to 36 months with a mean of 10 months were noted by Hacker *et al.* [13]. Whether this is due to fear or ignorance on the patients' part or delay in clinical

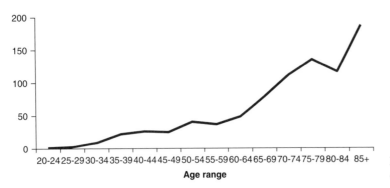

Fig. 52.1 Age distribution of vulval cancer: number of cases in England in 2000.

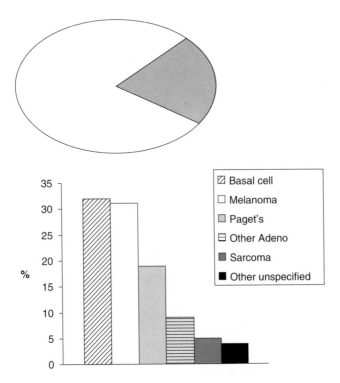

Fig. 52.2 Histological variants of vulval cancer.

examination by her primary carers is unknown but large tumours still present. The reasons for presenting have been analysed by Podratz *et al.* [14].

Assessment

There are two phases of investigation. First, confirming the diagnosis and extent of disease (Stage). Second, assessing the patient's fitness and possibility of concurrent disease that might influence management.

Examination

The clinical assessment of a vulval malignancy should document both the size and location(s) of all the lesions. Care

should be taken to assess any involvement of the vagina, urethra, base of bladder or anus. Palpation is important with large tumours to determine whether the tumour is infiltrating deep to the pubic and ischial bone. Discomfort and tenderness are often associated with large tumours necessitating examination under general anaesthesia. The presence or absence of groin lymphadenopathy should also be noted.

Diagnosis

Diagnosis is based upon a representative biopsy of the tumour that should include an area where there is a transition of normal to malignant tissue. Biopsies should be of a sufficient size to allow differentiation between superficially invasive and frankly invasive tumours and orientated to allow quality pathological interpretation. Occasionally an alternative strategy might be considered. In certain situations where the clinical diagnosis is apparent and the patient very symptomatic, that is heavy bleeding and or pain, definitive surgery to the vulval lesion may be performed but biopsy with frozen section is recommended prior to proceeding with any radical procedure.

Because of the potential for other genital tract malignancy, the vagina and cervix should also be thoroughly assessed and biopsied as necessary.

Spread

The tumour spreads both locally and by the lymphatics to the regional lymph nodes. Local spread may involve the vagina, perineum and anal canal, urethra, clitoris and in late disease involvement of bone may occur. The sites and extent of spread and the involvement of structures where function may be impaired (anal sphincter, urethra, clitoris etc.) are of extreme importance when planning treatment. Skin beyond the vulva may also become involved (Plate 52.1, *facing p. 562*), particularly over the mons onto the lower abdominal wall and laterally to involve the skin of the thighs. Lymphatic drainage of the

Table 52.1 Histological types of vulval cancer

Histotype	Comments
Squamous cell Carcinomas	Account for 90% of malignant vulvar neoplasms
	They metastasize to the local lymph nodes, primarily the superficial and deep inguinal nodes and they may be involved bilaterally
	The risk of nodal disease varies with location and degree of invasion
	They usually present with a nodule or ulcer and may cause pruritus or soreness and pain. Bleeding and an offensive odour may be present with larger lesions
Veruccous and basal cell carcinomas	Squamous variants and rarely if ever metastasize locoregionally
	Verrucous carcinomas present as slow growing wart like lesions with a tendency to local recurrence after excision
	Basal cell carcinomas usually present as an ulcerated nodule on the labia. They do not metastasize and can be managed by local excision or radiation. Up to 20% recur locally after treatment
Malignant melanoma	Has a poor prognosis and is generally managed as for cutaneous melanomas at other sites
	The overall 5-year survival ranges between 8 and 50% and appears to be worse than for cutaneous melanomas elsewhere
	Three patterns of vulval melanoma are identified – mucosal lentinginous (commonest), superficial spreading and nodular. Breslow's thickness of invasion (invasion greater than 1.75 mm has a high risk of recurrence), ulceration and amelanosis are significant prognostic factors. Surgical excision of the lesion with wide margins remains the mainstay of the treatment
Adenocarcinomas	Are exceedingly rare and are more likely to represent metastases from another site. There is an association with vulvar Paget disease
Carcinoma of the Bartholin gland	Is also rare and may be either squamous, adenocarcinoma or an adenoid cystic carcinoma. They occur more often in younger, premenopausal women and overall have a survival of about 35% at 5 years
	They usually present as a solid mass in the region of Bartholin's gland with intact overlying skin. Surgical management is similar to squamous cell carcinoma
Sarcomas	Are very uncommon and in general are biologically similar to soft-tissue sarcomas at other sites. Generally there is poor prognosis after the appearance of regional or distant relapse. Wide local excision appears to offer the best chance of preventing local recurrence. Elective treatment of the regional nodes is not indicated and there is no advantage in resecting metastatic nodes. The role of adjuvant radiation and chemoradiation has not been assessed largely because of its rarity
Metastatic tumours	Are rare and account for about 8% of all vulvar neoplasms. Cervix, endometrium and renal carcinomas have been the most frequently documented primary sites
Paget disease	Presents as a crusty, erythematous, dark pink/red eczematous 'glazed' area on the vulva. It is an intraepithelial malignancy in 90%. Up to 10–15% of vulval Paget's disease is associated with underlying adenocarcinoma, which may be of the breast, stomach, bowel and bladder. Fluorescein dye has been used to detect the lateral extent of disease spread. Wide local excision with closure of large defects with advancement flaps is required to manage this condition

vulva is initially to the superficial inguinal nodes, thence to the deep inguinofemoral chain and on to the pelvic (iliac) nodes. In general, central vulvar structures drain bilaterally whereas lateral structures drain to the ipsilateral nodes primarily. Deep pelvic node involvement in the absence of inguinal node disease is rare. Overall, about 30% of operable patients have nodal spread, 10–15% with FIGO stage I and II tumours and greater for higher stage tumours (Table 52.1) [15–20].

Haematogenous spread can also occur but is uncommon and tends to be associated with large tumours that have already involved the regional nodes.

Premalignant and malignant change in the vagina and cervix is not infrequently seen in association with vulvar cancers. This is not necessarily a metastatic process but may indicate a common aetiological event such as oncogenic HPV infection that can render the whole lower genital tract vulnerable to neoplastic transformation.

Staging

Vulval cancer is staged surgico-pathologically using the International Federation of Gynaecology and Obstetrics (FIGO) staging system last updated in 2000. FIGO staging employs the familiar four categories with substages (Table 52.2). An alternative is the TNM system, which as in other organs is a composite of primary tumour, nodal and metastatic status. Both systems employ nodal status to allocate stage. Many studies to date have demonstrated the fallibility of clinical determination of nodal status and thus while of value in comparative studies, management

Table 52.2 Presenting symptoms in vulvar carcinoma

Symptoms	Frequency (%)
Pruritus	71
Vulvar lump or swelling	58
Vulvar ulceration	28
Bleeding	26
Pain or soreness	23
Urinary tract symptoms	14
Discharge	13

Table 52.3 Relationship of depth of invasion to risk of nodal disease [20]

Invasion depth (mm)	Percent node positive (%)
<1	0
1.1–2	7.7
2.1–3	8.3
3.1–5	26.7
>5	34.2

planning must take other factors into account, particularly the size, site and spread of the vulvar lesion.

Prognostic factors

The 5-year survival in cases with no lymph node involvement is in excess of 80% falling to less than 50% if the inguinal nodes are involved and 10–15% if the iliac or other pelvic nodes are involved. Nodal status and primary lesion diameter, when considered together, are the only variables associated with prognosis [21]. Several other factors may also impact on outcome and need to be taken into consideration when formulating a plan of treatment.

Site of the tumour. Central tumours located close to midline structures such as the clitoris, urethra, vagina and anus are at a higher risk of bilateral inguinal nodal spread than tumours located on the lateral surface. In practice the distance from the midline is somewhat arbitrary although if the excision margin around the tumour is planned to be 2 cm and this would cross the midline, then this is defined as a centrally placed tumour. If these tumours are invasive then bilateral groin node dissection is required compared to unilateral groin nodes for lateral tumours.

Tumour size. Tumours larger than 2 cm in diameter have a greater chance of being frankly invasive and metastasizing to the lymph nodes.

Depth of invasion. Invasion less than 1 mm (superficially invasive or stage Ia) is associated with negligible risk of lymph node involvement, but this rises to 8% for a depth of 1–2 mm, 11% for 2–3 mm, and over 25% for lesions of greater than 3 mm depth [22] (Table 52.3).

Lymphovascular space involvement. This factor along with tumour border pattern (infiltrating versus pushing) and perineural invasion although not included in the surgicopathological staging of vulvar cancer is associated with an increased risk of metastasis [23, 24].

Lymph node involvement. One of the most important prognostic variables. The number of lymph nodes involved and the type of involvement also influence the prognosis. Metastasis to more than one node, involvement of multiple nodal sites and extracapsular spread of metastasis adversely influence the prognosis.

Lymph node status

The most important feature of vulvar cancer, and that, which influences the outcome more than any other, is the histological state of the lymph nodes. The overall survival for all cases of histologically proven groin node negative vulvar cancers is approximately 70–90% while that for node positive is between 25 and 40%. Those with positive pelvic lymph nodes rarely survive. Furthermore, recurrence in the groin is virtually always fatal whereas local vulvar recurrence may often be amenable to either surgical or non-surgical salvage (Plate 52.2, *facing p. 562*). It is therefore of vital importance that the risk of nodal disease is properly addressed at the outset.

It is well recognized that groin node dissection is associated with significant morbidity. Almost 50% of patients undergoing groin node dissection will suffer postoperative complications, most commonly wound infection, wound breakdown and lymphoedema [25]. For these reasons a pre-surgical investigation that could identify those at least risk could have a significant therapeutic benefit. Assessment by clinical palpation of the groins is inadequate; of patients with clinically normal lymph nodes, 16–24% have metastases, while 24–41% of those with clinically involved nodes are negative when examined histologically [26,27]. Even though the majority of vulval cancers are still assessed clinically, there is increasing interest in utilizing additional imaging, particularly of the regional node groups.

Groin node imaging

MRI

Magnetic resonance imaging (MRI) allows clear delineation of tissue planes and detailed anatomical assessment. MRI allows assessment of the depth of the tumour extension as well as clearly visualizing the involvement of adjacent pelvic structures (e.g. urethra, bladder, vagina and anal sphincters). MRI also allows the assessment of nodal involvement [28], which has a high specificity of 97–100% but low sensitivity of 40–50%. These findings may assist in the pre-operative staging of vulval cancer. Identifying nodal involvement is important pre-operatively, as this will clearly identify a group of patients who would benefit from groin lymphadenectomy. MR imaging is also important in recurrent disease to exclude distant metastases before any radical procedure such as exenteration.

MAGNETIC RESONANCE LYMPHOGRAPHY

In this technique ultra-small-iron-oxide-peroxide (USIOP) particles coated with dextran are administered intravenously. These particles are taken up by macrophages in the lymph nodes and effectively reduce the signal intensity on T1 and T2 weighted images. In metastatic nodes, however, where malignant cells have replaced macrophages, the signal intensity is not altered. This technique has improved the sensitivity of detecting involved lymph nodes from 55 to 89% [29].

SENTINEL NODE LYMPHOSCINTIGRAPHY

The sentinel node is defined as the first node in the lymphatic chain draining an anatomical area. If the sentinel node from the suspected lesion is negative for disease then the remainder of the nodes should also be free of the disease (Fig. 52.3). The sentinel node for vulval lesions can be identified by injecting methylene blue dye into the tumour edge or using immunoscintigraphy where a radiolabelled marker (technetium 99) is injected into and around the margins of the lesion. A hand-held gamma camera is used to identify the radioactive tracer uptake in the regional lymph nodes [30,31].

ULTRASOUND

Ultrasonography is relatively cheap and widely available [32,33]. It has also been shown to be of use in assessing groin nodes. Suspicious sonographic features include:
• Larger than 1 cm in size
• Loss of oval shape
• Hypoechoic cortex
• Loss of echogenic hilar sinus fat
• Irregular margin
• Increasing low attenuation of the cortex.
• Increased peripheral vascularity on colour Doppler (rather than a hilar perfusion in reactive nodes).

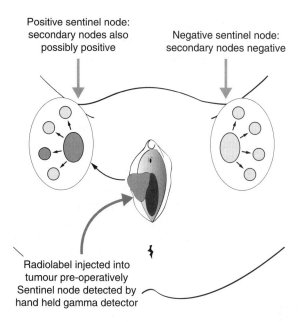

Fig. 52.3 Schematic of sentinel node sampling.

Ultrasound assessment of the nodes can be combined with fine needle aspiration cytology (FNAC) but has a low sensitivity of 58% due to sampling error. It is also associated with a failure to obtain an analysable sample [32], false negative histology [34] and a potential risk of metastatic spread.

CT SCAN

Has a limited role in the assessment of vulval cancers as its use has been superseded by MRI.

POSITRON EMISSION TOMOGRAPHY

This technique is useful for detecting extranodal disease. It is expensive and has limited availability; therefore, is not routinely used. In one prospective evaluation of this non-invasive technique it was found to have relatively poor accuracy rates [35] making it unfeasible for routine use. The reasons for this are unclear but may be related to a reduced metabolic activity associated with tumour necrosis.

Management of vulvar cancer

Managing the vulvar lesion

The objectives of managing the primary vulvar lesion are to remove the cancer, minimize the risk of local recurrence and preserve as much function as possible. These objectives have initially been addressed by modifications of the surgical approach and more latterly by considering combined modality management, especially combinations of surgery, radiotherapy and chemoradiation.

Surgical management of the primary vulvar lesion

The site, size and relation of the lesion to important functional structures will determine the most appropriate method to treat the vulvar lesion. Similarly, the clinical presence or absence of nodal or distant disease will affect the strategies designed to manage non-vulvar, and to a certain extent, vulvar disease. It would, for instance, be illogical to embark upon radical local treatment for the primary cancer in the presence of distant, untreatable metastases unless there was no other suitable form of palliation. Two broad categories of patient can be identified at the outset.

• Those who have small unifocal vulvar lesions with no clinical evidence of nodal involvement
• Those who have more advanced vulvar disease and have clinical evidence of nodal involvement.

For the purposes of further discussion, these will be termed early and late disease, respectively.

Surgical management of early vulvar cancer

Radical vulvectomy is excessive treatment for the majority of unifocal and early cancers. Wide local excision is usually sufficient for the majority of lesions between 1 and 10 mm tumours. The most important factor governing local recurrence is the margin of excision. The risk of recurrence increases as the disease free margins decrease (≥ 8 mm 0%; 8–4.8 mm 8%; <4.8 mm 54%) [23,36]. Because of shrinkage associated with fixing, this margin should be increased. Surgical excision should therefore be at least 15 mm on all the tumour dimensions. The excision should be taken to the depth of the fascia lata, which is coplanar with the fascia of the urogenital diaphragm. Lateral margins should not be compromised even if this would entail excision of a functional midline structure such as the anus, clitoris or urethra. In situations where this pertains, that is, early but midline cancers, radiotherapy may have a role in allowing local control without loss of function. Even if wide excision has been achieved, there may be other variables identified after examination of the specimen that some have suggested indicate a high risk of relapse. These include tumour thickness (or invasiveness) and capillary lymphatic space (CLS) involvement, but this suggestion requires further confirmation. In addition the adjacent epithelium, which may reflect the underlying oncogenic process, may influence recurrence. Differentiated VIN appears to have a higher rate of recurrence than basaloid or warty VIN although this is based on very small case series [37].

As one would expect, the local recurrence rate for wide local excision compares favourably with that following radical vulvectomy. Hacker and Van der Velden [36] have collated data from 12 published series including 530 patients. One hundred and sixty five were treated by radical local excision and 365 by radical vulvectomy. The local recurrence rates were 7.2 and 6.3% respectively.

Surgical management of advanced vulvar lesions

The reader should appreciate that 'advanced' in vulvar terms indicate that wide local excision would either be a radical vulvectomy and or would compromise function. The same principles apply here as with the smaller unifocal lesions in that the objective is to obtain clearance by at least 15 mm on all of the resection margins. As subsequent function and cosmesis are more likely to be affected, consideration should also be given to adjunctive treatment. It is important to consider the woman and her feelings when constructing the management plan. The elderly woman with extensive or multifocal disease with an associated symptomatic non-neoplastic epithelial disorder such as lichen sclerosus might well gain an overall benefit from radical vulvectomy with subsequent grafting. Conversely, the young woman with a clitoral cancer might initially be managed by radiotherapy, reserving surgery for failed local control. These types of cases form the basis for local management of advanced vulvar lesions. The prime objective is to maximize local control, closely followed by consideration of further function and cosmesis in that particular woman.

Lymph node disease

Patients with superficially invasive vulvar cancer are at minimal risk of nodal disease (Table 52.3). This is defined as a depth of invasion of less than 1 mm. Depth of invasion is closely related to the risk of nodal disease. It should be measured from the most superficial dermal papilla adjacent to the tumour.

Overall, about 30% of vulvar cancers will have inguinofemoral nodal disease and about one fifth of those with positive inguinofemoral nodes will have positive pelvic nodes (i.e. about 5% overall). It has been known for many years that pelvic nodes are rarely if ever involved if the inguinal nodes are negative. The low frequency of pelvic node involvement and the doubts surrounding the ability of surgery to control disease at this site have led most to conclude that the routine application of pelvic node dissection in vulvar cancer should be discontinued.

Some clinical factors can predict for the presence of lymph node disease although clinical examination of the nodes themselves is unreliable:

- Lesion size
- Whether or not the nodes are clinically suspicious
- Disease that involves both the labia minora and majora has a 50% chance of nodal involvement whereas with one of these structures only involved the risk is approximately 20%. Steheman *et al.* [38] also suggested that clitoral or perineal siting of the tumour carried an increased risk of nodal disease.

Others risk factors depend on histopathological assessment of the primary lesion and not surprisingly are similar to the general prognostic factors for outcome, they include:

- Tumour grade
- Capillary lymphatic space involvement
- Degree of invasion (tumour thickness) [27]
- Perineural invasion.

Management of the lymph nodes

Types of lymph node dissection

The primary lymphatic drainage of the vulva and distal vagina is to the inguinal (superficial femoral) and the nodes lying along the femoral vein. Efferent vessels from the superficial inguinal nodes drain to the deep inguinal or femoral nodes. The most cephalad femoral lymph node is the node of Cloquet. This is not a constant anatomical finding and has been noted to be absent in 54% of cadavers. The femoral nodes also receive some direct afferents particularly from the clitoris and anterior vulva thus explaining the observation of involved femoral nodes with uninvolved inguinal nodes. One prospective study [38] has suggested that superficial lymphadenectomy alone may be associated with a higher risk of groin relapse.

Laterality

Extensive crossover of lymphatic channels of the vulva may result in nodal involvement of the contralateral groins in addition to the ipsilateral groin nodes. Because of this, bilateral groin node dissection is usually required. However in small (<2 cm) lateral tumours only an ipsilateral groin node dissection need initially be performed. A lateralized lesion, agreed by consensus, is defined as one in which wide excision, at least 1 cm beyond the visible tumour edge, would not impinge upon a midline structure [consensus statement of the EORTC Vulva Group]. If the ipsilateral nodes are subsequently shown to be positive for cancer, the contralateral nodes should also be excised or irradiated as the nodes are more likely to be positive in this scenario.

Andrews *et al.* [39] noted that this was also the case for T_2 lesions despite a relatively high ipsilateral positivity rate of 34%. Exceptions have, however, been reported. For larger lateralized lesions the picture is more confused and until further data become available, bilateral node dissection would be advisable.

En bloc and separate groin incisions

The need for en bloc removal of the lymph nodes has received much attention, largely as it has been felt that this type of procedure accounts for a significant proportion of the morbidity (Plate 52.3, *facing p. 562*) and that the technique employing separate groin incisions (Plate 52.4, *facing p. 562*) results in a better cosmetic outcome. The triple incision technique was first described in 1965 although it only became popular in the 1980s. Those that have reported on its use have not shown any disadvantages in terms of survival or local relapse for early stage carcinomas and there have been quite marked improvements in the morbidity.

The anxiety relating to the triple incision is the possibility of relapse in the bridge of tissue left between the vulvectomy or local excision and the groin nodes. This tissue will contain lymphatic channels but whether lymphatic metastasis is an intermittent or embolic event or a continuous or permeation event remains uncertain. Certainly if the lymphatic channels contain malignant cells at the time of resection, then recurrence would seem to be a real possibility.

Current consensus would suggest that en bloc dissection of the nodes is probably best retained for large vulvar lesions and also in situations where there is gross involvement of the groin nodes (Plate 52.5, *facing p. 571*).

MANAGEMENT OF INVOLVED LYMPH NODES

Resection of the groin lymph nodes provides prognostic information and might also confer some survival benefit. There are varying degrees of positivity from microscopic deposits in one of many nodes to gross extracapsular spread in the entire group of nodes. As with overall stage, this spectrum is also associated with a spectrum of outcomes (Table 52.4) and requires different approaches to management. The most important variable influencing survival is extracapsular spread from the lymph nodes and for patients who have only one node involved the most important prognostic factor is the greatest dimension of the metastasis within the node (Table 52.5).

In the past, pelvic lymphadenectomy was considered appropriate if the inguinal-femoral nodes were involved. This practice has become increasingly uncommon as it has been well demonstrated in GOG protocol 37 [38] that in this situation, pelvic radiation confers a better outcome

Table 52.4 Survival in relation to nodal status and size of vulvar lesion [21]

Node status	Primary size	Survival (%)
Negative (N = 385)	2 cm or less	97.9
	2–3 cm	90.5
	>3 cm	75–80
	All	90.9
Positive (N = 203)	All	57.2
1 or 2 positive nodes		75
3 or 4		36
5 or 6		24
7 or more		0

Table 52.5 Management in relation to lymph node status

Groin nodes negative	No further treatment
Groin nodes positive after surgery	
One node only involved*	Observation only
Two or more nodes involved	Inguinal and pelvic radiation
Clinically positive prior to surgery	Resection followed by radiation
	Radiation followed by resection
	Radiation only

*In the situation where there is only one node involved but the node is either completely replaced by tumour or there is extracapsular spread, the author feels that adjuvant radiotherapy is justifiable.

Table 52.6 Complications of surgery

Groin dissection	Vulvar resection
Wound breakdown/cellulitis	Wound breakdown/cellulitis
Lymphocyst	Rectocoele
Lymphoedema	Urinary problems
	Psychological

than pelvic node dissection. Interestingly the survival difference appeared to reflect better control of disease in the groin and not pelvic or distant disease.

Complications of surgical treatment

The complications of vulval and groin surgery are listed in Table 52.6. Any major cancer procedure carries immediate morbidity such as haemorrhage, thromboembolism and infection and vulvar procedures are no exception to this. Prophylactic anti-embolic strategies are of value and should be used in all cases. Reducing the length of hospitalization and early mobilization indirectly enhances

such prophylaxis and may result from modifications of the radical approach.

Radical en-bloc dissection (radical vulvectomy and bilateral node dissection) results in lymphoedema in between 8 and 69% of cases. Wound breakdown is very common occurring in anything between 27 and 85% of cases and can become secondarily infected resulting in cellulitis. The average hospital stay in days for this radical procedure varies from 17 to 33 days. The triple incision technique has yielded significant improvements in operative blood loss and length of stay although high breakdown rates continue to be reported (22–52%) [39,40]. The occurrence of lymphocyst (Plate 52.5, *facing p. 562*) and lymphoedema does not seem to be significantly less than with the radical en bloc technique. Unilateral groin dissection does appear to lower the incidence of morbidity but there is no significant difference in morbidity when superficial is compared to deep groin node dissection.

Less radical approaches to the vulva have certainly improved cosmesis and subsequent function. Other surgical modifications [41] to reduce morbidity are sparing the saphenous vein at the time of surgery to reduce wound and lower limb complications although the data on outcome in terms of lymphoedema are inconclusive [42,43]. It has also been suggested that tissues most lateral in the groin need not be resected. Sartorius transposition to cover the femoral vessels in thin and emaciated patients also helps to reduce wound morbidity [43]. Wound healing is also improved by avoiding undermining of the skin edges, performing tension free closures, using wound drainage and administering prophylactic antibiotics. More recently surgeons have employed grafting techniques either at the time of initial surgery or as a second-stage procedure. The grafts employed successfully have been the gracilis and rectus muscle myocutaneous flaps and rotational full thickness skin flaps taken from the inner thigh or buttock (Plate 52.6, *facing p. 562*). The use of these flaps to fill considerable defects and a more conservative approach to excision have resulted in less scarring and more functional vulvas. It has not been possible to demonstrate as yet that this translates into improved psychological well-being although the psychological trauma of radical excision without reconstruction is well documented [44].

Management of complications

For lymphoedema, compression hosiery is prescribed along with rest and exercise, avoidance of trauma (skin care), simple gravity drainage and manual lymphatic drainage (MLD). For lymphocyst a conservative approach is adopted and drainage under antibiotic cover is recommended only for symptomatic cases, but they tend to reform.

Wound healing can be promoted with manuka honey dressing [45]. Recently there have been anecdotal reports of using tissue sealant to promote healing in groin wounds that have broken down [46]. Trials are ongoing to assess these techniques.

Radiotherapy and chemotherapy

The role of radiotherapy and chemotherapy in the treatment of vulvar cancer is less well defined than that for surgery. There are, however, data quite clearly indicating that squamous vulvar cancers are sensitive to both radiotherapy and chemotherapy.

Basal cell cancers are well recognized as being radiosensitive and radiotherapy may be the treatment of choice if surgery is likely to result in either functional or cosmetic impairment. Melanomas have not been shown to respond and verrucous cancers have been reported as becoming much more aggressive as a result of radiotherapy.

Adjuvant radiotherapy

The factors influencing the need for adjuvant radiotherapy are:
- Surgical margins
- Groin node positivity.

There is insufficient evidence to recommend adjuvant local therapy routinely in patients with sub-optimal surgical margins (<8 mm). Adjuvant treatment for positive margins is associated with improved survival when compared to observation alone [47].

Adjuvant radiotherapy should be considered when two or more lymph nodes are involved with microscopic metastatic disease or there is complete replacement and or extracapsular spread in any node [38,48,49]. Treatment should be to the groins and the pelvic nodes although there is no evidence to show whether treatment should be directed at both sides or to the involved side only.

Primary treatment

Radiotherapy with or without concurrent or sequential chemotherapy is being used more frequently in the management of advanced vulval cancer. Radiotherapy may, in certain circumstances be the sole treatment but more usually it is used pre-operatively with a view to allowing for sphincter preserving surgery. Radiotherapy may also be of use in place of surgery for histologically proven involved groin lymph nodes. Whether such irradiated nodes require removal after treatment remains unknown.

Radiotherapy and chemotherapy schedules

Most schedules are based upon those developed by the Toronto Group [50]. Fraction size is important with 1.7 Gy being close to tolerance although it is recognized that some centres may use slightly larger fractions (1.8 Gy). Doses will have to be reduced for radical treatment if fractions greater than 1.7 Gy are employed.

Radical treatment usually requires that a prophylactic dose (45–50 Gy) is delivered to the primary and nodal sites and the tumour then boosted by a second phase of treatment using electrons, conformal radiotherapy or brachytherapy to a total dose of 65 Gy. The total prescribed dose is determined by the clinical context.

A Cochrane review suggests that there is no evidence that prophylactic groin irradiation should be used in preference to surgery [51]. With regard to the use of concurrent chemotherapy and radiation therapy, there are no robust prospective data. Several small retrospective studies have suggested that there may be some improvement in local control in regimens employing cisplatinum and 5-fluorouracil, Mitomycin C and 5-fluorouracil and 5-fluorouracil alone.

When there is no obvious macroscopic disease and the sole intention is adjuvant treatment the total dose is 45–50 Gy with no concurrent chemotherapy.

Complications of radiotherapy

The reason for the limited application of radiotherapy in this disease lies in the poor record of tolerance and high levels of complications reported in the older series. This almost certainly relates to the type of treatments and techniques available in these series. More modern equipment and a greater understanding of its potential and applications have resulted in a marked improvement in tolerance and morbidity.

Most women will note erythema and some moist desquamation as a result of radiotherapy. With appropriate care and attention to local hygiene, such problems are rarely such as to result in a premature discontinuation of treatment. Radiation induced cystitis requires bladder irrigation and treatment of any infection. Proctitis is managed with steroid (Predfoam), normacol and loperamide.

More severe side effects include necrosis of bone (symphysis and femoral heads) and fistula formation. Careful planning of field sizes, dose and fractionation minimize such risks.

Recurrent disease

Between 15 and 30% of cases will develop recurrence. The most common site is the residual vulva (70%) with the groin nodes accounting for almost 25 and 15 and 18% of relapses occurring in the pelvis or as distant metastases, respectively [52].

Up to 80% of recurrences occur 2 years after primary treatment and close surveillance every 3 months in the first 2 years is usually practised. This is reduced to 6 monthly surveillance for a further 2–3 years and annually thereafter [53]. Additionally patients are encouraged to self-inspect and report any symptoms of pain, bleeding or discharge. It should be stated that this schedule for follow-up is empirical and is not evidence based.

Survival is poor following regional relapse; hence the efforts to prevent this at the outset. Skin bridge recurrence has been reported to be more likely to occur in patients with positive lymph nodes [54].

Treatment

The management of relapsed disease will depend on the site and extent of the recurrence [52]. Wide excision of local recurrences can result in a 5-year survival rate of 56% if the inguinal nodes are negative [55]. If excision would risk sphincter function radiotherapy should be considered as the first choice. If radiotherapy has already been given to maximum dose, then excision should be considered.

Groin recurrence has a much poorer prognosis and is difficult to manage. In patients who have not been treated previously with groin irradiation then radiotherapy (with or without additional surgery) would be the preferred option. The options are much more limited in those who have already been irradiated and palliation, which may include surgery, should be considered. There is no standard chemotherapy or other systemic treatment effective in patients with metastatic disease.

Vaginal cancer

Background

Vaginal cancer is rare and accounts for only 1–2% of all gynaecological malignancies. They arise as primary squamous cancers or are the result of extension from the cervix or vulva. Most authors report a wide age range (18–95 years) with the peak incidence in the 6th decade of life and a mean age of approximately 60–65 years. There would appear to be no relationship with race or parity.

Aetiology

The cause is unknown although several predisposing and associated factors have been noted. These include:
• Prior lower genital tract intraepithelial neoplasia and neoplasia (mainly CIN and/or cervical carcinoma)
• HPV infection (Oncogenic subtypes).

• Previous gynaecological malignancy. Several authors report approximately one out of four or as high as one out of three of patients as having had a previous gynaecological malignancy.

Large case-controlled studies have not been able to confirm pelvic radiotherapy, previous hysterectomy, long-term use of a vaginal pessary and chronic uterovaginal prolapse as causative factors.

Presentation

The symptoms at presentation will depend on the stage of tumour at presentation. The most common presenting features are:
• Vaginal bleeding. Accounts for more than 50% of presentations.
• Vaginal discharge
• Urinary symptoms
• Abdominal mass or pain
• Asymptomatic. Approximately 10% of tumours will be asymptomatic at the time of diagnosis.

Vaginal tumours may be overlooked during vaginal examination, particularly when a bivalve speculum is used. Careful inspection of the vaginal walls while withdrawing the speculum is necessary to avoid this as otherwise the blades of the speculum may obscure a tumour on the anterior or posterior vaginal wall.

PATHOLOGY

Eighty to ninety percent of tumours in the larger series are squamous. Other carcinomas include adenocarcinomas, adenosquamous carcinomas and clear cell adenocarcinomas. Other rarer primary vaginal cancers are discussed separately.

SITE AND SIZE

Tumours can occur at any site in the vagina. The upper third of the vagina is the site most frequently involved either alone or together with the middle third in approximately two out of three of cases. Approximately one in six will be found to involve the entire length of the vagina. There is no predilection for any particular wall of the vagina. Plate 52.7 (*facing p. 562*) demonstrates a well-localized lesion in the lower vagina but not originating from the vulva.

As with site the size of tumour shows great variation at presentation ranging from small ulcers less than a centimetre in diameter to large pelvic masses, although the majority of tumours are 2–4 cm in maximum diameter.

Staging and assessment

Any tumour classified as a primary vaginal carcinoma should not involve the uterine cervix. There should be no

Table 52.7 FIGO clinical staging of primary vaginal carcinoma

FIGO stage	Definition
0	Vaginal intraepithelial neoplasia III (Carcinoma in situ)
I	Invasive carcinoma limited to vaginal wall
IIa	Carcinoma involves sub-vaginal tissue but does not extend to parametrium
IIb	Carcinoma involves parametrium but does not extend to pelvic sidewall
III	Carcinoma extends to pelvic sidewall
IVa	Involvement of mucosa of bladder or rectum (bullous oedema does not qualify for stage IV) or direct extension beyond true pelvis
IVb	Spread to distant organs

clinical evidence that the tumour represents metastatic or recurrent disease. Staging should be carried out according to the classification FIGO. This classification is summarized in Table 52.7.

The staging process itself can present problems since it may be difficult to differentiate one stage from another. This applies particularly to stage I and II disease that may be hard to separate clinically and similarly it is difficult to separate stage IIa and b on purely clinical grounds. Differences also exist in interpretations of the significance of positive inguinal nodes and their effect on staging. The current staging does not indicate in which group such patients should be placed and some authors would assign these patients to stage III with others preferring IVa or IVb.

The majority of series report that stage II disease is most commonly found at presentation (approximately 50% of all cases). Stages I and II combined consistently comprise 70–80% of cases.

Assessment

This is best performed under general anaesthesia.
- The site and limits of the tumour can be accurately determined and a full thickness biopsy taken for histological analysis.
- Combined rectal and vaginal examination is helpful to determine if there is any extension of the tumour beyond the vagina and the extent of any spread.
- Cystoscopy and sigmoidoscopy are required to exclude or confirm the involvement of bladder or rectum.
- Chest X-ray.
- Intravenous urogram.
- More complex radiological investigations such as rectal ultrasound scanning or magnetic resonance imaging may be helpful in selected instances to define the dimensions and extension of the tumour.

Treatment

The majority of cases of vaginal carcinoma are treated using pelvic radiotherapy although surgical excision is an appropriate form of management in selected cases. Experimental chemotherapeutic regimes are being developed both alone and in conjunction with radiotherapy for advanced cases or recurrent disease.

Radiotherapy

The proximity of bladder and rectum means that, except in early cases, salvage of normal bladder and rectal function can only be achieved using radiotherapeutic techniques. Radiotherapy is certainly effective in treating vaginal cancer and survival rates have improved throughout the century as techniques have developed and improved. Techniques utilized have included:
- External beam radiotherapy (teletherapy)
- Brachytherapy (e.g. interstitial implants, intravaginal cylinders or vaginal ovoids)
- Combination of the two.

There is little place for using external beam therapy alone and the majority of tumours should be treated in combination with brachytherapy, with small early stage tumours being suitable for treatment by brachytherapy alone. The optimal dose remains unclear but the mid-tumour dose should be at least 75 Gy. Above this dose any survival benefit must be weighed against the increased toxicity of therapy and doses of 98 Gy or more have been shown to cause a higher incidence of severe side effects. Complication rates reported for radiotherapy vary according to dosage and techniques used and to the different grading systems used by different authors. Most report complications as occurring in 10–20% of patients. Life-threatening complications have been reported to occur in 6% of those undergoing radiotherapy for gynaecological malignancies and vaginal carcinoma is no exception.

Acute complications include
- Proctitis
- Radiation cystitis
- Vulvar excoriation or ulceration and even vaginal necrosis.

Significant long-term complications reported include:
- Vesico-vaginal or recto-vaginal fistulae
- Rectal stricture
- Vaginal stenosis.

In younger women, vaginal stenosis may be a long-term complication of great significance.

Surgery

There are relatively few reports of the use of surgery in vaginal cancer. Given what little information does exist, there are three general situations where surgery might be considered as first-line management. These are:

1 Patients presenting with a stage I tumour in the upper 1/3 of the vagina, particularly on the posterior wall where resection may be technically straightforward. These patients can be treated with radical hysterectomy (if uterus *in situ*), pelvic lymphadenectomy and vaginectomy.

2 Patients with small mobile stage I tumours low down in the vagina, which if amenable to excision can be treated by vulvectomy with inguinal lymphadenectomy.

3 Bulky lesions that are unlikely to be cured by primary radiotherapy may be considered for exenteration in a few carefully selected cases.

It is undoubtedly possible in many instances to remove a vaginal carcinoma by surgical means and there is little evidence to suggest that survival is improved following either treatment modality. The choice of treatment will depend on the potential toxicity of the proposed treatment in relation to an individual patient and an individual tumour. Surgery is problematic in this respect since, to achieve adequate margins around tumour, important structures (e.g. bladder or rectum) may be compromised.

The addition of lymphadenectomy would appear important as Stock *et al.* [56] reported that 10 (34%) out of 29 patients undergoing pelvic node dissection and all 3 of their patients subjected to inguinal lymphadenectomy had positive nodes. High rates of metastasis to inguinal nodes from tumours of the lower third of the vagina have been noted. Early reports suggested that morbidity after surgical treatment of vaginal cancer was both frequent and serious.

However, the majority of complications were seen in patients undergoing surgical management of post-irradiation recurrence or following exenterative surgery for advanced disease. Serious complications include urinary problems (stress and/or urge incontinence) and fistulae. Lastly, any procedure requiring removal of the entire vagina will render the patient apareunic although lesser degrees of vaginal excision usually allow subsequent sexual function.

Chemotherapy

There is little published work regarding the use of chemotherapy in vaginal cancer. Reports that exist concern combined chemoradiation as first-line treatment of advanced disease and the palliative use of chemotherapy for recurrent disease. In squamous vaginal cancer the use of chemotherapy should be regarded as experimental.

Survival

Overall 5-year survival rates are now in the region of 50% with rates of 39–66% reported. Survival is much higher in early stage disease. However, there is some inconsistency in the allocation of cases to stages I and II. Survival rates for stage I disease are consistently reported between 70 and 80%.

Prognostic factors

Stage, size, site, histological grade and type have all been proposed as factors that may influence survival. Only tumour stage and site, however, are consistently reported as being directly related to survival.

Recurrence

Recurrence occurs locally or within the pelvis in most instances with about 20% relapsing with distant metastasis. The majority of relapses occur soon after primary therapy. Stock *et al.* [56] found a median time to relapse of 0.7 years. The outlook after failure of primary therapy is poor and in the majority further treatment is unlikely to be successful. As with cervical carcinoma, those patients with purely pelvic recurrence are sometimes suitable for salvage surgery by anterior and posterior exenteration.

Uncommon vaginal tumours

Sarcomas

Leiomyosarcomas are most frequently diagnosed with other types reported including adenosarcoma and angiosarcoma. Primary therapy is surgical involving wide local excision of the tumour with free margins. Adjuvant radiotherapy has been advocated for high-grade tumours or in recurrent disease. Adjuvant chemotherapy has been utilized by some but has not been shown to confer a survival advantage in soft-tissue sarcomas of the extremities. The majority of women present with discomfort or bleeding.

Rhabdomyosarcoma (sarcoma botryroides)

Rhabdomyosarcoma accounts for <2% of vaginal sarcomas. It is the most common soft-tissue tumour in the genito-urinary tract during childhood. About 90% of cases occur in children less than 3 years of age and almost two out of three occur in the first 2 years of life although rare cases are reported in older women. Presentation is classically with a vaginal mass composed of soft 'grape-like' vesicles but others may present with vaginal bleeding, discharge, a single small polyp or occasionally, a black haemorrhagic mass.

Treatment involves conservative surgery (aimed at preserving function of the female pelvic organs) but depends largely on combination chemotherapy using vincristine, actinomycin-D and cyclophosphamide. Adjuvant surgery or radiotherapy may be added dependent on response to chemotherapy. Survival has been greatly improved by the advent of combination chemotherapy and over 90% of individuals have been reported to survive following treatment.

Clear cell adenocarcinoma

As suggested by its name, it displays characteristic histological features that include the presence of solid sheets of clear cells, or of tubules and cysts lined by hobnail cells. The median age at diagnosis is 19 years (range 7–42) and approximately 61% of patients have documented exposure to diethylstilboestrol (DES) or to a chemically related non-steroidal oestrogen *in utero*. Although the risk of developing a clear cell adenocarcinoma following exposure to such drugs *in utero* was thought to be considerable it is now appreciated that the risks are in fact very low at 0.014–0.14%. Highest risks are for exposure which occurs early in pregnancy, the risk after exposure in the first 12 weeks' gestation being threefold that at 13 weeks. The majority occur in the upper third of the anterior vaginal wall. Treatment is either by radical surgery or radiotherapy dependent on stage in a fashion akin to the management of cervical carcinoma.

Although the peak incidence of DES associated clear-cell carcinoma in the United States was in 1975 a recent report suggests that there may also be an association with the development of non-clear-cell adenocarcinomas occurring in older DES-exposed women [57].

Melanoma

Primary malignant melanoma of the vagina is an aggressive and rare gynaecological malignancy. Less than 200 cases have been reported worldwide to date but it is known that this disease has the worst prognosis of all gynaecological malignancies. Malignant melanoma of the vagina is 100-fold less common than melanoma of non-genital skin. The behaviour of this tumour also differs from that of melanomas found in other sites in that it is more aggressive than cutaneous melanomas (including vulvar melanoma) and that there is no difference in incidence between different races or skin types. The median age at presentation is around 66 years and the incidence increases with advancing age. The commonest presenting complaint is vaginal bleeding, but presentation may also be with a pelvic mass, vaginal discharge or dyspareunia. The optimal mode of treatment remains unclear but whatever method is used the outlook is bleak. Prognostic factors that have been proposed include age, stage, tumour diameter

depth of invasion and mitotic rate. As with squamous vaginal carcinoma the choice of treatment lies between surgery, radiotherapy or a combined approach. A number of recent articles support the use of radical surgery as a primary approach [58]. Radical surgery refers to either anterior or complete exenteration and it is suggested that although a 5-year survival is not necessarily increased by such measures, the median and disease-free survival may be prolonged.

Endodermal sinus tumour

Endodermal sinus tumours, which more commonly arise in the ovary or testis of infants, are also recognized in the vagina of very young girls. Approximately 50 cases have been reported with no patient aged over 3 years of age. Presentation will usually follow an episode of vaginal bleeding or discharge in a young girl who at examination is found to have a friable, polypoid, exophytic tumour.

Immunohistochemistry will reveal positive staining for alpha fetoprotein (αFP) and in some cases serum αFP levels are elevated.

The behaviour of the tumour is locally aggressive but metastasis will also occur via haematogenous or lymphatic spread. Most tumours arise on the posterior vaginal wall and, if untreated, patients are known to die within 2–4 months of diagnosis.

The emphasis for treatment has moved towards limited excisional surgery combined with pre- or post-operative chemotherapy. Multi-agent chemotherapy is used and is the same as that used for the successful treatment of ovarian endodermal sinus tumour.

Conclusions

The rarity of vaginal cancer means that many questions regarding its management remain unanswered. Many cases are amenable to treatment by more than one method with comparable results in terms of survival. Choice of treatment may, therefore, often be made in relation to the potential toxicities of different treatments and should be tailored to each individual patient.

References

1. ONS (Office of National Statistics) (2002) Cancer Statistics, registration in England 1999, Series MBI no. 30. London: The Stationary Office 2002.
2. MacLean AB, Buckley CH, Luesley D *et al.* (1995) Squamous cell carcinoma of the vulva: the importance of non-neoplastic epithelial disorders. *Int J Gynecol Cancer* **5**, 70.
3. Meffert JJ, Davis BM & Grimwood RE (1995) Lichen sclerosus. *J Am Acad Dermatol* **32**, 393–416.

4. Jones RW, Baranyai J & Stables S (1997) Trends in squamous cell carcinoma of the vulva: the influence of vulvar intraepithelial neoplasia. *Obstet Gynecol* **90**, 448–52.

5. Herod JJO, Shafl MI, Rollason TP, Jordan JA & Luesley DM (1996) Vulvar intraepithelial neoplasia: long term follow up of treated and untreated women. *Br J Obstet Gynaecol* **103**, 446–52.

6. Fishman DA, Chambers SK, Shwartz PE, Kohorn EL & Chambers JT (1995) Extramammary Paget's disease of the vulva. *Gynecol Oncol* **56**, 266–70.

7. Ragnarssonolding B, Johanson H, Rutgvist LE & Ringborg U (1993) Malignant melanoma of the vulva and vagina: trends in incidence, age distribution and long term survival among 245 consecutive cases in Sweden 1960–1984. *Cancer* **71**, 1893–7.

8. Bradgate M, Rollason TP, McConkey CC & Powe UJ (1990) Malignant melanoma of the vulva: a clinico-pathological study of 50 cases. *Br J Obstet Gynaecol* **97**, 124–33.

9. Ansink AC & Heintz AP (1993) Epidemiology and etiology of squamous cell carcinoma of the vulva. *Eur J Obstet Gynecol Reprod Biol* **48**, 111–5.

10. Tate JE, Mutter GL, Prasad CJ, Berkowitz R, Goodman H & Crum CP (1994) Analysis of HPV-positive and -negative vulvar carcinomas for alterations in c-myc, Ha-, Ki-, and N-ras genes. *Gynecol Oncol* **53**(1), 78–3.

11. Crum CP, McLachlin CM, Tate JE & Mutter GL (1997) Pathobiology of vulvar squamous neoplasia. *Curr Opin Obstet Gynecol* **9**(1), 63–9.

12. Monagham JM (1990) Management of vulval carcinoma. In: *Clinical Gynaecological Oncology*. Oxford: Blackwell Scientific Publications, 145.

13. Hacker NF, Leucher RS, Berek JS, Casaldo TW & Lagasse LD (1981) Radical vulvectomy and inguinal lymphadenectomy through separate groin incisions. *Obstet Gynecol* **58**, 574–9.

14. Podratz KC, Symmonds RE, Taylor WF & Williams TJ (1983) Carcinoma of the vulva: analysis of treatment and survival. *Obstet Gynecol* **61**(1), 63–74.

15. Ross M & Ehrmann RL (1987) Histologic prognosticators in stage I squamous cell carcinoma of the vulva. *Obstet Gynecol* **70**, 774–84.

16. Parker RT, Duncan I, Rampone J, & Creasman W (1975) Operative management of early epidermoid carcinoma of the vulva. *Am J Obstet Gynecol* **123**, 349–55.

17. Magrina JF, Webb MJ, Gaffey TA, Symmonds RE (1979) Stage I squamous cell cancer of the vulva. *Am J Obstet Gynecol* **134**, 453–9.

18. Iversen T, Abeler V & Aalders J (1981) Individualized treatment of stage I carcinoma of the vulva. *Obstet Gynecol* **57**, 85–9.

19. Boyce J, Fruchter RG, Kasambilides E, Nicastri AD, Sedlis A & Remy JC (1985) Prognostic factors in carcinoma of the vulva. *Gynecol Oncol* **20**, 364–77.

20. Hacker NF, Berek JS, Lagasse LD, Leuchter RS & Moore JG (1983) Management of regional lymph nodes and their prognostic influence in vulvar cancer. *Obstet Gynecol* **61**, 408–12.

21. Homesley HD, Bundy BN, Sedlis A *et al.* (1991) Assessment of current International Federation of Gynecology and Obstetrics staging of vulvar carcinoma relative to prognostic factors for survival (a Gynecologic Oncology Group study). *Am J Obstet Gynecol* **164**(4), 997–1003; discussion 1003–4.

22. Morrow CP, Curtin JP & Townsend DE (1993) Tumours of the vulva. In: *Synopsis of Gynaecologic Oncology*, 4th edn. 65–92. Edinburgh: Churchill Livingstone.

23. Heaps JM, Fu YS, Montz FJ, Hacker NF & Berek JS (1990) Surgical-pathologic variables predictive of local recurrence in squamous cell carcinoma of the vulva. *Gynecol Oncol* **38**(3), 309–14.

24. Hopkins MP, Reid GC, Vettrano I & Morley GW (1991) Squamous cell carcinoma of the vulva: prognostic factors influencing survival. *Gynecol Oncol* **43**(2), 113–7.

25. Gaarenstroom KN, Kenter CG, Trimbos JB *et al.* (2003) Postoperative complications after vulvaectomy and inguinofemoral lymphadenectomy using seperate groin incisions. *Int J Gynecol Cancer* **13**(4), 522–7.

26. Sedlis A, Homesley H & Bundy B (1987) Positive groin lymph nodes in superficial squamous vulvar cancer. *Am J Obstet Gynecol* **156**, 1159–64.

27. Homesley H, Bundy B & Sedlis A (1993) Prognostic factors for groin node metastasis in squamous cell carcinoma of the vulva. *Gynecol Oncol* **49**, 279–83.

28. Barton DP, Shepherd JH, Moskovic EC & Sohaib SA (2003) Identification of inguinal lymph node metastases from vulval carcinoma by magnetic resonance imaging: an initial report. *Clin Radiol* **58**(5), 409.

29. Sohaib SA & Moskovic EC (2003) Imaging in vulval cancer. *Best Pract Res Clin Obstet Gynaecol* **17**(4), 543–56.

30. Boran N, Kayikcioglu F & Kir M (2003) Sentinel lymph node procedure in early vulvar cancer. *Gynecol Oncol* **90**(2), 492–3.

31. Hullu JA & van der Zee AG (2003) Groin surgery and the sentinel lymph node. *Best Pract Res Clin Obstet Gynaecol* **17**(4), 571–89.

32. Hall TB, Barton DP, Trott PA *et al.* (2003) The role of ultrasound-guided cytology of groin lymph nodes in the management of squamous cell carcinoma of the vulva: 5-year experience in 44 patients. *Clin Radiol* **58**(5), 367–71.

33. Mohammad DKA, Uberoi R, Lopes ADB & Monaghan JM (2000) Inguinal node status by ultrasound in vulval cancer. *Gynecol Oncol* **77**, 93–6.

34. Moskovic EC, Shepherd JH, Barton DP, Trott PA, Nasiri N & Thomas JM (1999) The role of high resolution ultrasound with guided cytology of groin lymph nodes in the management of squamous cell carcinoma of the vulva: a pilot study. *Br J Obstet Gynaecol* **106**, 863–7.

35. Cohn DE, Dehdashti F, Gibb RK *et al.* (2002) Prospective evaluation of positron emission tomography for the detection of groin node metastases from vulvar cancer. Gynecol Oncol **85**(1), 179–84.

36. Hacker, NF & Van der Velden, J (1993) Conservative management of early vulvar cancer. Cancer **71**(4 Suppl), 1673–7.

37. Yang B & Hart WR (2000) Vulvar intraepithelial neoplasia of the simplex (differentiated) type: a clinicopathological study including analysis of HPV and p53 expression. *Am J Surg Pathol* **24**(3), 429–41.

38. Homesley HD, Bundy BN, Sedlis A & Adcock L (1986) Radiation therapy versus pelvic node resection for carcinoma of the vulva with positive groin nodes. *Obstet Gynecol* **68**, 733–40.

39. Berman M, Soper J, Creasman W, Olt G & DiSaia P (1989) Conservative surgical management of superficially invasive stage I vulval carcinoma. *Gynecol Oncol* **35**, 352–7.

40. Burke T, Stringer A, Gershenson D, Edwards C, Morris M & Wharton J (1990) Radical wide excision and selective inguinal node dissection for squamous cell carcinoma of the vulva. *Gynecol Oncol* **38**, 328–32.

41. Rouzier R, Haddad B, Dubernard G, Dubois P & Paniel BJ (2003) Inguinofemoral dissection for carcinoma of the vulva: effect of modifications of extent and technique on morbidity and survival. *J Am Coll Surg* **196**(3), 442–50.

42. Lin JY, DuBeschter B, Angel C & Dvoretsky PM (1992) Morbidity and recurrence with modifications of radical vulvectomy and groin dissection. *Gynecol Oncol* **47**, 80–6.

43. Paley PJ, Johnson PR & Adcock LL *et al.* (1997) The effect of sartorius transposition on wound morbidity following inguinal femoral lymphadenectomy. *Gynecol Oncol* **64**, 237–41.

44. Andersen BL (2000) Sexuality and quality of life for women with vulvar cancer. In: Luesley DM (ed.) *Cancer and Pre-cancer of the Vulva*. London: Arnold, 202–6.

45. Barton DP (2003) The prevention and management of treatment related morbidity in vulval cancer. *Best Pract Res Clin Obstet Gynaecol* **17**(4), 683–701.

46. Han LY, Schimp V, Oh JC & Ramirez PT (2004) A gelatin matrix-thrombin tissue sealant (FloSeal®) application in the management of groin breakdown after inguinal lymphadenectomy for vulval cancer. *Int J Gynecol Oncol* **14**, 621–4.

47. Faul CM, Mirmow D, Huang Q *et al.* (1997) Adjuvant radiation for vulvar carcinoma: improved local control. *Int J Radiat Oncol Biol Phys.* **38**, 381.

48. Paladini D, Cross P, Lopes A & Monaghan JM (1994) Prognostic significance of lymph node variables in squamous cell carcinoma of the vulva. *Cancer* **74**(9), 2491–6.

49. van der Velden J, van Lindert ACM, Lammes FB *et al.* (1995) Extracapsular growth of lymph node metastases in squamous cell carcinoma of the vulva. The impact on recurrence and survival. *Cancer* **75**(12), 2885–90.

50. Thomas G, Dembo A, DePetrillo A *et al.* (1989) Concurrent radiation and chemotherapy in vulvar carcinoma. *Gynecol Oncol* **34**(3), 263–7.

51. van Der Velden J & Ansink A (2000, 2001) Primary groin irradiation vs primary groin surgery for early vulvar cancer [Update in Cochrane Database Syst Rev. 2001;4, CD002224; PMID: 11687151]. Cochrane Database Syst Rev **3**, CD002224.

52. Piura B, Masotina A, Murdoch J, Lopes A, Morgan P & Monaghan J (1993) Recurrent squamous cell carcinoma of the vulva: a study of 73 cases. *Gynecol Oncol* **48**(2), 189–95.

53. Oonk MH, de Hullu JA, Hollema H *et al.* (2003) The value of routine follow-up in patients treated for carcinoma of the vulva. *Cancer* **98**(12), 2624–9.

54. Rose PG (1999) Skin bridge recurrences in vulvar cancer: frequency and management. *Int J Gynecol Cancer* **9**, 508–11.

55. Hopkins MP, Reid GC & Morley GW (1990) The surgical management of recurrent squamous cell carcinoma of the vulva. *Obstet Gynecol* **75**(6), 1001–5.

56. Stock RG, Chen ASJ & Seski J (1995) A 30-year experience in the management of primary carcinoma of the vagina: Analysis of prognostic factors and treatment modalities. *Gynecol Oncol* **56**, 45–52.

57. Hatch E, Herbst A, Hoover R *et al.* (2000) Incidence of squamous neoplasia of the cervix and vagina in des-exposed daughters. *Ann Epidemiol* **10**(7), 467.

58. Miner TJ, Delgado R, Zeisler J *et al.* (2004) Primary vaginal melanoma: a critical analysis of therapy. *Ann Surg Oncol* **11**(1), 34–9.

Chapter 53: Benign diseases of the vagina, cervix and ovary

D. Keith Edmonds

Vagina

The vagina is the lowest part of the internal genital tract of the female. Frequently it is ignored by the clinician as it merely allows the passage of the fetus from its *in utero* existence to the outside world, or as it is bypassed with both the speculum and vaginal fingers to gain access to the cervix and uterus during pelvic examination.

The vagina consists of a non-keratinized squamous epithelial lining supported by connective tissue and surrounded by circular and longitudinal muscle coats. The muscle coat is attached superiorly to the fibres of the uterine cervix, and inferiorly and laterally to the pubococcygeus, bulbospongiosus and perineum. The lower end of the epithelium joins, near the hymen, the mucosal components of the vestibule, and superiorly extends over the uterine cervix to the squamocolumnar junction. The vaginal epithelium has a longitudinal column in the anterior and posterior wall, and from each column there are numerous transverse ridges or rugae extending laterally on each side. The squamous epithelium during the reproductive years is thick and rich in glycogen. It does not change significantly during the menstrual cycle, although there is a small increase in glycogen content in the luteal phase and reduction immediately premenstrually. The prepubertal and postmenopausal epithelium is thin or atrophic.

Vaginal infection

Between puberty and the menopause the presence of lactobacilli maintains a pH between 3.8 and 4.2. This protects against infection. Before puberty and after the menopause the higher pH and urinary and faecal contamination increase the risks of infection. The other time when vaginal atrophy is noted is in the post-partum period or associated with lactation. Normal physiological vaginal discharge consists of transudate from the vaginal wall, squames containing glycogen, polymorphs, lactobacilli, cervical mucus and residual menstrual fluid, and a contribution from the greater and lesser vestibular glands. Vaginal discharge varies with oestrogen levels and does not automatically mean infection. Non-specific vaginitis may be associated with sexual trauma, allergy to deodorants or contraceptives and to chemical irritation from topical antimicrobial treatment. Non-specific infection may be further provoked by the presence of foreign bodies, for example, ring pessary, continual use of tampons and the presence of an intrauterine contraceptive device.

BACTERIAL VAGINOSIS

Bacterial vaginosis has been previously associated with organisms of the *Corynebacterium* or *Haemophilus* species and more recently with the organism *Gardnerella vaginalis*. It is now believed to be due to a *Vibrio* or comma-shaped organism named *Mobiluncus*. These organisms are believed to be sexually transmitted. Usually the vagina is not inflamed and therefore the term vaginosis is used rather than vaginitis. Nearly half of 'infected' patients will not have symptoms [1]. Examination will reveal a thin grey white discharge and a vaginal pH increased to greater than 5; and a Gram stain of collected material will show 'clue cells' which consist of vaginal epithelial cells covered with microorganisms and the absence of lactobacilli. The diagnosis can also be confirmed by adding a drop of vaginal discharge to saline on a glass slide and adding one drop of 10% potassium hydroxide. This releases a characteristic fishy amine smell. There are claims that bacterial vaginosis is associated with increased risk of preterm labour [2], endometriosis, pelvic inflammatory disease and postoperative pelvic infection [3,4]. The treatment of bacterial vaginosis is with metronidazole, either as 200 mg three times a day for 7 days or as a single 2 g dose. Alternatively, clindamycin can be used as a vaginal cream.

TRICHOMONIASIS AND GENITAL CANDIDIASIS

For a description of infection due to *Trichomonas vaginalis* (Plate 53.1) and fungal infection associated with

Candida albicans see Chapter 42. (Plates 53.1–53.16 *facing p. 562*)

SYPHILITIC LESIONS OF THE VAGINA

Syphilis is uncommon among women in the UK. However, unusual vaginal lesions must be considered, particularly if the patient or partner has recently travelled overseas.

The primary lesion may be in the vagina or on the vulva or cervix. There is usually a single painless well-demarcated ulcer with indurated edges, associated with lymphadenopathy. Secondary lesions include condyloma lata, mucous patches and snail-track ulcers.

Diagnosis is based on identification of the causative organism, *Treponema pallidum*, on dark ground microscopy, or by serological examination for syphilis, for example, enzyme-linked immunoabsorbent assay (ELISA). For further details, and details of treatment with Bicillin (i.e. procaine penicillin with benzyl-penicillin sodium), see [5].

GONOCOCCAL VAGINITIS

Gonorrhoea may infect the cervix or Bartholin's gland but not vaginal epithelium except in prepubertal girls or postmenopausal women. If there is suspicion of sexual abuse in a young child with a vaginal discharge, a swab for culture for *Neisseria gonorrhoeae* (see Chapter 42) should be taken.

VIRAL INFECTIONS

Lesions due to human papilloma and herpes simplex virus can be seen in the vagina. Further information is given in Chapter 42.

Toxic shock syndrome

This topic has been included because it is associated with the use of vaginal tampons during menstruation or less frequently in the puerperium [6]. Although there is a link between this syndrome and certain organisms found within the vagina of affected women, it is not a vaginal infection.

The syndrome was first described by Todd *et al.* [7] in seven children and teenagers (aged 8–17 years) with particular multisystem manifestations and similarities with other conditions produced by staphylococcal toxins. The sudden appearance in the early 1980s of a large number of similar cases in young women led to epidemiological investigation, with the resultant finding that 92% of reported cases were associated with menstruation, and 99% of these were in tampon users [8]. The majority of cases were seen in USA, but occasionally in the UK or elsewhere.

The characteristics of the syndrome are an abrupt onset of pyrexia equal to or greater than 38.9°C, myalgia, diffuse skin rash with oedema and blanching erythema, like sunburn, and subsequent (1–2 weeks later) desquamation of the palms and soles. Less commonly vomiting and diarrhoea symptomatic of hypotension is seen. Laboratory results include leucocytosis, thrombocytopaenia, and increased serum bilirubin, liver enzymes and creatine phosphokinase. *Staphylococcus aureus* can be identified frequently from the vagina but blood cultures are usually negative. It is believed that the syndrome is due to the systemic features of a toxin (TSST-1; toxic shock syndrome toxin) and subsequent release of bradykinin, tumour necrosis factor or other biological response mediators. Group A β haemolytic streptococci have also been implicated because they can release a similar toxin (erythrogenic toxin A) [9].

Initial studies [6] could find no association with the brand of tampon used, degree of absorbency as stated on the packet, frequency of tampon change, frequency of coitus or coitus during menstruation or type of contraception. Subsequent assessment has suggested that the inclusion of synthetic superabsorbent materials in certain brands of tampons was responsible. Removal of these brands from the market in the USA reduced the frequency of the syndrome from 17 per 100,000 menstruating women to only 1 per 100,000. However, this reduction also coincided with increased public education and greater care in tampon use including insertion.

Mortality rates from the syndrome were reported initially as high as 15% but fell to 3% by 1981 [8]. The high mortality was probably due to earlier under-reporting of less severe cases, but mortality fell with increasing awareness of the diagnosis and early effective treatment of the hypovolaemia in severe cases. Recommended treatment is as for any septicaemia (as outlined in Chapter 42) and includes intravenous fluids and, where necessary, inotropic support. The cause, where possible, should be eliminated and a β lactamase-resistant penicillin given parenterally. Relapse can occur with subsequent menstruation and it is recommended that tampons should not be used until *Staphylococcus aureus* has been eradicated from the vagina. Relapse has been described in the puerperium [10].

Vaginal atrophy

This is seen following the menopause, but also prior to puberty and during lactation. Examination shows loss of rugal folds and prominent subepithelial vessels, sometimes with adjacent ecchymoses. The patient may present with vaginal bleeding, vaginal discharge, or vaginal dryness and dyspareunia. Superficial infection, with Gram-positive cocci or Gram-negative bacilli, may be associated.

Treatment requires oestrogen to restore the vaginal epithelium and pH. This is usually by topical oestrogen cream, but care must be taken to avoid excessive absorption through the thinned mucosa. Vaginal cream inserted nightly for a week and repeated monthly should prevent atrophy. Alternatively in postmenopausal women, hormone replacement therapy can be used.

Vaginal trauma

This may follow coitus, with damage to the epithelium or less frequently vaginal muscle wall, or breaking down of adhesions at the vault following vaginal surgery (Plate 53.2 *facing p. 562*). It may be associated with parturition or be iatrogenic, for example, ulceration associated with the use of a ring pessary. Trauma may be associated with significant haemorrhage and occasionally will leave vesical or rectal fistulae.

Fistula

A fistula may be due to trauma, as described earlier, or it may be due to carcinoma or Crohn's disease. Fistula of the anterior wall is now uncommon in association with childbirth, but rectovaginal fistula may follow an obstetric tear or extension of an episiotomy, and an incomplete or inadequate repair. Fistulae involving ureter, bladder or rectum may follow gynaecological surgery.

Endometriosis

Occasionally deposits of endometriosis can be found beneath the vaginal epithelium, following surgery or episiotomy. They may cause abnormal vaginal bleeding (e.g. after hysterectomy) or pain. They are most easily identified while they are bleeding. Treatment can be by laser vaporization or excision, or by drug therapy as for endometriosis elsewhere.

VAGINAL INTRAEPITHELIAL NEOPLASIA

Vaginal intraepithelial neoplasia (VAIN) is seen coexisting with cervical intraepithelial neoplasia (CIN) in 1–6% of such patents (Plate 53.3). It is almost always in the upper vagina, and confluent with the cervical lesion [11]. It is uncommon to find VAIN in the presence of a normal cervix but Lenehan *et al.* [12] reported that 43% of their patients with VAIN after hysterectomy had a history of negative cervical smears and benign cervical pathology.

Imrie *et al.* [13] reported VAIN occurring in an artificial vagina in a woman who had congenital absence of vagina and cervix. VAIN may be present in vaginal vault or suture line after hysterectomy (Plate 53.4) (this may be residual after CIN has been treated) or may be distant from the vault and associated with multicentric intraepithelial neoplasia. Hummer *et al.* [14] reported a series of 66 patients with VAIN and showed that one third had developed within 2 years of their previous cervical lesion being treated. The longest time interval between the diagnosis of CIN and VAIN was 17 years; the age of patients with VAIN in that series ranged from 24 to 74 years with a mean age of 52 years.

The aetiology of VAIN is probably similar to that of CIN. Extension of the transformation zone into the fornices would seem responsible, even though no abnormality was recognized when the cervical lesion was treated. A higher incidence of VAIN has been noted in patients on chemotherapy or immunosuppressive therapy. The role of radiotherapy for carcinoma of the cervix some 10–15 years prior to the development of VAIN has been noted, particularly when a subsequent lesion is in the lower vagina. It is thought by some that a sublethal dose of radiation may induce tumour transformation and that VAIN or vaginal sarcoma may result.

As for cervical lesions VAIN I is equivalent to mild dysplasia, VAIN II moderate dysplasia and VAIN III severe dysplasia or carcinoma in situ. The disease is normally recognized as a result of abnormal cytology seen in a vaginal vault smear specimen. Townsend [15] recommended that vault smears should be performed annually for women after hysterectomy performed for CIN, and 3-yearly if the hysterectomy was for benign disease. Current teaching discourages the need for any subsequent smears in this latter group but recommends a follow-up of patients who have had hysterectomy for cervical lesions. Gemmell *et al.* [16] recommend that vault smears should be taken 6 months, 12 months and 2 years after hysterectomy; the patient should then return to 5-yearly screening.

Colposcopic assessment of patients with abnormal vault smears will delineate areas of aceto-white epithelium. Punctuation may be apparent in more that 50%, and areas of abnormality will often fail to stain following the application of Lugol's iodine solution (Plate 53.5). However, atrophic changes within the vagina may lead to extensive areas of non-Lugol's staining and difficulty in defining the limits of lesions. A preliminary 2-week course of oestrogen cream to correct oestrogen deficiency and then colposcopy examination 2 weeks following this will make definition of lesions better. Problems may be encountered in interpreting or getting access to areas of change disappearing into post-hysterectomy vaginal angles or suture line. Vaginal biopsies from the vault can usually be taken without anaesthesia but occasionally difficult access into vaginal angles may require the use of general anaesthesia and appropriate vaginal retractors.

No adequate study on the progression of VAIN to invasive disease has been reported. Among the series of patients reported by McIndoe *et al.* [17] were patients who had abnormal smears following hysterectomy; some of these patients were followed up for almost 20 years before developing invasive carcinoma while others progressed more rapidly.

There have been a wide variety of treatments used to treat VAIN. These include excision biopsy for smaller lesions and 5-fluorouracil cream or laser vaporization for more extensive lesions [18–20]. Experience with the use of 5-fluorouracil has been less in the UK than in the USA. Caglar *et al.* [21] claimed that the subsequent denudation of epithelium was specific for only abnormal epithelium. However, sometimes the epithelial ulceration is extensive, accompanied by severe vaginal burning and subsequent healing may take several months. Treatment failure is common. Use of the carbon dioxide laser is more likely to be successful in treating those women who have not had hysterectomy and where the full extent of the lesion can be demarcated. It must be noted that the vaginal wall may be thin in postmenopausal women and bladder and rectal mucosa less than 5 mm away. The advantage of the carbon dioxide laser over other forms of selective ablation, for example, diathermy or loop excision is that there should be greater control of the area and depth of the laser vaporization. Techniques using high-power density and rapid beam movement minimize carbonization and adjacent thermal necrosis to allow recognition of tissue architecture with removal of lesional epithelium down to the underlying stroma, thereby reducing the risk of bladder or bowel damage.

The difficult patient to treat is the one who has already undergone hysterectomy for a cervical lesion and returns with an area of abnormality in the suture line. Whether leaving the vault open at the time of hysterectomy avoids sequestration of vaginal mucosal above the usual suture line has not been proven. Ireland and Monaghan [22] found 9 of their 32 patients with VAIN had invasive carcinoma in the area of the suture line and they emphasized both the difficulty in assessing the vaginal vault and the need for obtaining adequate tissue for histological examination. They therefore advocated partial vaginectomy whenever abnormal epithelium is seen at the angles or suture line of the vault. This procedure [23] requires an abdominal approach after packing the vaginal vault and involves the mobilization of the ureters down to their insertion into the bladder, dissection of bladder and rectum from the vagina and sufficient mobilization to allow removal of the upper 1–2 from the top of the vagina.

Definition of just how much to remove is usually best achieved by commencing a mucosal dissection from below prior to packing the vagina. Occasionally more extensive disease will require total vaginectomy followed by either skin grafting or mobilization of a loop of bowel to reconstruct the neovagina. There are some who advocate a vaginal approach [24] but access may not be easy and occasionally brisk bleeding from vaginal arteries may be encountered [25]. The other option is to use radiotherapy by the intravaginal approach [26,27]. Concerns that such treatment may produce vaginal narrowing and interfere with coitus have not been realized but some younger women develop radiation-induced menopause and require hormone replacement therapy. The latter authors reported that all of their patients remained cytologically normal and free of disease at follow-up of more than 2 years; colposcopic appearances after radiotherapy may be complex (Plate 53.6). Soutter [25] suggested the management of VAIN after hysterectomy in young women is better by the surgical approach and recommended radiotherapy in older women. Such treatment may not be simple and referral to a centre with gynaecological oncology expertise is desirable.

Diethylstilboestrol and related vaginal lesions

Diethylstilboestrol (DES) was used from the mid-1940s for the treatment of recurrent or threatened abortion and unexplained fetal loss late in pregnancy, predominantly in the north-eastern states of the USA (where it is estimated that 2 million women were treated) and also Canada, Mexico, Western Australia and Western Europe.

Herbst and Scully [28] reported seven cases of clear cell adenocarcinoma of the vagina seen and treated in Massachusetts General Hospital, Boston, in young women aged between 14 and 22 years. A retrospective study by them linked these carcinomas with the intrauterine exposure of the patients to DES given to their mothers during pregnancy. The more extensive survey [29] looked at 346 cases of clear cell adenocarcinoma of the cervix and vagina. In 317 patients the maternal history was available and it was found that two thirds of the patients had been exposed *in utero* to DES or a similar non-steroid oestrogen given to the mothers during pregnancy. In a further 10% drugs of doubtful origin were given, but in 25% no history of maternal hormone therapy could be obtained. They found that the age incidence for clear cell adenocarcinoma of the vagina in young women began at age 14 years, peaked at 19 years and then subsequently declined. They estimate that the probable risk of development of clear cell carcinoma in women exposed to DES *in utero* to be 0.14–1.4 per 1000 women. DES produced various other vaginal and cervical lesions. Vaginal adenosis was often seen in combination with cervical eversion or ectropion. The patients often had a ridge between the vaginal and cervical tissue referred to as a collar, a rim or a 'cock's comb cervix'. Such appearances occurred in approximately 25% of exposed patients. The adenosis can affect the anterior and posterior vaginal walls and lateral vaginal fornices, but is usually restricted to the upper third of the vagina. Sometimes there will be cytological abnormality, extensive immature metaplasia and CIN. Originally it was recommended that women who were known to have been DES exposed *in utero* should be screened from the age of 14 years with both cytology and colposcopy. DES exposure was uncommon in the UK and associated vaginal changes will be seen infrequently. Such patients should be managed by annual cervical and vaginal cytological surveillance and colposcopic assessment. It is still not known if the risk of adenocarcinoma persists, for example, after the menopause.

Benign vaginal tumours

These are uncommon but occur within the vaginal wall and include myoma, fibromyoma, neurofibroma, papilloma, myxoma and adenomyoma.

Cystic lesions may be found within the vagina, usually laterally and occasionally extending from the fornix down to the introitus. These are usually of Gartner's or Wolffian duct origin. They may increase to such a size as to interfere with coitus or tampon use. They can usually be managed by de-roofing but care must be taken in the fornices to avoid large uterine and vesical vessels.

Cervix

Benign lesions

POSITION OF THE SQUAMOCOLUMNAR JUNCTION
AND CHANGES WITHIN THE TRANSFORMATION ZONE

It is known that the uterine cervix increases in size in response to oestrogens; because the cervix is anchored at the fornices the end result of any enlargement is eversion to expose the columnar epithelium of the endocervical canal. This occurs dramatically in the neonate and under the influence of maternal oestrogens, at puberty under the influence of rising oestrogen levels, during the use of the combined oral contraceptive pill and during the first pregnancy (Plate 53.7, *facing p. 562*). Ectopy is the preferred term for this display of columnar epithelium (rather than 'erosion'); colposcopic examination demonstrates the folding of the epithelium into villi (Plate 53.8). Upon withdrawal of oestrogen, for example, in the puerperium or at the menopause, the squamocolumnar

junction approaches the external os once more and indeed may be found within the endocervical canal.

In approximately 5% of women there will be extension of the squamocolumnar junction into the anterior and posterior fornices so that on subsequent examination an extensive area of change will be noted – the so-called congenital transformation zone. The presence of this may not be apparent to the naked eye but can be demonstrated following the application of Lugol's iodine. Biopsy will show no evidence of intraepithelial neoplasia but delayed or immature metaplasia.

CERVICAL METAPLASIA

Exposure of the columnar epithelium to low pH as found within the vagina promotes a series of physiological changes, known as metaplasia. It is believed that reserve cells lying within the monolayer of columnar epithelium will proliferate giving a multilayered epithelium with the columnar cells left perched on the surface (Plate 53.9). These cells will initially appear immature and undifferentiated but with the passage of time will show the usual differentiation to resume a squamous epithelium with glycogenation of the superficial squamous cells. This process occurs at the squamocolumnar junction, or transformation zone, starting in the neonate and continuing until well after the menopause. Examination of the endocervix will show a series of longitudinal ridges with columnar cells lining both the tops of the ridges and extending down into the depths or crypts (Plate 53.10). Metaplasia usually occurs initially in the ridges and may well bridge over these leaving a squamous cover with columnar epithelium remaining within the crypts. If a crypt cannot expel the mucus produced from the columnar epithelium a retention cyst or Nabothian follicle will occur (Plate 53.11); sometimes these follicles are large and extensive across the transformation zone. They are entirely benign and are not associated with infection, that is they are not a sign of cervicitis.

ENDOCERVICAL POLYPS

The recognition of endocervical polyps at the time of taking a cervical smear is common and usually increases with age up to the menopause (Plates 53.12, 53.13). Occasionally these polyps will be symptomatic producing heavy vaginal discharge or bleeding upon coital contact. Histology of these polyps will show that they consist of columnar epithelium sometimes with metaplastic squamous epithelium across the tip. Malignant change is most unusual. However, if these polyps are removed, for example by polypectomy, tissue should be sent for histology, recognizing that some 15% of uterine tumours will be polypoidal and occasionally will extrude through the external os.

CHRONIC CERVICITIS

There was previous enthusiasm for treating by cautery or diathermy those patients who complained of chronic watery vaginal discharge and were found to have an 'erosion'. As explained earlier, these areas of ectopy or everted columnar epithelium are not pathological and the term cervicitis is not appropriate.

However, some women with *Chlamydia trachomatis* (and rarely with *Neisseria gonorrhoeae*) will present with symptoms of discharge and an abnormal cervix will be noted. Brunham *et al.* [30] described 'mucopurulent cervicitis' in association with *Chlamydia*, and Hare *et al.* [31] the colposcopy appearances of 'follicular cervicitis' (see Chapter 54). Providing these organisms have been excluded by appropriate microbiology, 'cervicitis' does not require treatment except by increasing vaginal acidity (Aci-jel) to promote squamous metaplasia.

Ovaries

Benign disorders

ANATOMY

The ovaries are attached to the lateral pelvic side walls by the suspensory ligament containing the ovarian vessels, and to the cornua of the uterus by a ligamentous condensation of the broad ligament. Each ovary is $3 \times 2 \times 1 \text{ cm}^3$ in size in the resting or inactive state, but will increase in size during physiological stimulus; they will shrink after the menopause. The surface is covered by a flattened monolayer of epithelial cells, and beneath this are the ovarian follicles, with oocyte, granulosa layer and surrounding theca. Beneath this cortical layer are a stromal medulla and a hilum where the vessels enter through the mesovarium. The events that are associated with follicular development and ovulation are described elsewhere (Chapter 35). The size and position of the ovaries varies between puberty and menopause – the mean volume, as assessed by transvaginal ultrasound scan of a premenopausal ovary is 6.8 cm^3 (upper limit of normal 18 cm^3) compared to a mean postmenopausal size of 3 cm^3 (upper limit 8 cm^3) [32].

OVARIAN ENLARGEMENT

Ovarian enlargement will occur in response to follicle-stimulating and luteinizing hormones. Follicular and luteal cysts can occur, and theca lutein cysts up to 15 cm in size will develop in response to very high levels of chorionic gonadotrophin as seen with trophoblastic disease. Hyperstimulation syndrome can occur, with massive enlargement of the ovaries and development of ascites, in response to doses of gonadotrophin injections during fertility treatment.

POLYCYSTIC DISEASE

Polycystic enlargement of the ovaries has been described under a variety of names. Stein and Leventhal [33] described seven cases of amenorrhoea or irregular menstruation with enlarged polycystic ovaries demonstrated by 'pneumoroentgenography', and restoration of normal physiological function after wedge resection. Judd *et al.* [34] demonstrated that the mildly elevated androgen levels found in this syndrome were of ovarian origin. The changes in gonadotrophin ratios and androgen levels are not always consistent with the appearances of the ovaries and increasingly the diagnosis of polycystic ovarian disease is based on ultrasound findings of peripheral distribution of 10 or more follicles of 2–8 mm in diameter, with increased ovarian volume (see Chapter 39).

OVARIAN PREGNANCY

Ovarian ectopic pregnancy is uncommon, with an estimated incidence of 1 per 25000 of all pregnancies, although Grimes *et al.* [35] reported an incidence of 1 per 7000 deliveries in their Chicago series. There appears to be an association with intrauterine contraceptive device use [36] or tubal pathology and infertility [35]. Patients usually present with features of an extrauterine pregnancy or bleeding from a corpus luteum. The Spiegelberg criteria [37] to fulfil the diagnosis are as follows:

1 that the tube including the fimbria is intact and separate from the ovary;

2 that the gestation sac definitely occupies the normal position of the ovary;

3 that the sac be connected with the uterus by the ovarian ligament; and

4 that unquestionable ovarian tissue be demonstrated in the walls of the sac.

OVARIAN ENDOMETRIOSIS

Ovarian enlargement may be found secondary to endometriosis, that is, endometriomas. Endometriomas of more than 10 cm in diameter will not respond to medical management alone, and either require laparotomy with the risks of eventually having to perform oophorectomy, or laparoscopic cyst aspiration, 3-months treatment with luteinizing hormone releasing hormone analogue, and then laparoscopic dissection of the cyst lining or destruction with, for example, a KTP (potassium-titanylphosphate) laser [38].

OVARIAN TUMOURS

There is a large list of benign ovarian tumours (cystic, solid or a mixture of both) contained within the World Health Organization Committee on the Nomenclature and Terminology of Ovarian Tumour Classification. Common benign tumours include mature cystic teratomas (Plate 53.14, *facing p. 562*), epithelial (serous or mucinous) cystadenoma and various soft tissue tumours not specific to the ovary, for example, fibroma (Plate 53.15).

These cysts may be asymptomatic and found coincidentally or until their size increases the abdominal girth or causes bladder or bowel symptoms. Pain due to rupture, haemorrhage into a cyst, venous congestion or torsion may be of sudden onset, or of a more chronic nature. Haemorrhage from a cyst, for example, corpus luteum, may be dramatic and cause hypovolaemia in association with the resulting haemoperitoneum. Torsion of the ovary is often colicky in nature with pain referred to the sacroiliac joint or onto the upper medial thigh, before the development of ischaemia (from occlusion of the artery), and initially causes localized and then more generalized peritonism – systemic signs of pyrexia and tachycardia will develop along with nausea, vomiting and bowel upset, and may be confused with acute pyelonephritis or appendicitis. At surgery the tube may also be involved, and there may be no viable ovarian tissue to salvage (Plate 53.16). Further description of ovarian tumours and their malignant counterparts is found in Chapter 55.

References

1. Thomason JL, Gelbart SM, Anderson RJ, Watt AK, Osypowski PJ & Broekhuizen FF (1990) Statistical evaluation of diagnostic criteria for bacterial vaginosis. *Am J Obstet Gynecol* **162**, 155–60.
2. McDonald HM, O'Loughlin JA, Jolley P *et al.* (1991) Vaginal infection and preterm labour. *Br J Obstet Gynaecol* **98**, 427–35.
3. Paavonen J, Teisala K, Heinonen PK *et al.* (1987) Microbiological and histopathological findings in acute pelvic inflammatory disease. *Br J Obstet Gynaecol* **94**, 454–60.
4. Eschenbach DA, Hillier S, Critchlow C, Stevens C, De Rouen T & Holmes KK (1988) Diagnosis and clinical manifestations of bacterial vaginosis. *Am J Obstet Gynecol* **158**, 819–28.
5. Roberts J (1990) Genitourinary medicine and the obstetrician and gynaecologist. In: MacLean AB (ed.) *Clinical Infection in Obstetrics and Gynaecology.* Oxford: Blackwell Scientific Publications, 237–54.
6. Shands KN, Schmid GP, Dan BB *et al.* (1980) Toxic shock syndrome in menstruating women. Association with tampon use and *Staphylococcus aureus* and clinical features in 52 cases. *N Engl J Med* **303**, 1436–42.
7. Todd J, Fishant M, Kapral F & Welch T (1978) Toxic shock syndrome associated with phage-group-1 staphylococci. *Lancet* ii, 1116–18.
8. Reingold AL, Hargreett NT, Shands KN *et al.* (1982) Toxic shock syndrome surveillance in the United States, 1980 to 1981. *Ann Int Med* **96**, 875–80.
9. Sanderson P (1990) Do streptococci cause toxic shock? *Br Med J* **301**, 1006–7.
10. Tweardy DJ (1985) Relapsing toxic shock syndrome in the puerperium. *J Am Med Assoc* **253**, 3249–50.
11. Nwabineli NJ & Monaghan JM (1991) Vaginal epithelial abnormalities in patients with CIN: clinical and pathological features and management. *Br J Obstet Gynaecol* **98**, 25–9.
12. Lenehan PM, Meffe F & Lickrish GM (1986) Vaginal intraepithelial neoplasia: biologic aspects and management. *Obstet Gynecol* **68**, 333–7.
13. Imrie JEA, Kennedy JH, Holmes JD & McGrouther DA (1986) Intraepithelial neoplasia arising in an artificial vagina. Case report. *Br J Obstet Gynaecol* **93**, 886–8.
14. Hummer WA, Mussey E, Decker DC & Docherty MB (1970) Carcinoma *in situ* of the vagina. *Am J Obstet Gynecol* **108**, 1109–16.
15. Townsend DE (1981) Intraepithelial neoplasia of vagina. In: Coppleson M (ed.) *Gynaecologic Oncology.* Edinburgh: Churchill Livingstone, 339–44.
16. Gemmell J, Holmes DM & Duncan ID (1990) How frequently need vaginal smears be taken after hysterectomy for cervical intraepithelial neoplasia? *Br J Obstet Gynaecol* **97**, 58–61.
17. McIndoe WA, McLean MR, Jones RW & Mullins PR (1984) The invasive potential of carcinoma *in situ* of the cervix. *Obstet Gynecol* **64**, 451–8.
18. Petrilli ES, Townsend DE, Morrow CP & Nakao CY (1980) Vaginal intraepithelial neoplasia: biologic aspects and treatment with topical 5-fluorouracil and the carbon dioxide LASER. *Am J Obstet Gynecol* **138**, 321–8.
19. Woodman CBJ, Jordan JA & Wade-Evans T (1984) The management of vaginal intraepithelial neoplasia after hysterectomy. *Br J Obstet Gynaecol* **91**, 707–17.
20. Stuart GCE, Flagler EA, Nation JG, Duggan M & Robertson DI (1988) Laser vaporization of vaginal intraepithelial neoplasia. *Am J Obstet Gynecol* **158**, 240–3.
21. Caglar H, Hertzog RW & Hreschchyshyn MM (1981) Topical 5-fluorouracil treatment in vaginal intraepithelial neoplasia. *Obstet Gynecol* **58**, 580–3.
22. Ireland D & Monaghan JM (1988) The management of the patient with abnormal vaginal cytology following hysterectomy. *Br J Obstet Gynaecol* **95**, 973–5.
23. Monaghan JM (1986) Operations on the vagina. In: Monaghan JM (ed.) *Bonney's Gynaecological Surgery.* London: Baillière Tindall, 138–42.
24. Curtis EP, Shepherd JH, Lowe DG & Jobling T (1992) The role of partial colpectomy in the management of persistent vaginal neoplasia after primary treatment. *Br J Obstet Gynaecol* **99**, 587–9.
25. Soutter WP (1988) The treatment of vaginal intraepithelial neoplasia after hysterectomy. *Br J Obstet Gynaecol* **95**, 961–2.

26. Hernandez-Linares W, Puthawala A, Nolan JF, Jernstrom PB & Morrow CP (1980) Carcinoma *in situ* of the vagina: past and present management. *Obstet Gynecol* **56**, 356–60.

27. Woodman CB, Mould JJ & Jordan JA (1988) Radiotherapy in the management of vaginal intraepithelial neoplasia after hysterectomy. *Br J Obstet Gynaecol* **95**, 976–9.

28. Herbst AL & Scully RE (1970) Adenocarcinoma of the vagina in adolescence; a report of seven cases including six clear cell carcinomas (so-called mesonephromas). *Cancer* **25**, 745–57.

29. Herbst AL, Norvsis MJ, Rosenow PJ *et al.* (1979) An analysis of 346 cases of clear cell adenocarcinoma of the vagina and cervix with emphasis on recurrence and survival. *Gynecol Oncol* **7**, 111–22.

30. Brunham RC, Paavonen J, Stevens CE *et al.* (1984) Muco-purulent cervicitis: the ignored counterpart in women of urethritis in men. *N Engl J Med* **311**, 1–6.

31. Hare MJ, Toone E, Taylor-Robinson D *et al.* (1981) Follicular cervicitis-colposcopic appearances in association with *Chlamydia trachomatis. Br J Obstet Gynaecol* **88**, 174–80.

32. van Nagell JR, Higgins RV, Donaldson ES *et al.* (1990) Transvaginal sonography as a screening method for ovarian cancer. *Cancer* **65**, 573–7.

33. Stein IF & Leventhal ML (1935) Amenorrhea associated with bilateral polycystic ovaries. *Am J Obstet Gynecol* **29**, 181–91.

34. Judd HL, Barnes AB & Kliman B (1971) Long-term effect of wedge resection on androgen production in a case of polycystic ovarian disease. *Am J Obstet Gynecol* **110**, 1061–5.

35. Grimes HG, Nosal RA & Gallagher JC (1983) Ovarian pregnancy: a series of 24 cases. *Obstet Gynecol* **61**, 174–80.

36. Majumdar DN & Ledward RS (1982) Primary ovarian pregnancy in association with an intra-uterine conceptive device *in situ. J Obstet Gynaecol* **3**, 131–2.

37. Novak ER & Woodruff JD (1979) Ovarian pregnancy. In: *Novak's Gynecologic and Obstetric Pathology*, 8th edn. Philadelphia: Saunders, 556–60.

38. Sutton CJG (1993) Minimally invasive surgical approach to endometriosis and adhesiolysis. In: Studd S & Jardine Brown C (eds) *Yearbook of the Royal College of Obstetricians and Gynaecologists*. London: RCOG Press, 117–25.

Chapter 54: Premalignant and malignant disease of the cervix

Mahmood I. Shafi

Introduction

Carcinoma of the cervix is the second commonest cancer among women worldwide, with only breast cancer occurring more commonly. Worldwide, cervical cancer accounts for about 500,000 new cases diagnosed and 250,000 deaths every year. Of the new cases, 80% occur in the less developed countries and in some of these countries, cervical cancer is the commonest cancer in women. This situation is compounded by the fact that in underdeveloped countries 75% present with an advanced stage, which is the converse of presentations in the developed countries where 75% present early and cure can be realistically expected. This is partly due to education and empowerment of women so that in developed countries they present early because of symptoms and as part of screening programmes for cervical cancer.

While the natural history of breast cancer is poorly understood, cervical cancer is a preventable condition and considerable effort goes into detecting and treating the preinvasive disease, primarily in the developed countries. This should have a direct effect on incidence and mortality from this condition.

The National Health Service cervical screening programme (NHSCSP) established in 1988 has made significant inroads into the toll from cervical cancer in the United Kingdom. Cervical cancer incidence fell by 42% between 1988 and 1997 in England and Wales. The cervical screening programme is estimated to save approximately 4,500 lives per year in England. For the first time ever, death rates from cervical cancer have fallen below 1,000 in England – in 2002, 927 deaths were registered. One anticipates that the falling incidence and mortality will continue but several areas of the screening programme could be refined further (Fig. 54.1).

One of the areas that has greatly contributed to the overall success of the programme has been the wide coverage of the at-risk population. In England and Wales, women between the ages of 25 and 64 are offered cervical cytology screening every 3–5 years (Table 54.1) [1]. Prior to the introduction of the national programme, the target age coverage was 42% and this has increased to 82% by 2002.

Historical perspective

Preinvasive lesions of the cervix have been recognized for over 100 years. In 1886, Sir John Williams presented the Harveian Lectures at which he described eight cases of cervical cancer, one of which was equivalent to carcinoma in situ or CIN 3 [2]. In his lecture he stated that 'this is the earliest condition of undoubted cancer of the portio vaginalis that I have met with, and it is the earliest condition which is recognizable as cancer. It presented no distinct symptoms, and was discovered accidentally'.

In the mid-1920s the basic principles of colposcopy were described [3]. A system of low power magnification and illumination of the cervix was developed. Hinselmann hoped that with this system he would be able recognize the earliest lesions of the cervix that were invisible to the naked eye. Schiller described the Schiller iodine test a few years later. Schillers iodine solution when applied to the cervix stained normal squamous epithelium rich in glycogen but failed to stain columnar epithelium and abnormal epithelium which contained little or no glycogen. Colposcopic technique was further developed by the introduction of a green filter which enhanced recognition of vascular patterns. Colposcopy went into decline when cervical cytology was first described for the screening and detection of premalignant lesions of the cervix [4]. The realization that the techniques were complementary rather than being competitive led to the resurgence of colposcopy and its widespread introduction worldwide.

Cervical cytology classification

The NHSCSP has developed guidance on laboratory reporting for cervical cytology [5]. The cytology report should consist of a concise description of cells in precisely defined and generally accepted cytological terms. This

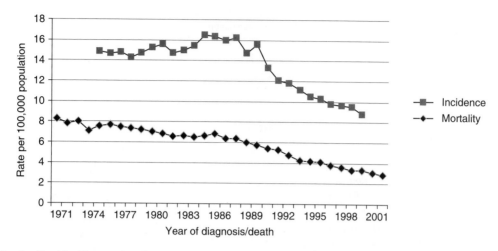

Fig. 54.1 Age standardized incidence of, and mortality from, cervical cancer, Great Britain, 1971–2002.

Table 54.1 Screening intervals for national cervical screening programme [11]

Age group (years)	Frequency of screening
25	First invitation
25–49	Three yearly
50–64	Five yearly
65+	Only screen those who have not been screened since age 50 or those who have had recent abnormal tests

may be followed, if appropriate, by a prediction of the histological condition based on the overall picture and should include a recommendation for further management of the patient. In North America and many other countries, the Bethesda reporting system has been adopted [6]. The classification consists of a statement of adequacy, general categorization (normal, epithelial cell abnormality or other) and descriptive diagnoses (organisms, other). The classification uses the term squamous intraepithelial lesion (SIL) to encompass all grades of CIN. SIL is further subdivided into two categories – low grade which includes cellular changes associated with human papilloma virus (HPV) infection and CIN 1, and high-grade SIL which includes CIN 2 and 3. The atypical squamous cells have two subcategories – atypical squamous cells of undetermined significance (ASC-US) and atypical squamous cells that cannot exclude high-grade SIL (ASC-H).

Management of abnormal cervical smears

Ideally all women with abnormal cervical cytology should have colposcopic assessment (Fig. 54.2). The aim of colposcopy is first to exclude an invasive process and secondarily to identify the extent of the abnormality and its likely grade which may allow a more conservative approach to management. For adequate colposcopy, the whole of the transformation zone (TZ) needs to be visualized. If the TZ is not fully visualized, then colposcopy is deemed unsatisfactory. This inability to visualize the squamocolumnar junction (SCJ) may be an indication for excisional biopsy of the cervical transformation zone.

Classification of CIN

The CIN classification has almost universally replaced the World Health Organization classification; CIN 1, 2 and 3 corresponding to mild, moderate and severe dysplasia/carcinoma in situ, respectively. A revised classification has been introduced with high-grade lesions (CIN 2 and 3) that are likely to behave as cancer precursors and low-grade lesions (CIN 1 and HPV associated changes) with unknown but a likely low progressive potential [7]. Whichever classification is used, there is intra- and inter-observer variation in the histopathological reporting.

Progressive potential of CIN

The progressive potential of high-grade lesions or CIN 3 is not questioned [8]. The progressive potential has been calculated to be 18% at 10 years and 36% at 20 years. Women with continuing abnormal cytology after initial management of carcinoma in situ of the cervix were almost 25 times more likely to develop invasive carcinoma than women who have normal follow-up cytology. When compared with the population at large, the chances of women with normal follow-up cytology developing

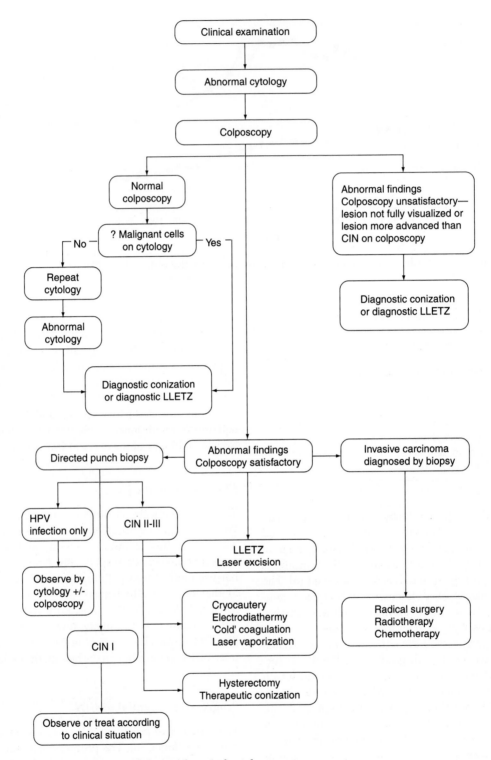

Fig. 54.2 Flow diagram for management of abnormal cervical cytology.

invasive cervical or vaginal vault carcinoma increase threefold over women who have never had carcinoma in situ of the cervix. As a result, there appears to be complete unanimity for the immediate treatment of CIN 3 lesions once diagnosed.

Colposcopy

Various parameters of the colposcopic assessment are studied including the vascular patterns, the degree of acetowhite epithelium, the border characteristics,

Table 54.2 Clinico-Colposcopic Index (CCI) – Shafi and Nazeer [9] – maximum score = 10

Variable	Score		
	Zero points	One point	Two points
Index cytology	Low grade	–	High grade
Smoking status	No	–	Yes
Age	≤30 years	>30 years	–
Acetowhitening	Slight	Marked	–
Surface area of lesion	≤1 cm^2 (small lesion)	>1 cm^2 (large lesion)	–
Intercapillary distance	≤350 μm (fine/no mosaic or punctation)	>350 μm (coarse mosaic or punctation)	–
Focality of lesion	Unifocal or multifocal	Annular	–
Surface pattern	Smooth	Irregular	–

the surface pattern and the surface area of the lesion under study. Using these variables an assessment of the likely nature of the lesion can be gauged. Various grading systems are advocated and one of these has been developed [9] using clinical and colposcopic parameters (Table 54.2). Using the clinico-colposcopic index (CCI) to devise a score for each individual patient helps in predicting the histological abnormality and management options. The CCI takes into account the important prognostic factors and for each patient a maximum score of 10 can be achieved. Those scoring 0–2 on this scale invariably have insignificant lesions. Those scoring 6–10 on this scale generally have high-grade disease present. In those scoring between 3 and 5, the histological pattern is mixed with a tendency of the lesion to harbour CIN grade 1 or 2.

If the transformation zone is fully visualized, biopsy of the worst atypical epithelium may be undertaken. Excisional methods such as laser excision or diathermy loop provide considerably more histopathological material than a punch biopsy. If the whole of the transformation zone is not visualized, then colposcopy is deemed to be unsatisfactory making a colposcopically directed punch biopsy of the worst area impossible. In this situation, recourse to a cone biopsy or an extended diathermy loop procedure is recommended.

If the woman is pregnant at the time of colposcopic assessment, a conservative approach is usually employed and treatment undertaken after delivery. If cancer is suspected, then a large biopsy, usually a wedge biopsy, is taken under general anaesthesia as there is a risk for significant haemorrhage.

Treatment of CIN

In an ideal world, all women with truly premalignant lesions destined to develop cancer could be selected and treated with a simple, rapid, non-morbid and effective office technique. The two main methods of treatment are ablative or excisional techniques (Table 54.3). Cure rates

Table 54.3 Methods for treatment of CIN

Excisional methods	Ablative methods
Loop TZ excision (LLETZ/LEEP)	Cryocautery
Laser TZ excision	Electrodiathermy
Knife cone biopsy	Cold coagulation
Laser cone biopsy	Carbon dioxide laser
Loop cone biopsy	
Hysterectomy	

for both ablative and excisional techniques are in excess of 90% [10]. Recently there has been a tendency towards using excisional methods. This allows better histopathological interpretation of the excised specimen and in certain circumstances allows a 'see and treat' strategy if the colposcopic assessment is consistent with a lesion requiring local treatment and the patient is agreeable to treatment under local anaesthetic at the initial visit. This policy can lead to overtreatment of insignificant lesions [11] and with this realization a 'select and treat' strategy is employed in most colposcopy units. The CCI scoring system described is a useful aid in this management strategy.

The treatment method used is subjective influenced. An important aspect is the depth of destruction of any local treatment modality. Studies to assess the depth of crypt involvement with CIN suggest that a depth of destruction to 3.8 mm would eradicate premalignant disease in 99.7% of cases. However, some gland crypts with involvement by CIN to 5 mm in depth were observed, and therefore a destructive depth greater than this is desirable. Ablation to a depth of 5–8 mm has been recommended. If depth of destruction is inadequate, then this deep-seated component may be a source of residual or recurrent disease.

Ablative techniques

Cryocautery destroys tissue by freezing using probes of various shapes and sizes and is probably best reserved for small lesions. While lesion size is important in determining success or failure using any of the treatment modalities [12], it is especially important with cryocautery. When using cryocautery, a double freeze-thaw-freeze technique is advocated to minimize failure rates. With larger lesions, multiple applications may be necessary. The depth of destruction is approximately 4 mm and this may be inadequate for some of the CIN lesions. Depth of destruction cannot be accurately gauged and incomplete eradication of disease may lead to regenerating epithelium covering the residual disease.

While electrodiathermy destroys tissue more effectively than cryocautery, it does require general, regional or local anaesthesia. Under colposcopic control, it is possible to destroy up to 1 cm depth using a combination of needle and ball electrodes. An extension of this technique using a wire loop allows electrodiathermy to be used in an excisional mode.

Cold coagulation was a term coined by Kurt Semm, the inventor of the instrument in 1966. Heat is applied to tissue using a Teflon-coated thermosound. Using overlapping applications of the thermosound for 20 s at 100°C, the whole of the transformation zone may be treated. The procedure does not usually require analgesia. Measurement of the depth of destruction is difficult. Depth of destruction is approximately 2.5–4 mm or more after treatment at 100°C for 30 s and always exceeds 4 mm after treatment at 120°C for 30 s.

Laser is an acronym for Light Amplification by Stimulated Emission of Radiation. A micromanipulator attached to the colposcope is used to manipulate the laser and treatment is conducted under direct vision. As the technique is precise, it allows good control of the depth of destruction, good haemostasis and excellent healing as there is minimal thermal damage to the adjacent tissue. The technique is particularly useful for treating premalignant disease with vaginal involvement. As there are no gland crypts in the vaginal epithelium, destruction to 2–3 mm depth is adequate.

Excisional methods

Transformation zone excision has been developed as a conservative excisional technique. Both the laser and diathermy loop have been used for this purpose. Laser excision is technically more demanding than laser vaporization and requires a high-power density beam with a small spot size that can function in a cutting mode. Both methods can also be used to fashion cone biopsies of the cervix. Diathermy loop excision using low power voltage apparatus is now widely practised [13]. The technique is referred to as large loop excision of transformation zone (LLETZ) in Europe and as loop electrosurgical excision

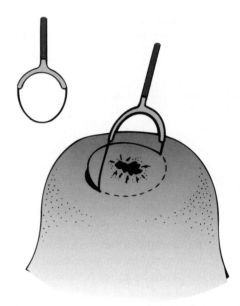

Fig. 54.3 Diagrammatic representation of large loop excision of the transformation zone (LLETZ).

procedure (LEEP) in North America (Fig. 54.3). Using this technique, a 'see and treat' management strategy for women with abnormal cervical smears can be adopted, whereby women are treated at their first visit to the colposcopy clinic. Strict guidelines need to be adhered to as this policy will undoubtedly lead to overtreatment in some women and will also result in an increased histopathological workload compared to processing punch biopsies. While histopathology workload is increased, this also results in excisional techniques providing considerably more material for assessment allowing a more reliable interpretation.

Success rates following local excisional techniques is similar to those quoted for laser ablation and cold coagulation. There appears to be no adverse effect on fertility and the outcome of subsequent pregnancies.

Cone biopsy and hysterectomy still retain a place in the management of CIN. Hysterectomy may need to be contemplated if CIN is present in a woman with other gynaecological conditions such as fibroids, menorrhagia or prolapse. Prior to operation, colposcopy will identify the extent of the lesion and avoid incomplete excision which may result in vaginal intraepithelial neoplasia (VAIN). If the lesion is seen to extend on to the vagina, this may be excised as part of the hysterectomy procedure. An alternative is to ablate the vaginal extension of CIN (using laser or diathermy) and then proceed to excision or hysterectomy as indicated.

The size and shape of the cone biopsy is governed by the colposcopic findings. The internal os and as much of the endocervical canal are left intact as is possible within the confines of disease eradication. This limits haemorrhagic morbidity and fertility will be little compromised.

Histological incomplete excision at the time of cone biopsy represents a management dilemma. Cervical cytology may in fact be a more useful prognostic guide to residual disease than excision cone margins. In this study no patient had residual disease if the post-cone smear was negative. In those women with severe cervical stenosis, hysterectomy may be contemplated. The risk of invasive disease following incomplete excision is related to the presence of cytological abnormality following treatment. A persistent cytological abnormality after cone biopsy is a good indicator of residual disease; such women warrant further treatment.

Treatment failures

The primary objective of treating women with CIN is to prevent invasive cervical cancer. If invasive disease develops or indeed if there is residual CIN, the initial treatment is deemed a failure.

Women who have undergone treatment of CIN remain at higher risk for invasive cervical disease. Those women that have abnormal cervical cytology following treatment are at much increased risk compared to those with normal cytology after treatment [8]. Therefore women who have been treated for CIN need long-term follow-up. Reports of invasive disease after local destructive therapy have been reviewed and many, but not all, of the invasive carcinomas are as a result of inappropriate selection for treatment and a failure to recognize early invasive disease at the time of initial assessment. Invasive disease following transformation zone excision has also been reported. It is suggested that the use of excisional procedures should further reduce the small risk of invasive carcinoma developing after treatment for CIN. Cytological abnormality following treatment, no matter how minor, should be regarded as an indication for colposcopic reassessment.

Colposcopic assessment is technically more difficult in those that have undergone previous treatment. Islands of CIN and indeed invasive disease can be buried under an apparently normal surface epithelium. For failures of initial treatment, it is generally recommended that an excisional method of treatment be used in preference to ablative techniques.

Human papilloma virus

Cervical cancer is a rare outcome of human papilloma virus (HPV) infection. HPV is a common and mainly sexually transmitted infection. It can be found in almost all cases of cervical cancer. However, most HPV infections will not progress to CIN or cancer. The invasive disease does not develop unless there is persistence of HPV DNA and it has been proposed as the first ever identified 'necessary cause' of a human cancer. Out of the 80 known HPV genotypes, 30 are known to infect the genital tract. Out of these 20 have been identified as carcinogenic with types 16 and 18 found most commonly in malignant lesions.

The common types are classified according to their oncogenic potential as follows:
- Low risk : 6, 11, 41, 44
- Intermediate risk : 31, 33, 35,
- High risk : 16, 18, 45, 56

There are many proposals to include HPV subtyping into management protocols for abnormal cervical cytology. Commercially available kits are available that will test for the common oncogenic virus subtypes. Although the use of such techniques has shown considerable promise in cross-sectional studies, this has not been translated into any meaningful longitudinal results with regards to progressive potential. Evaluation of the HPV/LBC (liquid based cytology) cervical screening pilots in the United Kingdom have concluded that caution be exercised in implementing HPV testing to triage women with minor cervical cytological abnormalities [1].

Currently, vaccines against HPV are being evaluated. In theory, cervical cancer can be prevented and treated by HPV vaccine therapy. Important progress has been made towards producing recombinant, type specific, vaccines both, preventive and therapeutic. Studies have shown significant effect on prevention of cervical cytological abnormalities and CIN and these are now moving to the next phase in terms of evaluation [14,15]. The conclusion from these studies is that vaccination could substantially reduce incidence of cervical cancer.

Non-treatment and serial colposcopy

The progressive potential of low-grade lesions is unknown and cannot be predicted from cytological, colposcopic or histological criteria. Many of these low-grade lesions will regress, but others will persist or progress. National recommendations for the United Kingdom allow CIN 1 lesions to be treated or kept under close surveillance [11]. However, some women are unlikely to accept even a low risk of malignancy and would prefer treatment. Also in a transient population, early intervention may be the preferred option as women are unlikely to adhere to a surveillance programme. The introduction of digital imaging colposcopy and video colposcopy allows scope for close surveillance and will allow serial colposcopy to be performed with comparison of the colposcopic images easily undertaken [16,17].

Cervical cancer presentation

Women may present asymptomatically when their disease is detected as a result of abnormal cervical cytology. In more advanced lesions, there are usually symptoms raising the possibility of cervical cancer. These include post-coital bleeding, postmenopausal bleeding and offensive blood-stained vaginal discharge. If there is abnormal bleeding during pregnancy, then a cervical lesion needs to be excluded. In some women presenting with late disease, there may be backache, leg pain/oedema, haematuria, bowel changes, malaise and weight loss.

Diagnosis

A full history and clinical examination is undertaken. If the referral is due to cervical cytology suspicious of invasion, then a colposcopic examination should be performed. Suspicious features at colposcopy include intense acetowhiteness, atypical vessels, raised/ulcerated surface, contact bleeding and atypical consistency on bimanual examination. Diagnosis is based on histology and appropriate biopsies should be taken. This biopsy should be either wedge or cone shaped to obtain sufficient material for histological assessment. Once cancer has been diagnosed, it is important to stage the disease so that treatment can be planned appropriately. The staging will also give an idea of prognosis and facilitates exchange of information between treatment centres.

Staging

Staging should include an assessment of disease extent and sites of spread (Table 54.4). Staging of cervical cancer is clinical although early cancers are staged according to the surgical specimen. All women with stage Ib or worse should have a chest X-ray (CXR) and an intravenous urogram (IVU) to exclude distant metastasis and complete the staging process by looking for obstructive uropathy and therefore disease extending to the pelvic side wall.

Staging should include:
- Examination under anaesthetic which should include a combined recto-vaginal assessment.
- Biopsy of the suspicious area. This should be suitably large to make a definitive diagnosis.
- Cystoscopy should be considered.
- Sigmoidoscopy should be considered.
- CXR and IVU.
- Other imaging as indicated and according to facilities available. These might include computerized axial tomography (CT) scan and Magnetic Resonance Imaging (MRI) scan.

Table 54.4 FIGO staging of cervical cancer (1994)

Stage	Features
0	Carcinoma in situ, intraepithelial carcinoma (cases of stage 0 should not be included in any therapeutic statistics for invasive carcinoma)
I	Carcinoma strictly confined to the cervix (extension to the corpus should be disregarded)
Ia	Preclinical carcinoma of the cervix, i.e. diagnosed by microscopy
Ia1	Minimal microscopically evident stromal invasion <3 mm in depth and a horizontal spread ≤7 mm
Ia2	Lesions with a depth of invasion >3 mm and no more than 5 mm, and horizontal spread ≤7 mm
Ib	Clinical lesions confined to the cervix or preclinical lesions greater than stage Ia
Ib1	Clinical lesions <4 cm in diameter
Ib2	Clinical lesions ≥4 cm in diameter
II	The carcinoma extends beyond the cervix, but has not extended on to the pelvic wall; the carcinoma involves the vagina but not as far as the lower third
IIa	No obvious parametrial involvement
IIb	Obvious parametrial involvement
III	The carcinoma has extended on to the pelvic wall; on rectal examination there is no cancer-free space between the tumour and the pelvic wall; the tumour involves the lower third of the vagina; all cases with a hydronephrosis or non-functioning kidney should be included unless they are known to be due to another cause
IIIa	No extension to the pelvic wall, but involvement of the lower third of the vagina
IIIb	Extension onto the pelvic wall or hydronephrosis or non-functioning kidney
IV	The carcinoma has extended beyond the true pelvis or has clinically involved the mucosa of the bladder or rectum
IVa	Spread of the growth to adjacent organs
IVb	Spread to distant organs

In the United Kingdom, it has become common practice to omit the IVU and place more reliance on MRI assessment.

Survival

Survival is stage dependent and the advanced stages are associated with a poor outlook. The national 5-year relative survival rate for all women treated for invasive cervical cancer is 61% [18]. The 5-year relative survival rates is 79% for stage I, 47% for stage II, 22% for stage III and 7% for stage IV.

Histology

The majority of cervical cancers are squamous (80–85%) and the remainder have an adenocarcinoma element.

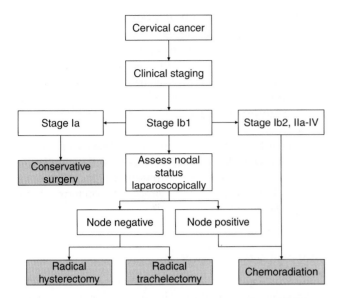

Fig. 54.4 Flow chart showing management options available with suspicion of cervical cancer incorporating minimal access surgery.

The proportion containing adenocarcinoma elements has been rising. Rarer histological types include clear cell, lymphomas and sarcomas.

Management

The management options to be considered include surgery, radiotherapy, chemotherapy and combinations of these modalities (Fig. 54.4). Age in itself is not a barrier to full assessment and definitive treatment. The women should be divided into those in whom the treatment is curative or palliative. For those with early stage cervical cancer curative intent with surgery or radiotherapy needs to be contemplated. In those with more advanced disease, chemoradiotherapy is the optimal method of management but surgery may have a role in a palliative setting.

Stage Ia

Stage Ia disease presents a paradox, in that they breach the basement membrane yet are rarely associated with metastasis. It is now considered appropriate for such cases to be managed by simple hysterectomy or even cone biopsy in the majority of cases. This dilemma is only pertinent in those young women wishing to retain fertility. A suitably planned cone biopsy may be both diagnostic and therapeutic. The entire abnormality must be included in the pathological specimen. If the cone biopsy margins are positive for CIN or invasive disease, this is a significant risk factor for finding residual invasive disease in the re-excision specimen. The risk of distant spread is <1% in stage Ia1 and <5% in stage Ia2 disease. Some authorities recommend a more aggressive surgical procedure with pelvic node dissection and a modified radical hysterectomy depending on the volume of the tumour. Tumours with less than 420 mm^3 have virtually no risk of metastases. Lesions that invade beyond 5 mm in depth should be considered stage Ib carcinoma and undergo radical surgery or radiotherapy.

No generally accepted definition exists for microinvasive adenocarcinoma. At present the preferred term for a small invasive adenocarcinoma is 'early invasive adenocarcinoma'. It is very difficult to differentiate extensive high-grade cervical glandular intraepithelial neoplasia (CGIN) from early invasive disease and borderline cases should probably be treated as invasive.

Stage Ib1

For those with stage Ib1 disease, the options lie between radical surgery (radical hysterectomy with bilateral pelvic lymphadenectomy with or without oophorectomy) or radical radiotherapy. The optimal therapy is that which has the highest cure rates with the least associated morbidity. For young women, surgery also offers the opportunity to preserve the ovaries, reduces the risk of sexual dysfunction and is not associated with the late sequelae seen with radiotherapy. The small but definite risk of radiation carcinogenesis is also avoided. The nodal status impacts long-term survival – the 5-year survival rate is approximately twice as good in node negative patients (90%) as in node positive patients (46%). For those women offered surgical treatment, this should be undertaken by appropriately trained doctors in the context of full support services.

Radical radiotherapy is preferred in those centres where surgical expertise is not available or in women who are not medically fit for surgery. Contraindications to surgery are relative, and some of the factors may also compromise delivery of the radiotherapy schedule (e.g. obesity). Radical radiotherapy aims to control the primary tumour and also to treat any lymphatic spread. Usually a combination of intracavitary (to treat the primary tumour) and external beam therapy (to treat pelvic lymph nodes) is used. Planned combinations of radiotherapy and surgery are not advocated as this increases morbidity with no attendant gain in cure or survival rates. As a general rule, intracavitary brachytherapy is given with the addition of external beam therapy. Using modern after loading techniques with the high dose regimens (HDR) reduces both the patient morbidity and exposure of staff.

Adjuvant chemoradiotherapy is not routinely indicated but should be offered to those with pelvic lymph node spread, tumour at the excision margins and other risk factors that make a recurrence likely. Neither the overall response rate nor the complete response rate has been reproducibly improved by adding other drugs to cisplatinum. The attendant morbidity is highest when surgery is combined with chemoradiotherapy.

While the incidence of ovarian involvement is <1% in squamous cell cancers, the incidence rises to 5–10% in adenocarcinomas. In the latter an oophorectomy is usually recommended if the surgical option is taken.

Stage Ib2-IVa

For those with stage Ib2-IVa disease, chemoradiotherapy is preferred [19]. Several studies indicate overall survival advantage for cisplatin-based chemotherapy in conjunction with radiotherapy.

Radiotherapy may be given either as radical or in a palliative setting. Radical radiotherapy is given with the intent of cure whereas palliative radiotherapy does not prolong survival but can control symptoms, especially pain.

Stage IVb

No 'standard' therapeutic protocol applies. The treatment is individualized according to location and extent of disease.

Minimal access surgery

An important factor in outcome for women with cervical cancer is whether there is lymphatic spread at the time of diagnosis. This has a significant effect on survival figures and current imaging modalities are unable to identify accurately those individuals with metastatic disease to the lymph nodes. Several surgical centres now routinely assess the lymph nodes surgically prior to planning treatment. This can either be done using minimal access surgery or using an extraperitoneal approach. Lymph node yield at laparoscopy is certainly equivalent to the open approach. Lymph nodes that are removed are submitted for histological and immunohistochemical assessment and further management planned. In those with negative nodes, surgical cure is feasible and these individuals proceed with radical or fertility sparing surgery. In those with metastatic disease, cure from surgery is not possible, and these women are offered chemoradiotherapy as their best option to attain cure (Fig. 54.4).

Fertility sparing surgery

In those women who wish to preserve fertility options, radical trachelectomy is a surgical option. This technique has evolved from the radical vaginal hysterectomy and involves removing the cervix, parametrium and upper one third of the vagina in those with histologically negative pelvic lymph nodes [20]. Cervical cerclage with a non-absorbable suture is inserted at the end of the surgical procedure to maintain closure of the uterine isthmus in the event of future pregnancy. Caesarean section is advocated for delivery.

Trachelectomy is not appropriate for those women that have completed their family as long-term data are being accrued. Those women with tumours of ≤2 cm are most suitable. In those achieving a pregnancy, preterm labour is a significant risk factor.

Recurrent cervical cancer

These women should be referred to those with expertise in managing this situation. This may involve the gynaecological, radiation or medical oncologist (Fig. 54.5). If further treatment is planned it should be conducted in centres suitably equipped and with appropriate support facilities including an intensive care unit.

Cases of pelvic recurrence are considered for the modality of treatment that has not previously been utilized. Recurrence after surgery is generally treated with radiotherapy (with some protocols including chemotherapy). In post-radiation failures where the disease is confined to the pelvis, pelvic exenteration is offered to those women who are surgical candidates. This should only be undertaken by those with the appropriate training in surgical gynaecological oncology working in centres with a multidisciplinary team.

No single treatment protocol exists for recurrent disease beyond the pelvis, or in those women who have failed radiotherapy and are not candidates for further surgery. In those where palliation is appropriate, early involvement of clinicians specializing in palliative care and Macmillan cancer relief nurses can be extremely beneficial, not only for the patient but also the family concerned.

Cervical cancer in pregnancy

The presentation is usually abnormal bleeding, though some 20% are asymptomatic. The survival figures are stage for stage the same as those for women who are not pregnant. It is now believed that the route of delivery does not affect the ultimate 5-year survival.

Cone biopsy can result in excessive bleeding and spontaneous abortion. The absolute indications for cone biopsy include a Pap smear suspicious for invasive cancer with no colposcopic proof, and colposcopic suspicion or directed biopsy indicating an invasive lesion.

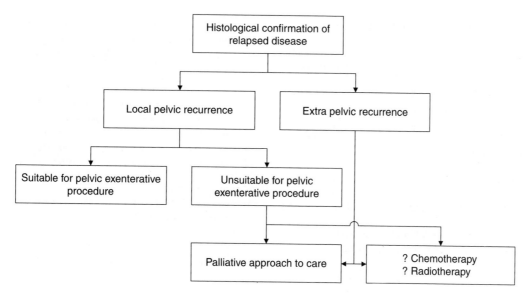

Fig. 54.5 Flow chart of management options with recurrence of cervical cancer.

Prior to 24 weeks, the treatment recommended is the same as for women who are not pregnant. If the treatment is radiotherapy, patients in the first trimester usually abort during the external beam therapy. In the second trimester, spontaneous abortion often is not the case, and the fetus must be removed surgically prior to radiation.

Radical hysterectomy and pelvic lymphadenectomy can be accomplished at any gestational age. When cancer is detected at the time of fetal viability, radical Caesarean hysterectomy can be offered or the fetus can be delivered and therapy instituted thereafter. The route of delivery has traditionally been Caesarean section, though this is more related to the possibility of increased bleeding, rather than the older concept of spread of disease if the vaginal route is chosen.

Patients diagnosed a few weeks prior to fetal viability, or those who refuse abortion based on moral or religious views present the greatest challenge. In such cases, with appropriate counselling, the fetus is carried to earliest viability and therapy then undertaken.

Key points

1 Colposcopic assessment of women with abnormal cervical cytology should be undertaken prior to any treatment.
2 Whichever local method is used for treatment, the depth of destruction should be at least 5–8 mm as gland crypts may be involved with CIN.
3 Success rates for local ablative and local excisional techniques are similar after a single treatment episode (90–95%).

4 After local treatment for CIN, women remain at a higher risk for development of invasive disease as compared to the general population. Those women that have continuing abnormal cervical cytology following treatment are at greatest risk of developing an invasive lesion.
5 Survival for cervical cancer is stage specific and volume of disease has a major influence on outcomes.
6 For early stage invasive disease (Ib1) there appears to be no difference in survival outcomes between radical surgery and radical radiotherapy.
7 For locally advanced cervical cancers (Ib2-IVa), chemoradiotherapy is the preferred management.

References

1. Sasieni P, Adams J & Cuzick J (2003) Benefits of cervical screening at different ages: evidence from the UK audit of screening histories. *Br J Cancer* **89**, 88–93.
2. Williams J (1886) *Cancer of the uterus. Harveian Lectures for 1886.* London: HK Lewis.
3. Hinselmann H (1925) Verbesserung der inspektionsmoglichkeit von vulva, vagina und portio. *Munchener medizinische Wochenschrift* **77**, 1733.
4. Papanicolaou GN & Traut HF (1941) The diagnostic value of vaginal smears in carcinoma of the uterus. *Am J Obstet Gynecol* **42**, 193–206.
5. Johnson J & Patnick J (2000) *Achievable Standards, Benchmark for Reporting, and Criteria for Evaluating Cervical Cytopathology,* 2nd edn. NHSCSP publication no. 1. London: Stationary Office, London.
6. Solomon D, Davey D, Kurman R *et al.*, The Forum Group Members & The Bethesda 2001 Workshop (2002) The 2001 Bethesda System: terminology for reporting results of cervical cytology. *J Am Med Assoc* **287**, 2114–9.

7. Richart RM (1990) A modified terminology for cervical intraepithelial neoplasia. *Obstet Gynecol* **75**, 131–3.

8. McIndoe WA, McLean MR, Jones RW & Mullins PR (1984) The invasive potential of carcinoma in situ of the cervix. *Obstet Gynecol* **64**, 451–8.

9. Shafi MI & Nazeer S (2004) Grading system for abnormal colposcopic findings. In: Bosze P & Luesley D (eds) *EAGC Course Book on Colposcopy*. Budapest: Primed-X Press.

10. Martin-Hirsch PL, Parakevaidis E & Kitchener H (2000) Surgery for cervical intraepithelial neoplasia. *Cochrane Database Syst Rev* **2**, CD001318.

11. Luesley DM & Leeson S (2004) *Colposcopy and Programme Management: Guidelines for the NHS Cervical Screening Programme*. NHSCSP publication no. 20. London: Stationary Office, London.

12. Shafi MI, Dunn JA, Buxton EJ, Finn CB, Jordan JA & Luesley DM (1993) Abnormal cervical cytology following large loop excision of the transformation zone: a case controlled study. *Br J Obstet Gynaecol* **100**, 145–8.

13. Prendiville W, Davies R & Berry PJ (1986) A low voltage diathermy loop for taking cervical biopsies: a qualitative comparison with punch biopsy forceps. *Br J Obstet Gynaecol* **93**, 773–6.

14. Koutsky LA, Ault KA, Wheeler CM *et al.*, Proof of Principle Study Investigators (2004) A controlled trial of a human papillomavirus type 16 vaccine. *N Engl J Med* **347**, 1645–51.

15. Harper DM, Franco EL, Wheeler C *et al.*, GlaxoSmithKline HPV vaccine study group (2004) Efficacy of a bivalent L1 virus-like particle vaccine in prevention of infection with human papillomavirus types 16 and 18 in young women: a randomised controlled trial. *Lancet* **364**, 1757–65.

16. Shafi MI, Dunn JA, Chenoy R, Buxton EJ, Williams C & Luesley DM (1994) Digital imaging colposcopy, image analysis and quantification of the colposcopic image. *Br J Obstet Gynaecol* **101**, 234–8.

17. Etherington IJ, Dunn J, Shafi MI, Smith T & Luesley DM (1997) Video colpography: a new technique for secondary cervical screening. *Br J Obstet Gynaecol* **104**, 150–3.

18. Cancer Research UK (2005) www.cancerresearchuk.org

19. Thomas GM (1999) Improved treatment for cervical cancer – concurrent chemotherapy and radiotherapy. *N Engl J Med* **340**, 1198–1200.

20. Dargent D, Brun JL, Roy M, Mathevet P & Remy I (1994) La Trachelectomie Elargie (TE). Une alternative a l'hysterectomie radicale dans le traitement de cancers infiltrants developpes sur la face externe du col uterin. *J Obstet Gynaecol* **2**, 285–92.

Further reading

Shafi Mahmood I, Luesley DM & Jordan JA (2000) *Handbook of Gynaecological Oncology*. London: Churchill Livingstone.

Luesley DM & Leeson S (2004) Colposcopy and Programme Management: Guidelines for the NHS Cervical Screening Programme. NHSCSP publication no. 20.

http://bethesda2001.cancer.gov/
www.cancerresearchuk.org/
www.cancerscreening.nhs.uk/cervical
www.nci.nih.gov/

Chapter 55: Epithelial ovarian cancer

Hani Gabra

Ovarian cancer is a common solid tumour and is the leading cause of death from gynaecological cancer. It is a serious disease particularly in advanced stages with a course that is punctuated by frequent tumour recurrence and negative impact on quality and length of life.

Disease progression and patient decline is typically due to locoregional peritoneal dissemination and its consequence rather than due to visceral metastatic disease and this brings opportunities for therapy research that cannot be contemplated for other types of cancer.

Some patients are cured completely even of advanced ovarian cancer with multimodality therapy and therefore research interest in reducing the incidence and improving the prognosis of the disease is intense.

Aetiology, epidemiology and genetics

The current lifetime risk is 1 per 48, the incidence being approximately 22 per 100,000 population. Epithelial ovarian cancer is a disease of older women, the incidence peaking at the age of 67.

There are about 7000 cases of ovarian cancer in the United Kingdom annually with about 5400 deaths, and in most centres the overall survival at 5 years is about 30%.

There is geographic variation of ovarian cancer, being commoner in northern Europe and in the United States and less common in Africa and Japan. The aetiology of ovarian cancer is incompletely understood.

Incessant ovulation is thought to be an important factor (ref fathalla). In large case-control studies, factors that interfere with ovulation are found to affect the incidence of ovarian cancer. Use of the oral contraceptive pill reduces the risk of ovarian cancer by 50% in some studies (refs). Other factors include early menarche, late menopause, pregnancy, childbirth, breastfeeding, infertility and the use of hyperovulating drugs.

However, the risk of ovarian cancer is seen to be reduced by mechanical sterilization and by hysterectomy, and there is an increased risk associated with inflammatory conditions such as pelvic inflammatory disease (PID) and perineal dusting with talc. This suggests that chronic inflammation has an important role in the aetiology of ovarian cancer. Factors such as cytokine and outside-in signalling molecule components may be of importance in this process.

Endometriosis is also known to be associated with endometrioid (and sometimes clear cell) Mullerian adenocarcinomas, and particularly so when present on the surface of the ovary.

Environmental factors are dominant in the aetiology of ovarian cancer. The daughters of Japanese migrants to the United States were noted to have an incidence of ovarian cancer approximating to that of the US population as a whole, as compared with much lower levels observed in Japan.

Genetic factors in ovarian cancer are important. However only 5–10% of ovarian cancer is associated with an autosomal dominant syndrome where there is an inherited defect in one of three gene classes; BRCA1, BRCA2 (site-specific ovarian cancer syndrome and breast-ovarian cancer syndrome) and the mismatch repair genes (identified in the type 2 Lynch syndrome or hereditary nonpolyposis colorectal cancer [HNPCC]). There is currently much controversy about the relevance of these genes to non-inherited breast cancer, and somatic methylation along with other epigenetic mechanisms may be important in inactivation of these genes in a substantial proportion of somatic (as opposed to familial) common epithelial ovarian cancers.

The molecular basis of sporadic ovarian cancer is slowly being unravelled. P53 mutation is a common molecular lesion in ovarian cancer, particularly in serous ovarian cancer. Although this is an important molecular lesion in the aetiology, its clinical significance is less certain with respect to diagnosis, prediction, prognosis or therapy. K-ras mutation and PTEN disruption are associated with clinical endometrioid ovarian cancer, and elegant mouse models show the multistep process that takes normal ovarian surface epithelium to endometriosis with K-ras mutation and then to endometrioid adenocarcinomas with

PTEN knockout. In fact, PTEN knockout represents an extremely important component of a disrupted PI3Kinase pathway. PI3K and AKT activation are both common lesions in ovarian cancer and form attractive targets for ovarian cancer treatment by inhibitors. Activation of tyrosine kinases is also common in ovarian cancer. This growth factor 'addiction' extends to members of the EGF receptor tyrosine kinase family commonly including EGFR and HER2. c-fms is also commonly upregulated in ovarian cancer. Doubtless this molecular classification will continue to grow with empirical scientific progress until a more complete understanding is achieved, and this is likely to be accompanied with recognition of redundancy and a better understanding of the therapeutic targets that will make a difference to the evolution of the disease.

Screening and prophylactic oophorectomy

Successful screening is defined as an intervention that results in reduction in the mortality of the screened population relative to the unscreened population. There is no evidence that screening of the general population or of targeted at-risk populations achieve reduction in mortality. Screening requires high sensitivity and specificity. High sensitivity maximizes the potential for influencing survival, whereas high specificity reduces the chances of false positives that result in unnecessary operations. These issues are compounded by the fact that ovarian cancer is a relatively rare condition; thus around 99.6% specificity is required to detect one case of ovarian cancer in every 10 women testing positive (10% positive predictive value). Lower specificity (e.g. 92% in BRCA1 mutant ovarian cancer), however, will achieve this level of positive predictive value in high-risk groups for ovarian cancer who have much higher incidence of the disease.

Important data demonstrates that prophylactic oophorectomy irrespective of screening in those with BRCA1 and BRCA2 germline mutations essentially abolishes the incidence of ovarian cancer and also markedly reduces the incidence of breast cancer in the oophorectomized population as compared with controls (NEJM article). This is increasingly considered the approach of choice where the high-risk patient is able to rationalize the cost/benefit equation. In general, where it is recommended, prophylactic bilateral salpingo-oophorectomy is performed with completion of childbearing and hormone replacement therapy is commenced thereafter until a point that appropriately corresponds to natural menopause, that is, around 50 years (JCO article Armstrong).

Large randomized controlled trials are now underway for screening in ovarian cancer. The endpoint in these trials is cause specific mortality reduction in the screened population.

In the United Kingdom, the large UKCTOCS trial is now underway. It seeks to recruit 200,000 women at average risk for ovarian cancer. There is a 3-way randomization to, first, a control unscreened group (group 3), to annual CA125 and, if abnormal, then subsequent transvaginal ultrasound (group 1) or annual transvaginal ultrasound and, if abnormal, then CA125 (group 2).

For those at higher genetic risk, the UKFOCSS study is investigating the benefit of screening for those with …5000 women are being recruited for this study where annual transvaginal ultrasound is performed, with CA125 at the time of TVS, and also 4 months preceding and following it. The endpoints are early detection and cancer mortality.

It is entirely unclear whether it will ever be feasible, effective or cost-effective to screen the general population for ovarian cancer. Furthermore, with the clear impact of prophylactic oophorectomy for targeted groups, it is also unclear whether screening of targeted groups even if effective will approach the definite benefits to be obtained by removal of ovaries after completion of childbearing.

Nevertheless, recent developments in proteomics have claimed specificities and sensitivities approaching 100% in diagnosis of ovarian cancer, and these may if correct alter the prospects of screening in both the general population and in targeted groups. However, a note of caution should be expressed in that the field of proteomics is currently controversial with many issues of sample quality control for both pre-analytical variables (sample collection and storage protocols) and analytical variables (day to day variation of complex machinery required for proteomics).

Clinical presentation

Ovarian cancer presents with non-specific symptoms. These symptoms include abdominal bloating and discomfort, and pressure symptoms such as nausea, early repletion or colicky abdominal pain. It is obvious that these symptoms may be due to advanced disease. More specific symptoms that are more likely to be associated with earlier stage diagnosis include postmenopausal bleeding (when associated with endometrial carcinoma) and significant pelvic pressure symptoms such as urinary frequency, pelvic pain due to torsion or haemorrhage of the ovary and rectosigmoid symptoms such as constipation or diarrhoea.

Signs include gaseous abdominal distension, a pelvic mass, abnormal bowel sounds, ascites, palpable abdominal masses, lymphadenopathy, pleural effusion, an umbilical mass (Sister Mary Joseph nodule) and, rarely, intra-abdominal organomegaly.

It is of interest that recent work (ref) suggests that it is not the nature of the symptoms themselves, rather their frequency after they commence that are associated with ovarian cancer as a diagnosis subsequently. However, this was a retrospective survey.

In retrospective analyses of General Practitioners' referrals, a variety of medical speciality destinations in response to the symptoms and signs described above ensured heterogeneity of routes to definitive management. However, it has not been established that these delays from primary care in any way affect the outcomes in ovarian cancer management. Many subsequent factors are unknown, for instance, is there a point at which the tumour may become inoperable, even if advanced but operable from the outset (see below)?

Despite not having complete answers to these issues, it is important to say that raising awareness among women and among health-care professionals is desirable to allow early appropriate referral of all stages of ovarian cancer, as this may yet ultimately be shown to impact on survival.

Pathobiology of epithelial ovarian cancer

The ovaries are covered by a polarized cuboidal epithelial monolayer that is in continuity with the rest of the peritoneal mesothelium. It is this surface that gives rise to epithelial ovarian cancer, either directly from the surface or from trapped surface epithelial cells within inclusion cysts (see below).

Is there an early ovarian cancer lesion?

Unlike cervical and colorectal cancer there are not defined anatomical steps in early tumour progression that allow screening of the preneoplastic or preinvasive states in ovarian cancer. There is considerable doubt that there exists anatomical stage progression and there is some evidence that malignant ovarian neoplasms arising on the surface of the ovary may disseminate to bulky stage III disease without stepwise FIGO stage progression. This introduces considerable uncertainty to the notion of screening by anatomical characteristics such as those currently performed for breast cancer. New and very interesting data suggest that at least some ovarian cancers arise from surface epithelial inclusion cysts, and if this data remains robust and is extended to most ovarian cancers arising in this way, there may be a feasible route to ovarian cancer prevention, having identified a precursor lesion.

Borderline lesions and invasive cancer: evolving concepts

Borderline epithelial tumours (tumours of low-malignant potential) of the ovary in general have differing characteristics to epithelial ovarian cancer. The hallmark of borderline tumours is the absence of basement membrane invasion. The conversion rate of borderline tumours to ovarian cancer is extremely low, and in general these lesions are compatible with prolonged survival even when disseminated either as a monoclonal or polyclonal process. It is possible that there is a biologically aggressive subgroup of borderline tumours and several studies have tried to define these characteristics, among them histological features of a 'proliferative state' and aneuploidy. Rarely some cases of borderline tumours do truly progress to invasive ovarian cancer, and therefore definitive protocols for dealing with this clinical entity are essential. Borderline tumours, particularly serous are also associated with a definite incidence perhaps as high as 10% of *de novo* primary peritoneal carcinoma.

Pathology of epithelial ovarian cancer

Most ovarian cancers have serous histology, which have histology reminiscent of fallopian tube origin, and often have characteristic psammoma bodies. Endometrioid adenocarcinomas and clear cell carcinomas are the next commonest histological type, and mucinous carcinomas are less common still. Uncommonly ovarian carcinosarcomas do present and are epithelial tumours with sarcomatous differentiation. There is evidence that clear cell and mucinous ovarian cancers are far less responsive to chemotherapy than serous and endometrioid ovarian cancers. An important feature of histological classification is the grade of the cancer, ranging from well differentiated (Grade 1) to moderately differentiated (Grade 2) to poorly differentiated (Grade 3). Borderline tumours are not regarded as cancers and in general have an excellent prognosis. These are not considered further here.

Patterns of spread of ovarian cancer

The FIGO classification for ovarian cancer is shown in Table 55.1, and is based on surgical staging. Like other malignant neoplasms, ovarian cancer can disseminate along locoregional, lymphatic and blood-borne routes. However there are patterns of dissemination that are characteristic of ovarian cancer, and also patterns that are characteristic of histological subtypes of ovarian cancer.

In the common serous ovarian carcinomas, the dominant pattern is that of transperitoneal locoregional dissemination resulting often in bulky intra-abdominal disease particularly involving the omentum as well as other peritoneal surfaces. This is often accompanied by malignant ascites. With the exception of malignant unilateral or bilateral pleural effusion, and involvement of the umbilicus due to tumour spread along the remnant of the umbilical vein, it is unusual to present with visceral metastatic disease, for example, visceral hepatic metastases, pulmonary,

Table 55.1 FIGO staging for ovarian cancer

Stage	
I	Growth limited to the ovaries
Ia	Tumour in one ovary; no ascites, capsule intact, no tumour on surface
Ib	As in Ia but tumour in both ovaries
Ic	Tumour either as in Ia or Ib, but ascites with cancer cells, or capsule ruptured or tumour on surface, or positive peritoneal washings
II	Growth on one or both ovaries with peritoneal implants within the pelvis
IIa	Extension or metastases to uterus or fallopian tubes
IIb	Extension to other pelvic organs
IIc	Tumour either IIa or IIb, but with findings as in Ic
III	Tumour in one or both ovaries with peritoneal implants outside the pelvis, or retroperitoneal node metastases
IIIa	Tumour grossly limited to the true pelvis; negative nodes, but microscopic implants on abdominal peritoneal surfaces
IIIb	As in IIIa, but abdominal implants are <2 cm in diameter
IIIc	Abdominal implants >2 cm, ± retroperitoneal lymph node metastases
IV	Tumour involving one or both ovaries with distant metastases, e.g. malignant pleural fluid, parenchymal liver metastases

cerebral or bone metastases that are so common in other gynaecological tumours such as breast or cervical cancer. Lymph node involvement (which stages the patient as stage IIIc) is relatively common.

Diagnosis

The diagnosis of ovarian cancer is histopathological, and most large centres will require the fine details of histopathological diagnosis to manage the patient rationally. Histopathological type, Tumour Grade and FIGO stage are all determined by adequate biopsy obtained by procedures such as radiologically guided core biopsy, laparoscopic biopsy, and formal staging laparotomy. In general, many centres would regard a CA125, CEA and cytological diagnosis from a sample of ascites as inadequate for management of the patient with ovarian cancer, and that is certainly the case for the West London Gynaecological Cancer Centre.

CA125, a glycoprotein serum marker is neither a diagnostic nor a screening marker for ovarian cancer. It is elevated in a variety of benign and malignant conditions. It is helpful in prognostication about 3 months into chemotherapeutic; however, its main role is in evaluating

response not in initial therapy but in treatment for relapsed disease.

Prognostic factors

The majority of patients with ovarian cancer will relapse and ultimately die from their disease. While the prognosis in stage I ovarian cancer is excellent with earlier lower grade stages having a cure rate of greater than 90%, overall, prognosis leaves much room for improvement, with 1-year survival of 70%, 2-year survival of 50%, 5-year survival of 30% and 10-year survival of 20%.

Analysing large cohorts of newly diagnosed patients with carefully collected clinical data has revealed prognostic factors that have been subsequently validated in other clinical datasets. Important factors that predict survival include performance status, FIGO staging, tumour grade, surgical debulking status, histological subtype, age at diagnosis and albumin. Heterogeneity in the sample populations with respect particularly to treatment effects has limited extrapolation to real cohorts of patients. Ongoing research is now applying whole genome molecular profiling analysis as well as individual characterized molecular targets to the refinement of predictive and prognostic models.

For patients with recurrent ovarian cancer, there are several factors that predict favourable response to platinum retreatment. These include serous histology, disease bulk of less than 5 cm, and number of tumour sites (<3). A conventional definition of this platinum sensitivity that closely correlates with residual disease bulk is that of an interval since last chemotherapy of greater than 6 months.

Treatment of newly diagnosed ovarian cancer

Integrated multidisciplinary care of ovarian cancer

Ovarian cancer is best managed in centralized integrated multidisciplinary teams. This has been shown to improve outcomes in this disease. In general, the team consists of a surgical oncologist and a non-surgical oncologist, a radiologist and a pathologist specialized in ovarian cancer management. The team crucially also requires a specialist nurse who acts as glue and conduit between the patient and the multidisciplinary team and is available for the patient throughout his or her journey. Palliative care specialist input may be required in all phases of the disease. Increasingly multidisciplinary teams are developing integrated care pathways for patients with ovarian cancer that bring together hospital and community services within one framework.

SURGERY

The aim of surgery is total macroscopic debulking of tumour. The purpose of this is to minimize the volume of tumour prior to further non-surgical treatment.

The procedure is really only valuable if the disease is debulked to less than 2 cm maximum diameter in terms of impact of survival, and is a powerful independent prognostic variable in ovarian cancer outcome (Griffiths). Optimal cytoreduction is feasible variably according to surgical effort and experience, and if one compares chemotherapy studies with similar entry criteria the proportion optimally debulked can vary from 30% (ICON 3) up to 85% in some studies and series, with apparently acceptable operative morbidity. There have been various definitions of what constitutes 'optimal debulking'. At the West London Gynaecological Cancer Centre the definition is <1 cm maximum diameter.

Where the surgeon regards macroscopic debulking as a realistic objective for a patient, a midline incision is performed. After evaluation, the surgeon performs bilateral salpingo-oophorectomy, total abdominal hysterectomy and omentectomy. Removal of all visible deposits is also undertaken. If the surgeon is not able to achieve total macroscopic debulking, it may nevertheless be possible to achieve optimal debulking (Wharton and Herson).

Is surgery important?

This is an important question. There has been no randomized trial of surgery versus no surgery; however, the survival of patients with advanced ovarian cancer receiving no surgery in the pre-chemotherapy era was of the order of 12–14%, and several small retrospective studies implied a relationship between optimal debulking and better survival. In an influential study by Van Den Berg (ref) and colleagues, patients achieving suboptimal debulking were randomized to interval debulking surgery or not. Those patients receiving interval debulking had better survival. Although this study has been criticized, it is important in that it shows a survival benefit associated with surgery in a randomized setting. An important recent study was the surgical study within the SCOTROC1 chemotherapy trial. In SCOTROC 1 all post-operative patients received carboplatin and were randomized to either Paclitaxel or Docetaxel, with progression-free survival as an endpoint. Surgical data was collected from this trial, and 2 out of 3 of patients were from the United Kingdom, with 1 out of 3 from outwith. This allowed comparison of surgical practice and of relationship of surgery to outcome since the case-mix and chemotherapy were identical in all countries where patients were operated on. In the United Kingdom although similar rates of TAH BSO and omentectomy were performed, there were

significantly less bowel resections and para-aortic/pelvic lymphadenectomy procedures performed, particularly in those patients who were optimally debulked. Furthermore the United Kingdom had significantly inferior complete debulking rates compared with non-UK centres. It was found that the United Kingdom had significantly less operating time per patient than non-UK centres across all stages. As an independent prognostic variable with respect to progression-free survival, residual disease (>2 cm) carries an adverse hazard ratio of 1.6; however, this depends on the extent of pre-surgical disease. In less extensive disease, optimal debulking is associated with a large survival benefit, whereas with more extensive disease the benefit was much less. However, UK patients who were completely debulked (as opposed to optimally) did much less well than those who were completely debulked overseas (HR 2). However, in those optimally (as opposed to completely) or suboptimally debulked there was no such adverse effect of being operated in the United Kingdom (Crawford *et al.* JCO 2005).

Lymphadenectomy in ovarian cancer

The role of lymphadenectomy in ovarian cancer remains debatable. In the UK lymphadenectomy is not performed routinely for ovarian cancer and this is the case whether the ovarian cancer is early (limited) or advanced stage.

Lymphadenectomy in early (limited) stage ovarian cancer

The general argument is that lymphadenectomy in early ovarian cancer carries additional morbidity and confers no therapeutic survival advantage to the patient, and the chances of upstaging a patient who does not have a Grade 3 tumour is relatively low. In the United States, Australia and Europe it is generally the rule that lymphadenectomy is undertaken. This of course provides better staging for the patient; however, there is no evidence of an ensuing survival advantage. In the ICON1/ACTION studies of immediate versus delayed carboplatin in early ovarian cancer, it was found that no subgroup overall failed to benefit from chemotherapy, and this has been interpreted as 'all early ovarian cancer patients should generally receive chemotherapy; therefore, there is no advantage in selection of higher risk groups by lymphadenectomy, and therefore it should not be performed'. However, chemotherapy carries significant morbidity and mortality risks also. In subgroup analysis of the ACTION study (which was a parallel European study to ICON1) it was found that those who had complete debulking including lymphadenectomy appeared not to benefit from chemotherapy. Therefore there is an argument to be made that patients with stage Ia and Ib disease which is surgically fully staged (i.e. lymphadenectomy), where there is no room for doubt that the case might be stage IIIc and where the patient has Grade 1 or Grade 2 carcinoma could be spared chemotherapy. This approach is the one utilized at the West London Gynaecological Cancer Centre.

Lymphadenectomy in advanced ovarian cancer

Lymphadenectomy for advanced ovarian cancer is generally not regarded as important in the United Kingdom; however, recent data from the SCOTROC1 surgical study (Crawford *et al.*) suggest that it may have an influence on patient outcome and this area needs to be looked at more closely. In our centre this procedure is not routinely performed in advanced ovarian cancer unless there are overtly involved bulky nodes.

Interval debulking

In patients who have been suboptimally debulked, a single European study has demonstrated benefit for re-operating after three cycles of chemotherapy, so-called interval debulking surgery. In the trial conducted, patients had an approximately x month survival advantage. In a subsequent study, no benefit was seen for interval debulking if the initial surgical procedure was performed by a specialist gynaecological oncologist; therefore, the value of this approach is controversial.

ADVANCED OVARIAN CANCER

Front-line chemotherapy post-surgery: benefit and toxicity

The chemotherapy debate for advanced ovarian cancer is constantly shifting and in doing so is constantly attempting to address the balance between toxicity and benefit.

There are some relatively stable facts now about ovarian cancer chemotherapy that lay down the framework for the current debates. First, systemic platinum agents given after surgery are the single best and most important drugs in ovarian cancer either alone or in combination. Second, systemic therapy carboplatin is as effective as cisplatin but with an improved toxicity profile. Third, cisplatin with paclitaxel as a chemotherapy regime is definitely better than cisplatin with cyclophosphamide (but not than platinum alone necessarily) as systemic therapy. Almost everything else in ovarian cancer chemotherapy is a debate currently.

Carboplatin and paclitaxel as front-line therapy

Where a patient is fit, lacking in co-morbidities (especially those exacerbated by the treatment or its supportive therapies) and able to cope with combination chemotherapy, particularly when optimally debulked, our standard of care is carboplatin and paclitaxel. The evidence for this is based on two seminal studies, the GOG111 study reported in 1996 and the OV10 study reported in 2000. These studies virtually replicate each other with almost identical survival curves and demonstrate beyond any doubt that cisplatin with cyclophosphamide is inferior to cisplatin and paclitaxel. The AGO study in 1999 demonstrated that carboplatin and paclitaxel was equivalent to cisplatin and paclitaxel, so at least for systemic therapy of advanced ovarian cancer, carboplatin and paclitaxel is the regime of choice.

It is important to note that there are differences in response rate between histological types. In serous and endometrioid ovarian cancers the response rates are relatively high ($\sim$ 70–80%) with carboplatin and paclitaxel, and not dissimilar with single-agent carboplatin and cisplatin. However, for advanced mucinous and clear-cell cancers, the response rate to single-agent platinum in the front-line setting is particularly low, of the order of 12–14% overall response rate in several series, and carboplatin–paclitaxel have a higher response rate of 23–25%. Currently therefore single-agent platinum is not an attractive option for patients with these unusual and prognostically poorer histologies in advanced disease.

THE TOXICITIES OF CARBOPLATIN–PACLITAXEL COMBINATION CHEMOTHERAPY

There are significant toxicities from this standard combination. Alopecia occurs early and is inevitable but reversible. Patients do not generally retain their hair using the pre-chemotherapy 'cold cap' although interestingly in a few anecdotal cases they have managed to do so. All other toxicities are not inevitable but may be severe and debilitating. Due to the hypersensitivity potential of the cremaphor vehicle necessitating the use of dexamethasone there is potential for significant weight gain for the patient and worsening of diabetic control (if a concurrent co-morbidity) that may have significant consequences if there is additional neutropenic sepsis as part of the toxicity profile. With the use of paclitaxel there is a risk of neurotoxicity, mainly peripheral sensory neuropathy in fingers and toes which occurs in about a third of patients, but is usually mild and generally settles after the end of chemotherapy; however, in a small proportion of patients neurotoxicity is severe and may interfere with function substantially with patients left unable to use their hands accurately and with sufficient power. Rarely the paclitaxel neuropathy is permanent and does not resolve. Another adverse toxicity of paclitaxel is the joint-pain syndrome that comes on typically 3 days after chemotherapy and lasts typically 3 days. This usually affects the small joints of the hand, and the knees as well as the small joints of the feet. It can be severe and sometimes the duration extends beyond 3 days. Its severity may necessitate the use (pre-emptively) of analgesics such as paracetamol and ibuprofen at full dose. Although emesis is unusual with this regimen, nausea can be a problem, particularly with younger patients. Neutropenic sepsis is also a risk of this combination chemotherapy.

Single agent carboplatin as front-line therapy

In most European, Australasian and North American countries, standard treatment is considered to be carboplatin and paclitaxel. The basis for this was the superior outcomes seen for the paclitaxel and cisplatin arms in the GOG111 and OV10 studies. However, the control arm for these studies was cyclophosphamide and cisplatin, and in the influential meta-analysis by Parmar, this control arm was clearly inferior to the single-agent platinum-control arms seen in GOG132 and ICON3 randomized trials. These latter trials showed no difference between platinum and platinum plus Taxol. Hence, this leads to the current NICE guidelines that suggest discussion between doctor and patient and choice for the patient between single-agent carboplatin and carboplatin and paclitaxel. There are many centres in the United Kingdom that regard carbopatin as an appropriate standard of care for many patients. At the West London Gynaecological Cancer Centre currently around 60% of patients receive combination therapy with paclitaxel and carboplatin with 40% receiving single-agent carboplatin.

ARE HIGHER-DOSE INTENSITY OR MORE CYCLES BETTER?

Several studies have been conducted of more versus less cycles of chemotherapy (greater total dose) and higher versus lower doses (greater dose-intensity) and in general these studies have shown no benefit for either greater total dose or dose intensity. In terms of total dose, Bertelsen in 1993 showed no difference for 6 versus 12 cycles and led by this institution, Lambert and colleagues in 1997 showed no difference for five versus eight cycles, with a smaller study also showing no difference for five versus ten cycles (Hakes 1992). With respect to dose intensity, eight trials have compared differing dose intensities, all of these essentially comparing one dose intensity with double that dose intensity, and with the exception of two trials there was no difference in survival (refs). Furthermore, two randomized controlled trials of high-dose chemotherapy have been performed and the mature data show no difference in survival for standard versus high-dose chemotherapy

(Cure *et al.*, Ledermann *et al.*). Dose density, however, remains an issue to be explored. This is where the interval between cycles of chemotherapy is reduced to less than the 3 weeks typically utilized in standard regimens. For breast and cervical cancer, this increase of dose density is seen to improve survival of patients and this remains an open question in ovarian cancer.

NEOADJUVANT SYSTEMIC THERAPY AND PRIMARY MEDICAL TREATMENT OF OVARIAN CANCER

The gold standard for treating ovarian cancer has long been held to include upfront surgery. However, there is no doubt that if there is no adverse impact on survival it would be desirable to treat patients with neoadjuvant chemotherapy as this would make the delayed primary operation much easier and more complete as a result of control of the disease by chemotherapy prior to surgery. This is currently the subject of the CHORUS and EORTC trials. However, a note of caution is indicated, which is to say that wholesale adoption of neoadjuvant chemotherapy should not be adopted until these trials report. There are theoretical considerations that chemotherapy may be less effective in a high tumour burden environment and that surgical debulking may enhance the chemotherapy effect by debulking chemo-resistant clones and also by creating a cytokine environment that drives cells into cycle making them more sensitive to chemotherapy, and these potential consequences need to be considered.

INTRAPERITONEAL THERAPY

Ovarian cancer is principally a disease of locoregional peritoneal dissemination within the abdominal cavity. Control of locoregional dissemination is the top priority in the control of advanced ovarian cancer. The idea of intraperitoneal therapy is an old one, having been performed for 30 years or more. Over the last 10 years there have been seven randomized trials comparing intraperitoneal (IP) chemotherapy intravenous intravenously (IV). The common factor is that all included platinum, and most added a second drug. Metanalysis of these trials shows a significant reduction in hazards of 0.78 with confidence intervals of 0.69–0.89 and an improvement in median overall survival of about 12 months over IV-chemo beyond an expected median survival of this optimally debulked group of 4 years.

The most recent of the three large trials, GOG 172 showed the largest difference ever in a randomized ovarian cancer trial with median overall survival of 67 months against the IV control arm of 49 months, the improvement being 17.4 months with a hazard ratio of 0.71. This regimen utilized IV paclitaxel on day 1, IP cisplatin on day 2 and IP taxol on day 8, on a 21-day cycle for six cycles. However, IP chemotherapy was associated with enhanced toxicities including neuropathy, gastrointestinal toxicity and myelotoxicity. It is likely that this approach will become a standard option for women with optimally debulked ovarian cancer in the near future.

The treatment of recurrent ovarian cancer

Recurrent ovarian cancer is currently an incurable clinical state, although survival improvement can still be realized by utilizing appropriate chemotherapy and overall multidisciplinary clinical effort. Nevertheless, palliation and optimization of quality of life are important considerations in this clinical scenario utilizing aggressive symptom management, chemotherapy radiotherapy and surgery, with palliative care in the community and hospice provision being important components in this phase of disease. Limitation of treatment toxicity is a major aim too when considering treatment in this clinical scenario.

The timing of reintroduction of therapy in ovarian cancer recurrence is a controversial issue which will hopefully be addressed by an important trial, MRC-OVO5, which is now closed to recruitment and will report in the future. In this trial, ovarian cancer patients in complete remission with a normal CA125 are monitored with CA125 levels blinded to physician and patient. When CA125 levels reach twice the upper limit of normal the patients are randomized to either immediate treatment by informing the physician or not informing the physician until clinical recurrence demands treatment. The current UK guidance is to not treat until symptomatic recurrence of ovarian cancer, since there is no evidence that this improves outcome and may interfere with what otherwise is excellent quality of life in asymptomatic marker recurrence, for instance. At the West London Gynaecological Cancer Centre, our current policy is to try and avoid treatment until early symptomatic progression, but this demands fairly intensive watchful waiting and can generate considerable anxiety for patients. Upon early symptomatic progression or if there is evidence that the recurrence may cause significant anatomical damage if unchecked ('prophylactic palliation') palliative treatment can be instituted and this typically consists of chemotherapy, although sometimes multimodality therapy including surgery or radiotherapy may be required. Recurrent ovarian cancer may be considered as platinum refractory, resistant or potentially sensitive. Platinum-refractory ovarian cancer represents an extremely poor situation of primary non-response to chemotherapy, and implies that it is unlikely that these patients will respond to further standard chemotherapy agents. These patients often have aggressive disease and poor prognosis. They can be considered for phase I, and some phase II trials if sufficiently fit.

Chemotherapy

PLATINUM-SENSITIVE RECURRENCE

Platinum-sensitive recurrence has several definitions. A pragmatic definition is that of recurrence of ovarian cancer requiring treatment occurring more than 6 months after last chemotherapy. These patients are potentially platinum sensitive, and the likelihood of overall response to rechallenge with platinum-based chemotherapy is a function of time, with those relapsing more than 18 months after previous chemotherapy having up to a 94% chance of response to subsequent platinum-based therapy (as compared with 10% response rate in those relapsing within 6 months of last platinum therapy) from the findings of Blackledge.

Eisenhauer and colleagues looked at factors predicting response to subsequent chemotherapy in platinum pretreated ovarian cancer using data from 13 randomized trials of 6 chemotherapy agents (not just platinum). They found that serous histology, tumour bulk (<5 cm) and number of disease sites (<3) were significant factors; yet treatment-free interval was not, a feature at first sight at odds with Blackledge's findings. These biological predictors of subsequent response were the main determinants of response, with the treatment-free interval correlating closely with tumour size.

A seminal randomized clinical trial, MRC ICON4, was conducted in patients relapsing more than 6 months after last chemotherapy requiring chemotherapy. This trial asked if the addition of paclitaxel to carboplatin improved survival in platinum-resistant disease. This study was extremely important because the MRC ICON3 study had shown no improvement in survival for carboplatin and taxol as front-line chemotherapy in advanced ovarian cancer. In the ICON4 trial, addition of paclitaxel significantly improved survival in platinum-sensitive recurrent ovarian cancer with a hazards ratio of 0.82, an absolute survival advantage at 2 years of 7% and an improvement to median survival of 5 months, in other words, benefit of similar magnitude to the addition of chemotherapy in front-line ovarian cancer. There were no real differences in patient perceived toxicity and, in general, where there are not reasons to avoid paclitaxel (e.g. previous severe neuropathy, concurrent medical co-morbidity especially advanced diabetes etc.) it can be recommended for patients relapsing > 12 months from last chemotherapy. However, this trial does have some cautions in that more trials are needed in the 6–12 month group, and in those who previously received paclitaxel–carboplatin, where the benefits in survival are not completely clear.

In patients who are platinum sensitive but platinum allergic, pegylated liposomal doxorubicin (Caelyx) can be considered as it has been shown to have a survival advantage in platinum-sensitive disease in comparison to topotecan, a commonly used topoisomerase I inhibitor.

At the West London Gynaecological Cancer Centre we offer combination chemotherapy to all platinum-sensitive recurrent patients if it is not medically contraindicated, although we do make it clear that carboplatin monotherapy is an effective and low-toxicity alternative.

PLATINUM-RESISTANT RECURRENCE

There are various definitions of platinum-resistant recurrence; however, a pragmatic definition is one of recurrent disease requiring treatment within 6 months of completing last chemotherapy. In this group of patients it is unlikely that re-challenge with conventional schedules of platinum will result in response (<10% chance of response). These patients appear to benefit (or fail to benefit) equally from all conventionally dosed and scheduled chemotherapeutic agents. These monotherapies all have a 10–20% overall response rate, and combination chemotherapy in conventional dose and schedule has not been shown to improve survival or response rate. Agents that can be considered in this indication include Caelyx, topotecan, oral etoposide, paclitaxel and gemcitabine. Where oestrogen and progestin receptors are strongly positive, disease stabilization may be achieved by the use of endocrine therapy, usually tamoxifen or a progestin.

It is important to note that this platinum-resistant group of patients should be strongly considered for phase II and some phase I clinical trials.

Where patients are platinum resistant, symptomatic and exceptionally fit The Rustin/Van der Berg regime can be considered. This regime increases dose density and dose intensity of platinum to overcome clinical platinum resistance, delivering 60–70 mg/m^2 cisplatin weekly (double the conventional dose intensity of 25–33 mg/m^2) for six cycles over 7 weeks, with daily oral etoposide. Using this regime, in two studies, platinum-resistant patients achieved a 46% response rate which is a significant improvement over the conventionally dosed monotherapies (10–20%) and a much higher response than would be expected with conventional platinum (<10%) in this group.

SURGERY AND RADIOTHERAPY

The use of surgery in recurrent ovarian cancer is controversial and lacking in a strong evidence base. Patients with malignant bowel obstruction should not be given chemotherapy in general, and these patients may benefit from a palliative surgical procedure to correct their bowel obstruction and then continue with chemotherapy.

Occasionally solitary recurrence can be resected fully and in these cases individual outcomes can be good. The German AGO group is currently validating a model of factors that predict for successful secondary debulking and this evidence-based approach will more clearly define the role of surgery in this context. Radiotherapy is in general reserved for palliation of symptomatic disease particularly symptomatic pelvic recurrence, cutaneous and intracerebral disease.

Future developments

CYTOTOXIC REGIME DEVELOPMENTS

The further development and refinement of cytotoxic chemotherapy combinations continues. Recent trials of adding a third drug, epirubicin, to paclitaxel and carboplatin have shown no benefit, and the outcome of the ICON5/GOG trial is awaited which compares several combination regimens. The toxicity of triple therapy is significant and feasibility studies of four cycles of carboplatin monotherapy followed by doublet chemotherapy consisting of paclitaxel and gemcitabine are being explored currently. Increasingly, it is becoming clear that the histological heterogeneity of ovarian cancer has therapeutic importance with significantly inferior response outcomes observed for clear cell and mucinous carcinomas of the ovary. The same is also true for carcinosarcoma of the ovary. The Gynaecological Cancer Intergroup (GCIG) has commenced a phase III clinical trial comparing cisplatin and irinotecan versus paclitaxel–carboplatin in advanced clear cell carcinoma of the ovary. A similar trial of chemotherapy for advanced mucinous carcinoma of the ovary is in discussion and this is likely to utilize bowel cancer-type chemotherapy in a randomized setting against paclitaxel–carboplatin.

The intriguing results of intraperitoneal therapy will continue to ensure that this will be a growth area in terms of understanding the biology and immunology of the peritoneum as well as developing chemotherapy intraperitoneally.

Biotherapeutic targets

Antiangiogenic agents are an attractive target for ovarian cancer treatment. Bevacizumab will shortly be integrated with paclitaxel–carboplatin in a front-line randomized ovarian cancer trial against chemotherapy alone (MRC-ICON 7).

Lung cancer studies have demonstrated interesting data as to likely responders and survivors by mutation and expression status respectively of EGF receptor tyrosine kinase with the EGF receptor tyrosine kinase inhibtors Tarceva and Iressa.

Manipulating the PTEN/AKT pathway will be likely to provide rich therapeutic benefits ultimately. The PI3Kinase pathway is very frequently disrupted in different ways in different histological subgroups and treatment states of ovarian cancer. PTEN disruption is very frequent in endometrioid and clear cell ovarian cancer, PI3K and AKT activation is frequent in serous carcinomas of the ovary. PI3Kinase activation is involved in clinical platinum resistance in ovarian cancer. PI3K, AKT and mTOR inhibitors will therefore find indications once successfully integrated with chemotherapy. The wealth of new targeted agents to use singly or in combination is astounding, and the challenge will be how to integrate these molecular therapies with chemotherapy both systemic and intraperitoneal over the next few years to further improve the prognosis of ovarian cancer; but I would predict that realistically we stand on the threshold of significant numerically substantial improvement in survival at least for optimally debulked patients over the next 5–10 years, but whether such substantial improvements will occur for suboptimally debulked patients remains uncertain at this time.

References

1. Boyle P & Ferlay J (2005) Cancer incidence and mortality in Europe, 2004. *Ann Oncol* **16**(3), 481–8.
2. Parkin DM, *et al.* (2005) Global cancer statistics, 2002. *CA Cancer J Clin* **55**(2), 74–108.
3. Fathalla MF (1971) Incessant ovulation–a factor in ovarian neoplasia? *Lancet* **2**(7716), 163.
4. Greer JB, *et al.* (2005) Short-term oral contraceptive use and the risk of epithelial ovarian cancer. *Am J Epidemiol* **162**(1), 66–72.
5. Ness RB & Cottreau C (1999) Possible role of ovarian epithelial inflammation in ovarian cancer. *J Natl Cancer Inst* **91**(17), 1459–67.
6. Ness RB (2003) Endometriosis and ovarian cancer: thoughts on shared pathophysiology. *Am J Obstet Gynecol* **189**(1), 280–94.
7. Herrinton LJ, *et al.* (1994) Ovarian cancer incidence among Asian migrants to the United States and their descendants. *J Natl Cancer Inst* **86**(17), 1336–9.
8. Sogaard M, Kjaer SK & Gayther S (2006) Ovarian cancer and genetic susceptibility in relation to the BRCA1 and BRCA2 genes. Occurrence, clinical importance and intervention. *Acta Obstet Gynecol Scand* **85**(1), 93–105.
9. Baldwin RL, *et al.* (2000) BRCA1 promoter region hypermethylation in ovarian carcinoma: a population-based study. *Cancer Res* **60**(19), 5329–33.
10. Hall J, Paul J & Brown R (2004) Critical evaluation of p53 as a prognostic marker in ovarian cancer. *Expert Rev Mol Med* **2004**, 1–20.
11. Dinulescu DM, *et al.* (2005) Role of K-ras and Pten in the development of mouse models of endometriosis and endometrioid ovarian cancer. *Nat Med* **11**(1), 63–70.
12. Sherbet GV & Patil D (2003) Genetic abnormalities of cell proliferation, invasion and metastasis, with special reference to gynaecological cancers. *Anticancer Res* **23**(2B), 1357–71.
13. Sharma A & Menon U (2006) Screening for gynaecological cancers. *Eur J Surg Oncol*.
14. Kauff ND, *et al.* (2002) Risk-reducing salpingo-oophorectomy in women with a BRCA1 or BRCA2 mutation. *N Engl J Med* **346**(21), 1609–15.
15. Ransohoff DF (2005) Lessons from controversy: ovarian cancer screening and serum proteomics. *J Natl Cancer Inst* **97**(4), 315–9.
16. Goff BA, *et al.* (2004) Frequency of symptoms of ovarian cancer in women presenting to primary care clinics. *Jama* **291**(22), 2705–12.
17. Leitao MM Jr., *et al.* (2004) Clinicopathologic analysis of early-stage sporadic ovarian carcinoma. *Am J Surg Pathol* **28**(2), 147–59.
18. Kurman RJ & Trimble CL (1993) The behavior of serous tumors of low malignant potential: are they ever malignant? *Int J Gynecol Pathol* **12**(2), 120–7.
19. Kaern J, *et al.* (1993) DNA ploidy; the most important prognostic factor in patients with borderline tumors of the ovary. *Int J Gynecol Cancer* **3**(6), 349–358.
20. Fox H & Buckley CH (1992) The female genital tract and ovaries., in Oxford Textbook of Pathology, N.A. Wright, Editor. Oxford University Press.: Oxford. 1563–1640.
21. Sugiyama T, *et al.* (2000) Clinical characteristics of clear cell carcinoma of the ovary: a distinct histologic type with poor prognosis and resistance to platinum-based chemotherapy. *Cancer* **88**(11), 2584–9.
22. Hess V, *et al.* (2004) Mucinous epithelial ovarian cancer: a separate entity requiring specific treatment. *J Clin Oncol* **22**(6), 1040–4.
23. Clark TG, *et al.* (2001) A prognostic model for ovarian cancer. *Br J Cancer* **85**(7), 944–52.
24. Eisenhauer EA, Vermorken JB & van Glabbeke M (1997) Predictors of response to subsequent chemotherapy in platinum pretreated ovarian cancer: a multivariate analysis of 704 patients [seecomments]. *Ann Oncol* **8**(10), 963–8.
25. Vasey PA (2003) Resistance to chemotherapy in advanced ovarian cancer: mechanisms and current strategies. *Br J Cancer* **89** Suppl 3, S23–8.
26. Junor EJ, *et al.* (1999) Specialist gynaecologists and survival outcome in ovarian cancer: a Scottish national study of 1866 patients. *Br J Obstet Gynaecol* **106**(11), 1130–6.
27. Griffiths CT & Fuller AF (1978) Intensive surgical and chemotherapeutic management of advanced ovarian cancer. *Surg Clin North Am* **58**(1), 131–42.
28. van der Burg ME, *et al.* (1995) The effect of debulking surgery after induction chemotherapy on the prognosis in advanced epithelial ovarian cancer. Gynecological Cancer Cooperative Group of the European Organization for Research and Treatment of Cancer. *N Engl J Med* **332**(10), 629–34.

29. Crawford SC, *et al.* (2005) Does aggressive surgery only benefit patients with less advanced ovarian cancer? Results from an international comparison within the SCOTROC-1 Trial. *J Clin Oncol* **23**(34), 8802–11.

30. Trimbos JB, *et al.* (2003) International Collaborative Ovarian Neoplasm trial 1 and Adjuvant ChemoTherapy In Ovarian Neoplasm trial: two parallel randomized phase III trials of adjuvant chemotherapy in patients with early-stage ovarian carcinoma. *J Natl Cancer Inst* **95**(2), 105–12.

31. van der Burg ME & Vergote I (2003) The role of interval debulking surgery in ovarian cancer. *Curr Oncol Rep* **5**(6), 473–81.

32. McGuire WP, *et al.* (1996) Cyclophosphamide and cisplatin compared with paclitaxel and cisplatin in patients with stage III and stage IV ovarian cancer. *N Engl J Med* **334**(1), 1–6.

33. Piccart MJ, *et al.* (2000) Randomized intergroup trial of cisplatin-paclitaxel versus cisplatin-cyclophosphamide in women with advanced epithelial ovarian cancer: three-year results. *J Natl Cancer Inst* **92**(9), 699–708.

34. du Bois A, *et al.* (2003) A randomized clinical trial of cisplatin/paclitaxel versus carboplatin/paclitaxel as first-line treatment of ovarian cancer. *J Natl Cancer Inst* **95**(17), 1320–9.

35. Enomoto T, *et al.* (2003) Is clear cell carcinoma and mucinous carcinoma of the ovary sensitive to combination chemotherapy with paclitaxel and carboplatin? in Proc Am Soc Clin Oncol.

36. Sandercock J, Parmar MK & Torri V (1998) First-line chemotherapy for advanced ovarian cancer: paclitaxel, cisplatin and the evidence. *Br J Cancer* **78**(11), 1471–8.

37. Muggia FM, *et al.* (2000) Phase III randomized study of cisplatin versus paclitaxel versus cisplatin and paclitaxel in patients with suboptimal stage III or IV ovarian cancer: a gynecologic oncology group study. *J Clin Oncol* **18**(1), 106–15.

38. Paclitaxel plus carboplatin versus standard chemotherapy with either single-agent carboplatin or cyclophosphamide, doxorubicin, and cisplatin in women with ovarian cancer: the ICON3 randomised trial. Lancet, 2002. **360**(9332), 505–15.

39. Guidance on the use of paclitaxel in the treatment of ovarian cancer., in Technology Appraisal No. 55, Issue date: January 2003 Review date: July 2003.

40. Bertelsen K, *et al.* (1993) A prospective randomized comparison of 6 and 12 cycles of cyclophosphamide, adriamycin, and cisplatin in advanced epithelial ovarian cancer: a Danish Ovarian Study Group trial (DACOVA). *Gynecol Oncol* **49**(1), 30–6.

41. Lambert HE, *et al.* (1997) A randomized trial of five versus eight courses of cisplatin or carboplatin in advanced epithelial ovarian carcinoma. A North Thames Ovary Group Study. *Ann Oncol* **8**(4), 327–33.

42. Hakes TB, *et al.* (1992) Randomized prospective trial of 5 versus 10 cycles of cyclophosphamide, doxorubicin, and cisplatin in advanced ovarian carcinoma. *Gynecol Oncol* **45**(3), 284–9.

43. Muggia FM (2004) Relevance of chemotherapy dose and schedule to outcomes in ovarian cancer. *Semin Oncol* **31**(6 Suppl 15), 19–24.

44. Cure H, *et al.* (2004) Phase III randomized trial of high-dose chemotherapy (HDC) and peripheral blood stem cell (PBSC) support as consolidation in patients (pts) with advanced ovarian cancer (AOC): 5-year follow-up of a GINECO/FNCLCC/SFGM-TC study. in ASCO Annual Meeting 2004: Journal of Clinical Oncology, ASCO Annual Meeting Proceedings (Post-Meeting Edition).

45. Ledermann JA, *et al.* (2005) A phase III randomised trial of sequential high dose chemotherapy (HDC) with peripheral blood stem cell support or standard dose Chemotherapy (SDC) for first-line treatment of ovarian cancer. in ASCO Annual Meeting. 2005: Journal of Clinical Oncology, ASCO Annual Meeting Proceedings.

46. Armstrong DK, *et al.* (2006) Intraperitoneal cisplatin and paclitaxel in ovarian cancer. *N Engl J Med* **354**(1), 34–43.

47. Hamilton CA, Berek JS (2006) Intraperitoneal chemotherapy for ovarian cancer. *Curr Opin Oncol* **18**(5), 507–15.

48. Markman M & Walker JL (2006) Intraperitoneal chemotherapy of ovarian cancer: a review, with a focus on practical aspects of treatment. *J Clin Oncol* **24**(6), 988–94.

49. Blackledge G, *et al.* (1989) Response of patients in phase II studies of chemotherapy in ovarian cancer: implications for patient treatment and the design of phase II trials. *Br J Cancer* **59**(4), 650–3.

50. Parmar MK, *et al.* (2003) Paclitaxel plus platinum-based chemotherapy versus conventional platinum-based chemotherapy in women with relapsed ovarian cancer: the ICON4/AGO-OVAR-2.2 trial. *Lancet* **361**(9375), 2099–106.

51. Gordon AN, *et al.* (2001) Recurrent epithelial ovarian carcinoma: a randomized phase III study of pegylated liposomal doxorubicin versus topotecan. *J Clin Oncol* **19**(14), 3312–22.

52. Meyer T, *et al.* (2001) Weekly cisplatin and oral etoposide as treatment for relapsed epithelial ovarian cancer. *Ann Oncol* **12**(12), 1705–9.

53. de Jongh FE, *et al.* (2002) Dose-dense cisplatin/paclitaxel. a well-tolerated and highly effective chemotherapeutic regimen in patients with advanced ovarian cancer. *Eur J Cancer* **38**(15), 2005–13.

54. Pfisterer J, *et al.* (2005) The role of surgery in recurrent ovarian cancer. *Int J Gynecol Cancer* **15** Suppl 3, 195–8.

Chapter 56: Benign disease of the uterus

Mary Ann Lumsden

Introduction

Benign disease of the uterus is an important problem for many women and their gynaecologists. The commonest condition in this category is fibroids but adenomyosis and uterine polyps are also of importance. Both fibroids and endometrial polyps are very common and although asymptomatic in many women, they can cause considerable morbidity for others.

This chapter will discuss each of these conditions and consider the aetiology, pathogenesis, presenting symptoms and treatment with inclusion of new developments, particularly in the treatment of fibroids.

Adenomyosis

Definition

Adenomyosis is defined as the benign invasion of endometrium into the myometrium. Both endometrial glands and endometrial stroma must be present and some pathologists also consider that these should be surrounded by hypertrophic, hyperplastic musculature. Since the endometrial myometrial border is irregular, the definition usually includes depth of penetration that may vary from 2.5 to 5 mm or, it can be determined in terms of microscope fields, one low power field being equivalent to 1 cm [1]. Since the symptoms appear to be related to the depth of penetration, then it would seem reasonable to include only those with a greater degree of invasion. The result is enlarged uteri in which the adenomyosis may be either diffuse or present as focal deposits or adenomyomas.

Incidence

Because of the difficulties in definition as outlined above, the incidence of adenomyosis reported in the literature varies considerably from between 8 and 61%, the preoperative diagnosis usually being less than 10%. It is a post-hysterectomy diagnosis and some discrepancy is likely to result from the difference with which pathologists will search for it.

Clinical presentation

The commonest presentation is that of heavy menstrual bleeding associated with worsening dysmenorrhoea, the latter being worse in deep, infiltrating disease [2]. The condition is characteristic of the 5th decade with the age of 45 being the commonest age of presentation and is very rare in nulliparous women [3].

Aetiology

The ectopic endometrium is responsive to steroid hormones and gene polymorphisms have been identified in the oestrogen receptor with mutations of the oestrogen receptor alpha; therefore, bleeding will occur each month. It is possible that this contributes to the symptom of dysmenorrhoea. In addition, there is abnormal prostaglandin production and this could contribute to both the pain and the heavy bleeding. These symptoms are associated with a gradually enlarging uterus although this is unlikely to be picked up clinically unless repeated vaginal examinations are performed.

The diagnosis is normally made on histological examination of the uterus after hysterectomy. However, magnetic resonance imaging (MRI) has been shown to be more accurate than ultrasound in diagnosing adenomyosis (Fig. 56.1) [4]. This modality enables the clinician to distinguish adenomyosis from other pathologies such as uterine fibroids that might also present with an enlarged uterus. Early diagnosis can impact significantly on the treatment offered to an individual patient.

Treatment

Treatment is likely to be hysterectomy since this is the only method of curing the problem. Endometrial ablation is relatively contraindicated since it will fail to remove deeply

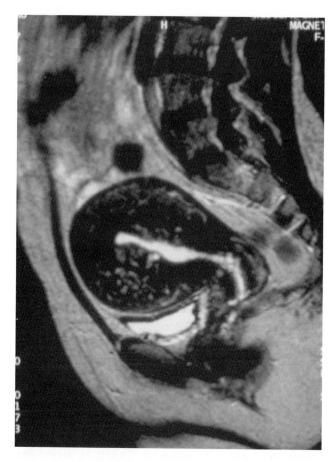

Fig. 56.1 Diffuse adenomyosis of the uterus. By kind permission of Dr Nigel McMillan, Consultant Radiologist, The Western Infirmary, Glasgow.

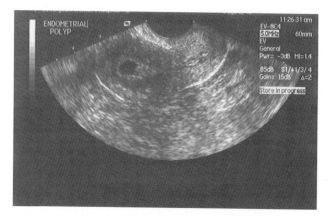

Fig. 56.2 An ultrasound scan demonstrating an endometrial polyp. By kind permission of Dr Justine Clark, Consultant Gynaecologist, Birmingham Women's Hospital.

infiltrating glands and is unlikely to be successful. In fact, it has been suggested that it is a common cause of failure of this procedure. It is possible that modalities such as the levonorgestrel-releasing intrauterine system or uterine artery embolization may be useful in this context although few data are yet published concerning these possibilities.

Endometrial polyps

Endometrial polyps are discreet outgrowths of the endometrium that contain a variable amount of gland stroma and blood vessel. They are attached to the endometrium by a pedicle and they may be pedunculated or sessile. It would appear that they are relatively insensitive to cyclical hormonal changes and so are not shed at the time of menstruation. In addition, they may contain hyper plastic foci particularly in those that are symptomatic.

Epidemiology

The presence of endometrial polyps is being increasingly recognized since the widespread adoption of transvaginal ultrasound and outpatients hysteroscopy. It is probable that they are present in 25% of women with abnormal vaginal bleeding although at least 10% of asymptomatic women are also likely to have polyps. They are particularly common in women taking preparations such as tamoxifen.

Presentation

Unscheduled vaginal bleeding or spotting is the commonest presentation for endometrial polyps. They are frequently found in association with women experiencing abnormal bleeding while taking hormone replacement theory (HRT) or tamoxifen. In the latter case, the whole endometrial surface may appear polypoid.

Diagnosis

Endometrial polyps are frequently missed with blind endometrial sampling such as performed at the time of dilatation and curettage. Uterine imaging is more sensitive in diagnosing these focal lesions, particularly transvaginal ultrasound, which might identify them singly or as part of abnormally thickening endometrium (Fig. 56.2). However, studies have noted marked inter-observer variation in interpretation of the ultrasound images. Intrauterine injection of saline can markedly increase the diagnostic performance of transvaginal ultrasound.

Hysteroscopic characteristics

The best method for diagnosing polyps is hysteroscopy; so it is a possibility that they might then be treated at the same time (Plate 56.1, *facing p. 562*). They can be pedunculated or sessile single or multiple but can be distinguished from pedunculated fibroids since they have fewer vessels over the surface. Malignant polyps are more likely to be irregular, vascular or friable. Biopsy should be carried out to confirm the diagnosis since appearance is not sufficient.

Treatment

In the symptomatic women, treatment will normally be performed under general anaesthesia. However, they can also be treated in the outpatients setting either by removal under direct vision or by treatment with specially developed diathermy instrumentation. One possibility is to separate the polyp at the base and then remove the whole lesion intact. Alternatively, the lesion can be cut up into small pieces and removed using direct vision.

Uterine leiomyomata (fibroids)

These common tumours are clinically apparent in 20% of women of reproductive age and maybe present in as many as 70% of uteri removed at hysterectomy. Their incidence is increased in women of Afro-Caribbean origin [5]. The incidence is decreased with prolonged use of the oral contraceptive pill as well as with increasing numbers of term pregnancies.

Fibroids consist of varying proportions of smooth muscle and fibroblasts. They may be single or multiple and can occur anywhere in the uterus (Fig. 56.3). The assumption is often made that only those impinging on the uterine cavity cause symptoms (other than size related). However, data suggest that even subserosal lesions may lead to menstrual problems. They also vary in size from less than 1 cm to over 30 cm in diameter. What determines the final size is unknown.

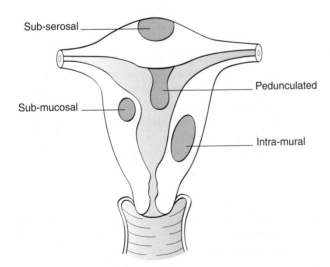

Fig. 56.3 The position of fibroids in the uterus.

Aetiology

Clonality studies using the homozygosity of glucose-6-phosphate dehydrogenase forms show that multiple tumours in the same uterus are derived from individual myometrial cells and not through a metastatic process. This, together with the high prevalence suggests that initial development arises from a frequently occurring event, the nature of which is currently unknown. Growth of fibroids is partly dependent on the ovarian steroids, as is discussed later, that act through receptors present on both fibroid and myometrial cells. It is likely that the control of growth is due, in part, to alterations in apoptosis. Bcl-2, an inhibitor of apoptosis is significantly increased in cultured leiomyoma cells and, moreover, is influenced by the steroid hormone milieu.

Cytogenetic abnormalities occur in 50% of uterine fibroids. Most commonly, these involve translocation within or deletion of chromosome 7, translocations of chromosome 12 and 14 and, occasionally, structural aberrations of chromosome 6 [6]. These cytogenetic abnormalities are not observed in normal myometrial tissue and may not be present in all the fibroids in a single uterus, depending on their site [7]. In addition, mutations in the gene encoding fumarate hydratase (an enzyme of the tricarboxylic acid cycle) were shown to predispose women to multiple fibroids in association with cutaneous leiomyomata and renal cell carcinoma. This is an interesting example of a mutation in a gene with a general function causing disease in a highly restricted range of tissue. Whether this is relevant to fibroids in general is unknown.

Malignancy in uterine fibroids is extremely uncommon. Leiomyosarcoma is a disease largely occurring in the seventh decade whereas fibroids tend to occur in women 20 to 30 years younger. The cytogenetic profile is completely different between the two conditions and there is the possibility that their origins are separate. However, gynaecologists with an interest in this area will all have anecdotal examples of malignancy occurring in younger women and so the possibility must be considered in fibroid disease that differs from the norm in presentation or response to treatment.

Myometrium and fibroids consist of spindled cells arranged in fasicles with abundant eosinophilic cytoplasm and uniform nuclei. A malignant leiomyosarcoma is hypercellular and consists of atypical smooth muscle cells with hyperchromatic, enlarged nuclei. Increased mitotic figures and necrosis occur commonly. However, benign fibroids may have one or more of these characteristics and prediction of malignant potential is extremely difficult [8].

Abnormalities in uterine blood vessels and angiogenic growth factors are also involved in the pathobiology of uterine fibroids. The myomatous uterus has increased

Uterine artery embolization

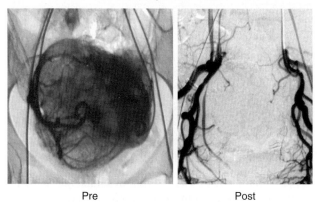

Pre   Post

Fig. 56.4 The left hand image shows an angiogram of the uterine arteries illustrating the vascularity of the fibroid. The right hand image is post uterine artery embolization and little flow is seen.

numbers of arterioles and venules as well as venule ectasia. It was thought that this was due to pressure from the large tumours but it could also be due simply to increased numbers of vessels. However, there are no mature vessels running through uterine fibroids even though they have a well-developed blood supply (Fig. 56.4, pre-embolization). This feature might be useful in trying to distinguish clinically between a benign and malignant lesion as a sarcoma may have large vessels running through it that could be identified using colour Doppler. The angiogenic fibroblast growth factor is also present in higher amounts in fibroid than the surrounding myometrium.

Growth factors may also be of importance in the control of growth of fibroids and composition. The function of transforming growth factor β, granulocyte-macrophage colony-stimulating factor, and epidermal growth factor, among others has been shown to differ between fibroid and normal myometrium [8].

CONTROL OF GROWTH

More information is available on the control of the growth of uterine fibroids than on their aetiology. Since fibroids have not been identified in pre-pubertal girls and usually shrink at the time of the menopause, it has long been assumed that they are dependent on the presence of the sex steroid oestrogen and progesterone. Much of the research has concentrated on this area that has been exploited for the purposes of developing novel medical treatments for fibroids.

The sex steroids act via receptors. The steroid combines with the receptor that is then translocated to the nucleus of the cell. Studies have identified that steroid receptors are present in higher concentrations in the fibroid than in surrounding myometrium and that the concentration of receptors is significantly affected by administration of agents that alter circulating oestradiol concentration. Further work has centred on the relationship between steroid hormones and growth factors such as epidermal growth factor and insulin like growth factor and it would appear that these are important, possibly as mediators for oestrogen action. The role of progesterone is less clear. The number of progesterone receptors is greater in fibroids than the surrounding myometrium. Like oestrogen it has an impact on epidermal growth factor (EGF) receptor content and also suppresses apoptosis. From studies using antiprogestins, progesterone receptor modulators and also administration of progestogens to hypoestrogenic women, it has been inferred that progesterone may stimulate fibroid growth as will be discussed more fully later in the chapter in the section on treatments. The relative contribution of oestradiol and progesterone is unclear.

Symptoms associated with uterine fibroids

Uterine fibroids commonly present with menstrual problems particularly heavy menstrual bleeding [9]. In women with dysfunctional uterine bleeding, at least half of those who complain of heavy menstrual loss have a blood loss in the normal range on objective assessment. This is not so for uterine fibroids where a vast majority are likely to have objectively confirmed menorrhagia, sometimes with more than a litre being lost with every period. This is then likely to be associated with anaemia and also, considerably impacts on lifestyle. Dysmenorrhoea can be an additional problem leading to misery for the women affected. Menorrhagia is not just confined to those who have submucous fibroids but can also be associated with subserosal lesions as mentioned above. However, it is probable that those with intracavity fibroids are more likely to get unscheduled bleeding and menorrhagia, possibly due to the surface vessels of the fibroid and the increased area of the uterine cavity. There has been much speculation over the years as to why the heavy bleeding occurs and abnormalities of endometrial function are still considered to be a likely option [3,10].

Not all women will present with a menstrual problem. Some experience symptoms related purely to the size of the fibroid. This may be a feeling of dragging or pressure in the pelvis or simply that of abdominal swelling. In a young woman, a 32-week size fibroid uterus can cause considerable embarrassment particularly in those who are slim. The relationship of fibroids with fertility is unclear [9]. It is often assumed that fibroids cause infertility since pregnancies do occur after myomectomy and other treatments

Table 56.1 Presenting symptoms of uterine fibroids

Menstrual problems
   Menorrhagia
   Dysmenorrhoea
Abdominal discomfort
   Feelings of pressure
Abdominal distension
Urinary problems
   Frequency of micturition
   Urinary retention
Bowel problems
Subfertility
   Difficulty in conceiving
   Pregnancy loss
   Intrapartum bleeding (particularly Caesarian section)

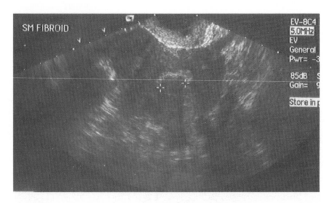

Fig. 56.5 An ultrasound scan showing an intrauterine fibroid. By kind permission of Dr Justine Clark, Consultant Gynaecologist, Birmingham Women's Hospital.

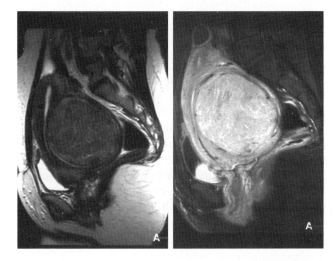

Fig. 56.6 An MRI image of a uterine fibroid. The fibroid is enhanced in the right hand image using gadolinium that provides an indication of the vascularity of the lesion. By kind permission of Dr Alan Reid, Consultant Radiologist, Glasgow Royal Infirmary.

where the fibroids are removed. However, there are no randomized data of, for example, myomectomy and no treatment and it is well known to all those involved in obstetric practice that women sometimes with very large fibroid uteri containing many fibroids do become pregnant. The best data to support a direct association comes from the study of success rates in assisted conception since fibroids adversely affect the outcome. However, whether this applies only to intracavity and submucosal is not clear. This is an important issue since many myomectomies are carried out where fibroids are subserosal or intramural and it would be of value to know if this does improve the outcome of future pregnancies.

It would appear that there is a definite association between fibroids and difficulty in conceiving and thus, the suggestion of surgical treatments that may result in hysterectomy can cause considerable distress. Consequently, non-surgical options have been developed as will be discussed below and their impact on fertility is discussed by Olive and colleagues [11].

As mentioned at the beginning of this chapter, approximately 50% of fibroids are asymptomatic and it is unclear as to why some do produce symptoms and others do not [3].

Other possible presenting symptoms, such as urinary and bowel problems, are outlined in Table 56.1, Urinary retention is the presenting symptom for fibroids although some will only be identified on routine examination, for example, at the time of having a cervical smear or when pregnant.

Diagnosis

The uterus is often found to be enlarged on abdominal examination. However, it may be difficult to distinguish between an enlarged uterus and an ovarian mass and so further imaging is mandatory. Ultrasonography is very

useful as a first line (Fig. 56.5), unless the uterus is very large or distorted leading to difficulty in visualizing the ovaries. Under these circumstances an MRI scan can give excellent visualization of the uterus and ovaries. In addition, enhancement with gadolinium gives an indication of the vascularity of the uterus (Fig. 56.6). Biopsy of the fibroid is not commonly undertaken.

Treatment of uterine fibroids

The treatment of fibroids has historically been surgery, usually hysterectomy. Myomectomy is an option in women wishing to maintain fertility and for those desiring to keep their uterus. However, with the shift of emphasis of gynaecological practice towards medical therapies, research has been made over the past 20 or 30 years for effective medical options.

Medical treatments do not cure the problem but are designed to bring symptom relief. The most established medical option is administration of the gonadotrophin releasing hormone agonists (GnRH agonists). These drugs lead to downregulation of pituitary receptors that results initially in stimulation of gonadotrophin release but within 2–3 weeks of initiation of treatment, gonadotrophin output decreases and consequently, that of ovarian steroids (Fig. 56.6). The decreased output of ovarian steroids continues while treatment is ongoing. This is usually given by monthly depot injections as the most convenient option although other methods of administration such as the nasal spray are available. Fibroid shrinkage occurs rapidly in the first 3 months but then tends to slow down with little further decrease. The reason for this is likely to be related to the alteration in the blood supply to the uterus that occurs with GnRH agonist administration. The principal disadvantages of administration of these agents are that the fibroids grow again when treatment has stopped and also, they are associated with postmenopausal type side effects. These consist of hot flushing and vaginal dryness but what is more important from a public health perspective is that they can lead to significant bone loss. It is possible to counteract these side effects by administration of low-dose hormone replacement therapy. The fibroids do not appear to re-grow, the symptoms do not occur and side effects are halted. This is an option that is available if a woman is unsuitable for surgery possibly due either to multiple previous abdominal operations, medical problems or morbid obesity.

GnRH agonists are also useful prior to surgery [12,13] and have a license for use in the UK in women with severe anaemia. Their administration results in amenorrhoea and this is associated with a significant increase in haemoglobin. They also enable more procedures to be carried out vaginally, with or without laparoscopic assistance, or through a small transverse incision and blood loss at the time of surgery is decreased when compared with a group who do not receive agonists. Consequently, although they are not widely used preoperatively, they can be very useful for large fibroids or if they are in a particularly awkward position. GnRH agonists may be useful prior to myomectomy for the same reasons although the chance of recurrence of fibroids is increased. However, it is also noted that the plane of cleavage between the fibroid and the surrounding myometrium can be masked and this can make the surgery significantly more difficult. Despite these benefits, GnRH agonists are not thought to be cost-effective [14] and therefore should be used in highly selected, anaemic patients only.

Progesterone receptor modulators

Although the antiprogestins have been shown to lead to the shrinkage of uterine fibroids, they are not widely used in clinical practice. However, further development of new preparations that affect the progesterone receptors have led to the testing of the progesterone receptor modulators. These drugs are still in the research domain but are likely to become an important treatment option for uterine fibroids. When administered to women, they cause amenorrhoea in a vast majority of cases without causing anovulation, that is, they have a direct effect on the endometrium and it is thought that the main site of action is the endometrial vasculature. In addition, preliminary data suggest that fibroid shrinkage occurs associated with a significant decrease in vaginal bleeding. Short-term administration appears to be safe and they are likely to have a profound effect on the treatment of this common problem [15].

Levonorgestrel-secreting intrauterine system

This device has revolutionized the treatment of dysfunctional uterine bleeding and evidence suggests that it may be one of the reasons why the hysterectomy rate has declined over recent years. However, the use of the device in women with fibroids has not been widely studied in that it has been deemed a relative contraindication. This may partly be due to the fact the device is more likely to be expelled during a very heavy menstruation and also because of the presence of a very distorted cavity as is often found with uterine fibroids. Intuitively, if the cavity is normal then a trial with the device maybe appropriate although it should be checked after a very heavy menstruation. It is well known that this device is associated with irregular bleeding for many months after insertion in many women. However, it is not known if this problem is worsened in those with fibroids.

Other treatments used for uterine fibroids are usually those involving the induction of amenorrhoea when patients may be satisfied with their treatment although the fibroids have not themselves decreased in size. Data are available to support this in relation to administration of progestogens and also, some women find the oral contraceptive pill beneficial. Danazol and gestrenone are also possible ways of achieving amenorrhoea but are not widely used.

Surgical treatment of uterine fibroids

The commonest option for the treatment of uterine fibroids is still hysterectomy. Since a common presentation is that of heavy menstrual bleeding, then this operation is associated with a high likelihood of success. However, major complications occur with hysterectomy and data from a recent large UK audit (the VALUE audit) suggest that complications are all increased in the presence of uterine fibroids [16]. In addition, many women do not wish to lose their uterus, either because they wish to maintain their fertility or because they feel that this is not an appropriate option for them. In these women, uterine sparing options must be considered. The first of these is obviously that of myomectomy, which involves removing the fibroids only. This can be carried out as an open, laparoscopic or as a hysteroscopic procedure. Small pedunculated intracavity fibroids lend themselves to hysteroscopic removal and this has been documented as being associated with decreased blood loss and improved fertility although randomized data are lacking for the latter. The main problem with myomectomy is that fibroids are often multiple and therefore, it is extremely difficult to remove them all at surgery. Also, bleeding can be heavy and this may lead in a small number of cases to the need for hysterectomy to stop the bleeding. Also, it is very difficult to achieve perfect haemostasis after myomectomy and adhesion formation maybe a major problem. These issues are likely to be even more significant when laparoscopic myomectomy is considered to be the best treatment option. Rupture of the uterus is also a possibility although it is much less common than the risk after lower segment Caesarean section. Myomectomy is thus not the perfect answer for someone wishing to maintain their fertility and, therefore, other options have been sought.

Uterine artery embolization

This option has been offered in specialist units over the last 10 years. Pelvic arterial embolization has been used in the treatment of massive obstetric haemorrhage for a long time but it was not until a French gynaecologist, Ravina, published a paper suggesting that it might be useful in the treatment of uterine fibroids that this became reasonably widespread. Uterine artery embolization involves the canulation of the femoral artery and a small plastic tube is fed around the aortic arch through the iliac vessels and into the uterine artery of the contra lateral side. Embolization material is then injected down into the artery until flow ceases. This procedure is then carried out on the other side. For poorly understood reasons, the blood supply to the normal myometrium renews itself via collateral circulation with the ovarian vessels and those supplying the vagina. However, the fibroids do not usually revascularize to the significant extent. This leads to shrinkage of the fibroids that, unlike with GnRH agonists, continues in some cases for as long as follow-up has occurred. In addition, observational data suggest that there is a significant beneficial effect on menstrual blood loss and patient satisfaction with the procedure seems high [17].

There has been much discussion in the literature of the pros and cons of uterine artery embolization (UAE) [18]. Personal series have been reported with promising early and midterm results [17]. The advantages of embolization are that although procedure is painful and opiate analgesia is required post-procedure, the stay in hospital is usually short and most patients are discharged within 24 h. Recovery time is also shorter than with hysterectomy or myomectomy and the uterus is conserved. The average uterine shrinkage is 40% although in some instances this can be greater (Fig. 56.7). A cervical or submucosal fibroid may also pass vaginally resulting in an anatomically normal uterus (Fig. 56.8). On the other hand, complications do occur (Table 56.2) and these may be serious particularly if severe sepsis occurs. There is no guarantee that the

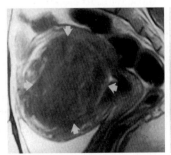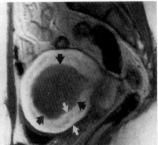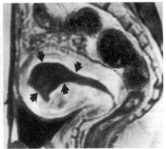

Pre-embolization
(GAD enhanced)

3 months post embolization
(GAD enhanced)
71% vol reduction

1 year post embolization
(GAD enhanced)
88% vol reduction

Fig. 56.7 These MRIs were taken before (left hand image), 3 months (middle image) and 12 months after uterine artery embolization. Fibroid shrinkage is continuing even up to 1 year. By kind permission of Dr Nigel McMillan, Consultant Radiologist, The Western Infirmary, Glasgow.

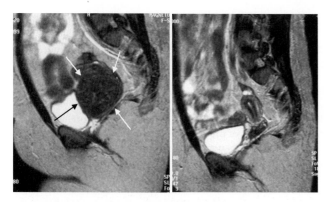

Fig. 56.8 This image illustrates a cervical fibroid that was passed after uterine artery embolization leaving a normal uterus. By kind permission of Dr Nigel McMillan, Consultant Radiologist, The Western Infirmary, Glasgow.

Table 56.2 The complications of uterine artery embolization

Sepsis
Vaginal discharge
Groin injury
Non-target embolization
    Ovary
    Bowel or bladder
Amenorrhoea
    Premature ovarian failure
    Endometrial atrophy
    Intrauterine adhesions
Post-embolization syndrome
Treatment failure
    Failed canulation of uterine artery
    Further surgery required

procedure will work and revascularization of fibroids does occur. In addition, a significant number of women require further treatment either with hysterectomy, myomectomy or a repeat embolization. The recurrence rate for fibroids after embolization is as yet unknown although it is likely to occur as is well documented with myomectomy.

There are further problems that are specific to embolization. The first of these is post-embolization syndrome that occurs 7–10 days after the procedure and consists of a flu-like illness with a mild pyrexia, raised white count and general malaise. This is not as a result of infection but cytokine release at the time of necrosis of the fibroid. However, it is often very difficult to distinguish from infection and that is another significant problem resulting from embolization that has led to the death of at least one woman. The second problem is premature ovarian failure that probably occurs following non-target embolization of the ovarian vessels. This occurs in 5–10% of women but is significantly more likely in those over the age of 45. Consequently, care must be taken when considering carrying out this procedure in those wishing to conceive in the future.

There are few studies reported in the literature of pregnancies but those available suggest that the outcome is not adversely affected [19]. However, it is clear that long-term studies must be carried out to ensure that this is a safe option for woman. In addition, randomized data are needed to allow appropriate comparison with the currently available options.

Comparisons are now being made with other treatments such as myomectomy or hysterectomy [18,20] although no randomized studies have yet been reported. Cost-effectiveness has been discussed [21] but no firm conclusions can be drawn without randomized data.

Other radiological techniques

Laser ablation of fibroids can be carried out at surgery either using a hysteroscope or a laparoscope depending on the position of the fibroids. Laser can also be used with MRI or ultrasound guidance.

These techniques allow target treatment and lead to significant fibroid shrinkage and decrease in menstrual blood loss [22]. MRI guided laser treatment requires an open MRI machine and few are available in the United Kingdom. However, ultrasound guided laser does not require such sophisticated equipment and is an interesting option for the future. Alternatively MRI guidance can be used to focus ultrasound and fibroid necrosis occurs without significant adverse outcomes.

Endometrial ablation

Endometrial ablation is a popular option with women with menorrhagia and a successful outcome is obtained in approximately 75%. A number of the studies carried out where ablation has been evaluated have included women with small fibroids. Overall, provided that the cavity is not too enlarged or distorted, then this is a successful option. It would appear that microwave endometrial ablation may be the best of the second generation techniques although randomized data looking at fibroids in particular are not available. Endometrial ablation may be performed with or without myomectomy and is associated with a high rate of amenorrhoea.

Conclusions

Benign gynaecological disease causes women many problems, some of which can have a significant impact on quality of life. Although medical treatments for adenomyosis and endometrial polyps are lacking, new modalities are being sort for uterine fibroids. This together with work studying the aetiology and pathogenesis of this common problem should lead to progress and the development of new treatment options.

References

1. McElin T & Bird C (1974) Adenomyosis of the uterus. *Obstet Gynecol Ann* **3**, 425–41.

2. Bird C, McElin T & Manalo-Estella F (1972) The elusive adenomyosis of the uterus – revisited. *Am J Obstet Gynecol* **112**, 583–93.

3. Buttram VC Jr & Reiter RC (1981) Uterine leiomyomata: etiology, symptomatology, and management. [Review] [71 refs]. *Fertil Steril* **36**(4), 433–45.

4. Ascher SM, Jha RC & Reinhold C (2003) Benign myometrial conditions: leiomyomas and adenomyosis. [Review] [61 refs]. *Top Magn Reson Imag* **14**(4), 281–304.

5. Kjerulff KH, Langenberg P, Seidman JD, Stolley PD & Guzinski GM (1996) Uterine leiomyomas. Racial differences in severity, symptoms and age at diagnosis. *J Reprod Med* **41**(7), 483–90.

6. Andersen J (1998) Factors in fibroid growth. [Review] [100 refs]. *Baillieres Clin Obstet Gynaecol* **12**(2), 225–43.

7. Brosens I, Deprest J, Dal Cin P & Van den BH (1998) Clinical significance of cytogenetic abnormalities in uterine myomas. *Fertil Steril* **69**(2), 232–235.

8. Stewart EA (2001) Uterine fibroids.[see comment]. [Review] [71 refs]. *Lancet* **357**(9252), 293–8.

9. Lumsden MA & Wallace EM (1998) Clinical presentation of uterine fibroids. [Review] [88 refs]. *Baillieres Clin Obstet Gynaecol* **12**(2), 177–95.

10. Stewart EA & Nowak RA (1996) Leiomyoma-related bleeding: a classic hypothesis updated for the molecular era. *Hum Reprod Update* **2**(4), 295–306.

11. Olive DL, Lindheim SR & Pritts EA (2004) Non-surgical management of leiomyoma: impact on fertility. [Review] [35 refs]. *Curr Opin Obstet Gynecol* **16**(3), 239–43.

12. Lumsden MA, West CP, Thomas E *et al.* (1994) Treatment with the gonadotrophin releasing hormone-agonist goserelin before hysterectomy for uterine fibroids. *Br J Obstet Gynaecol* **101**(5), 438–42.

13. Lethaby A, Vollenhoven B & Sowter M (2002) Efficacy of pre-operative gonadotrophin hormone releasing analogues for women with uterine fibroids undergoing hysterectomy or myomectomy: a systematic review. [Review] [16 refs]. *Br J Obstet Gynaecol* **109**(10), 1097–108.

14. Farquhar C, Brown PM & Furness S (2002) Cost effectiveness of pre-operative gonadotrophin releasing analogues for women with uterine fibroids undergoing hysterectomy or myomectomy. [see comment]. [Review] [15 refs]. *Br J Obster Gynaecol* **109**(11), 1273–80.

15. Chwalisz K, DeManno D, Garg R, Larsen L & Mattia-Goldberg C (2004) Therapeutic potential for the selective progesterone receptor modulator asoprisnil in the treatment of leiomyomata. *Semin Reprod Med* **22**(2), 113–9.

16. McPherson K, Metcalfe MA, Herbert A *et al.* (2004) Severe complications of hysterectomy: the VALUE study. *Br J Obstet Gynaecol* **111**(7), 688–94.

17. Walker WJ & Pelage JP (2002) Uterine artery embolisation for symptomatic fibroids: clinical results in 400 women with imaging follow up. *Br J Obster Gynaecol* **109**(11), 1262–72.

18. Lumsden MA (2002) Embolization versus myomectomy versus hysterectomy: which is best, when? [Review] [65 refs]. *Hum Reprod* **17**(2), 253–9.

19. Goldberg J, Pereira L, Berghella V *et al.* (2004) Pregnancy outcomes after treatment for fibromyomata: uterine artery embolization versus laparoscopic myomectomy. *Am J Obstet Gynecol* **191**(1), 18–21.

20. Broder MS, Goodwin S, Chen G *et al.* (2002) Comparison of long-term outcomes of myomectomy and uterine artery embolization. *Obstet Gynecol* **100**(5:Pt 1), t-8.

21. Beinfeld MT, Bosch JL, Isaacson KB & Gazelle GS (2004) Cost-effectiveness of uterine artery embolization and hysterectomy for uterine fibroids. [Review] [28 refs]. *Radiology* **230**(1), 207–13.

22. Law P, Gedroyc WM & Regan L (1999) Magnetic-resonance-guided percutaneous laser ablation of uterine fibroids. *Lancet* **354**(9195), 2049–50.

Chapter 57: Cancer of the uterine corpus

Henry C. Kitchener

Introduction

Cancers of the uterine corpus include endometrial cancers, by far the commonest and accounting for 95%, carcinosarcomas and sarcomas. Overall cancers of the corpus rank second in incidence among gynaecological cancers in the European Union at 13/100,000 per year and the death rates of 2.5/100,000 per year, lower than cervical cancer which has a low incidence. This relatively low death rate of 20% ranks endometrial cancer among the most curable, which is due primarily to its early presentation. In the last century, there was a fair amount of complacency about endometrial cancer because its management was relatively straightforward and successful. There is now considerably increased interest because its incidence is rising and there is a need to improve treatment for advanced and recurrent disease. Recently reported randomized trials and research in progress are adding to the evidence based on which the most effective treatment protocols can be developed. This chapter will review investigation and current treatment strategies and will conclude with some future perspectives for the next 5–10 years.

Aetiology

The precise nature of endometrial carcinogenesis is far from understood, but there are a number of epidemiological observations that indicate a link with hyperoestrogenism for the endometrial cancers at least, which constitute the large majority. For many years obesity and related co-morbidity such as diabetes and hypertension have been associated with endometrial cancer. There is no doubt that trends in affluent countries, for example, Northern Europe and North America, have seen increases in obesity related morbidity and it is, therefore, not surprising that the highest incidence of endometrial cancer is seen in North America and Northern Europe. The incidence in Japanese women is low but women of Japanese origin living an altered lifestyle in Hawaii have exhibited an increased incidence. This epidemic of obesity over the past 30 years has been accompanied by an increase in the incidence of endometrial cancer.

The obese woman experiences increased circulating oestrogen from conversion of androgens in peripheral fat, which provides a plausible link between obesity and endometrial changes. A number of unrelated gynaecological conditions such as polycystic ovary syndrome and granulosa cell tumours, both of which can produce hyperoestrogenism are frequently associated with endometrial hyperplasia. Indeed this may be so marked that cytological atypia develops, which is widely acknowledged as a premalignant condition. Corroborative evidence is available from reports linking unopposed oestrogen replacement therapy with increased rates of endometrial cancer.

If oestrogen and oestrogenic effects can imitate cytological atypia other factors are probably required for promotion to cancer, because while some women acquire cancer from a background of cytological atypia, the majority do not.

Another factor involved in the rising incidence of endometrial cancer, and probably also carcinosarcoma, is tamoxifen, an antioestrogenic drug widely used as an adjuvant therapy in breast cancer. Tamoxifen exerts pro-oestrogenic effect in the endometrium and 5 years use of tamoxifen induces a relative risk of around 6.0 of developing endometrial cancer. Importantly though any potential mortality from endometrial cancer is greatly outweighed by the protective effect from recurrent breast cancer.

There are groups of women who are genetically predisposed to endometrial cancer, particularly those with hereditary non-polyposis colon cancer (HNPCC). These women carry a lifetime risk of up to a 30% chance of developing endometrial cancer. In this case it is clear that genetic mutations are responsible, possibly with oestrogen as a cofactor. Other evidence pointing to a different pathway from the endometrial tumours are the papillary serous tumours, a high proportion of which exhibit mutant p53, a potent tumour suppressor gene.

Pathology

Although endometrioid carcinoma contributes about 90% of tumours, other histotypes are found and their

Table 57.1 Classification of differentiation for endometrial cancer

Well differentiated, G1	≥5% of non-squamous or non-morula solid growth pattern
Moderately differentiated, G2	6–50% of a non-squamous or non-morula solid growth pattern
Poorly differentiated, G3	>50% of a non-squamous or non-morula solid growth pattern

Significant nuclear atypia raises the grade by one

Table 57.2 Endometrial cancer histotypes; WHO classification

Endometrioid adenocarcinoma, not otherwise specified (NOS)
    Variants
        Ciliated cells
        Secretory cells
Adenocarcinoma, NOS, with squamous differentiation
Mucous adenocarcinoma
Serous adenocarcinoma
Clear cell carcinoma
Squamous carcinoma
Undifferentiated carcinoma (large and small cell type)
Mixed carcinoma
Metastatic carcinoma

Table 57.3 Incidence of pelvic lymph node involvement as a function of tumour grade and myometrial invasion in clinical stage I endometrial cancer – results of a prospective Surgicopathological study

Depth of invasion	Grade		
	G1	G2	G3
Endometrium only	0/44 (0%)	1/31 (3%)	0/11 (0%)
Inner 1/3rd	3/96 (3%)	7/131 (5%)	5/54 (9%)
Middle 1/3rd	0/22 (0%)	6/69 (9%)	1/24 (4%)
Deep 1/3rd	2/18 (11%)	11/57 (19%)	22/64 (34%)

(Creasman *et al.* (1987) Cancer **60**:2035).

Table 57.4 FIGO surgicopathological staging for carcinoma of the uterine corpus

Stage I	Tumour is confined to the corpus uteri	
	Stage IA	Tumour limited to endometrium
	Stage IB	Invasion to less than half of the myometrium
	Stage IC	Invasion to greater than half of the myometrium
Stage II	Tumour involves the corpus and the cervix, but has not extended outside the uterus	
	Stage IIA	Endocervical glandular involvement only
	Stage IIB	Cervical stromal invasion
Stage III	Tumour extends outside of the uterus but is confined to the true pelvis	
	Stage IIIA	Tumour invades serosa and/or adnexae and/or positive peritoneal cytology
	Stage IIIB	Vaginal metastases
	Stage IIIC	Metastases to pelvic and/or para-aortic lymph nodes
Stage IV	Tumour invades bladder or bowel mucosa or metastasis to distant sites	
	Stage IVA	Tumour invasion of the bladder and/or bowel mucosa
	Stage IVB	Distant metastases, including intra-abdominal and/or inguinal lymph nodes

importance often lies in their worse prognosis. Papillary serous, clear cell carcinoma and carcinosarcoma are all associated with higher rates of metastases at presentation, and are also more resistant to conventional therapy.

In addition to the histotype, there are other pathological features of importance at least for endometrial cancer. These include the degree of differentiation and the extent of myometrial infiltration. The power of the differentiation and the deeper the myometrial infiltration, the greater the risk of extrauterine disease particularly lymph node metastases, which is the key prognostic factor in most cases of corpus cancer, where there is otherwise no evidence of distal spread.

The classification of differentiation for endometrial cancer is shown in Table 57.1 and the World Health Organization classification of endometrial cancer histotypes is listed in Table 57.2.

The pattern of spread in endometrial cancer is generally through the myometrial thickness to the serosal surface of the uterus and then involvement of the ovaries and fallopian tubes. At any point lymph node metastases may occur but the majority of lymph node metastases are found in association with deeper involvement of the myometrium. The association of lymph node involvement with myometrial invasion and degree of differentiation is shown in Table 57.3. It is clear that the large majority of node involvement is seen with G3 (polydifferentiated)

disease and outer involvement of the myometrium. Conversely women with G1 (well differentiated) disease and inner myometrial involvement have a very low risk of lymph node involvement. This is important for treatment planning (see p. 647). Staging is important in endometrial cancer and the FIGO staging rules are shown in Table 57.4.

Investigation including staging

Tissue diagnosis

The diagnosis of endometrial cancer is usually made following the clinical presentation of post-menopausal bleeding. The definitive diagnosis requires a biopsy but ultrasound, which is a useful first screen for PMB, is capable of demonstrating not only a likely tumour but also myometrium invasion. A critical review of the management of PMB is outside the scope of this chapter and the role of hysteroscopy will not be discussed. However it is obtained, whether by an outpatient procedure using devices such as Endocell or Pipelle or by formal curettage, there needs to be an adequate biopsy for the pathologist to be able to distinguish between severe atypia and invasive disease. Without stroma it may be impossible to distinguish severe cytological atypia and well differentiated intraendometrial carcinoma. Furthermore, invasive disease, unsampled by the biopsy, may occur within a field of cytological atypia. Therefore, there needs to be an index of suspicion that severe cytological atypia may be associated with invasive cancer.

The histopathology report should clearly indicate the histotype of invasive disease and the degree of differentiation which are the minimum data required to plan management. Examples of some different tumours are shown in Plate 57.1a–f (*facing p. 562*).

Radiological investigation

Because of surgical management, it is desirable to stage the disease at least radiologically, prior to surgery. The principal reasons for this are:
1 to determine whether a full surgical staging is required;
2 if surgical staging is warranted, referral should be made to a gynaecological oncologist.
The optimal method of radiological assessment is MR scan, which although not superior to CT scanning at identifying nodal involvement, is superior at assessing both myometrial invasion and cervical involvement, and direct extension of tumour outside the uterus. Examples of MR scans are shown in Fig. 57.1a–c.

Pre-anaesthesia assessment

In addition to radiological assessment of the tumour, careful investigation of associated co-morbidity is extremely important. As previously mentioned many of these women are elderly and obese, with a high prevalence of ischaemic heart disease, hypertension and chronic obstructive airways disease. This means that a careful preoperative assessment is essential. Full haematological and biochemical screening is essential, together with ECG and

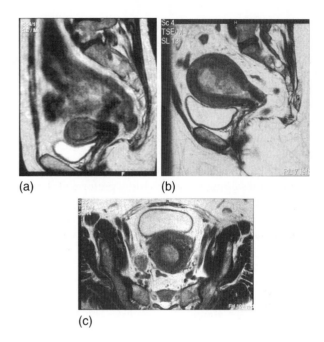

(a)　　　　　　　　(b)

(c)

Fig. 57.1 (a) Sagittal section showing a uterine cavity filled with tumour. (b) Sagittal section showing cervical involvement. (c) Transverse section showing grossly involved pelvic nodes (with thanks to Dr. J Hawnaur).

chest X-ray, which is also required to exclude pulmonary metastases. It may be that although a woman would normally benefit from full surgical staging, the presence of co-morbidity means that it would be more judicious simply to remove the uterus. Such decisions should be discussed by the multidisciplinary team, including the anaesthetist.

Treatment

The principal treatment for endometrial cancer is surgery, and because endometrial cancer usually presents when the disease is confined to the uterus, surgical excision is curative in the majority of cases. In high-risk cases, adjuvant therapy is employed and in a minority of cases, either advanced disease or in the presence of extreme co-morbidity, non-surgical treatment needs to be considered. Less common histotypes such as papillary serous tumours and carcinosarcoma merit special consideration.

Endometrioid tumours

Early disease

Ninety percent of uterine tumours are endometrioid endometrial cancer and of these 80% present in the absence of obvious extrauterine disease. The standard management is governed largely by prior allocation of the case to either high or low risk. Low risk would include cases comprising well and moderately differentiated tumours with less than 50% myometrial invasion on radiological assessment. Tumours that are poorly differentiated or with greater than myometrial invasion and/or suspicion of pelvic node involvement in MR scan would be classed as high risk. While low-risk cases can safely be managed by general gynaecologists, high-risk cases should be referred to gynaecological oncologists because of the requirements for full surgical staging.

Low-risk tumours can be managed by total abdominal and bilateral salpingo oophorectomy performed through a vertical incision. A thorough palpation of the contents of the peritoneal cavity should be made including the pelvic and para-aortic nodes. The omentum should be visualized and any suspicious mass should be sampled.

A staging laparotomy is often performed for high risk tumors. A full pelvic lymphadenectomy and is performed if there is a suspicion of involved pelvic or para-aortic nodes the latter should be sampled. The role of peritoneal washings is controversial because interpretation can be difficult and there is debate as to whether positive cytology would affect adjuvant treatment decisions in the absence of other relevant features such as positive nodes or evidence of serosal involvement and whether high- or low-risk tumours, thromboprophylaxis and prophylactic antibiotics should be used.

The decision to undertake lymphadenectomy may be moderated by the presence of co-morbidity leading to anaesthetic risk and a desire to undertake the least complex surgery possible and discretion by the operating surgeon need to be exercised.

The uterus should not be opened prior to fixation because this can lead to distortion and present difficulty to the pathologist. Some have advocated opening the uterus and assessing whether the depth of invasion suggests the need for lymphadenectomy; however, proper pre-operative evaluation should avoid the need for this. A full pathological assessment is crucial for further management decisions, in particular differentiation, degree of myometrial invasions, lymph/vascular channel involvement, histotype and involvement of fallopian tubes, ovaries, cervix and nodes needs to be documented.

The two principal controversies in the management of endometrial cancer have been the role of lymphadenectomy and that of adjuvant radiotherapy. While everyone agrees that a thorough lymphadenectomy, not sampling, should be a part of FIGO staging, there is little evidence as to whether this has any therapeutic benefit. Lymphadenectomy could be therapeutically effective either (1) indirectly, if it directed subsequent effective adjuvant therapy or (2) directly, if removal of involved nodes improved survival. There is not yet strong evidence that either of these is true, but the MRC ASTEC trial which will report late 2005 was designed to answer the question of therapeutic benefit by randomizing women to either lymphadenectomy or no lymphadenectomy without the result influencing the decision to give radiotherapy. Earlier studies have reported cohorts who have received lymphadenectomy or no lymphadenectomy with some evidence of improved survival but these results could be confounded by surgeon skill, case mix, co-morbidity and stage shift, i.e. staging renders stage 1 of lower risk than unstaged "stage 1", which will include some occult stage 3 disease.

Adjuvant radiotherapy

Until recently there was little consensus regarding adjuvant radiotherapy. In North America and Australia the general approach by gynaecological oncologists was to reserve adjuvant radiotherapy (meaning following complete surgical excision) for those in whom staging had demonstrated extrauterine disease, usually involving nodes. In Europe, the approach has placed emphasis on, pathological criteria to determine the use of adjuvant radiotherapy. This was certainly the situation in the United Kingdom and many other countries in the European Union until the late 1990s, with rates of radiotherapy reaching 40%. This was despite a randomized trial reported from Norway in 1980, which showed no survival benefits for adjuvant radiotherapy in stage I endometrial cancer. Although it did show fewer pelvic relapses in irradiated women, more irradiated women developed distal disease.

More recently the PORTEC study has begun to influence the use of adjuvant radiotherapy. In this trial women with intermediate risk disease (G1/outer invasion; G2/any invasion; G3/inner invasion) were again randomized to receive adjuvant external beam radiotherapy. Again there was evidence of improved pelvic control but no overall survival benefit, although there was a benefit for women over 60 years compared with younger women. These data have resulted in fewer women receiving radiotherapy.

ASTEC has also randomized women, for all risk categories to receive radiotherapy or no radiotherapy, independent of the lymph node status, and these results expected in 2007, will include the effect on high-risk disease. Brachytherapy has been widely used in the past to reduce the risk of vault recurrence.

Until further data are available radiotherapy should be offered to women with nodal involvement and those with poorly differentiated tumours extending to the outer half of the myometrium or any degree of differentiation with serosal or tubal/ovarian involvement. Women with intermediate risk disease over 60 years may be offered radiotherapy.

If the endocervix is affected with very superficial stroma involvement radiotherapy is probably not required but significant stromal involvement would be an indication for radiotherapy. If MR scanning indicates significant cervical involvement pre-operatively, a radial hysterectomy can be considered as a potentially curative procedure.

Advanced disease

Where disease has spread beyond the uterus but is considered potentially resectable, surgery should be attempted to debulk a tumour that may be resistant to other forms of treatment. Following surgery, residual disease, if confined to the pelvis, can be treated by additional radiotherapy. If disease has spread beyond the pelvis then chemotherapy should be considered. Active agents doxorubicin and cisplatin in combination are associated with at least short-term response rates of 30–40% but with significant haematological toxicity. There is now increasing use of carboplatin in combination with paclitaxel, which is better tolerated although no large randomized trials of its use have been reported.

Hormone therapy in the form of progestogens has been widely used in the past and although it has been shown not to be effective as a routine adjuvant following primary treatment, there is a response rate in recurrent disease. There are now new hormonal therapies available, for example, anastrozole and tamoxifen and there is a need to evaluate those formally in clinical trials. Another group of drugs showing promise in a variety of tumours is the biological agents or small molecules which block key molecular pathways, and these are now being considered for clinical trials. Unfortunately due to tumour resistance, most women with advanced disease will die within 2 years.

Recurrent disease

The situation with recurrent disease is similar in some respects for advanced disease. The most straightforward category of recurrence is central disease confined to the vagina in non-irradiated women. In these cases there is a salvage rate of up to 70% with radiation alone. In all cases of pelvic recurrence without prior radiation, women should be offered radiotherapy although salvage rates for disease involving the pelvic side wall are around 30%. When there is disease outside the pelvis, radiotherapy can be offered as outlined for advanced disease but response in previously irradiated tumours is low, and the prospects for salvage is poor. Hormone therapy may be used using megestrol acetate 100–200 mg BD.

Less common histotypes

The most common non-endometrial carcinomas arising on the endometrium are uterine papillary serous carcinoma (UPSC), clear cell carcinoma (CCC) and carcinosarcoma formerly known as mixed mullerian tumours. These tumours, which account for about 10% of all endometrial cancers, are important because they carry a far higher death rate compared with endometrioid. Endometrioid tumours have an overall 5-year survival of around 75% compared with 42% and 27% for CCC and UPSC respectively. This is largely due to stage at presentation. Whereas 80% of endometrioid tumours are Stage I at presentation, corresponding figures for CCC and UPSC have been reported at 58 and 26% respectively. UPSC tumours behave rather like serous ovarian tumours in terms of spread. This makes surgical staging important for these tumours because the risk of extrauterine disease is so high.

Uterine papillary serous carcinoma. In fully surgical staged patients, with no evidence of extrauterine disease following hysterectomy, there is no proven benefit for adjuvant therapy. Radiotherapy is not effective for UPSC and a 5-year survival in a GOG randomized trial of whole abdominal radiotherapy is only 35%. Chemotherapy is the accepted modality with either cisplatin/adriamycin or carboplatin/paclitaxel combinations. In advanced or recurrent disease chemotherapy is again recommended with a platinum-based combination.

Carcinosarcoma. This tumour behaves rather like a high-grade endometrial carcinoma which spread via lymph nodes, though at a higher rate than high-grade endometrioid. Management relies on surgical staging and additional treatment on the form of radiotherapy and chemotherapy. There have been few trials in carcinosarcoma with little evidence of benefit from radiotherapy. In the absence of other proven effective therapy, when extrauterine disease is confined to the pelvis, radiotherapy is reasonable. When there is disease spread beyond the pelvis chemotherapy may be offered. Again the most commonly used regiment is a combination of cisplatin/adriamycin and ifosfamide may be added though this triplet is rather toxic. The prognosis for women with extrauterine disease at presentation is poor.

Uterine leiomyosarcoma. This is rare accounting for about 1% of all corpus tumours. Treatment which relies on surgical excision is possible and chemotherapy is recommended for node positive or residual disease. Chemotherapy regiment of ifosfamide and doxorubicin is usually used and the response rates are around 30–40% but with poor survival rates.

Endometrial stromal sarcoma. This is another rare tumour but is far more indolent than leiomyosarcoma. If the disease is confined to the uterus, hysterectomy is usually curative. If there is residual disease following hysterectomy, it is usually resistant to radiotherapy or chemotherapy, and recurrences are best treated by repeated surgical excision.

Future perspectives

The management of endometrial cancer has become more evidence based in recent years. Future research will focus on chemotherapy designed to treat advanced and recurrent disease, including new hormone and biological therapy. There will be increased interest in trying to understand the molecular pathogenesis of endometrial cancer, which will offer insights into possible strategies for biological therapy. Recent data suggests, for example, that targeting c-Kit, abl and platelet-derived growth factor receptor may be relevant. The drug imatimib mesylate (Gleevec, Novartis) targets some of these kinases suggesting a possible strategy for treatment. HNPCC, which is associated with mutation of the mismatch repair (MMR) gene, is the subject of increasing interest and we need to know how we can reduce the risk of endometrial cancer in these women, for example, by screening with ultrasound and hysteroscopy or even by a progestogen intrauterine system (IUCD).

With a rising incidence, endometrial cancer may become the commonest gynaecological tumour over the next 20 years. Improved forms of treatment are required for advanced/recurrent disease.

Chapter 58: Sexual dysfunction

Fran Reader

Introduction

The sex drive is not about individual survival, but survival of the species. However, sexual expression has a far broader role than procreation. It is used recreationally to confirm bonding in an environment of trust and affection. On the 'darker side' it may also be used or withheld to dominate or humiliate.

Human sexual behaviour became a legitimate topic for research beginning with *Kinsey* in 1948 and extended by *Masters & Johnson* in the 1950s. Greater expectations of sexual fulfilment followed this knowledge. A normal physiological response to sexual arousal will occur when there is physical and psychological health, so that a couple can choose and enjoy a full range of mutually agreed sexual behaviours. However, when there are problems it can be devastating for the individual and the relationship. Studies suggest that 40–45% of women have at least one sexual dysfunction, low desire is the most frequent presentation with the prevalence increasing with age, followed by orgasmic dysfunction [1]. Women are more likely to present for help than men.

The sexual response

The biological function of sexual intercourse is to ensure that sperm are released into the woman's vagina so they can fertilize the egg. Vaginal penetration is just one form of sexual expression. Couples may enjoy giving or receiving oral sex, anal intercourse or non-penetrative mutual masturbation. The Kama Sutra lists 64 elements in love play and 41 positions in copulation.

Slang words used to describe sexual intercourse usually depict the act as being male active and female passive. However, both partners can enjoy being active or passive and may change roles during the same sexual encounter.

Understanding the stages of the human sexual response cycle

All humans possess a biological sex drive. The stages of sexual response cycle arise from this drive beginning with desire progressing through arousal to orgasm and ending with resolution.

Imagine the journey from desire to orgasm is like going upstairs (Fig. 58.1). Ground level is non-sexual. Step 1 – is

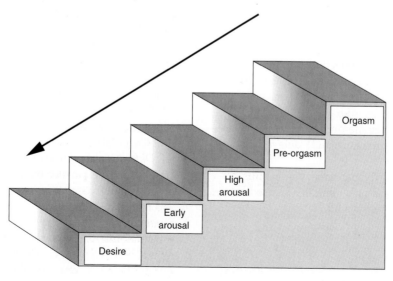

Fig. 58.1 The arousal staircase.

desire without any physical change. Step 2 – early arousal begins and the man's penis begins to get firm, but not firm enough for penetration, and the woman begins to lubricate. Step 3 – arousal progresses to give the man a firm erection that could penetrate and a woman lubricates more and the inner part of the vagina lengthens and widens. Step 4 – orgasm is recognized as being imminent. Step 5 – orgasm itself. Sliding down the banisters is the process of returning back to the ground. With this analogy you can understand that you can climb on to the banister from any step on the staircase. As you slide down you take with you all the thoughts and feelings surrounding that particular sexual encounter. It is normal for both men and women to spend time going up and down some of the steps and not to go directly to Step 5 in one dash.

Men and women often progress up the stairs at different rates. Physiologically a man on Step 3 can penetrate a woman who could still be on Step 1. The reverse is impossible. The important concept for both partners to understand is that each is responsible for their own progression up the staircase and the point they choose to step off. The man is responsible for his orgasm and the woman for hers. Communication and respect for each other's needs is therefore essential. There is no need to aim for synchronicity or even to make orgasm the goal. It is important that each individual is comfortable with their progress and that the thoughts and feelings that are around when returning down the banister are of fulfilment and contentment, not anger, resentment or a sense of failure.

Sexual dysfunctions

Sexual dysfunctions can be primary, secondary, situational or global, organic (including physiological or iatrogenic) or non-organic (psychosocial).

Classification – based on ICD-10

- Sexual desire disorders – hypoactive sexual desire disorder, sexual aversion disorder, hyperactive sexual desire.
- Sexual arousal disorders – female sexual arousal disorder (FSAD), male erectile disorder
- Orgasmic disorders – female orgasmic disorder, male orgasmic disorders (1) premature; (2) delayed and (3) retrograde
- Sexual pain disorders – dyspareunia, vaginismus
These definitions are based on a genitally focused model and are currently under revision [2].

Aetiology

1 Physiological
  (a) Menstrual cycle
  (b) Childbirth
  (c) Menopause
  (d) Ageing process
2 Organic or iatrogenic
  (a) Affecting the sexual response, e.g. diabetic neuropathy
  (b) Affecting genital autonomy, e.g. vulvectomy
  (c) Affecting mobility, e.g. cerebrovascular accident
  (d) Limited by pain, e.g. arthritis, angina
  (e) Limited by genital pain, e.g. endometriosis
  (f) Limited by fatigue or chronic illness, e.g. renal failure
  (g) Side-effect or medication
  (h) Combinations of the above
3 Psychosocial
  (a) *Lack of or incorrect information about sex.* Even in this day and age sex education may be inadequate and lack of knowledge lead to guesswork, incorrect information from peers, dirty jokes or medical sensationalism.
  (b) *Sexual myths and taboos.* Sexual beliefs, attitudes and value systems develop within our family, social, cultural and religious experiences. What is acceptable sexual behaviour to one person may trigger guilt in another.
  Example of sexual myths:
  - Performance is everything
  - Nice women do not initiate sex or ask for what they want
  - Good sex is always spontaneous
  - The man is responsible for the woman's climax
  - The woman is responsible for the man's erection
  - The man automatically mind reads what the woman wants 'if he really loves me'
  - Sex equals intercourse
  - Women need penetration to climax
  - A woman cannot be sexually satisfied without a climax
  (c) *Communication problems.* It may be sexual communication that is the problem. Alternatively unresolved general relationship problems may lead to anger, resentment or guilt that sour the sexual relationship.
  (d) *Predisposing and precipitating factors.* Related to past experiences or life events can contribute to sexual problems (Table 58.1).
  (e) *Differing and unrealistic expectations.* Problems can arise when one partner wants sex more than the other or unrealistic expectations lead to performance pressure and fear of failure.
  Examples of unrealistic expectations:
  - Sexual interest will stay unchanged by tiredness, illness, bereavement, childbirth or ageing
  - Simultaneous orgasm should happen on every occasion.

Table 58.1 Common predisposing and precipitating factors

Predisposing factors	Precipitating factors
Physical, emotional or sexual abuse in childhood	Parenthood
Restrictive upbringing	Illness
Lack of information	Random failure
Poor self-esteem	Life stresses
Poor body language	Performance pressure
Communication problems	Sexual trauma
Uncertain sexual identity	Loss of trust in relationship
Psychiatric illness	

Assessment

Taking a sexual history

Talking about a sexual problem can be embarrassing. It is therefore important that health professionals are trained to develop an open non-judgemental style that encourages talking about delicate matters such as sexual orientation, masturbation, fantasies and infidelities. It is important to be confident about the use of sexually explicit words. It can be helpful to check out the understanding of words to ensure they will be understood and help the patient feel comfortable when talking about their sexual problem.

Sexual history taking

BACKGROUND

- Family and important relationships
- Education, culture and religion
- Attitudes to sexuality, intimacy and expression of emotion
- Traumatic sexual or other life experiences.

ADOLESCENT EXPERIENCES

- Sex education
- Experience of puberty – periods, wet dreams, etc.
- Sexual opportunities, masturbation, non-coital and coital experiences
- Traumatic sexual and other experiences
- Ease of transition to adult identity.

ADULT EXPERIENCES

- Past relationships
- Traumatic life events.

CURRENT EXPERIENCES

- History of the presenting problem
- Details of the current sexual dysfunction

- Present sexual practices and preferences including masturbation
- Present relationship(s)
- Sexual orientation
- The use of fantasy, erotic material or sex aids.

MEDICAL HISTORY

- Past medical and surgical history
- Past obstetric and gynaecological history – especially factors that may affect sexual responsiveness such as, endometriosis, chronic pelvic infection, pelvic floor obstetric damage, pelvic organ prolapse, urinary or faecal incontinence
- Drug history both social and therapeutic
- Contraception/infertility
- Sexually transmitted infections
- Dermatological problems
- Vulva and vaginal hygiene – possible irritants (Table 58.2).

Examination

Examining patients with a sexual problem needs to be done sensitively particularly for the patient with a past history of sexual abuse. Privacy must be guaranteed and a chaperone must always be offered and should be present when a man is examining a woman.

General examination

Check secondary sexual characteristics and look for signs of:
- Anaemia
- Thyroid disease
- Cardiovascular disease
- Central nervous system disorders
- Dermatological conditions
- Any chronic illness.

Genital examination

How a woman approaches a genital examination will give non-verbal or verbal clues to how comfortable she is with her sexuality.

VULVAL INSPECTION

- Anatomical appearances, e.g. juvenile external genitalia, large labia minora
- Dermatological problems, e.g. lichen sclerosis, lichen planus, eczema, psoriasis

Table 58.2 Examples of drugs that can affect sexual function

Cardiovascular	Mental health	Hormonal	Other	Recreational
Antihypertensives	Antidepressants	Antiandrogens	Antiemetics	Alcohol
Beta blockers	Anxiolytics	Steroids	Antiepileptics	Canabis
Diogoxin	Antipsychotics	Hormonal contraception	Antihistamines	Opiates/cocaine/amphetamines

See recommended reading – Sexual pharmacology fast facts.

- Sexually transmitted infections, e.g. genital ulceration (herpes, syphilis), warts
- Changes suspicious of benign or malignant lesions
- Scar tissue.

VAGINAL INSPECTION

- Anatomical abnormalities, e.g. vaginal septum
- Atrophic changes
- Pelvic organ prolapse
- Discharge suggestive of candida or bacterial vaginosis or sexually transmitted infection.

VAGINAL EXAMINATION

- High tone in the pubococcygeus muscle indicating vaginismus
- Tenderness anteriorly (possible bladder pathology)
- Posteriorly (possible ouch of Douglas or rectal pathology)
- Right fornix (possible pathology in right adnexae)
- Left fornix (possible pathology in sigmoid colon or left adnexae)
- Size, shape, position, mobility and tenderness of the uterus.

Investigations

Specific sexual problems

LACK OR LOSS OF DESIRE

Personal problems or relationship difficulties often present in this way. Chronic physical illness frequently leads to low desire because of fatigue, loss of self-esteem, altered body image or as a side-effect of medication. It is possible for low desire to exist in isolation, but it may be secondary to other sexual problems because of fear of failure.

Recently there has been research interest in the difference between desire in men and women. Desire may be biological and innate, or responsive and linked to maintaining self-esteem and a contented sexual partnership. It appears that for women the responsive desire is more important, especially after the menopause when fertility has ended [2]. Women report that they initiate sex

Table 58.3 Investigations for specific sexual problems

Low desire	Prolactin
	Thyroid function tests
	Testosterone, estradiol, follicle stimulating hormone (FSH)/ luteinizing hormone (LH)
	Full blood count (FBC), B12, urea and electrolyte (U&E), liver function tests (LFT) – if clinically indicated
Arousal problems/ orgasmic problems	Similar tests as for desire, also fasting blood sugar and lipid profile
Superficial dyspareunia	Test for sexually transmitted infections (STIs) and other vaginal or urinary infections
Deep dyspareunia	As for superficial dyspareunia plus ultrasound scan, diagnostic laparoscopy

less frequently when innate desire fades but they can still experience responsive desire at the same time as arousal.

Physical options

- Look for physical factors. If they exist, treat them and recognize their significance to the maintenance of the sexual problem
- Change medication if this might be contributing to the problem (see Table 58.3) and recommended reading
- Oestrogen dominant combined oral contraception for women who are hypooestrogenic, e.g. low body mass index from an eating disorder or excessive exercise
- Hormone replacement therapy (HRT) if menopausal (Tibilone is licensed for treatment of low desire)
- Testosterone implants (licensed) or gel (unlicensed) for postmenopausal women, especially if the menopause occurs prematurely through iatrogenic loss of ovarian function
- Treat depression
- Treat hypoprolactinaemia.

Psychosexual options

- Individual or couple therapy as appropriate
- Treat any preceding sexual problem

- 'Homework' exercises to improve understanding and communication of sexual needs.

SEXUAL AVERSION AND LACK OF SEXUAL ENJOYMENT

Sexual avoidance, aversions and phobias often stem from some traumatic experience such as childhood sexual abuse or rape. They may also stem from receiving strongly negative messages about sex that leads to feelings of guilt or shame. Sexual aversion may mimic low desire because frequency of sexual activity is low. Sexual aversion and phobis can be total (in which case all sexual activity is avoided) or situational when specific sexual activities may trigger the phobic response. A woman who needs to remain in control may panic when she feels aroused especially if childhood conditioning has enforced the idea that sexual pleasure is wrong.

Psychosexual options

- Individual therapy to help to discover the predisposing or precipitating factors
- Abuse resolution work before dealing with the sexual problem
- Gradual desensitization to sexual activities that lead to the aversive response.

Physical options

- Serotonin re-uptake inhibitors (SSRIs) can reduce the physical phobic response.

FEMALE SEXUAL AROUSAL DISORDER

The physiological arousal response in the female is invisible, unlike the male erection. Most men and women know that vaginal lubrication indicates arousal, but have no knowledge of the pelvic congestion and ballooning of the inner two thirds of the vagina that occurs with high arousal.

It is uncommon for women to present with arousal problems in isolation. They are usually linked to low desire, sexual avoidance or orgasmic dysfunction. FSAD has been subdivided into 'genital arousal disorder', 'subjective sexual arousal disorder' and 'combined genital and subjective arousal disorder' [2]. Genital arousal problems often present as painful sex. Lack of lubrication makes penetration sore and lack of vaginal ballooning can lead to the woman experiencing deep dyspareunia. The problem is rarely a true inability to become aroused, but rather that her partner is ahead of her in his arousal and penetrated her too soon and the woman is unable to communicate the problem.

Psychosexual options

- 'Homework' exercises to improve understanding and communication of sexual needs
- Use of fantasy, erotic material or sex aids (see 'Useful websites')
- Reading self-help books (see 'Further reading').

Physical options

- Change medication if appropriate
- HRT or vaginal oestrogen – if oestrogen deficiency is a factor in failure of lubrication
- Artificial lubricants
- Sildenafil or other 5 phophodiesterase inhibitors may be worth trying on an unlicensed basis. There is evidence that they may help, especially in premenopausal women with no desire disorder [3]
- Zestra [4]
- Eros clitoral therapy device [5].

ORGASMIC DYSFUNCTION

Studies suggest that about 25% of women experience orgasmic dysfunction [6]. Women tend to climax less readily compared to men and can feel sexually satisfied without an orgasm. Biologically they do not need to reach a climax to achieve a pregnancy. Of the women who are orgasmic 50% will orgasm through manual, rather than vaginal, stimulation. When there is a problem it is usually psychosexual and related to either inadequate stimulation or to difficulty in letting go and losing control. It is often situational so that orgasm may occur with masturbation but not with a partner. When anorgasmia is secondary it is important to consider physical causes. The most common cause being a side effect of an SSRI used to treat depression. Other physical causes to exclude are neurological such as diabetic neuropathy or multiple sclerosis.

Psychosexual options

- Exploring the use of fantasy, erotic material and sexual aids
- Reading self-help books (see 'Further reading')
- Using nipple stimulation during sexual arousal to enhance orgasmic response due to oxytocin release.

Physical options

- Change medication if appropriate
- Sildenafil to assist arousal may help orgasmic release.

VAGINISMUS

In this condition the woman has an involuntary spasm of the pubococcygeus muscle. The muscle tightens in anticipation of physical or emotional pain. The vaginal spasm may also be accompanied by spasm of the adductor muscles of the thigh. The reasons for vaginismus are various, such as traumatic past experiences, or growing up with negative messages about sex leading to fear or intimacy or loss of control.

Psychosexual options

• Give information about genital anatomy and the female sexual response
• Individual therapy to explore and resolve predisposing factors
• Couple therapy where couples collude to maintain the problem
• Gradual desensitization using such items as fingers, tampon covers, specifically designed vaginal Amielle dilators – plus plenty of synthetic lubrication.
• Gradually move to penile penetration with the woman maintaining control.

DYSPAREUNIA

In women there are many physical causes for superficial and deep dyspareunia that need to be treated appropriately; however, for some there will be no obvious underlying disease process. Sometimes the disease process has been cured but the woman had developed a secondary vaginismus in response to anticipated dyspareunia. Emotional pain can also be expressed as genuine physical pain that has the unconscious gain of avoiding intimacy with a partner.

Physical options

• Treat vulvovaginal infections
• Topical steroids may help dermatological problems
• Topical oestrogens may improve atrophic changes
• Topical local anaesthetic
• Amitryptiline or gabapentin for neuropathic pain.

Psychosexual options

• The management is similar to vaginismus
• Adaption of sexual positions may minimize pain.

Specific issues

Puberty

The physical changes that occur at puberty are welcomed by most young women, but can be disturbing for young women who are in conflict about their emerging adult sexuality, gender identity or sexual orientation [7]. Adolescence is also a time of separation from parents and authority figures to find ones personal identity. Achieving this separation involves experimentation and risk taking, which may also be of a sexual nature. Low self-esteem or poor body image may manifest itself in sexual hyperactivity as the young woman seeks reassurance about her attractiveness. Adolescent identity crises may present as menstrual problems, contraceptive problems, unintended pregnancy or sexually transmitted infections. It can be difficult to remain non-judgemental when confronted by an 'irresponsible teenager with attitude' presenting yet again with a vaginal discharge or unintended pregnancy. It is important to build rapport with these young women and treat them respectfully. It could be the first time they experience respect.

PARENTHOOD

The transition to motherhood involves enormous changes to a woman's lifestyle, roles and career opportunities. This can be another time of crisis as she adds the role of mother to wife/partner and lover. Conflict over parenting roles may arise leaving her partner feeling marginalized and jealous. The pregnancy or birth experience may lead to sexual avoidance because of a fear of repeating a traumatic experience. Her body is likely to have changed, which may lead to doubts about physical/sexual activeness. If she is breastfeeding high prolactin levels will reduce sex drive and low oestrogen levels contribute to vaginal dryness. Sleepless nights and exhaustion put the final nail in the coffin for sexual activity [8].

The typical sexual problems that occur post-natally are either loss of interest or sexual avoidance. Both present with reduced frequency of sexual activity.

Infertility

Sexual problems may cause infertility or infertility may trigger sexual problems. Taking a good sexual history is important in infertility work to pick up low frequency of sexual activity from loss of interest or sexual avoidance, dyspareunia, vaginismus or male factors, such as erectile dysfunction, premature ejaculation, retarded or retrograde ejaculation.

Finally it is important to never assume what a couple mean by 'having sex'. Even in the twenty-first century some couple remain naïve. Anal sex, umbilical sex or mutual masturbation may be the couples' sexual activity and they may not understand that sperm cannot meet the egg without vaginal penetration [9].

Menopause and beyond

Most women report relief or neutral feelings towards the menopause. The main physical factors linked to negative feelings are physical symptoms of persistent hot flushes, night sweats and vaginal dryness. Pelvic organ prolapse and incontinence may also contribute. Declining hormone levels may be responsible for depression and loss of sexual interest around the menopause, but so too may life events involving loss or role change, such as children leaving home, death of parents, redundancy or retirement.

It is therefore best to take a holistic approach to managing sexual problems that occur around the menopause. The increasing use of successful oral treatments for age-related erectile dysfunction is leading to an increased presentation of older women with sexual problems [10].

Genital cancers

Loss of genital anatomy or physiological responsiveness occurs with treatment for most female genital cancers. This may have a profound effect on the individual or couple. Counselling and support may be helpful as well as practical support such as vaginal dilators to help maintain vulval patency or vaginal depth [11].

References

1. Lewis R, Kersten S *et al.* (2004) Epidemiology/risk factors of sexual dysfunction. *J Sex Med* **1**, 35–9.
2. Basson R, Leiblum S *et al.* (2004) Revised definitions of Women's sexual dysfunction. *J Sex Med* **1**, 40–8.
3. Caruso S, Intelisano G *et al.* (2001) Pre-menopausal women affected by sexual arousal disorder treated with sildenafil: a double-blind, cross-over, placebo-controlled study. *Br J Obstet Gynaecol* **108**, 623–8.
4. Ferguson D, Singh G *et al.* (2003) Randomised, placebo-controlled, double-blind, cross-over design trial of the efficacy of Zestra for women with and without sexual arousal disorder. *J Sex Marital Therapy* **29**, 33–44.
5. Billups K, Berman L *et al.* (2001) Non-pharmacological vacuum therapy for female sexual dysfunction. *J Sex Marital Ther* **27**, 435–41.
6. Meston C, Hull E *et al.* (2004) Disorders of orgasm in women. *J Sex Med* **1**, 82–6.
7. Aggleton P, Ball A & Purnima G (2002) Young people, sexuality and relationships. *Sex Relat Ther* **17**, 253–60.
8. Reader F (2004) Is there sex after childbirth? *J Assoc Chartered Physiotherapists Women's Health* **96**, 35–40.
9. Read J (1995) *Counselling and Fertility Problems*. London: Sage.
10. Myskow L (2000) Perimenopausal issues in sexuality. *Sex Relat Ther* **15**, 213–20.
11. Kew F, Nevin J & Cruikshank D (2002) Psychosexual impact of gynaecological malignancy. *Obstet Gynaecol* **4**, 193–6.
12. Basson R, Althof S *et al.* (2004) Summary recommendations on sexual dysfunctions in women. *J Sex Med* **1**, 24–34.
13. Kinsey A, Pomeroy W *et al.* (1953) *Sexual Behaviour in The Human Female*. Philadelphia: Saunders.
14. Masters W & Johnson V (1966) *Human Sexual Response*. New York: Little Brown.

Further reading

For professionals

John Tomlinson (ed.) (2004) *ABC of Sexual Health*. London: BMJ Books.
Skrine R & Montford H (eds) (2001) *Psychosexual Medicine. An Introduction*. London: Arnold.
Seagraves RT & Balon R (2003) *Sexual Pharmacology Fast Facts*. London: WW Norton.
Cooper E & Guillebaud J (1999) *Sexuality and Disability*. Oxford: Radcliffe Medical Press.

For self help

Quilliam S 2003 *The Woman's Complete Illustrated Guide to Sex*. Gloucester Massachusetts: Fairwinds Press.
Heiman J & LoPiccolo J (1992) *Becoming Orgasmic*. New York: Simon & Schuster.
Goodwin A (1998) *A Woman's Guide to Overcoming Sexual Fear & Pain*. Oakland: New Harbinger.
Cole J & Sampson V (2004) *How to Have Great Sex for the Rest of Your Life*. London: Piatkus.

Useful websites

British Associations for Sexual and Relationship Therapy (basrt) www.barst.org.uk.
Institute of Psychosexual Medicine (IPM) www.ipm.org.uk
British Society for Sexual Medicine (BSSM) www.bssm.org.uk
Sexual Dysfunction Association www.sda.uk.net
Vulval Pain Society www.vulvalpainsociety.org
For Amielle dilators, lubricants and sex aids, www.fpsales.co.uk
For sex aids and self-help advise www.emotionalbliss.co.uk

Chapter 59: Ethical dilemmas in obstetrics and gynaecology

Gordon M. Stirrat

Introduction

Those who aspire to practice Obstetrics and Gynaecology accept several necessary characteristics shared by all medical practitioners. There is, for example, a tradition of practice based on a body of knowledge. Not only is it necessary that this body of knowledge be continually updated on the best available evidence, but also each of us must keep abreast of the aspects of that knowledge required for best practice. In addition practitioners must meet required standards of competence, care and conduct so that we are, at all times, striving to make best use of our skills and knowledge.

Unfortunately self-motivation is not sufficient to guarantee minimum, let alone high, standards of practice. That is why one of the defining characteristics of a profession is that it is regulated by a body to which all who practice it must belong. The Royal College of Obstetricians and Gynaecologists (RCOG) in the UK (and comparable organizations elsewhere) is central to the setting, achieving and maintaining standards of care to improve women's health. It is not, however, a regulatory authority. In the UK this is the statutory responsibility of the General Medical Council (GMC) for the profession as a whole and similar bodies exist in other countries. The GMC's stated vision is 'to be recognised as delivering and safeguarding the highest standards of medical ethics, education and practice, in the interests of patients, public and the profession'. In 'Duties of a Doctor' [1] they state, 'Patients must be able to trust doctors with their lives and well-being. To justify that trust, we as a profession have a duty to maintain a good standard of practice and care and to show respect for human life.' Those duties are further stated in Table 59.1 and are amplified in the GMC's document 'Good Medical Practice' [2] (http://www.gmc-uk.org/standards). They speak for themselves. The focus of this book is quite appropriately on clinical practice and the authors, all of whom are eminent in their field, have brought to you the current best available evidence on how to manage specific problems in our specialty. They tell you what *Can* be done and give some guidance on how to do it (the latter needs to

Table 59.1 Duties of a doctor [1]

As a doctor you must:
- Make the care of your patient your first concern
- Treat every patient politely and considerately
- Respect patients' dignity and privacy
- Listen to patients and respect their views
- Give patients information in a way they can understand
- Respect the rights of patients to be fully informed in decisions about their care
- Keep your professional knowledge up to date
- Recognize the limits of your professional competence
- Be honest and trustworthy
- Respect and protect confidential information
- Make sure that your personal beliefs do not prejudice your patients' care
- Act quickly to protect patients from risk if you have good reason to believe that you or a colleague may not be fit to practise
- Avoid abusing your position as a doctor
- Work with colleagues in the ways that best serve patients' interests

In all these matters you must never discriminate unfairly against your patients or colleagues and you must always be prepared to justify your actions to them

be further developed by hands-on practice). They usually neither tell you what *Should* nor what *Ought* to be done (though they will, where necessary, make it clear what should not be done). The word 'can' makes a statement one of fact and nothing more. 'Should' and 'ought' are different – they both imply obligation but 'ought' is the stronger because it speaks of duty, which is definitely a moral action. One of the purposes of this chapter is to explore the ethical dimensions of the practice of obstetrics and gynaecology to increase ethical awareness and guide moral reasoning. In other words, it is a guide as to how to think ethically but it is not an ethical rulebook that tells you what to think or do in specific circumstances.

We have already noted that duty implies moral action but it goes further than this because it is the kind of moral action in which one is blameworthy if one does not perform it. In other words it is obligatory. An example of this would be if a woman collapsed on the antenatal ward and the on-call obstetrician, having received an urgent call to attend, failed to do so for no good reason. The doctor would have failed in the 'duty of care' and not only would be morally culpable but also would be liable for at least civil proceedings against him/her. A moral action can also be self-sacrificing, altruistic and an ideal 'beyond the call of duty'. The technical word for this is 'supererogatory'. An example of this might be a junior doctor who voluntarily stays on the ward when off duty to help a colleague who is finding it difficult to cope with their workload.

In its stated purpose, which we have noted above, the GMC gives medical ethics precedence over education and practice. In addition, if we look carefully at the 'Duties of a Doctor' [1] (see Table 59.1) there are several words that have a strong moral sense. Among them are honesty, trust and trustworthiness; respect (for human life, dignity and privacy, rights of the patient and confidentiality); and avoidance of unfair discrimination. Thus, ethics is at the very heart of being a doctor (let alone a good doctor). This includes an absolute commitment to these duties and, of course, one will be held to account if one fails to meet them.

The basis for ethics

Ethics (or moral philosophy) is the discipline that underpins moral judgements when we are faced with such fundamental questions as 'How do we know what is good?', 'What is the right thing to do?' or 'What is justice?' It attempts to provide a rational framework for understanding the complexities of moral judgement [3]. Morals are not only the specific judgements, codes or beliefs of particular groups or societies but also the actions that follow from them. Ethics and morals can, perhaps be better understood if we compare them with DNA and the cell proteins coded for in the genome (Fig. 59.1). Ethics can be seen as a system of thought encompassing the actions of people in society which, if adhered to, is most likely to lead to the welfare, health and happiness of the individual and the society in which he or she lives. Table 59.2 outlines some essentials of medical ethics [4].

Ethics is often said to be nothing more than 'common sense' based on experience but one of the problems with common sense is that it is not so common! But how does one determine what ought to be done? This is considered below. Let us also put common sense to the test in a hypothetical clinical example.

CASE 1

Mrs AB, aged 34, having failed to conceive for 6 years, becomes pregnant with triplets following assisted conception. An ultrasound scan shows that she has a major degree of placenta praevia and the potential implications of this are discussed with her. Both she and her husband have a devout religious objection to blood transfusion and they make it clear in writing that she is not to be given blood under any circumstances. She is admitted for long-term stay in hospital after several episodes of vaginal bleeding. A major antepartum haemorrhage occurs at 34 weeks that is of such severity that it is considered necessary to proceed to delivery by Caesarean section under general anaesthatic (GA) and she gives her consent. She repeats her absolute refusal to allow blood transfusion despite being told the risk that she might die without it if bleeding cannot be controlled. All three babies are delivered in good condition but she continues to bleed. The possibility that she might die as a result of this decision is again made clear to her husband. He supports his wife's prior decision despite the potential outcome.

What do you think the ordinary man or woman would say? Would it be 'Here is a couple who have been trying to have a family for 6 years and have gone to the lengths of assisted conception to do so. If she dies the three babies will be left motherless. Surely no one in their right mind would wish to die under these circumstances? Her objection to receiving blood must be irrational! Surely common sense suggests that she must be given blood!' If you share that 'common sense' view you might say, 'Let's give her the blood – she doesn't even need to know we have done so!' The problem with that pragmatic approach is that, despite acting in what clearly seems to be in the best interests of herself, her husband and the three babies, a transfusion would not only contravene desires clearly expressed when she was fully competent but it would also technically be an assault. So there is more to resolution of this problem than common sense.

CASE 1: Outcome

You consult with the hospital legal department and advise them that, if the woman's life is to be saved, there is not enough time for the case to be taken to court. The lawyer advises that the woman was competent (see Table 59.3) when she made her original decision and that, in his opinion, blood cannot legally be given. You comply with this view. The bleeding cannot be halted. Mrs AB dies.

In light of the outcome was that ethically the 'right' or 'wrong' decision?

The late Professor Gordon Dunstan [5] suggested that the criteria for the practice of Ethics in Medicine are:

- Good moral theories;
- The elucidation of principles to which implicit or explicit appeal can be made;
- The discipline of logic for the framing of good arguments and the exposure of bad ones;

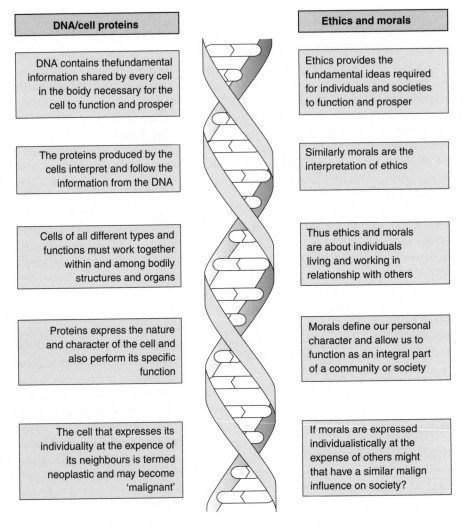

DNA/cell proteins	Ethics and morals
DNA contains thefundamental information shared by every cell in the boidy necessary for the cell to function and prosper	Ethics provides the fundamental ideas required for individuals and societies to function and prosper
The proteins produced by the cells interpret and follow the information from the DNA	Similarly morals are the interpretation of ethics
Cells of all different types and functions must work together within and among bodily structures and organs	Thus ethics and morals are about individuals living and working in relationship with others
Proteins express the nature and character of the cell and also perform its specific function	Morals define our personal character and allow us to function as an integral part of a community or society
The cell that expresses its individuality at the expence of its neighbours is termed neoplastic and may become 'malignant'	If morals are expressed individualistically at the expense of others might that have a similar malign influence on society?

Fig. 59.1 The similarities between ethics/morals and DNA/cell proteins.

- Learning the art of moral reasoning;
- Discipline in the use of words without clichés;
- And wisdom above all.

This transcends 'common sense' and the aim of this chapter is to guide you to an understanding of ethical theory to assist you in making appropriate moral judgements in clinical situations such as that of Mrs AB.

Diversity of moral theory

Dealing with uncertainty is difficult and can be stressful in both clinical medicine and, indeed, life itself. It is a defining characteristic of *Homo sapiens* that we try to make sense out of uncertainty by classification and codification of what we think we know. As a result, a multiplicity of theoretical approaches to ethics has arisen. It has been suggested [3] that the diversity of ethical theories is about as wide as that of the ways we understand the relationship between the human race and our environment. Thus, in the same way that mariners need charts as they travel across the oceans, we need frameworks as reference points to allow us to progress through our lives as individuals in society. Thus, while principles provide an indispensable general guiding direction, other features of the problem must be taken into consideration as the passage from moral question to moral answer is navigated [6].

The two most frequently referred to systematic accounts of what makes actions morally right or wrong (or 'theories of obligation') are *Deontological theories* (or 'duties in action') [7] and *Consequentialist theories* [8]. These are summarized in Tables 59.4 and 59.5. Clearly these theories are not, of themselves, sufficient for the resolution of clinical problems in real life and several other views have been developed to try to deal with their inherent problems.

Table 59.2 Some essentials of medical ethics

Ethics is for something and must be translatable into moral action
- It has to work in real life

Each one of us is required to think ethically and act morally (i.e. we are all 'moral agents')
- This is not an optional extra

Ethics is about individuals living and working in community
- It is not just about 'me' and 'mine'

Individuals not only have rights but also duties/obligations towards others

The fundamental principles underpinning medical ethics are (or should be) those of society in general

We as doctors in the UK have special obligations or duties to our patients that are clearly laid down by the General Medical Council

Clinical medicine, ethical analysis and moral action cannot be practiced in isolation from one another
- Ethics is a necessary part of good clinical practice

Reproduced from Stirrat [4]. With the permission of the Royal College of Obstetricians and Gynaecologists.

Table 59.3 Competence – a brief guide

Men and women over the age of 16 years are presumed to have the capacity (i.e. be competent) to make decisions including those involving proposed medical interventions unless this can be shown not to be so. The doctor proposing the treatment can usually assess the patient's competence. Specialist advice (e.g. from a psychiatrist) should be sought if there is any doubt or if, for example, the procedure proposed is associated with significant risks

The following is a brief guide to the criteria to be considered. Fuller information can be found in 'Further reading'

A person has the capacity to decide if she can:
- Understand when explained in simple language
  — what the medical treatment is
  — its purpose and nature and
  — why it is needed
- Understand the main benefits, risks and alternatives
- Understand in broad terms what will be the consequences of not receiving the proposed treatment
- Retain the information for long enough to make an effective decision
- Properly assess the information given
- Make her choice free from pressure by others (including yourself)

Full contemporary and signed notes should be made of all such consultations.

The *Four Principle Approach* [9] (otherwise known as 'Principlism' (*sic*)) – was formulated as a basis for working out practical solutions for problems in Medical Ethics. The four main principles and the associated obligations

Table 59.4 Deontological theories or 'Duties in Action'

Deontology derives from a Greek word meaning 'that which is obligatory'

This theory of obligation is 'backward looking' because it holds that an action is made right or wrong by a criterion prior to the action

The essence of Kant's ethics is that
- Certain kinds of acts are intrinsically right and others intrinsically wrong determined by a set of rules
- The rules must be universally applicable, coherent (i.e. not contradictory) within what Kant called 'a rational system of nature' and capable of being freely adopted by 'a community of rational beings'
- Among the rules are 'do not kill, cause pain, disable, deprive of freedom or pleasure'; and 'do not deceive, break promises, cheat, break laws or neglect one's duty'
- Each of us has a set of obligations or duties to our fellow men and women
- He set these out in a series of 'maxims' one of the most important of which is to 'act so that you treat humanity, whether in your own person or in that of any other, always as an end, and never as a means only' [7]
- An action should not be judged to have been right or wrong by its consequences in individual situations

  Kant's dismissal of consequences as totally irrelevant ('Do your duty though the heavens may fall!') has been modified to consider that consequences are one factor among many relevant to obligation

No theory is without problems and the main difficulties with Kant are defining the meaning of 'rational' and agreeing on universally applicable rules. Superficial analysis suggests that it also removes incentives to act morally. As also noted in Table 59.5 the present day use of the word 'pleasure' makes it problematic

This is based on the work of the eighteenth-century philosopher Immanuel Kant [7].

are shown in Table 59.6. We may feel much more comfortable with these because the obligations attached to the principles are familiar to us as part of our daily practice as obstetricians and gynaecologists. Perhaps because of this, they are often used uncritically and are assumed to provide an easy answer to every problem. This they neither can nor were designed to do. When specific clinical problems are considered later in the chapter we will discover that the principles can often be in conflict with one another.

The concept of autonomy requires some further consideration. Dunstan suggested that the currently dominant view of autonomy is that it confers a right to act on one's own judgment about matters affecting one's life, without interference by others [5]. There is an increasing body of thought [10–12] that this so-called individualistic version of autonomous choice is fundamentally flawed. Medical ethics, properly understood, should always be set in the

Table 59.5 Consequentialist and utilitarian theories [7]

Consequentialism is a 'forward-looking' theory of obligation in which the rightness or wrongness of an action is totally determined by the action's consequences.

• Consequentialist theories differ over what is the nature of the good consequences arising from 'right' actions (e.g. 'pleasure' or biological survival, etc.) and also against whose good rightness is to be measured. At one extreme some base it on what produces good for the individual ('egoistic'): at the other extreme the criterion is those right actions that produce good for everyone affected by it ('universalistic').

• The most popular consequentialist theory of 'universal ethical hedonism' or '*Utilitarianism*' was developed in the nineteenth century by Jeremy Bentham, John Stuart Mill and Henry Sidgwick. They argued that the maximization of pleasure or happiness was what made acts right. This has been summarized as 'the greatest happiness of the greatest number'. The word 'pleasure' is now problematic and it has been replaced by the opaque phrase 'preference satisfaction'.

• Consequentialist theories can be further divided. 'Act consequentialism' holds that the right action is the one that produces the most good. In 'rule consequentialism' the test is whether an action accords with a set of rules whose general acceptance would result in the most good.

• Many versions have become mechanistic requiring that goods and ills be measured, added and subtracted according to some agreed scale. This has proved to be unsatisfactory.

Among the problems with consequentialism are that although consequences are undoubtedly important in moral judgments and actions:

• We are rarely capable of predicting the long-term outcomes of our actions.

• Happiness is highly subjective and what is good (let alone the 'greatest good') is not always easy to determine.

• Benefiting the majority could result in ignoring vulnerable minorities.

　　— Where do the seriously disadvantaged in our society such as the very pre-term infant, the severely disabled child, the terminally ill or the elderly with dementia fit with this philosophy?

　　— A rule to protect the vulnerable could be set aside if it did not promote general happiness.

Table 59.6 The Four Principles [9]

Principle	The obligation/duty
Beneficence	To do what is in the patient's best interests To provide benefits balanced against risks
Non-maleficence	Not to cause harm and, indeed, seek to prevent it
Autonomy ('self-rule')	To respect the right of the individual to make choices about her own life in the context of equal respect for everyone else involved
Justice	To treat patients fairly and without unfair discrimination Fairness in the distribution of benefits and risks

context of relationships and community [5]. An alternative, 'principled', version of patient autonomy has been proposed that is well founded in moral philosophy and, it is suggested, fits better the optimal patient/doctor relationship [11,12]. In this model patients with the capacity to make a settled choice about medical interventions on themselves do so responsibly in a manner considerate to others having been provided with sufficient and understandable information and adequate space for reflection. Thus, *principled autonomy* implies a settled view of the individual reached by deliberation as to what is in his or her own long-term best interests. It is also to be balanced with the interests and autonomy of others, including, in this context, medical staff caring for a patient.

Unfortunately there is no such thing as a single, comprehensive theory that can be applied to all cases. Sherwin [13] finds it preferable to view different theoretical perspectives as providing a set of lenses. Thus, by using the appropriate lens, one can get a clearer view of complex moral problems. One lens will provide clearer understanding than others in any given situation. Whatever one's criticisms of the Four Principles, they can provide a useful framework for analysing ethical problems if one recognizes their shortcomings and incorporates some other 'lenses' such as:

Narrative ethics. This takes account of the patient's and the clinician's context, emotions and relationships [14,15].

Virtue ethics. Instead of asking, 'How should I act?' this asks 'How should I live?' [16]. This system tries to define 'excellences' of character or behaviour to which individuals or groups should aspire. One aspect is caring *about* someone rather than just caring *for* him or her and it can provide a useful perspective in, for example, those faced with chronic and/or serious illness or disability.

Feminist approaches to ethics. One aspect of feminist ethics considers that women have been and continue to be oppressed and that such oppression is morally and politically unacceptable [17]. Feminist ethics also attempts to balance the dominant masculine ethos of traditional ethics with a more feminine perspective. The ethics is one of caring for individuals and, although caring resolutions may be different in their outcomes, they are linked by personal regard and respect given to individuals [18].

Making ethical judgements

Medical ethics is not solely a matter of moral theory: it is 'an ethics of relation and practice' [5].

Some of the ethical issues we face can be dealt with relatively straightforwardly. Others are highly complex and may be intractable – true dilemmas. How then do we go about making ethical judgements in the clinical context?

Table 59.7 The nature of ethical judgements in medicine

Ethical judgements are integral to the clinical process	We have been making ethical decisions every day since we qualified perhaps without recognizing it!
The process must be carried out sincerely and honestly 'making the care of your patient your first concern'	Whatever method is used it must fit with the realities of the clinical setting
There is no magic formula (beware those who suggest that there is) and each case is different from any other	There is seldom an absolutely 'right' or 'wrong' decision. One is often trying to balance the greater good or the lesser evil!
This does NOT mean that ethical decision making is arbitrary	Although some decisions must be reached quickly, the process of decision making should be no less rigorous
Criteria for rigorous ethical reasoning [20]	
Clarity	Terms and concepts must have precise meaning
Consistency	Those terms must always be used with that precise meaning: reasoning must be free of contradiction
Coherence	Ethical deliberations must be internally consistent
Applicability	The process results in comprehensive and clinically relevant judgements
Adequacy	These judgements allow ethical conflicts to be identified, managed or, preferably, prevented

Reproduced from Stirrat [4]. With the permission of the Royal College of Obstetricians and Gynaecologists.

Table 59.8 Making ethical judgements – 1: analysis

Define the problem(s)

Analyse the problem(s)

What are its elements? – e.g. medical, ethical, legal etc.

What parties are involved? – the patient, her family, statutory authorities (e.g. social workers, police), health-care professionals etc.

How do their perspectives fit together or conflict and, if the latter, what are the appropriate mechanisms for resolution?

What is its context? – e.g. social, economic (within this may be issues about 'rationing')

Consider the underlying principles involved

It may be useful to start with the 'Four Principles' (see Table 59.6)

- What is in the patient's best interests?
- How can I balance this with the avoidance of harm?
- Is the patient competent? If so:
  — Is she expressing her 'settled' view on what she wants?
  — Am I respecting her right to make choices about her own life?
  — Does this conflict with the autonomy of others and, if so, how is this to be resolved?
- If she is not competent (e.g. a minor or an unconscious adult) or if this is open to question (e.g. a child aged 12–13) how is this to be dealt with?
- Are there any issues of justice? e.g.
  — Is the patient being unfairly discriminated against?
  — Is there any conflict between what I consider to be in the patient's best interest and what can be provided in the NHS?

What other perspectives could assist in resolution?

- Have the patient's social context, emotions and relationships been adequately considered?
- Am I sure that I am treating the patient as a person?
- Are we both 'caring for' and 'caring about' the patient?

Reproduced from Stirrat GM [4]. With the permission of the Royal College of Obstetricians and Gynaecologists.

Some necessary characteristics of ethical judgements and the guiding criteria for rigorous ethical analysis are shown in Table 59.7 [4]. A practical mechanism for moving from ethical analysis to clinical action is shown in Tables 59.8 and 59.9 [4]. It must, however, be emphasized that this is not a mathematical exercise in which 'plusses' and 'minuses' can determine the correct decision. Each problem must be dealt with in its context and with empathy for all involved. The establishment of clinical ethics committees by some hospital has helped both in dealing with

Table 59.9 Making ethical judgements – 2: action

Move towards recommending actions that best meet the above criteria
  What are the proposed objectives? e.g. cure, relief of symptoms (e.g. pain and suffering) or prevention of disease?
  • Which objectives are essential and which desirable?
  • What alternatives are available (including doing nothing)?
  • What are the risks of acting (or failing to act) and what is their probability and severity?
  • Do the expected benefits outweigh the potential risks?
      — Has the patient been properly informed of the available options?
  • Is she competent to give consent?
      — If so, has the consent been obtained properly?
      — *If yes, put chosen option into effect*
      — If she is not competent who, if anyone, can legally give consent?

Dealing with potential or actual conflict:
This difficult area cannot be dealt with comprehensively here but examples include
  The patient refuses to accept the recommended interventions
  • If competent, she has the right to do so even if it leads to harm of herself (or unborn child). *Do not coerce her.* Among the things to do are:
      — If junior, inform more senior colleagues: if senior, seek advice through clinical governance channels
      — Make sure that full contemporaneous notes are made
She requests intervention that informed medical opinion suggests is not justified or in her best interests
  • You are not bound to do as she asks particularly if it is contrary to your principles
  • Offer referral for another opinion or, if needs be, transfer care to another team. (If the patient is requesting TOP you are obliged to refer to another practitioner)
  • (And then as above)
Another party tries to intervene inappropriately, e.g.
  • A member of the family tries to influence the patient in her decision making contrary to the former's autonomous choice
  • The family or another third party asks for confidential information
      — The presumption is that confidentiality must be kept (see Table 59.11).
      — Any breach can only be justified in 'exceptional circumstances'
          • It is preferable that this be with the knowledge of the patient
          • However, if, for example, it is judged that the patient would be seriously harmed by knowing that her illness is terminal but that it would be in her best interests that a close relative should know about it, information may be divulged without consent. Do not make this decision without appropriate consultation
  • The family asks that the patient be not told the truth of her illness
      — The assumption (possibly rebuttable with good grounds – see example above) must be to tell the truth at all times
      — Not to do so can have regrettable consequences, e.g. who is she to trust when she discovers any deception?
      — Remember that your primary duty of care is to your patient and not her family
Good communication skills in general and knowing how to impart bad news in particular are central to being a good doctor

Review the outcome
  Ethical issues do not lend themselves easily to audit but it may be useful to record and review major cases from time to time
  In individual cases remember that a good or bad outcome does not necessarily mean that the intervention was 'right' or 'wrong'

Reproduced from Stirrat [4]. With the permission of the Royal College of Obstetricians and Gynaecologists.

particularly difficult problems (e.g. end of life decisions) and the development of guidelines for good practice in dealing with them.

The impact of law on ethics

Chapter 60 describes current legislation as it affects the practice of obstetrics and gynaecology and tries to predict what further developments might be expected in the future particularly in the context of human rights legislation. What then is the relationship between ethics and the law? We have already noted that ethics is to do with moral judgement; the law, however, concerns public policy. At one level it defines what one can/cannot or must/must not do to avoid risk of legal penalty: for example, practitioners must at all times comply with the law on induced abortion. The usage of the words 'should' and 'ought' in a legal context implies an obligation that can be enforced by law. We have already noted that when used in an ethical sense they imply 'duty' – a moral action that is not necessarily prescribed or proscribed in law. For example, failure to tell a patient the truth about her condition may not be illegal but, in most instances, it is unethical. Thus ethics encompasses much more than the law. Ethics can help determine what is 'right' in the sense that it is 'good': the intention of the law is to define what is 'right' in the sense that it is or is not permitted. We can, therefore, conclude that not only is 'determining that something is unethical neither a necessary nor a sufficient reason to make it illegal' [21] but also that determining that something is lawful does not necessarily make it good ethics. In practice there are many occasions in which the law assists clinical decision making (see, for example, 'Contraception', below) by setting parameters that help both the patient and the clinician.

Specific issues in obstetrics and gynaecology

'Reproduction differs from many other areas of medical practice because of its complexity and because tension can sometimes arise between the rights of women to make decisions about their own bodies and the moral duties owed to unborn children' [22]. We have already alluded to the diversity of moral theory in general let alone in public opinion on issues in reproductive issues. It is, therefore, perhaps not surprising that some of the issues that obstetricians and gynaecologists face 'can never be resolved to the satisfaction of all sections of society but will be the subject of continuing ethical debate' [22]. Table 59.10 outlines some of the general principles relevant to the issues about to be discussed that have been derived from the Handbook of Ethics and Law [22].

Table 59.10 General principles that apply to reproductive ethics [22]

The confidentiality of all patients, including those aged under 16, should be respected except in exceptional cases

Young people who are sufficiently mature to understand the nature and implications of the treatment requested are able to give valid consent, but parental involvement should be encouraged

No treatment may be provided to a competent adult without valid consent

Adults are presumed to be competent unless there is clear evidence to the contrary. (Being in labour does not, in itself, render a woman incompetent to make decisions)

Women should be encouraged to participate to the greatest possible extent in decisions about their pregnancy

A woman who plans to carry her fetus to term has special moral responsibilities towards the unborn child, but neither health professionals nor society can force her to fulfil those duties

Discussion about reproduction inevitably focuses primarily on women, but the role of men should not be undermined

Contraception and sexual health are the responsibility of both sexes

Is there a 'right' to procreate?

To address this, one must consider the difference between a negative right (or liberty) and a positive right. The former involves not being prevented from procreating by, for example, forced sterilization. Thus Article 12 of the European Convention on Human Rights [24] states, 'Men and women of marriageable age have the right to marry and found a family according to the national laws governing the exercise of this right'. This is a liberty or negative right. But does Article 12 describe a positive right that places a corresponding obligation on health services or the State to fulfil this right in, for example, those who find themselves unable to have children without assistance? Warnock [25] concludes that procreation is neither a fundamental right nor a universal need generating a right. In addition, courts in the UK have, up to the time of writing, consistently decided that no such legal obligation exists.

Consideration of a series of topics that pose ethical dilemmas across the broad range of our specialty follows. They are intentionally not comprehensive but are meant to both indicate the nature of the issues they raise and also provide guides to their resolution. Resolution of the problems should be assisted by reference to Tables 59.8 and 59.9. Most of the topics are illustrated by hypothetical cases for consideration. The suggested resolutions are not necessarily the only ethical outcomes and further reflection and, perhaps, discussion with colleagues is encouraged.

Contraception

CASE 2: Contraception for BC, a girl aged under 16

You are working in a Family Planning Clinic. A 14-year-old girl consults you to request oral contraception. She is already in an active sexual relationship with an 18-year-old man. She wants to keep her parents from knowing about this consultation and she does not wish her general practitioner (GP) to know either because 'I don't trust him not to tell my parents.'

What ethical considerations influence your clinical decision?

The three main issues here are competence (see Table 59.3), confidentiality (see Table 59.11) and 'best interests'. In a legal judgement made in 1985 [26] it was determined that a patient, though a minor, is deemed competent if the doctor involved decides, after careful consideration, that she has maturity to understand the nature of the consultation and of the treatment proposed. That being so her autonomy and confidentiality should be respected. The doctor should, of course, try to persuade the patient to agree to parental involvement but, if she

Table 59.11 Confidentiality [1, 23]

Confidentiality is the basis of trust between doctor and patient

The GMC [1] states 'Patients have a right to expect that you will not disclose any personal information which you learn during the course of your professional duties, unless they give permission.'

Breaches of confidentiality can lead to:
- Breakdown of the patient–doctor relationship
- Lack of confidence and trust in other doctors
- Failure by patient to seek future medical treatment as a result of which their health may suffer
- Disciplinary action by the GMC
- Civil action for compensation

Confidentiality may be breached in exceptional circumstances but only when that can be justified and preferably with the patient's knowledge
- Requests to disclose patient information to the media must be treated with the greatest care and the usual rules of confidentiality apply. Advice should be sought from hospital legal services departments
- Confidential information should not be disclosed over the telephone without the express consent of the patient. The person to whom you are speaking may not be who he or she claims to be!

Disclosure of confidential information in the 'public interest'

Occasionally disclosure is 'essential to prevent or lessen a serious and imminent threat to public health or the life or health of another individual' [23]
The BMA [23] advise that, when considering; disclosing information to protect the public interest, doctors must:
- Consider how the benefits of making the disclosure balance against the harms associated with breaching a patient's confidentiality
- Assess the urgency of the need for disclosure
- Consider whether the person could be persuaded to disclose voluntarily
- Inform the person before making the disclosure and seek his or her consent, unless to do so would enhance the risk of harm
- Reveal only the minimum information necessary to achieve the objective
- Seek assurances that the information will be used only for the purpose for which it was disclosed
- *Be able to justify the decision*

In addition full contemporary notes must be made

Advice on all of these issues can be sought from medical defence organizations and professional or regulatory authorities (e.g. the GMC)

---

refuses, there is a duty to maintain the confidentiality of the consultation.

The Fraser Guidelines (named after one of the judges in the case) derive from the above case. These state [22]:

'Before providing contraception to young people, health professionals must:
- Consider whether the patient understands the potential risks and benefits of the treatment
- Consider whether the patient understands the advice given
- Discuss with the patient the value of parental support (Doctors must encourage young people to inform parents of the consultation and explore the reasons if the patient is unwilling to do so. It is important for persons aged under 16 who are seeking contraceptive advice to be aware that, although the doctor is obliged to discuss the value of parental support, he or she will respect their confidentiality)
- Take into account whether the patient is likely to have sexual intercourse without contraception

- Assess whether the patient's physical and/or mental health are likely to suffer if the patient does not receive contraceptive advice or treatment
- Consider whether the patient's best interests would require the provision of contraceptive advice or treatment or both without parental consent'.

The British Medical Association (BMA) Handbook [22] advises that, 'even if the doctor is unwilling to supply contraception on the grounds of the patient's immaturity, he or she still maintains a general duty of confidentiality (see Table 59.11) unless there are exceptional reasons for disclosing information without consent. Such reasons could occur when, for example, the request for contraception arises in the context of sexual exploitation, incest, or other sexual abuse. In such exceptional cases the doctor has a duty to protect the patient and this may eventually involve a breach of confidentiality, although with counselling and support the patient may feel able to agree to disclosure. Nevertheless, it is important that doctors avoid making completely unconditional promises about secrecy to individual young people, while at the same time making it clear that confidentiality as a general principle extends to all consultations' [27,28].

CASE 2: Outcome

You decide that the benefits of prescribing an oral contraceptive pill outweigh the risks for BC. You strongly advise that she discuss it with her parents but she refuses. You also request that you be allowed to inform her GP and you give her your reasons for doing so. She also refuses. You comply with both wishes and arrange to see her again in 6 weeks with the long-term objective of maintaining a good clinical relationship with her. You consider that, in this case, your pledge of confidentiality outweighs any responsibility to inform the police about BC being involved in under-age sexual intercourse.

Sterilization

CASE 3: Sterilization of women with learning difficulties

A GP refers CS, a 26-year-old woman with severe learning difficulties, to your gynaecological clinic for consideration of sterilization. A formal assessment of her competence has been performed and she has the mental capacity of a 5-year-old child. She also has an atrial septal defect (ASD).

Her widowed mother, who is incapacitated because of severe rheumatoid arthritis, attends the clinic with her. CS is currently living at home but on weekdays attends a day centre for people with learning difficulties. She has a social worker assigned to her there. CS is very friendly and naïve but she is also sexually aware. She has already had sexual advances from young men with similar learning difficulties in the day centre. Although her mother does not wish to deprive her of 'intimate relationships', she is, for several understandable reasons, 'terrified' that CS might become pregnant. CS's menstrual cycle is very erratic and the bleeding is quite heavy. She also becomes so agitated during her menses (including smearing the walls of the house with blood) that her mother finds it impossible to cope. The mother thinks that sterilization will stop her periods and, thus, would solve both problems.

The GP has already tried to prescribe a combined oral contraceptive pill but CS would not take them. He also suggested using a long-acting depot for contraception and menstrual regulation but, despite several attempts, she would not allow the nurse or doctor to give her the injection.

Consider how you would proceed and what ethical/legal considerations would influence your clinical decision.

The first principle to be considered is that people with learning difficulties should be encouraged to make decisions for themselves, the implications of which they broadly understand and with which they are happy. In this context let us assume that you discover that she is incapable of understanding what you are saying even when expressed as simply as possible.

People with learning disabilities are also considered to have the right to enjoy sexual relationships in private and, in this case CS's mother does not wish to deprive her daughter of this. The first clinical problem to consider, therefore, is that of contraception. Therefore, the second principle to be considered is 'contraceptive services for people with learning difficulties should not impede the exercise of autonomy more drastically than is essential to protect against an unwanted pregnancy' [22]. Given the previous experience of the referring GP, your room for manoeuvre is limited. An intrauterine device is not thought clinically appropriate because of the difficulties with fitting and the problems associated with menstruation.

You therefore proceed to discuss tubal occlusion. Sterilization of women (or men) who lack the capacity to give valid consent is controversial. The case of Re F in 1989 [29] set out the legal conditions to be filled in the medical treatment of adults who are unable to consent for themselves. It confirmed that the courts cannot, in fact, give consent on behalf of an adult and that, in all cases any proposed treatment must be in the patient's 'best interest'. This means that the treatment must be:

• Necessary to save the life of the person; or either ensure improvement/prevent deterioration in her physical or mental health and
• 'In accordance with a practice accepted at the time by a responsible body of medical opinion skilled in the particular form of treatment in question'.

Unless carried out for 'therapeutic reasons' such interventions must not be performed without applying for permission from the court. This is because of the intention to deprive the person permanently of the right to bear a child contravenes Article 12 of the European Convention on Human Rights ([24] and see Chapter 60).

In the case of CS you would, for example:

• Explain to her mother all of the aspects of the procedure as in any other case including, of course, the small failure rate and the fact that it will not make the menstrual problems any easier;
• Consider whether any proposed intervention was clearly in her best interests with the benefit clearly outweighing any risk;
• Consider whether you would be acting more in the interests of her mother and other carers than of CS.

CASE 3: Outcome

- The consultation ends there because you need to consult with the hospital legal department; seek further information from CS's GP and social worker (including any perceived added risk of CS being exposed to sexual abuse following sterilization); and consider any additional peri-operative risks as a result of her general condition and ASD.
- The result of the assessment is that:
  — It is deemed that sterilization would be in CS's best interests.
  — Her GP confirms that menstruation causes CS such distress that it would also be clearly in her best interests not to have menses.
  — The social worker states that, in her opinion, there would be no added risk of sexual abuse.
  — The anaesthetist considers that laparoscopy is contraindicated.
- Application is made to the court and, following careful consideration, you are permitted to perform such interventions as you consider to be in CS's best interests.
- In light of the above you see CS and her mother again and discuss the option of performing a subtotal hysterectomy.
- Subtotal hysterectomy is subsequently performed uneventfully.

In your opinion was this procedure ethically justified?

Moral status of the human embryo and fetus

It is necessary to provide a brief guide to this important matter prior to considering further specific issues in reproductive ethics. It is not possible to consider in full the different views, often firmly held and vehemently defended (the 'Further reading' and 'Reference' lists provide the sources for more detailed study). An additional level of complexity is often provided by the question of the moral status of the embryo/fetus being posed as 'when do persons come into existence?' Unfortunately the use of the word 'person' by those arguing for their viewpoint tends to support Humpty Dumpty's statement 'When I use a word it means just what I choose it to mean – neither more nor less' [30]. Although exploration of what is meant by a person is not insignificant, the emphasis in this section focuses more on moral status per se. It also asks 'How ought we to treat the embryo/fetus?' or 'When is the embryo/fetus to be regarded as a patient?' [31]. The main philosophical positions on the questions of if and when the conceptus achieves significant or full moral status can be summarized as follows:

1 The conceptus has full moral status from the time of fertilization.

2 Full moral status is gained at one of several points during development or at birth.

3 Moral status gradually increases throughout pregnancy.

THE CONCEPTUS HAS FULL MORAL STATUS FROM THE TIME OF FERTILIZATION

One of the defining characteristics of full moral status is that it confers on the individual a right to life. In the view expressed above moral status derives from the fact that the conceptus is fully (and never anything other) than human from fertilization. Finnis [32], one of the most cogent exponents of this position, argues, 'On all biologically and philosophically pertinent criteria (fertilisation) marks substantial change and no subsequent development or event can be identified plausibly as a genuine substantial change'. One consequence of this view is that from fertilization the embryo must be treated as one would a mature human. Finnis [32] recognizes that 'our imagination balks at equating the intelligent adult with a one-cell zygote'. He argues, 'reason can find no event or principle or criterion by which to judge that the typical adult or newborn child or full-term or mid-term unborn child is anything other than one and the same individual human being as the one-cell, 46 chromosome zygote whose emergence was the beginning of the personal history of that same child and adult. In short, science and philosophy concur in the conclusion: every living human individual must be regarded as a person' (i.e. with full moral status). Iglesias [33] distinguishes between development *into* a person and development *of* a person believing that there is no stage of the pregnancy when the conceptus/fetus is not a person. She too concludes that, even at the earliest stage in development, they should be accorded absolute respect. Given the premise that biological continuity is to be seen as the same as personal identity, the argument may be consistent but, despite Finnis's [32] appeal to reason, it inevitably causes unreasonable moral dilemmas in the real clinical world. Consider the following cases.

CASE 4: Ectopic pregnancy

Mrs FW, a 40-year-old nulliparous woman presents to the early pregnancy unit with 8 weeks' amenorrhoea, left-sided lower abdominal pain, and slight vaginal bleeding. She is desperately anxious to have a child having been trying for 10 years. She is a devout Roman Catholic. A strong clinical suspicion of a left tubal ectopic pregnancy is confirmed. A beating heart is seen in the embryo.

You recommend that laparoscopy be undertaken to remove the ectopic pregnancy. You also explain to her the risks (including those to her life) if, as could well occur, the tube ruptures. You recommend that, in her best interests,

Table 59.12 The principle of double effect

This applies when the primary intention of one's actions is to produce a good effect but that this also contributes to or brings about a secondary unintended bad effect
The principle permits one to perform such acts if the bad effect is:
  Truly unintended,
  Not disproportionate to the intended good effect, and
  Unavoidable if the good effect is to be achieved

laparoscopy be carried out immediately. She asks about the chances of the pregnancy continuing to viability and you explain that they are infinitesimally small. Despite this she remains concerned that this would be seen as killing the embryo.

According to the conservative position described on p. 668 Mrs FW and the living embryo have equal moral status. However remote the possibility of a good outcome would be, the embryo would have to be given a chance of life and laparoscopy could not be morally justified at this time. In fact most who hold that conservative position would allow the laparoscopy to take place in the mother's interests. This scenario cannot properly be justified by the 'principle of double effect' (see Table 59.12). The only possible rational reason is that, while holding that the embryo has moral worth, the value of the life of the mother takes precedence over that of the early embryo.

Let us consider another scenario that has been adapted from Strong [34].

CASE 5

You are walking past the Reproductive Medicine laboratory in your hospital and notice smoke coming through the open door. In the laboratory there is a container that holds fifty embryos intended for transfer to the maternal uterus at some time in the future. You raise the alarm and go in to be immediately faced with smoke and flames. You first notice the container that holds the embryos but you also see a technician, who has been overcome by the smoke, lying unconscious on the floor. Both the container and the technician are close to being engulfed in the flames. You must choose between saving the technician or the embryos but cannot do both. Which would you choose to save?

Surely the only morally correct choice is to save the technician? However, if one held that the embryos and the technician had equal moral status then one would be driven to the inescapable conclusion that it would be better to save 50 embryos than one technician.

Do the intuitive moral responses to Cases 4 and 5 not suggest that, when a choice has to be made between them, the life of the mother and the technician respectively have

greater moral worth than that of the early embryo? This is discussed further later when the issue of potentiality is considered.

SIGNIFICANT MORAL STATUS IS GAINED AT ONE OF SEVERAL POINTS DURING DEVELOPMENT OR AT BIRTH

It has been suggested that moral status depends on the acquisition of *sentience* defined as the capacity for feeling and perception. Singer [35], for example, considers that the conceptus is a 'thing' with no moral rights until the onset of brain function. Unfortunately any decision about when this occurs can only be arbitrary. The range of suggestions for the onset of brain development sufficient for sentience ranges from 6 to 28 weeks' gestation [36]! Strong [33] considers that sentience is a necessary but not sufficient defining characteristic of personhood.

The capacity for *self-consciousness* is a more demanding standard for full moral status. In this view, expounded for example by Tooley [37] and Singer [35] and see 'Further reading', full moral status depends on the being having the recognizable ability to reflect on what it is to be himself or herself. Thus, since according to the stated definition the embryo/fetus are not, 'self-conscious', they cannot have full moral status. Singer [35] suggests that we should 'accord the life of the fetus no greater value than the life of a non-human animal at a similar level of rationality, self-consciousness, awareness, capacity to feel, etc'. He goes on to describe an inescapable consequence of this view; namely that, since an infant is not, in his terms, a rational and self-conscious being, 'if the fetus does not have the same claim to life as a person it appears that the newborn baby does not either'. According to this argument, since patients with severe dementia or in a persistent vegetative state have lost self-consciousness, they must also have lost all moral worth. It is here that the law backs up the moral consensus of our society that infants, elderly people with dementia and patients in a persistent vegetative state (legal cases relating to patients in a persistent vegetative state have been determined on the best interests of the patient and not on whether he or she still had moral and legal status as a person) have full moral interests that demand protection. Thus the argument for self-consciousness as the defining criterion for full moral status inevitably fails.

This argument focuses one's mind on some important issues. For example, it is universally agreed that everyone who is self-conscious has full moral standing because of that capacity. However, the clear acceptance of moral status of infants shows that one does not have to be self-conscious to have moral standing [34]. Second, if one accepts that the infant has such standing what can the morally significant difference be between it and itself as a fetus a few days or even weeks before birth?

Birth, of course, marks a categorical dividing line in the life of the viable fetus/infant and is the legally defining moment for personhood. However, Singer [35], in questioning birth as the moral defining point at which a right to life is gained, points out that 'the fetus/baby is the same entity, whether inside or outside the womb, with the same human features (whether we can see them or not) and the same degree of awareness and capacity for feeling pain'. Given that a pre-term infant born at, say, 28 weeks is less well developed than the 34 weeks fetus it cannot be logical to give the latter greater moral status and, therefore, much more protection than the former. As Singer argues, the location of a being – inside or outside the womb – should not define his or her right to life.

Potential viability has also been suggested as the time when the fetus acquires full moral status. It, at least, resolves the issue of the suggested moral difference between the fetus before and the infant after birth. Although the capacity for at least some degree of independent existence is technology dependent, it is the point at which obstetricians generally accept that the fetus is to be regarded as a patient and tends to put it into a different category from the pre-viable fetus. Viability is not, however, an absolute criterion for the fetus as a patient as shown by interventions that treat pre-viable fetuses (e.g. intrauterine transfusion for Rhesus haemolytic disease and an increasing ability to carry out surgery on some pre-viable fetuses). Thus, like self-consciousness, viability may be a significant criterion for full moral standing but the fetus does not have to be viable to have moral standing.

MORAL STATUS GRADUALLY INCREASES THROUGHOUT PREGNANCY

This viewpoint has been well expressed by Campbell *et al.* [36]. It, they say, recognizes the fact of the continuum of biological development, and does not draw arbitrary lines to denote the acquisition of full moral status with all of the flaws associated with them noted above. They suggest, 'There is no point in development, regardless of how early, when the embryo or foetus fails to display the potential for personhood – no matter how rudimentary. This bestows upon the conceptus and the fetus some claim to life and respect. This claim, however, becomes stronger as development proceeds, so that by some time in the third trimester the claim is so strong that the consequences of killing a foetus may be the same as those of killing an actual person – whether child or adult. Consequently, the fetus in the last trimester should be treated as a 'patient'. This reflects most people's responses in ordinary life, where we recognize a difference between the accidental loss of an

embryo or early foetus and the birth of a stillborn child' [36]. They realize that this 'potential person position' satisfies neither the conservative view because it is too liberal nor the liberal view because it is too conservative. However, they consider that 'its gradualist emphasis strikes a chord with many people, on biological, philosophical, intuitive, and pragmatic grounds'. It also can act as a guide for tackling the specific ethical issues raised in this chapter.

Induced abortion and pregnancy reduction

Induced abortion is one of the most polarized and divisive ethical issues that we face. It is as though there are two armies in conflict: each carries a banner, one labelled 'pro-life' and the other 'pro-choice'. Neither is willing to listen to the other, so convinced are they of the absolute correctness of their own position. Thus 'the vast complexity of the moral discourse is whittled down to a simple decision – either an absolute stance in favour of the unborn or an absolute stance in favour of the mother's right to self-determination' [36]. Both arguments are simplistic and such polarization can never be the basis for good clinical practice. All doctors have both a duty of care towards their patients and also responsibilities towards colleagues who have different and sincerely held value systems. The BMA Handbook of Ethics and Law [22] has set down the main arguments relating to those positions and also that of the middle ground. The ethical principles underpinning them have been outlined in Moral Status of the human embryo and fetus, (see p. 668) and the intention of this section is to attempt to navigate a way through the minefield by providing a framework with which most if not all readers can agree. What are the specific ethical factors that need to be taken into account in considering the ethics of requests for termination of pregnancy? The first principle is that all must work within the confines of the law (see Chapter 60). Campbell *et al.* [35] suggest that among the other factors are the wishes of the pregnant woman, the ethical demands made on us by the fetus, the stage of fetal development and the conflicting ethical assessments of abortion within society.

ETHICS AND THE LAW ON INDUCED ABORTION

There are several things that need to be noted about the law in this context. First, the law tells one what is permitted; not necessarily what is the good or best thing to do. Indeed, one is usually trying to determine the lesser of two evils in each tragic case. Second, although the law does not provide a comprehensive ethical position on any subject let alone induced abortion (see 'The impact of law on ethics', p. 664), it undoubtedly influences public opinion. Without any real change in the ethical arguments for or against induced abortion, the 1967 Abortion Act in the UK led to it becoming more socially acceptable although serious conflicting ethical assessments of abortion remain within society. Third, the law is open to interpretation and this process must be undertaken with ethical integrity. For example, termination on the grounds of fetal sex alone is not included within the current abortion legislation in Great Britain and the British Medical Association [22] advise that termination of pregnancy on the grounds of fetal sex alone (save in cases of severe sex-linked disorders) is normally unethical and unlawful.

Let us now consider the example of a request for termination of pregnancy after 24 weeks in Great Britain under the Abortion Act (1990). One ground on which this is permitted is if there is 'a substantial risk that if the child were born it would suffer from such physical or mental abnormalities as to be seriously handicapped': but what do 'substantial risk' and 'seriously handicapped' mean? Neither is defined in the Abortion Act. Consider the following example.

CASE 6

You request an ultrasound scan for assessment of fetal growth on Ms BN who is 34 weeks pregnant. This shows an appropriately grown fetus but detects a left-sided talipes. All other assessments (including an amniocentesis for fetal karyotype) are normal.

You reassure BN about the likely good outcome for an isolated 'club foot'. Despite this she requests termination of pregnancy on the grounds that she and her partner consider a club foot to be a 'serious handicap' and that, if surgery is required, it will cause her child to suffer; and, also, you cannot guarantee that there is nothing else wrong with her baby.

The word substantial means of real significance, important, sizeable, fairly large, real, or having substance [38]. Thus, since the talipes was clearly evident, it is real. What then is 'a serious handicap?' Although the meaning has not, at the time of writing, been decided by case law, practical guidance from the RCOG [39] suggests some criteria for the assessment of the seriousness of a handicap that must be considered. They are shown in Table 59.13.

Application of the best available criteria therefore suggest in this hypothetical case that termination of the pregnancy would be both morally wrong and illegal and should not be performed whatever the wishes of the pregnant woman.

Such cases arise rarely but when they do it would be wise to consult with senior colleagues and with the legal department in your hospital. Full note keeping is also mandatory.

THE WISHES OF THE PREGNANT WOMAN

The importance of the principle of autonomy has been discussed in 'Diversity of moral theory' (see p. 660) where it was defined as a settled view of the individual reached by deliberation as to what is in his or her own long-term best interests balanced with the interests and autonomy of others. In this context the relevant interests are those of the embryo/fetus. What should happen if a third party tries to influence a woman to have a termination of pregnancy? Consider the following case.

CASE 7

KM, a 23-year-old unmarried woman, attends an antenatal clinic at 16 weeks in her first pregnancy. A midwife asks her 'do you want the test to see if your baby is normal'? On that basis alone she has a combined test carried out. The result suggests a greater than expected risk of Down syndrome and she is referred to a fetal medicine specialist. After appropriate counselling she says that 'she wishes to know the answer one way or another' but 'she doesn't agree with abortion'. She is found to be carrying a fetus with Down syndrome and a congenital cardiac defect. Despite this KM states that she does not wish to have a termination of pregnancy. Her mother tries to persuade her to do so because she does not think that KM could cope with 'a handicapped baby' with the result that she, the mother, would have to carry the burden. She also thinks that KM is being irresponsible in 'bringing such a baby into the world'. KM is referred back to your clinic with a view to her having an induced abortion. In discussion it is clear that KM's views have not actually changed but she is afraid that her mother will not give her the support that she badly needs. What should you do?

The first point in this hypothetical case is that it could probably have been avoided if proper counselling had been carried out before the combined test was carried out. However, as we shall find again later, one has to deal with the situation as it is, not as it might have been. Let us assume that you agree with KM's mother that termination of pregnancy is the 'correct decision' for her to make. It would be unethical and unlawful for you to try to coerce her. You must, therefore, not only support her decision to continue with the pregnancy but also work to ensure that she has support following the birth of the baby (e.g. by referral to a social worker).

What, however, of the autonomy of the woman who attends requesting termination of pregnancy? If you have willingly accepted the responsibility of being involved in counselling or contributing to such a service for your patients, the only ethically consistent approach is to make it clear to the woman from the very beginning that, if her request falls within the terms of the Abortion Act, she will

Table 59.13 Assessment of seriousness of a 'handicap'

RCOG criteria [39]	Possible comments re. case of BN
The probability of effective treatment either *in utero* or after birth	This was clearly available after birth in this case
The child's probable degree of self-awareness and of ability to communicate with others	Neither of these should be impaired
The suffering that would be experienced (both by the child when born or by the people caring for the child)	The child would undoubtedly experience some physical pain if surgery were required. She may also be teased by other children if there was any residual problem with her foot. Does the severity of either of these mean that it would be preferable if she were born dead? Would any parental suffering be of such a different order to warrant termination?
The extent to which actions essential for health that normal individuals perform unaided would have to be provided by others	Not relevant in this case
The probability of being able to live alone and to be self-supporting as an adult	Unimpaired

be the one who decides whether or not to proceed. Respect for her autonomy does not necessarily mean that you need to agree with her choice.

THE ETHICAL DEMANDS MADE ON US BY THE FETUS AND THE STAGE OF FETAL DEVELOPMENT

Mature reflection surely suggests 'abortion demands serious ethical assessment of the situation of both woman and fetus' [36]. Campbell *et al.* [36] argue that the degree of protection afforded to the fetus should increase as pregnancy progresses and this fits with the view, considered above, that moral status gradually increases throughout pregnancy. Thus, a 28-week fetus merits significantly greater protection than a 3-day-old embryo. There will be occasions on which when the interests of the mother and the fetus will conflict and 'criteria have to be formulated for taking seriously the welfare of both' [36], any irresolvable conflict of interests should, they argue, be settled in favour of the mother.

Let us now reconsider Case 6 with one significant difference – the talipes has been discovered at 20 weeks. What difference would this make to the decision and on what grounds? In practice, BN's request at 20 weeks is much more likely to result in the pregnancy being terminated. This cannot be on the grounds of risk to the life of the woman nor have the criteria about substantial risk of serious handicap changed in any way. It would have to be on the basis that 'the continuance of the pregnancy would involve risk, greater than if the pregnancy were terminated, of injury to the physical or mental health of the pregnant woman'. Whether it can be ethically justified or not, this clause is currently liberally interpreted particularly in the context of first trimester induced abortions.

Based on what we have considered above, I leave you to reflect on what the morally significant difference between the fetus may be at 20 compared with 34 weeks' gestation in this case.

SELECTIVE REDUCTION OF MULTIPLE PREGNANCY

This procedure involves the killing of one or more fetuses *in utero* to provide the remaining fetus or fetuses with a greater chance of a better outcome. The same legal considerations apply as to the termination of a singleton pregnancy. The commonest indication is in high-order multiple pregnancies (triplets and greater) that are known to be associated with a greatly increased risk of perinatal death or severe handicap. Thus one or more fetus must die in the interests of the survivor(s). This is an ethical dilemma that can only be resolved pragmatically usually by making a random choice however unsatisfactory that may seem. It would normally be unethical to select on the basis of fetal sex alone (save in cases of sex-linked disorders) [22]. Consider the following hypothetical case.

CASE 8

Miss TD, aged 22, was born with a serious congenital cardiac defect that required surgical correction. She has no insight into the severity of her condition and her current cardiac status is poor partly because of her failure to comply with medical advice or take necessary medication. She has no contact with her family.

TD has been desperately trying to become pregnant for the past 3 years and has been found to have bilateral tubal occlusion due to chronic pelvic inflammatory disease. She has sought *in vitro* fertilization (IVF) from several centres because she considers that 'she has a right to have a child' but this has been refused partly because of her cardiac status. However, one centre agrees to carry out IVF and three embryos are transferred (for the purposes of this case it is assumed it took place when transfer of three embryos was an acceptable practice). All three embryos implant.

She is referred to your antenatal clinic at 14 weeks with a triplet pregnancy and on the verge of cardiac failure. What should you do?

This scenario is set out to show, once more, that one has to deal with the clinical situation as it is, not as it might or even should have been. You are faced with several dilemmas in this case. In your opinion, backed by that of a cardiologist with a special interest in congenital cardiac disease, her medical condition is such that even a single-ton pregnancy will be hazardous and continuation of a triplet pregnancy has a significant risk of maternal death and a poor chance of good fetal outcomes. You wish to act in TD's best interests.

CASE 8: (*contd*)
The cardiologist and yourself discuss at great length with her the risks associated with triplet pregnancy to her and the fetuses. You raise the possibility of selective reduction to a singleton fetus. The potential benefits and risks of this are fully discussed. She refuses to consider it. At 18 weeks she is admitted with cardiac failure and for the first time she fully realizes the seriousness of her condition. Following treatment her cardiac status is improved and she agrees to selective reduction. You perform this at 20 weeks. Unfortunately her membranes subsequently rupture and she develops chorio-amnionitis. As a result of this she miscarries and develops septicaemia for which admission to ITU is necessary. Her condition is critical for several days but she survives albeit with further deterioration in her pre-pregnancy cardiac status. Contact is lost with her once she is discharged from hospital.

If you were to be faced with such a case, the tragic outcome would understandably make you question the correctness of your advice. We have already noted in Table 59.8 that a bad outcome in individual cases does not necessarily mean that the intervention was 'wrong'. Given that you acted in what was felt by yourself and colleagues to be the clear best interests of both TD and the randomly selected surviving fetus, selective reduction was ethically justified. It would be wise to subject the whole case to detailed review particularly in relation to the technique used for selective reduction. The IVF clinic should also be fully informed of the outcome. This is discussed again later.

CONSCIENTIOUS OBJECTION TO INDUCED ABORTION

Doctors are legally permitted to refuse to participate in termination of pregnancy services but should they see a woman requesting termination of pregnancy they must enable her to see another doctor without delay. Consider the following situation.

CASE 9
You are clinical director of an Obstetrics and Gynaecology unit in a District General Hospital. Dr SP, one of the senior house officers (SHOs) asks to see you. She states that she has a conscientious objection to termination of pregnancy but that her consultant is pressurizing her to clerk women being admitted for termination and to be involved in the theatre list. He argues that her refusal to be involved in the clerking is unfair to her colleagues and that she needs to attend the list as part of her training. What should you do?

It is inappropriate for the consultant to pressurize SP to attend the theatre list and observe terminations being performed and you advise him of this. However, the BMA considers [22] that clerking of the woman is incidental to the procedure and, therefore, not covered by the conscience clause. You discuss this with SP and, after further consultation with the other SHOs, you suggest that she perform other work for her colleagues in return for them clerking the women being admitted for termination. SP and her colleagues agree to this.

Two weeks later Sister in the gynaecological ward advises you that SP had refused to treat a woman who was bleeding vaginally after having had a termination of pregnancy because of SP's conscientious objection. Another SHO attended and the woman came to no harm. What should you do now?

Neither the conscience clause nor one's 'duty of care' permit doctors to refuse to provide emergency treatment to a woman who has had an induced abortion. Not to do so contravenes the General Medical Council's 'duties of a doctor' [2] that state that care of the patient must be one's first concern and that personal beliefs must not prejudice patient care. You advise SP that, despite the fact that the woman came to no harm, her refusal was a failure of duty of care and that, unless she guarantees that this will never happen again, she will face disciplinary action.

Assisted reproduction

The clinical and legal aspects of assisted reproduction have been considered elsewhere but some of the profound ethical issues raised will be considered briefly here. Once more the 'References' and the 'Further reading' provide opportunities for their further and deeper study. The highly relevant questions of 'is there a right to procreate?' and 'what is the moral status of the human embryo/fetus?' have been considered in 'Is there a "right" to procreate' (see p. 665) and 'Moral status of the human embryo and fetus' (see p. 668), respectively. The BMA Handbook [39] points out that interventions such as donated gametes or surrogacy challenge, for example, our basic concepts of personal identity, family and inter-family relationships, and definitions of 'mother' and 'father'. 'Techniques that were originally developed to help people to overcome some pathology that meant they were unable to reproduce are increasingly being used to allow people greater choice in their reproductive decisions' [40]. One consequence is that some women can have children long beyond the natural span of their reproductive ability. This revives the 'can v. ought' question raised in 'Introduction' (see p. 658) and makes some people consider whether barriers have been reached that society should not breach.

WHO SHOULD OR SHOULD NOT BE TREATED USING ASSISTED REPRODUCTION TECHNIQUES?

It has already been argued in 'Is there a "right" to procreate' (see p. 665) that procreation is neither a fundamental right nor a universal need generating a right [25]. However, Warnock also argues [25] 'the infertile who want to conceive are entitled to expect that they will be given the medical assistance they need, even if they have to pay for it'. This entitlement cannot be unconditional and judgements are still required about who should or should not be treated. These fall into two main categories – clinical and non-clinical. The hypothetical Case 8 in which Miss TD was provided with IVF despite her poor cardiac status shows that even clinical judgements have ethical components. It can be argued that the fertility specialist's acquiescence to a strongly desired intervention contrary to reasonable clinical judgement on the basis that he was honouring 'patient autonomy' was actually an abrogation of his duty as a doctor.

The BMA [22] suggests some general principles for making judgements as to who should or should not be treated by assisted conception techniques. The two most relevant to this discussion are:
• Doctors who help to initiate a pregnancy have legal and ethical duties to address the welfare of any future child. This principle is enshrined in British law under the

Table 59.14 Human Fertilisation and Embryology Act [41]

A woman shall not be provided with treatment services unless account has been taken of the welfare of any child who may be born as a result of the treatment (including the need of that child for a father), and of any other child who may be affected by the birth

Human Fertilisation and Embryology Act (HFEA) – 1990 (Table 59.14).
• All people are entitled to a fair and unprejudiced consideration of their request for treatment, so individual cases should be considered and blanket restrictions should not be applied to certain groups.
Although at first glance, the first of these guiding principles seems entirely reasonable, it requires that the state of existence and non-existence ('any future child') be compared with one another. This is rather like trying to add (or subtract) any number from infinity. However, to change the metaphor, in clinical practice it is a circle that must be squared. Hope and McMillan [41] quote Derek Parfit as referring to it as the 'non-identity' problem. Several philosophers and bio-ethicists argue [43–45] that, since existence must in almost all circumstances be a benefit over not existing, any life is invariably better than no life. Murray [46] suggests that uncritical acceptance of that view could be used to justify ethically any novel reproductive technology. What is more, if existence is indeed invariably better than non-existence, the argument must be applied equally to end of life decisions in the context of, for example, euthanasia.

There has been considerable debate about whether duties can be owed to a 'potential person'. Whereas many individuals experiencing pain, abuse, neglect, or other substantial disadvantages are nevertheless glad to have been born, most people regard it as axiomatic that it would be wrong to generate a pregnancy knowing that the future child would be harmed.

Warnock [47] suggests that refusal to treat on grounds other than clinical unfitness should happen rarely with each case being judged on its own merits and the grounds for refusal being openly declared. Clinics providing these services should have ethics committees to advise them on such matters.

As in other areas of medicine, focus on rights without any discussion of duties and responsibilities is both incomplete and inappropriate. In many circumstances, however, doctors' duties are primarily focused on the patient before them, whereas in assisted reproduction there is another party to be considered, that is, the child born as a result of medical intervention. Disputes continue about the ethical obligations, if any, owed to the unborn child. The BMA [40] suggests that the fetus deserves respect but does not have absolute claims that can override those of an autonomous person, usually the mother. In the case of any form of assisted reproduction, however, the 'person' to whom a duty is owed is not only unborn, but also not yet conceived. The BMA Handbook of Ethics and Law [40] states, 'In the BMA's view, as well as in the view of the law, doctors who are asked to intervene to help to generate a pregnancy have particular duties to consider the welfare of any resulting children. The child is the most vulnerable party and doctors' obligations are held to be significantly greater than in any case in which the doctor assumes management of an already existing pregnancy'.

The HFEA [48] provides guidance on what kind of factors should be taken into account when assessing whether people should be accepted for assisted reproduction. These should include:

• Their commitment to having and bringing up a child or children
• Their ability to provide a stable and supportive environment for any child produced as a result of treatment
• Their personal and family medical histories
• Their health and consequent future ability to look after or provide for a child's needs
• Their ages and likely future ability to look after or provide for a child's needs
• Their future ability to meet the needs of any child or children who may be born as a result of treatment, including the implications of a possible multiple birth
• Any risk of harm to the child or children who may be born, including the risk of inherited disorders or transmissible diseases, problems during pregnancy and of neglect or abuse
• The effect of a new baby or babies upon any existing child of the family.

Such judgements are very difficult to make and, to avoid any claim of unfair discrimination, it would be wise for clinics to refer to their ethics committee cases in which doubt as to suitability arises. It is argued that no such limitations are placed on couples who conceive naturally so why should they apply to couples requesting assisted conception? The key difference is that, in the latter case, the responsibility for bringing children into the world is shared by the parents and the health care professionals involved in the treatment. In essence the biological parents have the autonomous right to be irresponsible: health care professionals have a duty of care not to abrogate that responsibility.

GAMETE DONATION

CASE 10

AL and her partner, MF (both aged 29 years) attend your infertility clinic having been trying unsuccessfully to conceive for 3 years. Investigations suggest that AL is potentially fertile but that MF has azoospermia following severe mumps orchitis as a child. After appropriate counselling, they elect to proceed with donor insemination (DI). You discuss with them the issue of telling any child arising from DI how he or she was conceived. They promise to think about it but would rather wait to see if the DI is successful first. The sperm donor has consented to being identifiable.

AL conceives and the pregnancy progresses normally to the full-term normal delivery of a healthy male infant. They inform you that they have decided not to tell the child how he was conceived. The reasons they give are:
• 'There really isn't any need to tell him – what good will it do? The news would be too upsetting for him'.
• MF thinks it would make people think he 'wasn't quite a man' and it could cause problems between him and 'his son'.
• The donor should be protected.

Gamete donation per se no longer seems to raise major ethical concerns. The main focus of interest is the anonymity of donors. The main arguments for removing anonymity include:

• It is important to know one's genetic heritage for both emotional and medical reasons.
• It contravenes Articles 8 and 14 of the Human Rights Act (24). These respectively confer 'the right of respect for private and family life' and prevent 'discrimination in the enjoyment of that right'. (This was the main argument for the recent non-retrospective change in English law.)
• If adopted children are able, in law, to have access to information about their birth parents why should it be different for those conceived by gamete donation?
• Secrecy in a family is, generally, a bad thing.
The main arguments against removing anonymity are:
• The effect on the number of donors. However, experience in those countries in which anonymity has been removed suggests that, after an initial fall in numbers, they were replaced but with a different kind of sperm donor. He was more likely to be altruistically motivated, older and married [49].
• It implies a presumption that there *should* be a relationship between the donor and any donor children.
• As noted above, consistent application of any human rights argument must arguably allow retrospective disclosure even when anonymity was guaranteed.

The arguments for and against anonymity are 'finely balanced' [40]. However, although knowledge of one's genetic parents may be desirable, the argument that it is a fundamental right in this context but not others is illogical. For example, as previously noted, not only does a human rights based argument necessarily mean that disclosure would also have to be retrospective (despite previous donors being guaranteed anonymity) but the same right would have to be afforded to all offspring no matter how conceived! Such arguments are, of course, rendered redundant in the hypothetical case presented above because the couple decided not to tell the child about his origins. Not only is this consistent with experience reported from around the world [40] in which 70 to 80% of parents decided not to tell children born after donor insemination of the manner of their conception but the reasons given by the couple are those most commonly reported. Thus, another argument against involvement of the Human Rights Act in this context is that it would inevitably mean that such decisions could not be left to parental discretion!

Fuller discussion on this can be found in 'Further reading'.

SURROGATE MOTHERHOOD

Although in practice requests for surrogacy arrangements are uncommon they raise profound questions. Indeed, in 1984 the Committee of Inquiry into Human Fertilisation and Embryology [50] opined, 'it is inconsistent with human dignity that a woman should use her uterus for financial profit and treat it as an incubator for someone else's child'. Furthermore the separation of the carrying and social roles of motherhood deeply challenges both emotional and legal concepts of what a mother is. Baroness Warnock, who chaired the above Committee, while continuing to accept that 'surrogacy is an extremely risky enterprise and liable to end in tears', now suspects on pragmatic grounds that the legislation following the report of her Committee may have been mistaken [51]. However rational the arguments and despite the understandable wish of couples who cannot have a child by any other means, can the deliberate breaking of the fundamental (and not yet fully understood) relationship between the birth mother and the child ever be justified? The fact that the surrogate mother usually does so for financial gain adds to the concern. Although the use of another family member (e.g. sister or even mother) as the surrogate may remove the financial incentive it adds another extremely complex dynamic to family relationships.

The BMA accepts surrogacy as 'a treatment of the last resort' when it is 'impossible or highly undesirable for medical reasons for the intended mother to carry a child herself'. Details of the current regulatory framework for surrogacy arrangements can be found on p. 299 of the BMA handbook of ethics and law [50].

Preimplantation and prenatal testing for genetic or other reasons

The clinical aspects of this subject have been dealt with elsewhere and they illustrate the dramatic rise in our knowledge of genetically determined conditions and in the sophistication of the technology at our disposal to detect them. It is likely that many, if not all, of the readers of this book who practice obstetrics and gynaecology will either have faced, or will almost certainly have to face in the future, clinical and ethical dilemmas relating to genetic testing or therapy.

THE PURPOSE OF PREIMPLANTATION AND PRENATAL TESTING

Although these topics do not, of themselves, raise new ethical issues they lift them to new levels of complexity that need to be addressed. The purpose of this section is to allow those of us in this field to stand back and reflect on our practice.

The focus of current preimplantation and prenatal testing is mainly, but not solely, on serious genetic disorders. In his book, the Worth of a Child, Murray wrote in 1996, 'Prenatal testing (if written today he would probably have included preimplantation testing) was created as a means for adults to avoid the birth of children with problems ranging from significant to absolutely devastating. In practice, the barriers of invasiveness and risk were too high to tempt prospective parents to use prenatal testing to detect anything less than severe health problems with their fetuses. Now that the barriers are on the verge of crumbling and the menu of genetic information about to grow exceedingly long, the time has come to take a hard look at the moral foundations of prenatal testing. Can the current understanding of the ethics of prenatal testing guide us through the thicket of increased demand for prenatal testing for a potentially massive list of human genes, many of which may have nothing to do with disease or disability? The answer, I fear, is no' [52].

It is likely that, in the relatively near future further advances will, for example, lead to:

- Genetic testing of the fetus from cellular or free DNA in maternal plasma
- Increased ability to test future risk of common diseases (e.g. diabetes, heart disease or an increasing number of cancers)
- The ability to predict a series of non-disease characteristics, e.g. height, athleticism and, possibly, intelligence.

Further in the future lies the prospect of beneficial, effective, and safe somatic cell gene transfer. This does not fall within the compass of this chapter and is considered only briefly. Somatic gene transfer uses vectors (usually viruses) to carry the required human gene in an attempt to make the cells of the individual express the gene. Germ line gene therapy involves transfer of a gene to gametes and, unlike somatic therapy, would affect the genome for all future generations. The risk of harm for all future generations by interfering with the genome is so great that germ line gene transfer is ethically absolutely contraindicated. Currently the use of viruses as vectors is associated with a series of major risks [53] including an observed incorporation of the new gene in the germ line, unquantified effects on gene expression and the immune system, and long-term pathological effects from possible latency of viral vectors. The ethical issues arising as a result of the possibility of genetic enhancement of children should gene transfer ever be found to be safe and effective are similar to those dealt with in 'The quest for the perfect child' (see p. 679) and have also been discussed by Tong [54].

Murray [52] suggests, 'In concert with some of the values implicit in alternative reproductive technologies, prenatal' (and now preimplantation) 'testing makes children increasingly the product of explicit adult choices. Prenatal testing involves the choice whether or not to have *this particular child* rather than the choice whether to have *a child*'.

WHAT KIND OF CHILD DO PARENTS WANT?

At one level the answer is obvious – they want a child who is 'normal' by which they usually mean not having any disabilities. This raises two different kinds of questions. The first is about the meaning of the words 'normal' and 'disability'. The second is the role of health care professionals in helping them to achieve their desires. Neither of these questions can be dealt with extensively here but the following two hypothetical scenarios (based on Hope and McMillan [42]) are relevant to them.

CASE 11: Deafening an embryo

A couple, EF and GM, who both have a known genetic condition causing deafness wish to have a child who is also deaf. This is so that the child is part of the deaf community. They also consider that being deaf is not to be 'disabled' but to be 'alternatively enabled'. The woman becomes pregnant. They attend your clinic requesting genetic testing to determine whether the fetus has the gene causing deafness. They provide literature from the Internet about a drug that, if taken by a pregnant woman, will cause a normal fetus to become deaf. It has no other effect and is otherwise safe for embryo and mother. They state that, if testing suggested that the fetus is likely to become a hearing child they wish you to prescribe this drug to make it deaf.

Harming a fetus is clearly a moral wrong where harm is defined as any action that detracts from 'species-typical functioning' [55]. In the above case, whereas it may arguably be appropriate to accede to the request to perform genetic testing to determine whether the child would or would not be deaf, it would be morally wrong both for you to harm the fetus by prescribing the drug to cause deafness and for the couple to take it. This is both because it is typical for human beings to be able to hear and because the drug would be 'identity-altering' [42]. Now consider the following somewhat different scenario.

CASE 12: Choosing a deaf embryo

A couple, HJ and FS, with the same genetic condition causing deafness as EF and GM attend your fertility clinic requesting assisted conception and preimplantation diagnosis to determine whether the embryos carry the deafness gene. They further request that only an embryo that carries the deafness be implanted for the same reasons as EF and GM.

Would you accede to their request? If 'yes' why and if 'no' why not?

Hope and McMillan [42] postulate that the main difference in the two scenarios is that, even though the outcome would be the same, in the first case the fetus had an identity and would be harmed and in the second they contend that it did not have an identity and could, therefore, not be harmed (whether one agrees with this or not is not pertinent to the current argument). On the basis of what they consider to be a 'non-identity problem' (see 'who should or should not be treated using assisted reproduction techniques', p. 648) and the great weight given to parental reproductive choice, they argue that the request should be acceded to. Although the following scenario (adapted from Murray [21]) may stretch one's imagination, it illustrates a point that questions their recommendation.

CASE 13

A terrorist conceals a time bomb in a nursery school with the intention of harming the children who are all 3 years of age or under. His intention is that it goes off in 4 days. He is apprehended and the bomb is both discovered and defused.

He is clearly morally culpable and should be punished accordingly.

The same terrorist conceals the bomb in the nursery school and, for reasons known only to him, sets it to detonate in 4 years time. Once more he is apprehended and the bomb is both discovered and defused. The children who would have been in the nursery at that time have not yet been conceived.

Is his moral culpability different in this scenario? The answer is surely 'no' despite the fact that the children who would have been harmed have not yet been conceived and, therefore, do not have an identity. Thus it is actually possible to apply concepts of morality and even harm to those not yet conceived let alone born. Applying the same line of thought to Cases 11 and 12 it can, perhaps, be argued that, since the end result is the same in both (namely that the child is deaf), it is no more or less justifiable to produce a 'non-species typical' deaf fetus in the latter as it is in the former. Harris [44] argues that it would, in fact be morally wrong to create a life that is likely to have more suffering than other possible lives. The above is far from being the last word on the subject but it is intended to give food for thought.

PREIMPLANTATION GENETIC DIAGNOSIS AND 'SAVIOUR SIBLINGS'

Preimplantation genetic diagnosis (PGD) is currently permitted in the UK for the determination of sex in the context of a risk of sex-linked disorders; the detection of single gene defects (e.g. cystic fibrosis); and for chromosomal translocations, inversion and deletions (but not aneuploidy). Robertson [56] considers that its use can be ethically justified for the identification of genes indicating susceptibility to, and the late onset of, disease and HLA matching. Its use to detect non-medical characteristics is more questionable and he suggests that this 'depends on the parental needs served and the harm posed to embryos, children and society'. This consequentialist argument has to be considered in the context of other factors such as those discussed below.

The term 'saviour siblings' is an emotive term to describe the use of PGD to select a matched donor for a seriously ill child (but not a parent). As doctors we obviously wish to do all we can to help those families in this terrible predicament. Many of us would do the same in their position! The main ethical arguments about it surround the best interests of the 'saviour sibling' and the risk of 'using an unborn child as a commodity' (see Table 58.3). Boyle and Savalescu [57] deal with these and other lesser points and ask, 'Who is harmed by allowing PGD to be performed solely for the benefit of a relative? Not the couple who wish to produce an embryo: nor the child who would not otherwise have existed: nor the person who receives the stem cell transplant that might save his or her life'. They conclude, 'We must avoid the trap of interfering with individual liberty by preventing such procedures for no good reason'. The following case, however, shows that there may be more to the issue than this. It is loosely based on Jodi Picoult's novel 'My Sister's Keeper' [58].

CASE 14

Kate develops a rare form of leukaemia at 2 years of age. She requires a bone-marrow transplant but no suitable donor can be found. Her parents, Brian and Sara, decide to go ahead with IVF and PGD to provide an embryo that is an exact HLA match. Anna is conceived and born. Umbilical cord cells are taken to provide stem cells.

Unfortunately the stem cell infusion is only temporarily effective. Over the next few years Anna provides a series of donations of bone marrow. Her parents love her for herself but she increasingly becomes aware of the purpose for which she was conceived. Brian and Sara seem to assume

that she would always consent to be a donor for her sister but it is never discussed with her and her consent is assumed.

Kate has to undergo a series of treatments with cytotoxic drugs as a result of which she develops renal failure when she is 16 years of age. The only remedy is a renal transplant. Anna is now 13 years old and her parents, once again, assume that she will willingly be a kidney donor because she is a perfect match. What ethical issues does this raise in your mind?

The rest of the story, and particularly the complex family dynamics involved, are compellingly told in the novel but the above illustrates that the role of the 'saviour sibling' does not end with umbilical cord blood donation. This is seldom considered. The novel also shows the burden that Anna has to bear in relation to whether her sister dies or lives and we can learn from this in real life too.

SEX SELECTION FOR NON-MEDICAL REASONS

In 1999, the Ethics Committee of the American Society of Reproductive Medicine (ASRM) concluded, 'The initiation of IVF with pre-implantation diagnosis solely for sex selection holds even greater risk of unwarranted gender bias, social harm and the diversion of medical resources from genuine medical need. It therefore should be discouraged' [59]. They were concerned that the emphasis that gender selection places on a child's genetic characteristics rather than his or her inherent worth tends to treat the fetus as a commodity rather than an end in itself (see Table 59.4). In addition, if sex were to be allowed as a sole criterion for choice, then selection for other characteristics (e.g. intelligence, beauty, sporting prowess etc.) would be permissible should the techniques for doing so become available.

In 1994 the International Federation of Gynecology and Obstetrics (FIGO) recommended that sex selection 'could be justified on social grounds in certain cases with the objective of allowing children of the two sexes to enjoy the love and care of parents. For this social indication to be justified, it must not conflict with other society values where it is practiced' [60]. In 2001 the ASRM modified their position to state, 'If – methods of preconception gender selection are found to be safe and effective, physicians should be free to offer (them) in clinical settings to couples who are seeking gender variety in their offspring if the couples (1) are fully informed of the risks of failure, (2) affirm that they will fully accept children of the opposite sex if the preconception gender selection fails, (3) are counseled about having unrealistic expectations about the behavior of children of the preferred gender, and (4) are offered the opportunity to participate in research to track and access the safety, efficacy and demographics of preconception gender selection. Practitioners offering assisted reproductive services are under no legal or ethical obligation to provide non-medically indicated preconception methods of gender selection' [61].

There are arguably only two internally consistent and logical ethical positions on sex selection for non-medical reasons. The first would not allow it under any circumstances enforced by law. The second is that expressed by the ASRM in which, as long as the techniques are safe and effective, physicians should be free to offer preconception gender selection within the very clear parameters they suggest and with the proviso that they were under no legal or moral obligation to do so. If it were to be permitted it should be regulated by a statutory licensing authority.

THE QUEST FOR THE PERFECT CHILD

Murray [52] defines the quest for the perfect child as 'the desire to attain something that is wholly without flaw'. He points out that 'the quest for perfection in Western culture is an ancient one, with roots in Greek philosophy long before Socrates. Through most of Western history the quest for perfection took the shape of a spiritual or metaphysical striving. More recently the search for human perfectibility allied itself with the ideas of science and of progress'. He continues, 'The quest for perfection was primed and ready to meet modern science in the form of genetics' and 'is now poised to enlist in its service the ever-growing power of genetic technology'. Bromage [62] suggests, 'Through a lens forged in post-modern society we may see these new obstetric technologies as one method of "aesthetic normalisation", aimed at satisfying the post-modern predilection for faultlessness'.

Tong [54] hopes that 'the public has the courage to answer honestly the question of why so many parents want to have "perfect" babies'. She considers that 'the quest for the "perfect child" is, at root, not a quest to make sure that all children have an equal opportunity to lead a normal and meaningful life, but a quest to guarantee that one's own child will have what it takes to get more pieces of the pie than one's neighbour's child'.

Murray [52] suggests that modern parents, with so much at stake in their children, might want to protect themselves against the hurt and disappointment that they fear a child with a disability or disfigurement might bring. But, he asks, 'Is the worth of the parent–child relationship to be judged by how successfully it avoids unpleasantness and totes up its pleasures? The more we come to see our children's characteristics as the product of choice, the more vulnerable we become to the likelihood – indeed the near certainty – of disappointment'.

ATTITUDES TOWARDS DISABILITY

The BMA [63] state, 'A challenge for society as a whole is to help people who want to avoid passing on a genetic disorder to future children while providing unambiguous respect and proper support for those who suffer disabling genetic conditions'. Newell [64] wrote, 'The voices of those with disability, and those utilising social and human rights approaches to disability, have particular value in assisting us to critique the project which is bioethics'. Parens and Asch [65] argue in their Disability Rights Critique of Prenatal Genetic Testing that 'prenatal genetic testing followed by selective abortion is morally problematic and that it is driven by misinformation'. The moral problems are, they suggest, twofold. 'First, selective abortion expresses negative or discriminatory attitudes not merely about a disabling trait, but about those who carry it. Second, it signals an intolerance of diversity not merely in the society but in the family, and ultimately it could harm parental attitudes towards children'. The second problem is that 'prenatal testing depends on a misunderstanding of what life with a disability is like for children with disabilities'. They assert, 'Recent studies suggest that many members of the health professions view childhood disability as predominantly negative for children and their families, in contrast to what research on the life satisfaction of people with disabilities and their families has actually shown'. They also point out that families that include disabled children fare, on average, no better or worse than families in general'. Others, however, agree with Gillam [66] that discrimination against people with disabilities is neither an inevitable result of prenatal diagnosis, nor is it a necessary conceptual part of it. She accepts that there is the potential for significant negative effects on people with disabilities and 'if prenatal diagnosis is to proceed in an ethically acceptable way, these negative effects must be recognised, acknowledged and countered as far as possible'. Parens and Asch [65] write, 'It is crucial that prospective parents are offered both information about disability and the opportunity to explore the values and dreams that enter into deciding what to do with prenatal genetic information. Equally crucial is that professionals honor both acceptances and refusals of those offers'.

There is a moral, ethical and professional obligation of doctors to honestly and unbiasedly impart information to couples and not to bias towards termination of pregnancy.

Obstetric interventions

Clinical aspects of obstetric interventions are considered in their respective chapters. The issue of the illegality of performing a Caesarean section on a competent woman without her consent no matter what the outcome for herself and her baby is dealt with in Chapter 58. Legal decisions are based on such an intervention being an assault and focus on whether the woman is competent when making her decision. This is not considered further here.

REQUEST FOR CAESAREAN SECTION IN THE ABSENCE OF MEDICAL INDICATIONS

The current guidelines on Caesarean section from the National Institute for Clinical Excellence in the UK [67] state that 'maternal request is not on its own an indication for caesarean section'. Other authors have argued that it should be so [68–70]. The following illustrates an ethical dilemma surrounding such a case.

CASE 15
CJ is 32 years of age and in her second pregnancy. Her first child, a boy, is now 3 years old and was born at term after an uneventful pregnancy and normal labour and delivery. His birth-weight was on the 60th centile.

She is referred to your hospital at 37 weeks not having felt fetal movements for two days. There is no history of, for example, abdominal pain or vaginal bleeding. She is not in labour. Her blood pressure is normal and there is no other evidence of a causative factor such as pre-eclampsia. Intrauterine fetal death is confirmed.

She requests delivery by Caesarean section under general anaesthesia because she 'doesn't want to deliver a dead baby' or 'spoil the wonderful experience of her last delivery'.

Would you accede to her request? If so why and if not why not? Your decision should be based on the balance between the exercise of her autonomy and what you consider to be in her best interests from your clinical experience. The very strong likelihood is that, if labour were to be induced, she would labour normally. She would also be able to go home soon afterwards which would not be possible after Caesarean section. Delivery by Caesarean section under general anaesthesia (or regional block) would be associated with greater risk for her without any balancing benefit to the fetus. The uterine scar would also add to risk in any future pregnancy. There is no absolutely right or wrong answer to this dilemma but let us assume that you advise against Caesarean section and that she ultimately accepts this.

Labour is induced and, 5 hours later, she delivers a stillborn male infant. There is no obvious cause of death although he is small for gestational age. She goes home within a few hours of delivery. She returns in 2 weeks to discuss the pregnancy and thanks you for 'not doing as she asked because if you had it would have been treating my dead baby as a tumour'.

Of course, the fact that she now feels what happens was appropriate does not of itself make your decision right or wrong. How would you have responded on this situation? In twin articles on the 'unethics' and 'unfacts' of request Caesarean section, Bewley and Cockburn [71,72] state, 'taking women's views seriously is ordinary good practice but it is not the over-riding consideration in decision making'. This has been already discussed in 'Diversity of moral theory', (see p. 660). Balancing the current clinical evidence they conclude that elective Caesarean section has not been shown to be safer than labour.

Gynaecological oncology

CASE 16
Mrs LW is a 58-year-old woman who had surgery and chemotherapy 4 years ago for ovarian carcinoma. The tumour has recurred and is now widespread. She is admitted and you present the options for treatment including a new course of aggressive chemotherapy. You also tell her that the treatment would probably make her feel very unwell and that the likelihood of success is limited. You do not tell her that the chemotherapy is very expensive.

LW states that she does not want another course of chemotherapy but wishes to go home and receive palliative treatment as it becomes necessary. Let us assume that you consider this to be the 'correct decision'.

A few days later she returns to see you to say that, following discussions with her husband, her older sister and her three children she has changed her mind and wishes to receive chemotherapy.

What should you do?

You must now judge between two alternatives. First, that LW's initial decision reflected her true state of mind but she has been influenced inappropriately by her family to make her change her mind. Second, in the initial consultation she perceived that you felt she should not have the treatment and she thought that 'you probably knew best'. It was only when she consulted with her family that she really understood her true preferences. In the context of a busy ward or clinic it may be more difficult to perceive the importance of the latter. Her General Practitioner might be able to help here but, unfortunately, she might not know LW and the family much better than you do! This case emphasizes the importance of the patient's narrative (see 'Diversity of moral theory' p. 634) and the risk of rushing too soon to ethical judgement.

Conclusion

If it were not so before, it should be clear by now that ethical judgements are integral to all aspects of clinical practice. This chapter aimed to emphasize the importance of rigorous, clear, consistent, coherent and relevant ethical reflection and analysis in your practice. You may, perhaps, feel that you have been provided with as many (or more) questions than answers. You should, however, also have the wherewithal to answer those questions either directly by what is written in the text or in the 'Further reading' section.

References

1. General Medical Council (2005) *Duties of a Doctor*. Available from www.gmc-uk.org/standards. Accessed April 15, 2005.
2. General Medical Council (2005) *Good Medical Practice*. Available from www.gmc-uk.org/standards. Accessed April 15, 2005.
3. Campbell AV (1972) *Moral Dilemmas in Medicine*. Edinburgh: Churchill Livingstone.
4. Stirrat GM (2003) How to approach ethical issues – a brief guide. *Obstet Gynaecol* **5**, 130–5.
5. Dunstan G (1994) Should philosophy and medical ethics be left to the experts? In: Bewley S & Ward RH. *Ethics in Obstetrics & Gynaecology* (eds) London: RCOG Press.
6. Jonsen A (1994) Clinical ethics and the four principles. In: Gillon R (ed.) *Principles of Healthcare Ethics*. Chichester and New York: John Wiley & Sons, 13–21.
7. Baron MW (1997) Kantian ethics. In: Baron MW, Pettit P & Stone M (eds) *Three Methods of Ethics: a Debate*. Oxford: Blackwell Publishers, 3–91.
8. Pettit P (1997) The Consequentialist Perspective. In: Baron MW, Pettit P & Stone M (eds) *Three Methods of Ethics: a Debate*. Oxford: Blackwell Publishers, 92–174.
9. Beauchamp TL (1994) The 'Four Principles Approach'. In: Gillon R (ed.) *Principles of Healthcare Ethics*. Chichester and New York: John Wiley & Sons, 3–12.
10. Schneider CE (1998) The practice of autonomy: patients, doctors and medical decisions. New York: Oxford University Press, xi, 3, 9,10, 226–31.
11. O'Neill O (2002) *Autonomy & Trust in Bioethics*. Cambridge: Cambridge University Press. 30, 83–85.
12. Stirrat GM & Gill R (2005) Autonomy in medical ethics after O'Neill. *J Med Ethics* **31**, 127–30.
13. Sherwin S (1999) Foundations, frameworks and lenses. In: *The Role of Theories in Bioethics*. Oxford: Blackwell, 198–206.
14. Brody H (1994) The four principles and narrative ethics. In: Gillon R (ed.) *Principles of Healthcare Ethics*. Chichester and New York: John Wiley & Sons, 207–15.
15. Murray TH (1996) Why do adults have children? The importance of context. In: *'The Worth of a Child'*. Berkeley: University of California Press, 6–7.
16. Campbell AV (1998) The 'ethics of care' as virtue ethics. *Adv Bioeth* **4**, 295–305.
17. Cook RJ (1994) Feminism and the four principles. In: Gillon R (ed.) *Principles of Healthcare Ethics*. Chichester and New York: John Wiley & Sons, 193–206.
18. Tong R (ed) Feminist ethics. In: *Concise Routledge Encyclopaedia of Philosophy*. London and New York: Routledge, 278. Online Encyclopaedia, www.rep.routledge.com
19. Percival T (1987) *Medical ethics. Classics in Medical Literature*. Lederle laboratories from the Collection of the Yale University Medical Historical Library.
20. McCullough LB & Chervenak FA (1994) A framework for ethics in a clinical setting. In: *Ethics in Obstetrics and Gynecology*. New York and Oxford: Oxford University Press, 3–81.
21. Murray TH (1996) Moral obligations to the not-yet-born child. In: *The Worth of a Child*. Berkeley: University of California Press, 96–112.
22. British Medical Association Ethics Department (2004) Contraception, abortion and birth. *Medical Ethics Today*, 2nd edn. London: BMJ books, 224–68.
23. British Medical Association Ethics Department (2004) Confidentiality. *Medical Ethics Today*, 2nd edn. London: BMJ books, 165–97.
24. Human Rights Act 1998. Available form www.pfc.org.uk/legal/hra98.htm accessed on April 15, 2005.
25. Warnock B (2002) *Making Babies. Is There a Right to Have Children?* Oxford: Oxford University Press, 54.
26. Gillick v West Norfolk and Wisbech AHA [1985] 3 All Er 402.
27. British Medical Association, Brook, General Practitioners Committee, Medical Defence Union, Royal College of General Practitioners, Royal College of Nursing (2000) *Confidentiality and young people. Improving teenagers' uptake of health advice. A toolkit for general practice, primary care groups and trusts*. London: RCGP and Brook.
28. Teenage Pregnancy Unit (2000) Best practice advice on the provision of effective contraception and advice services for young people. Department of Health.
29. Re F (mental patient: sterilisation) sub nom F v West Berkshire Health Authority [1989] 2 All ER 545:566.
30. Carroll L (1984) Through the Looking Glass. London, Puffin Classics 87.
31. McCullough LB & Chervenak FA (1994) A framework for obstetric ethics in the clinical setting. In: *Ethics in Obstetrics and Gynecology*. New York and Oxford: Oxford University Press, 96–129.
32. Finnis J (1994) Abortion and health care II. In: Gillon R (ed.) *Principles of Healthcare Ethics*. Chichester and New York: John Wiley & Sons, 547–57.
33. Iglesias T (1984) *In vitro* fertilisation: the major issues. *J Med Ethics* **10**, 32–7.
34. Strong C (2002) Overview: a framework for reproductive ethics. In: Dickenson DL (ed.) Ethical Issues in Maternal-Fetal Medicine. Cambridge: Cambridge University Press, 17–35.
35. Singer P (1993) Taking life: the embryo and fetus. *Practical Ethics*, 2nd edn. Cambridge: Cambridge University Press, 135–74.
36. Campbell AV, Gillett G & Jones G (2001) Issues before birth. *Medical Ethics*, 3rd edn. Oxford: Oxford University Press, 98–114.
37. Tooley M (1983) *Abortion and Infanticide*. Oxford: Clarendon Press.
38. Sykes JB (ed.) *The Concise Oxford Dictionary of Current English*, 6th edn. Oxford: Clarendon Press.
39. Royal College of Obstetricians and Gynaecologists (1996) *Termination of Pregnancy for Fetal Abnormality in England, Wales and Scotland*. (1996) London, RCOG Press, 1.

40. British Medical Association Ethics Department (2004) Assisted reproduction. *Medical Ethics*, 2nd edn. London: BMJ books, 269–306.

41. Human Fertilisation and Embryology Authority Act 1990. Available from www.hfea.gov.uk accessed on 15 April 2005.

42. Hope T & McMillan J (2003) Ethical problems before conception. *Lancet* **361**, 2164.

43. Overall C (2002) Do new reproductive technologies benefit or harm children? . In Dickenson DL (ed) *Ethical Issues in Maternal-Fetal Medicine*. Cambridge: Cambridge University Press, 305–19.

44. Bennett R & Harris J (2002) Are there lives not worth living? When is it morally wrong to reproduce?. In Dickenson DL (ed.) *Ethical Issues in Maternal-Fetal Medicine*. Cambridge: Cambridge University Press, 321–34.

45. Robertson JA (1994) *Children of Choice*. Princeton: Princeton University Press.

46. Murray TH (1996) Families, the marketplace and values. In *The Worth of a Child*. Berkeley: University of California Press, 14–40.

47. Warnock B (2002) Making babies. May doctors refuse treatment? Oxford: Oxford University Press, 43–50.

48. Human Fertilisation and Embryology Authority (2001) *Code of Practice*, 5th edn. London: HFEA.

49. Widdows H (2002) The ethics if secrecy in donor insemination. In Dickeson DL (ed.) *Ethical Issues in Maternal-Fetal Medicine*. Cambridge: Cambridge University Press, 167–80.

50. The Committee of Inquiry into Human Fertilisation and Embryology (2005) Available from www.ncbi.nlm.nih.gov. Accessed April 15, 2005.

51. Warnock B (2002) *Making Babies. Are All Methods of Fertility Treatment Legitimate?* Oxford: Oxford University Press, 87–96.

52. Murray TH (1996) Prenatal testing and the quest for the perfect child. In *The Worth of a Child*. Berkeley: University of California Press, 115–41.

53. Kimmelman J (2005) Recent developments in gene transfer: risk and ethics. *Br Med J* **330**, 79–82.

54. Tong R (2002) Genetic screening: should parents seek to perfect their children genetically? In Dickenson DL *Ethical issues in maternal-fetal medicine*. Cambridge: Cambridge University Press, 87–100.

55. Daniels N (1986) *Just Health Care*. New York: Cambridge University Press.

56. Robertson JA (2003) Extending preimplantation genetic diagnosis: medical and non-medical uses. *J Med Ethics* **29**, 213–6.

57. Boyle RJ & Savulescu J (2001) Ethics of using preimplantation genetic diagnosis to select a stem cell donor for an existing person. *Br Med J* **323**, 1240–3.

58. Picoult J (2005) *My Sister's Keeper*. London: Hodder and Stoughton.

59. Ethics Committee of the American Society for Reproductive Medicine (1999) Preimplantation genetic diagnosis and sex selection. *Fertil Steril* **72**, 595–8.

60. FIGO Committee for the study of ethical aspects of human reproduction (1997) Sex selection. In: *Recommendations on Ethical Issues in Obstetrics and Gynecology*. London, FIGO, 10–11.

61. Ethics Committee of the American Society for Reproductive Medicine (2001) Preconception gender selection for non-medical reasons. *Fertil Steril* **75**, 861–864.

62. Bromage DI (2006) Prenatal diagnosis and selective abortion: a post-modern phenomenon? *J Med Humanit*. **32**, 38–42.

63. British Medical Association (1998) Ethics, Society and Genetics. In *Human Genetics; Choice and Responsibility*. Oxford: Oxford University Press, 11–26.

64. Newell C (2003) Disability: a voice in Australian bioethics. *N Z Bioeth J* **June**, 7–20.

65. Parens E & Asch A (1999) The disability rights critique of prenatal testing. Reflections and recommendations. Special Supplement. *Hastings Cent Rep* **29**, S1–22.

66. Gillam L (1999) Prenatal diagnosis and discrimination against the disabled. *J Med Ethics* **25**, 163–71.

67. National Institute for Clinical Excellence (2005) *Caesarean Section*; NICE guideline 13. Available from www.nice.org.uk. Accessed April 15, 2005.

68. Paterson-Brown S (1998) Should doctors perform an elective caesarean section on request? Yes, as long as the woman is fully informed. *Br Med J* **317**, 462–3.

69. Minkoff H & Chervenak FA (2003) Elective primary caesarean delivery. *N Eng J Med* **348**, 946–50.

70. Hannah ME (2004) Planned elective caesarean section: a reasonable choice for some women? *Can Med Assoc J* **170**, 813–4.

71. Bewley S & Cockburn J (2002) The unethics of request caesarean section. *Br J Obstet Gynaecol* **109**, 593–6.

72. Bewley S & Cockburn J (2002) The unfacts of request caesarean section. *Br J Obstet Gynaecol* **109**, 597–605.

Further reading

Ethics and medical ethics

English V (2004) Medical Ethics Today. The BMA's handbook of ethics and law. London: BMJ Publishing Group. A comprehensive, concise and authoritative guide to medical ethics.

Campbell A, Gillett G & Jones G (2005) An invaluable primer for the subject accessible to the non-expert. *Medical Ethics*, 4th edn. Oxford: Oxford University Press. An invaluable primer for the subject accessible to the non-expert.

Jonsen AR, Siegler M & Winslade WJ (2002) *Clinical Ethics*, 5th edn. New York: McGraw-Hill. Facilitates solutions to everyday ethical problems.

Gillon R (ed.) (1994) *Principles of Health Care Ethics*. Chichester/New York: John Wiley. A detailed in depth analysis of the field.

Beauchamp TL & Childress JF (2001) *Principles of Bio-Medical Ethics*, 5th edn. New York/Oxford: Oxford University Press. Another excellent source book.

O'Neill O (2002) *Autonomy and Trust in Bioethics*. Cambridge: Cambridge University Press. A must for anyone who wishes to understand the true nature of autonomy.

Baron MW, Pettit P & Slote M (1997) *Three Methods of Ethics*. Oxford: Blackwell Publishers. For those who wish to consider more deeply and contrast Kantian Ethics, Consequentialism and Virtue Ethics.

Obstetrics & gynaecology

Bewley S & Ward RH (eds) (1994) *Ethics in Obstetrics & Gynaecology*. London: RCOG Press. Despite its age it is still highly relevant and worth reading.

McCullough LB & Chervenak FA (1994) Ethics in Obstetrics and Gynecology. New York and Oxford: Oxford University Press. Looks particularly at ethical conflicts in practice and suggests frameworks for dealing with them.

Dickenson DL (ed.) (2002) *Ethical Issues in Maternal-Fetal Medicine*. Cambridge: Cambridge University Press. This book is a serious ethical analysis of very relevant issues. Highly recommanded.

Murray TH (1996) *The Worth of a Child*. Berkeley: University of California Press. This is an excellent book that asks very pertinent questions that demand an answer. A 'must read'.

Warnock B (2002) *Making Babies: Is there a Right to Have Children?* Oxford: Oxford University Press. A short paperback that raises real issues in a very accessible manner.

FIGO Committee for the study of ethical aspects of human reproduction (1997) *Recommendations on Ethical Issues in Obstetrics and Gynecology*. London, FIGO.

A compilation of the ethical issues considered between 1985 and 1997. Well worth reading.

Shenfield F, Sureau C (2006) Contemporary Ethical Dilemmas in Assisted Reproduction. London, Taylor and Francis. Provides a framework for discussing topical issues in assisted reproduction with patients.

Chapter 60: The law and the obstetrician and gynaecologist

Bertie Leigh

One plausible approach to the predicament of the law in managing society's expectations of your profession is to see it as a by-product of clinical success. The achievements of obstetrics over the last 60 years have been remarkable. The decline of maternal and infant mortality would have astonished our grandparents. The virtual elimination of mortality from anaesthesia and the achievement of safe and predictable remedies for a wide range of gynaecological diseases has naturally brought with it a process of adjustment. Where it used to be the case that a doctor sheltered behind the threat of disease and offered a possible and unreliable bridge over distinctly troubled surgical waters, now that the threat of the disease and the troubles of the waters have largely been eliminated there is inevitably a revaluation of the clinician. Paradoxically, the advent of a safe and predictable service has led to a diminution in confidence in the person who provides the service. Where safe and predictable clinical excellence can be produced, which means that service remains fallible, the human agency is regularly weighed in the balance and occasionally found wanting.

The rise of autonomy

Furthermore, because the service is safe and predictable, society demands that it be delivered on the patient's own terms. If the survival of mother and child is a hazardous matter the clinician who is responsible for the delivery may reasonably demand that it takes place on his own terms and at a place and in circumstances determined by him. If it is safe and easy to deliver a child, then it is comparatively easy to understand how it may be viewed as a 'lifestyle choice' in which the pleasure to be derived from the occasion is a higher priority than the elimination of an already very modest risk. Although society generally is more risk averse than ever before, it is also predisposed to doubt risks described by experts. It is odd that the first generation to embrace evidence-based medicine and to limit the ability of clinicians to introduce new therapies that have not been subjected to a double-blind trial, is also more willing than ever before to embrace complementary medicine and to advocate the woman's right to home delivery when that has never been subjected to any such gold standard evidence-based assessment of risk.

Much of this development is not confined to obstetrics and gynaecology. Most aspects of medicine have become safer and more predictable. As a consequence across medicine the relative strength of different ethical considerations and obligations of the doctor has changed. Twenty years ago when medical ethics was first recognized as having practical implications which should be utilized by mainstream clinicians, it was accepted that there were four different ethical obligations which it was the duty of the doctor to balance. The primary obligation was to do good, and that preoccupied the thoughts of the clinicians of the 1970s. They might say 'first of all do not harm', but in reality that usually meant take reasonable care and the aspiration to non-maleficence took second place since it was seen as being of less practical importance in most circumstances. Third was the obligation to act justly, since it was crucial in circumstances where doctors were more responsible for the management of the service and therefore the allocation of resources. For example, the modern reader of a 1970s textbook such as Ian Donald's *Practical Obstetric Problems* (1979) will be surprised by the extent of the advice on how to manage the labour ward effectively. The idea that the patient's autonomy should be respected enjoyed no primacy and was barely entitled to parity of esteem. It was seen as a good thing doubtless, and a part of good manners, but hardly a fundamental aspiration of the service. The 1970s woman took herself to a doctor for the treatment of an ailment rather than the exercise of her autonomy.

Today respect for the patient's autonomy has grown like a cuckoo in the nest and threatens to drive all other considerations to the margin. A vivid illustration of this was seen in a case involving spinal surgery which came to the House of Lords in 2004. The court found Miss Chester was not told that there was a 1% risk of significant morbidity associated with spinal surgery. The defence accepted that every reasonable surgeon would have warned of this risk, which is in itself a striking change since Sidaway's case failed on precisely that issue in 1985. She said that if she had been told she probably would have undergone the surgery in any event and very likely in the hands of the same surgeon, but only after obtaining a second opinion. On a conventional analysis this meant that Miss Chester could not prove that Mr Afshar had caused her any damage. However, the House of Lords felt that in these circumstances the plain meaning of the English language needed some trifling adjustment. It did so on a twofold basis.

First, that it was of vital importance that Miss Chester's autonomy be respected and in circumstances where she was contemplating spinal surgery this demanded that she must be told the risks that she was letting herself in for. Otherwise she would be stripped of her dignity as a human being when she disrobed on admission. Second, that if it was not held that the erring doctor became the insurer of the patient's damage, the duty would be emptied of its content. The law would not be upholding the duty. Thus to enforce the duty the law should hold that in these circumstances the doctor has caused the patient damage. Some felt that there would have been more logic about it if the House of Lords had invented a new tort of Showing Disrespect, or Dis for short, and said that in these circumstances they would order the surgeon to compensate the patient for the complete tort of advising and treating with disrespect; that would have the advantage of forcing the surgeon to compensate the patient for the insult he had rendered, whether or not she was unlucky enough to get a complication which sounded in damages. A minor solatium of £500 would uphold the duty and reflect society's real evaluation of the insult. Since he had not really caused the complication it seems illogical to pretend that the law is enforcing the duty to advise which is equally important whether the complication results or not.

Another oddity of the case was that Miss Chester was at no less risk if she had opted for conservative therapy. The evidence was conflicting, but some experts thought that she was at greater risk of long-term disability if she had not undergone surgery. Since she was in significant pain pre-operatively, she would need to persuade the court that she would have undergone surgery or recovered spontaneously to recover full compensation when her quantum was assessed.

The controversy surrounding the Judgment in *Chester v. Afshar* was not diminished a month later when the House of Lords had to deal with a member of the Bar who had failed to mention that there was a 50% chance that an application to get in a medical report might be turned down. Jacqueline Perry advised a claimant in a medical negligence case to turn down an offer of damages because she thought that she had a 50% chance of getting a crucial medical report in and that she thought that he could probably sue his solicitors afterwards if she failed, if he could find

the resources and stomach for a further bout of litigation. She did not trouble him with these details, simply advising him to turn down the payment into court. The House said that there was a respectable body of opinion that held that a client still paid an advocate for her advice and her opinion rather than her doubts. That it would be a sad day if an advocate in the heat of battle had to watch her own back. This demonstrates how the member of the Bar is still seen as delivering an uncertain service which cannot be based in evidence. She deals with an essentially human agency, the reaction of one judge to a set of facts and his impression of the witnesses who appear before him in deciding how to do justice. A doctor is seen as delivering a comparatively impersonal service that should be consistent. As the art progresses in the direction of certainty the artist becomes more of a cipher if not a technician.

The problem is more acute for obstetricians and gynaecologists than it is for other specialties for a number of different reasons. In gynaecology most procedures performed outside cancer are designed primarily to enhance the woman's comfort or reproductive choices. They are elective procedures, which the woman is free to accept or reject on her own terms. Many of them are seen as affecting her reproduction and control of her reproduction in a fashion that is held should be free for her to choose. In obstetrics the reduction of maternal mortality and the marginalization of infant mortality have meant that the woman feels that she should be put in a more powerful position. But it is in abortion that matters have reached the most unfortunate predicament.

Abortion

Doctors have been in the front line of the legal control of abortion since *R v Bourne* in 1938. They have consistently been seen as the servants of the law as well as their patients. Until the Abortion Act 1967 was passed the doctor who performed an abortion in most circumstances committed a professional offence as well as a criminal offence and would be struck off on conviction. The day after the Abortion Act was passed, the doctor who performed an abortion more or less on demand ceased to commit a crime. At the same time prosecutions of doctors for performing abortions before the General Medical Council (GMC) ceased as abruptly. This struck no one as odd because the law had been changed by the Queen in Parliament and if the abortions were going to be performed lawfully then the GMC had to permit them. The professional offence had been to break the law. Yet the change in GMC policy consequent upon the change in the law served to emphasize the fact that the GMC in this respect did not impose any distinct medical ethic or code of behaviour upon doctors, it simply reflected the law. It further served to demonstrate that in this respect at least there was no separate stream of medical law controlling the activities of doctors. In 1967 the change in abortion law was not that which was foreseen by Parliament when it passed the Act. When Parliament decided that it should be lawful to perform an abortion when the continuation of the pregnancy would be more hazardous to the health of the mother or other children in the family than the termination of the pregnancy, it did not appreciate that this in effect legalized abortion on demand since sufficient doctors believed that such a continuation would always be more hazardous.

The predicament of the obstetrician who is asked to treat a woman for an unwanted pregnancy was made more complicated in 1990. In essence MPs were faced with a widespread doubt about the wisdom of the existing law when the new Human Embryology and Fertilization Act was being debated. A sizeable group of MPs wished to bring down the upper limit for abortion, which was then when the fetus would be capable of being born alive. Others took a more liberal view. The compromise agreed upon was that up to 24 weeks' gestation, which probably means 26 weeks from the last menstrual period, abortion should be free on the existing criteria, which effectively meant abortion on demand. Over 24 weeks doctors should be free to perform abortions when there was a substantial risk that the child if born, would suffer from a significant handicap. The meaning of neither significant nor serious was discussed in detail. In essence what MPs who could not agree among themselves decided was that matters should be left to doctors and women to discuss between themselves. The doctor was given the power to decide in consultation with the patient when it would be appropriate to perform an abortion. A substantial risk is, generally speaking, regarded as one which is something of substance, to be taken into account in the organization of one's affairs. This implies that it means less than the balance of probabilities. If right, this would have the odd effect of making it lawful for a doctor to perform an abortion on a fetus, who on the balance of probabilities will be normal at any point up to delivery.

Parliament did not consider such questions as whether the child had to be abnormal at birth, so that it would not be lawful to terminate in the case of Huntington's chorea, which does not usually afflict a person until the fourth decade of life. Nor did it determine whether the surgical or medical remediability of the disability should be taken into account.

The intervening years have not been kind to a compromise based upon deference to the medical judgment of an individual clinician. Today with the rise of personal autonomy and the decline of medical authority there is little role for a doctor to decide what is best for a patient and there is much less role for a doctor to tell a patient what they must and must not do. If a medical service is available the assumption is that the doctor must provide it if the patient demands it and it is clinically appropriate. Something of a crunch point was reached in 2004 when a Curate of the Church of England recognized in the statistics issued by the Department of Health that a pregnancy had been terminated at 26 weeks where the indication given was a cleft palate. If the lesion was a part of a broader syndrome it was not apparent in the information published by the Department of Health. The Curate, Miss Jepson, complained to the Police who sought guidance from the Royal College of Obstetricians and Gynaecologists. The Police decided not to investigate further and Miss Jepson applied for Judicial Review of that decision. The Police agreed to reconsider matters and did investigate with a view to prosecution. Eventually they decided that the evidence available did not enable them to conclude that a prosecution would have a better than 50% chance of persuading a jury that the doctors did not bona fide believe that the circumstances of the Act were satisfied.

However, the case triggered a debate around several issues. The first is whether the compromise decided by Parliament was far more liberal than can be defended, particularly in view of intervening medical developments. Where advances in ultrasound have made it possible to visualize the unborn child more clearly than ever before, the difficulty in defending a decision to terminate on grounds of cleft lip and palate is harder to justify. As advances in neonatology have brought the age of viability down still further, the fetus that is being killed is more often capable of being born alive and of surviving than ever before.

This is something about which obstetricians may provide expert advice to the legislature but must remain essentially neutral. It is not the role of the Royal College or any other professional body as a whole to advance a corporate view as to the circumstances in which it should be lawful to perform an abortion. Doctors may express individual views as citizens and have a statutory right to decide whether they are prepared to be involved in this work, but the corporate view that society seeks from the profession should be rendered in neutral professional terms, simply explaining what is and what is not practical and helping the rest of society to understand the implications of a given decision.

However, there is a second underlying debate about the role of the clinician in these cases. Is the doctor expected to exercise a judgement about whether the procedure is in the patient's best interests? If so on what basis? The indication for the procedure is choice and how can or should the doctor second guess the patient? When Parliament said that it wanted the decision to be taken by doctors and patients together, did it mean that the patient should have complete freedom to decide if the doctor was satisfied that the unborn child would suffer from any recognizable handicap in the case of a post 24-week pregnancy? What is the extent to which it is proper to expect obstetricians to be put in the guise of judges at all in such circumstances? The assessment of the degree of handicap should surely be taken by those in another specialty: in some places such patients are referred to paediatric surgeons for advice, but perhaps the assessment of long-term handicap ought to involve a multidisciplinary assessment involving specialists in mental handicap, physiotherapists, speech therapists and occupational therapists, since the effect of a given physical lesion will vary greatly from case to case, depending on the personality of the victim and the resources available as well as the severity of the lesion. How can such an assessment be organized swiftly enough when the pregnancy is advancing?

The law here has to balance society's interest in protecting the autonomy of the pregnant woman and ensuring that she is not forced to carry to term a baby which she does not want. That right has to be balanced against the right of the unborn child. Few think it appropriate to provide women with an unqualified right to demand the destruction of a normal third trimester fetus. The need to balance these issues calls for a political and judicial assessment. Whereas doctors were placed in the front line, it is increasingly hard to understand what role society allots to them or how it equips them for this task. In few other areas of medicine are doctors asked to legislate between conflicting interests in this fashion and where they have been hitherto, that obligation is being removed.

In these circumstances the individual clinician needs to be aware of the conflicting obligations which are imposed by the law and patients. My own advice is that so far as possible obstetricians should ensure that they have objective advice from appropriate specialists on which to base their advice. In contentious cases I suspect that we will soon advise obstetricians to transfer the decision to the place where it should properly be made, Her Majesty's Judiciary. At least that way we will get some guidelines. It will be very unfortunate if the first time that any guidelines as to the law's assessment of the meaning of substantial risk of serious handicap comes to be decided is in the context of a criminal prosecution. Under the law until 1990 the reluctance of the police to intervene meant that no one attempted to find out what 'capable of being born alive' meant between its passage into law in 1929 and the advent of a negligence action in respect of an obstetrician's failure to advise a woman of the failure of an α-feto protein (AFP) test. The Court ducked the question then and was forced to determine it in 1989 when a radiologist was sued in respect of his failure to recognize spina bifida. Only then was it established that 'capable of being born alive' meant capable of maintaining life by means of one's own breathing, even though 60 years had elapsed since the Act was passed.

Professional discipline

Another feature of the landscape of which clinicians need to be more aware than in the past is the changing role of the GMC. After the profession suffered body blows in public esteem through a series of scandals such as those surrounding the sale of kidneys, the advent of second generation minimal access surgery, the career of Rodney Ledward and the Bristol Cardiac Babies, the GMC was reformed so as to make itself much tougher on the underperforming doctor. The innovations were surrounded with honeyed words about reform and rehabilitation, but in practice those doctors who have been identified as underperforming through the GMC processes have rarely found their way back into mainstream practice again. The National Clinical Assessment Authority was started in 1998 to help deal with the problem of the underperforming doctor. Again its hit rate for getting doctors back into practice once they have been identified as underperforming has not been good. These processes usually lead to the end of the clinician's career. It was also agreed by the profession that it should embark on some formal system of revalidation. Continuing professional education was instigated in the 1990s in response to the minimal access surgery furore and as a result the RCOG was the first College to instigate a system of formal recorded continuing professional education. But it was agreed revalidation needed to be something more, involving not only evidence of learning but also evidence of continuing ability.

Revalidation was going to be introduced by the GMC in 2005 when the powers that be were hit by a long-awaited exocet in the form of the Fifth Report from the Shipman Inquiry. Dr Shipman was a very good GP who happened to be a mass murderer. He poisoned his patients by giving them lethal doses of intravenous morphine and probably killed well over 200 people. Dame Janet Smith, a High Court Judge, ran an Inquiry which lasted over 5 years. In the course of this Inquiry she considered a series of measures designed to detect the underperforming doctor and found them wanting inter alia because they would not have prevented another Shipman. It was of course recognized that since Dr Shipman was not an underperforming doctor, it was unlikely that any such measures would have detected him. But such was the diminution in public esteem for the medical profession associated with the discovery that its goodwill and benevolent aspirations could not be taken for granted that there is a general cloud of uncertainty at the time of writing about the future of professional regulation. The GMC's proposals for revalidation have been withdrawn and are going to be redrafted in the light of the Shipman Inquiry's strictures. There are proposals afoot to make it impossible for any doctor who has been convicted of a criminal offence ever to practise again and the GMC is unlikely to retain much discretion in such cases. One cannot at the time of writing predict the future landscape, save to say that it will be more anti-medical, more unforgiving and more inflexible. Whether this will be a temporary phase it is hard to tell.

Post graduate training

Another problem which makes one concerned for the future of the profession arises from the developments in professional training over the last 10 years. The introduction of the working time directive in the UK has reduced the number of hours per week that the junior hospital doctor works by half. The introduction of the Calman Reforms and the Specialist Registrar Grade has reduced the number of years of experience in training grades that a newly appointed consultant can be expected to have achieved by a similar proportion. The result is that the newly minted consultant is to have about 25% of the clinical hours of experience of her predecessor 20 years ago.

In dealing with junior hospital doctors over the last 30 years one feels that the profession has squandered a monastic tradition of devotion and apprenticeship. Articles in the British Medical Journal (BMJ) report Senior House Officer's (SHO's) in surgery who have not learned to tie knots. Seniors report occasions when assistants have walked out at 17:00 sharp, although the operation has reached a critical point.

Furthermore, the experience of the junior doctor in each hour of experience that is gained is markedly reduced. Whereas a newly appointed Senior Registrar of the 1970s would be likely to have performed more surgical procedures on his own and to have experienced significant complications, such as venous bleeding, more often than the newly appointed consultant of today. At the moment the position is still being mitigated by the presence of senior consultants who benefited from the old fashioned model of training. Every year they retire and are replaced by colleagues who simply do not have the same sort of training. To some extent the problems can be mitigated in elective surgery by increasing sub-speciality and post-appointment higher training, but we are already encountering a brave new world of District General Hospitals in which there is no consultant who benefited from the old fashioned sort of training. The idea that junior consultants are going to acquire the experience and training that they need in the course of their early consultant years overlooks the fact that they are not in a training grade and

that increasingly there is no one there to train them if they do have the modesty to ask for help and guidance.

The conflict between the lack of training and the hostile environment

The combination of this crisis in professional training and the less forgiving professional environment in which doctors work means that the prospects for the individual doctor are ever gloomier. The basic premise of the reforms proposed by the Shipman Inquiry is that there is an almost unlimited supply of newly minted doctors available to replace those who are found not to have kept their professional skills up to date. This premise is profoundly mistaken and the unprincipled attempt to entice doctors to quit poorer countries cannot provide a sustainable solution. In defending doctors before the GMC we already find an unforgiving atmosphere and an assumption that someone must have done something wrong whenever a patient has died. Some aspects of the Shipman Report suggest that the idea that many complaints may be ill-founded would come as a surprise to the author. The notion of being just to the doctor who is the respondent to a complaint is low down on a set of priorities that are headed by making sure that the Service is 'safe' and giving satisfaction to somebody simply because they have complained.

Outside the portals of the GMC the complaints system within hospitals has been reformed and made similarly more hostile to the profession. The advice that one gives to professionals in these circumstances is much the same as it has always been. Spend time with patients, talking to them and listening to them; explain in detail what is proposed; recognize that the purpose of the consultation is to put your knowledge at the patient's disposal so that she can make her decision about what she wants to do. This explicitly involves an acceptance of the proposition that sometimes patients will make decisions which the doctor thinks are surprising, if not profoundly misconceived. The patient has an unfettered right to refuse surgery for good reason, bad reason or no reason. Make sure that the risks of inaction are spelled out as clearly as the risks of the intervention in question. The doctor's role is to advise and to recognize that while her skills are for her patient, her notes are for herself and her own protection. It is as important to make detailed records of what is said to and by the patient as it is to make records of the clinical history that is elicited and the signs that are found.

It must also be recognized that the patient's right to choose in effect must sometimes mean a right to demand therapy which the doctor thinks is contraindicated. This is an issue that the profession and the service are only beginning to grapple with. It found its first utterance in the NICE guidelines concerning Caesarean section. It might be unkind to summarize those guidelines with the proposition that maternal request is not on its own an indication for a Caesarean section, but the clinician should elicit the reason for the request and the woman's decision should be respected. The patient who demands an unfair share of resources in the form of a Caesarean section which the doctor thinks is not in their best interest should be offered referral elsewhere and the doctor is given a list of contraindications which may well exhaust the interval before a spontaneous delivery in many cases. As I say, that may be an unfair summary, but several hours could easily be spent in discussing the various contraindications that the professional should point out to the woman who is contemplating a Caesarean section which has no clinical indication other than her choice.

In other areas the Service operates on the premise that patients will not demand surgery which is not in their interests. How far that premise is well founded is unclear. We do have some experience of professionals being sued for unnecessary procedures in the context of dentistry. There is a long established line of cases in which patients have demanded extravagant, conservative restoration of teeth whose roots are unsuitable. The smile may be attractive at first but the life expectancy of the bridge is short. The Courts almost invariably criticize the dentist for having performed a procedure contrary to the patient's best interests as the professional saw them. The conventional advice to a professional is that when a patient demands a procedure which appears to be contrary to their best interests, the professional should decline to perform it and offer to refer to someone else. That conventional advice must still be good in 2005, but as professional autonomy advances the question must arise as to whether the patient's right to choose will sooner or later entitle them to demand surgery which the doctor thinks is contraindicated, with the same freedom as the waiter should accept my order for an unsuitable combination of dishes. If the autonomy of the patient is paramount and the playing field of knowledge of the implications of medical procedures becomes ever more level, it is difficult to understand how the status quo can be preserved indefinitely.

Cerebral palsy

All this is a long way from the core of the issues which were at the forefront of professional concern when I wrote this chapter's predecessor in 1999. Then, the concern of the obstetrician with the law, was as it had been since 1980 when the House of Lords gave Judgment in *Jordan v. Whitehouse* that they would be sued by children suffering from cerebral palsy who sought to blame their disability on the doctor. Although Mr Jordan's case resulted in a victory for the defence, the experience of the defence organizations was that plaintiffs at large remembered only that a claim had been brought in respect of a brain damaged child, not that it was lost. (See Litigation and Obstetrics & Gynaecology proceedings of 14th Study Group of the Royal College of Obstetricians and Gynaecologists May 1985, see p. 22 contribution of Dr R N Palmer of the MPS). Although the defence witness who gave evidence that the damage could not have been caused by the actions of which complaint was made, Professor Ronald Illingworth found his evidence rejected at trial. He subsequently wrote an influential article in the BMJ 'Don't Blame the Obstetrician' (BMJ 1979) which drew on work already being done by neonatologists in America and which over the succeeding 25 years has led to a much more measured assessment of causation in these cases.

To date it is still true that two thirds of the expenditure of the National Health Service Litigation Authority (NHSLA) which deals with claims against the service is devoted to cases of this sort. It is also true that the number of children in the population suffering from cerebral palsy has remained roughly constant despite the improvements in obstetrics and paediatrics, which have transformed the infant mortality and the prospects of survival of the child once delivered. It is also true that the expectations of Society for a perfect result have made it difficult for us to defend such cases save where the extremity of prematurity makes it clear that survival at all is astonishing.

Yet the problem is no longer at the forefront of professional thinking. There are a number of reasons for this. First and foremost, the advent of National Health Service (NHS) indemnity in 1990 has taken the financial burden of these sort of cases off the shoulders of the medical profession. Claim handling was centralized under the clinical negligence scheme for NHS Trusts in 2002 and the claims experience of the Trust does not affect the premium that trusts pay to be members of the scheme, so that there is an additional level of insulation between the individual doctor and the damage. Risk management and clinical governance demand ever higher and more intolerant standards, but the purely financial impact of these claims is well removed from the services delivered in the individual Trust. There was a period when a multimillion pound claim against the Trust would or could cause cash flow problems which sent the Chief Executive cap in hand to the Regional Office of the Department of Health. That has gone.

Other measures have been adopted in most other jurisdictions to limit the direct fiscal impact of these claims on the profession.

The state will provide

However, another reform is now coming into practice in England that may have an even greater effect. In 1999 a lady called Mrs Coghlan sued Devon Health Authority because they proposed to close the home in which she lived and she felt that they had given her a reasonable expectation that they would not do this. She won. This case triggered an appreciation that continuing care rendered in the community is of an unsatisfactory standard. The Department of Health issued Guidelines requiring individual Health Authorities, and Primary Care Trusts as they are now called, to publish Eligibility Criteria for continuing care. Similar obligations have been imposed on Social Services. Where a patient qualifies for complete care, then whatever the patient is ascertained to need by a multidisciplinary team is provided free of charge. This has been introduced first patchily and now up and down the country. The initial guidance from the Department of Health has been reinforced and tightened up as a result of a series of critical reports from the NHS Ombudsman. Every time the Department publishes a set of guidelines the Ombudsman finds a case which does not meet them and criticizes. The Department publishes tighter guidelines requiring a higher standard of care and the Ombudsman finds a case where those guidelines are not being met. The result of this process is that ever higher standards of continuing care in the community are being delivered up and down the country.

The extension of this pattern of care to children is more patchy but it is already happening. We are seeing cases coming to litigation where the Primary Care Trust (PCT) is already supplying packages of care to children in their homes costing over £100,000 a year. These are the real fiscal core of the negligence claims made against the service in respect of cerebral palsy children and as this pattern of care become widespread the justification for awarding such damages through the tort system becomes much harder to understand. Apart from anything else the judge can only assess a child's needs on the day when the decision is taken. The one thing that is clear is that those needs will not remain constant. The claimant in respect of a structured settlement has with effect, from 1 April 2005, acquired the right to seek a variation of their package when it becomes apparent that their condition has deteriorated but there is no obligation upon them to notify the erstwhile tortfeasor when their condition improves or their need for care is reduced until the point of death. By contrast the multidisciplinary team must reassess the client at regular intervals.

One unsatisfactory feature of the landscape which has not yet been resolved is that since care of this sort is free at the point of delivery and there is no means of testing its validity, there is nothing to stop a claimant from recovering damages through the tort system and then seeking to demand care from the local multidisciplinary teams. It may be possible for a PCT to argue that the claimant does not need any care because they are already receiving it from the package which they purchased but that will depend upon the detail of regulations.

Reforming the system: redress 1

The Department of Health produced a report entitled *'Making Amends'* in 2001 which proposed two Redress schemes. In the intervening 4 years there was a great deal of debate about the detail of these schemes. Broadly speaking Redress 1 will provide an alternative to the tort system to determine liability in small claims. Without needing to use lawyers, the claimant or complainant would make a claim to the Health Service which would assess it on the basis of a single expert and either make an offer in respect of claims worth up to £20,000 or up to £30,000 where it is thought there is liability. If the claimant chooses to accept the offer then they would forfeit their legal right to sue and compromise their claim. If they chose to reject the offer they could elect to use the tort system.

The principal objection to Redress 1 is that no evidence-based assessment of it has been done to ascertain what it will cost. It has been a characteristic of the service over recent years that massive reforms have been introduced without any controlled trial to assess the costs. This innovation will for the first time provide a financial incentive to patients to complain. Since complaints against various aspects of the NHS are running at about 10 times the rate that claims are made, it seems likely that there will be a prodigious expansion in the present bill for NHS damages. This may be no bad thing: at the moment the total bill for NHS damages each year is static at about £500 million. Ignoring the cerebral palsy babies, the figure comes down to about £200 million, which is a quarter of 1% of NHS turnover. The number of claims made to the NHSLA is falling steadily. At the moment it is at about 7000 per annum. By contrast although no centralized store of data is available, 19,000 Legal Aid certificates were issued in 1991 and it seems that the number of Certificates has fallen to one third of this figure over the last 15 years. This is partly as a result of reforms in the provision of Legal Aid: it is now difficult, if not impossible to get Legal Aid for small claims where a reasonable person would not spend their own money to bring litigation and one criterion which is being used to assess applications for Legal Aid is whether or not use has been made of the NHS complaints procedure. Given what we know of iatropathy in the service and hospital acquired infections it seems extraordinary that the number of claims should have fallen to this extent, and if the volume and value of claims were to rise substantially, it might well be thought appropriate. However, the scope to introduce a true compensation culture in which any trivial complication or delay while the person is in pain will be followed routinely by a claim threatens to introduce a true claims culture such as we have only seen in this country in the context of slipping claims against the Council in Liverpool where it is widely said that if you fall over at paving stones you will find five people queuing to fall over it after you before you can get up.

The second scheme, Redress 2, would have provided no fault care for brain damaged babies. That was abandoned area it was realised how unfair it would be to favour this group of disabled people rather than any other groups.

Chapter 61: Domestic violence and sexual assault

Maureen Dalton

The effects of domestic violence, rape, and child sexual abuse are seen daily in the practice of the obstetrician and gynaecologist. So it is important to be aware of the problems and the correct care of victims.

Domestic violence

Domestic violence (DV) is a major cause of maternal mortality and morbidity. One in four women is a victim of DV [1] and it is not just accident and emergency (A&E) that manages the aftermath. It is now being recognized that the consequences of DV are commonly seen in obstetrics and gynaecology. It is not always possible to spot the victim but it is important to try.

Domestic violence does not have to be physical violence. The threat of financial and psychological controls are also forms of DV [2].

Identification

The first step to identifying a victim is to think about the possibility that she is being abused. In the past professionals were either unaware of the problem or thought that DV was nothing to do with them, being between the patient and her partner or family. However, as it is health that picks up the consequences and, if the underlying abuse is missed, she will repeatedly re-present and be inappropriately investigated and treated, domestic violence has become a part of the 'diagnostic' aspect of medicine.

Domestic violence can occur in any social class and affects people of all educational abilities. However, the less well able are not as skilled at getting out of the situation and are more likely to turn to drink or drugs to numb the pain.

The importance of DV has been stressed in the latest CEMACH (3) report 'Why Mother's Die' and in the RCOG publication 'Violence Against Women' [2].

The abused woman has very low self-confidence and esteem. She feels ashamed of her situation and finds it difficult to ask for help. During their care all women should have the opportunity to have at least one consultation alone, without partner, friends or relatives, to allow inquiries about DV to be made. This may be very difficult to arrange in practice. There are standard questionnaires that can be handed out to women but they must be given when the woman is alone, filled out when she is alone and handed in when she is alone.

A simple but effective extra way of helping victims come forward is the 'red spot' system. Notices are placed in women's toilets in the clinics and wards, asking the questions 'Are You Living with Fear? You are not alone. 1 in 4 women are living with domestic violence. If you would like to talk to someone about your situation put a red spot on your urine sample and we will find a time to talk to you in confidence about this'. Plastic bags and some adhesive red spots must also be provided. It is unlikely anyone with the woman is going to realize that there was not a red spot on the sample before. The staff then have to find the time to see the woman alone and help her (Fig. 61.1).

The victims need to be asked specific questions not generalizations such as 'are things alright at home'. Women may be desperate to reveal what is going on but only if asked directly and with privacy. The woman needs to be seen in a room with closed windows and doors, in the absence of relatives or friends. Interpreters may be part of the same community even if not members of the family and so may inhibit the revelations.

> **'...Are You Living in Fear?**
> You are not alone 1 in 4 women are living with domestic violence. If you would like to talk to someone about your situation put a red spot on your urine sample and we will find a time to talk to you in confidence about this.'

Fig. 61.1 *...Are You Living with Fear?* You are not alone: 1 in 4 women are living with domestic violence. If you would like to talk to someone about your situation put a red spot on your urine sample and we will find a time to talk to you in confidence about this'.

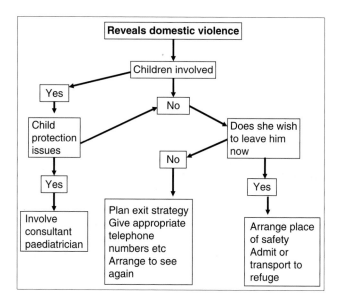

Fig. 61.2 Diagram of management of DV.

Drawing the curtains around a bed on a ward is definitely nota way to create privacy. Evidence suggests that repeated questioning helps. So it does not matter if someone else has already asked about DV.

Action when domestic violence is revealed (Fig. 61.2)

1 Acknowledge how difficult it has been for the woman to tell another person about it.

2 Reassure her that what has been done to her is absolutely wrong and that she did not 'deserve it'.

3 Assure her about confidentiality, about who will know, how much and show her or agree what is written in the notes to demonstrate trust. Remember she has a right of access to her notes but that in reality within a hospital set up many people have access to these notes. It is possible that someone who is connected to the perpetrator may be able to read what is in the notes.

4 Ask her what she wants to do. She may wish to return to her home despite what is happening. She may be worried about her children or afraid of her partner or she may hope he will change.

5 The woman should NOT be forced to leave home as this would be another form of bullying, controlling behaviour and would contribute to the abuse.

6 Advice on leaving the perpetrator should be given if she wishes to receive it, e.g. to give her the telephone numbers of national help lines and local women's refuge, the names of local solicitors interested in family law can be given.

Reassure her that the police now take DV seriously and changes in the law have strengthened what they can do.

7 WRITE CAREFUL NOTES.

Child protection issues

If there are children involved, there is a legal obligation to consider whether the children are significantly at risk. If this seems to be the case, the woman's wishes can be overruled. Often she will agree to some form of compromise if there are significant child protection issues. It is vital at this point to go down the agreed child protection protocols drawn up for the local area. Involve the consultant paediatrician on call. Hospital social work departments should also be contacted for advice. It is not appropriate or necessary to go down child protection protocols in every case of DV, but the possibility should always be considered.

Support for staff

Staff should be reassured that they have made successful use of their communication skills if they have uncovered upsetting levels of grim abuse. The woman trusted them enough to tell them the situation and was given a choice. Staff may find that they went back to the perpetrator, was severely injured or even murdered but IT WAS NOT THEIR FAULT. At least the woman had been given a chance to talk about changing her situation. On the other hand, never asking about DV and never giving the victim an opportunity to reveal what was happening would be a definite failure.

Health consequences

Research in this area is difficult. It is not possible to do double blind randomized control trials and even cohort studies in this area rely on the 'non-abused' cohort being genuinely non-abused rather than just too scared to reveal. The number of times seen by the researcher in privacy will increase the chance a woman will reveal DV. There is conflicting evidence therefore on the effects.

The following generalizations can probably be made.

Obstetrics

Pregnancy is a time when DV often starts or increases. It is highest among teenage pregnancies. There is an association with increased risk of:

Miscarriage
Low birth weight
Unintended pregnancy and increased terminate of pregnancy (TOP) requests
Preterm labour
Chorioamnionitis

The 'Why Mother's Die' [3] report confirms the tendency of women who were murdered to present late or to be frequent non-attendees. It must be remembered that this vulnerable group may not be able to attend hospital appointments because they are not allowed to. It is important to consider why a woman has failed to attend a clinic and give further appointments. A 'one strike and you are out' policy will only victimize the victims.

Partner's who perpetrate violence are often with their women the whole time with a noticeable controlling and dominating attitude.

Gynaecology (Table 61.1)

It is now being recognized that the consequences of DV are commonly seen in gynaecology as well as obstetrics. Women who are victims of DV are more likely to present complaining of:

Pelvic pain
Menstrual disturbances
Dyspareunia
Vaginal discharge
Sterilization
TOP requests
Pelvic inflammatory disease (PID)

The list is similar to that seen in a routine gynaecology clinic but they are also more likely to have:

Psychiatric problems
Irritable bowel syndrome

Table 61.1 Presentation of DV

Obstetrics
Miscarriage
    Low birth weight
    Unintended pregnancy and increased TOP requests
    Preterm labour
    Chorioamnionitis
Gynaecology
    Pelvic pain
    Menstrual disturbances
    Dyspareaunia
    Vaginal discharge
    Sterilization
    Top requests
    PID
General
They are also more likely to have
    Psychiatric problems
    Irritable bowel syndrome
    Asthma
    Chest pain
    Headache

Asthma
Chest pain
Headache
Alcohol or drug abuse problems.

Sexual assault (Fig. 61.3)

Any woman who is seen in Obstetric and Gynaecology clinics could have been a victim of sexual assault. The British Crime survey 4 found that 1 in 20 women had been sexually assaulted. After they have been assaulted they are more likely to perceive their health as poor or fair than good. They become heavy users of the health service, presenting more frequently than others with vaginal discharge, psychiatric problems, menstrual disorders, dyspareunia, abdominal pain, IBS and headache. It is therefore important to provide good initial care for a victim, that does not necessarily involve the police, to help with her long-term healthcare. This must be done sensitively and accurately to maximize possible forensic evidence.

They will often not have gone to the police for many reasons including:

Fear of not being believed,
Fear of the court process,
Fear of the assailant (especially as the assailant is usually known to the victim)
Embarrassment and fear of further examinations.

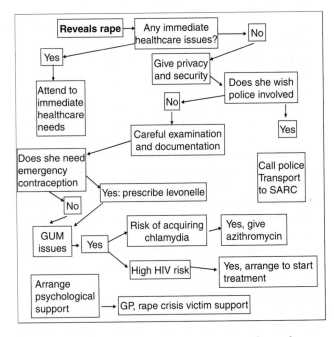

Fig. 61.3 Diagram of management of acute sexual assault.

The development of post-traumatic stress disorders and the fear of damage from the assault results in frequent visits to health care providers.

Initial action following a revelation of an acute sexual assault

The victim may reveal she has been recently assaulted during a consultation, when presenting to the Emergency department or during an admission for a supposed other problem.

Immediate health needs must obviously be checked first. If she is bleeding heavily, she needs a drip and appropriate resuscitation. When she is stable move her into a room where she can have some privacy and then ask if she wishes the police to be involved. Save any urine passed before the police arrive (they may wish to screen for drugs).

Check briefly whether there was forced oral sex. If yes, no drinks should be offered until the police can provide an early evidence kit that provides a mouth sample for sperm.

Sexual assault referral centres

Police forces around the country are being encouraged to collaborate with health services to develop Sexual assault referral centres (SARCs) such as the long-standing centres at St Mary' in Manchester and REACH in the northeast of England. The victim can go to the SARC for examination but also in addition counselling and support can be arranged. Most SARCs do not need the victim to have been to the police.

When initially seen in a SARC, the doctor has first to consider if the victim can consent to examination. If she has been drugged or is very drunk she may need more time before the examination can take place.

A general history, including asking for bleeding problems and psychiatric problems should be taken initially

The doctor's role is not to be the detective and decide if the woman has or has not been raped. The doctor must appear to believe her for the sake of her long-term recovery, BUT if a written statement is required for the court, it should be independent and NOT written on her behalf or that of the defendant.

The doctor will be seeing the woman before she has given a statement to the police and so should not ask too many questions about the incident as inadvertent suggestions may be made.

The examination (Table 61.2)

The advantage of examining in a SARC is that they are specially designed to minimize DNA contamination. If

Table 61.2 Management of sexual assault victim

Management of rape victim
Assess immediate health needs
Arrange privacy
Ask if wishes police involvement
Consent to examine
Examine from head to toe
Careful documentation
Swabs if appropriate
Emergency contraception
Infection prophylaxis
Psychological support

there is no alternative to examining the victim in a ward or emergency department contact with any people before examination should be minimized. Gloves should be worn and theatre clothes or gowns are less contaminated than ordinary clothes. A careful head to toe examination looking for bruises, scratches and grazes should be performed. Swabs dampened with sterile water taken from areas the perpetrator has kissed such as face and nipples, and even from areas where he has gripped if taken soon enough after the event, can reveal his DNA.

Most normally sexually active victims do not have genital injuries but may have other injuries, e.g. where she has been forcibly held down. Careful, accurate documentation is one of the most important parts of the examination; it is helpful to use body diagrams to show where the injuries are. Bruises need the size, shape and colour recorded. It is not possible to accurately age bruises.

Abrasions (scratches and grazes) also need the size and shape recorded. It is often possible to tell the direction of the force in a scratch and if fresh the loops of skin are present. These rub off once they have dried.

From April 2004 the Royal College of Paediatrics and Child Health & Association of Forensic Physicians (RCPCH&AFP) guidelines [5] for examination of victims of sexual assault under the age of 18, recommend the use a colposcope for genital examination. This should be considered best practice for all female victims. The injuries can be better recorded. All examinations in children should be totally recorded but for adults, when the majority do not have genital injuries, it is appropriate to use it to record injuries so that they can be discussed with another medical expert. A colposcope also allows intimate examination without invading the victim's personal space too much when looking and taking swabs. Using a magnifying glass and light close in between her knees is intrusive for the victim. In addition more injuries can be identified using a colposcope.

There must be consent for any photographs or videos taken and access must be restricted. They become part

Table 61.3 Persistence of sperm

Persistence of sperm	
Vagina	7 days
Anal canal/rectum	3 days
Mouth	Usually 6 h up to 2 days
Cervix	7–10 days
Skin/hair	Unknown but may persist after cleaning

of the medical records not the police notes. Photographs relating to an assault should only be revealed to a medical expert who must confirm they will not show them to any one else without the victim's permission or on the direction of a judge.

Unfortunately there have been occasions when these pictures have fallen into the wrong hands and if care is not taken women will not allow these useful records to be taken.

Swabs should be taken during the genital examination from outside in, that is, starting with the perineum, then the labia, introitus, lower vagina, higher vagina and then cervix.

The time since the assault and the details of the assault are important in deciding which swabs to take (see Table 61.3).

Aftercare

Once the examination is complete, the woman may take a shower or bath, as she is likely to feel dirty.

These are then the other issues to be discussed:

1 *Emergency contraception if appropriate.*
2 *Infection.* Azithromycin should be offered if there is any possibility of Chlamydia infection.
HIV prophylaxis. Is the perpetrator likely to have HIV? Is he an IV drug abuser or does he come from a high-risk area for HIV, were there multiple assailants, anal intercourse or many bleeding injuries? If so, HIV prophylaxis may be appropriate and most hospitals have a protocol for how to access the start of treatment out of hours.
Encourage victims to visit their local geneto urinary medicine (GUM) clinic within the following few days where HIV risk and hepatitis vaccination can be discussed further.
3 *Psychological support.* If the local SARC does not have access to counselling services early involvement of the GP should be encouraged as initial careful management reduces long-term health risks and it is the GP that will be in the first line when these problems arise. Everyone benefits from helping the victim initially.

Guilt feelings are part of a victim's psychological response, so it is useful to stress to her that she has done nothing wrong; the guilt and the shame lie with the perpetrator.

The statement

The duty is to provide a statement to the court, even if it is the police that ask for it. If a doctor is found to have misled the court with their evidence or statements this is taken seriously by the GMC.

In a 'professional' statement it should be made clear to the police, Crown prosecution service and, if necessary, to the judge that the doctor has just acted as a professional without the expertise to interpret the injuries.

An expert view considers the cause but must remember all reasonable possible alternative causations for each injury. Certainty of causation can be expressed on a scale of one to five where:

(1) – no suggestion that the injury is explained by (or relates to) any particular causation …
To:
(5) – certainty that the injury has been caused by …

Any statement must be accurate and look professional. Qualifications and experience should be stated. Conclusions should consider both causation and consistency with the history.

The statement should end with a phrase such as 'based on information given to me to date' as new information may come to light that means conclusions need to be reviewed. Help and advice in writing a statement may be available from the nurse or doctor designated for child protection in your hospital or area.

Child sexual abuse

Many women attending gynaecology clinics were sexually abused as children. Like the rape victim they present more commonly with gynaecological problems than the non-abused. They may find pelvic examinations difficult. It is helpful to allow her to feel in control. She may find it easier to pass the speculum herself. She may find a male doctor more frightening and get flashbacks to her abuse. This may result in her feeling violated and reluctant to return for further treatment.

She may not be suitable for outpatient procedures and day case admission and anaesthetic may be a better option for her.

There is evidence that child sex abuse (CSA) is another area that is underdiagnosed currently. When a gynaecologist sees any child it is appropriate to consider CSA. Clearly this does not mean that every child seen by the gynaecologist is abused but many of the presentations are similar and so it will frequently be part of the differential

> All examinations of children where there is a possibility of sexual assault should be combined with a paediatrician and involve two doctors

Fig. 61.4 All examinations of children where there is a possibility of sexual assault should be combined with a paediatrician and involve doctors.

diagnosis. Has the child seen in the emergency department really fallen astride a bicycle or is the injury a result of abuse. What about the child with a vaginal discharge?

A child who is old enough to talk will do so, if they feel safe in the environment, and are allowed to use their own terms, to give a relevant history. Often the right privacy for disclosure is not provided. Unlike physical abuse of a child, sexual abuse rarely presents acutely and the medical examination findings are usually only a small part of the evidence that decides a child has been abused. Often there are no clear indications of abuse on examination.

If a gynaecologist has any concerns about the possibility of sexual abuse it is essential to discuss this with a paediatrician who has expertise in this area or the on-call paediatric consultant. A joint examination with a paediatrician is best practice [5] so there are two people independently assessing the injuries (Fig. 61.4).

The initial examination should be the same as for any forensic examination. A head to toe examination, looking for bruising, scratches and other injuries that may support the allegation, must be performed. The stage of puberty must always be noted.

If the genitalia of a child in whom there may have been a history of abuse if needs to be examined. It should be a joint examination and a colposcope is a very useful way of recording the findings.

A young child may feel more secure sitting on her mother's knee. The interpretation of a normal hymen is difficult. Minor clefts or bumps may be normal and redundant folds of the hymen may hide significant tears. The hymen must be gently inspected all around. Posterior-lateral traction of the hymen may improve visualization as may gently 'floating' the hymen with warmed normal saline or water. Passing a small catheter into the vagina, then blowing up the balloon and gently retracting may also allow the whole hymen to be visualized. It is now appreciated that the size of the hymenal orifice varies considerably especially in obese children and so great significance should not be placed on measurements of its size.

When examining the anus care must be taken to avoid too much pressure for too long or venous suffusion by the separation process can be produced.

Many sexually abused children do not have abnormalities, even when the perpetrator has admitted full penetration. As in adult assault the finding of no injury does not mean nothing has happened.

Summary

The gynaecologist will see a number of women who have been sexually assaulted as children or an adult and this must be remembered as it may have a significant influence on the presenting problem and how she should be examined and managed. Domestic violence is common and victims may not attend clinics but are high-risk patients who should not be rapidly discharged. When they are pregnant they are at a greater risk of complications and maternal death.

References

1. Dalton M (ed.) (2004) *Forensic Gynaecology*. London: RCOG Press.
2. Bewley S, Friend J & Mezey G (eds) (1997) *Violence against Women*. London: RCOG Press.
3. Lewis G (2004) Chapter 14 Coincidental deaths and domestic violence. In: Lewis G & Drife J (eds) *Why Mothers Die 2000–2002. Sixth Report of the Confidential Enquiries into Maternal Deaths*. London: RCOG Press. www.afpweb.org.uk.
4. British Crime Survey (2002) www.homeoffice.gov.uk/rds/bcs1.html
5. The Royal College of Paediatrics & Child Health and the Association of Forensic Physicians Guidelines on paediatric forensic examinations in relation to possible child sex abuse. http://www.rcpch.ac.uk/publications/recent.publication/PaediatricForensicExaminations.pdf

Index

Page numbers in *italics* represent figures, those in **bold** represent tables.